T0337449

Core Curriculum

WOUND MANAGEMENT

SECOND EDITION

Wound, Ostomy, and Continence Nurses Society™ (WOCN®)

Core Curriculum

WOUND
MANAGEMENT

SECOND EDITION

EDITED BY

Laurie L. McNichol, MSN, RN, CNS, GNP, CWOCN, CWON-AP, FAAN
Clinical Nurse Specialist and WOC Nurse
Cone Health
Greensboro, North Carolina

Catherine R. Ratliff, PhD, RN, GNP-BC, CWOCN, CFCN, FAAN
Nurse Practitioner
Heart and Vascular Center
UVA Health
Charlottesville, Virginia

Stephanie S. Yates, MSN, RN, ANP-BC, CWOCN
Nurse Practitioner
Duke University Hospital Cancer Center
Durham, North Carolina

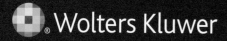
. Wolters Kluwer

Philadelphia • Baltimore • New York • London
Buenos Aires • Hong Kong • Sydney • Tokyo

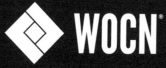
WOCN® Wound, Ostomy, and Continence Nurses Society®

Acquisitions Editor: Jamie Blum
Development Editor: Maria M. McAvey
Editorial Coordinator: Anthony Gonzalez/Linda Christina
Production Project Manager: Kim Cox
Design Coordinator: Teresa Mallon/Stephen Druding
Manufacturing Coordinator: Kathleen Brown/Beth Welsh
Marketing Manager: Linda Wetmore
Prepress Vendor: SPi Global

Second Edition

Cataloging-in-Publication Data available on request from the Publisher

ISBN: 978-1-9751-6459-1

PREVIOUS EDITION CONTRIBUTORS

Ashwin Agarwal, BS

Lizabeth E. Andrew, MS

Elizabeth A. Ayello, PhD, RN, ACNS-BC, CWON, ETNN, MAPWCA, FAAN

Sharon Baranoski, MSN, RN, CWCN, APN-CCNS, FAAN

Barbara M. Bates-Jensen, PhD, RN, FAAN

Carole Bauer, MSN, RN, ANP-BC, OCN, CWOCN

Janice M. Beitz, PhD, RN, CS, CNOR, CWOCN, CRNP, MAPWCA, FAAN

Phyllis A. Bonham, PhD, MSN, RN, CWOCN, DPNAP, FAAN

David M. Brienza, PhD

C. Tod Brindle, MSN, RN, CWOCN, Clin IV

Ruth A. Bryant, RN, MS, CWOCN

Michele (Shelly) Burdette-Taylor, PhD, RN-BC, MSN, CWCN, CFCN

Joanna J. Burgess, BSN, RN, CWOCN

Adela Rambi G. Cardones, MD

Linda J. Cowan, PhD, ARNP, FNP-BC, CWS

Suzanne Creehan, MSN, RN, CWON

David R. Crumbley, MSN, RN, CWCN

Barbara A. Dale, BSN, RN, CHHN, CWOCN

Becky Dorner, RD, LD, FAND

Dorothy B. Doughty, MN, RN, CWOCN, FAAN

Kevin R. Emmons, DrNP, RN, AGPCNP-BC, CWCN

JoAnn Ermer-Seltun, MS, RN, ARNP, FNP-BC, CWOCN

Jane Fellows, MSN, RN, CWOCN

Bonny Flemister, MSN, RN, CWOCN, ANP, GNP-BC

Lynn Fong, BSN, RN, CWOCN

Elizabeth Friedrich, MPH, RD, CSG, LDN, FAND

Kelly A. Jaszarowski, MSN, RN, CNS, ANP, CWOCN

Jan Johnson, MSN, ANP-BC, CWOCN

Lee Ann Krapfl, BSN, RN, CWOCN

Carolyn Lund, RN, MS, FAAN

Dianne Mackey, MSN, RN, CWOCN

Morris A. Magnan, PhD, RN

JoAnn Maklebust, MSN, RN, APRN, AOCN, FAAN

Laurie L. McNIchol, MSN, RN, GNP, CWOCN, CWON-AP

The names and credentials are listed as they were printed during the time of the previous edition publication.

Yvette Mier, BSN, RN, CWOCN

Susan S. Morello, BSN, RN, CWOCN, CBN

Asfandyar Mufti, BMSc

Rose W. Murphree, DNP, RN, CWOCN, CFCN

Debra S. Netsch, DNP, APRN-CNP, FNP-BC, CWOCN

Denise Nix, MS, RN, CWOCN

C. W. J. Oomens, PhD, Ir

Benjamin F. Peirce, RN, CWOCN

Barbara Pieper, PhD, RN, CWOCN, ACNS-BC, FAAN

Mary Ellen Posthauer, RD, CD, LD, FAND

Janet M. Ramundo, MSN, RN, CWOCN

Laurie M. Rappl, PT, DPT, CWS

Michelle C. Rice, MSN, RN, CWOCN

Bonnie Sue Rolstad, MS, RN, CWOCN

Barbara Rozenboom, BSN, RN, CWON

Gregory Schultz, PhD

R. Gary Sibbald, BSc, MD, Med, FRCPC(Med), FRCPC(Derm), MACP, FAAD, MAPWCA

Charleen Singh, MSN/Ed, RN, FNP-BC, CWOCN

Joyce K. Stechmiller, PhD, ACNP-BC, FAAN

Debra M. Thayer, MS, RN, CWOCN

Freya van Driessche, BS, MS

Lia van Rijswijk, MSN, RN, CWCN

Myra Varnado, BS, RN, CWOCN, CFCN

Carolyn Watts, MSN, RN, CWON

Dot Weir, RN, CWON, CWS

Stephanie S. Yates, MSN, RN, ANP-BC, CWOCN

The names and credentials are listed as they were printed during the time of the previous edition publication.

CONTRIBUTORS

Ashwin G. Agarwal, MD, FAAD
Dermatologist and Dermatologic Surgeon
Dallas Dermatology and Aesthetics
Plano, Texas

Lizabeth E. Andrew, BS
Gerontology
Retired
Newnan, Georgia

Elizabeth A. Ayello, PhD, MS, BSN, ETN, RN, CWON, MAPWCA, FAAN
Co-Editor in Chief
Advances in Skin and Wound Care Journal
LWW
Philadelphia, Pennsylvania
Faculty Emeritus
Excelsior College School of Nursing
Albany, New York

Barbara M. Bates-Jensen, PhD, RN, WOC Nurse, FAAN
Professor of Nursing and Medicine
School of Nursing and David Geffen School of Medicine
University of California Los Angeles
Los Angeles, California

Carole Bauer, MSN, RN, ANP-BC, OCN, CWOCN
Wound and Ostomy Nurse Practitioner
Beaumont Health
Troy, Michigan

Janice M. Beitz, PhD, RN, CS, CNOR, CWOCN-AP, CRNP, ANEF, FNAP, FAAN
Professor
School of Nursing
Rutgers University Camden
Camden, New Jersey

Tara Beuscher, DNP, RN-BC, GCNS-BC, ANP-BC, CWOCN, CFCN, NEA-BC
Nurse Practitioner
Podiatry
Doctors Making Housecalls
Charlotte, North Carolina

Phyllis Bonham, PhD, MSN, RN, CWOCN, DNAP, FAAN
Professor Emerita
College of Nursing
Medical University of South Carolina
Mount Pleasant, South Carolina

Kathleen Borchert, MS, RN, APRN, CNS, CWOCN, CFCN
WOC Program Manager
University of Minnesota Health
Minneapolis, Minnesota

David M. Brienza, PhD
Professor
Department of Rehabilitation Science and Technology
Associate Dean of Technology and Innovation
School of Health and Rehabilitation Sciences
University of Pittsburgh
Pittsburgh, Pennsylvania

Tod Brindle, PhD, MSN, RN, CWCN
United States Medical Director
Medical Affairs
Mölnlycke Healthcare
Norcross, Georgia

Glenda Brunette, MSN, RN, CWON
Wound and Ostomy Care Nurse
Medical University of South Carolina
Charleston, South Carolina

Ruth A. Bryant, PhD, MS, RN, CWOCN
Director of Nursing Research
Abbott Northwestern Hospital
Minneapolis, Minnesota

Joanna J. Burgess, BSN, RN, CWOCN
Clinical Support Nurse
ConvaTec
Bridgewater, New Jersey

Adela Rambi Cardones, MD, MHSc
Associate Professor of Dermatology
Duke University School of Medicine
Durham, North Carolina

Sue Creehan, MSN, RN, CWON
Independent Consultant
Wound & Ostomy
Midlothian, Virginia

David R. Crumbley, MSN, RN, CWCN
Associate Clinical Professor
School of Nursing
Auburn University
Auburn, Alabama

Barbara A. Dale, BSN, RN, CWOCN, CHHN
Director of WOC Services
Quality Home Health and Hospice
Hilham, Tennessee

Becky Dorner, RDN, LD, FAND
President
Becky Dorner & Associates
Dunedin, Florida

Laura Edsberg, PhD
Professor of Natural Sciences and Director of Center for
    Wound Healing Research
Daemen College
Amherst, New York

**Kevin R. Emmons, DrNP, RN, APN, AGPCNP-BC,
    CWCN, CFCN**
Clinical Associate Professor
School of Nursing
Rutgers University Camden
Camden, New Jersey

**JoAnn M. Emer-Seltun, MS, RN, ARNP, FNP-BC,
    CWOCN, CFCN**
President, Co-Director and Faculty
WEB WOC Nursing Education Programs
Minneapolis, Minnesota
MercyOne North Iowa Continence Clinic & Vascular and
    Wound Center
Mason City, Iowa

Jane Fellows, MSN, RN, CWOCN-AP
Wound and Ostomy Clinical Nurse Specialist
Duke University Hospital Cancer Center
Durham, North Carolina

**Elizabeth Friedrich, MPH, RDN, CSG, LDN, FAND,
    NWCC**
President
Friedrich Nutrition Consulting
Salisbury, North Carolina

**Susan Gallagher, PhD, MA, MSN, RN, CBN, HCRM,
    CSPHP**
Senior Clinical Consultant
The Celebration Institute
Sierra Madre, California

Kelly Jaszarowski, MSN, RN, CNS, APN, CWOCN
Assistant Director
WOC Nursing Education Program
Cleveland Clinic
Washington, Illinois

Teresa J. Kelechi, PhD, RN, CWCN, FAAN
Professor
College of Nursing
Medical University of South Carolina
Charleston, South Carolina

Lee Ann Krapfl, BSN, RN, CWOCN
Wound/Ostomy Nurse Specialist
MercyOne Dubuque Medical Center
Dubuque, Iowa

Kimberly LeBlanc, PhD, RN, NSWOC, WOCC(C), IIWCC
Chair
Wound Ostomy Continence Institute
Association of Nurses Specializing in Wound Ostomy
    and Continence Nursing
Ottawa, Ontario

Carolyn Lund, MS, RN, FAAN
Clinical Nurse Specialist
Neonatal Intensive Care Unit
UCSF Benioff Children's Hospital Oakland
Oakland, California

Dianne Mackey, MSN, RN, CWOCN
Wound/Skin Coordinator
Kaiser Permanente
San Diego, California

Khalad Maliyar, BA
Fourth year medical student
Faculty of Medicine
University of Toronto
Toronto, Ontario

**Laurie L. McNichol, MSN, RN, CNS, GNP, CWOCN,
    CWON-AP, FAAN**
Clinical Nurse Specialist and WOC Nurse
Cone Health
Greensboro, North Carolina

Yvette Mier, BSN, RN, CWON
Clinical Supervisor
Outpatient Wound Care
WellStar Kennestone Hospital
Marietta, Georgia

Asfandyar Mufti, MD, BMSc
Division of Dermatology
Department of Medicine
University of Toronto
Toronto, Ontario

Rose W. Murphree, DNP, RN, CWOCN, CFCN
Assistant Professor
Emory University Nell Hodgson Woodruff School of Nursing
Atlanta, Georgia

Debra Netsch, DNP, APRN, FNP-BC, CNP, CWOCN-AP, CFCN
Co-Director and Faculty
WEB WOC Nursing Education Program
Advanced Practice WOC Nurse Practitioner
Ridgeview Wound & Hyperbaric Healing Center
Ridgeview Medical Center
Waconia, Minnesota

Denise Nix, MS, RN, CWOCN
Wound, Ostomy, Continence Nurse
M Health Fairview
Edina, Minnesota

Jennifer O'Connor, PhD, RN, CFCN, CNE
Assistant Teaching Professor
Sinclair School of Nursing
University of Missouri
Columbia, Missouri

Danielle Pecone, MD
Internal Medicine
Greenville, North Carolina

Benjamin F. Peirce, BA, RN, CWOCN
Consultant
Wound Care
Hollywood, Florida

Barbara A. Pieper, PhD, RN, ACNS-BC, CWOCN, FAAN
Professor Emerita
College of Nursing
Wayne State University
Detroit, Michigan

Joyce Pittman, PhD, RN, ANP-BC, FNP-BC, CWOCN, FAAN
Associate Professor
College of Nursing
University of South Alabama
Mobile, Alabama

Mary Ellen Posthauer, RDN, LD, FAND
President
MEP Healthcare Dietary Services, Inc.
Evansville, Indiana

Janet Ramundo, MSN, RN, CWOCN, CFCN
Clinical Instructor
Emory WOC Nursing Education Program
Nurse Specialist WOC Nursing
Houston Methodist Hospital
Houston, Texas

Laurie Rappl, PT, DPT, CWS
Director
Rappl & Associates, LLC
Simpsonville, South Carolina

Catherine R. Ratliff, PhD, RN, GNP-BC, CWOCN, CFCN, FAAN
Nurse Practitioner
Heart and Vascular Center
UVA Health
Charlottesville, Virginia

Michelle Rice, MSN, RN, CWOCN
Wound and Ostomy Clinical Nurse Specialist
Duke University Hospital
Durham, North Carolina

Leanne Richbourg, MSN, RN, APRN-BC, CWON-AP, CCCN
Wound Ostomy Clinical Nurse Specialist
Duke University Hospital
Durham, North Carolina

Bonnie Sue Rolstad, MS, RN, CWOCN
Faculty and Program Administrator
Web WOC Nursing Education Program
Minneapolis, Minnesota

Barbara J. Rozenboom, BSN, RN, CWON
Wound and Ostomy Nurse
UnityPoint at Home
West Des Moines, Iowa

Gregory Schultz, PhD
Professor
Department of Obstetrics and Gynecology
University of Florida
Gainesville, Florida

R. Gary Sibbald, BSc, MD, DSc (Hons), MEd, FRCPC, FAAD, MAPWCA
Professor
Medicine and Public Health
University of Toronto
Toronto, Ontario

Charleen Singh, PhD, RN, FNP-BC, CWOCN
Assistant Professor
Betty Irene Moore School of Nursing
University of California Davis
Sacramento, California

Debra Thayer, MS, RN, CWOCN
Lead Technical Service Specialist
Medical Solutions Division Laboratory
3M
St. Paul, Minnesota

Lia van Rijswijk, DNP, RN, CWCN
Associate Dean Undergraduate Programs
W. Cary Edwards School of Nursing
Thomas Edison State University
Trenton, New Jersey

Myra F. Varnado, BS, RN, CWOCN, CFCN
Director of Clinical Services
Corstrata
Savannah, Georgia

Carolyn Watts, MSN, RN, CWON
Clinical Nurse Specialist (Retired)
Vanderbilt University Medical Center
Nashville, Tennessee

Dorothy Weir, RN, CWON, CWS
Clinician
Center for Wound Healing and Hyperbaric Medicine
Saratoga Hospital
Saratoga Springs, New York

Sarah Wolfe, MD
Associate Professor of Dermatology
Duke University Hospital
Durham, North Carolina

Stephanie S. Yates, MSN, RN, ANP-BC, CWOCN
Nurse Practitioner
Duke University Hospital Cancer Center
Durham, North Carolina

FOREWORD

I t is an honor to be invited to write the foreword to the *Wound, Ostomy, and Continence Nurses Society™ (WOCN®) Core Curriculum*, 2nd edition. Having served 22 years as a Wound, Ostomy, and Continence (WOC) Nursing Program Director, I can attest as to how valuable a resource these books will be to students, faculty, preceptors, and all clinicians caring for people with wounds, ostomies, and incontinence.

Terms currently popular in health care refer to patient-centered and patient-focused care. For those of you entering the wonderful WOC nursing specialty, know this: the patient has always been the focus of WOC nursing! In fact, our specialty grew from a need identified by patients themselves. As colorectal and urologic surgeries advanced, so did the number of people living with ostomies. In 1958, Akron, Ohio, native Norma N. Gill joined her surgeon, Rupert B. Turnbull Jr, MD, in founding what was then coined by Dr. Turnbull as enterostomal therapy (ET).

Beginning in 1948, when she was a 28-year-old mother of two young children, Norma began a long odyssey battling mucosal ulcerative colitis. She manifested all the gastrointestinal symptoms, including massive bouts of bloody diarrhea associated with this disease, along with many of the extraintestinal manifestations, such as uveitis, iritis, and extensive pyoderma gangrenosum on her face, chest, abdomen, and legs. During a brief remission in 1951, much to the amazement of Norma and her husband Ted, she became pregnant. The pregnancy was fraught with complications, the need for numerous blood transfusions, and fear for the lives of both mother and child throughout. Despite all of these life-threatening occurrences, in June 1952, Norma gave birth to a healthy baby girl. The complications continued after her baby's birth, and Norma's response to treatment was spotty at best. In October 1954, she was admitted to the Cleveland Clinic, and there her life was saved, and history forever changed. Dr. Turnbull operated to remove Norma's colon and create an ileostomy. Her postoperative course after ileostomy was rocky, and she had to undergo some additional operations to remove her rectum and have plastic surgery performed on her face.

Despite all of this, Norma began to feel better—incredibly better. As she was resuming her role as a wife and mother, she felt the need, as we now say, to "pay it forward." Norma wanted to help others who were facing the same challenges she had endured and emerged stronger than she had been before her illness. Her journey began with the Akron physicians and hospital she had come to know well during her illness. Norma started from scratch and cobbled together an inventory of the limited equipment available at the time. Soon she had many referrals from the surgeons and knew she had found her calling. In 1958, during an appointment with Dr Turnbull, she told him what she was doing in Akron to help people with new ostomies and fistulae. He was impressed and called her a couple of months later to offer her a job at the Cleveland Clinic.

August 1958 is when the seeds for the modern specialty of WOC nursing were planted. It was not long before the word was out, and surgeons began requesting that their staff come to train with Norma and Dr. Turnbull. The R.B. Turnbull Jr., School of Enterostomal Therapy (now WOC Nursing) was established. After her long work day in Cleveland, Norma would return to Akron and see patients in hospitals there before heading home to her family and doing it all again the next day.

There was a child in an Akron hospital born with exstrophy of the bladder after years of urinary incontinence, reflux, and renal stones whose family made the lifesaving decision to have her undergo a urinary diversion. She always remembered her first encounter with Norma. Here was a woman who commanded respect. The surgeon, head nurse, and staff nurses, as well as the girl's mom, crowded around the bed as Norma taught the proper way to care for a new ileal conduit. The equipment at that time was very primitive. Heavy stoma plates, rubber pouches with complex assembly secured with cement and a belt and a prayer! Norma never gave up attempting to help her patients and along with Dr. Turnbull urged industry to develop better, more secure pouching systems. Thanks to a great family and the one and only Norma Gill, the child in that Akron hospital grew up well adjusted to her new stoma that child grew up to be me! I knew I wanted to "pay it forward" just like Norma. The baby who was predicted never to be born to Norma and Ted is Sally Gill-Thompson—one of my best friends and a famous ET practitioner in her own right.

After establishment of the formal program in Cleveland, other ET schools soon opened, and graduates from the United States and abroad spread the word across the globe. Professional organizations were established, and admission criteria became more stringent as health care became more complex. ET nurses became well respected for their skills and experience caring for people with complex ostomies and fistulae. It was a natural extension of our practice to embrace wound and continence care. In the 1990s, we bid good-bye to our ET designation and became known as WOC nurses to better reflect our practice. After 38 years, I have retired from clinical practice but my passion for WOC nursing is not diminished. As you embark on your studies of WOC nursing, take time to reflect and appreciate the wonderful legacy you are continuing with your specialty practice. Your actions will have an immeasurable impact improving the lives of your patients through direct care and advocacy, educating your colleagues, expanding research to support our evidence-based practice. I know our future is in good hands.

Norma (and I) will be watching!

Paula Erwin-Toth, MSN, RN, FAAN

PREFACE

The WOCN Society has funded development and publication of the WOC Nursing Core Curriculum to support both WOC nursing education and WOC nursing practice. The content is based on the curriculum blueprint developed by the WOC Nursing Education Program Directors and approved by the WOCN Society's Accreditation Committee and Board of Directors. The content is organized in a manner to support learning by the novice practitioner or student in a wound care program. The textbook begins with the characteristics of normal skin, the physiology of wound healing, and principles of wound assessment and wound management, and then moves to skin and wound care for specific patient populations and for specific types of wounds. The text is also designed to support the knowledgeable wound care clinician. There are chapters on thermal wounds, surgical wound management, oncologic lesions, palliative care, and fistula management, in addition to in-depth content related to pressure injury prevention and management and the pathology and management of venous, arterial, and neuropathic wounds.

The chapters in the wound text are predominately written by clinicians, many of whom are wound care nurses. Each chapter begins with curriculum objectives addressed in the specific chapter, and a topical outline to give the reader a quick overview of the content covered in that chapter. Throughout the chapters, key points are embedded to highlight core concepts. Each chapter also includes multiple illustrations, tables, and boxes to facilitate understanding. Finally, there are questions and answers at the end of each chapter to support the individual's self-assessment of knowledge.

ACKNOWLEDGMENTS

The Wound, Ostomy, and Continence Nurses Society™ (WOCN®) wishes to thank all of the clinical experts who generously shared their time and expertise to create the second edition of this textbook. The Society would like to especially acknowledge the consulting editors, Laurie McNichol, Catherine Ratliff, and Stephanie Yates, for their inspiration, knowledge, and unwavering commitment to the development of this resource and to the field of wound, ostomy, and continence nursing.

The WOCN Society would like to acknowledge Hollister Incorporated for providing a commercially supported educational grant for the development of this textbook.

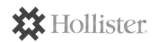

CONTENTS

CHAPTER 1

PROFESSIONAL PRACTICE FOR WOUND, OSTOMY, AND CONTINENCE NURSING

Rose W. Murphree and Kelly Jaszarowski

OBJECTIVES

1. Define the nursing specialty of wound, ostomy, and continence nursing and describe the key role components.
2. Identify the WOC nurse's specific scope of practice based upon licensure:
   a. WOC registered nurse
   b. WOC graduate registered nurse
   c. Advanced practice (APRN)
3. Describe the tri-specialty role of WOC nursing.
4. Name the various populations served by the WOC nurse.
5. List the WOC nurse practice settings.

TOPIC OUTLINE

WOUND, OSTOMY, AND CONTINENCE NURSING SPECIALTY

Wound, ostomy, and continence (WOC) nursing is a multifaceted, evidence-based practice that incorporates a unique body of knowledge to enable nurses to provide excellence in prevention of wound, ostomy, and/or continence problems and complications (WOCN, 2018). Also included in the scope of WOC nursing is health maintenance, therapeutic intervention, and rehabilitative and palliative nursing care to persons with select disorders of the gastrointestinal, genitourinary, and integumentary systems. The WOC nurse directs efforts at improving the quality of care, life, and health of health care consumers with wound, ostomy, and/or continence care needs. WOC nursing is a complex nursing specialty that encompasses the care of individuals of all ages, in all health care settings, and across the continuum of care.

HISTORY AND EVOLUTION OF WOC NURSING

WOC nursing originated as a lay practice to address the unmet needs of health care consumers with an ostomy. During the 1940s and 1950s, surgical techniques developed rapidly with an increase in ostomy surgeries (WOCN, 2010). Stoma construction was often poor, there were few pouching systems available, and hospitals lacked support systems to help the affected individuals deal with the life-altering surgeries. To fill the gap in ostomy care, one particular individual with an ostomy began the quest to improve ostomy care and services (WOCN, 2010). In 1955, Norma Gill Thompson had surgery at Cleveland Clinic (Ohio) with Dr. Rupert Turnbull that resulted in the creation of an ileostomy. During one of her post-op follow-up visits, she spoke with Dr. Turnbull about her rehabilitation with her ostomy care. He was impressed with her adaptation, willingness to help others, and attitude toward life with an ostomy that he asked her to become an ostomy technician (the role became known as enterostomal therapist) for Cleveland Clinic. In 1961, they opened the first formal Enterostomal Therapy School to provide rehabilitative care and psychological support to individuals with ostomies. The following chronology highlights, adapted from the WOCN Scope and Standards (Wound, Ostomy and Continence Nurses Society™, 2018), documents some of the top defining moments in the history of WOC nursing.

- 1958: Norma Gill became the first "ostomy technician" at Cleveland Clinic.
- 1961: The first enterostomal therapy (ET) program was established at Cleveland Clinic.
- 1968: The first professional specialty organization was founded (American Association of Enterostomal Therapists), which later became known as the International Association for Enterostomal Therapy (IAET).
- 1976: Registered nurse licensure was required for entry into ET nursing education programs, which are now known as WOC nursing education programs.
- 1979: Certification in the specialty was first offered by the Enterostomal Therapy Nursing Certification Board, founded in 1978, which is a separate entity from the WOC nursing society and is now known as the Wound, Ostomy and Continence Nursing Certification Board.
- 1982: The scope of practice was expanded to include the care of individuals with wounds and urinary and fecal continence disorders.
- 1985: A baccalaureate degree was implemented as the minimum educational requirement for admission to the WOC nursing education programs and eligibility for certification in the specialty.
- 1992: The International Association of Enterostomal Therapy evolved into the Wound, Ostomy and Continence Nurses Society: An Association of ET Nurses, which is now known as the Wound, Ostomy and Continence Nurses Society™.
- 2010: Wound, ostomy, and continence nursing was recognized as a nursing specialty by the American Nurses Association.

KEY COMPONENTS OF THE WOC NURSE ROLE

Core values that guide the professional practice of the WOC nurse include integrity, leadership, and knowledge. These values are demonstrated by the following beliefs and behaviors (WOCN, 2018):

- Integrity: WOC nurses are uncompromised in their dedication to being a trusted, unbiased, and credible source of evidence-based information, care, and expertise.
- Leadership: WOC nurses are stewards of excellence with a common passion for mutual respect, shared experiences, and lifelong learning.
- Knowledge: WOC nurses demonstrate a continued commitment to education and research to generate and disseminate knowledge that improves patient outcomes.

WOC nursing integrates art and science using creativity and innovation and assimilates evidenced-based practices to manage patients with wounds, abdominal stomas, fistulas, percutaneous tubes/drains, and continence problems. WOC nurses are often called on to create new products, modify therapies, use innovative approaches for topical therapies or products, and orchestrate interdisciplinary resources to provide treatment plans for individuals or groups of health care consumers to achieve optimum health and independence (WOCN, 2018). In addition to providing unique and creative clinical skills, WOC nurses address other problems that patients experience such as limited access to supplies, lack of support, and teaching family, caregivers, and staff. Essential to the practice of WOC nursing is the establishment of a relationship with the patients and their families/caregivers to gain trust, to help set goals, and to move the patient toward an optimal state of health.

PROFESSIONAL PRACTICE GOALS

Throughout the process of care, key goals for WOC nurses are to promote safe, patient-centered, quality, effective, equitable, efficient, timely, evidence-based, and cost-effective care for health care consumers (WOCN, 2018). WOC nurses contribute to achieving these goals through a variety of activities including, but not limited to, the following (WOCN, 2018):

- Collaborating with the health care consumer, family members, and other health care providers to develop individualized care plans and outcomes
- Implementing and marketing the role
- Providing evidence-based care to promote quality, effective and safe care and practice, and optimal outcomes for health care consumers who are culturally, socioeconomically, and geographically diverse
- Preventing complications and reducing readmissions
- Using proactive risk management strategies to reduce health care–acquired injuries such as the following: surgical site and wound infections, catheter-associated urinary tract infections, medical adhesive–related skin injuries, pressure injuries, and medical device–related skin injuries, etc.
- Educating staff to improve the quality, effectiveness, and safety of care; and staff productivity, competency, and efficiency
- Using advanced technology for prevention, diagnosis, and treatment of wound, ostomy, and/or continence problems
- Coordinating care to promote continuity across health care settings
- Translating research into practice
- Developing metrics for quality outcomes
- Establishing standards for documentation and practice
- Developing formularies for supply management
- Developing protocols for cost-effective utilization of resources (e.g., pressure redistribution support surfaces, negative wound pressure therapy)
- Engaging in advocacy efforts for reimbursement of supplies and services
- Participating in/or conducting trials and evaluations of new products and treatments

LEVELS OF THE WOC NURSING PRACTICE

WOC REGISTERED NURSE

The WOC nurse is a registered nurse with a baccalaureate degree or higher, with at least 1 year of clinical nursing experience following RN licensure. To attend an accredited WOC Nursing Educational Program (WOCNEP), the applicant must have current clinical nursing experience within 5 years prior to applying to WOCNEP. Applicants can choose from several accredited WOCN Educational Programs, and the structure of each program is diverse. Programs follow the curriculum blueprint that is part of the WOCN accreditation of the educational program; all programs contain a didactic and clinical component. Upon completion of the educational program in wound, ostomy, and/or continence, the nurse is awarded a certificate designating WOC nurse or specialty status, and the graduate is qualified to take national board examinations to become board certified in wound, ostomy, and/or continence care.

Those nurses not attending a WOCNEP, that have advanced their knowledge through additional studying in the specialty area(s) as well as through clinical practical experience. It is the inclusion of a clinical practicum with an approved Certified Wound Ostomy Continence Nurse (CWOCN) preceptor, which sets the WOC nurse apart. Certification is through the WOC Nursing Certification Board (WOCNCB®), an organization that is separate and distinct from the WOCN® Society.

WOC GRADUATE DEGREE REGISTERED NURSE

The WOC graduate degree RN is licensed as an RN within the state of practice and has a masters or doctoral degree but is not a graduate of an APRN educational program. They have attended an accredited WOCNEP or sought additional focused education and practical experience.

ADVANCED PRACTICE WOC REGISTERED NURSE

Advanced practice registered nurses (APRNs) have completed the educational requirements for licensure as an advanced practice nurse, either at the masters or doctoral level and are licensed in the state or states that they practice as APRNs. They have obtained education in one, two, or all three specialty areas through an accredited WOC Nursing Education Program (WOCNEP) or through additional study focused in the specialty or specialties including focused practical experience. Certification is through the WOC Nursing Certification Board (WOCNCB®). The WOC APRN may practice independently or in collaboration with a physician, which depends on the state board of nursing, where the nurse practices.

 THE TRI-SPECIALTY OF WOC NURSING

WOUND SPECIALTY

WOC nurses provide care to health care consumers across the continuum of care with varied types of acute or chronic wounds due to pressure; venous, arterial, or diabetes/neuropathic disease; trauma; thermal injury; surgery; and/or other disease processes (e.g., cancer, infection, vasculitis, sickle cell disease, calciphylaxis, etc.). Wounds can have devastating effects on the health care consumer with increased morbidity and mortality due to complications. Pain, bleeding, odor, drainage, necrosis, infection, sepsis, and limb loss are some of the complications associated with wounds. Throughout the process of care, WOC nurses collaborate and coordinate with other health care providers in developing and implementing wound treatment plans.

OSTOMY SPECIALTY

Health care consumers undergoing ostomy surgery require intensive physical and emotional care and continued support to return to their normal lives. For health care consumers with fecal or urinary diversions, fistulas, or percutaneous tubes/drains, WOC nurses (regardless of the practice setting) provide specialized care to maximize the individual's independence in self-care and adaptation to the life-altering changes in their body image and function. According to the American Society of Colon and Rectal Surgeons, "... all patients who have ostomies should have access to an ostomy nurse for follow-up care, as needed and wherever possible" (Hendren et al., 2015).

After ostomy surgery, individuals are faced with life-altering changes that can be overwhelming and devastating without proper care and education. The selection and fitting of an ostomy pouching system requires a specially educated nurse who is qualified and skilled to assess and determine the unique medical and physical needs of each individual.

The need for specialized ostomy care continues well beyond the immediate surgical period. WOC nurses are needed to provide long-term support and follow-up care to health care consumers with ostomies.

CONTINENCE SPECIALTY

Living with fecal or urinary dysfunction and incontinence places a great burden on affected individuals and their families or caregivers. Loss of continence can cause skin and wound care complications and may contribute to individuals being prematurely placed in long-term care facilities (WOCN, 2013b). Unfortunately, many individuals, family/caregivers, and health care providers do not intervene in continence issues believing that loss of continence is a normal part of the aging process (WOCN, 2016). Successful outcomes for individuals with continence problems require specialized care, and WOC nurses play an important role in the management of fecal and urinary continence issues.

COMPLEX PROBLEMS

A fistula is an abnormal tract that develops between a body cavity or organ or an organ and the skin (Bryant & Best, 2016). Some of the most difficult fistulas that WOC nurses care for are enterocutaneous fistulas that develop an opening from the small intestine to the skin, enteroatmospheric fistulas that open into the base of a wound, and multiple fistulas (Bryant & Best, 2016). An interdisciplinary team is required to manage an individual with a fistula, and WOC nurses are essential members of the team. WOC nurses utilize a variety of creative and adaptive techniques for both pouching and nonpouching modalities to achieve the goals for topical management of fistulas: skin protection, containment and accurate measurement of drainage, odor control, comfort and mobility of the individual, and cost containment (Bryant & Best, 2016).

WOC nurses are also often consulted to assist in management of complications due to percutaneous tubes/drains (i.e., gastrostomy, jejunostomy, nephrostomy, biliary). Percutaneous tubes/drains are placed to provide drainage, relieve an obstruction and maintain an opening into an organ, and/or for administration of fluids, medications, or feedings. Multiple complications occur with enteral tubes/drains that include irritant dermatitis from leakage around the tube, device-related pressure ulcers/injuries from inappropriate stabilization of the tube, fungal infections, cellulitis, and hypertrophic granulation tissue (Fellows & Rice, 2016).

 WOC NURSE ROLES

WOC nurses serve in a variety of roles including clinician, educator, consultant, researcher, and administrator, and they may engage in dual or multiple roles.

CLINICIAN

The WOC nurse provides care to individuals in multiple practice settings. The WOC nurse may also evaluate individuals and their care via telehealth services. To achieve optimal outcomes, the WOC nurse uses the nursing process when caring for health care consumers. Each plan of care is individualized to complement the developmental age of the health care consumer and their caregiver and achieve the best outcomes (ANA, 2010, 2015a).

EDUCATOR

Education is an integral component of every WOC nurse's role. The WOC nurse provides education directly to health care consumers, caregivers, nurses, clinical staff, and other health care providers. WOC nurses provide staff education through orientation, on-the-job training, in-service education, and development of protocols and/or guidelines (WOCN, 2013a).

WOC nurses may also provide formal education in academia or other organized continuing education programs that focus on one or more aspects of wound, ostomy, or continence care (WOCN, 2013a). Educational webinars are examples of some of the numerous continuing education programs provided by WOC nurses and the WOCN® Society. These programs extend the reach of the WOC nurse and the WOCN® Society to areas and settings that lack a WOC nurse.

CONSULTANT

In a direct consultant role, the WOC nurse partners with the health care consumer and other members of the health care team (WOCN, 2013a). The WOC specialty nurse has unique skills to coordinate individualized care based on assessment of the needs of the health care consumer, knowledge of current best practices, and an ongoing evaluation of outcomes. Collaboration with other health care providers and groups is also an essential part of the WOC nurses consultant's role. Some WOC nurses serve as independent consultants with contractual arrangements for the delivery of wound, ostomy, and/or continence care services in various settings. WOC nurses may also utilize their expertise in other practice areas such as legal nurse consulting.

RESEARCHER

In the role of researcher, the WOC nurse advances the science and art of wound, ostomy, and/or continence care. Varied types of research are conducted using different methodologies (e.g., applied research/clinical trials, problem-focused research, exploratory research, etc.). WOC nurse researchers are active in all settings where WOC nurses practice including academia, industry, and direct patient care areas (WOCN, 2013a). At the clinical level, WOC nurses assist in the translation of research and evidence-based guidelines into practice to enhance the delivery of quality care.

ADMINISTRATOR

The WOC nurse may also assume the role of an administrator. As an administrator, the WOC nurse's duties and responsibilities include management and oversight of clinical staff and the delivery of services across a broad spectrum of care (WOCN, 2013a). Other activities involved in administration include program development and efforts to ensure quality outcomes. The WOC nurse manager may be responsible for developing and overseeing operating budget for their department/unit.

PRECEPTOR

A WOC nurse can assume the role of preceptor for students. The most common role of preceptor is for either graduate nursing students (if the WOC nurse is an advanced degree nurse) or WOC nurse students. The WOCNEP have a clinical component of 40 hours per specialty, and a WOC nurse who has completed the WOCNEP and is certified with an active practice can become a preceptor.

DUAL/MULTIPLE ROLES

Often WOC nurses assume dual or multiple roles, depending on their educational preparation and setting. In addition, WOC graduate-level prepared registered nurses and WOC advanced practice registered nurses contribute to the specialty and profession by delivering direct care as providers, examining systems, spearheading research, and providing clinical leadership in WOC nursing.

POPULATIONS SERVED BY WOC NURSES

Although the basic principles of wound, ostomy, and continence care are the same regardless of population or practice setting, certain populations may be at greater risk for wound, ostomy, and/or continence problems and complications. Also, they may require adaptation or modifications in their care to address their unique needs including, but not limited to, the following patient populations: pediatric patients (neonates, infants, children, adolescents), older adults, patients needing palliative or hospice care, and obese patients. WOC nurses have expertise in caring for individuals with wound, ostomy, and/or continence needs across the spectrum of ages and developmental stages, including those at end of life and others with unique or special needs.

PEDIATRIC POPULATION

Key concepts in effective management of the pediatric population include development of rapport with the patient, family, and caregivers; interdisciplinary collaboration and coordination of care; patient and family education; and ongoing follow-up, support, and positive reinforcement by the WOC nurse to promote cooperation and adherence to the treatment plan (Jinbo, 2016). Education must always be presented that is appropriate for the cognitive abilities of the child.

OLDER ADULTS

It is important for WOC nurses to collaborate and coordinate care with the patient, family and caregivers, and members of the interdisciplinary team to assess needs and provide appropriate, dignified care for the older adult with wound, ostomy, and/or continence needs. The assessment must include the preferences for care and personal goals of the older adult. Coordination of care with other disciplines (e.g., physical and occupational therapists, dieticians, social workers, etc.) is needed to provide comprehensive care to manage frail older adults and those with comorbid conditions.

PALLIATIVE/HOSPICE CARE

Increasing numbers of infants, children, adolescents, and adults are living with serious or critical illnesses or injuries (ANA & Hospice & Palliative Nurses Association [HPNA], 2017). Palliative care that includes hospice care is provided by an interdisciplinary team, and WOC nurses contribute in wound care (prevention or management of pressure injuries, malignant wounds), continence issues (fecal or urinary incontinence), and in management of fecal and urinary diversions.

WOC NURSE PRACTICE SETTINGS

The majority of WOC nurses work in the acute care setting. In addition, WOC nurses have the opportunity to practice in other settings such as outpatient care, home health care, long-term care, nursing homes, industry, academia, private practice, etc. WOC nurses may practice in multiple clinical settings that are affiliated with/or part of a large organization or health care system, or they may function as an independent consultant to several settings.

The following descriptions provide a brief overview of WOC nursing practice in some of the most common settings (WOCN, 2010).

ACUTE CARE

In the acute care setting, WOC nurses care for health care consumers with a wide variety of medical, surgical, and/or trauma diagnoses. The WOC nurse may provide services in one or more areas of the tri-specialty practice to health care consumers across the lifespan from newborns to the elderly. Health care consumers with wound, ostomy, and/or continence needs may be found in any level of care within the hospital setting including the emergency department, intensive/critical care units, operating room, and medical–surgical units.

OUTPATIENT CARE

WOC nurses may practice in outpatient care settings that include private practice settings, hospital-based outpatient clinics, and freestanding ambulatory care centers. WOC nurses may work in conjunction with physicians and surgeons (e.g., urologists, vascular specialists, colorectal surgeons) to optimize management of health care consumers with wound, ostomy, and/or continence disorders. WOC advanced practice registered nurses may also serve as providers within these practices.

HOME HEALTH CARE

In the home care setting, WOC nurses provide direct care and consultation to health care consumers with wound, ostomy, and/or continence concerns. The prospective payment system in home care has fueled an increased demand for WOC nursing expertise to help streamline services, educate caregivers and staff, and contain costs. WOC nurses can develop protocols for care and product formularies to reduce costs while maintaining quality care. In addition to serving as a direct care provider, the WOC nurse's responsibilities often include educating other home health nurses and clinical staff to promote quality, evidence-based care for management of health care consumers with wound, ostomy, and/or continence needs. WOC nurses are integral members of interdisciplinary teams and work closely with rehabilitation staff to facilitate self-care and independence in the home environment. Additionally, the WOC nurse may serve as a case manager/care coordinator to facilitate care delivery.

LONG-TERM/EXTENDED CARE

In long-term care and extended care settings, WOC nurses may monitor, direct, or assist with care and/or provide education to facilitate care by other registered and/or licensed practical/vocational nursing staff and nursing assistants. WOC nurses must be knowledgeable about the regulatory and risk management issues and assessment and documentation requirements that are unique to the setting. The WOC nurse may serve as an independent consultant or an employee of the facility.

REHABILITATION

Services in skilled nursing facilities focus on care that enables health care consumers to achieve maximum independence in self-care. WOC nurses, with their emphasis on optimizing self-care and strong educations skills, are able to meet the challenges posed by individuals who need rehabilitative services and have wound, ostomy, and/or continence issues. WOC advanced practice registered nurses who practice in this setting may be able to receive third-party reimbursement for their services.

INDUSTRY

WOC nurses may practice in one or more areas of the tri-specialty, depending on the industry's focus. The WOC nurse in this setting may function primarily as a researcher and/or educator to investigate and develop new products and teach the end users. The WOC nurse in industry may serve as a resource to direct care providers and provide research evidence about the clinical effectiveness of products for wound, ostomy, and/or continence care and can offer guidance about the appropriate indications and use of products.

ACADEMIA

The WOC nurse in academia may function as an educator, researcher, administrator, or department head. The WOC nurse may provide formal education for one or more areas of the tri-specialty, or the content may be incorporated into other graduate or undergraduate courses. In addition to an academic appointment, a WOC nurse faculty member may have an active clinical practice as part of their role. Academic accreditation standards for nursing programs dictate faculty educational standards; therefore, the WOC nurse in this practice area will have an advanced degree.

RESEARCH CONSUMER AND EVIDENCE-BASED PRACTICE

Health care consumers and providers, including agencies such as the Centers for Medicare & Medicaid Services (CMS) and the health care insurance industry, expect care to be delivered based on the best available research and evidence. Many agencies and groups utilize and publish evidence-based clinical practice (EBP) guidelines, including the WOCN Society®. WOC nurses use all types of research and evidence to influence the quality of patient care that is provided while practicing in the full scope of WOC specialty nursing.

There are many roles for a WOC nurse in research and EBP, such as consumer and developer of EB guidelines and standards of care, investigator in a scientific research trial, as well as evaluator of products.

The WOC nurse can contribute to the development of evidence-based care in many ways without assuming the role (or responsibility) of a primary investigator such as by participating in the following activities:

Surveys or polls
Clinical trials or product evaluations (see section on product evaluation)
Data collection for pressure injury prevalence and incidence studies or continuous quality improvement projects/studies that relate to WOC care or foot and nail care

The components of EBP include a systematic search and appraisal of evidence to answer the clinical question(s), integration of the expertise, and experience of the WOC nurse as well as consideration of the patient's preference, values, and concerns. As part of the critical appraisal process, it is necessary to be able to discern the level and quality of the evidence. There are levels and criteria for rating research evidence utilized by the WOCN® Society in developing clinical practice guidelines.

CARE COORDINATION AND COLLABORATION BY WOC NURSE

The WOC nurse works collaboratively with other health care disciplines to provide comprehensive care. Successful collaboration between the WOC nurse, physicians, and other health care members increases member's awareness of each other's type of knowledge and skills that will lead to improvement in patients' treatment plan and successful outcome. In order to coordinate individualize patient care, the WOC nurse should partner with members of the health care team, patient's families/caregivers, and other health care providers across the continuum of care (WOCN, 2018). Collaboration and coordinating of care requires skill to ensure that the patient receives quality care.

The WOC nurse coordinates care for complex cases, utilizing their expertise, skills, and resources in various practice settings. The WOC APRN can provide additional services: order and interpret diagnostic and laboratory tests, prescribe pharmacological and nonpharmacological agents, and treatments for wound, ostomy, and continence complications (WOCN, 2018).

HEALTH CARE REIMBURSEMENT

Health care reimbursement has a direct effect on the amount and type of care provided to patients by all health care providers, including WOC nurses. Payment for health care in the United States involves several mechanisms, including self-pay by the consumers, insurance companies, and government agencies. The federal government is the single largest payer through Medicare, Medicaid, and the Department of Veterans Affairs (Sherman, 2012). Medicare is a federally provided health insurance program that is administered by the U.S. Department of Health and Human Services through CMS. Medicare provides coverage for individuals over the age of 65, younger than 65 with disabilities, and with end-stage renal disease at any age.

Medicare Part A covers hospital and hospice visits, stays in skilled nursing facilities, and home health. Medicare Part B covers 80% of expenses incurred with outpatient visits/care, some home health, and durable medical equipment. Medicare Part C provides insurance coverage by private-run insurance companies. Medicare Part D helps cover the cost of prescriptions. More information about Medicare can be found on the CMS Web site.

Medicaid is a joint state and federal health insurance program for low-income individuals. States establish and administer their own Medicaid programs and determine the type, amount, duration, and scope of services within broad federal guidelines. Medicaid provides health coverage to pregnant women, seniors and individuals with disabilities, and nonelderly, low-income parents or caretaker relatives and varies from state to state.

The Wound, Ostomy and Continence Nurses Society™ has developed two fact sheets about reimbursement for its members and are available on the Web site (http://www.wocn.org) in the Public Policy and Advocacy section. The fact sheet, *Reimbursement of Advanced*

Practice Registered Nurse Services, provides information about reimbursement opportunities and challenges for the advanced practice RN (WOCN® Society, 2019a). In addition, the fact sheet, *Understanding Medicare Part B Incident to Billing*, provides some insight into cases where a nonadvanced practice WOC nurse might bill in the outpatient setting. "Incident to" is a billing mechanism for Medicare that allows services provided in an outpatient setting to be delivered by auxiliary personnel and billed under the provider's national provider identification (NPI). For example, under the incident to provision, a physician or APRN could develop the plan of care and a non-APRN could provide the care and bill under the provider's NPI (WOCN® Society, 2019b).

CONTINUOUS PROFESSIONAL DEVELOPMENT

Continued professional development is critical for the practicing WOC nurse. There are many opportunities through the WOCN® Society for the WOC nurse to maintain current, evidence-based practice. This can be accomplished by reading the *Journal of Wound Ostomy and Continence Nursing*, attending conferences and working within the WOCN® Society as a volunteer. The WOCN offers an annual conference, that provides current research, topics related to the wound, ostomy, and continence practice. WOCN regions and affiliates offer on-site conferences. The WOCN® Society also provides live streaming/webcasts of sessions presented at the annual conference. Throughout the year, there are webinars available that provide continuing education credits. WOC nursing practice requires lifelong learning.

Involvement in professional activities can provide professional growth where opportunities are available to become a committee member to work on important projects, develop strategies to enhance care delivery, as well as opportunities to develop relationships with other WOC nurse specialists. Examples of organizations that are within the scope of WOC practice include WOCN® Society, World Council of Enterostomal Therapists, and National Pressure Injury Advisory Panel.

Certification

Wound, Ostomy and Continence Nursing Certification Board (WOCNCB) is a national-certified organization that provides credentials based on valid and reliable testing process. The WOCNCB is a separate and distinct organization from the WOC Nursing Society. WOCNCB validates the specialized knowledge, skills, and expertise of nurses who meet the requirements for certification. Certification is voluntary, however recommended as it provides assurance to patients and employers of a safe and competent practice. WOCN certification is granted for 5 years. Compliance must be demonstrated every 5 years by either reexamination or development of a professional growth program portfolio. Advance practice nursing certification in wound, ostomy, and continence nursing is

TABLE 1-1 WOCNCB'S WOUND, OSTOMY, AND CONTINENCE CERTIFICATION CREDENTIALS	
CWOCN	Certified Wound, Ostomy, and Continence Nurse
CWCN	Certified Wound Care Nurse
COCN	Certified Ostomy Care Nurse
CCCN	Certified Continence Care Nurse
CWON	Certified Wound Ostomy Nurse
Advanced Practice Certifications Credentials	
CWOCN-AP	Certified Wound, Ostomy, and Continence Nurse–Advanced Practice
CWCN-AP	Certified Wound Care Nurse–Advanced Practice
COCN-AP	Certified Ostomy Care Nurse–Advanced Practice
CCCN-AP	Certified Continence Care Nurse–Advanced Practice
CWON-AP	Certified Wound Ostomy Nurse–Advanced Practice

available through WOCNCB (see **Table 1-1** on credentials). For more information on WOCNCB and certification requirements, see their Web site www.wocncb.org.

 ## ETHICS IN WOC NURSING

WOC nursing as a specialty practice embraces the provisions of the *Code of Ethics for Nurses with Interpretive Statements* (ANA, 2015b). WOC nurses are obligated to "adhere to standards of ethical practice established by the WOCN Society and to conduct themselves in a manner that upholds the highest professional standards" (WOCN, 2018). The *Code of Ethics for Nurses*:

Provision 1. The nurse practices with compassion and respect for the inherent dignity, worth, and unique attributes of every person.

Provision 2. The nurse's primary commitment is to the patient, whether an individual, family, group, community, or population.

Provision 3. The nurse promotes, advocates for, and protects the rights, health, and safety of the patient.

Provision 4. The nurse has authority, accountability, and responsibility for nursing practice; makes decisions; and takes action consistent with the obligation to promote health and to provide optimal care.

Provision 5. The nurse owes the same duties to self as to others, including the responsibility to promote health and safety, preserve wholeness of character and integrity, maintain competence, and continue personal and professional growth.

Provision 6. The nurse, through individual and collective effort, establishes, maintains, and improves the ethical environment of the work setting and conditions of employment that are conducive to safe, quality health care.

Provision 7. The nurse in all roles and settings advances the profession through research and scholarly inquiry, professional standards development, and the generation of both nursing and health policy.

Provision 8. The nurse collaborates with other health professionals and the public to protect human rights, promote health diplomacy, and reduce health disparities.

Provision 9. The profession of nursing, collectively through its professional organizations, must articulate nursing values, maintain the integrity of the profession, and integrate principles of social justice into nursing and health policy.

For interpretive statements specific to WOC nursing are available in the full scope and standards document (WOCN, 2018).

CONCLUSION

WOC nurses are professionals dedicated to individuals with WOC care needs. It is the goal of the WOC nurse to enhance delivery of wound, ostomy, and continence care directly and indirectly to those persons in need of such care.

REFERENCES

American Nurses Association. (2010). *Nursing's social policy statement: The essence of the profession* (3rd ed.). Silver Spring, MD: Author.

American Nurses Association. (2015a). *Nursing: Scope and standards of practice* (3rd ed.). Silver Spring, MD: Author.

American Nurses Association. (2015b). *Code of ethics for nurses with interpretive statements*. Silver Spring, MD: Author.

American Nurses Association & Hospice and Palliative Nurses Association. (2017). Call for action: Nurses lead and transform palliative care. Retrieved August 21, 2017, from http://nursingworld.org/MainMenu-Categories/ThePracticeofProfessionalNursing/Palliative-Care-Call-for-Action/Draft-PalliativeCare-ProfessionalIssuesPanel-CallforAction.pdf

Bryant, R., & Best, M. (2016). Management of draining wounds and fistulas. In R. Bryant & D. Nix (Eds.), *Acute & chronic wounds* (5th ed.). St. Louis, MO: Elsevier.

Fellows, J., & Rice, M. (2016). Nursing management of the patient with percutaneous tubes. In J. E. Carmel, J. C. Colwell, & M. T. Goldberg (Eds.), *Wound, Ostomy and Continence Nurses Society™ Core curriculum: Ostomy management* (pp. 220–230). Philadelphia, PA: Wolters Kluwer.

Hendren, S., Hammond, K., Glasgow, S. C., et al. (2015). Clinical practice guidelines for Ostomy surgery. *Diseases of the Colon and Rectum, 58*(4), 375–387. doi: 10.1097/DCR.0000000000000347.

Jinbo, A., & Bliss, D. (2016). Facilitators and barriers to adherence to prescribed bowel management programs by adolescents with neurogenic bowel conditions. Conference poster, WOCN 2016 Conference, Montreal, Canada.

Sherman, R., & Bishop, M. (2012). The business of caring: What every nurse should know about cutting costs. *American Nurse Today, 7*(11), 32–34.

Wound, Ostomy and Continence Nurses Society (WOCN). (2010). *Wound, ostomy, and continence nursing: Scope & standards of practice*. Mt. Laurel, NJ: Author.

Wound, Ostomy and Continence Nurses Society. (2013a). *Professional practice manual* (4th ed.). Philadelphia, PA: Wolters Kluwer/Lippincott Williams & Wilkins. Retrieved April 11, 2020, from the Lippincott Nursing Center at http://www.nursingcenter.com/journalarticle

Wound, Ostomy and Continence Nurses Society. (2013b). A quick reference guide for managing fecal incontinence. Retrieved April 3, 2017, from http://www.wocn.org/?page=QuickRefGuide

Wound, Ostomy and Continence Nurses Society. (2016). Reversible causes of acute/transient urinary incontinence: Clinical resource guide. Retrieved April 3, 2017, from http://www.wocn.org/?page=RevAcuteTransientUI

Wound, Ostomy and Continence Nurses Society. (2018). *Wound, ostomy and continence nursing scope & standards of practice* (2nd ed.). Mt. Laurel, NJ: Author.

Wound, Ostomy and Continence Nurses Society. (2019a). *Reimbursement of advanced practice registered nurse services: A fact sheet*. Mt. Laurel, NJ: Author.

Wound, Ostomy and Continence Nurses Society. (2019b). *Understanding Medicare Part B incident to billing: A fact sheet*. Mt. Laurel, NJ: Author.

QUESTIONS

1. Medicare Part B covers
  A. Hospice visits
  B. Durable medical equipment
  C. Prescriptions
  D. Hospital visits

2. When designing and implementing a WOC nurse role, it is important to
  A. Practice according to the WOCN® Scope and Standards
  B. Read the *Journal of WOC Nursing*
  C. Practice in all roles of the WOC nurse
  D. Provide annual reports to administration

3. Completion of an accredited WOCNEP to become a WOC nurse requires
  A. Didactic, special project, and passing final examination
  B. Didactic and 40 hours of clinical experience
  C. Didactic and acceptance of previous wound experience
  D. Didactic and 120 clinical hours with an approved CWOCN preceptor

4. As an educator, the WOC nurse is responsible for
  A. Providing staff nurse orientation
  B. Conducting clinical trials of products
  C. Developing protocols and guidelines
  D. Collecting data for quality improvement

5. Data collection for the WOC nurse should be
  A. Purposeful and outcome oriented
  B. Filled with everything the WOC nurse does
  C. Provided to administration annually
  D. Created by the WOC nurse only

6. As a research consumer, the role of the WOC nurse is
  A. Primary investigator for rigorous research studies
  B. Evaluator of WOC patient products
  C. Required to show proof of education in research
  D. Developer of evidence outside the scope of practice

7. The components of evidence-based practice include all of the following *except*
  A. Appraisal of evidence
  B. Systematic search of the literature
  C. Integration of the expertise of WOC nurse
  D. Work independently of others

8. Best practice documents provide which type of evidence?
  A. Randomized clinical trials
  B. Expert opinion
  C. Quasi-experimental studies
  D. Task force reviews

9. The first program for WOC nursing (previously enterostomal therapy) was located in
  A. Minneapolis
  B. New York City
  C. Cleveland
  D. Boston

10. Name two of the most common roles of the WOC nurse practices in acute care setting.
  A. Clinician and research
  B. Clinician and educator
  C. Educator and administrator
  D. Educator and preceptor

ANSWERS AND RATIONALES

1. B. Rationale: Medicare Part B covers durable medical equipment. Medicare Part A covers hospice and hospitals and Medicare Part D covers prescriptions.

2. A. Rationale: The WOCN® Scope and Standards is the foundation to incorporate into the WOC nursing practice.

3. D. Rationale: Requirements to complete a WOCNEP are didactic and 120 clinical hours (40 hours each specialty in wound, ostomy, and continence) with an approved CWOCN preceptor.

4. A. Rationale: As an educator, the WOC nurse has the responsibility to provide orientation to staff nurses. Conducting clinical trials of products and developing guidelines is an example of the role in research. In the role of a clinician, the WOC nurse is responsible for quality improvement projects related to the specialty.

5. A. Rationale: Data collection is important to the WOC nurse's practice. It should be purposeful and outcome oriented to validate the role and position of the WOC nurse.

6. B. Rationale: The WOC nurse can contribute to research by evaluating WOC products.

7. D. Rationale: The components of evidence-based practice do not include work independently of others.

8. B. Rationale: Best practice documents level of evidence is from expert opinion.

9. C. Rationale: Cleveland was the first site for an enterostomal therapy program (WOCN Program).

10. B. Rationale: Clinician and educator are the two major roles of the WOC nurse in the acute care setting. The role of a consultant is also a major role for the WOC nurse.

CHAPTER 2

ANATOMY AND PHYSIOLOGY OF THE SKIN

Asfandyar Mufti, Khalad Maliyar, Elizabeth A. Ayello, and R. Gary Sibbald

OBJECTIVES

1. Describe the anatomy and physiology of the skin and soft tissue, changes across a lifespan, and implications for maintenance of skin health.

2. Describe common skin conditions to include pathology, presentation, and management.

3. Use accurate dermatologic terminology to describe skin lesions and wounds.

TOPIC OUTLINE

INTRODUCTION

The skin is the largest organ in the human body and serves the critical barrier function between the internal and external environments. Anatomically, the skin is divided into two major components: the epidermis and dermis. The epidermis is the outermost layer of the skin, and the dermis is deep to the epidermis. The subcutaneous fat tissue lies beneath the dermis and is sometimes known as the hypodermis, although it is not a primary skin layer (see **Fig. 2-1**).

ANATOMY AND PHYSIOLOGY OF THE SKIN

The skin itself is divided into two major layers, the epidermis and dermis; each layer has unique structures and functions.

EPIDERMIS

The epidermis is a stratified squamous epithelial structure, with four to five distinct and well-defined stratified layers.

The layers are, from the base to external environment, as follows: stratum basale (also known as stratum germinativum), stratum spinosum, stratum granulosum, stratum lucidum (present only in areas of thicker skin including the palms/soles), and stratum corneum (see **Fig. 2-1**). The layers of the epidermis contain migrating epithelial cells (keratinocytes) that are undergoing differentiation and proliferation cycles. This migration provides a continuous renewal of the epidermis and helps to prepare an effective barrier once the epidermal cells reach the skin surface (stratum corneum). At the epidermal surface, the cells that become corneocytes eventually undergo programmed cell death and are sloughed away. These cells will eventually be replenished by continuously dividing cells in the stratum basale. In addition to keratinocytes, the epidermis contains other cell types that are important for both the structural integrity and function of the skin: melanocytes, Langerhans cells, and Merkel cells.

Stratum Basale

The deepest layer of the epidermis is known as the *stratum basale* or *stratum germinativum* and ranges from

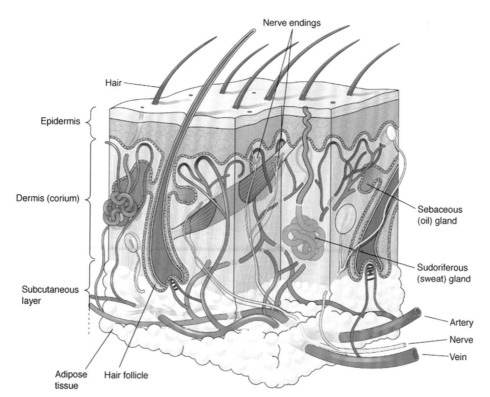

FIGURE 2-1. Cross Section of Skin and Soft Tissue. (Reprinted with permission from Cohen, B. J., & Taylor, J. (2005). *Memmler's structure and function of the human body* (8th ed.). Philadelphia, PA: Lippincott Williams & Wilkins.)

one to three cells in thickness. It is separated from the deeper dermis by the basement membrane (basal lamina) and is attached to the basement membrane via hemidesmosomes. The *stratum basale* is the reproductive layer of the epidermis and is characterized by proliferating keratinocytes. When a basal cell divides, one cell begins upward migration and the other cell remains in the basal layer to continue the reproductive cycle. As these keratinocytes migrate toward the stratum corneum (outermost epidermal layer), they undergo a maturation process involving several morphological and biochemical changes; this is known as *terminal differentiation* or *keratinization*. Once terminal differentiation is complete, all that remains is a layer of tightly packed dead cells (corneocytes).

The stratum basale also contains melanocytes, which are responsible for producing the pigment *melanin*. Morphologically, melanocytes have dendrites extending from their cell bodies and contain organelles known as melanosomes. As the name suggests, melanosomes contain melanin that is produced from the amino acid tyrosine. In addition to being responsible for everyone's unique skin color, melanin also has photoprotective properties; it can absorb harmful ultraviolet (UV) light and protect cells against DNA damage. Migrating keratinocytes in the *stratum spinosum* are protected from harmful UV light by the melanosomes. These organelles move along the dendrites of the melanocytes to the periphery providing enhanced pigment dispersion and photoprotection (as evidenced by hyperpigmentation or tanning).

Stratum Spinosum

Above the *stratum basale* lies the *stratum spinosum*. This layer is 8 to 10 cells in thickness that contains irregular, polyhedral cells with cytoplasmic processes that expand toward nearby neighboring cells and contact them through desmosomes. In addition to keratinocytes, this cell layer contains immune cells known as *Langerhans (LH) cells*. These LH cells are dendritic in nature and are usually classified as phagocytic and *antigen-presenting cells* (APCs) responsible for contact allergic reactions.

Stratum Granulosum

Moving further toward the surface of the epidermis, the next cell layer is the *stratum granulosum* that is three to five cells thick. The stratum granulosum is composed of flattened keratinocytes that have distinct darkly staining keratohyalin granules. The cells within this epidermal layer contain organelles known as *Odland bodies* that contribute significantly to the barrier function of the epidermis. Odland bodies contain lipids and enzymes that are discharged into the extracellular space. These lipids and enzymes form a lipophilic layer between the stratum granulosum and the stratum corneum that acts as a barrier to water loss. Defects in this lipophilic barrier are now

hypothesized to be the major defect in atopic dermatitis, which is characterized by structural abnormalities or lower levels of normal lipids including ceramides.

Keratinocytes in the stratum granulosum layer release lipids including ceramide lipids that help to maintain the normal brick and mortar skin barrier function. The stratum granulosum cells also contain glycolipids that when released function to act as a glue, holding the cells together.

Stratum Lucidum

This layer is found between the stratum corneum and the stratum granulosum and is two to three cells thick. The stratum lucidum consists of translucent cells seen present on the palms and soles and not on thinner skin in other body regions.

Stratum Corneum

The outermost layer of the epidermis is known as the *stratum corneum* and is 20 to 30 cells thick. The cells in this layer are terminally differentiated keratinocytes, also known as corneocytes; they are flat, keratinized, and dead, with no nuclei or organelles. The stratum corneum varies in thickness, depending on the region of the body. It is thickest on the palms and soles.

Retained nuclei in the stratum corneum are present only when the cells from the basal layer of the skin migrate more quickly to the skin surface. For example, in active psoriasis, transit time is cut in half (from the usual 28 to 14 days); this results in reduced differentiation of the keratinocytes and retained nuclei with the abnormal silver white scale characteristic of psoriatic plaque.

New skin cells (keratinocytes) are produced in the basal layer with one cell migrating to the surface and the second cell left to repopulate the basal layer. The migrating epidermal cells lose their nuclei and undergo terminal differentiation to enable them to provide an effective surface barrier.

DERMIS

Below the epidermis, there is a major connective tissue component known as the *dermis*. The dermis is connected to the epidermis via rete ridges. These ridges are sawtooth projections of the epidermis into the dermis that allow the two layers to interlock with each other. This pattern adds mechanical strength and reduces the risk of skin tears. The interface between dermal papillae and epidermal rete ridges is known as the dermal–epidermal junction (see **Fig. 2-1**).

Papillary Dermis

The dermis is composed of two distinct layers: reticular and papillary. The papillary layer is the uppermost layer of the dermis and the layer immediately below the epidermis that extends between the rete ridges. This layer of the dermis is composed primarily of loose areolar connective tissue, capillary loops, and nerve terminals including Meissner corpuscles (mechanoreceptors). One of the main functions of the papillary layer is to supply nutrients to the avascular epidermis through the overlying *stratum basale* layer. The capillary loops of the papillary dermis provide perfusion required to support epidermal cell mitosis and the differentiation of keratinocytes required for normal barrier function.

Reticular Dermis
The reticular layer is the bottom layer of the dermis. This layer contains most of the connective tissue proteins that give the skin its strength and elasticity. These proteins, such as collagen and elastin fibers, are embedded in a glycosaminoglycan (mucopolysaccharide) network. As is true of the epidermis, the dermis contains several different cells that are often concentrated in the reticular layer.

Key cells include the fibroblasts, mast cells, and macrophages. Fibroblasts are responsible for the synthesis of connective tissue and extracellular matrix, specifically the production of collagen (dermal building blocks) and elastin (tensile strength). In addition, laminin, a key component of basement membrane, and fibronectin, which binds extracellular matrix proteins, are both produced by fibroblasts.

Mast cells are granulated immune cells that are situated throughout the dermis. They are responsible for the release of histamine, leukotrienes, prostaglandins, and various chemotactic agents. Excessive release of histamine and other inflammatory mediators can cause hives (urticaria) in the skin along with allergic rhinitis of the nose and upper respiratory tract and asthma in the lower respiratory tree.

Lastly, the dermis contains macrophages, a key component of the innate immune system. The macrophages normally function to remove extracellular debris and engulf pathogens as an essential role in normal wound healing. In addition to a rich vascular network of arteries, arterioles, capillaries, venules, and veins, the dermis has an extensive lymphatic system and multiple sensory nerves.

In conclusion, the dermis is critical to tensile strength of the skin, contains the cutaneous blood vessels as well as migrating cells that are critical to immune function.

Epidermal Appendages
The hair follicles, sweat glands, and sebaceous glands are anatomically basal layer lined extensions of the epidermis branching from the surface of the epidermis to deep in the dermis and may extend into the subcutaneous fat. The epidermal and dermal structures are capable of reproduction throughout life; however, the epidermal appendages are not capable of reproduction. If an injury extends past the hair follicles, sebaceous glands, and sweat glands, those structures cannot be reproduced.

Epidermal structures and most dermal structures are capable of regeneration; the epidermal appendages, subcutaneous tissue, and muscle do *not* have the ability to regenerate, and wounds involving loss of these structures will heal by scar formation. However, if deep remnants of hair follicles are left, they can produce reepithelialized islands of epidermal tissue within the wound base.

SUBCUTANEOUS TISSUE
Underneath the dermis is a layer of subcutaneous fat, often referred to as the *hypodermis*. It provides insulation and acts to separate the skin from underlying muscle, tendons, bone, and joints. The subcutaneous tissue also plays a critical role in pressure redistribution. Individuals who have very minimal subcutaneous tissue are at much higher risk for pressure injury development especially if they become bedbound or chairbound.

Persons who are morbidly obese that develop a pressure injury or other wound may be at a higher risk for impaired healing. This is because the excess subcutaneous tissue increases interface pressures between the skin and the bed or chair, and subcutaneous tissue is poorly perfused and therefore slow to heal. The EPUAP/NPIAP/PPPIA (2019) guideline references the 2008 study by Bergstrom et al. that states that having obesity adversely influences healing times. A particularly harmful feature of severe obesity is maceration, inflammation, and tissue/skin necrosis, especially in large and deep skin folds. An increased tissue weight exerts additional load on dependent tissues resulting in vascular occlusion and tissue deformation. These changes in conjunction with a fragile vascular and lymphatic framework combined with an increased diaphoresis are responsible for additional skin and tissue complications in individuals who are obese (Bergstrom et al., 2008; EPUAP, NPIAP, PPPIA, 2019). Subcutaneous tissue lacks the capacity for reproduction; if a wound extends to the subcutaneous tissue layer, the defect will heal with scar formation.

MUSCLE
The layer of soft tissue deep to the hypodermis and immediately adjacent to the bone is the muscle layer. This layer has a higher metabolic rate than either the skin or subcutaneous tissue and is the layer most impacted by unrelieved pressure over a bony prominence. Current evidence suggests that most pressure injuries begin at the muscle–bone interface (EPUAP/NPIAP/PPPIA, 2019). "Muscle tissues are more susceptible to damage than skin tissues": (EPUAP/NPIAP/PPPIA, 2019). This is because the skin is stiffer than muscle or fat and deforms to a lesser degree in most clinically relevant scenarios including bodyweight forces during prolonged sitting or lying in bed (EPUAP NPIAP PPPIA, 2019).

FUNCTIONS OF THE SKIN AND SOFT TISSUE

The most critical function of the skin is its role as a barrier between the internal and external environments; however, it has several additional functions, and each of these is briefly described.

THERMOREGULATION AND REGULATION OF CUTANEOUS BLOOD FLOW

The ability of the skin to control blood flow is vital for thermoregulation and maintenance of physiologic body temperature. For humans, core temperature is maintained at approximately 37°C (98°F to 99°F). There are normal temperature fluctuations that can occur throughout the day (circadian rhythm), throughout the month (e.g., menstrual cycle), and throughout one's life (aging). Cutaneous blood flow is primarily controlled by the sympathetic nervous system with noradrenaline and adrenaline being the primary vasoconstricting neurotransmitters (Charkoudian, 2003). Increased local temperature is sensed through primary somatosensory afferent nerves in the skin. The release of noradrenaline or adrenaline leads to vasoconstriction that decreases cutaneous blood flow. When the levels of noradrenaline and adrenaline are reduced, the result is vasodilation and an increase in cutaneous blood flow.

The skin responds rapidly to restore thermal equilibrium when there is an increase or decrease in core body temperature. For example, during exercise or episodes of severe hyperthermia, blood flow to the skin can increase over 20 times the baseline flow rate to as much as 6,000 to 8,000 mL/min (Johnson & Proppe, 2011; Rowell, 2011; Taylor et al., 1984). In comparison, resting blood flow to the skin is approximately 250 to 300 mL/min (Johnson et al., 1986; Johnson & Proppe, 2011). Cutaneous vasodilation provides for increased heat dissipation returning core body temperature toward normal. We have the capacity to increase cutaneous blood flow to 30 times baseline, but these changes in disease states including erythroderma (red skin on 90% or more of the body) can lead to high-output cardiac failure.

The opposite is true for severe cold exposure and hypothermia. The resulting cutaneous vasoconstriction significantly decreases blood flow to the skin and subsequently limits heat dissipation. If a compensatory mechanism is insufficient to restore thermal homeostasis, shivering begins. The contraction of skeletal muscles involved in shivering generates heat that helps to maintain core body temperature (Charkoudian, 2003).

INSULATION

Insulation and conservation of heat is another very important function of the skin. In nonobese individuals, ≥80% of the total body adipose tissue is stored in the hypodermis. Due to the decreased perfusion and water content of adipose tissue, it does not conduct heat as efficiently and thus acts as a very efficient insulating layer.

IMMUNE SURVEILLANCE

The skin is exposed to a wide variety of pathogens and foreign bodies. One of the skin's major functions is to maintain a barrier against pathogenic invasion and consequently infection host with compromised host resistance. An intact stratum corneum provides a mechanical barrier to pathogenic invasion. In addition, the skin produces *antimicrobial peptides (AMPs)* that provide a second level of protection should the barrier be breached (Goodarzi et al., 2007). Over 20 different AMPs have been identified to date, and different AMPs are effective against bacteria, viruses, and fungi. Most AMPs have unique mechanisms of action; however, they can be categorized into general categories. For example, some AMPs disrupt the cell membranes of pathogens without harming human cell membranes, while others stimulate the host immune system via chemotactic and angiogenic agents (Gallo, 2008). Moreover, several studies have shown an increased production of AMPs in psoriasis, and reduced production in atopic dermatitis that may partially explain why superinfections are extremely uncommon in the former disease and more prevalent in the latter.

Langerhans Cells

For immune surveillance, Langerhans cells (LCs) are found mainly in the *stratum spinosum* layer of the epidermis. They are dendritic in morphology and act as *antigen-presenting cells*. In addition to their phagocytic properties, they present foreign antigens to lymphocytes, thus activating the cell-mediated immune system. Interaction with the T lymphocytes results in activation of the LCs themselves that triggers the release of different chemotactic agents (Bennett et al., 2007). Although LCs are primarily found in the epidermis, once they are activated by a foreign antigen, they move to local lymph nodes via the lymphatic vessels in the dermis. In the lymph nodes, T lymphocytes specific to the foreign antigen undergo clonal proliferation that leads to an extensive cell-mediated immune response (Burns et al., 2008). The presence of LCs in the skin accounts for the high incidence of contact allergic dermatitis caused by topical medications, especially in persons with leg ulcers. Chemicals in direct contact with the skin are more likely to cause an allergic response as compared to those given via the oral or parenteral routes.

SENSORY PERCEPTION

The skin possesses several afferent sensory receptors that respond to various environmental stimuli. These receptors are spread throughout the different layers of the skin and can detect touch, pressure, temperature, pain, and itch. Touch and pressure sensations are mediated by a class of receptors known as *mechanoreceptors*. There are four different mechanoreceptors in the skin: Merkel receptor (light tactile or resolve fine special details), Meissner receptor (touch), Pacinian corpuscle (pressure), and Ruffini corpuscle (deep tension in skin/fascia). Merkel receptors are primarily located in the basal layer of the epidermis, whereas Meissner receptors are predominantly found in the dermal papillae (Halata et al., 2003; Winkelmann, 1959).

BARRIER FUNCTION/PROTECTION

One of the main functions of the skin is to maintain a barrier between the internal and external environments, thus protecting against invasion by external pathogens and environmental irritants. The skin barrier prevents excessive losses including water, electrolytes, and other molecules. Moreover, it protects us from toxic contact irritant or allergic materials and UV radiation (Biniek et al., 2012; Menon et al., 2012). This barrier function is dependent on both an intact stratum corneum and on normal lipid production. Lipids found in the extracellular matrix of the stratum corneum are secreted by Odland bodies located primarily in the upper stratum spinosum and stratum granulosum. Odland bodies are concentrated with polar lipids, glycosphingolipids, free sterols, and phospholipids. The Odland bodies are secreted by the keratinocytes during the process of terminal differentiation. The lipids released by Odland bodies serve to fill the gaps between the corneocytes (terminally differentiated keratinocytes) into a characteristic lamellar structure. This process contributes the "mortar" to the brick and mortar configuration of the intact stratum corneum (the corneocytes are the bricks). The skin lipids also bind water, normally maintaining skin water content at 10% or higher. An intact barrier both excludes pathogens and contact irritants/allergens while retaining epidermal and dermal water content. The barrier function of the skin is usually measured objectively by transepidermal water loss (TEWL). When the barrier function of the skin is compromised, TEWL rises (Fluhr et al., 2006).

Normal barrier function is dependent on intact keratinocytes and on normal levels of skin lipids.

Protection against pathogenic invasion is also supported by the acidic pH of the skin, the AMPs, and the immune components of the skin. The pH of the skin is normally 4 to 6.5 in healthy people; this "acid mantle" inhibits pathogenic growth. The acid mantle of the skin may be compromised with the use of alkaline antibacterial soaps and the mechanical action of removing the surface cells with vigorous cleansing routines. In addition, the AMPs and the immune system of the skin provide additional "secondary" protection against pathogenic invasion. The corneocytes (terminally differentiated keratinocytes) embedded in the extracellular matrix also

contribute to the mechanical rigidity and the protection from skin surface frictional forces.

VITAMIN D AND THE SKIN

Vitamin D is responsible for bone strength with a deficiency leading to thin and brittle bones. Vitamin D also appears to play a role in insulin production and immune function with the link to heart disease and cancer a subject of continued investigation and debate. An essential element of the innate immune response to injury is the capacity to recognize microbial invasion and stimulate production of AMPs. Vitamin D may play an important role in activating these antimicrobial peptides.

Although the amount of vitamin D adults get from their diets is often less than what's recommended, exposure to sunlight can make up for the difference. For most adults, vitamin D deficiency is not a concern. However, some groups—particularly people who are obese, who have dark skin, and who are older than age 65—may have lower levels of vitamin D due to their diets, little sun exposure, or other factors. Vitamin D comes in two forms (D_2 and D_3), which differ chemically in their side chains. These structural differences alter their binding to the carrier protein vitamin D binding protein (DBP) and their metabolism. In general, the biologic activity of their active metabolites is comparable. For complete coverage of this and related areas in endocrinology, visit free webbooks, www.endotext.org, and www.thyroidmanager.org.

In the presence of UV-B radiation from the sun, the skin can synthesize provitamin D_3 from 7-dehydrocholesterol. It is believed that over 90% of the vitamin D is produced in this manner. The precursor to vitamin D, 7-dehydrocholesterol, is abundantly present in the skin (Crissey et al., 2003). Vitamin D is further metabolized in the liver and finally activated in the kidney (Holick et al., 1987).

Vitamin D deficiency has been documented in individuals who lack UV exposure, including elderly individuals residing in nursing homes and individuals living in northern climates. The vitamin D levels should be checked and supplementation provided for individuals who are unable to obtain sun exposure and who have a documented vitamin D deficiency. It should be noted that the amount of UV exposure required for vitamin D metabolism can be obtained with minimal outdoor exposure. There are concerns that vitamin D deficiency may become more common due to the increased use of sunscreen, especially products with sun protection factors (SPFs) over 15 to 30 that block most of the photoactivated vitamin D_3 production (Institute of Medicine, US Committee to Review Dietary Reference Intakes for Vitamin D and Calcium, 2011). It has been reported that an experimental model of cutaneous application of sunscreen with a SPF of 30 can reduce vitamin D production of up to 95% (Matsuoka et al., 1987). Sunscreens also provide beneficial effects by blocking the cutaneous absorption of UV-B radiation preventing sun burning, premature aging, and cancer of the skin. However, a recent literature examined the associations between sunscreen use and vitamin D_3 concentration through the photoproduction of 25(OH)D. The review concluded that there is little evidence that suggests sunscreen decreases 25(OH)D concentration when used in real-life settings, suggesting that any concerns about vitamin D deficiency should not negate the use of sunscreen for skin protection (Neale et al., 2019). Routine use of sunscreen should be promoted in all situations where there is the risk of burning and subsequent increased risk of skin cancer development. Most individuals should be encouraged to have a limited amount of sun exposure to assure adequate vitamin D metabolism (Holick et al., 1995; Marks, R., et al., 1995).

Supplementary amounts of vitamin D can also come from animal and plant sources including fortified milk, fish oil, salmon, tuna, and shrimp. While the role of vitamin D in bone health and calcium and phosphorus absorption is well known, it has other roles of equal importance. These include immunocompetence, protection against some cancers, and genome control of cell proliferation and differentiation during the wound healing process (Berger et al., 1988; Kaminski & Drinane, 2014; Matsumoto et al., 1991; Norman, 1998). However, a recent large randomized controlled trial (RCT) with 25,871 patients published in the *New England Journal of Medicine* concluded that "Supplementation with vitamin D did not result in a lower incidence of invasive cancer or cardiovascular events than placebo" (Manson et al., 2019).

Vitamin D is also believed to express genes in keratinocytes that code for antimicrobial receptors and cathelicidin, an AMP that eradicates microbes found on wound surfaces (Bikle, 2000; Kaminski & Drinane, 2014; Norman, 2008; Schauber et al., 2007; Segaert, 2008).

Wound healing is a complex process that is influenced by multiple systemic factors, including nutritional status. Dai et al. (2019) conducted a systematic review and meta-analysis of the association of vitamin D levels and diabetic foot ulcers. Four studies were identified that reported data on severe vitamin D deficiency. Severe vitamin D deficiency was reported in 216/441 patients (48.98%) with diabetic foot ulcers (DFUs) and 108/474 (22.78%) persons with diabetes without DFU. The authors concluded that severe vitamin D deficiency [25-(OH)D < 10 ng/mL] was significantly associated with an increased risk of DFU (OR 3.22, 95% CI 2.42 to 4.28; $p = 0.64$, I2 = 0%).

Smart and colleagues, working in the Kingdom of Bahrain, documented a case series of 80 persons with wounds (Smart et al., 2019). Traditional clothing is associated with low UV exposure with 91% of females and 84% of males having a vitamin D_3 deficiency with a severe deficiency detected in 85% of the sample. Diabetes was present in 90% of the patients (the country incidence

is estimated between 8.2% and 20%). Only 3.8% of the study population had vitamin D levels above 50 ng/mL (175 nmol/L). Examining the patients with both diabetes mellitus and a vitamin D deficiency, there was delayed healing in 36.7% and deteriorating wounds in 39.7% with only 23.6% having wounds healing at the expected rate. The authors concluded that "adequate vitamin D supplementation coupled with improved HbA1c levels and adherence to regional treatment factors may improve the foot ulcer healing of persons with diabetes" (Smart et al., 2019). Further studies are needed to clarify the relationship of vitamin D levels, diabetic control, and the outcomes for healing of DFUs.

Worldwide reports have highlighted a variety of vitamin D insufficiency and deficiency diseases. Despite many publications and scientific meetings reporting advances in vitamin D science, a disturbing realization is growing that the newer scientific and clinical knowledge is not being translated into better human health. Over the past several decades, the biological sphere of influence of vitamin D_3, as defined by the tissue distribution of the vitamin D receptor (VDR), has broadened at least ninefold from the target organs required for calcium homeostasis (intestine, bone, kidney, and parathyroid). Now, research has shown that the pluripotent steroid hormone 1alpha,25(OH)(2)D(3) initiates the physiologic responses of more than 36 cell types that possess the VDR. In addition to the kidney's endocrine production of circulating 1alpha,25(OH)(2)D(3), researchers have found a paracrine production of this steroid hormone in more than 10 extrarenal organs. As a consequence, the nutritional guidelines for vitamin D_3 intake defined by serum hydroxyvitamin D_3 concentrations should be reevaluated. Future supplementation recommendations should be related to clinical outcomes.

● SKIN CHANGES THROUGHOUT LIFE

There are a number of skin changes that occur across the lifespan that impact on skin health and wound healing.

INFANTS AND CHILDREN

While the structural components of the skin remain similar across the age continuum, specific characteristics and functions are not as well developed in the newborn compared to an adult. For example, the stratum corneum of a newborn is thinner with lower levels of natural moisturizing factors. Moreover, the skin of a newborn is more permeable than adult skin, and there is a higher ratio of surface area to total body weight (Kelleher et al., 2013). These changes place infants at higher risk for fluid loss compared with adult (Jarvis, 2012) and for increased systemic absorption of topically applied substances. Topically applied agents that are absorbed through the skin can cause systemic effects throughout the body and may cause neurotoxicity, structural damage, and potential death (Rutter, 1987). The newborn infant's skin is not a complete barrier to the absorption of externally applied agents, particularly if it is damaged, diseased, or immature. Immaturity is the most important factor that determines percutaneous absorption. Very immature infants in the early neonatal period have a poorly developed epidermis that is readily permeable to drugs. The main consequences of percutaneous absorption are hazardous. Topically applied agents are absorbed, causing toxic systemic effects that may result in illness and even death without the cause being recognized. No drug or antiseptic agent should be applied to the premature infant's skin without consideration of the effects that might result from percutaneous absorption. On a more optimistic note, the relatively permeable skin could be an advantage to the preterm infant by providing an alternative method of drug administration. The drug theophylline, for example, can be absorbed and produce therapeutic blood levels for up to 3 days after a single topical application. There is a need for the development of transdermal drug delivery systems for the newborn infant similar to those currently used for therapy in adults (Rutter, 1987).

Temperature regulation is less effective among infants and children, often resulting in higher fevers, than adults. In addition, the eccrine sweat glands' ability to increase heat-induced sweat production is only minimally developed in children (Jarvis, 2012). It is reported that the capacity to sweat is correlated with the gestational age of the child. Moreover, there is a propensity for complete anhidrosis in the preterm infant in the first days of life (Oranges et al., 2015). The subcutaneous layer is thinner and less developed, and infants and children are less able to shiver; thus, they need to be protected from the cold (Jarvis, 2012). At puberty, the skin becomes more mature, the epidermis thickens, and there is increased oil and sweat production (Jarvis, 2012). See Chapter 13 for more detailed information on the care of Skin and Wounds for the Neonatal and Pediatric Populations.

KEY POINT

Infant skin is thinner, which places them at greater risk for systemic absorption of topically applied substances.

When assessing the skin of an infant, it is important to differentiate between normal skin color variations and bruises that could suggest child abuse. For example, African American, Asian American, Indian, and Hispanic newborns may exhibit dermal melanocytic lesions (commonly known as "Mongolian spots"). These lesions are areas of a blue-black coloration most typically found on the buttocks. Similar lesions can occur around the eye (nevus of Ito) and in the shoulder region (unilateral nevus of Ito). Another skin color variation is café au lait, an oval

patch of light brown pigmentation; while limited café au lait spots are considered normal, the presence of five or more is associated with increased incidence of neurofibromatosis. Another congenital color variation is portwine stain (nevus flammeus), a flat dark red-blue-purple patch usually found on the face or the scalp. Infants and children with Down syndrome (trisomy 21) may have cutis marmorata, a reticulated red or blue pattern of mottling seen on the extremities that is more prominent when the child is in a cooler environment (Jarvis, 2012). Infants may also present with pigmentary mosaicism (patterned dyschromatosis) that refers to regions of the skin that are hypopigmented or hyperpigmented. These areas of skin are genetically differentiated by late somatic mosaic genetic mutations in the skin cell progenitors. Patients may also present with extracutaneous abnormalities that involve the central nervous system and the musculoskeletal system (Kromann et al., 2018).

OLDER ADULTS

Aging is associated with multiple changes in the structure and function of the skin (see also Chapter 14, Skin and Wound Care for Geriatric Population). A summary is presented in **Table 2-1.**

Skin functions that decline with aging will be briefly discussed.

Thermoregulation

As individuals age, both endogenous and exogenous factors lead to changes in thermoregulation. Body heat is generated by endogenous factors such as metabolic heat production, physical activity, shivering (via skeletal muscle tremor), and nonshivering thermogenesis. As muscle mass is lost (also known as sarcopenia) and physical activity decreases, there is a decline in metabolism and energy production. This results in a decreased ability to maintain thermal homeostasis, specifically a slower and/or incomplete adaptation to temperature change

TABLE 2-1 STRUCTURAL CHANGES IN AGING SKIN	
SKIN LAYER	STRUCTURAL CHANGE
Epidermis	• ↓ Melanocytes • ↓ Langerhans cells • Flattening of dermal–epidermal junction • ↓ Epidermal thickness
Dermis	• ↓ Fibroblasts • ↓ Mast cells • ↓ Papillary capillary network • ↓ Collagen • ↓ Elastin

Sources: Fenske, N. A., & Lober, C. W. (1986). Structural and functional changes of normal aging skin. *Journal of the American Academy of Dermatology, 15*(4 Pt 1), 571–585. doi: 10.1016/s0190-9622(86)70208-9; Montagna, W., & Carlisle, K. (1979). Structural changes in aging human skin. *The Journal of Investigative Dermatology, 73*(1), 47–53. doi: 10.1111/1523-1747.ep12532761.

compared with their younger counterparts. Elderly individuals have thinner skin and most also lose body fat, resulting in less insulation against cold and less ability to radiate metabolic heat. Even in the summer months, the elderly may wear a sweater or need a blanket. As individuals age, they are also much more prone to heat stroke as aging skin has fewer sweat glands and the skin temperature regulation is decreased. In addition, elderly skin is drier, requiring moisturizers after bathing and avoiding extremes in temperatures. To compensate for reduced metabolic rate among the elderly, a high-protein meal can increase the metabolic rate by 30% or more, whereas a high-carbohydrate meal will only increase energy production by 4% (Guyton, 1991). When the ambient temperature changes, the skin's thermoreceptors detect changes at the skin surface and adjust the firing rate of the afferent fibers. It has been shown that thermal perception decreases with advancing age, leading to decreased heat and cold sensitivity and a longer response time to temperature changes (Natsume et al., 1992).

Cell Turnover Time

Aging is also associated with an increase in time required for renewal of the stratum corneum, due to a reduced rate of epidermal mitosis; specifically, renewal of the stratum corneum takes an average of 30 as opposed to 20 days. In octogenarians, the epidermal turnover rate has been reported to be 50% lower (Levine, 2020; Tobin, 2017). Wound healing is also prolonged in the middle-aged and elderly adult.

KEY POINT

Aging is associated with prolonged time required for replacement of the stratum corneum by new cells, due to slower rate of epidermal mitosis resulting in thinner skin and delayed healing.

COMMON SKIN CONDITIONS IN THE ELDERLY

There are several skin conditions, both benign and malignant, that are much more common in the elderly.

PHOTOAGING

Photoaging is a major cause of premature aging in persons who have experienced chronic UV radiation from excessive sun exposure (Zhang & Duan, 2018). Benign changes in the skin caused by photoaging include wrinkling, telangiectasia (thread-like blood vessels), thinning of the skin (atrophy of the dermis and epidermis), and pigmentary changes (hyper- and hypopigmentation). Collectively, these changes are often referred to as poikiloderma (telangiectasia, pigment change, atrophy).

This type of change is more common in persons with blonde or red hair, blue eyes, and skin that burns rather than tans. There are four white skin types based on the skin's response to UV radiation (Fitzpatrick, 1975, 1986). The four Fitzpatrick classes of skin color are as follows:

- Category 1 (always burns, never tans)
- Category 2 (usually burns, tans slightly)
- Category 3 (sometimes burns, tans uniformly)
- Category 4 (rarely burns, always tans)

Two other skin types were subsequently added to the Fitzpatrick classification (Fitzpatrick, 1988);

- Category 5 (brown skin)
- Category 6 (deeply pigmented black skin)

Changes in skin pigmentation are common among the elderly; some are due to natural "intrinsic" aging, but many are due to photoaging. Intrinsic aging refers to the inescapable physiologic changes to the skin cells and tissues that take place with time and are impacted by genetic and hormonal factors (Levine, 2020; Montagna et al., 1989). These changes include decreased collagen production, decreased blood flow to the skin, and lower amounts of lipids (Montagna et al., 1989). Intrinsically aged skin is characterized as dry, pale skin with fine wrinkles, diminished reparative capacity, and reduced elasticity. The difference in natural aging and photoaging can be easily illustrated, by comparing the skin on the buttocks (which is rarely if ever exposed to the sun) to the skin on the face, in terms of wrinkling, pigmentary changes, telangiectasia, and enlarged sebaceous glands (sebaceous hyperplasia). In addition to the mottled pigmentation caused by photodamage, there is hypopigmentation related to reduced numbers and function of melanocytes and increased risk of bruising due to capillary fragility. Purpuric lesions (bruises caused by minor trauma) are indicative of increased risk for skin tears. In addition, hypopigmentation related to diminished melanocyte function is indicative of increased risk for melanoma and its precursors.

ACTINIC KERATOSIS

Those individuals with Celtic-type skin (Fitzpatrick types 1 and 2) are much more prone to precancerous and cancerous changes in the skin, including palpable scaly red papular areas known as actinic keratosis (solar keratosis) (see **Fig. 2-2**). The presence of these premalignant lesions should alert the clinician to also inspect the skin carefully for cancerous lesions. Actinic keratoses typically develop in sun-exposed areas of the body such as the balding scalp, head, neck, forearms, and dorsal surface of the hands. Moreover, the number of sunburns during childhood is associated with an increased likelihood of developing actinic keratoses in the future

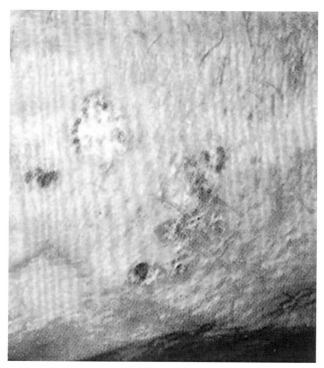

FIGURE 2-2. Actinic Keratosis. (Reprinted with permission from Sauer, G. C. (1985). *Manual of skin diseases* (5th ed.). Philadelphia, PA: JB Lippincott.)

(Traianou et al., 2012). The risk of developing actinic keratoses rises with increasing age and is significantly more common in the elderly (Eder et al., 2014; Flohil et al., 2013).

BASAL CELL CARCINOMA

The most common human skin cancer is basal cell carcinoma (BCC), which often presents as a "pearl-like" translucent papule with potential central ulceration (see **Fig. 2-3**). There is also frequently a surface telangiectasia (small thread-like blood vessel) traversing the edge of the lesion. These lesions are common on sun-exposed areas of the face, especially the nose, forehead, and ears. Less common variants of BCC include superficial BCC (often surface telangiectasias, translucent skin often without a surface scale), sclerosing BCC, morpheaform BCC, and pigmented BCC. Risk factors for developing BCCs include UV radiation exposure, light hair and eye color, inability to tan, and northern European ancestry (Rubin et al., 2005).

KEY POINT

The most common type of skin cancer is BCC, which presents clinically as a "pearl-like" translucent papule with central ulceration. The second most common type is squamous cell carcinoma (SCC), which presents clinically as an enlarging keratotic papule.

SQUAMOUS CELL CARCINOMA

The second most common human skin cancer is squamous cell carcinoma (SCC). These lesions begin as keratotic papules that gradually enlarge in an irregular way and may become painful (see **Fig. 2-4**). They are most common around the lips (especially the lower lip, as a result of sun damage or smoking), the ears, other areas on the face, or exposed skin on the back of the hands or arms. The incidence of SCC is rising, with a reported increase of 50% to 200% over the past three decades. The rise has been largely credited due to a greater lifetime UV radiation exposure as a result of increasing lifespan, the depletion of the ozone layer, and an increase in voluntary exposure to UV radiation (Karia et al., 2013). Both SCCs and BCCs may appear on the legs in the elderly and may be mistakenly diagnosed as skin ulcers (venous and mixed arterial/venous ulcers). For this reason, the wound care nurse must maintain a high index of

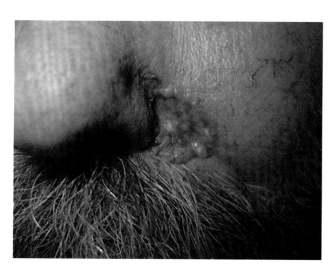

FIGURE 2-3. Basal Cell Carcinoma. (Image provided by Stedman's.)

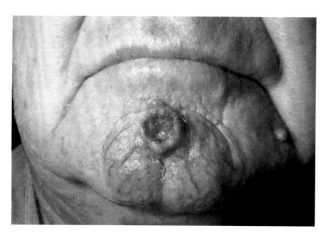

FIGURE 2-4. Squamous Cell Carcinoma. (Reprinted with permission from Weber, J. R. N., & Kelley J. R. N. (2003). *Health assessment in nursing* (2nd ed.). Philadelphia, PA: Lippincott Williams & Wilkins.)

suspicion and should not hesitate to obtain a biopsy of a nonhealing wound. Previous studies have documented that wounds that are healable and are appropriately managed should demonstrate a 30% reduction in size by week 4 of treatment (and potentially heal by week 12). Wounds that fail to demonstrate appropriate progress should have a biopsy at the wound margin to rule out skin cancer (Falanga & Sabolinski, 1999). Other nonhealing ulcer etiologies including inflammatory and infectious etiologies must also be considered. Clinical lesions suspicious of SCCs around the lips, on the nose, or on the ears should also be biopsied and treated accordingly.

SCCs on the legs may arise from old burn scars, osteomyelitis sinuses, the edge of previous skin grafts, or old radiotherapy sites (radiation dermatitis). Chronic inflammatory disorders of the mucosal tissue and skin can predispose one for SCC development; these conditions include hypertrophic actinic keratosis, lichen sclerosis, and discoid lupus erythematosus (Alam & Ratner, 2001). Early diagnosis is critical because failure to accurately diagnose the lesion can result in locally invasive or metastatic disease. An accurate differential diagnosis is therefore critical to avoid the tragic consequences of often long-term treatment of a cancerous leg lesion as a venous or mixed arterial/venous ulcer. For more information on accurate assessment of leg wounds, see Chapters 23 to 26 on venous, arterial, and neuropathic wounds, differential assessment of lower extremity wounds and Chapter 27 and 31 on atypical wounds and oncology-related wounds.

> **KEY POINT**
>
> Both BCC and SCC may occur on the legs in the elderly and may be mistaken for a venous or another chronic ulcer etiology.

CUTANEOUS HORN

Another common lesion in the elderly is the cutaneous horn (**Fig. 2-5**). These are caused by an irregular and often densely compacted vertical growth of keratin over a tissue base that varies in terms of pathology. They may range in size from a few millimeters to several centimeters. The lesions may be hard and *can* become painful. Cutaneous horns may have a thick or very narrow tapered keratotic column (the "horn"). About 60% of these lesions are benign with a wart or seborrheic keratosis (SK) at the base. Another 20% are premalignant, with an actinic keratosis histologically at the base. Unfortunately, the remaining 20% are frankly malignant. The malignant lesions are most commonly caused by Bowen disease (SCC that spreads horizontally without vertical invasion) or an early SCC (Copcu et al., 2004; Korkut et al., 1997). Horns that present on an invasive SCC base tend to be more painful, have a wider base versus

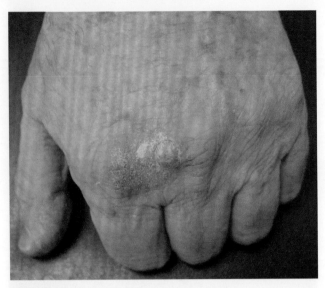

FIGURE 2-5. Cutaneous Horn.

height and more surrounding erythema than nonmalignant cutaneous horns (Pyne et al., 2013).

SEBORRHEIC KERATOSES

Seborrheic keratoses are common but benign skin lesions in the elderly that have the appearance of a "stuck-on barnacle" (Hafner & Vogt, 2008; Noiles & Vender, 2007) (**Fig. 2-6**). The lesions contain keratin with horn cysts that, if examined closely or viewed under the dermatoscope (instrument with illuminated magnification equivalent to an ophthalmoscope), often displays a grains of sand-like appearance within the surface. The lesions may be small and white (often referred to as stucco keratosis); these are more common on the lower

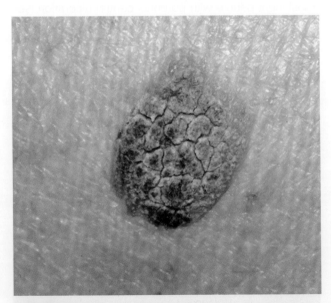

FIGURE 2-6. Seborrheic Keratosis. (Reprinted with permission from Goodheart, H. P. (2003). *Goodheart's photoguide of common skin disorders* (2nd ed.). Philadelphia, PA: Lippincott.)

legs, head, neck, distal hands, or arms (Yeatman et al., 1997).

SKs may also present as large, pigmented eruptive lesions that commonly occur on the trunk but can also occur on the face, backs of the hands, or other areas that are socially visible and can be potentially disfiguring. These lesions most commonly present in middle-aged and older adults. They have been reported to be more common in the white population and are found equally in both men and women (Verhagen et al., 1968).

NEVI (MOLES)

Moles are very common, typically benign lesions, especially among individuals with light skin tones (**Fig. 2-7**). Most nevi develop in late childhood or the teen years, although new lesions can occur up to approximately age 50. Acquired "normal" melanocytic nevi can occur anywhere on the body but are most commonly located on the posterior trunk, followed by the legs, arms, head, and neck. These nevi are extremely common within the pediatric population, with a mean nevus count of approximately 15 to 30 in White children, and 5 to 10 in children of Black, Asian, and American Indian ancestry by the end of the first decade of life. These nevi can enlarge and become more pigmented in the late teen years to around age 40. Between ages 40 and 60, nevi often become lighter and elevate from the surface of the skin. The number of nevi increases with more sun exposure in childhood. Excessive sun exposure can make preexisting nevi darker.

In addition to normal nevi, some individuals have slightly larger and irregular dysplastic nevi. They evolve in childhood and early adult life, are characterized by a much more irregular, indistinct surface, and can develop into melanoma. Dysplastic nevi when fully developed are slightly larger than normal nevi (e.g., larger than the size of an eraser on the end of a pencil) and have irreg-

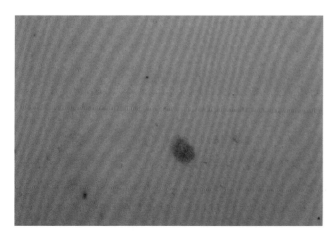

FIGURE 2-7. Benign Nevus (Mole). (Reprinted with permission from Goodheart, H. P. (2003). *Goodheart's photoguide of common skin disorders* (2nd ed.). Philadelphia, PA: Lippincott Williams & Wilkins.)

ular pigmentation (e.g., light brown and/or dark brown with often pink-red coloration with the pink-red coloration being more common in very fair individuals). Black pigmentation is more commonly associated with melanoma (Elder, 2006). The risk of melanoma increases in the presence of dysplastic nevi. One large meta-analysis reported that sporadic dysplastic nevi are associated with a 10-fold increased risk for melanoma (Gandini et al., 2005). The more nevi present, the greater the risk of malignant transformation or the de novo appearance of a melanoma. Individuals can be classified as having a few nevi, an average of 30 to 50 nevi, a moderately increased number of nevi with approximately 50 to 100, or markedly increased number of nevi with more than 100 nevi. In addition to a genetic predisposition, the cumulative sun exposure in childhood is linked to the number of nevi that form on the arms of adults (Gallagher & McLean, 1995).

Congenital melanocytic nevi are less common moles that are present on the skin at birth. They are benign proliferation of epidermal melanocytes that develop due to abnormal growth, development, or migration of melanocyte precursors called melanoblasts (Shah et al., 2016). As an individual grows, the congenital nevi may become more darkly pigmented, but the growth and pigmentation are regular and even (Schaffer, 2015). Clinically, congenital nevi are usually divided into three categories defined by their maximal projected diameter in adulthood. When these nevi are under 1.5 cm in diameter, they are referred to as "small," and the risk of malignant transformation is extremely low. When the size of these lesions is 1.5 to 19.9 cm in diameter, they are referred to as "medium," but the risk of malignant transformation remains low (Bittencourt et al., 2000; Habif, 2004). When the diameter of these lesions exceeds 20 cm, they are classified as "large," and the risk of malignant transformation is more significant (Egan et al., 1998; Zaal et al., 2005). The lesions in these individuals are mostly on the trunk, and they may have a number of other melanocytic nevi elsewhere on the body. The cumulative 5-year life-table risks for developing melanoma and neurocutaneous melanocytosis (NCM) were calculated. The relative risk for developing melanoma, using a control general population reference group, was determined (Bittencourt et al., 2000).

MELANOMA

The presence of dysplastic nevi, more than 100 normal nevi, along with blistering sun burns, blue eyes, and fair hair all predispose individuals to melanoma. Melanoma is more common if a first-degree relative had a melanoma (mother, father, brother, sister, aunt, uncle).

A melanoma is a malignant tumor that arises from melanocytes and is commonly cutaneous in origin but can arise on mucosal surfaces and within the uveal tract of the eye or the mucosa in the nose. Due to its metastatic potential, melanoma is the cause of over 90% of skin cancer deaths. It is also believed that melanoma is more common in individuals who have intermittent but intense sun exposure (e.g., sun exposure related to tropical holidays), as opposed to the prolonged but moderate amount of sun exposure experienced by the farmer or fisherman.

The most common melanoma is superficial spreading malignant melanoma (SSMM—70%). These lesions start as a flat nonpalpable lesions often with a rainbow of colors or an atypical black lesion. Seborrheic keratoses can often be black, but they are elevated and palpable. These lesions are often referred to dermatologists erroneously as a suspected melanoma. A melanoma can occur at any age but is diagnosed most frequently between 40 and 60 years and usually occurs on the backs of males and lower legs of females (**Fig. 2-8**). The lesions typically begin as a brown macule with color variations and irregular borders. The lesion will first slowly grow horizontally (radial) and is limited to the epidermis. Afterward, it will grow more rapidly in the vertical dimension and present clinically as a papule or nodule. The characteristics of a melanoma can be remembered best by the letters ABCDE. This includes the following:

A = asymmetry (one side does not look like the other)

B = irregular border (blurred, uneven, or "notched" edges)

C = variable and uneven color (black is too much melanin, blue is due to the Tyndall effect dermal melanin gives a scattered pattern on the skin surface, white is an area of regression, and pink relates to an area of active inflammation)

D = diameter >6 mm (the size of an eraser on the end of a pencil) requires more attention

E = evolving lesion (is worth further evaluation) (Abbasi et al., 2004; Rigel et al., 2005)

Approximately 20% to 50% of superficial spreading melanomas arise in existing nevi and 50% to 80% on what appears to be clinically normal skin; however, it is important to remember that abnormal melanocytes exist throughout the body, although they are concentrated in existing nevi. Removing all the existing nevi does not prevent all melanomas!

The second most common melanoma is the lentigo maligna melanoma (LMM). This type of melanoma accounts for 10% to 15% of melanomas and is seen on chronically sun-damaged skin, most commonly on the face, with a preference for the nose and cheeks. However, it can occasionally be involved on other exposed body areas. It is seen more commonly in the elderly, and, in this case, sun exposure is both the initiator and promoter of the malignancy. These melanomas do *not* arise within preexisting nevi but rather occur de novo. Early lesions are often undetected because they typically arise within a background of severely sun-damaged skin and can be confused with solar lentigines (freckles from sun damage that are larger than the usual freckles seen in young individuals) or a large flat SK.

Nodular melanomas (NMM) are relatively uncommon, accounting for about 10% to 15% of melanomas; these lesions lack a vertical growth phase, are invasive almost from their onset, and are elevated above the level of the skin (Kelly et al., 2003). These lesions can be darkly pigmented and quickly growing or may present without pigment or as an ulcer (**Fig. 2-9**). NMM are more frequently observed in men than in women. They typically present as a blue to black but occasionally as amelanotic pink

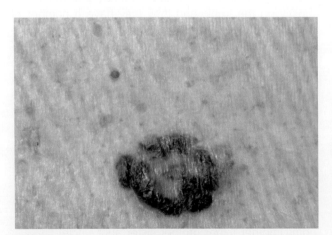

FIGURE 2-8. Superficial Spreading Melanoma. (Reprinted with permission from Goodheart, H. P. (2003). *Goodheart's photoguide of common skin disorders* (2nd ed.). Philadelphia, PA: Lippincott.)

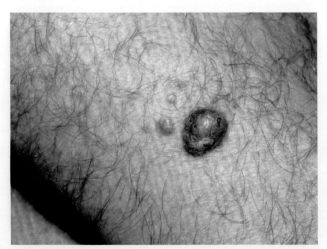

FIGURE 2-9. Nodular Melanoma. (Reprinted with permission from Goodheart, H. P. (2003). *Goodheart's photoguide of common skin disorders* (2nd ed.). Philadelphia, PA: Lippincott.)

to red lesions. NMM can be confused with other ulcerative lesions that again underscore the importance of early biopsy for any wound that has an atypical location or appearance especially if it is also not healing at the expected rate.

The least common melanocytic malignancy is an acrolentiginous melanoma (ALM) often found under the nail plate in a subungual location (Levit et al., 2000). They may also occur on the palms and soles, account for approximately 5% to 10% of all melanomas but represent up to 70% of melanomas found in individuals with darkly pigmented skin (Cress & Holly, 1997). A disproportionately high percentage of patients with ALMs are diagnosed at a late invasive stage. This is likely due to the difficulty in clinically distinguishing early lesions of the ALM variant from traumatic skin changes and other benign skin lesions. Again, a high index of suspicion is critical, because these lesions tend to metastasize early.

SKIN IMMUNE SYSTEM

The skin is the most efficient immune organ in the body. Allergic reactions to drugs applied topically are much more likely and more common than allergic reactions to drugs ingested systemically. A key component of the skin's immune system is the LCs; these cells are located in the epidermis where they are responsible for processing antigens (Bos & Kapsenberg, 1993). The LCs then "present" the antigen to the lymphocytes and migrate to regional lymph nodes, where they continue to process antigens and recruit activated T cells, triggering a more generalized inflammatory response.

ALLERGIC CONTACT DERMATITIS

Poison ivy (*Toxicodendron radicans*) and poison oak (*Toxicodendron diversilobum*) both from the *Toxicodendron* genus are two of the most potent known contact allergens (Gladman, 2006; Lee & Arriola, 1999). When the skin is exposed to one of these agents, a type 4 allergic hypersensitivity reaction occurs that is similar to the reaction that occurs with a tuberculin skin test that is evaluated 48 hours after the intradermal challenge with the antigen. If the allergen exposure is an initial (sensitizing) exposure, the rash is typically delayed, sometimes for up to 3 weeks (depending on the level of response by the LCs). If the person has already been sensitized, very small amounts of the allergen are required to elicit the dermatitis, and once exposed, blistering can occur at the site of contact within a few hours. External allergens usually cause linear types of blistering erythematous papules and vesicles where the plant has brushed the skin. Both poison ivy and poison oak most commonly contact the lower legs or arms where the skin is relatively thin and often unprotected in hot weather. The areas that are involved commonly have sharp margins, linear configurations, and geographic outlines. A single blind randomized paired comparison with 211 patients documented that a pretreatment of the skin with quaternium-18 bentonite lotion was effective in preventing or diminishing experimentally produced poison ivy and poison oak allergic contact dermatitis (Marks et al., 1995). The allergens responsible for poison ivy and poison oak are contained within the resinous sap material, known as urushiol. Urushiol is composed of a combination of a class of chemicals called catechols (Kim et al., 2019). *Toxicodendron* dermatitis is initiated when the urushiol catechols becomes actively fixed to and penetrates the skin within a few minutes. The dermatitis can spread to other parts of the body through contact with inanimate objects contaminated with the resin including exposed parts of a bicycle, clothing, or tools. The urushiol catechols are oxidized to quinone intermediates and are processed by lymphocytes and LCs at the site of skin contact in the epidermis and dermis. The sensitized lymphocytes then migrate to the regional lymph nodes and recruit other lymphocytes that become sensitized; these lymphocytes have the potential to migrate to distal skin sites, thus causing the rash to become generalized. Contact with inanimate objects can cause new skin sites to react; these objects should be washed thoroughly with a surface-active agent to remove the remaining reactive resin (Gladman, 2006; Lee & Arriola, 1999).

IMPACT OF AGING

Aging is associated with a diminution of the skin's immune system responsiveness. The decrease in cell-mediated immunity is a probable contributing factor to the increased risk of viral infections and malignancy among older individuals. One example would be varicella (chickenpox) and herpes zoster (shingles) that is caused by the varicella–zoster virus. When chickenpox is acquired at a young age, the child's immune system typically handles the virus very effectively. However, if primary infection occurs at an older age (e.g., in an individual over 20 years of age), the acute varicella illness is often much more severe. Therefore, varicella vaccination is recommended for individuals without evidence of previous chickenpox, especially immigrants moving to northern climates, where the indoor winter habitat facilitates the spread of varicella. Aging reduces immunity to the varicella virus and allows activation of the previously dormant virus, which results in outbreaks of varicella zoster (shingles) along a nerve pathway (dermatome). During a herpes zoster infection, the varicella–zoster virus will continue to replicate within the dorsal root ganglion and produce a painful ganglion. The elderly individual who develops shingles is also at greater risk for nerve damage resulting in painful postherpetic neuralgia that intensifies as the virus spreads peripherally down the sensory nerve. This excruciating neuropathic pain has a very negative effect on quality of life and requires prompt intervention (Woo et al., 2008). The severity and incidence of developing herpes zoster increases significantly with increasing age. In the United States and Europe, it has been shown that the annual incidence of herpes zoster is 2.5/1,000 persons between ages 20 and 50 years, 5.1/1,000 between ages 51 and 79 years, and 10.1/1,000 in those older than 80 years of age (Hope-Simpson, 1965). The aging process and the skin's diminished immunocompetence are key factors contributing to the increased risk for shingles (varicella–zoster) among the elderly.

PERMEABILITY AND DERMAL ABSORPTION

The permeability of the skin to topically applied agents varies, depending on the age of the person and the anatomic area and characteristics of the skin. At the extremes of life, the skin of infants and elders is thin and fragile with increased permeability to some but not all chemicals. Clinicians need to use caution when recommending topical medications that can be systemically absorbed.

All body sites are not equally permeable, with percutaneous absorption varying depending on the anatomic site. For example, if the absorption of topical steroids on the forearms is 1 as a reference baseline, the absorption rate on the palmar surface of the hand is 0.83, and the absorption rate on the plantar aspect of the foot is 0.14. This means that the absorption rate on the forearm is six times that on the plantar surface of the foot. The potency of a topical corticosteroid is the amount of drug needed to produce a desired therapeutic effect. There are seven classes of corticosteroid potencies, with class I super-potent and class VII being the least potent (Jacob & Steele, 2006). A lower potency steroid could be used on the forearm to obtain the same results as a much greater potency steroid on the plantar surface of the foot. Using the same comparator, the cheeks and forehead are much more permeable than the forearms, absorbing 8 to 13 times the amount of steroid, due in part to increased vascularity and in part to the thinner skin. The number of hair follicles in the area is another factor to consider, due to increased absorption along the hair follicle. An extreme example of high absorptive capacity is the scrotum. It will absorb 42 times the amount compared to the forearm, because the skin surface is very thin with a large surface area (due to folds), there is a prominent vascular network, and there are a large number of hair follicles facilitating absorption. In addition, proximity to the inner thighs and external genitalia creates a relatively occlusive environment for the scrotum (Feldmann & Maibach, 1967).

Percutaneous absorption of medications including topical steroids depends on the anatomic site. Current data and clinical experience indicate that one can crudely rank the regional permeability as follows: nail ≪ palm/sole < trunk/extremities < face/scalp ≪ scrotum.

● SKIN ASSESSMENT

While most clinicians would agree that skin assessment is part of a physical examination, there is a lack of consensus as to what should be included in a basic skin assessment. Common practice might include the following five components: skin color, temperature, turgor (flexible, rigid), moisture status, and integrity. In addition to the general physical assessment and specific skin assessment, factors that impact on skin health should be assessed including skin type/sun exposure, bruising, and other comorbidities (acute and chronic disease, vitamin and mineral deficiencies) and smoking.

SKIN COLOR

One of the most important features of a lesion other than the primary morphology is its color. Normal variations in skin color have already been described earlier in this chapter in relation to the continuum of aging from birth to death. Skin color assessment must be based on the individual's normal skin color, with attention to areas in which there are color changes. We have (EAA, RGS) developed a photo guide for assessing brown (Fitzpatrick category 5 dark brown) skin for changes related to moisture-associated skin damage (MASD), specifically incontinence-associated dermatitis or IAD, which can be downloaded from www. WoundPedia.com (Ayello et al., 2014).

Changes in skin color, either darkening or lightening, can be indicative of pathology. For example, a brownish gray discoloration of the lower limb(s) may be caused by hemosiderin staining in persons with venous disease and frequently precedes the development of a venous ulcer (**Fig. 2-10**). Atrophie blanche (**Fig. 2-11**) is manifested as white star-shaped patches (scars) just above the medial malleolus in the patient with vascular disease (typically chronic venous insufficiency) or occlusion of the surface capillaries of the skin with a vasculopathy (noninflammatory thrombosis of small vessels). In contrast, pallor with leg raising or cyanosis and dependent rubor are characteristic of arterial insufficiency. Other colors, such as red (also known as erythema) may result from inflammation leading to hyperemia (subtle vascular dilation). A more saturated red to purple can indicate vascular congestion (also known as rubor), and an even more saturated red to purple can lead to the development of malformed blood vessels or extravasated red blood cells (petechiae or purpura). Other colors and their histopathological correlations include yellow, which may indicate pus, lipid, or bilirubin; green, which can be seen in deep hemosiderin or pyocyanin pigment associated with local pseudomonas colonization or infection; and black, which

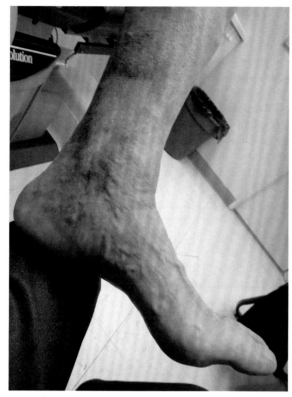

FIGURE 2-10. Hemosiderin Staining. (Courtesy of Dr. Afsaneh Alavi.)

is seen with dense melanin accumulation, necrosis, and intraepidermal hemorrhage.

SKIN TEMPERATURE

Normal skin is "warm to touch"; ischemic skin is typically cool to touch, and areas of trauma, deep and surrounding infection, and deep inflammation are frequently warmer than adjacent skin. The use of an infrared thermometer can also detect skin temperature elevation

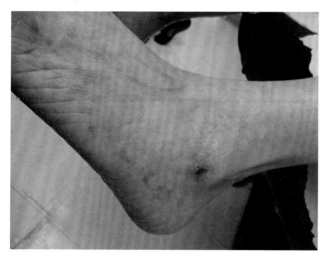

FIGURE 2-11. Atrophie Blanche. (Courtesy of Dr. Afsaneh Alavi.)

due to periwound infection that can contribute to prompt detection and treatment of the infection (Sibbald et al., 2015). Elevated skin temperature was the individual criterion most indicative of periwound infection involving the deep and surrounding wound tissues. A recent validation of the less expensive (under $100) infrared thermometers, commercially available as equivalent to the gold standard DermaTemp® thermometer was performed (Mufti et al., 2015). These findings support the validity of low-cost thermometers as appropriate diagnostic tools for clinicians in everyday practice. The authors recommend that these devices should be included in every wound care nurse's toolkit. See Chapter 11 for further discussion of the assessment and management of superficial and deep wound infections.

The clinical mnemonic STONEES defines seven clinical signs of deep and surrounding wound infection. Two additional criteria must be present in addition to temperature increase of greater than 3°F (>3°F or 1.7°C) at wound margin when compared to mirror image skin. STONEES criteria (Sibbald et al., 2006; Woo & Sibbald, 2009) include the following:

- **S**ize of the wound increased
- **T**emperature increase of >3°F or 1.7°C between wound margin compared to mirror image skin
- **O**s—Latin for bone—probing or exposed bone
- **N**ew areas of breakdown—often around the wound margins
- **E**xudate increase
- **E**rythema/**E**dema—swelling associated with cellulitis, but the erythema may be difficult to identify in darkly pigmented skin (brown, black)
- **S**mell—usually occurs in the presence of gram-negative or anaerobic organisms

Routine assessment of plantar surface temperature using a dermal thermometer can identify persons at immediate risk for diabetic or other neurotropic foot ulcers due to repetitive trauma. RCTs provide evidence that routine assessment (by the patient and by clinicians) can reduce the incidence of ulcers in persons with diabetes mellitus and neuropathy as outlined in three RCTs comparing daily monitoring of plantar foot temperatures compared to diabetic education or enhanced foot screening practices. See Chapter 20 for further discussion of plantar surface temperature monitoring in the management of the patient with neuropathy (Arad et al., 2011; Armstrong & Lavery, 1997; Armstrong et al., 2007; Houghton et al., 2013; Lavery et al., 2004, 2007; Sibbald et al., 2015). Patient self-monitoring of skin temperature reduces the risk for DFUs. If a temperature increase of 4°F is detected in one of six spots on the foot compared to a mirror image on the other foot, the patient should limit walking to avoid the risk of local skin breakdown and foot ulceration.

SKIN TURGOR

Skin turgor refers to the skin's resiliency and ability to quickly return to its original state. The clinician uses two fingers to gently lift a portion of the patient's skin, ideally over the sternum. The rate at which the skin returns to its original state reflects skin turgor. Failure of the skin to rapidly resume its original state is a common sign of dehydration; however, altered skin turgor is also a common finding in relatively healthy elders.

MOISTURE STATUS

As mentioned earlier in this chapter, one of the functions of skin is maintenance of moisture balance; normally, the stratum corneum has a water content that ranges from 10% to 15% (Dealey, 2009). When TEWL is excessive (>15%), the result is dry skin (xerosis) (Dealey, 2009). Dry skin is believed to be more vulnerable to damage and local injury from pressure and shear. Conversely, skin that is too moist is also more vulnerable to pressure injury as well as moisture-associated skin damage (MASD) (see Chapters 20 and 18 on pressure ulcers/injuries and MASD).

The simplest way to assess skin for moisture content is by visual inspection; dry skin frequently appears flaky and dull, while overhydrated skin appears moist and may be lighter in color or macerated compared to the surrounding skin. Touch can also be used to detect skin that is overly dry or overly moist. In the future, instruments may be available at the bedside to assess subepidermal moisture levels. There is emerging evidence that higher subepidermal moisture levels may be indicative of increased risk for pressure injury development, especially in individuals with darkly pigmented skin. It has been shown that the risk of pressure injury formation increases fivefold as a result of the moisture buildup from perspiration due to systemic fevers, or incontinence of urine and feces (Olesen et al., 2010). Research is ongoing to verify the significance of these findings and to develop simple tools that would allow the clinician to measure subepidermal moisture at the bedside (Bates-Jensen et al., 2009; EPUAP/NPIAP/PPPIA, 2019; O'Brien et al., 2018; Kim et al., 2018). The international pressure injury clinical guideline includes a recommendation to consider using a subepidermal moisture/edema measurement device as an adjunct to routine clinical skin assessment (EPUAP/NPIAP/PPPIA, 2019).

SKIN INTEGRITY

A critical element of skin assessment is prompt identification of any breaks in skin integrity. If there are any lesions or ulcerations, the clinician needs to determine the type of damage/cause of the lesion that will facilitate treatment of the causative factors (the critical first step in management of any wound) (Schultz et al., 2003; Sibbald et al., 2011). The wound nurse or other health care professional should base diagnosis/classification of any lesion or wound on a comprehensive history and physical examination as well as any indicated diagnostic studies. The correct classification system should be used for the type of chronic wound identified. For example, in the United States, the NPIAP pressure injury staging system (see Chapter 20) should only be used for pressure injuries and not for skin tears (see Chapter 18 for the International Skin Tear Advisory Panel [ISTAP] Classification system).

Skin status is also affected by micronutrient deficiencies, and the signs of micronutrient deficiency are not always recognized. Kaminski and Drinane (2014) have provided a succinct summary of some of the micronutrient deficiencies that can impact wound healing and that are manifested by skin changes; these are outlined in **Table 2-2**. See Chapter 7 on nutritional assessment and support for more detailed description of the role that vitamins and minerals play in skin and tissue integrity and wound healing.

The clinician should carefully describe the morphology of any skin lesion using standardized dermatologic terminology (**Table 2-3**).

KEY POINT

It is critical for the wound care nurse to use standard dermatologic terminology when documenting skin lesions and wound status.

 ## PRINCIPLES FOR USING SKIN CARE PRODUCTS

The skin has an acid mantle that needs to be maintained for proper barrier function. Skin care products and skin care routines should be designed to maintain this acidic pH. For example, use of alkaline soaps and cleansers should be avoided; pH-balanced no-rinse cleansers are generally the preferred agent for routine bathing. Overly frequent bathing should also be avoided, especially with hot water, due to the potential for dehydration of the stratum corneum and depletion of the normal lipid levels of the skin (with resultant compromise of the barrier function of the skin). After showering or bathing, moisturizing products (emollient and humectants) should be applied to the skin while the skin is still damp but not wet within 1 to 3 minutes of bathing rather than allowing it to dry completely. Emollients provide lipids to fill in the gaps between the skin cells and to retard water loss, helping to maintain the moisture content of the stratum corneum within the normal range of 10% to 15%. They also help relieve pruritus, particularly if it is related to xerosis or contact irritant eczema. The most effective emollients are water-free ointments, water-in-oil emollients, and creams. Emollients have a

TABLE 2-2 SKIN CHANGES RESULTING FROM MICRONUTRIENT DEFICIENCIES

VITAMIN DEFICIENCIES

VITAMIN	CLINICAL PRESENTATION	CHARACTERISTICS
B_2		Angular stomatitis is a moist crack in the mucosa at the angle of the upper and lower lips. It is a sign of vitamin B_2 deficiency, usually accompanied by magenta-colored glossitis.
B_3		(A) Pellagra is a vitamin B_3 deficiency. Early signs are a crepe paper appearance to the skin, as illustrated here. Thin islands of the epidermis are separated by rivulets. (B) Advanced pellagra is the typical alligator skin noted in sun-exposed areas of niacin-deficient individuals. In the past, farmers working with an open collar developed these legions on their superior chest/inferior neck.
C		Profound chronic scurvy leaves the skin susceptible to a typical triangular skin tear. This may be a sign of scurvy and not a condition in itself; the patient should be assessed for other indicators of vitamin C deficiency and treatment should be initiated.
C		Chronic scurvy can be staged by observing the thickness of the dermis and its transparency. Early stages prevent direct observation of the tendrils of extensor tendons and the venous plexus over the tendon sheath. The skin becomes progressively transparent with stage IV, featuring a slightly opaque, transparent epidermis revealing an unobstructed view of the deeper anatomy. (A) Normal dermis; (B) +1; (C) +2; (D) +3; and (E) +4.

MINERALS AND OTHER MICRONUTRIENTS

NAME	CLINICAL PRESENTATION	CHARACTERISTICS
Zinc		Zinc rash is a seborrheic-like reddish, flakey condition best seen along the lateral eyebrow (A) and the nasal labial folds (B).

(Continued)

TABLE 2-2 SKIN CHANGES RESULTING FROM MICRONUTRIENT DEFICIENCIES (*Continued*)

Fatty acids		Essential fatty acid deficiency presents as a large "snowflake" exfoliated condition of the epidermis. It typically starts with the anterior area of the lower extremities. It can progress to involve the entire body. These "snowflakes" can be released by gentle rubbing and gathered off the surface of the mattress.
Glucosamine		A deficiency in glucosamine and other intracellular constituents responsible for local hydration results in prolonged tenting of the skin despite normal hydration on physical examination.

Reprinted with permission from Kaminski, M. V., Jr., & Drinane, J. J. (2014). Learning the oral and cutaneous signs of micronutrient deficiencies. *Journal of Wound Ostomy & Continence Nursing, 41*(2), 127–135.

TABLE 2-3 COMMON DERMATOLOGIC TERMINOLOGY, LESIONS

GROUP	LESION TYPE	DEFINITION
Flat	Macule	A flat, generally <0.5 cm area of skin or mucous membranes with different color from surrounding tissue. Macules may have nonpalpable, fine scale (Fig. 3-1).
	Patch*	A flat, generally >0.5 cm area of skin or mucous membranes with different color from surrounding tissue. Patches may have nonpalpable, fine scale.
Raised and smooth	Papule	A discrete, solid, elevated body usually <0.5 cm in diameter. Papules are further classified by shape, size, color, and surface change (Fig. 3-3).
	Plaque	A discrete, solid, elevated body, usually broader than it is thick, measuring more than 0.5 cm in diameter. Plaques may be further classified by shape, size, color, and surface change (Fig. 3-4).
	Nodule	A dermal or subcutaneous firm, well-defined lesion usually >0.5 cm in diameter (Fig. 3-5).
	Cyst	A closed cavity or sac containing fluid or semisolid material. A cyst may have an epithelial, endothelial, or membranous lining (Fig. 3-6).

TABLE 2-3 COMMON DERMATOLOGIC TERMINOLOGY, LESIONS (*Continued*)

GROUP	LESION TYPE	DEFINITION
Surface change 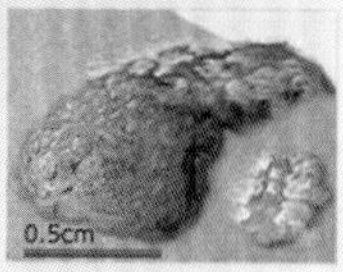	Crust 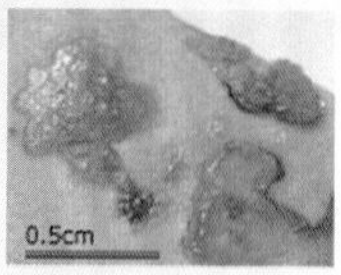	A hardened layer that results when serum, blood, or purulent exudate dries on the skin surface. Crusts may be thin or thick and can have varying color. Crusts are yellow-brown when formed from dried serum, green or yellow-green when formed from purulent exudate, or red-black when formed by blood (Fig. 3-7).
	Scale 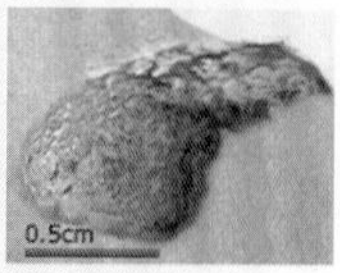	Excess stratum corneum accumulated in flakes or plates. Scale usually has a white or gray color (Fig. 3-8).
Fluid filled 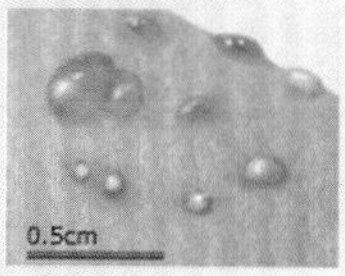	Abscess 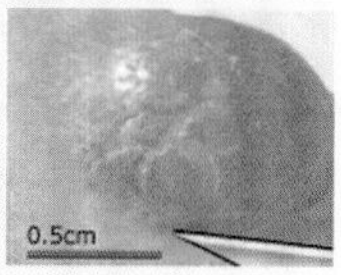	A localized accumulation of pus in the dermis or subcutaneous tissue. Frequently red, warm, and tender (Fig. 3-9).
	Bulla 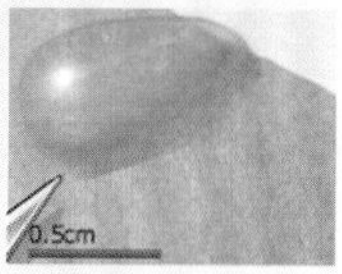	A fluid-filled blister >0.5 cm in diameter. Fluid can be clear, serous, hemorrhagic, or pus filled (Fig. 3-10).
	Pustule 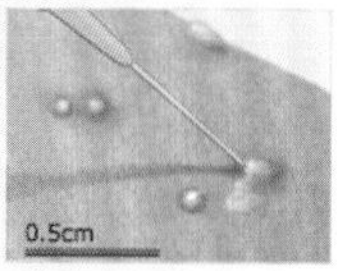	A circumscribed elevation that contains pus. Pustules are usually <0.5 cm in diameter (Fig. 3-11).
	Vesicle 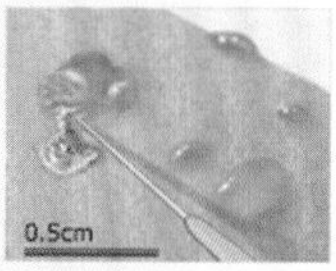	Fluid-filled cavity or elevation <0.5 cm in diameter. Fluid may be clear, serous, hemorrhagic, or pus filled (Fig. 3-12).
Red blanchable 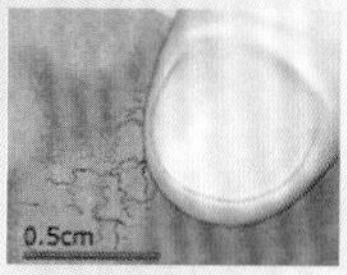	Erythema 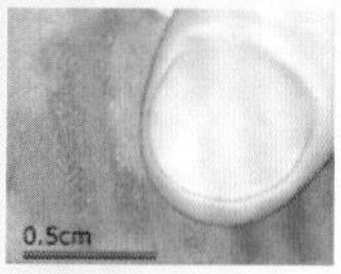	Localized, blanchable redness of the skin or mucous membranes (Fig. 3-13).
	Erythroderma 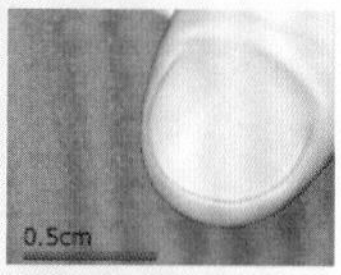	Generalized, blanchable redness of the skin that may be associated with desquamation (Fig. 3-14).
	Telangiectasia 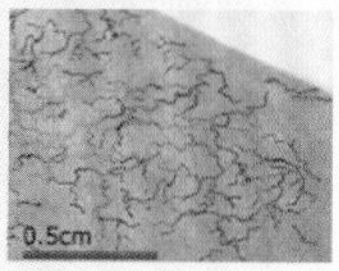	Visible, persistent dilation of small, superficial cutaneous blood vessels. Telangiectasias will blanch (Fig. 3-15).

TABLE 2-3 COMMON DERMATOLOGIC TERMINOLOGY, LESIONS (*Continued*)

GROUP	LESION TYPE	DEFINITION
Purpuric	Ecchymosis	Extravasation of blood into the skin or mucous membranes. Area of flat color change may progress over time from blue-black to brown-yellow or green (Fig. 3-16).
	Petechiae	Tiny 1–2 mm, initially purpuric, nonblanchable macules resulting from tiny hemorrhages (Fig. 3-17).
	Palpable purpura	Raised and palpable, nonblanchable, red or violaceous discoloration of skin or mucous membranes due to vascular inflammation in the skin and extravasation of red blood cells (Fig. 3-18).
Sunken	Atrophy	A thinning of tissue defined by its location, such as epidermal atrophy, dermal atrophy, or subcutaneous atrophy (Fig. 3-19).
	Erosion	A localized loss of the epidermal or mucosal epithelium (Fig. 3-20).
	Ulcer	A circumscribed loss of the epidermis and at least upper dermis. Ulcers are further classified by their depth, border/shape, edge, and tissue at its base (Fig. 3-21).
Gangrene	Gangrene	Necrotic, usually black, tissue due to obstruction, diminution, or loss of blood supply. Gangrene may be wet or dry (Fig. 3-22).
Eschar	Eschar	An adherent thick, dry, black crust (Fig. 3-23).

ˈWhen used to describe an early clinical stage of cutaneous T-cell lymphoma (mycosis fungoides), the term patch may include fine textural change such as "cigarette paper" thinning, poikilodermatous atrophy, or slickness secondary to follicular loss (Fig. 3-2).
From Craft, N., & Fox, L. P. (2010). *VisualDx: Essential adult dermatology*. Philadelphia, PA: Lippincott Williams & Wilkins.

softening and moisturizing effect on the skin; this category includes products containing silicone, dimethicone, lanolin, and ceramides.

Humectants are substances that actively attract water to the skin and are designed for use with very dry rough skin (xerosis). Humectants are ideal to hydrate the skin from the local environment when the ambient humidity exceeds 70%. Moreover, humectants help to enhance the smoothness of dry/xerotic skin by causing corneocytes to swell (Purnamawati et al., 2017). Humectants are made up of agents that are part of the natural moisturizing factor of the stratum corneum including urea, lactic acid, glycerin, propylene glycol, sorbitol, pyrrolidone carboxylic acid, gelatin, hyaluronic acid, and some other vitamins and proteins. For patients at risk for or who have MASD, moisture barrier products are an essential element of care; these products (zinc oxide ointment, petrolatum, or film-forming liquid acrylates) are discussed in detail in Chapter 18.

When selecting skin and wound care products, the wound care nurse must remember that the skin plays an important role in immunity and the skin is very susceptible to allergic reactions. It is important to avoid using products on the skin that have ingredients that are known sensitizers (likely to cause allergic reactions). For example, neomycin and polymyxin are two of the ingredients in some triple antibiotic creams and ointments. The third ingredient in triple antibiotic ointment is bacitracin (former allergen of the year for the American Academy of Dermatology) instead of gramicidin in the cream formulations. Neomycin has two sensitizers, with 60% of the allergic reactions due to the neomycin sugars and 40% of the allergic reactions caused by the deoxystreptamine backbone (Chung & Carson, 1975; Menezes de Pádua et al., 2005; Schorr & Ridgway, 1977). This backbone is common to all aminoglycoside antibiotics from the same class: gentamicin, amikacin, and tobramycin. The development of an allergy to the deoxystreptamine backbone eliminates other aminoglycosides as systemic antibiotic choices as well as other topical formulations with gentamicin, amikacin, or tobramycin. Common sensitizers other than neomycin include bacitracin, lanolin, and Pentalyn H®, an adhesive in some hydrocolloid dressings (Katz & Fisher, 1987; Wakelin et al., 2001).

Natural lanolin is found in some emollient creams and moisturizers and is a common sensitizer in persons with chronic leg ulcers; chemically modified lanolin may be less likely to cause a sensitivity reaction. Pentalyn H® is found in the adhesives of some ostomy skin barriers, and its allergic potential cross-reacts with colophony, a resin from pine trees. In addition to avoidance of sensitizing agents, it is best to avoid topical antibiotic agents with a systemic counterpart due to the development of resistant organisms that eliminate the effectiveness of the related systemic agent. If a patient is being treated with a topical antimicrobial and there is no improvement in wound status within 2 weeks, the patient and wound should be assessed for bacterial resistance or a deep and surrounding infection.

CONCLUSION

An assessment of the multiple functions and appropriate care of the skin is an important competency for wound care nurses. In this chapter, we have provided an overview of skin functions as well as the normal attributes of the skin including changes from birth to old age. Elements of a skin assessment include the five components of physical assessment: skin color, temperature, turgor, moisture status, and integrity. Factors to consider in a holistic assessment of a person at risk for skin injury have been reviewed.

Skin care treatment plans need to be based on the normal characteristics of the skin including maintaining the acidic pH, managing moisture balance, protecting the skin from barrier disruption, and avoidance of skin sensitizers. The remaining chapters in this book will build on this foundation as specific skin and wound conditions are presented in more detail.

REFERENCES

Abbasi, N. R., Shaw, H. M., Rigel, D. S., et al. (2004). Early diagnosis of cutaneous melanoma: Revisiting the ABCD criteria. *JAMA, 292*(22), 2771–2776. doi: 10.1001/jama.292.22.2771.

Alam, M., & Ratner, D. (2001). Cutaneous squamous-cell carcinoma. *The New England Journal of Medicine, 344*(13), 975–983. doi: 10.1056/NEJM200103293441306.

Arad, Y., Fonseca, V., Peters, A., et al. (2011). Beyond the monofilament for the insensate diabetic foot. *Diabetes Care, 34*(4), 1041–1046. doi: 10.2337/dc10-1666.

Armstrong, D. G., Holtz-Neiderer, K., Wendel, C., et al. (2007). Skin temperature monitoring reduces the risk for diabetic foot ulceration in high-risk patients. *The American Journal of Medicine, 120*(12), 1042–1046. doi: 10.1016/j.amjmed.2007.06.028.

Armstrong, D. G., & Lavery, L. A. (1997). Predicting neuropathic ulceration with infrared dermal thermometry. *Journal of the American Podiatric Medical Association, 87*(7), 336–337. doi: 10.7547/87507315-87-7-336.

Ayello, E. A., Sibbald, R. G., Quiambao, P. C. H., et al. (2014). Introducing a moisture-associated skin assessment photo guide for brown pigmented skin. *World Council of Enterostomal Therapists Journal, 34*(2), 18.

Bates-Jensen, B. M., McCreath, H. E., & Pongquan, V. (2009). Subepidermal moisture is associated with early pressure ulcer damage in nursing home residents with dark skin tones: Pilot findings. *Journal of Wound, Ostomy, and Continence Nursing: Official Publication of The Wound, Ostomy and Continence Nurses Society, 36*(3), 277–284. doi: 10.1097/WON.0b013e3181a19e53.

Bennett, C. L., Noordegraaf, M., Martina, C. A. E., et al. (2007). Langerhans cells are required for efficient presentation of topically applied hapten to T cells. *Journal of Immunology, 179*(10), 6830–6835. doi: 10.4049/jimmunol.179.10.6830.

Berger, U., Wilson, P., McClelland, R. A., et al. (1988). Immunocytochemical detection of 1,25-dihydroxyvitamin D receptors in normal human tissues. *The Journal of Clinical Endocrinology and Metabolism, 67*(3), 607–613. doi: 10.1210/jcem-67-3-607.

Bergstrom, N., Smout, R., Horn, S., et al. (2008). Stage 2 pressure ulcer healing in nursing homes. *Journal of the American Geriatrics Society, 56*(7), 1252–1258. doi: 10.1111/j.1532-5415.2008.01765.

Bikle, D. (2000). Vitamin D: Production, metabolism, and mechanisms of action. In K. R. Feingold, B. Anawalt, G. Boyce, et al. (Eds.), *Endotext.* Retrieved from http://www.ncbi.nlm.nih.gov/books/NBK278935/

Biniek, K., Levi, K., & Dauskardt, R. H. (2012). Solar UV radiation reduces the barrier function of human skin. *Proceedings of the National Academy of Sciences of the United States of America, 109*(42), 17111–17116. doi: 10.1073/pnas.1206851109.

Bittencourt, F. V., Marghoob, A. A., Kopf, A. W., et al. (2000). Large congenital melanocytic nevi and the risk for development of malignant melanoma and neurocutaneous melanocytosis. *Pediatrics, 106*(4), 736–741. doi: 10.1542/peds.106.4.736.

Bos, J. D., & Kapsenberg, M. L. (1993). The skin immune system: Progress in cutaneous biology. *Immunology Today, 14*(2), 75–78. doi: 10.1016/0167-5699(93)90062-P.

Burns, T., Breathnach, S., Cox, N., et al. (2008). *Rook's textbook of dermatology* (7th ed., Vol. 2). Oxford: Blackwell Publishing.

Charkoudian, N. (2003). Skin blood flow in adult human thermoregulation: How it works, when it does not, and why. *Mayo Clinic Proceedings, 78*(5), 603–612. doi: 10.4065/78.5.603.

Chung, C. W., & Carson, T. R. (1975). Sensitization potentials and immunologic specificities of neomycins. *The Journal of Investigative Dermatology, 64*(3), 158–164. doi: 10.1111/1523-1747.ep12533314.

Copcu, E., Sivrioglu, N., & Culhaci, N. (2004). Cutaneous horns: Are these lesions as innocent as they seem to be? *World Journal of Surgical Oncology, 2*, 18. doi: 10.1186/1477-7819-2-18.

Craft, N., & Fox, L. P. (2010). *VisualDx: Essential adult dermatology.* Philadelphia, PA: Lippincott Williams & Wilkins.

Cress, R. D., & Holly, E. A. (1997). Incidence of cutaneous melanoma among non-Hispanic whites, Hispanics, Asians, and blacks: An analysis of California Cancer Registry data, 1988–93. *Cancer Causes & Control, 8*(2), 246–252. doi: 10.1023/a:1018432632528.

Crissey, S. D., Ange, K. D., Jacobsen, K. L., et al. (2003). Serum concentrations of lipids, vitamin d metabolites, retinol, retinyl esters, tocopherols and selected carotenoids in twelve captive wild felid species at four zoos. *The Journal of Nutrition, 133*(1), 160–166. doi: 10.1093/jn/133.1.160.

Dai, J., Jiang, C., Chen, H., et al. (2019). Vitamin D and diabetic foot ulcer: A systematic review and meta-analysis. *Nutrition & Diabetes, 9*(1), 8. doi: 10.1038/s41387-019-0078-9.

Dealey, C. (2009). Skin care and pressure ulcers. *Advances in Skin & Wound Care, 22*(9), 421–428; quiz 429–430. doi: 10.1097/01. ASW.0000360255.92357.ad.

Eder, J., Prillinger, K., Korn, A., et al. (2014). Prevalence of actinic keratosis among dermatology outpatients in Austria. *The British Journal of Dermatology, 171*(6), 1415–1421. doi: 10.1111/bjd.13132.

Egan, C. L., Oliveria, S. A., Elenitsas, R., et al. (1998). Cutaneous melanoma risk and phenotypic changes in large congenital nevi: A follow-up study of 46 patients. *Journal of the American Academy of Dermatology, 39*(6), 923–932. doi: 10.1016/s0190-9622(98) 70264-6.

Elder, D. E. (2006). Precursors to melanoma and their mimics: Nevi of special sites. *Modern Pathology, 19*(Suppl 2), S4–S20. doi: 10.1038/ modpathol.3800515.

European Pressure Ulcer Advisory Panel, National Pressure Injury Advisory Panel, and Pan Pacific Pressure Injury Alliance [EPUAP/ NPIAP/PPPIA]. (2019). In E. Haesler (Ed.), *Prevention and treatment of pressure ulcers/injuries: Clinical Practice Guideline*. The International Guideline.

Falanga, V., & Sabolinski, M. (1999). A bilayered living skin construct (APLIGRAF) accelerates complete closure of hard-to-heal venous ulcers. *Wound Repair and Regeneration, 7*(4), 201–207. doi: 10.1046/j.1524-475x.1999.00201.x.

Feldmann, R. J., & Maibach, H. I. (1967). Regional variation in percutaneous penetration of 14C cortisol in man. *The Journal of Investigative Dermatology, 48*(2), 181–183. doi: 10.1038/jid.1967.29.

Fenske, N. A., & Lober, C. W. (1986). Structural and functional changes of normal aging skin. *Journal of the American Academy of Dermatology, 15*(4 Pt 1), 571–585. doi: 10.1016/s0190-9622(86)70208-9.

Fitzpatrick, T. B. (1975). Soleil et peau (Sun and skin). *Journal de Médecine Esthétique, 2*, 33–34.

Fitzpatrick, T. B. (1986). Ultraviolet-induced pigmentary changes: Benefits and hazards. *Current Problems in Dermatology, 15*, 25–38. doi: 10.1159/000412090.

Fitzpatrick, T. B. (1988). The validity and practicality of sun-reactive skin types I through VI. *Archives of Dermatology, 124*(6), 869–871. doi:10.1001/archderm.1988.01670060015008.

Flohil, S. C., van der Leest, R. J. T., Dowlatshahi, E. A., et al. (2013). Prevalence of actinic keratosis and its risk factors in the general population: The Rotterdam Study. *The Journal of Investigative Dermatology, 133*(8), 1971–1978. doi: 10.1038/jid.2013.

Fluhr, J. W., Feingold, K. R., & Elias, P. M. (2006). Transepidermal water loss reflects permeability barrier status: Validation in human and rodent in vivo and ex vivo models. *Experimental Dermatology, 15*(7), 483–492. doi: 10.1111/j.1600-0625.2006.00437.x.

Gallagher, R. P., & McLean, D. I. (1995). The epidemiology of acquired melanocytic nevi. A brief review. *Dermatologic Clinics, 13*(3), 595–603.

Gallo, R. L. (2008). Sounding the alarm: Multiple functions of host defense peptides. *The Journal of Investigative Dermatology, 128*(1), 5–6. doi: 10.1038/sj.jid.5701073.

Gandini, S., Sera, F., Cattaruzza, M. S., et al. (2005). Meta-analysis of risk factors for cutaneous melanoma: I. Common and atypical naevi. *European Journal of Cancer, 41*(1), 28–44. doi: 10.1016/j. ejca.2004.10.015.

Gladman, A. C. (2006). Toxicodendron dermatitis: Poison ivy, oak, and sumac. *Wilderness & Environmental Medicine, 17*(2), 120–128. doi: 10.1580/pr31-05.1.

Goodarzi, H., Trowbridge, J., & Gallo, R. L. (2007). Innate immunity: A cutaneous perspective. *Clinical Reviews in Allergy & Immunology, 33*(1–2), 15–26. doi: 10.1007/s12016-007-0037-4.

Guyton, A. C. (1991). *Textbook of medical physiology* (8th ed.). Philadelphia, PA: Saunders.

Habif, T. P. (2004). Nevi and malignant melanoma. In *Clinical dermatology: A color guide to diagnosis and therapy* (4th ed., pp. 776–777). Edinburgh, UK: Mosby.

Hafner, C., & Vogt, T. (2008). Seborrheic keratosis. *Journal der Deutschen Dermatologischen Gesellschaft, 6*(8), 664–677. doi: 10.1111/j.1610-0387.2008.06788.x.

Halata, Z., Grim, M., & Bauman, K. I. (2003). Friedrich Sigmund Merkel and his "Merkel cell", morphology, development, and physiology: Review and new results. *Anat Rec A Discov Mol Cell Evol Biol, 271*(1), 225–239. doi: 10.1002/ar.a.10029.

Holick, M. F., Matsuoka, L. Y., & Wortsman, J. (1995). Regular use of sunscreen on vitamin D levels. *Archives of Dermatology, 131*(11), 1337–1339. doi: 10.1001/archderm.131.11.1337.

Holick, M. F., Smith, E., & Pincus, S. (1987). Skin as the site of vitamin D synthesis and target tissue for 1,25-dihydroxyvitamin D3. Use of calcitriol (1,25-dihydroxyvitamin D3) for treatment of psoriasis. *Archives of Dermatology, 123*(12), 1677–1683a.

Hope-Simpson, R. E. (1965). The nature of herpes zoster: A long-term study and a new hypothesis. *Proceedings of the Royal Society of Medicine, 58*(1), 9–20.

Houghton, V. J., Bower, V. M., & Chant, D. C. (2013). Is an increase in skin temperature predictive of neuropathic foot ulceration in people with diabetes? A systematic review and meta-analysis. *Journal of Foot and Ankle Research, 6*, 31. doi: 10.1186/1757-1146-6-31.

Institute of Medicine (US) Committee to Review Dietary Reference Intakes for Vitamin D and Calcium. (2011). In A. C. Ross, C. L. Taylor, A. L. Yaktine, et al. (Eds.), *Dietary Reference Intakes for Calcium and Vitamin D*. Retrieved from http://www.ncbi.nlm.nih.gov/books/ NBK56070/

Jacob, S. E., & Steele, T. (2006). Corticosteroid classes: A quick reference guide including patch test substances and cross-reactivity.

Journal of the American Academy of Dermatology, 54(4), 723–727. doi: 10.1016/j.jaad.2005.12.028.

Jarvis, C. (2012). *Physical examination and health assessment* (6th ed.). St. Louis, MO: Elsevier.

Johnson, J. M., Brengelmann, G. L., Hales, J. R., et al. (1986). Regulation of the cutaneous circulation. *Federation Proceedings, 45*(13), 2841–2850.

Johnson, J. M., & Proppe, D. W. (2011). Cardiovascular adjustments to heat stress. In American Physiological Society, *Handbook of Physiology: Environmental Physiology,* (pp. 215–243). doi:10.1002/cphy. cp040111.

Kaminski, M. V., & Drinane, J. J. (2014). Learning the oral and cutaneous signs of micronutrient deficiencies. *Journal of Wound, Ostomy, and Continence Nursing, 41*(2), 127–135; quiz E1–E2. doi: 10.1097/ WON.0000000000000012.

Karia P. S., Han J., & Schmults, C. D. (2013). Cutaneous squamous cell carcinoma: Estimated incidence of disease, nodal metastasis, and deaths from disease in the United States, 2012. *Journal of the American Academy of Dermatology, 68*(6), 957–966. doi: 10.1016/j. jaad.2012.11.037.

Katz, B. E., & Fisher, A. A. (1987). Bacitracin: A unique topical antibiotic sensitizer. *Journal of the American Academy of Dermatology, 17*(6), 1016–1024. doi: 10.1016/s0190-9622(87)70292-8.

Kelleher, M. M., O'Carroll, M., Gallagher, A., et al. (2013). Newborn transepidermal water loss values: A reference dataset. *Pediatric Dermatology, 30*(6), 712–716. doi: 10.1111/pde.12106.

Kelly, J. W., Chamberlain, A. J., Staples, M. P., et al. (2003). Nodular melanoma. No longer as simple as ABC. *Australian Family Physician, 32*(9), 706–709.

Kim, Y., Flamm, A., ElSohly, M. A., et al. (2019). Poison ivy, oak, and sumac dermatitis: What is known and what is new? *Dermatitis, 30*(3), 183–190. doi: 10.1097/DER.0000000000000472.

Kim, C., Park, S., Ko, J., et al. (2018). The relationship of subepidermal moisture surrounding pressure ulcers in persons with a spinal cord injury: By visual skin assessment. *Journal of Tissue Viability, 27*(3), 130–134. doi: 10.1179/2045772313Y.0000000193.

Korkut, T., Tan, N. B., & Oztan, Y. (1997). Giant cutaneous horn: A patient report. *Annals of Plastic Surgery, 39*(6), 654–655. doi: 10.1097/00000637-199712000-00019.

Kromann, A. B., Ousager, L. B., Ali, I. K. M., et al. (2018). Pigmentary mosaicism: A review of original literature and recommendations for future handling. *Orphanet Journal of Rare Diseases, 13.* doi: 10.1186/ s13023-018-0778-6.

Lavery, L. A., Higgins, K. R., Lanctot, D. R., et al. (2004). Home monitoring of foot skin temperatures to prevent ulceration. *Diabetes Care, 27*(11), 2642–2647. doi: 10.2337/diacare.27.11.2642.

Lavery, L. A., Higgins, K. R., Lanctot, D. R., et al. (2007). Preventing diabetic foot ulcer recurrence in high-risk patients: Use of temperature monitoring as a self-assessment tool. *Diabetes Care, 30*(1), 14–20. doi: 10.2337/dc06-1600.

Lee, N. P., & Arriola, E. R. (1999). Poison ivy, oak, and sumac dermatitis. *Western Journal of Medicine, 171*(5–6), 354–355.

Levine, J. A. (2020). Clinical aspects of aqinq skin: Considerations for the wound care practitioner. *Advances in Skin & Wound Care, 33*(1), 1. doi: 10.1097/01.ASW.0000616268.46423.cb.

Levit, E. K., Kagen, M. H., Scher, R. K., et al. (2000). The ABC rule for clinical detection of subungual melanoma. *Journal of the American Academy of Dermatology, 42*(2 Pt 1), 269–274. doi: 10.1016/S0190-9622(00)90137-3.

Manson, J. E., Cook, N. R., Lee, I. M., et al.; VITAL Research Group. (2019). Vitamin D supplements and prevention of cancer and cardiovascular disease. *The New England Journal of Medicine, 380*(1), 33–44. doi: 10.1056/NEJMoa1809944.

Marks, R., Foley, P. A., Jolley, D., et al. (1995). The effect of regular sunscreen use on vitamin D levels in an Australian population. Results of a randomized controlled trial. *Archives of Dermatology, 131*(4), 415–421.

Marks, J. G., Fowler, J. F., Sheretz E. F., et al. (1995). Prevention of poison ivy and poison oak allergic contact dermatitis by quaternium-18 bentonite. *Journal of the American Academy of Dermatology, 33*(2 Pt 1), 212–216. doi: 10.1016/0190-9622(95)90237-6.

Matsumoto, K., Azuma, Y., Kiyoki, M., et al. (1991). Involvement of endogenously produced 1,25-dihydroxyvitamin D-3 in the growth and differentiation of human keratinocytes. *Biochimica et Biophysica Acta, 1092*(3), 311–318. doi: 10.1016/s0167-4889(97)90006-9.

Matsuoka, L. Y., Ide, L., Wortsman, J., et al. (1987). Sunscreens suppress cutaneous vitamin D3 synthesis. *The Journal of Clinical Endocrinology and Metabolism, 64*(6), 1165–1168. doi: 10.1210/jcem-64-6-1165.

Menezes de Pádua, C. A., Schnuch, A., Lessmann, H., et al. (2005). Contact allergy to neomycin sulfate: Results of a multifactorial analysis. *Pharmacoepidemiology and Drug Safety, 14*(10), 725–733. doi: 10.1002/pds.1117.

Menon, G. K., Cleary, G. W., & Lane, M. E. (2012). The structure and function of the stratum corneum. *International Journal of Pharmaceutics, 435*(1), 3–9. doi: 10.1016/j.ijpharm.2012.06.005.

Montagna, W., & Carlisle, K. (1979). Structural changes in aging human skin. *The Journal of Investigative Dermatology, 73*(1), 47–53. doi: 10.1111/1523-1747.ep12532761.

Montagna, W., Kirchner, S., & Carlisle, K. (1989). Histology of sun-damaged human skin. *Journal of the American Academy of Dermatology, 21*(5 Pt 1), 907–918. doi: 10.1016/s0190-9622(89)70276-0.

Mufti, A., Coutts, P., & Sibbald, R. G. (2015). Validation of commercially available infrared thermometers for measuring skin surface temperature associated with deep and surrounding wound infection. *Advances in Skin & Wound Care, 28*(1), 11–16. doi: 10.1097/01. ASW.0000459039.81701.b2.

Natsume, K., Ogawa, T., Sugenoya, J., et al. (1992). Preferred ambient temperature for old and young men in summer and winter. *International Journal of Biometeorology, 36*(1), 1–4. doi: 10.1007/bf01208726.

Neale, R. E., Khan, S. R., Lucas, R. M., et al. (2019). The effect of sunscreen on vitamin D: A review. *The British Journal of Dermatology, 181*(5), 907–915. doi: 10.1111/bjd.17980.

Noiles, K., & Vender, R. (2007). Are all seborrheic keratoses benign? Review of the typical lesion and its variants. *Journal of Cutaneous Medicine and Surgery, 12*(5), 203–210. doi: 10.2310/7750.2008.07096.

Norman, A. W. (1998). Sunlight, season, skin pigmentation, vitamin D, and 25-hydroxyvitamin D: Integral components of the vitamin D endocrine system. *The American Journal of Clinical Nutrition, 67*(6), 1108–1110. doi: 10.1093/ajcn/67.6.1108.

Norman, A. W. (2008). From vitamin D to hormone D: Fundamentals of the vitamin D endocrine system essential for good health. *The American Journal of Clinical Nutrition, 88*(2), 491S–499S. doi: 10.1093/ajcn/88.2.491S.

O'Brien, G., Moore, Z., Patton, D., et al. (2018). The relationship between nurses assessment of early pressure ulcer damage and sub epidermal moisture measurement: A prospective explorative study. *Journal of Tissue Viability, 27*(4), 232–237. doi: 10.1016/j.jtv.2018.06.004.

Olesen, C. G., de Zee, M., & Rasmussen, J. (2010). Missing links in pressure ulcer research—An interdisciplinary overview. *Journal of Applied Physiology (Bethesda, MD: 1985), 108*(6), 1458–1464. doi: 10.1152/japplphysiol.01006.2009.

Oranges, T., Dini, V., & Romanelli, M. (2015). Skin physiology of the neonate and infant: Clinical implications. *Advances in Wound Care, 4*(10), 587–595. doi: 10.1089/wound.2015.0642.

Purnamawati, S., Indrastuti, N., Danarti, R., et al. (2017). The role of moisturizers in addressing various kinds of dermatitis: A review. *Clinical Medicine & Research, 15*(3–4), 75–87. doi: 10.3121/cmr.2017.1363.

Pyne, J., Sapkota, D., & Wong, J. C. (2013). Cutaneous horns: Clues to invasive squamous cell carcinoma being present in the horn base. *Dermatology Practical & Conceptual, 3*(2), 3–7. doi: 10.5826/ dpc.0302a02.

Rigel, D. S., Friedman, R. J., Kopf, A. W., et al. (2005). ABCDE—An evolving concept in the early detection of melanoma. *Archives of Dermatology, 141*(8), 1032–1034. doi: 10.1001/archderm.141.8.1032.

Rowell, L. B. (2011). Cardiovascular adjustments to thermal stress. *American Physiological Society, Handbook of Physiology: The Cardiovascular System, Peripheral Circulation and Organ Blood Flow* (pp. 967–1023). https://doi.org/10.1002/cphy.cp020327

Rubin, A. I., Chen, E. H., & Ratner, D. (2005). Basal-cell carcinoma. *The New England Journal of Medicine, 353*(21), 2262–2269. doi: 10.1056/NEJMra044151.

Rutter, N. (1987). Percutaneous drug absorption in the newborn: Hazards and uses. *Clinics in Perinatology, 14*(4), 911–930.

Schaffer, J. V. (2015). Update on melanocytic nevi in children. *Clinics in Dermatology, 3*(33), 368–386.

Schauber, J., Dorschner, R. A., Coda, A. B., et al. (2007). Injury enhances TLR2 function and antimicrobial peptide expression through a vitamin D–dependent mechanism. *Journal of Clinical Investigation, 117*(3), 803–811. doi: 10.1172/JCI30142.

Schorr, W. F., & Ridgway, H. B. (1977). Tobramycin-neomycin cross-sensitivity. *Contact Dermatitis, 3*(3), 133–137. doi: 10.1111/j.1600-0536.1977.tb03627.x.

Schultz, G. S., Sibbald, R. G., Falanga, V., et al. (2003). Wound bed preparation: A systematic approach to wound management. *Wound Repair and Regeneration, 11*(Suppl 1), S1–S28. doi: 10.1046/j.1524-475x.11.s2.1.x.

Segaert, S. (2008). Vitamin D regulation of cathelicidin in the skin: Toward a renaissance of vitamin D in dermatology? *The Journal of Investigative Dermatology, 128*(4), 773–775. doi: 10.1038/jid.2008.35.

Shah, J., Feintisch, A. M., & Granick, M. S. (2016). Congenital melanocytic nevi. *Eplasty, 16*, ic4.

Sibbald, R. G., Goodman, L., Woo, K. Y., et al. (2011). Special considerations in wound bed preparation 2011: An update©. *Advances in Skin & Wound Care, 24*(9), 415–436; quiz 437–438. doi: 10.1097/01.ASW.0000405216.27050.97.

Sibbald, R. G., Mufti, A., & Armstrong, D. G. (2015). Infrared skin thermometry: An underutilized cost-effective tool for routine wound care practice and patient high-risk diabetic foot self-monitoring. *Advances in Skin & Wound Care, 28*(1), 37–44; quiz 45–46. doi: 10.1097/01.ASW.0000458991.58947.6b.

Sibbald, R. G., Woo, K., & Ayello, E. A. (2006). Increased bacterial burden and infection: The story of NERDS and STONES. *Advances in Skin & Wound Care, 19*(8), 447–461; quiz 461–463. doi: 10.1097/00129334-200610000-00012.

Smart, H., AlGhareeb, A. M., & Smart, S. A. (2019). 25-Hydroxyvitamin D deficiency: Impacting deep-wound infection and poor healing outcomes in patients with diabetes. *Advances in Skin & Wound Care, 32*(7), 321–328. doi: 10.1097/01.ASW.0000559614.90819.45.

Taylor, W. F., Johnson, J. M., O'Leary, D., et al. (1984). Effect of high local temperature on reflex cutaneous vasodilation. *Journal of Applied Physiology: Respiratory, Environmental and Exercise Physiology, 57*(1), 191–196. doi: 10.1152/jappl.1984.57.1.191.

Tobin, D. J. (2017). Introduction to skin aging. *Journal of Tissue Viability, 26*(1), 37–46. doi: 10.1016/j.jtv.2016.03.002.

Traianou, A., Ulrich, M., Apalla, Z., et al.; EPIDERM Group. (2012). Risk factors for actinic keratosis in eight European centres: A case-control study. *The British Journal of Dermatology, 167*(Suppl 2), 36–42. doi: 10.1111/j.1365-2133.2012.11085.x.

Verhagen, A. R., Koten, J. W., Chaddah, V. K., et al. (1968). Skin diseases in Kenya. A clinical and histopathological study of 3,168 patients. *Archives of Dermatology, 98*(6), 577–586. doi: 10.1001/archderm.98.6.577.

Wakelin, S. H., Smith, H., White, I. R., et al. (2001). A retrospective analysis of contact allergy to lanolin. *The British Journal of Dermatology, 145*(1), 28–31. doi: 10.1046/j.1365-2133.2001.04277.x.

Winkelmann, R. K. (1959). The erogenous zones: Their nerve supply and its significance. *Proceedings of the Staff Meetings Mayo Clinic, 34*(2), 39–47.

Woo, K. Y., Harding, K., Price, P., et al. (2008). Minimising wound-related pain at dressing change: Evidence-informed practice. *International Wound Journal, 5*(2), 144–157. doi: 10.1111/j.1742-481X.2008.00486.x.

Woo, K. Y., & Sibbald, R. G. (2009). A cross-sectional validation study of using NERDS and STONEES to assess bacterial burden. *Ostomy/Wound Management, 55*(8), 40–48.

Yeatman, J. M., Kilkenny, M., & Marks, R. (1997). The prevalence of seborrhoeic keratoses in an Australian population: Does exposure to sunlight play a part in their frequency? *The British Journal of Dermatology, 137*(3), 411–414.

Zaal, L. H., Mooi, W. J., Klip, H., et al. (2005). Risk of malignant transformation of congenital melanocytic nevi: A retrospective nationwide study from The Netherlands. *Plastic and Reconstructive Surgery, 116*(7), 1902–1909. doi: 10.1097/01.prs.0000189205.85968.12.

Zhang, S., & Duan, E. (2018). Fighting against skin aging. *Cell Transplantation, 27*(5), 729–738. doi: 10.1177/0963689717725755.

QUESTIONS

1. Which structure of the skin provides the body with photoprotective properties by absorbing harmful ultraviolet light?
   A. Melanin
   B. Langerhans cells
   C. Odland bodies
   D. Stratum lucidum

2. What is a unique function of the layer of the epidermis known as the stratum basale?
   A. Providing immunity via Langerhans cells
   B. Producing new epithelial cells
   C. Releasing lipids to help maintain normal brick and mortar skin configuration
   D. Protecting the palms of the hands and soles of the feet

3. Which cells located in the dermis produce collagen (dermal building blocks) and elastin (tensile strength) critical to immune function and healing?
   A. Leukotrienes
   B. Prostaglandins
   C. Macrophages
   D. Fibroblasts

4. Which patient's wound would the wound care nurse expect to heal by scar formation?
   A. A head wound extending beyond the hair follicles
   B. A shallow wound on the hand
   C. A stage 2 pressure injury
   D. A first-degree burn

5. Which of the following statements accurately describes how the skin functions as a barrier between the internal and external environments?
   A. The skin lipids bind water, normally maintaining skin water content at 20% or higher.
   B. When the barrier function of the skin is compromised, transepidermal water loss (TEWL) decreases.
   C. Protection against pathogenic invasion is supported by an acidic pH of the skin.
   D. Merkel receptors embedded in the extracellular matrix contribute to the mechanical rigidity and frictional resistance protection of the skin.

6. The wound care nurse assessing the skin of patients in a nursing home keeps in mind the structural changes that occur in aging skin. What is one of these changes?
   A. Increase in melanocytes
   B. Rounding of dermal–epidermal junction
   C. Increase in mast cells
   D. Decrease in collagen

7. The wound care nurse uses the acronym ABCDE to distinguish a melanoma from a benign nevus. Based on this acronym, what is a distinguishing characteristic of melanoma?
   A. Regular border
   B. Consistent red or black color
   C. Diameter >4 mm
   D. Evolving lesion

8. On which body site would the transdermal application of a medication obtain the greatest percutaneous absorption?
   A. Plantar surface of the foot
   B. Forearm
   C. Forehead
   D. Hand

9. Which principle of skin care product use would the wound care nurse include in a teaching plan for a patient with a leg wound?
   A. Use alkaline soaps and cleansers to neutralize acidic skin.
   B. Do not use products on the skin that have known sensitizers.
   C. Bathe frequently using water that is as hot as tolerated.
   D. Allow skin to dry completely before applying moisturizers.

10. Which layer of skin contains cells that release lipids such as ceramides to maintain the normal "brick and mortar" skin barrier function.
   A. Stratum germinativum
   B. Stratum basale
   C. Stratum spinosum
   D. Stratum granulosum

ANSWERS AND RATIONALES

1. A. Rationale: In addition to being responsible for everyone's unique skin color, melanin also has photoprotective properties; it can absorb harmful ultraviolet light and protect cells against DNA damage.

2. B. Rationale: The stratum basale is the reproductive layer of the epidermis and is characterized by proliferating keratinocytes.

3. D. Rationale: Fibroblasts are responsible for the synthesis of connective tissue and extracellular matrix, specifically the production of collagen (dermal building blocks) and elastin (tensile strength).

4. A. Rationale: The epidermal appendages, subcutaneous tissue, and muscle do not have the ability to regenerate, and wounds involving loss of these structures will heal by scar formation.

5. C. Rationale: The pH of the skin is normally 4 to 6.5 in healthy people; this "acid mantle" inhibits pathogenic growth.

6. D. Rationale: Intrinsic aging refers to the physiologic changes to the skin cells and tissues that take place with time and are impacted by genetic and hormonal factors. These changes include decreased collagen production, decreased blood flow to the skin, and lower amounts of lipids.

7. D. Rationale: ABCDE includes the following:

A = asymmetry (one side does not look like the other)

B = irregular border (blurred, uneven, or "notched" edges)

C = variable and uneven color

D = diameter >6 mm

E = evolving lesion

8. C. Rationale: Current data indicate that one can crudely rank the regional permeability as follows: nail ≪ palm/sole < trunk/extremities < face/scalp ≪ scrotum. As part of the face, the forehead would be the most permeable of the choices for both sexes.

9. B. Rationale: It is important to avoid using products on the skin that have ingredients that are known sensitizers (likely to cause allergic reactions).

10. D. Rationale: Keratinocytes in the stratum granulosum layer release lipids including ceramide lipids that help to maintain the normal brick and mortar skin barrier function. The stratum granulosum cells also contain glycolipids that when released, function to act as a glue, holding the cells together.

CHAPTER 3

WOUND HEALING

Janice M. Beitz

OBJECTIVES

1. Differentiate between acute and chronic wounds to include implications for management.

2. Describe the physiology of partial-thickness and full-thickness wound healing and identify implications for nursing management.

3. Describe risk factors for nonhealing wounds.

INTRODUCTORY CONCEPTS

A wound represents a disruption in the normal structure and function of the skin and underlying soft tissues and can be related to a variety of etiologies (e.g., trauma, surgery, sustained pressure, vascular disease, infection, etc.). Human beings sustain wounds across their lifespan that range from a simple knee abrasion to a major surgical incision. With most acute wounds (abrasions, lacerations, or surgical incisions), there is little cause for concern since humans are "programmed" to heal and acute injury triggers the repair process. However, when an acute wound fails to heal normally or a wound develops as a result of a chronic condition (e.g., a venous or arterial ulcer), the patient's quality of life can be profoundly affected, and the costs of care can increase substantively. Since both acute and chronic wounds affect millions of people internationally, it is critical for contemporary clinicians to have a good understanding of wound healing mechanisms and the pathogenesis of chronic wounds. This chapter provides an overview of the processes and components of wound healing, describes the various types and phases of healing, distinguishes between the repair processes for acute and chronic wounds, and describes factors affecting wound healing.

PHASES OF WOUND HEALING

In an acute wound such as a surgical incision, wounding generates a cellular response. This response involves activation of specialized cells including platelets, macrophages, keratinocytes, fibroblasts, and endothelial cells. Simultaneously, cytokines (nonantibody proteins) and growth factors are released that coordinate and control the activities of the cells responsible for repair, thus promoting wound healing. Under normal conditions, bleeding will be quickly controlled and the wound will heal in an orderly, effective manner. The repair process for acute wounds involves four major phases: hemostasis, inflammation, proliferation or regeneration, and maturation (remodeling) (**Fig. 3-1**) (Armstrong & Meyr, 2019a).

> **KEY POINT**
>
> In an acute wound such as a surgical incision, the "order of repair" is a brief inflammatory phase, epithelial resurfacing and granulation tissue formation, and remodeling.

HEMOSTASIS

The hemostasis phase commences immediately following wounding. Small vessels in the wound constrict, and activated platelets aggregate within the damaged blood vessels, triggering the clotting cascade. The activated platelets release a myriad of growth factors and cytokines that control and expedite the wound healing process (e.g., platelet-derived growth factor [PDGF]); the activated platelets also help to create the fibrin structure that serves as the scaffold for cell migration during the initial repair process. Notably, larger blood vessels do not constrict, and additional measures are typically required to stop the bleeding from these vessels (e.g., manual pressure, electrocautery, suturing, etc.) (Armstrong & Meyr, 2019a, 2019b, 2019c).

> **KEY POINT**
>
> With acute injury, bleeding and clotting cause release of growth factors, which initiates the repair process.

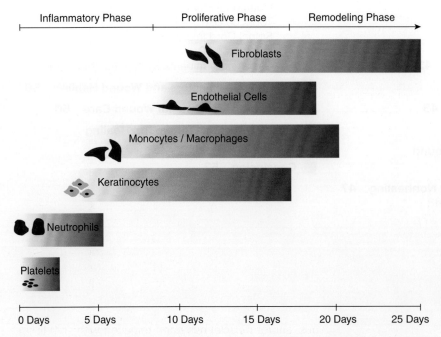

FIGURE 3-1. Phases of Healing with Associated Cellular Activity. Note that in this model, hemostasis and inflammation are considered one phase.

INFLAMMATION

Once the fibrin matrix has been established and bleeding has been controlled, the cytokines and growth factors initiate the inflammatory phase. The goal of the inflammatory phase is establishment of a clean wound bed (i.e., elimination of necrotic tissue and establishment of bacterial control). During this phase, neutrophils and monocytes are chemoattracted to the wounded area. Initially, neutrophils are predominant, and their primary effect is elimination of bacteria via enzymatic activity. As the inflammatory process continues, the number and activity of neutrophils decrease and the number and activity of macrophages (derived from tissue monocytes) increase; macrophages eliminate the dead bacteria, neutrophils, and cellular debris. In addition, macrophages release other cytokines that promote transition from the inflammatory phase into the proliferative phase of repair (e.g., vascular endothelial growth factor [VEGF], which promotes development of new blood vessels, or neoangiogenesis, and PDGF, which promotes fibroblast activity and synthesis of collagen and other connective tissue proteins, also known as fibroplasia). Macrophages are essential during the early phases of repair, and impaired macrophage activity, as seen in uncontrolled diabetes, is associated with impaired wound healing (Canedo-Dorantes & Canedo-Ayala, 2019). In contrast, normal macrophage activity contributes to rapid resolution of the inflammatory phase, followed by transition into the proliferative phase with formation of healthy durable scar tissue (Goodarzi et al., 2019).

PROLIFERATION

The proliferation or regeneration phase begins with fibroblast migration to the area, which occurs in response to cellular signaling; this is followed by formation of a new extracellular matrix (ECM) (granulation tissue). Fibroblasts are the cells responsible for synthesis of new connective tissue proteins; they are normally found primarily in the dermal layer of uninjured tissue, and their usual function is to repair any damage to the connective tissue, also known as the ECM. They are summoned to the specific wound site by the growth factors and cytokines released during the inflammatory phase: PDGF, interleukin-1 beta (IL-1β), and tumor necrosis factor alpha (TNF-α). These chemoattractants actually direct the fibroblast to the correct area by binding to specific areas on the cell surface; this helps the fibroblasts to orient themselves within the wound (Canedo-Dorantes & Canedo-Ayala, 2019). Once on-site and correctly oriented within the wound bed, the fibroblasts work to synthesize connective tissue proteins such as collagen, which is the most abundant family of proteins in the body (Bootun, 2013). The newly formed granulation tissue is composed primarily of newly formed blood vessels and provisional collagen (type III collagen), which lacks tensile strength and acts primarily as a filler and scaffold.

At the same time collagen is being synthesized, angiogenesis is occurring, which provides the new blood vessels that are essential to cellular activity and wound healing. Angiogenesis actually begins immediately after injury, because the activated platelets trigger angiogenic growth factors such as VEGF. However, there is another cell that also plays a vital role in neoangiogenesis. Endothelial progenitor cells (EPCs), normally located in the bone marrow, are recruited via the circulation to the area bordering the wound; they are then incorporated into the tissue and contribute to growth of new blood vessels (Canedo-Dorantes & Canedo-Ayala, 2019). EPC activity is mediated by substances that are well known to affect wound healing including nitric oxide, VEGF, matrix metalloproteinases (MMPs), and insulin-like growth factor. Some authors have suggested that it is deficiencies in these intermediate signaling substances that contribute to wound chronicity in diseases like diabetes (Davis et al., 2018).

Angiogenesis is quite vigorous during the proliferative phase of wound healing, which results in vessel density that far exceeds that needed by normal tissue. During the final phase of repair (the remodeling/maturation phase), most of the newly formed vessels disappear; the blood vessel bed is essentially "pruned back" to normal vascular density (Canedo-Dorantes & Canedo-Ayala, 2019). (This explains the change in the color of the scar tissue, from bright red to pale pink or white.) The ability to stimulate and control angiogenesis is predicted to be an important therapeutic option in the future for pathologic conditions like diabetic foot ulcers (Davis et al., 2018).

Another component of repair for full-thickness wounds closing by secondary intention is wound contraction. This process is dependent on specialized fibroblasts known as myofibroblasts. Myofibroblasts are specialized cells with characteristics of both fibroblasts and smooth muscle cells. Because they generate contractile force, they are able to pull the edges of the wound together to reduce the size of the defect (Canedo-Dorantes & Canedo-Ayala, 2019).

MATURATION

The final phase of wound healing is the maturation or remodeling phase. As the provisional collagen matrix is replaced with a stronger form of collagen (type 1), the cells responsible for collagen synthesis and angiogenesis undergo apoptosis. Wound strength increases significantly during the remodeling phase as the type 3 collagen is replaced with type 1 collagen (from minimal tensile strength at 21 days' postacute wounding to 60% or more at 2 to 3 months' postacute wounding). In a normally healing wound, 80% of original tensile strength will be achieved, and this is the maximum strength that can be obtained; 100% tensile strength is not a possibility because the normal soft tissue (dermis, subcutaneous, and/or muscle) has been replaced with scar tissue

(Gantwerker & Hom, 2012). In an open full-thickness wound, the contraction that began during the proliferative phase will also continue; contraction contributes to healing by reducing the size of the defect. Normally, there is a fine balance between the proliferation of new (type 1) collagen and breakdown of the old (type 3) collagen; however, in some situations, there is insufficient breakdown of the old collagen or overproduction of the new collagen, resulting in a hypertrophic scar or a keloid. Conversely, if the proliferation of new (type 1) collagen is impaired by factors such as cancer chemotherapy, diabetes mellitus, malnutrition, or steroids, the wound is at high risk for dehiscence or recurrent breakdown (because the "old" type 3 collagen lacks tensile strength) (Davis et al., 2018; Goodarzi et al., 2019).

KEY POINT

Remodeling occurs after the wound is closed at the surface and involves conversion of type 3 collagen to type 1 collagen, which provides tensile strength.

It is noteworthy that scar formation is not part of the wound healing process in utero. Early-gestation fetuses repair cutaneous wounds without scar formation. Full understanding of why this occurs is not yet available, but it is known that fetal wounds are associated with a very minimal inflammatory response and that there are higher levels of antifibrotic cytokines as compared to adult wounds (Yagi et al., 2016).

While the four phases have been discussed separately for the sake of simplicity, the wound healing process is highly complex with overlapping phases. In acute wounds, hemostasis begins immediately after wounding and lasts 1 to 2 days; inflammation begins shortly after wounding, typically peaks at days 3 to 5 postwounding, and is usually complete by day 10; proliferation begins at day 1 postinjury and is typically complete by days 21 to 30. Remodeling actually begins during the proliferative phase and can last for up to 2 years (Canedo-Dorantes & Canedo-Ayala, 2019). The time frame for the phases of wound healing differs substantially for chronic wounds.

KEY POINT

Maximum tensile strength for a full-thickness wound healing by scar tissue formation is 80% of original tissue strength.

⬤ MECHANISMS OF WOUND HEALING

Three main mechanisms typify the healing process: connective tissue deposition (also known as granulation tissue formation), contraction, and epithelialization. Whether all three mechanisms are necessary depends on the type and nature of the wound. For example, an acute surgical wound that is closed by a surgeon using sutures and clips up to skin level (called primary intention) will close by migration of epithelial cells (epithelial resurfacing) across the minimal gaps in the skin surface (concurrent with the inflammatory phase) and by formation of enough granulation tissue to knit the tissue layers together. No tissue contraction is necessary or possible, because all tissue layers have been approximated. In contrast, a large open chronic wound such as a dehisced incision or full-thickness pressure ulcer requires formation of a substantial amount of granulation tissue, and contraction can play a critical and beneficial role in healing by reducing the size of the defect. This wound closing by secondary intention will also require significant epithelial resurfacing once it has filled with granulation tissue. This type of wound is likely to have a broader scar when closed (**Fig. 3-2**).

KEY POINT

The "order of repair" for an open wound healing by secondary intention is a (sometimes prolonged) inflammatory phase, then granulation tissue formation followed by epithelial resurfacing, and finally remodeling.

Superficial (partial-thickness) wounds such as abrasions or skin graft donor sites heal by regeneration as opposed to scar formation, because the structures in the epidermis and the superficial dermis can replace themselves. This means that partial-thickness wounds heal by reepithelialization; granulation tissue formation is not needed and does not occur nor does contraction. If the wound extends into the dermis, the fibroblasts normally present in that skin layer will repair the dermal defect at the same time that epithelialization is occurring at the wound surface (Canedo-Dorantes & Canedo-Ayala, 2019). Partial-thickness wound healing involves two major phases; the first phase is epithelial resurfacing, which involves a marked increase in the rate of keratinocyte mitosis and changes in cell structure and function that permit lateral migration. Once the wound surface has been reepithelialized, lateral migration ceases due to a phenomenon known as contact inhibition, and vertical migration resumes, which gradually reestablishes normal epidermal thickness. It should be noted that the neoepidermis in all humans is bright pink in color but gradually repigments to match the surrounding skin (**Fig. 3-3**).

KEY POINT

Superficial (partial-thickness) wounds heal by epithelial resurfacing and reestablishment of normal skin thickness; there is no scar formation.

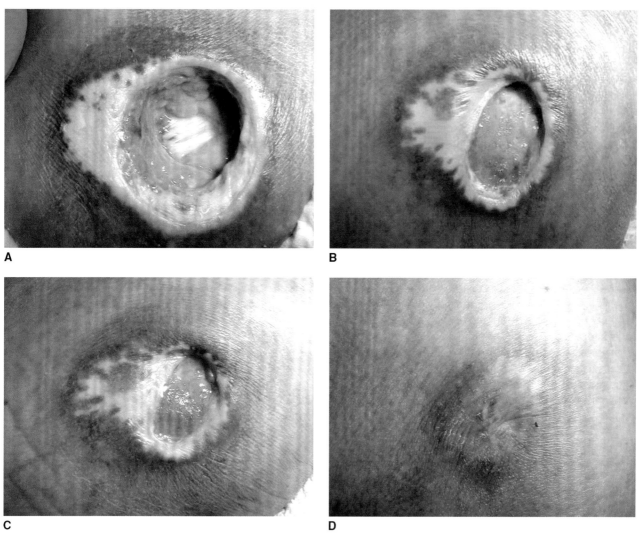

FIGURE 3-2. Series of Photos Showing Progress in Full-Thickness Wound Healing: **(A)** contraction, **(B, C)** granulation tissue formation, and **(D)** epithelialization. (Photos copyright © B. M. Bates-Jensen.)

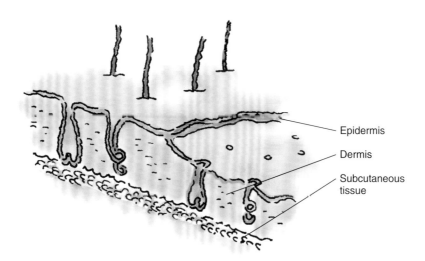

Epidermis

Dermis

Subcutaneous tissue

FIGURE 3-3. Partial-Thickness Wound.

As discussed, all wounds heal through some combination of the three critical processes: epithelialization, granulation tissue formation, and contraction. Interestingly, the factors that promote normal healing are essential for each of these processes and are the same as those identified by Winter (1962) in his seminal work on wound epithelialization in porcine models: (1) wound hydration, (2) blood supply, and (3) infection minimization. Moist wound healing is the foundation of modern wound care and is essential for maintenance of cellular viability and for cell migration. A dry wound bed compromises cell viability by eliminating the interstitial fluid environment critical to normal cellular function and also makes it much more difficult for cells to migrate across the wound surface. Normal perfusion is equally important, since all phases of wound repair are oxygen dependent and since blood flow is also the vehicle for delivery of the nutrients required for repair; thus, vascular health and neoangiogenesis are critical to wound healing. A third "essential element" of wound management is control of bacterial loads; infection is a major impediment to repair due to the negative effects of bacteria and their toxins on the repair process (Gantwerker & Hom, 2012; Ludolph et al., 2018). In summary, wound healing is facilitated by a wound bed that is free of dead tissue and debris, well vascularized, uninfected, and moist (Armstrong & Meyr, 2019a, 2019c).

> **KEY POINT**
>
> Moist wound healing is the foundation of modern wound care and is essential for maintenance of cell viability and cell migration.

TYPES OF WOUND CLOSURE

Specific terminology is used to describe the various ways in which full-thickness wounds heal, with surgical wounds as the reference point. Primary closure or primary intention refers to wounds closed by sutures or skin staples at the time of surgery. All layers of tissue are approximated, which means that minimal amounts of granulation tissue and new epithelium are required for healing. Secondary closure or intention involves closure of an abdominal wound to fascia level and intentionally leaving upper layers open to granulate in over time. Secondary intention can also refer to nonsurgical wounds filling in over time such as full-thickness pressure injuries. While the "primary intention or closure" process proceeds fairly quickly and predictably, secondary closure usually involves weeks of requisite granulation tissue deposition and wound contraction, followed by eventual slow epithelialization. The scar in secondary closure is often wider than primary closure (Armstrong & Meyr, 2019a; Chetter et al., 2019). Wounds that are considered dirty or contaminated with foreign debris or bacteria >10^5/g of tissue may be left open to heal by secondary intention to reduce the risk of deep wound infection (Chetter et al., 2019) (**Fig. 3-4**). A recent prospective cohort study of 393 patients with secondary intention surgical wounds followed them for 12 months and noted a median healing time of 86 days. Complications and adverse events were more common with negative impact on patients' quality of life (Boudreaux & Simmons, 2019; Chetter et al., 2019) suggested that preoperative optimization of modifiable risk factors for poor healing may improve surgical outcomes.

A third option is tertiary intention or closure. If a wound is too contaminated or infected to permit primary closure, the surgeon may keep the wound at secondary closure level until antibiotic therapy and manual cleansing reduce the bacterial burden to <10^5 organisms/g of tissue. The wound is then closed via delayed primary closure (Salcido, 2017) (**Fig. 3-5**).

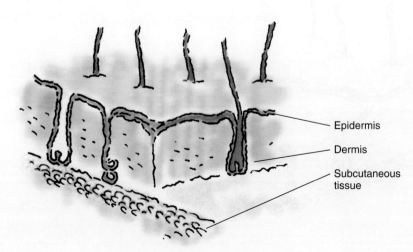

Epidermis

Dermis

Subcutaneous tissue

FIGURE 3-4. Full-Thickness Wound.

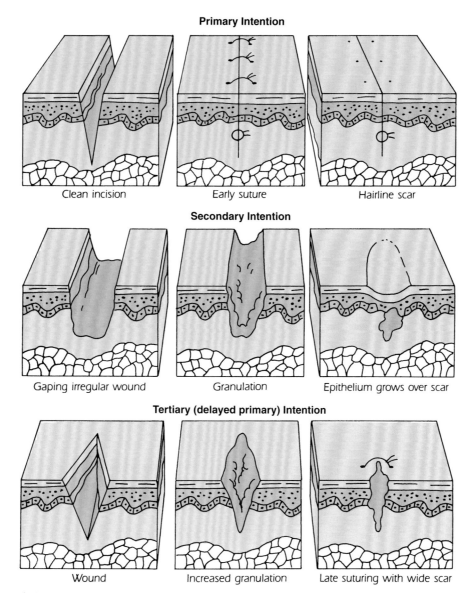

FIGURE 3-5. Types of Wound Healing/Closure: Primary, Secondary, and Tertiary Intention. (Adapted from Smeltzer, S. C., Bare, B. G., Hinkle, J. L., et al. (2010). *Brunner & Suddarth's textbook of medical–surgical nursing* (12th ed., p. 474). Philadelphia, PA: Lippincott Williams & Wilkins.)

ACUTE VERSUS CHRONIC WOUNDS

Differing definitions of acute versus chronic wounds are available from various authors and professional wound societies; however, a common core of descriptors is discernable upon review. It is first important to realize that the primary difference is in the nature of the repair process as opposed to a specific time frame (Armstrong & Meyr, 2019b, 2019c). An acute wound is a wound that heals in an orderly, timely, and durable manner and that does not require long-term follow-up. In general, acute wounds have a clearly identifiable mechanism of injury such as trauma or surgery (Armstrong & Meyr, 2019a). Some sources suggest that the trajectory for acute wound healing is complete within 4 weeks. Whatever the exact time frame, acute wounds quickly and efficiently proceed through the phases of wound healing: hemostasis, inflammation, fibroplasia (granulation tissue formation), epithelialization, and maturation (Armstrong & Meyr, 2019a). Risk factors for delayed healing are typically minimal, and the wound proceeds to a predictable state of tissue repair (Canedo-Dorantes & Canedo-Ayala, 2019).

> **KEY POINT**
>
> Acute wounds heal in a predictable and durable fashion, while chronic wounds frequently plateau or "stall."

Chronic wounds are characterized by descriptors that are the "opposite" of those just used for acute wounds. A chronic wound does not progress through healing in an orderly and timely manner; they commonly plateau or "stall" at some point due to various pathologic conditions, and as a result, predictable tissue repair does not occur (Armstrong & Meyr, 2019b, 2019c). Common features typifying chronic wounds include a prolonged or excessive inflammatory phase (due to large volumes of necrotic tissue or high bacterial loads), persistent or recurrent infection, the formation of drug resistant biofilms, and/or the failure of fibroblasts, endothelial cells, and keratinocytes to produce the new vessels and tissues required for durable closure of the defect (Davis et al., 2018). Biofilms are a commonly encountered impediment to repair; they are composed of complex communities of bacteria that work together to generate an extracellular polymeric substance that shields them from host defenses, most antiseptics, and antibiotics. Biofilms frequently present as a recurrent film or thin layer of slough and must be promptly recognized and effectively managed if wound healing is to progress (Metcalf & Bowler, 2019; Mori et al., 2019; Tyldesley et al., 2019) (**Fig. 3-6**).

Chronic wound types include venous ulcers, arterial ulcers, pressure injuries, neuropathic (diabetic) ulcers, malignant ulcers, and hypertensive (Martorell) ulcers, among others (Armstrong & Meyr, 2019b; Canedo-Dorantes & Canedo-Ayala, 2019). The percentage of adults with chronic wounds is predicted to increase with the increasing numbers of elderly individuals and the concomitant increase in chronic illness-related comorbidities. Since physical functioning, psychological health, social interaction, and financial stability are impacted by a chronic wound, it is critical that we focus our attention and resources on prevention of chronic wounds and amelioration of the underlying processes to the greatest degree possible (Armstrong & Meyr, 2019b, 2019c; Ayello et al., 2019; Imran et al., 2018). When dealing with a chronic wound, it is essential for the wound care nurse to accurately determine the etiologic factors and to address the cause of the wound as well as the wound itself (Armstrong & Meyr, 2019b).

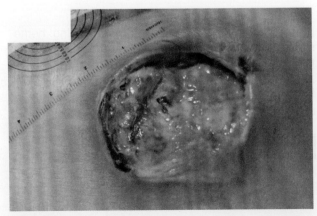

FIGURE 3-6. Chronic Wound with Yellow Slough. (Copyright © C. Sussman.)

Clinical differences between acute and chronic wounds can be explained in part by differences in the local wound environments. Acute wounds have higher mitogenic activity, while chronic wounds are characterized by higher levels of proinflammatory cytokines, elevated levels of MMPs, and greater numbers of senescent cells (i.e., cells that do not respond normally to the cytokines and growth factors regulating the repair process). MMPs deserve special mention. MMPs are enzymes produced by the body; there are 23 types of human MMPs organized into 8 categories, with the specific category determined by the domain structure. MMPs are *necessary* for normal healing; they function to degrade abnormal ECM components such as damaged collagen, and they promote the migration of immunologic cells (neutrophils and macrophages) into the injured tissue. Normal healing is characterized by high MMP levels during the inflammatory phase and markedly reduced levels during the proliferative phase. In contrast, chronic wounds are frequently characterized by persistently high MMP levels, which contribute to breakdown of growth factors and impaired collagen synthesis (Tardaguila-Garcia et al., 2019). One focus of ongoing wound-related research is methods to control and modify MMP levels throughout the repair process (Tardaguila-Garcia et al., 2019); currently available therapies for MMP modification will be discussed in Chapters 9 and 12.

Another characteristic of the chronic wound microenvironment is insufficient expression of fibronectin, chondroitin sulfate, and tenascin, all of which are critical to normal cell migration. In addition, chronic wounds are characterized by alterations in the ECM that can result in matrix instability and impaired synthesis of collagen and other connective tissue proteins. For example, hyperglycemia can increase MMP production, cause degradation of the ECM, and reduce the cell-to-cell interaction that is critical to normal repair (Davis et al., 2018).

One strategy that is sometimes used to convert a "chronic" wound into an "acute" wound is surgical debridement (Lavery et al., 2019; Young, 2019). Used for centuries, debridement induces acute tissue injury and bleeding, which results in hemostasis and activation of the many regulatory processes that normally control repair (White, 2019). However, it is equally important to address the systemic factors that caused the chronic wound if healing is to occur and recurrence is to be prevented (**Fig. 3-7**). A notable finding about prognostic factors for delayed healing was identified by Jenkins et al. (2019). In a scoping review, the researchers noted significant nonhealing factors: size of ulcer, duration of ulcer, age (older), gender, diabetes, smoking, and history of deep vein thrombosis. If a wound is present for a long time, its chronicity becomes a risk factor.

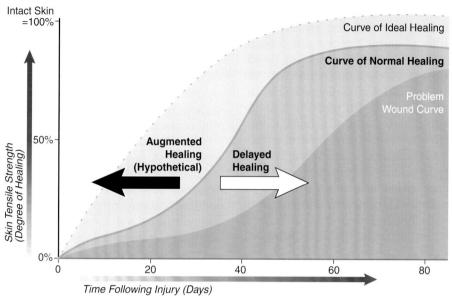

FIGURE 3-7. Healing Trajectories of Normal, Problem, and Hypothetical "Ideal" Wounds.

 AGING AND WOUND HEALING

While age is commonly noted as a potential risk factor for poor wound healing, it is clear from the literature that *age itself* is not a risk factor for failure to heal. In general, wound healing in healthy older adults may be delayed but is not defective. For example, healing of acute surgical wounds is not problematic for most older patients. Indeed, fibroblast activity in response to cytokines is not affected by age, and tensile wound strength seems to be unaffected in elders. "The accumulation of collagen in wounds does not seem to differ with age. In fact, the formation and quality of scarring may *improve* with age" (Thomas & Burkemper, 2013). Conversely, other authors (Bonifant & Holloway, 2019) noted that there are structural changes that occur with aging including flattening of the dermal–epidermal junction (DEJ) increasing fragility of the skin, decreased fibroblasts, mast cells, and macrophages in the dermis and lessened ECM components such as collagen. In addition to these structural issues are the life experiences of patients. Long-standing sun exposure, occupational hazards, and environmental toxins can differ among individuals affecting skin health. It appears that any problems with wound healing associated with advanced age are likely due to the multiple comorbidities and life circumstances that affect some older adults (Bonifant & Holloway, 2019).

 PARTIAL- VERSUS FULL-THICKNESS WOUND HEALING

Another perspective on wound healing relates to the depth of affected tissue. The deeper the tissue layers affected, the greater number of wound healing mechanisms required. From this perspective, wounds are classified as either partial or full thickness. More specifically, wounds confined to the epidermal and dermal layers are considered to be partial thickness, while wounds that extend through the dermis are considered full thickness. As previously noted, partial-thickness wounds heal by epithelialization alone; in contrast, full-thickness wounds require granulation tissue formation to fill the soft tissue defect and may require contraction to reduce the size of the defect, followed by epithelial resurfacing.

As an example, a stage 2 pressure injury is by definition a partial-thickness wound that heals by epithelialization, while a stage 3 or 4 pressure injury is a full-thickness lesion that requires granulation, contraction, and epithelialization. Deep tissue pressure injury (purple-maroon discoloration under intact skin) and unstageable pressure injuries most often represent full-thickness damage. Because the repair process for full-thickness wounds is quite extensive and may require months or even years for completion, the goal is always to either prevent the pressure injury or to prevent worsening of existing pressure injuries.

WOUND HEALING: RISK FACTORS FOR NONHEALING

Wounds that fail to heal normally are labeled "chronic," and, as noted, these wounds are associated with marked alterations in the patient's quality of life and with increased morbidity and even mortality. There is usually not one single factor that results in impaired healing; rather, it is a constellation of factors that interact to impair chemotaxis, tissue oxygenation, myofibroblast and fibroblast activity, development of provisional and mature collagen, and epithelialization (Armstrong & Meyr, 2019c).

The factors known to impede wound healing can be categorized as intrinsic and extrinsic factors. Intrinsic factors include factors such as advanced age, immune compromise (either innate or induced), psychological stress, hereditary skin disorders (e.g., epidermolysis bullosa), and disease states/comorbidities (e.g., diabetes and neuropathy, chronic obstructive pulmonary disease [COPD], cardiovascular disease, peripheral arterial disease, acute and chronic kidney disease, liver failure, alcoholism, malignant disease, and spinal cord disease). Extrinsic factors include factors such as infection (local and systemic), malnutrition, insufficient perfusion/oxygenation, smoking, chemotherapy, radiation therapy, and selected medications (e.g., steroids, anticoagulants, angiogenesis inhibitors) (Antonopoulos et al., 2019; Armstrong & Meyr, 2019c; Gantwerker & Hom, 2012) (**Table 3-1**). Since immunosuppressive agents such as steroids and antirejection drugs are commonly administered for inflammatory bowel disease, rheumatoid arthritis, and organ transplant, these disease states have also been associated with impaired wound healing (Beitz, 2017). The phenomenon of delayed wound healing is so pressing that researchers are seeking to validate assessment instruments or tools to accurately predict degree of risk for chronic and surgical wounds (Edwards et al., 2018; Peart, 2019; Sandy-Hodgetts et al., 2019).

KEY POINT

Failure to heal is frequently due to systemic factors such as impaired perfusion, malnutrition, smoking, and poor glycemic control.

TABLE 3-1 FACTORS AFFECTING WOUND HEALING

INTRINSIC	EXTRINSIC
• Age	• Smoking
• Alcoholism	• Radiation
• Immunosuppression	• Chemotherapy
• Hereditary skin disease	• Infection (local or systemic)
• Chronic disease:	• Poor nutritional intake
• COPD	• Insufficient oxygenation
• CAD	• Medication therapy
• CVD	• Anticoagulants
• Liver failure	• Cyclosporine
• Renal failure	• Steroids
• Renal insufficiency	• Immobility (e.g., SCI)
• Diabetes mellitus	
• Peripheral vascular disease	
• Chronic venous disease	
• Sickle cell disease	
• Vasculitic/thrombotic disorders	
• Pain	
• Psychological stress	

Sources: Adapted from Armstrong and Meyr (2019c), Antonopoulos et al. (2019), Avila et al. (2012), Beitz (2017), Boudreaux and Simmons (2019), Gantwerker and Hom (2012), Tehan et al. (2019), Woo (2012a, 2012b).

PERFUSION AND OXYGENATION

Though the list of intrinsic factors (those relating to the patient's health) and extrinsic factors is formidable, some risk factors are particularly important. For example, adequate perfusion and oxygenation are critical for normal wound healing. Oxygen is required for inflammation, angiogenesis, collagen synthesis, and epithelialization. Any alterations in oxygenation due to arterial disease, vasoconstriction, hypotension, vasopressors, advanced lung disease, severe anemia, or edematous states such as anasarca can be deleterious to wound healing. Any condition associated with impaired perfusion results in reduced delivery of critical cells and nutrients to the injured tissues and compromised removal of metabolic wastes (Armstrong & Meyr, 2019b, 2019c; Gantwerker & Hom, 2012), *in addition to* the adverse effects on tissue oxygenation. The critical role of oxygen in wound healing has been observed by mountain climbers who noted the inability to clear skin infections at high altitude. In addition, Tyldesley et al. (2019) pointed out that the most common chronic wounds (arterial, venous, neuropathic, and pressure) develop or are perpetuated due to inadequate tissue oxygen levels (Davis et al., 2018). Not surprisingly, delivery of high concentrations of oxygen (hyperbaric oxygen therapy [HBOT]) is an effective treatment for chronic wounds caused or perpetuated by hypoxia, so long as there is sufficient plasma flow to deliver the oxygen to the wound site (Golledge & Singh, 2019). Adequate tissue oxygen levels are also needed for maintenance of normal nitric oxide (NO) levels, and abnormal NO levels are associated with excessive inflammation and impaired collagen synthesis (Bishop, 2019).

GLYCEMIC CONTROL

Another factor critical to wound healing is glycemic level. Hyperglycemia can impair every major aspect of the repair process, specifically inflammation, granulation tissue formation, development of tensile strength, and epithelial resurfacing. Thus, tight glucose control is an essential element of care for the wound care nurse. Tight glycemic control has been associated with reduced wound complications in cardiovascular surgery patients, and tight glucose control is somewhat easier to maintain in the acute care setting; the staff can control dietary intake, medication administration, and glucose monitoring and can increase the frequency of glucose monitoring and implement insulin drips if needed. In the home care and outpatient setting, the wound care nurse must work with the patient as well as other members of the health care team to establish appropriate goals for glycemic control and to consider short-term contracts for adherence to the patient-controlled elements of the management plan. For diagnosis of diabetes, the American Diabetes Association (2019a) notes that fasting plasma glucose (FPG) or 2-hour plasma glucose level (2-H PG) or hemoglobin A1c can be used. The A1c is more highly recommended due to convenience and greater stability of analysis. The American Diabetes Association (2019b) suggests an A1c goal of 6.5 to 7.0 (random glucose 140 to 154 mg/dL) for individuals with long life expectancy, no significant cardiovascular disease, and no significant problems with hypoglycemia and an A1c goal of <8.0 (random glucose 183 mg/dL) for patients with limited life expectancy, history of severe hypoglycemia, and major comorbidities. Recent epidemiologic research supports that glycemic index, specifically the Hgb A1c, is a good predictor of nonhealing lower extremity ulcers (Moore et al., 2018). In addition to the issues with hyperglycemia, diabetes is important because it is associated with vasculopathy, neuropathy, and immune dysfunction. Diminished macro- and microvascular blood supply, diminished sensory awareness of acute or repetitive injury/infection, and cellular dysfunction (especially macrophage dysfunction) in the presence of prolonged hyperglycemia increase the risk for both wound development and impaired healing.

COMORBIDITIES

Other chronic disease states can have a profound and negative impact on wound healing. Cardiovascular disease (coronary artery disease [CAD] and associated heart failure and lower extremity arterial disease [LEAD]) can significantly reduce the amount of blood delivered to the distal extremities, resulting in chronic tissue ischemia. Conversely, venous insufficiency can impair venous return, resulting in chronic edema and changes in the soft tissues that increase vulnerability to minor trauma; the chronic edema then impairs delivery of oxygen to the traumatized tissues, which delays healing. Advanced COPD can also reduce tissue oxygen levels to a degree that impairs wound healing (Armstrong & Meyr, 2019c).

MEDICATIONS

Although some medications can augment wound healing (e.g., vitamins A and C, zinc, hormones like estrogen, prostaglandins), many drugs can impair wound healing through multiple phases of repair. Some drug can actually cause wounds by damaging skin integrity through adverse integumentary events.

Medications reported to delay wound healing include anticoagulants, antineoplastic drugs, antirheumatoid drugs (e.g., methotrexate), antigout drugs (e.g., colchicine), and some antimicrobials. Because of their common usage, two classes are noteworthy: steroids and nonsteroidal anti-inflammatory drugs (NSAIDs). Steroids inhibit wound healing across all phases but especially in the inflammatory phase. NSAIDs, especially high dose, long-term use therapy, can impair bone and ligament healing (Beitz, 2017). Another newer category of drug used primarily as an anticancer agent is the antiangiogenesis drugs. For example, bevacizumab, a monoclonal antibody, is used to attack tumors in patients with colon cancer. However, its negative impact on blood vessel growth is associated with delayed wound healing (Ahn et al., 2019).

Medications that are usually benign or even helpful to wound healing can be problematic in selected surgical wound healing settings. For example, corticosteroids, which may be necessary for neurosurgical patients to reduce cerebral edema, can impair wound healing. Vitamin A, which can restore the inflammatory response and promote epithelialization and collagen synthesis in the presence of steroid use, is contraindicated in this setting as retinoids may markedly increase intracranial pressure (Berry et al., 2019).

Recent research supports that medications can be part of a constellation of risk factors for perioperative morbidity in surgical wound healing. Farshad et al. (2018) conducted a retrospective case series of 1,009 spine surgical patients. Risk factors associated with an irregular postoperative course (including wound healing problems and infection) were elevated preoperative creatinine levels, greater blood loss, and systemic steroid use.

NUTRITIONAL STATUS

Malnutrition, especially inadequate protein intake, is a major risk factor for impaired healing. Malnourished individuals lack the available nutrients to synthesize the connective tissue proteins (such as collagen) required for wound repair. Nutritional management must address intake of sufficient calories and protein to promote healing but must also include attention to critical micronutrients (key vitamins and minerals). For example, ascorbic acid (vitamin C) plays an important role in all phases of wound healing; in addition to its antioxidant properties, it is a cofactor in collagen synthesis and helps to regulate normal cellular apoptosis (Bishop et al., 2018). Other nutrients that contribute to wound healing include trace elements such as magnesium, copper, zinc, and iron; specific amino acids such as arginine and glutamine; and possibly vitamins A and E (Bishop et al., 2018).

TOBACCO USE

Tobacco use is profoundly detrimental to wound healing. Cigarette smoking promotes prolonged vasoconstriction through the effects of nicotine and other noxious substances. The impact is especially negative for patients with lower extremity wounds, since arterial insufficiency is a common causative factor for these wounds; for these patients, smoking cessation is sometimes the factor that determines whether the wound will heal or whether amputation will be required. However, smoking also has a significant detrimental effect in trunk wounds of relatively healthy patients. This is illustrated by the findings of a retrospective chart review of 597 caesarean deliveries with 30 cases of wound dehiscence; smoking was independently and significantly associated with wound complications (OR 5.32, 95% CI: 1.77 to 15.97, p < 0.01) (Avila et al., 2012). A recent literature review on smoking effects on bone healing supports that smoking is associated with low bone mineral density, delayed fracture union, peri-implant bone loss, and implant failure (Beahrs et al., 2019).

Renal and hepatic failure can also increase risk for failure to heal, and advanced renal failure is also sometimes associated with the development of severe chronic wounds (e.g., calciphylaxis). The poor healing associated with advanced kidney and liver disease may be due to retention of metabolic wastes or to aberrations in mineral and electrolyte levels.

SPINAL CORD INJURY

Spinal cord injury is another comorbidity that increases both the risk for skin breakdown and the risk of impaired healing. The immobility and sensory loss associated with cord injury markedly increase the risk for pressure injury development, and for many patients, it is difficult to commit to the offloading typically required for wound healing. In addition, there are studies showing that healing below the level of injury is impaired as compared to healing above the level of injury; these differences and the implications for care are discussed further in Chapter 16.

INFECTION

Infection, especially if occult and/or untreated, can cause severe inhibition of wound healing; high levels of bacteria can cause additional tissue damage, and the inflammatory mediators and toxins associated with bacterial infections result in prolongation of the inflammatory phase of repair and delay in collagen synthesis and epithelial resurfacing (Ludolph et al., 2018). An effective management program for any wound requires prompt identification and effective treatment of any wound infection. It should be noted that topical therapies such as antimicrobial dressings are insufficient therapy for invasive infection. Newer technology like negative pressure wound therapy with instillation can help lower bacterial load and facilitate wound closure (Ludolph et al., 2018).

SOCIAL DETERMINANTS/SYSTEM FACTORS

A very different perspective about wound healing and therapy is emerging providing a more macroscopic perspective. Smit (2018) supported that a "super-system" of independent but interrelated structures and processes results in successful wound healing. He suggested that pathological factors inhibiting wound healing exist from the molecular to the population level. Smit described four levels of factors: general factors (social, demographic,

general health, comorbidities), local factors (wound location, dimensions, duration, local skin), systemic factors (cardiovascular system, immune, endocrine, renal, connective tissue systems), and molecular/cellular factors (genetics, epigenetics, signaling factors, migration, and proliferation, etc.). He believed the larger view of pathologic factors and promoted a more holistic map of the processes involved in wound healing. This "larger" perspective has become a component of a wound care–focused mnemonic: TIMERS (Tissue, Infection, Moisture, Edge, Regeneration/Repair, Social Factors) (Atkin & Tettelbach, 2019).

 ## PSYCHOLOGICAL FACTORS AND WOUND HEALING

The effect of psychological health on wound healing deserves special attention. Known psychological influences on wound healing include stress, coping style, positive affect, environmental enrichment, and social support. Psychological factors exert physiologic effects on conditions such as vessel size and leukocyte distribution through mediators such as oxytocin, vasopressin, epinephrine, and cortisol (Broadbent & Koschwanez, 2012). Chronic stress in particular has been shown to have immunosuppressive effects and to compromise wound healing (Lucas et al., 2018; Wynn & Holloway, 2019). Recent reviews have suggested that psychological interventions such as relaxation can help promote wound healing via a mind–body connection known and utilized for centuries (Waters, 2017).

Pain is another factor with profound impact on wound healing. In response to painful stimuli, pain fibers release pain neuropeptides (e.g., substance P and neurokinin A) that activate immunoactive cells and trigger release of proinflammatory cytokines. The stress response that is associated with pain also triggers release of glucocorticoid hormones, and cortisol can reduce signaling for and production of growth factors (Woo, 2012a, 2012b; Woo et al., 2018). A recent systematic review looked at preoperative interventions (anxiety reduction, psychological interventions, relaxation therapy) on postoperative wound healing. They were shown to be beneficial in improving wound healing and scar formation (Geers et al., 2018).

IMPLICATIONS FOR OPTIMAL WOUND CARE

The wound care nurse's understanding of the intrinsic and extrinsic factors affecting wound healing is critical because it provides a basis for intervention. The factors impeding prompt wound healing must be addressed and eradicated or ameliorated to the extent possible. Comorbidities must be well managed. For example, good and consistent glycemic control is imperative for the patient with diabetes, any cardiovascular or pulmonary disease must be addressed, and renal and hepatic function must be optimized.

Measures to optimize perfusion are critical. For persons who are smokers, smoking cessation programs and nicotine replacement therapy may be essential interventions. Persons with arterial compromise need to understand the importance of using requisite therapies *and* not smoking. Conversely, venous insufficiency clients need to understand why compression is critical to optimal healing and need to faithfully adhere to ambulation, compression, and elevation therapies.

Nutritional repletion is also essential; the wound care nurse must obtain or complete a baseline assessment of nutritional status and must monitor nutrient intake, weight trends, and relevant laboratory findings (such as albumin and prealbumin) (Jimenez et al., 2019). Baseline interventions include provision of adequate protein, calories, and micronutrients; if these interventions are insufficient, additional measures should be considered, such as protein supplements. In selected challenging situations, anabolic steroids such as oxandrolone may be considered for promotion of weight gain and wound healing (Osmolak et al., 2019). Chapter 7 addresses the nutritional aspects of wound healing and wound management in detail.

Wound healing is also dependent on maintaining a moist but balanced wound environment to support the cellular activities essential to repair. A variety of wound dressings can address the objective of maintaining appropriate moisture levels in the wound bed (Hall, 2018). A recent Cochrane Review could not identify if any specific type of dressing is better than others in preventing surgical site infections (Dumville et al., 2016). A more recent meta-analysis on topical treatments in healing of pressure injuries noted that topical and foam dressings and active wound dressings (e.g., collagen, hydroactive dressings [e.g., hydrocolloid, hydrogel], growth factors) were significantly better than basic dressings (e.g., saline gauze) in healing rates (Furuya-Kanamori et al., 2019). The researchers suggest that basic saline moist dressings should be replaced with these "newer" categories. Specific options and considerations are discussed in detail in Chapter 9. Individuals who are immunosuppressed may require additional interventions to promote healing; for example, a trial of topical vitamin A may be warranted for a patient who requires chronic corticosteroid therapy and whose wound is not progressing or progressing very slowly. Immunocompromised persons may also benefit from the use of dressings with antimicrobial and anti-inflammatory effects, since they are at high risk for both superficial and invasive wound infection; products to be considered include but are not limited to silver dressings, cadexomer iodine dressings, dressings impregnated with polyhexamethylene biguanide, dressings impregnated with methylene blue and crystal violet, and dressings with

Manuka honey (Hall, 2018). Prevention and management of wound infection is addressed in detail in Chapter 11.

Attention to psychological state is also vitally important; clinical depression and other psychological conditions have been associated with self-induced wounding (factitious wounds) that often require surgical intervention (David et al., 2018). Clinical psychologists, psychiatrists, or psychiatric advanced practice nurses should be consulted, since effective use of pharmacologic and cognitive therapies can help interrupt the cycle of wounding and improve healing outcomes.

As noted in Chapter 5, the goal for wound care is dependent on the ability to substantially correct the etiologic factors and the systemic factors affecting healing. In situations where these factors can*not* be corrected, the goal for wound care should be modified to focus on maintenance or simply on symptom management.

FUTURE DIRECTIONS FOR WOUND HEALING THERAPIES

Our understanding of the wound repair process and the factors controlling healing continue to evolve and to inform our clinical practice. A major area for future research related to wound healing is epigenetic regulation. Epigenetics may play a role in the development of risk factors for wounds *and* cellular activity in wound healing processes once diseases develop. Epigenetics is the study of the interaction between environmental factors and the genome of the individual cell; these interactions involve cell signaling, which produces persistent and heritable changes in gene expression even though the DNA is not changed. Epigenetics is relevant to wound care, because disease states can affect epigenetic processes in ways that contribute to chronic wounds (Lewis et al., 2014). Recent literature based on decades of population-focused research about adverse childhood experiences (ACEs) suggests that biologic embedding of childhood adversity is associated with substantially higher rates of adult chronic illnesses including diabetes, vascular disease, obesity, depression, and notable adult risk behaviors (smoking, alcohol abuse, substance abuse). The biologic connection is being mediated through epigenetic alteration of gene expression (Bryan, 2019; Bryan & Beitz, 2019). Epigenetic processes in wound healing (e.g., DNA methylation, histone protein modification) need further scrutiny. The science of epigenetics requires major development in disease causation and illness prevention. Current data suggest that stem cell therapy and gene therapy may be one approach to alteration of epigenetic signaling in a way that promotes improved wound healing (Cheng & Fu, 2018; Ti et al., 2014).

Another focus of study is the role of microRNAs in the regulation of wound healing. It is known that these substances act as key regulators of gene expression and that they therefore impact on wound healing. Ongoing research may provide the basis for development of microRNA-targeted wound healing therapies (Den Dekker et al., 2019; Goodarzi et al., 2019).

An additional area of investigation is related to the influence of the intestinal microbiome on wound healing and resilience to infections. Direct bacterial infection from intestinal microorganisms plays a role in surgical site infections but intestinal microbes also affect wound healing indirectly. Hypotheses being tested suggest that wound healing is positively affected by probiotic members of the intestinal microbiome via a gut–brain axis where intestinal microbiome imbalances can slow wound healing by diminishing proinflammatory properties of neutrophils or up-regulate the response with probiotic supplementation. Further research is needed to elucidate specific mechanisms (Krezalek & Alverdy, 2018).

The microbiome of the skin is also being scrutinized for its influence on potential mechanisms promoting chronic nonhealing wounds. Research is examining the role that skin microflora plays on up-regulating or synergistic effects on other microorganisms inhibiting or supporting pathogenic microbial growth (Pang et al., 2019).

● CONCLUSION

This chapter has addressed the major physiologic processes involved in wound repair (hemostasis, inflammation, granulation tissue formation and contraction, and epithelialization) and has compared and contrasted the repair process for acute and chronic wounds and for full-thickness and partial-thickness wounds. Systemic factors affecting healing have been addressed, along with implications for provider intervention.

REFERENCES

Ahn, J., Shalabi, D., Correa-Selm, L., et al. (2019). Impaired wound healing secondary to bevacizumab. *International Wound Journal, 16*, 1009–1012.

American Diabetes Association. (2019a). Classification and diagnosis of diabetes: Standards of medical care in diabetes-2019. *Diabetes Care, 42*(Suppl 1), S13–S28.

American Diabetes Association. (2019b). Standards of medical care in diabetes-2019. *Diabetes Care, 37*(Suppl 1), S14–S80.

Antonopoulos, C. N., Lazaris, A., Venermo, M., et al. (2019). Predictors of wound healing following revascularization for chronic limb-threatening ischemia. *Vascular and Endovascular Surgery, 53*(8), 649–657.

Armstrong, D. G., & Meyr, A. J. (2019a). Basic principles of wound management. *UpToDate*. Retrieved January 31, 2019, from www.uptodate.com/contents/basic-principles-of-wound-management

Armstrong, D. G., & Meyr, A. J. (2019b). Clinical assessment of wounds. *UpToDate*. Retrieved September 15, 2019, from www.uptodate.com/contents/clinical-assessment-of-wounds

Armstrong, D., & Meyr, A. (2019c). Risk factors for impaired wound healing and wound complications. *UpToDate*. Retrieved September 5, 2019, from www.uptodate.com/contents/risk-factors-for-impaired-wound-healing-and-wound-complications

Atkin, L., & Tettelbach, W. (2019). TIMERS: Expanding wound care beyond the focus of the wound. *British Journal of Nursing, 28*(20), S34–S37.

Avila, C., Bhangoo, R., Figuerua, R., et al. (2012). Association of smoking with wound complications after cesarean delivery. *Journal of Maternal-Fetal and Neonatal Medicine, 25*(8), 1250–1253.

Ayello, E., Levine, J., Langemo, D., et al. (2019). Re-examining the literature on terminal ulcers, SCALE, skin failure, and unavoidable pressure injuries. *Advances in Skin & Wound Care, 32*(3), 109–121.

Beahrs, T. R., Reagan, J., Bettin, C. C., et al. (2019). Smoking effects in foot and ankle surgery: An evidence-based review. *Foot and Ankle Surgery, 40*(10), 1226–1232.

Beitz, J. (2017). Pharmacological impact of medications on wound healing and wound generation: How drugs can "break bad". *Ostomy Wound Management, 61*(3), 42–46.

Berry, J., Miulli, D., Lam, B., et al. (2019). The neurosurgical wound and factors that can affect cosmetic, functional, and neurological outcomes. *International Wound Journal, 16*, 71–78.

Bishop, A. (2019). Hyperbaric oxygen therapy for problem wounds: An update. *Wounds UK, 15*(4), 26–31.

Bishop, A., Witts, S., & Martin, T. (2018). The role of nutrition in successful wound healing. *Journal of Community Nursing, 32*(4), 44–50.

Bonifant, H., & Holloway, S. (2019). A review of the effects of ageing on skin integrity and wound healing. *British Journal of Community Nursing, 24*, S28–S33.

Bootun, R. (2013). Effects of immunosuppressive therapy on wound healing. *International Wound Journal, 10*, 98–104.

Boudreaux, A. M., & Simmons, J. W. (2019). Prehabilitation and optimization of modifiable patient risk factors: The importance of effective preoperative evaluation to improve surgical outcomes. *AORN Journal, 109*(4), 500–507.

Broadbent, E., & Koschwanez, H. E. (2012). The psychology of wound healing. *Current Opinion in Psychiatry, 25*(2), 135–140.

Bryan, R. H. (2019). Getting to why: Adverse childhood experiences' impact on adult health. *Journal for Nurse Practitioners, 15*(2), 153–157.

Bryan, R. H., & Beitz, J. M. (2019). Connections among biologic embedding of childhood adversity; adult chronic illness, and wound care: A review of the literature. *Wound Management & Prevention, 65*(10), 18–28.

Canedo-Dorantes, L., & Canedo-Ayala, M. (2019). Skin acute wound healing: A comprehensive review. *International Journal of Inflammation, 2019*, 3706315. doi: 10.1155/2019/3706315.

Cheng, B., & Fu, X. (2018). The focus and target: Angiogenesis in refractory wound healing. *International Journal of Lower Extremity Wounds, 17*(4), 301–303.

Chetter, I. C., Oswald, A. V., McGinniss, E., et al. (2019). Patients with surgical wounds healing by secondary intention: A prospective, cohort study. *International Journal of Nursing Studies, 89*, 62–71.

David, J. A., Rifkin, W. J., & Chiu, E. S. (2018). Current management of self-inflicted wounds in surgery–A critical review. *Annals of Plastic Surgery, 81*(Suppl 1), S79–S88.

Davis, F. M., Kimball, A., Boniakowski, A., et al. (2018). Dysfunctional wound healing in diabetic foot ulcers: New crossroads. *Current Diabetes Reports, 18*(2), 8. doi: 10.1007/S11892-018-0970-Z.

Den Dekker, A., Davis, F. M., Kunkel, S. L., et al. (2019). Targeting epigenetic mechanisms in diabetic wound healing. *Translational Research, 204*, 39–50.

Dumville, J. C., Gray, T. A., Walter, C. J., et al. (2016). Dressings for the prevention of surgical site infection. *Cochrane Database of Systematic Reviews*, (12), CD003091. doi: 10.1002/14651858. CD0030091.pub4.

Edwards, H. E., Parker, C. N., Miller, C., et al. (2018). Predicting delayed healing: The diagnostic accuracy of the venous leg ulcer risk assessment tool. *International Wound Journal, 15*, 258–265.

Farshad, M., Bauer, D. E., Wechsler, C., et al. (2018). Risk factors for perioperative morbidity in spine surgeries of different complexities: A multivariate analysis of 1,009 consecutive patients. *The Spine Journal, 18*, 1625–1631.

Furuya-Kanamori, L., Walker, R. M., Gillespie, B., et al. (2019). Effectiveness of different topical treatments in the healing of pressure injuries. A network meta-analysis. *Journal of the American Medical Directors Association, 20*, 399–407.

Gantwerker, E. A., & Hom, D. B. (2012). Skin: Histology and physiology of wound healing. *Clinics in Plastic Surgery, 39*(1), 85–97.

Geers, N. C., Zegel, M., Huybregts, J., et al. (2018). The influence of preoperative interventions on postoperative surgical wound healing in patients without risk factors: A systematic review. *Aesthetic Surgery Journal, 38*(11), 1237–1249.

Golledge, J., & Singh, T. P. (2019). Systematic review or meta-analysis: Systematic review and meta-analysis of clinical trials examining the effect of hyperbaric oxygen therapy in people with diabetes-related lower limb ulcers. *Diabetic Medicine, 36*, 813–826.

Goodarzi, G., Maniati, M., & Oujeq, D. (2019). The role of micro RNAs in the healing of diabetic ulcers. *International Wound Journal, 16*, 621–633.

Hall, J. (2018). Dressed for success: Wound care dressing options have exploded, but deciding which material is best for which injury sometimes is an elusive quest for providers. No more. *McKnight's Long-Term Care News, 39*(6), 65–67.

Imran, I., Arisandi, D., Haryanto, S., et al. (2018). Effects of understanding well being on psychological aspects and wound healing in patients with diabetic foot ulcer recurrence: A pilot randomized controlled trial. *The Diabetic Foot Journal, 21*(2), 119–126.

Jenkins, D. A., Mohamed, S., Taylor, J. K., et al. (2019). Potential prognostic factors for delayed healing of common, non-traumatic skin ulcers: A scoping review. *International Wound Journal, 16*, 800–812.

Jimenez, C. B., Ovale, H. F., Moreno, M. F., et al. (2019). Under nutrition measured by the mini-nutritional assessment (MNA) test and related risk factors in older adults under hospital emergency care. *Nutrition, 66*, 142–146.

Krezalek, M. A., & Alverdy, J. C. (2018). The influence of the intestinal microbiome on wound healing and infection. *Seminars in Colon and Rectal Surgery, 29*, 17–20.

Lavery, L. A., Niederauer, M. Q., Papas, K. K., et al. (2019). Does debridement improve clinical outcomes in people with diabetic foot ulcers treated with continuous diffusion of oxygen? *Wounds, 31*(10), 246–251.

Lewis, C. J., Mararyeu, A. N., Sharov, A. A., et al. (2014). The epigenetic regulation of wound healing. *Advances in Wound Care, 3*(7), 468–475.

Lucas, V., McCain, N., Elslwick, R., et al. (2018). Perceived stress and surgical wound cytokine patterns. *Plastic Surgical Nursing, 38*(2), 55–72.

Ludolph, I., Fried, F. W., Kneppe, K., et al. (2018). Negative pressure wound treatment with computer-controlled irrigation/instillation decrease bacterial load in contaminated wounds and facilitates wound closure. *International Wound Journal, 15*, 978–984.

Metcalf, D., & Bowler, P. (2019). Perceptions of wound biofilm by wound care clinicians. *Wounds, 31*(3), E14–E17.

Moore, K. J., Dunn, E. C., Marcus, E. N., et al. (2018). Glycemic indices and hemoglobin A1C as predictors for non-healing ulcers. *Journal of Wound Care, 27*(4), S6–S11.

Mori, Y., Nakagami, G., Kitamura, A., et al. (2019). Effectiveness of biofilm-based wound care system on wound healing in chronic wounds. *Wound Repair and Regeneration, 27*, 540–547.

Osmolak, A. M., Klatt-Cromwell, C. N., Price, A. M., et al. (2019). Does perioperative oxandrolone improve nutritional status in patients with cachexia related to head and neck carcinoma? *Laryngoscope Investigative Otolaryngology, 4*(3), 314–318.

Pang, M., Zhu, M., Lei, X., et al. (2019). Microbiome imbalances: An overlooked potential mechanism in chronic non healing wounds. *International Journal of Lower Extremity Wounds, 18*(1), 31–41.

Peart, J. (2019). A tool to assess the risk of surgical site complications and suitability for incisional negative pressure wound therapy. *Wounds UK, 15*(1), 20–26.

Salcido, R. (2017). Healing by intention. *Advances in Skin and Wound Care, 30*(6), 246–247.

Sandy-Hodgetts, K., Carville, K., Santamaria, N., et al. (2019). The Perth surgical wound dehiscence risk assessment tool (PSWDRAT): Development and prospective validation in the clinical setting. *Journal of Wound Care, 28*(6), 332–344.

Smit, H. J. (2018). A five-level model for wound analysis and treatment. *Wounds, 14*(4), 24–29.

Tardaguila-Garcia, A., Garcia-Morales, E., Garcia-Alomino, J., et al. (2019). Metalloproteinases in chronic and acute wounds: A systematic review and meta-analyses. *Wound Repair and Regeneration, 27*, 415–420.

Tehan, P. E., Linton, C., Norbury, K., et al. (2019). Factors contributing to wound chronicity in diabetic foot ulceration. *Wound Practice and Research, 27*(3), 111–115.

Thomas, D. R., & Burkemper, N. M. (2013). Aging skin and wound healing. *Clinics in Geriatric Medicine, 29*(2), xi–xx.

Ti, D., Li, M., Fu, X., et al. (2014). Causes and consequences of epigenetic regulation in wound healing. *Wound Repair and Regeneration, 22*, 305–312.

Tyldesley, H. C., Salisbury, A., Chen, R., et al. (2019). Surfactants and their role in biofilm management in chronic wounds. *Wounds International, 10*(1), 20–24.

Waters, N. (2017). From ancient wisdom to modern science: Retracing knowledge of mind-body connections in wound healing. *Wounds International, 8*(1), 15–20.

White, E. (2019). Carl Von Reyher and the origins of debridement. *Wounds UK, 15*(3), 85.

Winter, G. (1962). Formation of the scab and the rate of epithelialization of superficial wounds in the skin of young domestic pig. *Nature, 193*, 293.

Woo, K. Y. (2012a). Chronic wound-associated pain, psychological stress, and wound healing. *Surgical Technology International, 22*(12), 57–65.

Woo, K. Y. (2012b). Exploring the effects of pain and stress on wound healing. *Advances in Skin and Wound Care, 25*(1), 38–44.

Woo, K., Santo, V. L. C. G., & Alam, T. (2018). Optimizing quality of life for people with non-healing wounds. *Wounds International, 9*(3), 6–14.

Wynn, M., & Holloway, S. (2019). The impact of psychological stress on wound healing: A theoretical and clinical perspective. *Wounds UK, 15*(3), 20–27.

Yagi, I., Watanuki, L., Isaac, C., et al. (2016). Human fetal wound healing: A review of molecular and cellular aspects. *European Journal of Plastic Surgery, 39*(4), 239–246.

Young, T. (2019). The role of surfactants in mechanical debridement. *Wounds UK, 15*(1), 72–74.

QUESTIONS

1. The incision of a postoperative cardiac surgery patient is in the inflammatory phase of wound healing. What is one mechanism of healing occurring in this phase?
  A. Neutrophils and monocytes are chemoattracted to the wounded area.
  B. Fibroblasts migrate to the area in response to cellular signaling.
  C. A new extracellular matrix (granulation tissue) is formed.
  D. Cells responsible for collagen synthesis and angiogenesis undergo apoptosis.

2. The wound care nurse is explaining the phases of wound healing to a patient who has a sutured laceration. Which statement accurately describes the typical time frame for proliferation to occur?
  A. 1 to 2 days
  B. 3 to 5 days
  C. 21 to 30 days
  D. 1 to 2 years

3. A patient has a full-thickness pressure injury on the back of the head. What order of healing would occur with this wound?
  A. Epithelial resurfacing—granulation tissue formation
  B. Reepithelialization—granulation tissue formation—remodeling
  C. Epithelial resurfacing—scar formation—remodeling
  D. Inflammatory phase—granulation tissue formation—epithelial resurfacing—remodeling

4. What process is the foundation of modern wound care and is essential for maintenance of cellular viability and cell migration?
  A. Dry wound preparation
  B. Moist wound healing
  C. Antibacterial soaks
  D. Aggressive surgical debridement

5. The wound care nurse is assessing a surgical wound that is too contaminated to permit immediate closure. What is the expected recommendation for treatment of this wound?
  A. Keep the wound at secondary closure level until bacterial burden is decreased to <10^5 organisms/g of tissue; then, close via delayed primary closure.
  B. Close the wound using sutures or skin staples at time of surgery; reopen the wound in 2 to 3 days and allow to heal by tertiary closure.
  C. Close the wound to fascia level, and intentionally, leave upper layers open to granulate in over time.

  D. Allow the wound to fill in naturally over time, and close the wound with stitches after granulation tissue forms if necessary.

6. A patient who has diabetes mellitus has chronic foot ulcers. What is a characteristic of the healing phase of these types of wounds?
  A. There is a shortened inflammatory phase in chronic wounds.
  B. Biofilms do not commonly occur in chronic wounds.
  C. Chronic wounds heal in an orderly, timely, and durable manner.
  D. Chronic wounds commonly plateau at some point in the healing process.

7. The wound care nurse is explaining the difference between acute and chronic wounds to a patient diagnosed with hypertensive ulcers. What is one clinical characteristic of a chronic wound?
  A. Higher mitogenic activity than acute wounds
  B. Lower levels of proinflammatory cytokines than acute wounds
  C. Elevated levels of matrix metalloproteinases (MMPs)
  D. Decreased numbers of senescent cells than acute wounds

8. Which patient would the wound care nurse consider most "at risk" for delayed wound healing?
  A. A 75-year-old female with a surgical incision
  B. A 60-year-old male with hypotension
  C. A 40-year-old female with multiple sclerosis
  D. A 5-year-old male with an unintentional wound

9. A surgical patient is receiving anticancer medication that has a mechanism of action that inhibits new blood vessel growth. For which perioperative complication is the patient at risk?
  A. Excessive inflammation
  B. Decreased white blood cells
  C. Scar formation
  D. Dehiscence

10. Social determinants potentially affecting wound healing progress may include?
  A. Past childhood experiences
  B. Health insurance and access
  C. Geographic location and transport
  D. All of the above

ANSWERS AND RATIONALES

1. A. Rationale: Neutrophils and monocytes are chemoattracted to the wounded area. Initially, neutrophils are predominant, and their primary effect is elimination of bacteria via enzymatic activity.

2. C. Rationale: Proliferation begins at day 1 postinjury and is typically complete by days 21 to 30.

3. D. Rationale: The "order of repair" for an open wound healing by secondary intention is a (sometimes prolonged) inflammatory phase, then granulation tissue formation followed by epithelial resurfacing, and finally remodeling.

4. B. Rationale: Moist wound healing is the foundation of modern wound care and is essential for maintenance of cell viability and cell migration.

5. A. Rationale: If a wound is too contaminated or infected to permit primary closure, maintain the wound at secondary closure level until antibiotic therapy and manual cleansing reduce the bacterial burden to $<10^5$ organisms/g of tissue. The wound is then closed via delayed primary closure.

6. D. Rationale: A chronic wound does not progress through healing in an orderly and timely manner; they commonly plateau or "stall" at some point due to various pathologic conditions, and as a result, predictable tissue repair does not occur.

7. C. Rationale: Chronic wounds are characterized by higher levels of proinflammatory cytokines, elevated levels of MMPs, and greater numbers of senescent cells (i.e., cells that do not respond normally to the cytokines and growth factors regulating the repair process).

8. B. Rationale: Adequate perfusion and oxygenation are critical for normal wound healing. Oxygen is required for inflammation, angiogenesis, collagen synthesis, and epithelialization.

9. D. Rationale: The negative impact of antiangiogenesis drugs on blood vessel growth is associated with delayed wound healing.

10. D. Rationale: Pathological factors inhibiting wound healing exist from the molecular to the population level. The four levels of factors inhibiting wound healing are general factors (social, demographic, general health, comorbidities), local factors (wound location, dimensions, duration, local skin), systemic factors (cardiovascular system, immune, endocrine, renal, connective tissue systems), and molecular/cellular factors (genetics, epigenetics, signaling factors, migration, and proliferation, etc.).

CHAPTER 4

ASSESSMENT OF THE PATIENT WITH A WOUND

Barbara M. Bates-Jensen

1. Conduct a comprehensive assessment of the patient with compromised skin or soft tissue integrity to include history, physical examination, and appropriate diagnostic studies.

2. Use assessment data to determine the following:
   a. Factors causing or contributing to the alteration in skin/soft tissue integrity
   b. Potential for healing and any systemic conditions that would interfere with healing
   c. Wound characteristics (to include phase of wound healing) and implications for wound management

3. Develop an individualized plan of care based on assessment data and current evidence-based guidelines that addresses each of the following factors:
   a. Correction or amelioration of etiologic factors
   b. Attention to systemic factors affecting repair process
   c. Evidence-based topical therapy
   d. Pain management and quality of life
   e. Patient and caregiver education
   f. Use data from serial wound assessments to identify wound deterioration or failure to progress

TOPIC OUTLINE

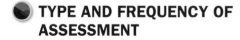
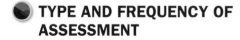
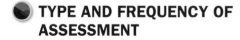
INTRODUCTION

Assessment of the patient with a wound includes assessment of the patient's overall health status and ability to heal including systemic diseases and medications, nutrition, and tissue perfusion and oxygenation, skin status, wound etiology and severity, and wound status, to include stage of healing. Assessment includes a focused history and physical examination, selected diagnostic studies when indicated, followed by interpretation and synthesis of the data, and communication of findings to other health care providers. Communication of wound assessment data is best accomplished using a standardized language and approach: use of standardized wound assessment tools, structured narrative wound notes, and/or photodocumentation. Multiple clinical practice guidelines for wound management include recommendations for the use of standardized wound assessment at baseline and at frequent intervals to determine wound treatment response and wound progress (Bolton et al., 2014; Bonham et al., 2016; EPUAP/NPIAP/PPPIA, 2019; Federman et al., 2016; Gould et al., 2016; Lavery et al., 2016; Marston et al., 2016; WOCN, 2016a, 2016b, 2019). An initial assessment of the wound provides the foundation for development of an appropriate management plan and provides the baseline data that permit determination of progress in healing during subsequent evaluations. In this chapter, aspects of assessment of the patient with a wound are presented including guidelines for skin inspection, guidelines for obtaining a focused history and review of systems, factors to be included in general physical examination and assessment of wound status and wound severity, pertinent laboratory values and diagnostic tests, use of biophysical measures in wound assessment, parameters to be included in assessment of wound-related pain, evaluation of progress in wound healing, and strategies for improving wound documentation, including photodocumentation.

TYPE AND FREQUENCY OF ASSESSMENT

There are two general types of wound assessment, initial or baseline assessment and serial or follow-up assessments. The initial baseline assessment provides the foundation for deciding treatment options and the plan of care and must include determination of wound etiology, assessment of systemic factors affecting the ability to heal, patient and caregiver goals, and wound status; the initial data permit comparison with follow-up data that allows caregivers to determine whether the wound is progressing or deteriorating. The baseline assessment should be performed when the wound is first observed or identified. The baseline assessment must be comprehensive, encompassing all aspects of the wound and the patient's ability to heal from a systemic perspective. Failure to address all aspects of wound development and wound status during the baseline assessment can compromise the appropriateness of the care plan and the ability to determine intermediary outcomes (progress vs. deterioration) during wound treatment. Follow-up assessments provide comparison data, which allow clinicians to determine wound response to treatment; these "serial" assessments should be performed at least weekly, with dressing changes, whenever a change occurs in the wound, or more frequently if so stipulated by health care facility policy. Follow-along assessments should be compared to either the baseline assessment data or the prior follow-along assessment.

Assessment should be performed by a licensed registered nurse, advanced practice nurse, physician's assistant, physical therapist, podiatrist, or physician with the requisite knowledge and skill in wound care. It should be noted that knowledge about wound assessment and wound healing has grown tremendously in the last 5 years, and the average nonspecialist clinician lacks current knowledge regarding clinical practice guidelines, correct wound-related terminology, and basic wound characteristics. A challenge for wound care nurses is providing continuous, timely, multidisciplinary education on wound assessment.

SKIN INSPECTION AND ASSESSMENT

Inspection is different from assessment. Inspection involves visually observing the skin and any wound sites for specific conditions and monitoring for any changes over time. Inspection can be performed by trained licensed practical or vocational nurses, physical therapy assistants, nurse aides, family members, home caregivers, and the patient. Skin inspection should occur whenever a patient is admitted to any health care organization and on a routine basis thereafter. Inspection occurs more frequently than assessments, usually daily or every shift. Because inspection occurs on a more frequent basis, it is a critical "first-line" tool for identifying early indicators of skin or wound deterioration that require further assessment. As an example, if a nursing assistant discovers a new reddened area over the sacrum while providing incontinence care, they should notify the registered nurse, who should assess the area and the patient to determine the etiology of the lesion and any changes needed in the existing care plan. Similarly, if a family caregiver notices increased wound drainage and odor from a surgical incision, the health care provider should be notified, and an assessment is scheduled to evaluate for possible infection.

SKIN INSPECTION

Skin inspection involves visually observing all body parts without the presence of clothing, undergarments, or shoes. Specific conditions to observe for include areas of skin loss, areas of redness or other skin discoloration, edema, rash, increased skin temperature or moisture, and, in the case of a wound, new or increased drainage. If a wound dressing is present and not due to be changed, the dressing should be observed for intactness and any signs of excess wound drainage, rash, or skin discoloration on the surrounding skin (Nix, 2016). If the dressing is dry and intact, dressing status should be documented, and it is not necessary to remove the dressing. The one exception to this is a protective dressing applied to the sacrococcygeal or heel locations; current guidelines stipulate that the protective dressing should be lifted daily or per facility protocol to permit skin inspection and then replaced (EPUAP/NPIAP/PPPIA, 2019).

Skin inspection can be accomplished as part of routine care. For example, the buttocks, sacrum, and perineal areas and sometimes the heels are easily inspected during incontinence care, during repositioning, when transferring the patient from bed to chair, or when getting the patient dressed. Inspection of the elbows and arms can occur when the intravenous site is checked or when dressing the patient. In acute care settings, head to toe skin inspection is typically performed at the beginning and ending of a shift, which allows team members to share findings between the outgoing and incoming team. Those who conduct the skin inspection must report any abnormalities in skin condition; at a minimum, skin status reports should include any change in skin condition, areas of discoloration, presence of rash, and wounds (Nix, 2016). In some institutions, this process is codified as part of the shift hand-off report and as part of required communication when transferring patients between areas. The Turn on Transfer (ToT) program involves both a verbal report of skin status and a brief visual inspection of the sacrum and heels by both delivering and receiving nurses. Routine skin and wound inspection coupled with standardized communication regarding skin and wound status is an essential baseline component of an effective skin and wound care program.

SKIN ASSESSMENT

Skin assessment involves palpation in addition to visual observations, considering interpretation of patterns and trends in the data. As with skin inspection, assessment should involve particular attention to bony prominences and the skin under medical devices, lower extremities and feet, skin folds and crevasses. In addition to inspecting for visible changes in color, integrity, and primary and secondary lesions, the clinician should gently palpate to identify areas of altered skin texture/roughness; callus formation; presence of induration; presence, severity, and type of edema; areas of skin temperature changes (using the backs of the fingers); and areas of tenderness. Skin turgor is a measure of skin hydration and is assessed by gently pinching a fold of skin (typically at the sternum or forehead) and noting how quickly it returns to baseline status. Palpation is also used to test for capillary refill (a measure of perfusion) and for blanchability of any erythematous areas; the examiner presses a finger firmly against the area of erythema for 5 seconds and then lifts the finger and observes the tissues for blanching followed by a return of color to the area (EPUAP/NPIAP/PPPIA, 2019). Nonblanchable erythema is indicative of tissue damage and inflammation involving the skin and soft tissues; nonblanchable erythema over a bony prominence or on the skin under a medical device is classified as a Stage 1 pressure injury (PrI) (EPUAP/NPIAP/PPPIA, 2019). For areas that are erythematous but blanchable, it is important to provide off-loading and to monitor the intensity of the erythema and the blanch response as an ongoing measure of treatment success. If the erythema progresses from blanchable to nonblanchable, it signifies worsening of skin and soft tissue condition.

Visually observe and palpate lower extremities and feet for skin changes including hemosiderosis/hemosiderin staining, venous eczema/dermatitis, hyperpigmentation, atrophie blanche, varicose veins, ankle flaring, scarring from previous ulcers, and lipodermatosclerosis, callus presence, fissures, muscle atrophy, in-grown toenails and deformities, and presence/absence of hair growth (Federman et al., 2016; Lavery et al., 2016; Marston et al., 2016). Palpate and observe for edema. Assess skin temperature (cool skin), capillary and venous refill, paresthesia, and color changes of the skin with elevation or dependency of the limb. Determine presence or absence of pedal pulses. Palpate both dorsalis pedis and posterior tibial pulses of each lower extremity. Presence of palpable pulses does not rule out lower-extremity arterial disease (LEAD); nor does absence of pulses indicate arterial disease, especially, in the presence of edema.

Examine skin under folds or crevasses for moisture-associated skin damage (MASD) and evidence of rash or excoriations. Typical rashes in skin folds and crevasses relate to fungal infections and involve red plaques and macules with satellite lesions often present.

SKIN ASSESSMENT IN PERSONS WITH DARK SKIN TONES

Assessment of skin discoloration in persons with dark skin tones is more complicated. Dark skin tones may not exhibit a visible blanch response, and it is difficult to detect changes in skin color, even for expert clinicians. Use of good lighting is essential for skin assessment of persons with dark skin tones. Moistening the skin may assist with assessment of skin discoloration (Black, 2018). The clinician should observe for a deepening of normal ethnic skin color or a purple, blue, or gray discoloration to the skin. Additional indicators of ischemic (pressure) damage include pain, change in skin texture (e.g., features similar to peau d'orange skin), edema, and increased warmth. In areas of previous full-thickness wounds, the scar tissue will be lighter in color as compared to the person's normal ethnic skin color as there are no melanocytes in the scar tissue. Assessment of skin status in the person with darkly pigmented skin must include palpation as well as inspection. Injured tissues may feel boggy or indurated when compared with adjacent healthy tissue.

KEY POINT

Assessment of skin status in the person with darkly pigmented skin must include palpation as well as inspection.

DOCUMENTATION OF SKIN STATUS

Assessment (and documentation) of any skin lesions should include location and distribution of any rash and use of appropriate terminology to describe primary and secondary skin lesions. Primary skin lesions are classified both by type of the lesion and size of the lesion. Macules and patches are erythematous flat skin discolorations (<1.0 cm and >1.0 cm, respectively), while papules or plaques are raised erythematous skin areas (<1.0 cm and >1.0 cm, respectively). Nodules and tumors represent solid areas of excess tissue growth, vesicles and bulla are clear fluid-filled blisters (<1.0 cm and >1.0 cm, respectively), and pustules are pus-filled blisters. Key secondary skin lesions include scale, lichenification, keloids, hypertrophic scars, erosions, fissures, excoriation, denudation, crusts, and atrophy. (See Chapter 2 for further discussion of common dermatologic lesions and appropriate dermatologic terminology.)

Documentation of the skin inspection must communicate any deviations from normal and may consist of a simple checklist or flow sheet, a body diagram, or narrative notes indicating "dressing intact" or "skin warm, dry, and intact; no lesions." **Figures 4-1 and 4-2** provide

Skin Observation Form

Name: _____ Date: _____ / _____ / _____

SKIN CONDITION check if present	BODY LOCATION See body diagrams below if unsure of location												
	SACRUM or COCCYX (Tailbone)	Right BUTTOCK	Left BUTTOCK	Right ISCHIUM (Bottom of Gluteal fold)	Left ISCHIUM (Bottom of Gluteal fold)	Right HIP	Left HIP	Right HEEL	Left HEEL	Right inner ANKLE	Left inner ANKLE	Right outer ANKLE	Right outer ANKLE
Normal Skin													
Redness													
Bruise													
Rash													
Blister													
Open wound													
Other:													

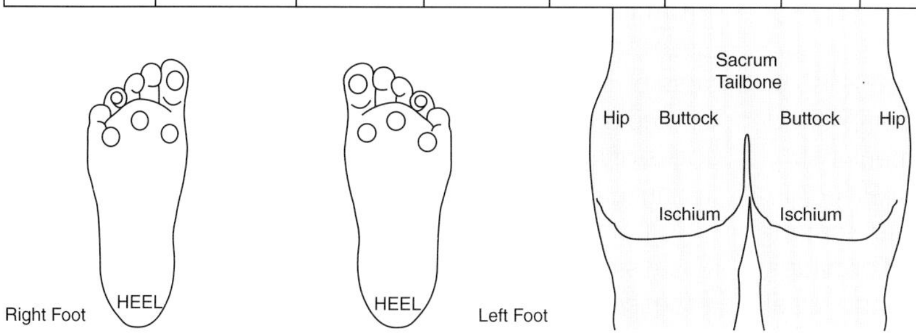

FIGURE 4-1. Sample of Skin Inspection Documentation Form.

Skin Observation Form—Instructions: Observe skin daily & record if condition is present

Name: _____ Month: _____ Year: _____

Body Location	Day:	1	2	3	4	5	6	7	8	9	10	11	12	13	14	15	16	17	18	19	20	21	22	23	24	25	26	27	28	29	30	31
	Skin Condition																																
Sacrum or Tailbone	Redness																																
	Bruise																																
	Wound																																
Right Buttock	Redness																																
	Bruise																																
	Wound																																
Left Buttock	Redness																																
	Bruise																																
	Wound																																
Right Ischium (At gluteal fold)	Redness																																
	Bruise																																
	Wound																																
Left Ischium (At gluteal fold)	Redness																																
	Bruise																																
	Wound																																
Right Hip	Redness																																
	Bruise																																
	Wound																																
Left Hip	Redness																																
	Bruise																																
	Wound																																
Right Heel	Redness																																
	Bruise																																
	Wound																																
Left Heel	Redness																																
	Bruise																																
	Wound																																
Other Locations:	Redness																																
	Bruise																																
	Wound																																

FIGURE 4-2. Another Sample of Skin Inspection Documentation Form.

examples of two types of skin inspection documentation forms. When findings differ from previous inspections, the changes must be communicated to other members of the health care team and documented in the patient's record.

An initial full body or head-to-toe skin assessment is particularly critical at the point of admission to a health care facility; a key responsibility of the admitting nurse is prompt identification of any existing wound or other skin condition. Documentation of pressure-related lesions that are "present on admission" is essential, because the Centers for Medicare and Medicaid Services (CMS) does not provide reimbursement and payment for full-thickness PrIs that develop while the patient is in the hospital (CMS, 2009).

 ## ASSESSMENT AND DOCUMENTATION OF WOUND STATUS

GENERAL CONCEPTS

Assessment and documentation of wound status is an important nursing responsibility and is best accomplished with the use of a standardized wound assessment instrument (Bates-Jensen & Sussman, 2012; EPUAP/NPIAP/ PPPIA, 2019). Use of a standardized wound assessment instrument guides the assessment process and provides continuity in communication about the wound. Initial documentation must include probable etiology, wound duration and previous treatments, and wound status, as well as documentation regarding systemic factors affecting ability to heal and the patient's concerns and goals, including wound-related pain. Documentation at each dressing change should include notations about wound location, appearance of the wound bed, volume and characteristics of exudate, and any evidence of infection, such as periwound erythema and induration (CMS, 2009).

A thorough documentation of wound status should be conducted at least weekly and must include wound dimensions and depth; undermining or pocketing and tunneling; description of wound base, wound edges, and surrounding tissues; amount and characteristics of exudate; and healing characteristics of the wound. Each of these parameters is discussed in greater depth later in this chapter. Maintaining wound assessment documentation in the same physical place in the electronic or paper medical record facilitates comparative evaluation and interpretation of serial assessment findings. Serial assessment data provide insight regarding wound progress or deterioration, which impact treatment plans. For example, as the amount of necrotic tissue decreases, the focus of topical therapy shifts from debridement to maintenance of a moist wound surface and exudate control.

Photography has also been used to enhance wound assessment and documentation and to provide visual assessment of wounds over time. Digital photography has been useful in diagnosing foot ulcers and pre-ulcers in persons with diabetes mellitus (DM) as part of telehealth home monitoring (Hazenberg et al., 2012, 2014). It is important to maximize the accuracy of wound photographs in order to ensure that they are meaningful (Russell Localio et al., 2006). Photography guidelines include the following:

- Place the patient in the same position for all photographs.
- Take the photograph from the same angle.
- Take a close-up photograph of the wound and then a second photograph showing the wound and the body part. Try to take the close-up photograph from a standard distance from the wound (e.g., use a string at the base of the camera to assure consistency in the distance of the close-up photograph).
- Include a ruler with centimeters and a color guide in the photograph.
- Include a label with date, anatomic location, and patient identification (ID) number (use a nonidentifiable ID that meets Health Insurance Portability and Accountability Act [HIPAA] regulations) in the photograph.
- Obtain patient authorization according to facility policy prior to photography.
- Use a digital camera with a density of at least 1.5 megapixels, but 3 megapixels or greater is better for picture clarity.
- Assure adherence to infection control policies. For example, prepare the wound for photography; then remove gloves, wash hands, retrieve the camera, and take the photograph without touching anything around the wound. Return the camera to a safe location, wash hands and don gloves, and complete wound care.
- Download the photographs to the patient's record and delete the photograph from the camera if applicable.

There are some nuances to wound photography for documentation purposes. Some facilities do not allow photographs for wound documentation. Most facilities require some level of individual patient consent for photography, though some organizations consider the consent for treatment to include consent for photography. Poor-quality photographs may be difficult to reconcile in the courtroom. A clear policy with guidelines for who can obtain wound photographs and how to photograph wounds is important for the facility. From a risk management perspective, it is useful, at a minimum, to obtain a photograph of the wound at admission and upon discharge from the organization.

A major benefit of wound photodocumentation is its use in telemedicine. Photography can increase access to expert wound care for people who live in rural areas or areas with limited access to wound experts, and it has been used to supplement wound assessment data. For example, photography has been used to reliably detect callus and foot ulceration and signs of foot infection in persons with diabetes, to quantify granulation tissue in healing wounds, and to enhance wound assessment by wound experts using telehealth modalities (Hazenberg et al., 2010, 2014; Houghton et al., 2000; Iizaka et al., 2013; Russell Localio et al., 2006). Some investigators have suggested that photography does not replace in-person assessment as they have not found strong agreement between assessments conducted in person compared to assessment by photograph (Terris et al., 2011). Others have found strong agreement between in-person and photographic approaches to wound assessment (Houghton et al., 2000; Jesada et al., 2013). Smart phone technology has made uploading wound photographs to electronic health records relatively easy. Examination of electronic health record wound photographs has shown bedside wound assessment of pressure injuries (PrIs) and assessment from photographs of PrIs have adequate agreement with PrI staging (Li et al., 2018). Serial wound photographs uploaded to electronic health records could be used with image processing technology programs to automatically calculate wound size and depth and potentially other wound characteristics (Li et al., 2018). There are also camera devices with lasers that measure the length, width, and depth of the wound and use these measurements to compute wound size. These devices provide more comprehensive photodocumentation and have been shown to improve accuracy and reliability of wound size measurements (Kecelj et al., 2008; Miller et al., 2012). An additional advantage to use of wound photographs may be motivating patients for self-care and wound treatment adherence. A majority of patients reported that photographing their wounds would help them to track the wound progress and would afford them more involvement in their own care (Wang et al., 2016). This is particularly relevant given most patients cannot visually observe their wounds.

KEY POINT

A clear policy with guidelines for who can obtain wound photographs and how to photograph wounds is important for the facility.

WOUND ETIOLOGY

An essential element of initial assessment for the patient with a wound is determination of wound etiology; this allows implementation of a treatment plan that includes measures to correct or ameliorate the causative factors. Critical clues to etiology of trunk wounds include wound location, wound depth and contours, and patient history (e.g., exposure to prolonged pressure and shear forces vs. exposure to moisture and/or friction). Critical clues to the etiology of lower extremity wounds include pain pattern, location, and appearance of wound bed and surrounding tissue. See **Table 4-1** for etiologic clues for common types of trunk wounds and leg ulcers.

TABLE 4-1 CLUES REGARDING WOUND ETIOLOGY

	PATHOLOGICAL FACTORS	TYPICAL LOCATION	TYPICAL CLINICAL MANIFESTATIONS
Pressure injuries	Any disease or condition that leads to limited mobility and/or exposure to shear force Skin and soft tissue compression by medical device	Sacrum, coccyx, buttocks, ischial tuberosities, trochanters, heels. Can occur over any bony prominence Most common locations: sacrum and heels Under medical devices	• Evidence of skin and tissue deformation and/or ischemic damage: red or purple discoloration of skin progressing to full-thickness skin loss surrounded by blanchable or nonblanchable erythema • Round ulcer; may be irregular if large • Tunneling/undermining or pocketing may be evident • Progression to a deep crater (subcutaneous tissue to the fascia) to exposure of the muscle, bone, or supporting structures (i.e., tendon) • Surrounding skin may appear with deepening of ethnic skin tone or erythema, induration, warmth, possible mottling
Incontinence-associated dermatitis (IAD)	Damage caused by maceration + friction or exposure to irritants and pathogens in urine or stool	Buttocks, coccyx, perineum, perianal area, and upper/inner thighs, linear breaks/wounds in gluteal cleft	• Diffuse, intense blanchable erythema • Superficial skin loss (patchy or extensive), often multiple lesions • Secondary candidiasis common (maculopapular rash with central patch or plaque formation and distinct satellite lesions at periphery)
Intertriginous dermatitis (ITD)	Maceration within body folds due to trapped moisture + friction or mechanical stretch	Linear breaks at the base of the body fold or matching lesions on either side of the body fold Natal cleft Under breast tissue Under pannus Axillae	• Linear break in the skin at the base of the body fold • Superficial "kissing" ulcers on opposing sides of skin folds

Venous leg ulcers	Compromised venous return resulting in soft tissue changes that render them vulnerable to ulceration	Lower extremity: calf superior to the medial or lateral malleolus, typically in the "gaiter" area	• Shallow ulcers with ruddy wound base (may also present with combination of red tissue and thin layer yellow film, i.e., fibrin)
			• Moderate to large amounts of exudate
			• If no coexisting arterial disease: warm feet, good pulses, ABI > 0.8
			• Surrounding skin may exhibit any or all of the following:
			  • Hemosiderin staining
			  • Edema
			  • Dermatitis (scaling, crusting, weeping, erythema, inflammation)
			• Pain typically worsened by dependency and relieved by elevation

Arterial leg ulcers	Lower extremity arterial disease causes severe tissue ischemia, resulting in spontaneous necrosis or nonhealing wounds (LEAD).	Tips of toes and/or forefoot Nonhealing wounds involving lower leg or foot	• Ulcers are full thickness, typically round, with punched-out appearance or a distinct border. • Ulcer base pale or necrotic • Typically minimal exudate • Pain worsened by activity and elevation and relieved by rest and dependency
Neuropathic ulcers (diabetic foot ulcers)	Damage to nerve endings results in sensory loss, foot deformities, very dry skin.	Plantar aspect of foot, metatarsal heads, areas of foot in contact with shoe	• Typically full-thickness ulcers with possible tunneling or undermining • Red wet base common but may also present with necrotic tissue • Commonly located within or under callus • May not be painful; may present with neuropathic ("pins and needles," "electric shock") pain that is frequently worse at night
Skin tears	Fragile skin with loss of normal cohesion between epidermal and dermal layers	Usually located on forearm or lower extremity (shin). May be present in other locations after falls	• Superficial injury/ulcer to the epidermis/dermis • May present with viable skin flap that covers the wound, partial skin flap, necrotic flap that has to be removed, or no flap • Bruising of surrounding skin common; bleeding also common • Fragile surrounding skin

Determination of wound etiology is a critical "first step" in wound assessment. If etiology is unclear, appropriate referrals and testing must be initiated.

SYSTEMIC HEALTH STATUS

In addition to determining wound etiology and wound status, the initial assessment must include assessment of the individual's overall health status, with particular attention to systemic factors and lifestyle factors affecting repair. This involves a focused history and physical examination. Data can be obtained from the patient, patient's family or significant others, caregivers, other health care providers, and the medical record.

Focused Patient History and Quality of Life

The patient history information is collected through an interview with key stakeholders (e.g., patient, family, significant others, and caregivers). A focused history is one that targets areas that are most pertinent to patients with wounds, that is, systemic factors and lifestyle factors affecting the repair process.

The interview usually begins with discussion of the "chief complaint," the problem that brought the individual to the clinic or provider, and the duration of the problem. The wound care nurse should investigate the patient's goals, understanding of the etiologic factors contributing to the wound and the interventions required to enhance healing, wound-related concerns, wound-related symptoms, and conduct a quality of life (QoL) assessment. Helpful questions to ask include the following:

- How did you hope I could help you today?
- When did you first notice the wound? How often have you had wounds?
- What do you think caused your wound? Why do you think it started when it did?
- Does the wound occur in a certain place or under certain circumstances? Is it associated with any specific activity?
- How long do you think the wound will last? What do you think will be required to get the wound to heal?
- What symptoms/problems are you experiencing related to the wound?

Specific questions to be asked in regard to wound-related symptoms include the following:

- What is the location and what are the characteristics of the symptom(s)? (Where do you feel the wound? Show me where it hurts. Do you feel it anywhere else? What does it feel like?)
- How severe is the symptom? When does the symptom appear/what is the timing of the symptom? What are the antecedents and consequences of the symptom(s)? What makes it better? Worse?

- How does the wound interfere with your usual activities? How bad is it?

Use of an instrument to measure quality of life with a wound is useful as a framework for identifying areas of most concern to the patient with a wound and measuring effectiveness of interventions to improve quality of life over time with patient reported outcomes. There are several tools available for assessment of quality of life that are specific for patients with wounds (Augustin et al., 2017a, 2017b; Blome et al., 2014; Engelhardt et al., 2014; Gorecki et al., 2011, 2013, 2014; Price & Harding, 2004; Sommer et al., 2017). Gorecki et al. (2013) developed a tool specific to PrI, the Pressure Ulcer-Quality of Life (PU-QOL) tool, which contains 10 scales for measuring symptoms, physical functioning, psychological well-being, and social participation specific to PrIs. Patients rate the amount of "bother" attributed during the past week on a 3-point response scale. Scale scores are generated by summing items, with lower scores indicating better outcome. The PU-QoL tool has also been modified, the Pressure Ulcer-Quality of Life-Prevention (PU-QoL-P) tool, for use in evaluating quality of life for persons at risk for developing a PrI (Rutherford et al., 2018). The PU-QoL-P tool consists of nine items, three symptoms and six function scales.

The Cardiff Wound Impact Schedule (CWIS) is a 47-item questionnaire to measure the impact of chronic wounds (leg ulcers and diabetic foot ulcers) on patient health-related QoL (HRQoL) and to identify areas of patient concern (Price & Harding, 2004). The CWIS contains items that focus on three domains: physical symptoms and daily living, social life, and well-being, as well as two questions on overall QoL. Most questions are rated on a 5-point Likert scale with 1 = not at all/not applicable and 5 = very much. The domain subscale scores can be summed for a total screening score (maximum score 245 points) with higher scores indicating poorer QoL (Price & Harding, 2004). The Wound Quality of Life (QoL) scale is a shorter questionnaire developed from three other longer tools including the CWIS (Gorecki et al., 2014). The Wound-QoL tool contains 17 items which can be attributed to three subscales on everyday life, body, and psyche with each item rated on a 5-point Likert scale. Condition-specific tools have advantages over generic QoL tools by examining items that are more relevant to the specific patient group and detecting small changes that are important to caregivers as well as patients.

The next component of the interview is a review of the patient's past health history. Information about management of and response to past problems provides an indication of the patient's potential response to current treatment of the problem. Much of this information may be available in the patient's medical record. If not available, the following general information should be obtained: past general health, accidents or injuries with any associated disabilities, hospitalizations, surgeries, major acute or chronic illnesses (specifically autoimmune diseases such as rheumatoid arthritis, uncontrolled vasculitis, or pyoderma gangrenosum, systemic sepsis, organ failure [hepatic, renal, respiratory, gut], major trauma/burns, diabetes, malignancy, cerebrovascular accidents (CVA), heart failure, renal failure, pneumonia) as all delay healing, medications (specifically immunosuppressive, nonsteroidal anti-inflammatory, steroids, chemotherapeutic drugs), and allergies. Current health information includes allergies (environmental, food, drug), habits, medications, and sleep and exercise patterns.

In conducting the health history, it is essential to ask about allergies, as there are a number of potential allergens in wound care products and topical antibiotics.

The wound care nurse should evaluate current and past habits, including alcohol, tobacco, substance, drug, and caffeine use. Alcohol, tobacco, and substance use, in particular, present significant problems for tissue perfusion and nutrition for wound healing. The patient should also be asked about nicotine patches or other common smoking cessation aides in use as these products may also affect tissue perfusion. A full medication profile must be obtained, including prescription, homeopathic or alternative products, and over-the-counter medications, to include names, dosages, frequency, intended effect, and adherence with the regimen.

It is important to assess the patient's usual routine and patterns of activity; one approach is to ask the patient to describe a usual day's activities. Exercise patterns influence wound healing and exercise and mobility are key factors for preventing many wounds. Usual daily (and weekend) activities provide insight into the patient's lifestyle and potential health risks. The wound care nurse should also ask about sleep patterns and whether the patient perceives the sleep to be adequate and satisfactory. The wound care nurse should ask the patient where they usually sleep; patients with severe arterial insufficiency may sleep sitting up in recliner chairs because of the pain associated with the disease. Patients with chronic obstructive pulmonary disease (COPD) may sleep sitting up because of difficulty breathing in the supine position.

The family health history provides information about the general health of the patient's relatives and family. Family health information is helpful in the identification of genetic, familial, or environmental illnesses. Specific areas to target are diabetes mellitus, heart disease, and stroke. Each of these diseases can impair wound healing in an existing wound and is a risk factor for further wounding. If the patient has a family history of these diseases, he or she may have early signs of the disease as yet undiagnosed and is at higher risk of eventual disease development.

It is important to ask about the patient's sociologic, psychological, and nutritional status. Sociologic data fall into seven areas: relationships with family and significant others, environment, occupational history, economic status and resources, educational level, daily life, and patterns of health care.

Relationships with family and significant others include gathering information on the patient's position and role in the family, the persons living with the patient, the persons to whom the patient relates, and any recent family changes or crises. The role of the patient within the family may dictate treatment decisions. For example, the truck driver with venous ulcers may also be responsible for financial security of the family; it is unrealistic to expect adherence with a care plan that includes restricted driving time. The family support system should be assessed by asking the following questions: Who will change the wound dressing and perform procedures? Who prepares meals? Who will transport the patient to the clinic?

Environment plays a significant role in the health and illness of individuals; the wound care nurse should ask about the home, community, and work environments. Home care patients present challenging environments for wound repair. For example, the homeless patient living alone with a dog on the street will require different management strategies than will the middle-aged man living with a spouse and family in a three-bedroom house in the suburbs. The community environment may provide additional resources for the patient, such as senior citizens' centers, health fairs, churches, or the neighborhood grocery store that delivers to the home. In contrast, the community may also pose significant hazards such as danger from street crime, fall risk because of poorly kept sidewalks or no sidewalks, and inadequate access to healthy food options (prolific fast food restaurants, no healthy options, limited access to fresh fruits/vegetables at local markets).

The work environment and occupational history provides information on the ability of the patient to eliminate certain risk factors for impaired healing. For example, the clerk whose job requires prolonged standing and who has a venous ulcer will need assistance with work setting modifications. Economic status and resources impact on the ability to obtain needed treatment and supplies; it is important to identify patients with inadequate resources (including inadequate health insurance) and to make appropriate referrals for financial assistance.

The educational level of the patient suggests potential health literacy level and learning style, and education is a critical component of wound care for every patient. Patients should be asked about their preferred learning approaches (written materials, audiovisuals, verbal explanations, or demonstrations). Assessment of usual health care and access provides insight into usual attention to health maintenance.

The psychological history includes an assessment of the patient's cognitive abilities (including learning style, memory, comprehension), responses to illness (coping patterns, reaction to illness), response to care (adherence), and cultural implications for care. If there are any concerns as to cognition, the clinician should administer a mental status examination to quantify cognitive status. Previous coping patterns and reactions to illness can be identified with questions such as the following: Have you had difficulties with wound healing in the past? Do you have a history of chronic wounds? A history of recurrent or nonhealing wounds may suggest potential problems with adherence to treatment regimens.

Assessment should also identify cultural issues that might impact care and adherence to recommended treatment regimens. The wound care nurse should ask about wound care beliefs and preferences and usual health care resources and providers. It is also important to determine the persons to be involved in the patient's care.

Nutrition plays a major role in wound healing (see Chapter 7 for Nutrition information). It is important to ask about the patient's usual nutritional intake and any recent unplanned weight loss. Queries regarding foods and fluids ingested during the past 24 hours are an effective means of determining nutritional intake patterns. The wound care nurse should pay particular attention to calorie and protein intake, fruit and vegetable consumption, and fluid intake, as well as ask about over-the-counter vitamin/mineral/nutritional supplements.

Review of Systems

The systems review portion of the patient history and the physical assessment of each system provide information important for wound diagnosis and on comorbidities that may impair wound healing. **Table 4-2** provides guidelines for systems review focused on factors affecting wound development and wound healing, and Chapters 7, 25, and 24 provide in-depth guidelines for assessment of nutritional status, arterial perfusion, venous return, and lymphatic function. The wound care nurse should consult physical assessment texts for more in-depth and comprehensive physical assessment parameters and guidelines.

KEY POINT

Wound healing is a systemic phenomenon; the assessment includes assessment of the many systems that impact on tissue integrity and wound healing.

TABLE 4-2 SYSTEMS REVIEW AND ASSESSMENT

SYSTEM	IMPACT ON REPAIR	FACTORS TO ADDRESS IN HISTORY TAKING	PARAMETERS TO INCLUDE IN PHYSICAL ASSESSMENT (IF INDICATED)
Respiratory	Responsible for oxygenation of blood (normal tissue oxygen levels essential for wound repair and infection control)	Cystic fibrosis COPD Lung cancer Pneumonia Post-op status Asthma (consider management/use of steroids/impact of steroids on repair) Current and past tobacco use (attempts to stop tobacco use, willingness to consider smoking cessation, etc.)	Color of mucous membranes/nail beds Lung sounds Pulse oximetry TcPO$_2$ levels if available Pulmonary function tests
Cardiac	Perfusion of tissues	CAD/history of MI Heart failure (to include medications and adherence to medication regimen) HTN (level of control; medications) Hyperlipidemia Cardiac surgery Current and past tobacco use (attempts to stop tobacco use, willingness to consider smoking cessation, etc.)	Pulses (brachial, radial, pedal) BP Heart sounds Edema (dependent vs. lower extremity—note dependent edema in patient on bed rest will be in sacral area; unilateral vs. bilateral; severity) Indicators of heart failure (bilateral edema, activity intolerance, shortness of breath, etc.) Advanced practice: auscultation for bruits
Gastrointestinal	Responsible for digestion/absorption of nutrients and fluids	Food and fluid intake (oral, enteral, TPN) Recent unplanned weight loss (% change in weight) Diarrhea (cause?) Fecal incontinence (especially if patient has trunk wound)	Weight and weight trends Indicators of vitamin and mineral deficiencies S/S dehydration (dry MM, reduced skin turgor) Perianal skin status
Genitourinary	Elimination of protein waste/excess fluid and electrolytes	ESRD and management approach (dialysis? protein restriction?) Coexisting DM and HTN? Urinary incontinence	Edema Perineal skin status if patient incontinent UA results BUN/creatinine

(Continued)

TABLE 4-2 SYSTEMS REVIEW AND ASSESSMENT (Continued)

SYSTEM	IMPACT ON REPAIR	FACTORS TO ADDRESS IN HISTORY TAKING	PARAMETERS TO INCLUDE IN PHYSICAL ASSESSMENT (IF INDICATED)
Peripheral vascular system	Delivers blood to tissues; returns venous blood and lymph to circulation	LEAD/PAD Vascular surgery (bypass procedures, stent placement, sclerotherapy, etc.) Amputations DVT Chronic venous insufficiency Past arterial or venous ulcers Lymphedema Claudication and level of activity associated with pain Pruritus	Peripheral pulses (femoral, popliteal, DP, PT)—presence and quality (0 = nonpalpable; 1+ = barely palpable; 2+ = normal; 3+ = full; 4+ = bounding) Ankle–brachial index Trophic changes in skin, hair, nails Symmetry of limbs/evidence calf muscle atrophy Elevational pallor or cyanosis/dependent rubor Temperature of skin on lower extremities Capillary refill Edema (unilateral vs. bilateral, pitting vs. nonpitting), severity using established scale (1+ = 2 mm induration; 2+ = 4 mm induration; 3+ = 6 mm induration; 4+ = 8 mm induration) Varicosities Ankle flare Hemosiderosis Lipodermatosclerosis Atrophie blanche Venous dermatitis Skin changes consistent with lymphedema (cobblestone texture, papillomatous lesions)
Musculoskeletal	Responsible for normal movement and ambulation	Spinal cord injury (level of injury and functional status; assess wheelchair cushion and sleep surface cushion) CVA Parkinson disease Arthritis MS	Gait and ambulatory stability ROM Deformities Ability to turn/move self in bed Ability to move extremities
Endocrine	Maintains normal glucose control	• DM • Type/duration • Management (diet, insulin, oral agents) • Control (HgbA1C levels, range of values for random glucose checks) • Complications (paresthesia, neuropathy, retinopathy, nephropathy) • Knowledge level/understanding of relationship between glycemic control and wound healing	Gait Results of monofilament testing of sensory function Deformities/callus formation Footwear (appropriateness of fit, abnormal wear patterns) Skin temperature Fissures (heels, between toes)
Medications/ therapies interfering with healing		History of radiation to the involved area Current or recently completed chemotherapy Steroids (>30 mg/day for more than 30 days)	

A review of systems with physical assessment guidelines is not inclusive; it provides a framework of those areas of most concern to the clinician managing patients with wounds. The wound care nurse must remember that wounds will not heal if there is inadequate systemic support; assessment of perfusion status, nutritional status, use of tobacco products, and glycemic control are of particularly critical importance. In addition, the wound care nurse must ask about all medications being taken and must ask specifically about steroids and agents known to be cytotoxic (such as chemotherapeutic or immunosuppressive agents). A past history of radiation to the area of the wound should be determined. Finally, the wound care nurse must conduct an open discussion of patient/caregiver goals in relation to the wound and their willingness to adhere to any required lifestyle modifications (such as smoking cessation, tight glycemic control, or consistent off-loading).

The wound care nurse can complete the general history, systems review, and physical assessment in about 30 to 40 minutes for a patient with a single wound. An experienced wound care nurse can perform a basic physical assessment in 10 to 15 minutes. Typically, not all information is gathered at the same time. Portions of the history and physical assessment may be gathered over a period of several days, during several clinic visits, or during multiple home visits.

WOUND HISTORY AND WOUND SEVERITY

The first step in assessing wound severity is to obtain a detailed wound history and determine how the wound occurred. The wound history should include questions about the onset, duration, and past treatment of the wound. (How long has the wound been present? Have you had previous wounds? How has the wound been treated? What was the response to treatment? What disciplines have been involved in the management of the wound?) It is very important to ask about previous therapy and response in order to avoid repetition of unsuccessful interventions. The patient should be queried regarding their understanding of the cause of the wound and their specific wound-related concerns (e.g., exudate, odor, and pain). Wound duration is an important assessment characteristic; evidence indicates that the longer the diabetic foot ulcer or leg ulcer has been present, the less likely it is to heal within a 12- to 20-week time frame (Kantor & Margolis, 1998, 2000a, 2000b, 2000c; Lantis et al., 2013; Margolis et al., 2002, 2003a, 2003b; Robson et al., 2000). Specifically, wounds older than 12 months were significantly less likely to heal within a 12- to 20-week time frame. Wound duration is also an important prognostic indicator for healing of PrIs. Brandeis et al. (1990) showed that PrI healing was most likely to occur during the first 3 months of therapy, with 32% of Stage 3 ulcers and 23% of Stage 4 ulcers healing during the 3-month time frame.

KEY POINT

Data indicate that wound duration is an indicator of potential for healing; the longer the duration of the wound, the less likely it is to heal.

Assessment of wound severity refers to the use of a classification system for diagnosing the severity of tissue trauma by determining the tissue layers involved in the wound. Classification systems such as determining partial- or full-thickness depth, staging PrIs, and grading diabetic ulcers provide objective communication regarding wound severity and the tissue layers involved in the injury. Determining wound severity involves evaluating the wound for depth of tissue involvement and classifying the wound according to an established and accepted system.

Open wounds are classified by depth and level of skin and tissue injury. Partial-thickness wounds involve the epidermis and part of the dermis. These lesions are shallow; present as a pink or red shallow ulcer, an abrasion, or a fluid-filled blister; and heal without scar tissue. Full-thickness wounds involve the epidermis, extend all the way through the dermis, and may involve subcutaneous fat tissues, muscle, and underlying structures such as tendons, ligaments, and bones. Full-thickness wounds may be divided into shallow full-thickness wounds (those involving epidermal, dermal structures, and subcutaneous tissues) and deep full-thickness wounds (those involving muscle and underlying structures). Once a wound is full thickness, it will heal with scar tissue formation. Depth of full-thickness wounds depends in part on the anatomic location of the wound; for instance, a full-thickness wound on the calyx of the ear can be very shallow and still involve the epidermis, dermis, and underlying tissues, while a full-thickness wound on the buttocks may be much deeper because the anatomy of the buttock includes adipose tissue and muscle, and the tissue layers in this area are thicker. To determine whether or not the wound is partial or full thickness, the wound care nurse should observe the wound bed for evidence of dermal appendages such as hair follicles, which appear as small red dots within a pale wound bed; the presence of dermal appendages is consistent with a partial thickness wound. The depth of the wound should be evaluated within the context of the anatomic location, recalling that the epidermis is the thinnest on the eyelids at 0.05 mm and the thickest on the palms of the hands and soles of the feet at 1.5 mm and the dermis also varies in thickness from 0.3 mm on the eyelid to 3.0 mm on the back. Average thickness of the epidermal dermal layers combined is 2 mm (0.2 cm); in general, a partial-thickness wound is <0.2 cm in depth and a full-thickness wound is >0.2 cm in depth. If the wound is deep full thickness, the wound care nurse should note the additional tissues and structures involved in the wound. Wounds of specific etiology are often further categorized. Pressure injuries are commonly classified according to grading or staging systems based on the depth of tissue destruction. The European Pressure Ulcer Advisory Panel (EPUAP)/National Pressure Injury Advisory Panel (NPIAP)/Pan Pacific Pressure Injury Alliance (PPPIA) staging classification system is most commonly used to describe depth of tissue damage (EPUAP/NPIAP/PPPIA, 2019). Staging systems measure only one characteristic of the wound, anatomic depth, and should not be viewed as a complete assessment independent of other wound characteristics. Staging systems are best used as a diagnostic tool for indicating wound severity. Chapter 20 presents PrI staging criteria according to the EPUAP/NPIAP/PPPIA.

PrI stage is determined by observing the level of visible tissue involvement where a Stage 1 PrI and deep tissue pressure injury (DTPI) are defined as discoloration of the skin over a bony prominence, erythema, or redness and maroon or purple, respectively. In persons with dark skin tones, the nurse should observe for a deepening of normal ethnic skin color or purple, blue, or gray skin discoloration. A Stage 2 PrI is a partial-thickness ulcer with damage to the epidermis and part of the dermis, and Stages 3 and 4 PrI represent full-thickness ulcers involving deeper tissues and structures such as subcutaneous fat, muscle, tendon, and bone. Diabetic foot ulcers are typically classified using one of two systems: the Wagner Ulcer Classification System (Wagner, 1981) or the University of Texas System (Armstrong, & Harkless, 1998) (see Chapter 26). The Wagner Ulcer Classification System is based on wound depth and the extent of tissue necrosis. The Wagner system includes six grades, progressing from 0 to 5 in order of severity of breakdown. The University of Texas System addresses ulcer depth and includes the presence of infection and ischemia (Armstrong & Harkless, 1998). Wounds of increasing grade and stage are less likely to heal without vascular repair or amputation (see Chapter 26).

ASSESSMENT OF WOUND STATUS

The physical examination of the wound is essential for determining baseline wound attributes for comparison with later, serial assessments to determine wound progress and response to treatment. Assessment of wound status also provides direction for treatment.

Location

The wound care nurse should first identify the location of the wound using accurate anatomical terms. Body diagrams are a frequently used and helpful tool for documentation of wound location. Location may also be identified by choosing the anatomic site from a list of anatomic locations. It is important to be specific with anatomic terminology. For example, documenting a wound on the "ankle" is not helpful as the wound could be located on the medial or lateral malleolus on either the right or left leg. Accurate documentation of wound location allows all clinicians to determine progress (or deterioration) of specific wounds over time and provides a clear (and legally defensible) record, whereas vague or inaccurate documentation of wound location in a patient with multiple wounds can result in confusion as to which wounds are improving and which are plateaued or deteriorating (**Fig. 4-3**). In addition, anatomic location of the wound is a key determinant of probable wound etiology:

- Wounds caused by arterial insufficiency generally occur at the tips of toes and distal foot, the areas most distal to the heart.

- Venous leg ulcers typically occur on the calf superior to the medial or lateral malleolus.
- Most PrIs occur over bony prominences with the sacral area and heels being the most common locations or under medical devices. Other pressure areas include right and left inner buttocks, ischial tuberosities, trochanters, knees, medial and lateral malleoli, shoulders, and occiput.
- Neuropathic ulcers typically develop on the plantar surface of the foot, most commonly over the metatarsal head of the great or second toe.
- Moisture-associated skin damage: Incontinence-associated dermatitis occurs over the perineal area, buttocks, groin, and possibly in the natal cleft.
- Moisture-associated skin damage: Intertriginous dermatitis occurs within skin folds where there is trapped moisture and may present as a linear break at the base of the fold or as "kissing lesions" on the opposing sides of the fold.
- Friction damage occurs over the fleshy prominences in contact with the seating or lying surface and is typically superficial (partial thickness).
- Skin tears typically occur on the forearms or shins.

Shape

Wound shape, which also helps to determine the overall size of the wound, is determined by evaluating the perimeter of the wound. Shape of the wound is related to wound contraction: As wounds heal, they often change shape and may begin to assume a more regular, circular/oval shape. Wounds that are butterfly shaped or mirror image lesions over the sacrum have been associated with rapid evolution and mortality in one study and have been suggested as a characteristic of terminal PrIs related to skin failure (Kennedy, 1989; Langemo & Brown, 2006; Levine, 2013; Sibbald et al., 2010). Shape of the wound is also associated with specific wound etiology. Wounds that are round, with a punched-out appearance, are often arterial in origin. Venous leg ulcers often have an irregular or an oval shape. Moisture-associated skin damage often presents on the buttocks area with "kissing" or matching lesions where two nearly identical wounds present on each buttock at the site where the buttocks touch each other and moisture is trapped, as a linear wound in the gluteal cleft or at the base of skin folds or crevasses.

Size

Wound size can be determined by measuring (in cm) the length and width (perpendicular to the length) of the wound surface that is visible; the wound care nurse can then determine surface area by multiplying the length by the width. It can be difficult to determine where to measure size on some wounds, because the edge of the wound may be hard to visualize or the edge may be irregular. Use of the same reference points for determining size improves the reliability and meaningfulness

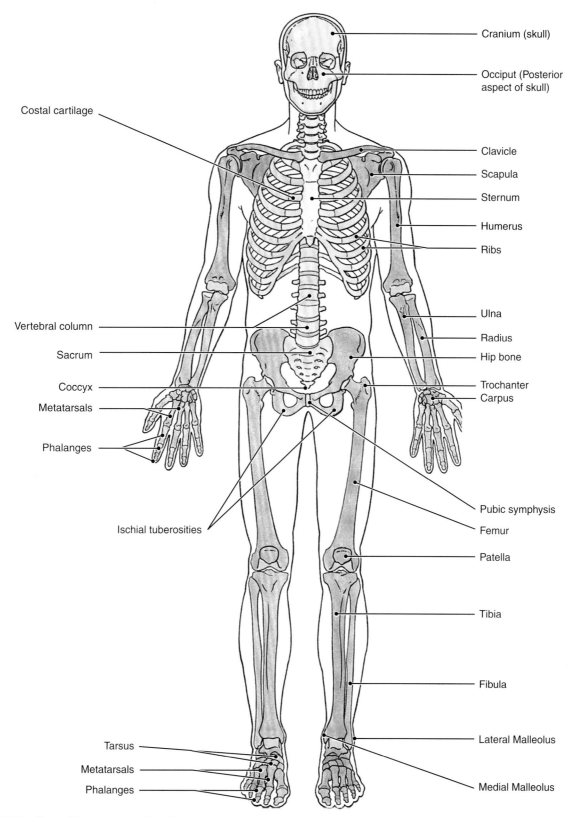

FIGURE 4-3. Chart of Anatomic Locations/Bony Prominences.

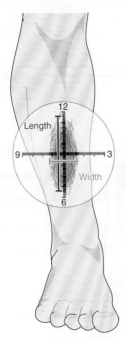

FIGURE 4-4. Wound Measurement (length × width).

of the measurements. In clinical practice, one of two reference points are used: the longest aspect of the wound and the widest aspect of the wound (perpendicular to the length), or the greatest length of the wound from head to toe (or using a clock face to represent the body, 12 o' clock—the head, to 6 o' clock—the feet) and the greatest width of the wound from side to side (or 3 o' clock to 9 o' clock) (**Fig. 4-4**). Depth is determined by placement of a cotton-tipped applicator or commercial measuring device at the deepest part of the wound. Kantor and Margolis (1998) have shown that simple wound measurements (length × width in cm for surface area) are highly correlated with more difficult planimetric wound area calculations. The use of simple wound measurements to monitor and predict healing can be used effectively and with confidence in the clinical setting.

Predicting Wound Healing

Multiple studies have demonstrated a clear and significant relationship between rate of change in wound size at 4 weeks and healing at 12 and 20 weeks (Cardinal et al., 2008, 2009a, 2009b; Edwards et al., 2005, 2018; Kantor & Margolis, 1998, 2000a, 2000b, 2000c; Lantis et al., 2013; Margolis et al., 2002, 2003a, 2003b; Robson et al., 2000; Van Rijswijk, 1993; Van Rijswijk & Multicenter Leg Ulcer Study Group, 1993; Van Rijswijk & Polansky, 1994; Warriner et al., 2011). Van Rijswijk (1993) showed that >30% reduction in surface area of venous leg ulcers at two weeks was a significant predictor of time required for healing. Kantor and Margolis (2000a, 2000b, 2000c) found that percent change in wound area in diabetic foot ulcers and venous ulcers during the first four weeks was

the best predictor for healing by 24 weeks. Other studies have confirmed that the percent change in wound area or wound trajectory during the first four weeks is a predictor of healing at 12 or 24 weeks for both diabetic foot ulcers and venous leg ulcers (Lantis et al., 2013; Margolis et al., 2002; Robson et al., 2000).

Other markers of size have also demonstrated ability to predict healing at 12 or 24 weeks. In addition to percent area reduction, healing rates of 0.11 cm/week or greater have been shown to be predictive of healing for both diabetic foot and venous leg ulcers. Venous ulcers with initial wound area <10 cm² and <12 months' duration have a 78% chance of healing at week 24 compared to those with initial wound area >10 cm² and longer than 12 months' duration, which have a 78% chance of nonhealing (Margolis et al., 2004).

Early work in this area found similar results and is the basis for conducting a comprehensive evaluation of the wound's response to therapy at least every 2 weeks. Two clinical studies found that full-thickness PrIs that decreased 47% and 39% in size during the first 2 weeks of treatment were much more likely to heal and were distinguishable from those that did not heal (Sheehan et al., 2003; Van Rijswijk, 1993; Van Rijswijk & Polansky, 1994). Other clinical studies of predictors of healing for leg ulcers found that a >30% reduction in ulcer area after two weeks of treatment was a significant predictor of healing (Arnold et al., 1994; Van Rijswijk, 1993). In addition, a retrospective study of prognostic factors for venous ulcer healing found that 40% healing by week 3 predicted more than 70% of the outcomes correctly. Kantor and Margolis report that the percentage of change in area over the first four weeks of treatment represents a practical and predictive measure of complete wound healing (Kantor & Margolis, 2000a, 2000b, 2000c). Sheehan et al. (2003) studied diabetic foot ulcers and found that 82% of ulcers with a documented 50% reduction in size at four weeks healed, whereas those with a percent change of 25% failed to heal. Of equal importance, the sensitivity of the finding of 50% reduction was 91%, and the negative predictive value was also 91%. (The high negative predictive value indicates that those who do not fall in the healer group have a high likelihood of failure to heal.) The findings related to the rate of reduction in wound size as a predictor of healing within a 12- to 20-week time frame are strong and consistent. The conclusion supported by these studies is that PrIs and leg ulcers (venous and diabetic) that fail to demonstrate a significant reduction in size (30% to 50%) during the first 2 to 4 weeks of therapy are much less likely to heal than ulcers that show a 30% to 50% reduction in wound area. Evaluation of the rate of wound area reduction should be part of all routine wound assessment to determine those wounds that require referral for more aggressive therapy.

Depth

The depth of the wound is measured using a cotton-tipped applicator, which is placed vertically at the deepest part of the wound; a pen is used to draw a line on the applicator at the parallel plane to the skin and then compared to a measuring device. Multiple measures of depth within the wound can increase reliability of depth evaluation.

Edges

Assessment of wound edges is one of the most important components of the wound assessment. When assessing wound edges, the nurse should use observation and palpation to determine the following:

- Are the edges clear and distinct, or indistinct and diffuse? (Edges are indistinct when there are areas where the normal tissues blend into the wound bed). Well-defined edges are clear and distinct from normal skin and can be outlined easily on a transparent piece of plastic.
- Are the edges attached or unattached to the wound bed? Edges that are even with the skin surface and the wound base are attached to the base of the wound; this means that the wound is flat at the edge, with no appreciable depth. Edges that are not attached to the base of the wound imply a wound with some depth of tissue involvement. The wound that is a crater or has a bowl/boat shape with sides and depth is a wound with edges that are not attached to the wound base.
- Are the wound edges open and proliferative, or closed and rolled under? (**Fig. 4-5**). The edges of chronic wounds frequently become rolled under and

thickened to palpation; the development of closed and rolled wound edges is termed epibole. Wounds of long duration may continue to undergo thickening and fibrosis of the wound edges, causing the edge to feel hard, rigid, and indurated to palpation. Hyperkeratosis is the callus-like tissue that may form around the wound edges; this is especially common with neuropathic diabetic foot ulcers. The chronic wound edge achieves a unique coloring over time due to hemosiderin deposits from breakdown of cells and tissues. The pigment turns a grayish brown hue in persons with both dark and light skin tones.

Undermining/Tunneling

Undermining, or pocketing, and tunneling represent the loss of tissue underneath an intact skin surface (**Figs. 4-6 and 4-7**). Undermining and tunneling are measured using a cotton-tipped applicator, which is gently inserted under the edge of the wound and, without undue pressure, advanced as far as possible; the tip of the applicator is then elevated so that it can be seen or felt on the surface of the skin, the surface is marked with a pen, and the distance from the mark on the skin to the edge of the wound is measured. This process is continued all around the wound. The extent of undermining is determined by noting the percent of the wound edge involved in the process and the distance the process extends from the wound edge; undermining (and tunneling) should be documented in terms of location (using a clockface) and extension from wound edge (e.g., undermining 3 to 6 o'clock extending 2 to 4 cm from wound edge).

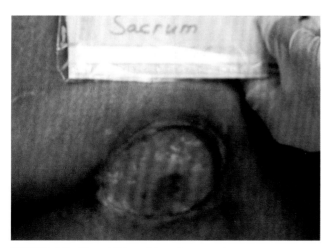

FIGURE 4-5. Wound Edges (closed vs. open).

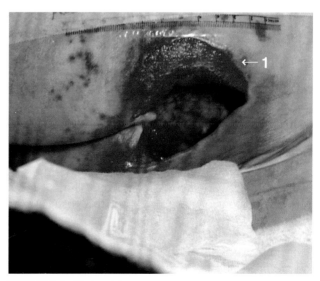

FIGURE 4-6. Undermining.

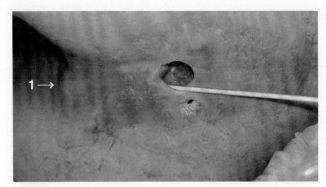

FIGURE 4-7. Tunneling.

Tunneling may occur at other sites besides the wound edge, such as the base of the wound. Tunneling presents as a narrow tract, whereas undermining presents as a lip or pocket.

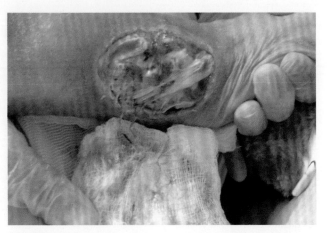

FIGURE 4-8. Slough.

KEY POINT

Undermining or tunneling should be documented in terms of location (by clockface) and extension from wound edge.

Necrosis

Necrosis is dead, devitalized tissue. Necrotic tissue should be assessed and documented in terms of amount, color, consistency or moisture content, and adherence to the wound bed. The amount of necrotic tissue present in the wound is evaluated by one of two methods. One method involves using clinical judgment to estimate the percentage of the wound covered with necrosis. (Picture the wound as a pie and divide it into four [25%] quadrants; look at each quadrant and judge how much necrosis is present; estimate the percentage of necrosis in each quadrant, and sum the percentages.) A second method involves actual linear measurements of the necrotic tissue. (Measure the length and width of the necrosis and multiply to determine surface area of necrosis.) Others have used a variety of methods for determining the area of necrotic tissue using computerized planimetry and portable wound measurement systems and have compared results obtained with these systems to visual estimation; data indicate that visual estimation is reliable and consequently a valid technique for daily practice (Laplaud et al., 2010).

The level and type of tissue death influence the clinical appearance of the necrotic tissue. For example, necrosis of the subcutaneous fat typically results in formation of stringy, yellow slough, while muscle necrosis results in dead tissue that may be thicker and more tenacious. Necrotic tissue is typically described based on the characteristics of color, consistency, and adherence. Color varies as necrosis worsens, from white/gray

nonviable tissue, to yellow slough, and finally to black eschar (**Figs. 4-8 and 4-9A and B**). Consistency refers to the cohesiveness of the debris (i.e., thin or thick, stringy or clumpy, moist or dry); typically, more advanced necrosis is thick and dry. *Adherence* refers to the adhesiveness of the necrotic debris to the wound bed tissues and the ease with which the two may be separated. The adherence of the necrotic tissue has major implications for best approaches to debridement, as discussed in Chapter 10. The characteristics of the necrotic tissue change with wound duration, additional trauma and tissue death, and debridement.

The terms *slough* and *eschar* refer to different levels of necrosis and are described according to color, consistency, and adherence. Slough is yellow or tan and may present as thin, mucinous, or stringy fibrin-like material scattered throughout the wound bed or clustered in the base of the wound. In contrast, eschar is associated with deeper tissue damage and is usually black, gray, or brown in color. It may be loosely or firmly adherent to the wound tissues and may be soggy, soft, hard, crusty, or leathery in texture. A soft, soggy eschar is usually strongly attached to the base of the wound but may be lifting from (and loose from) the edges of the wound. A hard, crusty leathery eschar is strongly attached to the base and edges of the wound and is sometimes mistaken for a scab. Evidence of underlying tissue necrosis may appear before a wound is apparent, for example, the purple or maroon skin discoloration in DTPI from pressure damage.

Exudate Type and Amount

Wound exudate (also known as wound fluid, wound drainage) is an important assessment feature, because the volume and characteristics of the exudate contribute to assessment for wound infection, appropriateness of topical therapy, and progress in wound healing. In the acute wound, exudate is tied to wound healing; the volume of exudate should be minimal progressing to none over days 1 to 4 postinjury, and the drainage should be

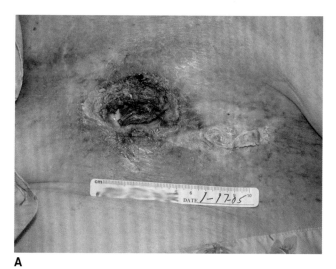

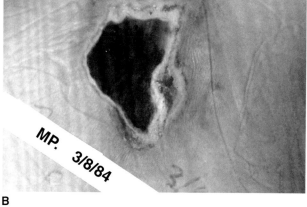

A

B

FIGURE 4-9. A, B. Eschar.

serosanguinous in nature. In chronic wounds, the presence of moderate to large amounts of drainage that persists even after necrotic tissue has been debrided and infection has been treated suggests prolonged inflammation with failure to move to the proliferative phase of wound healing. High volume drainage that is purulent or malodorous is one sign of infection, which retards wound healing, causes odor, and should be treated aggressively in most instances. (Normal exudate in the noninfected wound is usually serous or serosanguinous in nature.) In the infected wound, the exudate may thicken, become purulent, and persist in moderate to large amounts. Examples of exudate changes associated with wound infection include the thick, malodorous, sweet-smelling, green drainage associated with *Pseudomonas* infection or the ammonia-like odor characteristic of *Proteus* infection. Wounds with foul-smelling drainage are generally infected or filled with necrotic debris, and healing time is prolonged as tissue destruction progresses (Seiler & Stahelin, 1995). Proper assessment of wound exudate is also important because it affirms the body's brief, normal inflammatory response to tissue injury and is a key consideration in determination of appropriate wound therapy. However, the wound care nurse should be aware that exudate is one of the most distressing symptoms for patients with wounds (EPUAP/NPIAP/PPPIA, 2019; de Laat et al., 2005).

Accurate assessment of exudate volume and characteristics is frequently challenging, due to variability resulting from wound size and absorptive capacity of dressings being used. What might be considered a large amount of drainage for a smaller wound may be considered a small amount for a larger wound, making clinically meaningful assessment of exudate difficult. Evaluating exudate type is sometimes confusing, due to the fact that some dressing materials interact with or trap wound fluid to produce exudate with the color and consistency of purulent

drainage. For example, both hydrocolloid and alginate dressings mimic a purulent drainage on removal of the dressing. Assessment of exudate should be undertaken after removal of the wound dressing and wound cleansing with normal saline or water. To judge the amount of exudate in the wound, the wound care nurse should observe both the wound itself and the dressing removed from the wound. (Is the wound surface moist? Dry and desiccated? Macerated due to pooled exudate? Is the dressing completely saturated, 50% saturated, or minimally wet?) The wound care nurse must also take into consideration the absorptive properties of the dressing and the length of time the dressing has been in contact with the wound. For example, the wound care nurse might determine that the alginate dressing was 50% saturated following 24 hours of contact with the wound; based on these data, the wound care nurse might estimate the volume of exudate for this wound as "moderate." Clinical judgment of the amount of wound drainage requires some experience with expected volume of wound exudate in relation to phase of wound healing and type of wound as well as knowledge of absorptive capacity and normal wear time of topical dressings.

KEY POINT

Assessment of exudate type and volume is an important aspect of wound assessment but can be confounded by wound size, wound healing phase, and types of dressings.

Surrounding Skin Characteristics

The tissues surrounding the wound are often the first indication of impending further tissue damage; the wound care nurse should routinely assess the tissues within 4 cm of the wound edges for presence and extent of erythema, edema, induration, maceration, and denudement. Nonblanchable erythema or deep purple, blue, or black discoloration may herald impending extension of the wound due to additional ischemic, cell deformation or hypoxic damage; induration (abnormal firmness or hardness of the tissues) is another potential indicator of impending breakdown. To assess for periwound induration, the wound care nurse should gently palpate and "pinch" the tissues, moving from healthy tissue and toward the wound margins. It is usual to feel slight firmness at the wound edge itself. Normal tissues feel soft and spongy; induration feels hard and firm to the touch. The combination of erythema and induration extending circumferentially around the wound is typically indicative of invasive wound infection. Periwound edema presents an impediment to repair, because it interferes with tissue oxygenation; the wound care nurse should be alert to this finding and should undertake further assessment to determine the extent and severity of the edema, including palpation to determine whether the edema is pitting and to rule out crepitus. Crepitus is the accumulation of air or gas in tissues; is palpated as a grating, popping, or cracking sensation; and is usually indicative of anaerobic

infection. Macerated skin is a signal that wound exudate is not being effectively controlled and mandates a change in either dressing type or dressing change frequency. A positive (desired) finding is the extension of new epithelium from the wound edge toward the wound center; the new skin is pink and dry, lacks pigmentation, and typically mirrors the outline of the original wound.

Granulation Tissue and Epithelialization

Granulation and epithelial tissues are markers of wound health. They signal the proliferative phase of wound healing and usually foretell wound closure. Granulation tissue is the growth of small blood vessels and connective tissue into the wound cavity. The granulation tissue is healthy when it is bright, beefy red, shiny, and granular with a velvety appearance (**Fig. 4-10A and B**). The tissue looks "bumpy" and may bleed easily. Unhealthy granulation tissue, resulting from poor vascular supply or high bacterial loads, appears pale pink or blanched to a dull, dusky red. Usually, the first layer of granulation tissue to be laid down in the wound is pale pink, and, as the granulation tissue deepens and thickens, the color becomes bright, beefy red. The percentage of the wound that is

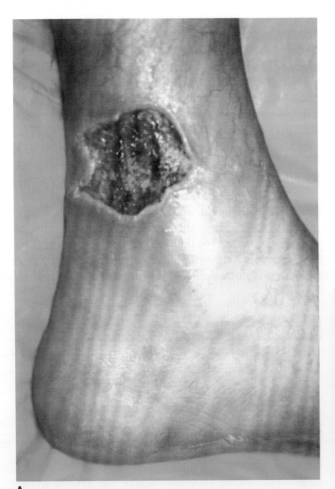

1/16   AL

A

B

FIGURE 4-10. A, B. Granulation Tissue.

filled with granulation tissue and the characteristics of the granulation tissue are indicators of wound health. The wound care nurse should estimate the percentage of the wound with granulation tissue; while this is easier when the same clinician is performing serial assessments, it is important even if this is the first time the wound has been seen, because it provides data that will be used for comparison at the next assessment.

It is critically important to differentiate between wounds with a pink/red but nongranulating base and wounds that are actively granulating; a pink red smooth base is frequently seen in wounds that have "plateaued" or wounds with muscle involvement, and are not healing, whereas granulation tissue is an indicator of healing. A viable but nongranulating wound requires further evaluation to determine the reasons for failure to heal (**Fig. 4-11**).

As explained in Chapter 3, partial-thickness wounds heal by epidermal resurfacing and regeneration, specifically the proliferation and migration of epithelial cells from the wound edges and the hair follicles distributed throughout the wound bed. In contrast, full-thickness wounds heal by scar formation: the tissue defect fills with granulation tissue, the edges contract, and the wound is resurfaced by epithelialization. Epithelialization may occur throughout the wound bed in partial-thickness wounds but only from the wound edges in full-thickness wounds. The new epithelium is pink and dry in people of all races (**Fig. 4-12**); progress in epithelialization is assessed by determining the percentage of the wound that is covered by new epithelium and the distance from the wound edge to which the new epithelium extends. A transparent measuring guide can be used to help determine the percentage of wound involvement and the distance to which the epithelial tissue extends across the wound.

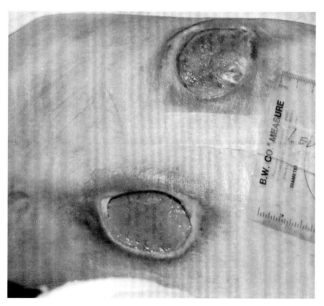

FIGURE 4-11. Viable Nongranulating Wound Bed.

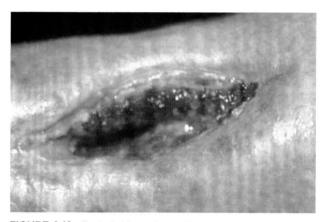

FIGURE 4-12. Epithelial Resurfacing. Note epithelial resurfacing at superior aspect of wound, where there is healthy granulation tissue. At the inferior aspect, there is minimal epithelial resurfacing because of poor quality granulation. At the left side of the wound, there is *no* epithelial resurfacing because there is no granulation tissue.

KEY POINT

Granulation tissue formation and reepithelialization are indicators of wound healing.

Wound Pain Assessment

Wound assessment would not be complete without an assessment of wound pain, to include the location, distribution, type, quality and intensity, and any aggravating or relieving factors (Krasner, 1995). Location of the pain may include the wound bed itself as well as surrounding skin and tissues. Distribution of the pain may be diffuse or specific to the wound area. The patient should be asked to describe the type of pain. Descriptors such as aching, throbbing, sharp, and dull are characteristic of nociceptive pain, while neuropathic pain is usually described as burning, tingling, "pins and needles," and "electric shock" in nature.

The wound care nurse should assess wound pain intensity using a valid pain severity assessment tool. Pain intensity is commonly measured quantitatively using a visual analog scale (VAS), FACES scale, numerical rating scale (NRS), or verbal descriptor scale (VDS) (Fink et al., 2019; Freeman et al., 2001). The VAS is a 0- to 100-mm numbered line with ratio scale properties. It has demonstrated high validity and reliability when used with hospitalized patients (Wewers & Lowe, 1990). It may be difficult for children and frail elders, with or without cognitive impairment, to follow the instructions for use of the VAS. The FACES scale consists of six cartoon faces ordered from smiling to crying (Bieri et al., 1990; Wong & Baker, 1988). The FACES scale has been used extensively with pediatric populations. A version for use with adults and cognitively impaired elders uses oval-shaped faces, without tears, that are more adult-like in appearance (Simon & Malabar, 1995; Stuppy, 1998; Taylor et al., 2003). Advantages of FACES scales are the ease and quickness of administration, simplicity, the correlation with VAS, and little mental energy required by the patient (Stuppy, 1998). The NRS uses two number anchors, most typically 0 and 10, in which 0 represents no pain and 10 represents the worst pain imaginable (Paice & Cohen, 1997). The NRS is administered verbally, allowing for use over the phone and with those who have visual or physical impairments such that use of other tools is difficult or not possible. The VDS uses adjectives that reflect extremes of pain and are ranked in order of severity (Manz et al., 2000). Each adjective is given a number that reflects the patient's pain intensity. In general, a VDS is easy to administer and understand. The patient must pick one word to describe his or her pain even if no word choice accurately describes it. Individuals with limited English and those who are illiterate may have difficulty with this tool (Fink et al., 2019).

In addition to assessing pain characteristics, assess the patient for factors that may place the patient at risk for high intensity pain during wound care procedures. Gardner et al. (2017) proposed a model of human and wound factors associated with increased pain that are easily available clinically and could be used to identify patients more likely to experience high intensity pain during wound care procedures and thus would benefit from aggressive early interventions. Human factors include gender, age, race/ethnicity, chronic pain conditions, repeated opioid administration, anxiety, depression, and pain catastrophizing. Female gender predisposes to higher intensity wound pain (Morin et al., 2000), and women have a higher prevalence of chronic diseases associated with increased pain intensity such as fibromyalgia. Stotts and colleagues (2004) showed that younger hospitalized patients have greater pain than older patients before and after wound care procedures suggesting that the younger the patient, the more pain and analgesia requirement. Stotts et al. (2004) also found that nonwhites had greater pain intensity than whites during wound care procedures, and racial/ethnic differences in pain perception exist across all types of pain (Green et al., 2003). Patients with comorbid conditions associated with changes to the central nervous system pain processing (e.g., fibromyalgia, irritable bowel syndrome) may have increased pain during wound care procedures (Gardner et al., 2017). Repeated administration of opioids can cause increased sensitivity to painful stimuli by initiating pain systems which increase the perception of pain. The amount of opioids taken prior to wound care procedures may influence the degree of pain experienced during and after the procedure (Gardner et al., 2017). Level of anxiety is related to anticipatory pain and pain experienced during procedures (Woo, 2008). Woo (2015) found that anticipation of pain triggers anxiety that can lead to increased pain during wound dressing procedures. Depression and pain are common co-morbidities that share biological pathways and neurotransmitters (Gardner et al., 2017; Sobol-Kwapinska et al., 2016). Pain catastrophizing is a negative response to pain involving magnification, helplessness, and pessimism and can amplify pain intensity and increase pain response (Richardson, 2012). Roth and colleagues (2004) found that patients with chronic wounds had a strong relationship between pain catastrophizing and pain intensity.

Wound factors to assess include recent injury/tissue loss, type of wound (acute or chronic), clinical inflammation, resting wound pain, and partial thickness wounds (Gardner et al., 2017). Early wound healing phases (hemostasis and inflammation) involve neutrophil release of cytokines which activate nociceptors in the injury site thus, increasing pain during wound care procedures. Wounds that are in the first phases of wound healing are more likely to be painful when procedures are performed (Gardner et al., 2017). Similarly, chronic wounds are known to have a prolonged inflammatory phase of wound healing compared to acute wounds, and patients with chronic wounds may exhibit increased pain during procedures (Price et al., 2008). Clinical inflammation is also positively associated with higher pain during procedures. Inflammation, which is a sign of vasodilation in the early phases of wound healing, chronic inflammation, or high wound bioburden may be associated with high pain intensity during wound care procedures (Gardner et al., 2001, 2014). Patients with high levels of wound pain at rest may experience greater pain during procedures as the pain at rest involves nociceptor sensitization (Gardner et al., 2014).

Partial thickness wounds and shallow full-thickness wounds may produce more pain during procedures because the skin is more densely innervated with nociceptors than deeper tissues. Determining the risk for high intensity pain during wound care procedures alerts the wound nurse to the need for more aggressive and earlier pain management interventions.

The pain assessment should include both procedural and nonprocedural resting wound pain. Procedural wound pain is pain experienced during procedures such as dressing changes, wound cleansing, patient repositioning or movement, and wound debridement (Krasner, 1995; Merskey & Bogduk, 1994). Nonprocedural pain is the pain associated with living with an open wound (Krasner, 1995; Merskey & Bogduk, 1994); it may be "around-the-clock" pain that interferes significantly with activities of daily living and QoL. The patient should also be asked about pain management strategies and should be queried regarding exacerbating and relieving factors. (What reduces or relieves wound pain? What makes the wound pain worse? How do you manage the pain?) A pain diary can pinpoint the time(s) of day and the activity(ies) associated with pain relief and aggravation, which assists the wound nurse to develop an effective plan for pain management. All pain management strategies, both behavioral and pharmaceutical, should be evaluated in terms of effectiveness. (Is the strategy/medication effective? For how long?) In general, procedural pain can be managed with premedication and with changes in wound care procedures and products. In contrast, around-the-clock pain typically requires around-the-clock analgesia, topical or systemic or both. A pain diary can be useful in monitoring and assessing treatment responses.

KEY POINT

Assessment of wound-related pain must include type of pain, severity, and exacerbating and relieving factors.

It should be noted that pain patterns and factors exacerbating or reducing the pain are an important aspect of differential assessment. Pain relief for painful venous ulcers typically occurs when the legs are elevated, and edema is lessened. In contrast, pain relief for arterial ulcers occurs when the legs are placed in a dependent position as this supports arterial blood flow. Intermittent claudication is characterized by reproducible pain or fatigue that is precipitated by a predictable level of activity or elevation and relieved by rest and dependency. Intermittent claudication may signal critical limb ischemia and portend poor healing outcomes. Patients with diabetic foot ulcers may complain of tingling or burning sensations, which signal neuropathic pain as compared to nociceptive pain.

Pain related to chronic wounds affects the patient's QoL, and pain is reported by patients with all types of chronic wounds (Roth et al., 2004; Woo, 2012). If pain is a significant factor for the patient and the goals of care are to improve QoL, conduct a QoL assessment. Pain is essential to assess as it negatively impacts wound healing outcomes (Gorecki et al., 2011; Woo, 2012) and yet, health care providers are not regular or consistent in assessing wound pain (Frescos, 2018).

Wound Inspection

Wound inspection involves observing the wound for signs of complications such as infection, deterioration, or increase in severity and can be conducted by caregivers, family members, the patient, and health care workers including licensed practical/vocational nurses, and nursing assistants/aides. Inspection for infection includes looking for increased wound drainage or purulent drainage, need for more frequent dressing changes due to increased volume of exudate, periwound erythema and induration, foul odor from the wound, and elevated patient temperature. Any increase in bleeding, wound

pain, wound size, visible depth, or necrotic tissue should be reported, as should evidence of foreign objects visible in the wound. The inspection findings should be reported to the registered nurse or provider for evaluation and determination regarding whether additional assessment is indicated.

Chronic wounds may exhibit signs of wound infection differently than acute wounds often due to immunosuppression of the patient. The classic signs of infection in acute wounds (redness, swelling or edema, pain, increase in temperature, and purulent exudate) are not always present in chronic wound infection. Signs of chronic wound infection include delayed healing or deterioration of the wound (despite appropriate treatment), pale or dark red and friable granulation tissue, pocketing or tunneling at the base of the wound, and foul odor (Gardner et al., 2001). Chronic wounds are all contaminated with microorganisms, and chronic wounds have been shown to heal in the presence of high levels of microorganisms in contrast to acute wounds; however, excessively high levels of bacteria may form a biofilm and impair healing and must be treated, typically with adequate repeated debridement and/or antimicrobial dressings (see Chapter 11). A robust assessment of wound characteristics is important in monitoring for infection.

SERIAL ASSESSMENTS

Performing a complete baseline assessment of multiple wound characteristics allows the development of an appropriate care plan. Baseline assessment and implementation of an appropriate management plan must be followed with ongoing serial assessments to determine responsiveness to therapy. Evaluation of the wound at scheduled intervals allows the provider to determine progress in healing versus a plateau or deterioration in wound status and to revise the treatment plan as appropriate; it often provides an indication of the patient's overall health as well. In many cases, the improvement or deterioration in wound status reflects a change in the patient's overall health status. Progressive monitoring of changes in wound characteristics is also important to determine whether the treatment is effective in meeting the goals for the patient—controlling odor, managing exudate, preventing infection, preparing a clean wound bed, reducing surface area, or minimizing pain. Serial assessment data involving multiple wound characteristics reflect the wound's progression through the wound healing phases. Wounds in the inflammatory phase have differing characteristics than those in the proliferative or remodeling phase of healing, and progress is measured differently for a wound in the inflammatory phase and a wound in the proliferative phase. Monitoring for specific wound characteristic changes as a measure of progression through the wound healing phases is important in providing treatment to support wound closure.

One way to monitor and interpret changes in wound characteristics over time is use of a standardized wound assessment tool. Use of a systematic approach with a comprehensive assessment tool is helpful for tracking and communicating findings and for organizing the assessment process. There are few tools available that encompass multiple wound characteristics to evaluate overall wound status and healing. Two available tools are the Pressure Ulcer Scale for Healing (PUSH) and the Bates-Jensen Wound Assessment Tool (BWAT).

The PUSH is a tool originally developed to measure PrI healing by the NPUAP (Bartolucci & Thomas, 1997; Stotts et al., 2001; Thomas et al., 1997). It has since been evaluated for use in assessment of venous and diabetic ulcer healing (Edwards et al., 2005; Gardner et al., 2011; Gunes, 2009; Hon et al., 2010; Ratliff, 2005).

The PUSH tool incorporates surface area measurements, exudate amount, and surface appearance. These wound characteristics were chosen based on principal component analysis to define the best model of healing (Bartolucci & Thomas, 1997; Thomas et al., 1997). The wound care nurse measures the size of the wound, calculates the surface area (length × width), and chooses the appropriate size category on the tool (0 to 10). Exudate is evaluated as none (0), light (1), moderate (2), or heavy (3). Tissue type choices include closed (0), epithelial tissue (1), granulation tissue (2), slough (3), and necrotic tissue (4). The three subscores are then summed for a total score. Total PUSH scores can be monitored over time for healing or wound degeneration. Aspects of the PUSH tool are included in the Minimum Data Set Assessment, the mandated multidomain assessment instrument used for persons admitted to any CMS-certified long-term care facility. The PUSH tool offers a quick assessment to predict healing outcomes (**Fig. 4-13**). The PUSH tool is best used as a method for predicting wound healing. Assessment of additional wound characteristics may still be needed, to develop a comprehensive treatment plan for wounds.

The BWAT includes additional wound characteristics that may be helpful in designing a plan of care for the wound. The BWAT (**Fig. 4-14**) was originally developed as the Pressure Sore Status Tool in 1990 by Bates–Jensen (Bates-Jensen & McNees, 1995, 1996; Bates-Jensen et al., 1992), using a Delphi iterative process with a multidisciplinary panel of experts in wound healing, and subsequently revised in 2001 and 2006. The tool requires evaluation of 13 macroscopic wound characteristics. The BWAT includes location and shape (nonscored items), size, depth, edges, undermining or pockets, necrotic tissue type and amount, exudate type and amount, surrounding skin color, peripheral tissue edema and induration, granulation tissue, and epithelialization. The 13 wound characteristic items appear with descriptors; nine characteristics are subjectively rated on a 1 to 5 scale,

with a value of 1 indicating the healthiest attribute and a value of 5 indicating the least healthy attribute of the characteristic. The remaining four characteristics (size, depth, edges, undermining) are rated from 0 to 5 with a value of 0 indicating "none present" and scored for wounds that have resolved. The 13 wound characteristic item scores can be summed (with no weighting) for a total score ranging from 9 (skin resurfaced) to 65 (profound tissue degeneration) (Bates-Jensen et al., 1992, 2019). It is recommended that wounds be scored initially for a baseline assessment and at regular intervals to evaluate therapy and healing progress. The BWAT is widely used in a variety of health care settings with all chronic wounds (Bolton et al., 2004; Carlson et al., 2017; de Laat et al., 2005; de Leon et al., 2009; Ebid et al., 2013)

An additional benefit associated with the assignment of numeric values to items on the BWAT is that it assists in setting interim wound healing goals. Clinical experience shows that not all wounds heal and certainly not always in the same setting. The BWAT allows for goal setting as appropriate to the health care setting and the individual patient and wound. For example, the patient with a large, necrotic, full-thickness wound in acute care will probably not be in the facility long enough for the wound to heal completely. The BWAT enables wound care nurses to set intermediate or secondary goals, such as "Necrotic tissue in the wound will decrease in amount and type." The BWAT allows for monitoring of improvement or deterioration in individual characteristics as well as the total score which enables assessment of the patient's response to specific treatments. For example, the characteristics of necrotic tissue type and amount may be tracked with exudate type and amount to evaluate the response to debridement or infection management. The ability to track wound symptoms such as exudate allows evaluation of interventions designed to alleviate distressing wound symptoms and as such is useful. Some investigators have also used subsets of BWAT characteristics to evaluate certain effects of treatments. For example, McCallon and Frilot (2015) used the BWAT total score and specific necrotic tissue characteristics to evaluate the effects of clostridial collagenase ointment and negative pressure wound therapy on healing of chronic PrIs. The BWAT has also been used by investigators to specifically profile wounds. For example, Paul (2013) used the BWAT to assess characteristics of wounds that itch and others have used the BWAT to examine characteristics of recurrent PrI (Bates-Jensen et al., 2009a, 2009b; Guihan et al., 2014).

There is also a pictorial guide for training health professionals in use of the BWAT (Harris et al., 2010). The BWAT Pictorial Guide includes 102 photographs of a variety of wound types, not just PrIs, illustrating each descriptor for each of the BWAT items. Validation of the photographic content was accomplished in a three-stage

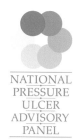

Pressure Ulcer Scale for Healing (PUSH)
PUSH Tool 3.0

Patient Name_____ Patient ID# _____

Ulcer Location _____ Date _____

Directions:

Observe and measure the pressure ulcer. Categorize the ulcer with respect to surface area, exudate, and type of wound tissue. Record a sub-score for each of these ulcer characteristics. Add the sub-scores to obtain the total score. A comparison of total scores measured over time provides an indication of the improvement or deterioration in pressure ulcer healing.

	0	1	2	3	4	5	Sub-score
LENGTH ✕ **WIDTH** (in cm²)	0	< 0.3	0.3 – 0.6	0.7 – 1.0	1.1 – 2.0	2.1 – 3.0	
		6	7	8	9	10	
		3.1 – 4.0	4.1 – 8.0	8.1 – 12.0	12.1 – 24.0	> 24.0	
EXUDATE AMOUNT	0 None	1 Light	2 Moderate	3 Heavy			Sub-score
TISSUE TYPE	0 Closed	1 Epithelial Tissue	2 Granulation Tissue	3 Slough	4 Necrotic Tissue		Sub-score
							TOTAL SCORE

Length ë Width: Measure the greatest length (head to toe) and the greatest width (side to side) using a centimeter ruler. Multiply these two measurements (length x width) to obtain an estimate of surface area in square centimeters (cm²). Caveat: Do not guess! Always use a centimeter ruler and always use the same method each time the ulcer is measured.

Exudate Amount: Estimate the amount of exudate (drainage) present after removal of the dressing and before applying any topical agent to the ulcer. Estimate the exudate (drainage) as none, light, moderate, or heavy.

Tissue Type: This refers to the types of tissue that are present in the wound (ulcer) bed. Score as a "4" if there is any necrotic tissue present. Score as a "3" if there is any amount of slough present and necrotic tissue is absent. Score as a "2" if the wound is clean and contains granulation tissue. A superficial wound that is reepithelializing is scored as a "1". When the wound is closed, score as a "0".

4 – **Necrotic Tissue (Eschar):** black, brown, or tan tissue that adheres firmly to the wound bed or ulcer edges and may be either firmer or softer than surrounding skin.

3   **Slough:** yellow or white tissue that adheres to the ulcer bed in strings or thick clumps, or is mucinous.

2 – **Granulation Tissue:** pink or beefy red tissue with a shiny, moist, granular appearance.

1 – **Epithelial Tissue:** for superficial ulcers, new pink or shiny tissue (skin) that grows in from the edges or as islands on the ulcer surface.

0 – **Closed/Resurfaced:** the wound is completely covered with epithelium (new skin).

www.npuap.org
11F

PUSH Tool Version 3.0: 9/15/98
©National Pressure Ulcer Advisory Panel

FIGURE 4-13. PUSH Tool. (Used with permission of the National Pressure Ulcer Advisory Panel, European Pressure Ulcer Advisory Panel & Pan Pacific Pressure Injury Alliance [NPUAP/EPUAP/PPPIA]. (2014). Prevention and treatment of pressure ulcers. In E. Haesler (Ed.), *Clinical Practice Guideline*. Perth, Australia: Cambridge Media.)

BATES-JENSEN WOUND ASSESSMENT TOOL
Instructions for use

General Guidelines:

Fill out the attached rating sheet to assess a wound's status after reading the definitions and methods of assessment described below. Evaluate once a week and whenever a change occurs in the wound. Rate according to each item by picking the response that best describes the wound and entering that score in the item score column for the appropriate date. When you have rated the wound on all items, determine the total score by adding together the 13-item scores. The HIGHER the total score, the more severe the wound status. Plot total score on the Wound Status Continuum to determine progress. If the wound has healed/resolved, score items 1, 2, 3 and 4 as = 0.

Specific Instructions:

1. **Size**: Use ruler to measure the longest and widest aspect of the wound surface in centimeters; multiply length × width. Score as = 0 if wound healed/resolved.

2. **Depth**: Pick the depth, thickness, most appropriate to the wound using these additional descriptions, score as = 0 if wound healed/resolved:

    1 =   tissues damaged but no break in skin surface.
    2 =   superficial, abrasion, blister or shallow crater. Even with, &/or elevated above skin surface (e.g., hyperplasia).
    3 =   deep crater with or without undermining of adjacent tissue.
    4 =   visualization of tissue layers not possible due to necrosis.
    5 =   supporting structures include tendon, joint capsule.

3. **Edges**: Score as = 0 if wound healed/resolved. Use this guide:

Indistinct, diffuse	=	unable to clearly distinguish wound outline.
Attached	=	even or flush with wound base, <u>no</u> sides or walls present; flat.
Not attached	=	sides or walls <u>are</u> present; floor or base of wound is deeper than edge.
Rolled under, thickened	=	soft to firm and flexible to touch.
Hyperkeratosis	=	callous-like tissue formation around wound & at edges.
Fibrotic, scarred	=	hard, rigid to touch.

4. **Undermining**: Score as = 0 if wound healed/resolved. Assess by inserting a cotton tipped applicator under the wound edge; advance it as far as it will go without using undue force; raise the tip of the applicator so it may be seen or felt on the surface of the skin; mark the surface with a pen; measure the distance from the mark on the skin to the edge of the wound. Continue process around the wound. Then use a transparent metric measuring guide with concentric circles divided into 4 (25%) pie-shaped quadrants to help determine percent of wound involved.

5. **Necrotic Tissue Type**: Pick the type of necrotic tissue that is <u>predominant</u> in the wound according to color, consistency and adherence using this guide:

White/gray non-viable tissue	=	may appear prior to wound opening; skin surface is white or gray.
Non-adherent, yellow slough	=	thin, mucinous substance; scattered throughout wound bed; easily separated from wound tissue.
Loosely adherent, yellow slough	=	thick, stringy, clumps of debris; attached to wound tissue.
Adherent, soft, black eschar	=	soggy tissue; strongly attached to tissue in center or base of wound.
Firmly adherent, hard/black eschar	=	firm, crusty tissue; strongly attached to wound base <u>and</u> edges (like a hard scab).

© 2001 Barbara Bates-Jensen

FIGURE 4-14. Bates-Jensen Wound Assessment Tool (BWAT). (Copyright © 2006 Barbara Bates-Jensen.)

6.   **Necrotic Tissue Amount**: Use a transparent metric measuring guide with concentric circles divided into 4 (25%) pie-shaped quadrants to help determine percent of wound involved.

7.   **Exudate Type**: Some dressings interact with wound drainage to produce a gel or trap liquid. Before assessing exudate type, gently cleanse wound with normal saline or water. Pick the exudate type that is <u>predominant</u> in the wound according to color and consistency, using this guide:

Bloody	=	thin, bright red
Serosanguineous	=	thin, watery pale red to pink
Serous	=	thin, watery, clear
Purulent	=	thin or thick, opaque tan to yellow or green may have offensive odor

8.   **Exudate Amount**: Use a transparent metric measuring guide with concentric circles divided into 4 (25%) pie-shaped quadrants to determine percent of dressing involved with exudate. Use this guide:

None	=	wound tissues dry.
Scant	=	wound tissues moist; no measurable exudate.
Small	=	wound tissues wet; moisture evenly distributed in wound; drainage involves ≤ 25% dressing.
Moderate	=	wound tissues saturated; drainage may or may not be evenly distributed in wound; drainage involves > 25% to ≤ 75% dressing.
Large	=	wound tissues bathed in fluid; drainage freely expressed; may or may not be evenly distributed in wound; drainage involves > 75% dressing.

9.   **Skin Color Surrounding Wound**: Assess tissues within 4 cm of wound edge. Dark-skinned persons show the colors "bright red" and "dark red" as a deepening of normal ethnic skin color or a purple hue. As healing occurs in dark-skinned persons, the new skin is pink and may never darken.

10.   **Peripheral Tissue Edema & Induration**: Assess tissues within 4 cm of wound edge. Non-pitting edema appears as skin that is shiny and taut. Identify pitting edema by firmly pressing a finger down into the tissues and waiting for 5 seconds, on release of pressure, tissues fail to resume previous position and an indentation appears. Induration is abnormal firmness of tissues with margins. Assess by gently pinching the tissues. Induration results in an inability to pinch the tissues. Use a transparent metric measuring guide to determine how far edema or induration extends beyond wound.

11.   **Granulation Tissue**: Granulation tissue is the growth of small blood vessels and connective tissue to fill in full thickness wounds. Tissue is healthy when bright, beefy red, shiny and granular with a velvety appearance. Poor vascular supply appears as pale pink or blanched to dull, dusky red color.

12.   **Epithelialization**: Epithelialization is the process of epidermal resurfacing and appears as pink or red skin. In partial thickness wounds it can occur throughout the wound bed as well as from the wound edges. In full thickness wounds it occurs from the edges only. Use a transparent metric measuring guide with concentric circles divided into 4 (25%) pie-shaped quadrants to help determine percent of wound involved and to measure the distance the epithelial tissue extends into the wound.

FIGURE 4-14 (*Continued*)

BATES-JENSEN WOUND ASSESSMENT TOOL   NAME

Complete the rating sheet to assess wound status. Evaluate each item by picking the response that best describes the wound and entering the score in the item score column for the appropriate date. If the wound has healed/resolved, score items 1,2,3, & 4 as =0.

Location: Anatomic site. Circle, identify right **(R)** or left **(L)** and use **"X"** to mark site on body diagrams:

____	Sacrum & coccyx	____	Lateral ankle
____	Trochanter	____	Medial ankle
____	Ischial tuberosity	____	Heel
____	Buttock	____	Other site: _____

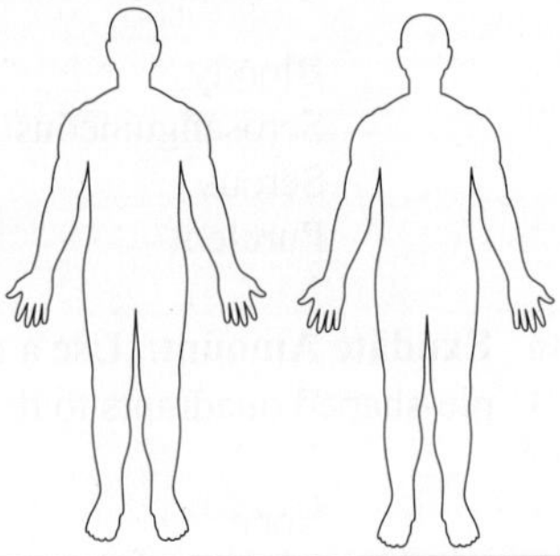

Shape: Overall wound pattern; assess by observing perimeter and depth.
Circle and <u>date</u> appropriate description:

____	Irregular	____	Linear or elongated
____	Round/oval	____	Bowl/boat
____	Square/rectangle	____	Butterfly Other Shape

Item	Assessment	Date Score	Date Score	Date Score
1. Size*	*0 = Healed, resolved wound 1 = Length x width <4 sq cm 2 = Length x width 4–<16 sq cm 3 = Length x width 16.1–<36 sq cm 4 = Length x width 36.1–<80 sq cm 5 = Length x width >80 sq cm			
2. Depth*	*0 = Healed, resolved wound 1 = Non-blanchable erythema on intact skin 2 = Partial thickness skin loss involving epidermis &/or dermis 3 = Full thickness skin loss involving damage or necrosis of subcutaneous tissue; may extend down to but not through underlying fascia; &/or mixed partial & full thickness &/or tissue layers obscured by granulation tissue 4 = Obscured by necrosis 5 = Full thickness skin loss with extensive destruction, tissue necrosis or damage to muscle, bone or supporting structures			
3. Edges*	*0 = Healed, resolved wound 1 = Indistinct, diffuse, none clearly visible 2 = Distinct, outline clearly visible, attached, even with wound base 3 = Well-defined, not attached to wound base 4 = Well-defined, not attached to base, rolled under, thickened 5 = Well-defined, fibrotic, scarred or hyperkeratotic			
4. Under-mining*	*0 = Healed, resolved wound 1 = None present 2 = Undermining <2 cm in any area 3 = Undermining 2–4 cm involving <50% wound margins 4 = Undermining 2–4 cm involving >50% wound margins 5 = Undermining >4 cm or Tunneling in any area			
5. Necrotic Tissue Type	1 = None visible 2 = White/grey non-viable tissue &/or non-adherent yellow slough 3 = Loosely adherent yellow slough 4 = Adherent, soft, black eschar 5 = Firmly adherent, hard, black eschar			
6. Necrotic Tissue Amount	1 = None visible 2 = <25% of wound bed covered 3 = 25% to 50% of wound covered 4 = >50% and <75% of wound covered 5 = 75% to 100% of wound covered			

FIGURE 4-14 (*Continued*)

Item	Assessment	Date Score	Date Score	Date Score
7. Exudate Type	1 = None 2 = Bloody 3 = Serosanguineous: thin, watery, pale red/pink 4 = Serous: thin, watery, clear 5 = Purulent: thin or thick, opaque, tan/yellow, with or without odor			
8. Exudate Amount	1 = None, dry wound 2 = Scant, wound moist but no observable exudate 3 = Small 4 = Moderate 5 = Large			
9. Skin Color Surrounding Wound	1 = Pink or normal for ethnic group 2 = Bright red &/or blanches to touch 3 = White or grey pallor orhypopigmented 4 = Dark red or purple &/or non-blanchable 5 = Black or hyperpigmented			
10. Peripheral Tissue Edema	1 = No swelling or edema 2 = Non-pitting edema extends <4 cm around wound 3 = Non-pitting edema extends >4 cm around wound 4 = Pitting edema extends <4 cm around wound 5 = Crepitus and/or pitting edema extends >4 cm around wound			
11. Peripheral Tissue Induration	1 = None present 2 = Induration, <2 cm around wound 3 = Induration 2–4 cm extending <50% around wound 4 = Induration 2–4 cm extending >50% around wound 5 = Induration >4 cm in any area around wound			
12. Granulation Tissue	1 = Skin intact or partial thickness wound 2 = Bright, beefy red; 75% to 100% of wound filled &/or tissue overgrowth 3 = Bright, beefy red; <75% & >25% of wound filled 4 = Pink, &/or dull, dusky red &/or fills ≤ 25% of wound 5 = No granulation tissue present			
13. Epithelialization	1 = 100% wound covered, surface intact 2 = 75% to <100% wound covered &/or epithelial tissue extends >0.5 cm into wound bed 3 = 50% to <75% wound covered &/or epithelial tissue extends to <0.5 cm into wound bed 4 = 25% to <50% wound covered 5 = <25% wound covered			
TOTAL SCORE				
SIGNATURE				

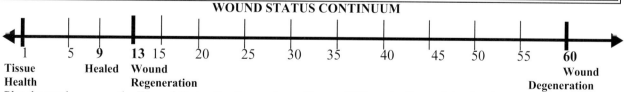

WOUND STATUS CONTINUUM

1   5   9   13   15   20   25   30   35   40   45   50   55   60

Tissue Health — Healed — Wound Regeneration — Wound Degeneration

Plot the total score on the Wound Status Continuum by putting an **"X"** on the line and the date beneath the line. Plot multiple scores with their dates to see-at-a-glance regeneration or degeneration of the wound.

FIGURE 4-14 *(Continued)*

consensus process working with nurses specializing in wound care.

In addition to being used to identify specific wound treatments, the BWAT has been used to describe characteristics of recurrent PrIs in persons with spinal cord injury as these ulcers have not been well described. Because the BWAT evaluates multiple wound characteristics, it is particularly well suited for describing specific wound characteristics in special populations or wounds. For example, recurrent PrIs in persons with spinal cord injury tend to occur at the same anatomic location as the original ulcer and present as full-thickness ulcers with a mean BWAT score of 33.63, with minimal exudate, and with nearly half presenting with undermining (48%) and necrotic slough (50%) (Bates-Jensen et al., 2009a, 2009b). The BWAT has also been used as an outcome measure examining the use of negative pressure wound therapy for PrIs in a long-term acute care setting (de Leon et al., 2009), and a change in total BWAT score at 1 week predicts 50% wound healing as evidenced by change in surface area (Bates-Jensen, 1999). The BWAT is incorporated into several health care organizational electronic medical records (EMR) and lends itself well to EMR in terms of data entry and data access for reports. The BWAT showed moderate to high reliability estimates (coefficients at or above r = 0.80) when used for assessment of PrIs of differing stages, at various anatomic locations, among different ethnicity/racial groups, and across all skin tones when used by non–health care workers (Bates-Jensen et al., 2019).

To assist clinicians in assessing wound bed preparation prior to application of advanced technology therapy, Falanga and colleagues developed the Wound Bed Score (WBS) to specifically address wound bed preparation (Falanga, 2008; Falanga et al., 2006). The WBS consists of a score for wound bed appearance (based on granulation tissue, fibrinous tissue, and presence of eschar) and a wound exudate score (based on exudate control, exudate amount, and dressing requirements). Additional items relating to the surrounding skin (healing edges, edema, periwound dermatitis, and callus) are also included. Each item receives a score from 0 (worst score) to 2 (best score) with all items summed for a total score. The WBS has been used in venous ulcers and correlated with healing (Falanga et al., 2006). The instrument can be used at the bedside to determine the likelihood that wound closure will occur. The higher the score, the more favorable the wound outcome and total scores are divided into four quartiles: scores up to 9, scores of 10 and 11, scores of 12 and 13, and scores of 14 to 16. For each quartile increase, there is a 22% increased chance of healing (Falanga et al., 2006).

Wound healing assessment tools provide a framework for assessment and documentation of wound healing, with an attempt at quantification of multiple wound characteristics. Thus, their use should promote more meaningful communication among health care professionals involved in wound care. An objective method of assessing wound healing and monitoring changes over time also allows for evaluation of the care plan and may be used to guide and direct therapy. For example, if a specific treatment modality is in use and the patient's wound status, as determined with the wound healing tool, has not changed in 2 weeks, reevaluation of the plan of care is warranted.

⬤ LABORATORY AND DIAGNOSTIC TESTS

Specific laboratory and diagnostic tests to be included in a comprehensive assessment include data on nutrition, glucose management, and tissue oxygenation and perfusion. Nutritional parameters typically include evaluation of serum albumin. Serum albumin is a measure of protein available for healing; a normal level is >3.5 mg/dL. Additional measures of nutrition include prealbumin levels and total lymphocyte count. Wound care nurses should evaluate laboratory values such as arterial blood gases and transcutaneous oximetry to assess tissue perfusion and oxygenation abilities. Review of laboratory values is also prudent in determining the level of diabetic control. Normal glucose levels are 80 to 120 mg/dL. Concentrations of 180 to 250 mg/dL or higher indicate that glucose levels are out of control. The goal is to maintain fasting blood glucose concentrations lower than 140 mg/dL and a glycosylated hemoglobin concentration (HgbA1C) lower than 7%. The HgbA1C helps to determine the level of glucose control the patient has had over the last 2 to 3 months. The wound care nurse should also evaluate hemoglobin and hematocrit for possible anemia; significant anemia compromises oxygen delivery to the tissues and mandates treatment in situations where the goal is wound healing. Wound culture and sensitivity is usually indicated when there is evidence of invasive infection and systemic antibiotic therapy is planned; the wound care nurse must assure that viable tissue is present in the wound bed and that the culture is obtained using accepted techniques (see Chapter 11).

Specific vascular studies should be reviewed for patients presenting with lower leg ulcers and diabetic foot ulcers (Bonham et al., 2016; Federman et al., 2016; Lavery et al., 2016; Marston et al., 2016; WOCN, 2019). Laser Doppler flow studies provide data on both arterial and venous systems and in particular microflow disorders (Belcaro et al., 2007; Ennis et al., 2012). For LEAD, arterial duplex scans, segmental pressures including toe pressures, pulse volume recordings, magnetic resonance angiography (MRA), and rapid sequence CT scans are noninvasive macrocirculation studies that may be ordered. An interventional angiogram and MRA are more specific diagnostic tests for LEAD.

Several diagnostic tests are available for evaluating patients with venous ulcer; the venous duplex scan to rule out venous reflux is essential and is the primary assessment tool (Ennis et al., 2012). Duplex scanning is a routine test used to rule out acute deep vein thrombosis in the hospital setting. Duplex scanning is noninvasive and portable, and accuracy is generally reported as over 90% for detecting femoral–popliteal thrombosis (Miller et al., 1996). There are four important components of all duplex scans, include visualization of the vein, compressibility of the vein wall, spontaneous venous flow, and the ability to augment flow with a compression force distal to the probe. Venous outflow can also be measured with impedance and/or strain gauge plethysmography (Hirai et al., 1985; Ting et al., 1999; WOCN, 2019).

BIOPHYSICAL SKIN AND TISSUE ASSESSMENT MEASURES

There are a variety of biophysical technology advances that enable clinicians to use devices in clinical practice for skin and tissue assessment. Use of biophysical measures may supplement and expand on visual and palpation assessment parameters. Use of thermography, ultrasonography, and subepidermal moisture measured with surface electrical capacitance have all demonstrated usefulness in skin and tissue assessment.

THERMOGRAPHY

Objective measure of skin and tissue temperature can be obtained using infrared imaging thermography devices. This technique can supplement skin temperature assessments. Cox and colleagues (2016) used infrared thermography to identify skin discoloration that advanced to deep tissue injury and necrosis. Discolored skin that was cooler in temperature was more likely to evidence necrosis within 7 days. Similarly, Farid et al. (2012) used a handheld infrared thermography device to supplement skin assessments and found lower temperatures in discolored skin compared to adjacent skin with normal coloration. Siah et al. (2019) used thermography to identify delayed healing in surgical wounds within 4 days after surgery and found a significant increase in wound temperature measured with infrared thermography for infected wounds compared to noninfected wounds. Others have also used thermography to detect inflammation and infection in patients with wounds (Chanmugam et al., 2017). Use of thermography to detect lower temperature at wound edges has been shown to predict undermining in PrIs (Kanazawa et al., 2016).

ULTRASONOGRAPHY

Ultrasound is a noninvasive biophysical measure that uses mechanical vibrations (acoustic therapy) to detect objects and measure distance. Ultrasound images have been used to measure tissue deformations and identify areas of pressure-induced tissue damage. Use of low frequency ultrasound has been used to identify deep tissue injury below intact skin, identifying muscle deformation associated with more severe PrI among elders at risk for PrI development admitted to the hospital via the emergency department (Scheiner et al., 2017).

Ultrasound has also been used as a noninvasive method of assessment of wound pockets to evaluate undermined tissues. Ultrasonography provides a visual picture of the impaired tissues and can be repeated to monitor for improvement (Ueta et al., 2011). Ultrasound has also been used to evaluate skin thickness over bony prominences in persons with spinal cord injury (Yalcin et al., 2013) and to detect heel PrIs in elders (Helvig & Nichols, 2012) and is responsive to changes in skin and tissues during PrI development (Kitamura et al., 2019). Key to using ultrasonography for skin and tissue assessment is access to someone with experience in obtaining and interpreting ultrasound images.

SUBEPIDERMAL MOISTURE

Subepidermal moisture (SEM) is a term coined in early studies of the relationship between edema and PrI development to describe edema present in tissues below the stratum corneum in order to differentiate from moisture on the surface of the epidermis (Bates-Jensen et al., 2007a, 2007b, 2008). The handheld instruments available to measure SEM do not differentiate the level at which the edema occurs in the tissues except as a reflection of the depth of tissue interrogation. These handheld devices detect and measure water or edema *below* the stratum corneum. Using dielectric parameters, high-frequency low power electromagnetic waves of 300 MHz are transmitted via an electrode that is manually placed on the skin. In the skin, the induced electrical field interacts mainly with water molecules closest to the electrode with depth of interaction depending on the diameter of the circular electrode on the wand (Alanen et al., 2004; Nuutinen et al., 2004; Zhang et al., 2014). The portion of the electromagnetic energy that is not absorbed by tissue water is reflected and measured by the same wand as used for wave transmission. Hydration of the skin and tissues is normal; however, inflammation associated with tissue damage increases SEM values. Gorelsky et al. (1995) used SEM measures to compare healing of split-thickness autografts to cultured skin substitutes in five patients with paired site comparisons. They showed that SEM values decreased as sites healed and epidermis matured, and SEM values approached levels seen for uninjured skin by 12 days. Mayrovitz and multiple colleagues demonstrated that SEM measures are useful to evaluate local tissue water and its change among healthy men and women of all ages, women with breast cancer awaiting surgery and with post breast cancer lymphedema, persons with and without diabetes mellitus and that it is only marginally responsive to changes in skin blood volume (Mayrovitz, 2007, 2010; Mayrovitz et al., 2008, 2013a, 2013b). Bates-Jensen and multiple colleagues have shown higher SEM values to be associated with and predictive of erythema and Stage 1 PrI damage at the trunk and heel locations among several populations including persons with dark skin tones and persons with spinal cord injury and using different devices to measure SEM (Bates-Jensen et al., 2007a, 2007b, 2008, 2009a, 2009b, 2017a, 2017b; Guihan et al, 2012). SEM has been used in hospitals to identify and predict PrIs and has decreased the incidence of hospital-acquired PrIs (Raizman, et al., 2018). SEM has been shown to identify PrI damage sooner than visual assessment or ultrasound evaluation (Gefen & Gershon, 2018; O'Brien et al., 2018).

Use of biophysical measures to supplement assessment of skin and tissues can provide important data on the health of skin and tissues as well as identify injury and damage that is unobservable visually. Biophysical measures have the advantage of not relying on the visual acuity or experience of the wound care nurse and provide objective reliable and actionable information.

 CONCLUSION

Accurate and comprehensive assessment of the individual with a wound is foundational to effective management. The initial assessment must include determination of wound etiology, assessment of the individual's ability to heal (systems review), determination of wound-related concerns and priorities from the perspective of the patient and caregiver, and in-depth assessment of wound status. Follow-up assessments focus on progress in wound healing. Structured wound assessment tools have been proven to be of significant benefit in objectively documenting progress (or deterioration) in healing.

REFERENCES

Alanen, E., Nuutinen, J., Nicklen, K., et al. (2004). Measurement of hydration in the stratum corneum with the Moisture Meter and comparison with the Corneometer. *Skin Research and Technology, 10*(1), 32–37.

Armstrong, D. G., & Harkless, L. B. (1998). Validation of a diabetic wound classification system. The contribution of depth, infection, and ischemia to risk of amputation. *Diabetes Care, 21*(5), 855–859.

Arnold, T., Stanley, J., Fellows, E., et al. (1994). Prospective multicenter study of managing lower extremity venous ulcers. *Annals of Vascular Surgery, 8*(4), 356–362.

Augustin, M., Baade, K., Heyer, K., et al. (2017a). Quality-of-life evaluation in chronic wounds: Comparative analysis of three disease-specific questionnaires. *International Wound Journal, 14*(6), 1299–1304.

Augustin, M., Conde Montero, E., Zander, N., et al. (2017b). Validity and feasibility of the wound-QoL questionnaire on health-related quality of life in chronic wounds. *Wound Repair and Regeneration, 25*(5), 852–857.

Bartolucci, A. A., & Thomas, D. R. (1997). Using principal component analysis to describe wound status. *Advances in Wound Care, 10*(5), 93–95.

Bates-Jensen, B. (1999). A quantitative analysis of wound characteristics as early predictors of healing in pressure sores. *Dissertation Abstracts International, 59*(11), Los Angeles: University of CA, Los Angeles.

Bates-Jensen, B., & McNees, P. (1995). Toward an intelligent wound assessment system. *Ostomy/Wound Management, 41*(Suppl 7A), 80–88.

Bates-Jensen, B. M., & McNees, P. (1996). The wound intelligence system: Early issues and findings from multi-site tests. *Ostomy/Wound Management, 42*(Suppl 7A), 1–7.

Bates-Jensen, B. M., & Sussman, C. (2012). Tools to measure wound healing. In C. Sussman, & B. M. Bates-Jensen (Eds.), *Wound care: A collaborative practice manual for health care practitioners* (4th ed.). Baltimore, MD: Lippincott Williams & Wilkins.

Bates-Jensen, B., Guihan, M., Garber, S. L., et al. (2009a). Characteristics of recurrent pressure ulcers in veterans with spinal cord injury. *The Journal of Spinal Cord Medicine, 32*(1), 34–42.

Bates-Jensen, B. M., McCreath, H. E., Harputu, D, et al. (2019). Reliability of the Bates-Jensen Wound Assessment Tool for pressure ulcer assessment: The pressure ulcer detection study. *Wound Repair and Regeneration, 27*(4), 386–395.

Bates-Jensen, B. M., McCreath, H. E., Kono, A., et al. (2007a). Sub-epidermal moisture predicts erythema and stage I pressure ulcers in nursing home residents: A pilot study. *Journal of the American Geriatrics Society, 55*, 1199–1205.

Bates-Jensen, B. M., McCreath, H., Pongquan, V. (2007b). Testing threshold values for sub-epidermal moisture: Identifying stage I pressure ulcers in nursing home residents. *L'escarre[French], 36*(4), 9–15.

Bates-Jensen, B. M., McCreath, H. E., Pongquan, V. (2009b). Sub-epidermal moisture is associated with early pressure ulcer damage in nursing home residents with dark skin tones: Pilot findings. *Journal of Wound, Ostomy, and Continence Nursing, 36*(3), 277–284.

Bates-Jensen, B. M., McCreath, H., Pongquan, V., et al. (2008). Sub-epidermal moisture differentiates erythema and stage I pressure ulcers in nursing home residents. *Wound Repair and Regeneration, 16*(2), 189–197.

Bates-Jensen, B. M., McCreath, H. E., Patlan, A. (2017a). Subepidermal moisture detection of pressure induced tissue damage on the trunk: The pressure ulcer detection (PUD) study outcomes. *Wound Repair and Regeneration, 25*(3), 502–511.

Bates-Jensen, B. M., McCreath, H. E., Nakagami, G., et al. (2017b). Sub-epidermal moisture detection of heel pressure injury: The Pressure Ulcer Detection study outcomes. *International Wound Journal, 15*(2), 297–309.

Bates-Jensen, B. M., Vredevoe, D., & Brecht, M. L. (1992). Validity and reliability of the pressure sore status tool. *Decubitus, 5*(6), 20–28.

Belcaro, G., Cesarone, M. R., Errichi, B. M., et al. (2007). Improvement of microcirculation and healing of venous hypertension and ulcers with Crystacide: evaluation with a microcirculatory model, including free radicals, laser doppler flux, and PO_2/PCO_2 measurements. *Angiology, 58*(3), 323–328.

Bieri, D., Reeve, R., Champion, G., et al. (1990). The Faces Pain Scale for the self-assessment of the severity of pain experienced by children: Development, initial validation, and preliminary investigation for ratio scale properties. *Pain, 41*, 139–150.

Black, J. (2018). Using thermography to assess pressure injuries in patients with dark skin. *Nursing, 48*(9), 60–61.

Blome, C., Baade, K., Debus, E. S., et al. (2014). The "Wound-QoL": a short questionnaire measuring quality of life in patients with chronic wounds based on three established disease-specific instruments. *Wound Repair and Regeneration, 22*(4), 504–514.

Bolton, L., Girolami, S., Corbett, L., et al. (2014). The Association for the Advancement of Wound Care (AAWC) Venous and Pressure Ulcer Guidelines. *Ostomy/Wound Management, 60*(11), 24–66.

Bolton, L., McNees, P., Van Rijswijk, L., et al.; Wound Outcomes Study Group. (2004). Wound-healing outcomes using standardized assessment and care in clinical practice. *Journal of Wound, Ostomy, and Continence Nursing, 31*(2), 65–71.

Bonham, P. A., Flemister, B. G., Droste, L. R., et al. (2016). 2014 Guideline for Management of Wounds in Patients With Lower-Extremity Arterial Disease (LEAD): An Executive Summary. *Journal of Wound, Ostomy, and Continence Nursing, 43*(1), 23–31.

Brandeis, G., Morris, J., Nash, D., et al. (1990). The epidemiology and natural history of pressure ulcers in elderly nursing home residents. *Journal of the American Medical Association, 264*(22), 2905–2909.

Cardinal, M., Eisenbud, D. E., & Armstrong, D. G. (2009a). Wound shape geometry measurements correlate to eventual wound healing. *Wound Repair and Regeneration, 17*(2), 173–178.

Cardinal, M., Eisenbud, D. E., Phillips, T., et al. (2008). Early healing rates and wound area measurements are reliable predictors of later complete wound closure. *Wound Repair and Regeneration, 16*(1), 19–22.

Cardinal, M., Phillips, T., Eisenbud, D. E., et al. (2009b). Nonlinear modeling of venous leg ulcer healing rates, *BMC Dermatology, 9*(1), 2.

Carlson, M., Vigen, C. L., Rubayi, S., et al. (2017). Lifestyle intervention for adults with spinal cord injury: Results of the USC-RLANRC pressure ulcer prevention study. *Journal of Spinal Cord Medicine, 17*, 1–18.

Centers for Medicare & Medicaid Services (CMS). (2009). Proposed Fiscal Year 2009 Payment, Policy Changes for Inpatient Stays in General Acute Care Hospitals. Retrieved from https://www.cms.gov/newsroom/fact-sheets/proposed-fiscal-year-2009-payment-policy-changes-inpatient-stays-general-acute-care-hospitals. Accessed January 27, 2020.

Chanmugam, A., Langemo, D., Thomason, K., et al. (2017). Relative temperature maximum in wound infection and inflammation as compared with a control subject using long-wave infrared thermography. *Advances in Skin & Wound Care, 30*(9), 406–414.

Cox, J., Kaes, L., Martinez, M., et al. (2016). A prospective, observational study to assess the use of thermography to predict progression of discolored intact skin to necrosis among patients in skilled nursing facilities. *Ostomy/Wound Management, 62*(10), 14–33.

de Laat, E. H., Scholte, O. P., Reimer, W. H., et al. (2005). Pressure ulcers: Diagnostics and interventions aimed at wound-related complaints: A review of the literature. *Journal of Clinical Nursing, 14*(4), 464–472.

de Leon, J. M., Barnes, S., Nagel, M., et al. (2009). Cost-effectiveness of negative pressure wound therapy for postsurgical patients in long-term acute care. *Advances in Skin & Wound Care, 22*(3), 122–127.

Ebid, A. A., El-Kafy, E. M., Alayat, M. S. (2013). Effect of pulsed Nd:YAG laser in the treatment of neuropathic foot ulcers in children with spina bifida: a randomized controlled study. *Photomedicine and Laser Surgery, 31*(12), 565–570.

Edwards, H., Courtney, M., Finlayson, K., et al. (2005). Improved healing rates for chronic venous leg ulcers: pilot study results from a randomized controlled trial of a community nursing intervention. *International Journal of Nursing Practice, 11*(4), 169–176.

Edwards, H. E., Parker, C. N., Miller, C., et al. (2018). Predicting delayed healing: The diagnostic accuracy of a venous leg ulcer risk assessment tool. *International Wound Journal, 15*(2), 258–265.

Engelhardt, M., Spech, E., Diener, H., et al. (2014). Validation of the disease-specific quality of life Wuerzburg Wound Score in patients with chronic leg ulcer. *VASA, 43*(5), 372–379.

Ennis, W. J., Borhani, M., &Meneses, P. (2012). Management and diagnosis of vascular ulcers. In C. Sussman, & B. M. Bates-Jensen (Eds.), *Wound care: A collaborative practice manual for health care practitioners* (4th ed.). Baltimore, MD: Lippincott Williams & Wilkins.

European Pressure Ulcer Advisory Panel, National Pressure Injury Advisory Panel, and Pan Pacific Pressure Injury Alliance [EPUAP/ NPIAP/PPPIA]. (2019). In E. Haesler (Ed.), *Prevention and treatment of pressure ulcers/injuries: Clinical Practice Guideline*. The International Guideline.

Falanga, V. (2008). Measurements in wound healing. *The International Journal of Lower Extremity Wounds, 7*(1), 9–11.

Falanga, V., Saap, L. J., Ozonoff, A. (2006). Wound bed score and its correlation with healing of chronic wounds. *Dermatologic Therapy, 19*, 383–390.

Farid, K. J., Winkelman, C., Rizkala, A., et al. (2012). Using temperature of pressure-related intact discolored areas of skin to detect deep tissue injury: An observational, retrospective, correlational study. *Ostomy/Wound Management, 58*(8), 20–31.

Federman, D. G., Ladiiznski, B., Dardik, A., et al. (2016). Wound Healing Society 2014 update on guidelines for arterial ulcers. *Wound Repair and Regeneration, 24*(1), 127–135.

Fink, R. M., Gates, R. A., Jeffers, K. D. (2019). Pain assessment. In B. R. Ferrell, & J. A. Paice (Eds.), *Textbook of palliative nursing* (5th ed.). New York, NY: Oxford University Press.

Freeman, K., Smyth, C., Dallam, L., et al. (2001). Pain measurement scales: A comparison of the visual analogue and faces rating scales in measuring pressure ulcer pain. *Journal of Wound, Ostomy, and Continence Nursing, 28*(6), 290–296.

Frescos, N. (2018). Assessment of pain in chronic wounds: A survey of Australian health care practitioners, *International Wound Journal, 15*(6), 943–949.

Gardner, S. E., Abbott, L. I., Fiala, C. A., et al. (2017). Factors associated with high pain intensity during wound care procedures: A model. *Wound Repair and Regeneration, 25*(4), 558–563.

Gardner, S. E., Blodgett, N. P., Hillis, S. L., et al. (2014). HI-TENS reduces moderate-to-severe pain associated with most wound care procedures: a pilot study. *Biological Research for Nursing, 16*(3), 310–319.

Gardner, S. E., Frantz, R. A., & Doebbeling, B. N. (2001). The validity of the clinical signs and symptoms used to identify localized chronic wound infection. *Wound Repair and Regeneration, 9*(3), 178–186.

Gardner, S. E., Hillis, S. L., & Frantz, R. A. (2011). A prospective study of the PUSH tool in diabetic foot ulcers. *Journal of Wound, Ostomy, and Continence Nursing, 38*(4), 385–393.

Gefen, A., & Gershon, S. (2018). An observational, prospective cohort pilot study to compare the use of subepidermal moisture measurements versus ultrasound and visual skin assessments for early detection of pressure injury. *Ostomy/Wound Management, 64*(9), 12–27.

Gorecki, C., Brown, J. M., Cano, S., et al. (2013). Development and validation of a new patient-reported outcome measure for patients with pressure ulcers: the PU-QOL instrument. *Health and Quality of Life Outcomes, 11*(1), 95.

Gorecki, C., Closs, S. J., Nixon, J., et al. (2011). Patient-reported pressure ulcer pain: A mixed-methods systematic review. *Journal of Pain and Symptom Management, 42*(3), 443–459.

Gorecki, C., Nixon, J., Lamping, D. L., et al. (2014). Patient-reported outcome measures for chronic wounds with particular reference to pressure ulcer research: A systematic review. *International Journal of Nursing Studies, 51*(1), 157–165.

Goretsky, M. J., Supp, A. P., Greenhalgh, D. G., et al. (1995). Surface electrical capacitance as an index of epidermal barrier properties of composite skin substitutes and skin autografts. *Wound Repair and Regeneration, 3*(4), 419–425.

Gould, L., Stuntz, M., Giovannelli, M., et al. (2016). Wound Healing Society 2015 update on guidelines for pressure ulcers. *Wound Repair and Regeneration, 24*(1), 145–162.

Green, C. R., Anderson, K. O., Baker, T. A., et al. (2003). The unequal burden of pain: confronting racial and ethnic disparities in pain. *Pain Medicine, 4*(3), 277–294.

Guihan, M., Bates-Jensen, B. M., Chun, S., et al. (2012). Assessing the feasibility of subepidermal moisture to predict erythema and stage 1 pressure ulcers in persons with spinal cord injury: A pilot study. *Journal of Spinal Cord Medicine, 35*(1), 46–52.

Guihan, M., Bombardier, C. H., Ehde, D. M., et al. (2014). Comparing multicomponent interventions to improve skin care behaviors and prevent recurrence in veterans hospitalized for severe pressure ulcers. *Archives of Physical Medicine and Rehabilitation, 95*(7), 1246–1253.

Gunes, U. Y. (2009). A prospective study evaluating the Pressure Ulcer Scale for Healing (PUSH tool) to assess stage II, stage III, and stage IV pressure ulcers. *Ostomy/Wound Management; 55*(5), 48–52.

Harris, C., Bates-Jensen, B., Parslow, N., et al. (2010). Bates-Jensen wound assessment tool: Pictorial guide validation project. *Journal of Wound, Ostomy, and Continence Nursing, 37*(3), 253–259.

Hazenberg, C. E., Bus, S. A., Kottink, A. I., et al. (2012). Telemedical home-monitoring of diabetic foot disease using photographic foot imaging—a feasibility study. *Journal of Telemedicine and Telecare, 18*(1), 32–36.

Hazenberg, C. E., Van Baal, J. G., Manning, E., et al. (2010). The validity and reliability of diagnosing foot ulcers and pre-ulcerative lesions in diabetes using advanced digital photography. *Diabetes Technology & Therapeutics, 12*(12), 1011–1017.

Hazenberg, C. E., van Netten, J. J., van Baal, S. G., et al. (2014). Assessment of signs of foot infection in diabetes patients using photographic foot imaging and infrared thermography. *Diabetes Technology & Therapeutics, 16*(6), 370–377.

Helvig, E. I. & Nichols, L. W. (2012). Use of high-frequency ultrasound to detect heel pressure injury in elders. *Journal of Wound, Ostomy, and Continence Nursing, 39*(5), 500–508.

Hirai, M., Yoshinaga M., & Nakayama, R. (1985). Assessment of venous insufficiency using photoplethysmography: A comparison to strain gauge plethysmography. *Angiology, 36*(11), 795–801.

Hon, J., Lagden, K., McLaren, A. M., et al. (2010). A prospective, multi-center study to validate use of the Pressure Ulcer Scale for Healing (PUSH(c)) in patients with diabetic, venous, and pressure ulcers. *Ostomy/Wound Management, 56*(2), 26–36.

Houghton, P. E., Kincaid, C. B., Campbell, K. E., et al. (2000). Photographic assessment of the appearance of chronic pressure and leg ulcers. *Ostomy/Wound Management, 46*(4), 20–30.

Iizaka, S., Kaitani, T., Sugama, J., et al. (2013). Predictive validity of granulation tissue color measured by digital image analysis for deep pressure ulcer healing: A multicenter prospective cohort study. *Wound Repair and Regeneration, 21*(1), 25–34.

Jesada, E. C., Warren, J. I., Goodman, D., et al. (2013). Staging and defining characteristics of pressure ulcers using photographs by staff nurses in acute care settings. *Journal of Wound, Ostomy, and Continence Nursing, 40*(2), 150–156.

Kanazawa, T., Kitamura, A., Nakagami, G., et al. (2016). Lower temperature at the wound edge detected by thermography predicts undermining development in pressure ulcers: A pilot study. *International Wound Journal, 13*(4), 454–460.

Kantor, J., & Margolis, D. J. (1998). Efficacy and prognostic value of simple wound measurements. *Archives of Dermatology, 134*(12), 1571–1574.

Kantor, J., & Margolis, D. J. (2000a). Expected healing rates for chronic wounds. *Wounds, 12*(6), 155–158.

Kantor, J., & Margolis, D. J. (2000b). A multicentre study of percentage change in venous leg ulcer are as a prognostic index of healing at 24 week. *British Journal of Dermatology, 142*, 960–964.

Kantor, J., & Margolis, D. J. (2000c). The accuracy of using a wound care specialty clinic database to study diabetic neuropathic foot ulcer. *Wound Repair and Regeneration, 8*(3), 169–173.

Kecelj Leskovec, N., Perme, M. P., Jezeršek, M., et al. (2008). Initial healing rates as predictive factors of venous ulcer healing: the use of a laser-based three-dimensional ulcer measurement. *Wound Repair and Regeneration, 16*(4), 507–512.

Kennedy, K. L. (1989). The prevalence of pressure ulcers in an intermediate care facility. *Decubitus, 2*(2), 44–45.

Kitamura, A., Yoshimura, M., Nakagami, G., et al. (2019). Changes of tissue images visualised by ultrasonography in the process of pressure ulcer occurrence. *Journal of Wound Care, 28*(Supp4), S18–S22.

Krasner, D. (1995). The chronic wound pain experience: A conceptual model. *Ostomy/Wound Management. 41*(3), 20.

Langemo, D. K., & Brown, G. (2006). Skin fails too: Acute, chronic, and end-stage skin failure. *Advances in Skin & Wound Care, 19*(4), 206–211.

Lantis, J. C., Marston, W. A., Farber, A., et al. (2013). The influence of patient and wound variables on healing of venous leg ulcers in a randomized controlled trial of growth-arrested allogeneic keratinocytes and fibroblasts. *Journal of Vascular Surgery, 58*(2), 433–439.

Laplaud, A. L., Blaizot, X., Gaillard, C., et al. (2010). Wound debridement: Comparative reliability of three methods for measuring fibrin percentage in chronic wounds. *Wound Repair and Regeneration 18*(1), 13–20.

Lavery, L. A., Davis, K. E., Berriman, S. J., et al. (2016). WHS guidelines update: Diabetic foot ulcer treatment guidelines. *Wound Repair and Regeneration, 24*(1), 112–126.

Levine, J. (2013). CMS recognizes the Kennedy Terminal Ulcer in long-term care hospitals. Retrieved from http://www.jeffreymlevinemd.com/unavoidable-kennedy-ulcer-in-long-term-care-hospitals/. Last accessed August 20, 2014.

Li, D., Mathews, C., Zhang, F. (2018). The characteristics of pressure injury photographs from the electronic health record in clinical settings. *Journal of Clinical Nursing, 27*(3–4), 819–828.

Manz, B. D., Moser, R., Nusser-Gerlach, M. A., et al. (2000). Pain assessment in the cognitively impaired and unimpaired elderly. *Pain Management Nursing, 1*(4), 106–115.

Margolis, D. J., Allen-Taylor, L., Hoffstad, O., et al. (2004). The accuracy of venous leg ulcer prognostic models in a wound care system. *Wound Repair and Regeneration, 12*(2), 163–168.

Margolis, D. J., Gelfand, J. M., Hoffstad, O., et al. (2003a). Surrogate end points for the treatment of diabetic neuropathic foot ulcers. *Diabetes Care, 26*, 1696–1700.

Margolis, D. J., Taylor, L. A., Hoffstad, O., et al. (2002). Diabetic neuropathic foot ulcer: The association of wound size, wound duration, and wound grade. *Diabetes Care, 25*, 1835–1839.

Margolis, D. J., Taylor, L. A., Hoffstad, O., et al. (2003b). Diabetic neuropathic foot ulcers: Predicting who will not heal. *The American Journal of Medicine, 115*, 627–631.

Marston, W., Tang, J., Kirsner, R. S., et al. (2016). Wound Healing Society 2015 update on guidelines for venous ulcers. *Wound Repair and Regeneration, 24*(1), 136–144.

Mayrovitz, H. N. (2007). Assessing local tissue edema in postmastectomy lymphedema. *Lymphology, 40*(2), 87–94.

Mayrovitz, H. N. (2010). Local tissue assessed by measuring forearm skin dielectric constant: Dependence on measurement depth, age and body mass index. *Skin Research and Technology, 16*(1), 16–22.

Mayrovitz, H. N., Davey, S., Shapiro, E. (2008). Local tissue water assessed by tissue dielectric constant: Anatomical site and depth dependence in women prior to breast cancer treatment-related surgery. *Clinical Physiology and Functional Imaging, 28*(5), 337–342.

Mayrovitz, H. N., Guo, X., Salmon, M., et al. (2013a). Forearm skin tissue dielectric constant measured at 300 MHz: Effect of changes in skin vascular volume and blood flow. *Clinical Physiology and Functional Imaging, 33*(1), 55–61.

Mayrovitz, H. N., McClymont, A., Pandya, N. (2013b). Skin tissue water assessed via tissue dielectric constant measurements in persons with and without diabetes mellitus. *Diabetes Technology & Therapeutics, 15*(1), 60–65.

McCallon, S. K., & Frilot, C. A. (2015). A retrospective study of the effects of clostridial collagenase ointment and negative pressure wound therapy for the treatment of chronic pressure ulcers. *Wounds, 27*(3), 44–53.

Merskey, H., & Bogduk, N. (1994). *Classification of chronic pain: Description of chronic pain syndromes and definitions of pain terms. IASP task force on taxonomy* (2nd ed.). Seattle, WA: IASP Press.

Miller, C., Karimi, L., Donohue, L., et al. (2012). Interrater and intrarater reliability of silhouette wound imaging device, *Advances in Skin & Wound Care, 25*(11), 513–518.

Miller, N., Satin, R., Tousignant, L., et al. (1996). A prospective study comparing duplex scan and venography for diagnosis of lower-extremity deep vein thrombosis. *Cardiovascular Surgery, 4*(4), 505–508.

Morin, C., Lund, J. P., Villarroel, T., et al. (2000). Differences between the sexes in post-surgical pain. *Pain, 85*(1–2), 79–85.

National Pressure Ulcer Advisory Panel, European Pressure Ulcer Advisory Panel & Pan Pacific Pressure Injury Alliance [NPUAP/EPUAP/PPPIA]. (2014). Prevention and treatment of pressure ulcers. In E. Haesler (Ed.), *Clinical Practice Guideline*. Perth, Australia: Cambridge Media.

Nix, D. P. (2016). Skin and wound inspection and assessment. In R. A. Bryant & D. P. Nix (Eds.), *Acute and chronic wounds: Current management concepts* (5th ed.). St. Louis, MO: Elsevier.

Nuutinen, J., Ikaheimo, R., & Lahtinen, T. (2004). Validation of a new dielectric device to assess changes of tissue water in skin and subcutaneous fat. *Physiological Measurement, 25*(2), 447–454.

O'Brien, G., Moore, Z., Patton, D., et al. (2018). The relationship between nurses; assessment of early pressure ulcer damage and sub epidermal moisture measurement: A prospective explorative study. *Journal of Tissue Viability, 27*(4), 232–237.

Paice, J. A., & Cohen, F. L. (1997). Validity of a verbally administered numeric rating scale to measure cancer pain intensity. *Cancer Nursing, 20*, 88–93.

Paul, J. (2013). Characteristics of chronic wounds that itch. *Advances in Skin & Wound Care, 26*(7), 320–332.

Price, P., & Harding, K. (2004). Cardiff Wound Impact Schedule: The development of a condition-specific questionnaire to assess health-related quality of life in patients with chronic wounds of the lower limb. *International Wound Journal, 1*(1), 10–17.

Price, P. E., Fagervik-Morton, H., Mudge, E. J., et al. (2008). Dressing-related pain in patients with chronic wounds: An international patient perspective. *International Wound Journal, 5*(2), 159–171.

Raizman, R., MacNeil, M., & Rappl, L. (2018). Utility of a sensor-based technology to assist in the prevention of pressure ulcers: A clinical comparison. *International Wound Journal, 15*(6), 1033–1044.

Ratliff, C. R. (2005). Use of the PUSH tool to measure venous ulcer healing. *Ostomy/Wound Management, 51*(5), 58–63.

Richardson, C. (2012). An introduction to the biopsychosocial complexities of managing wound pain. *Journal of Wound Care, 21*(6), 67–273.

Robson, M. C., Hill, D. P., Woodske, M. E., et al. (2000). Wound healing trajectories as predictors of effectiveness of therapeutic agents. *Archives of Surgery, 135*(7), 773–777.

Roth, R. S., Lowery, J. C., & Hamill, J. B. (2004). Assessing persistent pain and its relation to affective distress, depressive symptoms, and pain catastrophizing in patients with chronic wounds; a pilot study. *American Journal of Physical Medicine and Rehabilitation, 83*(11), 827–834.

Russell Localio, A., Margolis, D. J., Kagan, S. H., et al. (2006). Use of photographs for the identification of pressure ulcer in elderly hospitalized patients: Validity and reliability. *Wound Repair and Regeneration, 14*, 506–513.

Rutherford, C., Brown, J. M., Smith, I., et al. (2018). A patient-reported pressure ulcer health-related quality of life instrument for use in prevention trials (PU-QOL-P): Psychometric evaluation. *Health and Quality of Life Outcomes, 16*(1), 227.

Scheiner, J., Farid, K., Raden, M., et al. (2017). Ultrasound to detect pressure-related deep tissue injuries in adults admitted via the emergency department: A prospective, descriptive, pilot study. *Ostomy/Wound Management, 63*(3), 36–46.

Seiler, W. D., & Stahelin, H. B. (1995). Identification of factors that impair wound healing: A possible approach to wound healing research. *Wounds, 6*(3), 101–106.

Sheehan, P. J. P., Caselli, A., Gurini, J. M., et al. (2003). Percent change in wound area of diabetic foot ulcers over a 4-week period is a robust predictor of complete healing in a 12-week prospective trial. *Diabetes Care, 26*(6), 1879–1882.

Siah, C. R., Childs, C., Chia, C. K., et al. (2019). An observational study of temperature and thermal images of surgical wounds for detecting delayed wound healing within four days after surgery. *Journal of Clinical Nursing, 28*(11–12), 2285–2295.

Sibbald, R. G., Krasner, D. L., & Lutz, J. (2010). SCALE: Skin Changes at Life's End Final Consensus Statement: October 1, 2009©. *Advances in Skin & Wound Care, 23*(5), 225–236.

Simon, W., & Malabar, R. (1995). Assessing pain in elderly patients who can't respond verbally. *Journal of Advanced Nursing, 22*(4), 663–669.

Sobol-Kwapinska, M., Babel, P., Plotek, W., et al. (2016). Psychological correlates of acute postsurgical pain: A systematic review and meta-analysis. *European Journal of Pain, 20*(10), 1573–1586.

Sommer, R., Augustin, M., Hampel-Kalthoff, C., et al. (2017). The Wound-QoL questionnaire on quality of life in chronic wounds is highly reliable. *Wound Repair and Regeneration, 25*(4), 730–732.

Stotts, N. A., Puntillo, K., Morris, A. B., et al. (2004). Wound care pain in hospitalized adult patients. *Heart & Lung, 33*(5), 321–332.

Stotts, N. A., Rodeheaver, G. T., Thomas, D. R., et al. (2001). An instrument to measure healing in pressure ulcers: development and validation of the pressure ulcer scale for healing (PUSH). *The Journals of Gerontology. Series A, Biological Sciences and Medical Sciences, 56*(12), M795–M799.

Stuppy, D. J. (1998). The Faces Pain Scale: Reliability and validity with mature adults. *Applied Nursing Research, 11*(2), 84–89.

Taylor, L. J., Herr, K., & Paice, J. A. (2003). Pain intensity assessment: A comparison of selected pain intensity scales for use in cognitively intact and cognitively impaired African American older adults. *Pain Management Nursing, 4*(2), 87–95.

Terris, D. D., Woo, C., Jarczok, M. N., et al. (2011). Comparison of in-person and digital photograph assessment of stage III and IV pressure ulcers among veterans with spinal cord injuries. *Journal of Rehabilitation Research and Development, 48*, 215–224.

Thomas, D. R., Rodeheaver, G. T., Bartolucci, A. A., et al. (1997). Pressure Ulcer Scale for Healing: Derivation and validation of the PUSH tool. *Advances in Wound Care, 10*(5), 96–101.

Ting, A. C., Cheng, S. W., Wu, L. L., et al. (1999). Air plethysmography in chronic venous insufficiency: Clinical diagnosis and quantitative assessment. *Angiology, 50*(10), 831–836.

Ueta, M., Sugama, J., Konya, C., et al. (2011). Use of ultrasound in assessment of necrotic tissue in pressure ulcers with adjacent undermining. *Journal of Wound Care, 20*(11), 503–510.

Van Rijswijk, L. (1993). Full-thickness pressure ulcers: Patient and wound healing characteristics. *Decubitus, 6*(1), 16–21.

Van Rijswijk, L., & Multi-center leg ulcer study group. (1993). Full-thickness leg ulcers: Patient demographics and predictors of healing. *The Journal of Family Practice, 36*(6), 625–632.

Van Rijswijk, L., & Polansky, M. (1994). Predictors of time to healing deep pressure ulcers. *Ostomy/Wound Management, 40*(8), 40–48.

Wagner, F. E. W. (1981). The dysvascular foot: A system for diagnosis and treatment. *Foot & Ankle, 2*(2), 64–122.

Wang, S. C., Anderson, J. A., Jones, D. V., et al. (2016). Patient perception of wound photography. *International Wound Journal, 3*(3), 326–330.

Warriner, R. A., Snyder, R. J., & Cardinal, M. H. (2011). Differentiating diabetic foot ulcers that are unlikely to heal by 12 weeks following achieving 50% percent area reduction at 4 weeks. *International Wound Journal, 8*(6), 632–637.

Wewers, M. E., & Lowe, N. K. (1990). A critical review of visual analogue scales in the measurement of clinical phenomena. *Research in Nursing and Health, 13*, 227–236.

Wong, D., & Baker, C. (1988). Pain in children: Comparison of assessment scales. *Pediatric Nursing, 14*, 9–17.

Woo, K. Y. (2008). The relationship between anxiety, anticipatory pain, and pain during dressing change in the older population. *Journal of Wound, Ostomy, and Continence Nursing, 35*(3), S72.

Woo, K. Y. (2012). Exploring the effects of pain and stress on wound healing. *Advances in Skin & Wound Care, 25*(1), 38–44.

Woo, K. Y. (2015). Unravelling nocebo effect: The mediating effect of anxiety between anticipation and pain at wound dressing change. *Journal of Clinical Nursing, 24*(13–14), 1975–1984.

Wound, Ostomy, and Continence Nurses Society [WOCN]. (2016a). *Guideline for Prevention and Management of Pressure Ulcers (Injuries). WOCN clinical practice guideline series 2*. Mt. Laurel, NJ: Author.

Wound, Ostomy, and Continence Nurses Society [WOCN]. (2016b). *Pressure Ulcer Evaluation: Clinical Resource Guide*. Mt. Laurel, NJ: Author.

Wound, Ostomy, and Continence Nurses Society [WOCN]. (2019). *Guideline for Management of Wounds in Patients with Lower Extremity Venous Disease. WOCN clinical practice guideline series 2*. Mt. Laurel, NJ: Author.

Yalcin, E., Akyuz, M., Onder, B., et al. (2013). Skin thickness on bony prominences measured by ultrasonography in patients with spinal cord injury. *The Journal of Spinal Cord Medicine, 36*(3), 225–230.

Zhang, L., Liu, P., Dong, X., et al. (2014). A method for in vivo detection of abnormal subepidermal tissues based on dielectric properties. *Bio-Medical Materials and Engineering, 24*(6), 3455–3462.

QUESTIONS

1. A wound care nurse is performing a follow-up assessment of a patient's wound. What data would the nurse gather that is usually not included in the initial assessment?
   A. Wound etiology
   B. Systemic factors affecting the ability to heal
   C. Patient and caregiver goals
   D. Wound response to treatment plan

2. A wound care nurse gently pinches a fold of skin over the patient's sternum and notes how quickly it returns to normal. The nurse is assessing for
   A. Skin turgor
   B. Edema
   C. Capillary refill
   D. Erythema

3. The wound care nurse uses palpation to test a patient's skin for blanchability of an erythematous area. Which statement correctly identifies a key finding of this assessment?
   A. Blanchable erythema is indicative of some level of tissue damage and inflammation involving the skin and soft tissues.
   B. Blanchable erythema over a bony prominence is classified as a Stage 1 pressure injury.
   C. Erythema progressing from blanchable to nonblanchable signifies worsening skin condition.
   D. An area of erythema that is nonblanchable needs off-loading to monitor the intensity of the erythema.

4. Following a baseline skin assessment, a wound care nurse notes the following data: raised erythematous skin area on right forearm; lesions are 1.5 cm. What type of skin lesion would the wound care nurse document?
   A. Macule
   B. Patches
   C. Plaques
   D. Papules

5. The wound care nurse is documenting a pressure injury located on a patient's heel by using photography. Which of the following is a recommended guideline when using this technique?
   A. Take the photograph from different angles.
   B. Take a close-up photograph of the wound and a second showing the wound and body part.
   C. Place the patient in different positions for the photographs.
   D. Use a digital camera with a density of at least 6 megapixels.

6. A wound care nurse is assessing a patient who is receiving silver sulfadiazine as a topical therapy for a wound. For which adverse effect should the nurse monitor this patient?
   A. Allergic reaction
   B. Edema
   C. Erythema
   D. Fissures

7. The wound care nurse assesses a patient's wound as a shallow full-thickness wound. This classification indicates what type of tissue involvement?
A. Epidermis and part of the dermis
B. Epidermal, dermal structures, and subcutaneous tissues
C. Muscle and underlying structures
D. Epidermal tissue only

8. Which statement accurately describes a wound edge condition and its etiology?
A. Edges are distinct when there are areas where the normal tissues blend into the wound bed.
B. The edges of chronic wounds frequently are open and proliferative with thickening and fibrosis present.
C. Edges that are even with the skin surface and the wound base are attached to the base of the wound.
D. The wound that is a crater (bowl/boat shape with sides and depth) is a wound with edges that are attached to the wound base.

9. The wound care nurse is assessing tunneling in a patient's wound. Which step in the procedure is performed correctly?

A. The nurse inserts a cotton-tipped applicator under the edge of the wound and advances as far as possible.
B. The nurse uses a pen to make a mark on the applicator at the surface line of the wound.
C. The nurse determines undermining by noting the percent of the wound depth involved in the process and the distance the process extends from the wound base.
D. When documenting, the nurse distinguishes undermining as presenting with a narrow tract and tunneling presenting as a lip or pocket.

10. Which statement accurately describes the characteristics and implications of necrotic tissue in a wound bed?
A. Necrosis of muscle tissue typically results in the formation of stringy, yellow slough.
B. Consistency refers to the cohesiveness of the debris; typically more advanced necrosis is thin and wet.
C. A hard, crusty leathery eschar is not attached to the base and edges of the wound and is sometimes mistaken as a scab.
D. Color varies as necrosis worsens, from white/gray nonviable tissue, to yellow slough, and finally to black eschar.

ANSWERS AND RATIONALES

1. D. Rationale: Follow-up assessments provide comparison data, which allow clinicians to determine wound response to treatment.

2. A. Rationale: Skin turgor is a measure of skin hydration and is assessed by gently pinching a fold of skin (typically at the sternum or forehead) and noting how quickly it returns to baseline status.

3. C. Rationale: Nonblanchable erythema is indicative of tissue damage and inflammation involving the skin and soft tissues; nonblanchable erythema over a bony prominence or on the skin under a medical device is classified as a Stage 1 pressure injury.

4. C. Rationale: Macules and patches are erythematous flat skin discolorations (<1.0 cm and >1.0 cm, respectively), while papules or plaques

are raised erythematous skin areas (<1.0 cm and >1.0 cm, respectively).

5. B. Rationale: Take a close-up photograph of the wound and then a second photograph showing the wound and the body part. Try to take the close-up photograph from a standard distance from the wound.

6. A. Rationale: In conducting the health history, it is essential to ask about allergies, as there are a number of potential allergens in wound care products and topical antibiotics.

7. B. Rationale: Full-thickness wounds may be divided into shallow full-thickness wounds (those involving epidermal, dermal structures, and subcutaneous tissues) and deep full-thickness wounds (those involving muscle and underlying structures).

8. C. Rationale: Edges that are even with the skin surface and the wound base are attached to the base of the wound; this means that the wound is flat at the edge, with no appreciable depth.

9. A. Rationale: Undermining and tunneling are measured using a cotton-tipped applicator, which is gently inserted under the edge of the wound and, without undue pressure, advanced as far as possible; the tip of the applicator is then elevated so that it can be seen or felt on the surface of the skin.

10. D. Rationale: Color varies as necrosis worsens, from white/gray nonviable tissue, to yellow slough, and finally to black eschar.

CHAPTER 5

GENERAL PRINCIPLES OF WOUND MANAGEMENT: GOAL SETTING AND SYSTEMIC SUPPORT

Lee Ann Krapfl and Benjamin F. Peirce

OBJECTIVES

1. Use assessment data to determine the following:

   a. Factors causing or contributing to the alteration in skin/soft tissue integrity

   b. Potential for healing and any systemic conditions that would interfere with healing

   c. Wound characteristics (to include phase of wound healing) and implications for wound management

2. Establish appropriate wound care goals based on ability of the wound to heal and patient priorities.

3. Develop an individualized plan of care based on assessment data and current evidence-based

guidelines that addresses each of the following factors:

   a. Correction or amelioration of etiologic factors

   b. Attention to systemic factors affecting the repair process

   c. Evidence-based topical therapy

   d. Pain management

   e. Patient and caregiver education

4. Discuss challenges to seamless care and strategies to address those challenges.

TOPIC OUTLINE

● GOAL SETTING

Goal setting is a foundational first step in development of an effective plan of care. Goals should be established following comprehensive assessment and prior to care plan development. Redefining health care in terms of patient-centered goals focuses more on meaningful patient outcomes with greater emphasis on prevention. The role of patients within the wound care nurse-patient relationship would be strengthened with patient-centered goals which would improve quality of care (Mold, 2017). Patient and caregiver involvement in goal setting and care planning is essential, and patient involvement is mandated in various setting-dependent regulations. The reality is that patient involvement is often cursory; the result is that the wound care nurse's goals are not aligned with the patient's goals, and outcomes are compromised. Goals and care plan specifics must be mutual if the desired outcomes are to be achieved, because many components of the care plan are patient dependent and require the patient to modify lifestyle behaviors in order to manage the underlying disease process as well as the wound itself.

IMPACT OF CHRONIC DISEASE

Wounds are often manifestations of chronic disease. Goal setting and care planning must include measures to manage the chronic disease in addition to the wound. The first priority in wound management is correction of etiologic and contributing factors (Anderson & Hamm, 2014). For many of the most common and costly conditions associated with chronic wounds, patients need to modify and monitor behavior in three areas: medication management, diet, and lifestyle. Medications are important to managing the most common conditions including diabetes, cardiovascular conditions, and chronic obstructive pulmonary disease (COPD). Patients may be inconsistent with medication adherence due to socioeconomic issues. Osborn et al. (2017) surveyed 1,527 patients with acute coronary syndromes or acute decompensated heart failure to examine the relationships between financial strain, medication adherence, and self-rated health. In summary, having difficulty paying monthly bills determined medication nonadherence.

Dietary modifications related to caloric reduction, sodium and saturated fat restriction, and glycemic control can be challenging due to social and cultural pressures. Lifestyle modifications like increasing activity and smoking cessation involve altering long-term habits and maintaining new behaviors. While it is easy to prescribe lifestyle changes needed to improve health status, this approach is often unsuccessful. Changing these behaviors can be very challenging for patients and families. The wound care nurse should emphasize the impact of comorbid conditions on wound healing and negotiate realistic incremental goals with the patient according to patient priorities. For example, the patient with a neuropathic foot ulcer must be willing to consistently offload the ulcer. The patient is the sole support for the family and works as a chef. For this patient, making a living competes with the goal of offloading. The wound care nurse should establish an open and trusting relationship in order to assist the patient to prioritize goals and problem solve to establish realistic goals and a realistic care plan.

> **KEY POINT**
>
> Wounds are often manifestations of chronic disease; effective management requires a partnership between the wound care nurse and the patient.

One challenge in promoting effective self-management of chronic diseases is the insidious nature of disease progression and the cumulative and delayed effects of nonadherence to the plan of care. In general, nonadherence does not produce an immediate negative consequence. If the patient became violently ill following a deviation from the plan of care, that alone could prove to be a powerful motivator. In most cases, the negative effects of nonadherence manifest many weeks, months, or years later which can be a major barrier in getting patients to identify and change behavior. In the area of wound care, the effects of adherence or nonadherence may manifest quickly in terms of wound healing or deterioration. Setting short-term goals with the patient may be an effective strategy for wound healing. For example, the wound care nurse might conduct a thorough baseline assessment followed by a clear and open discussion with the patient regarding the elements of care required for wound healing. The wound care nurse might ask the patient if they would be willing to commit to 1 to 2 weeks of consistent compression to treat a venous ulcer. Within that time frame, there are signs of improvement such as less drainage and odor, decreased edema, and smaller wound measurements that reinforces the benefits of the recommended change in behavior.

> **KEY POINT**
>
> Working with patients to articulate realistic goals is both a science and an art. It requires knowledge of the various disease processes/comorbidities, effective communication skills, and the ability to educate and motivate in language the patient can understand.

TYPES OF GOALS

There are three types of goals related to wound management: wound healing, wound maintenance, and palliative care. When establishing a plan of care, it is essential to first determine whether or not wound healing is a realistic goal (Harries et al., 2016).

Healing

Wound care nurses are frequently confronted with wounds labeled as nonhealing, based on the fact that they have been open for a matter of weeks or months and have not closed using traditional strategies. The reasons for the failure to heal are varied but most often include failure to correctly identify and correct etiologic factors and/or inadequate attention to the systemic factors affecting the repair process. In most cases, when all of the etiologic factors have been accurately identified and addressed, systemic support provided, and topical care delivered, the wound will go on to closure.

Maintenance

Situations exist where the wound will never close, despite consistent appropriate management by the wound care nurse. This is usually due to inability to correct intrinsic or extrinsic factors (e.g., a spinal cord injured patient with a Stage 4 ischial pressure injury who seeks surgical closure but who refuses to stop smoking). A chronic wound determined to have a low probability of closure does not imply that the patient is at end of life. Patients and their caregivers can and do manage open wounds for years. For example, a wound with underlying osteomyelitis or a wound occurring in a previously radiated field may not close without surgical intervention. The patient who is at poor surgical risk or refuses surgical intervention needs to understand that wound closure is not a realistic goal. In these situations, wound healing is unlikely, and the goal becomes maintenance. The wound care nurse should work with the patient and caregiver to develop a plan of care that minimizes the risk of infection and prevent deterioration. This may be a lifelong issue for the patient and caregiver (Maida, 2013). Goals can be modified if there are changes in the patient's conditions; for example, changes in a patient's psychosocial situation may positively affect their ability and willingness to adhere to key elements of the management program.

Palliative Care

There are circumstances for which palliative care is the focus, such as when the chronic disease state is end stage and is no longer deemed responsive to medical treatment, or when the patient is terminally ill. In these situations, the focus of care should be based on the patient's and family's wishes for end-of-life care. In most cases, the primary goal of management becomes comfort; even if the patient retains some ability to heal, they may not live long enough to obtain wound closure. The individual may not wish to spend the final weeks of life focusing time, energy, and resources on their wound. An inappropriate focus on wound healing may result in expectations and care directives that adversely affect the patient's quality of life (Langemo et al., 2015). For example, frequent repositioning of an end-of-life patient may cause additional pain and distress for both the patient and family and may be contrary to the patient's and family's goals for end-of-life care. Wound care nurses should avoid establishing a healing goal without involving the patient and family in the goal-setting process. Wound care nurses are often asked to make recommendations for topical treatment when little healing potential exists. The wound care nurse should help the patient and caregiver set realistic

goals for palliative wound care including symptom management for pain, odor and drainage control. For additional information, see Chapter 35.

KEY POINT

There are three types of wound management goals: wound healing, wound maintenance, and palliative care.

When the wound care goal is maintenance or palliative, interventions should be focused on symptom alleviation (pain management, exudate containment, odor control, and bleeding prevention), prevention of infection, and establishment of simple, atraumatic care procedures. Expensive and complex treatment modalities are typically impractical and unnecessary. Select advanced wound care dressings might prove to be therapeutic in meeting palliative and maintenance goals by minimizing dressing changes, reducing pain, managing exudate, minimizing odor, reducing risk of infection, and minimizing bleeding and trauma (Woo, 2015).

Evaluation of the plan of care should be based on whether the symptoms are being successfully managed, rather than whether or not healing is occurring. While wound improvement or even healing does occasionally occur, it should not be the focus or the expectation of care in these situations. It is important for the wound care nurse to educate both the patient and caregiver that deterioration of the wound is not caused by any failure on the part of the patient or family, but on multiorgan failure. Reassurance by the wound care nurse that the patient is receiving quality care can lessen feelings of remorse.

KEY POINT

Even when wound healing is unlikely, it is possible to establish measurable goals and a plan of care that enhances quality of life.

 GENERAL PRINCIPLES IN TREATMENT PLANNING

Wound care is often focused primarily on topical treatment; this is only one element of comprehensive wound management. Some chronic wounds begin as minor traumatic injuries that would heal in a few days in a healthy individual but progress to serious nonhealing wounds in patients with underlying chronic disease (Demidova-Rice et al., 2012). Healing of these chronic wounds requires a comprehensive approach to management that includes correction of etiologic factors and attention to systemic factors that affect healing as well as topical therapy. Chronic wounds are complicated and challenging and are best managed with a holistic approach involving a variety of disciplines. A nonhealing wound is frequently indicative of underlying disease that is poorly controlled.

A comprehensive plan of care should address three areas: (1) correction of etiologic factors, (2) provision of systemic support for healing, and (3) topical treatment that creates and maintains an optimal healing environment. If all three areas are not addressed, healing will be jeopardized.

CORRECTION OF ETIOLOGIC FACTORS

Correctly identifying the etiology of the wound is key to developing a comprehensive management plan. Failure to adequately address the causative factor(s) will result in failure to heal, even if systemic support is provided and topical therapy is appropriate. Initial assessment and intervention must include identification of the etiologic factor(s) and initiation of measures to address those factors; for example, the most critical intervention in the management plan for a pressure injury is to eliminate or minimize the pressure that caused the wound. Typically, a thorough assessment of the wound and surrounding tissue provides definitive clues as to etiology, because most wounds present in a predictable location and with classic characteristics. It is important to obtain a detailed patient history when possible, because the patient history serves to confirm or correct initial impressions. In situations where the etiology is not clear, selected diagnostic tests or consults are necessary. **Table 5-1** provides a summary of the interventions required for the most commonly encountered wounds; the pathology, presentation, and management of each of these is covered in greater depth in upcoming chapters.

SYSTEMIC SUPPORT FOR HEALING

Wound healing is a systemic process that requires increased calorie, protein, and vitamin/mineral intake, sufficient blood flow and oxygenation to support the repair process, and relatively normal glycemic levels. Since many chronic wounds are associated with disease states impacting perfusion and oxygenation, nutritional status, and blood glucose levels, the body's ability to heal the wound may be significantly impaired; multiple poorly controlled comorbidities are also associated with compromised healing. Assessment and correction of systemic conditions that adversely affect repair is the second priority in wound management. **Box 5-1** lists factors to consider in providing systemic support for healing.

TABLE 5-1 CORRECTION OF ETIOLOGIC FACTORS	
ETIOLOGIC FACTOR	**INTERVENTIONS**
Pressure/shear	• Pressure redistribution surfaces for bed and chair • Routine repositioning to off-load bony prominences • Pad medical devices • Flotation of heels
Friction	• Gentle skin care and repositioning • Low friction coefficient (CoF) surface
Moisture-associated skin damage (MASD): • Incontinence-associated dermatitis (IAD) • Intertriginous dermatitis (ITD) • Periwound moisture-associated skin damage (PwMASD) • Peristomal moisture-associated skin damage (pMASD)	• Bladder/bowel management/toileting programs • Urine and stool containment (body worn absorbent products [BWAP], external collection devices [ECD]) • Skin care to include cleansing, moisturizing, and protection • Management of diaphoresis, skin fold management (intertrigo) • Management of microclimate
Lower extremity venous disease (LEVD)	• Leg elevation • Compression wraps/stockings • Increase activity/Walking program
Lower extremity arterial disease (LEAD)	• Vascular consult (revascularization) • Smoking cessation • Increase activity/walking program
Lower extremity neuropathic disease (LEND)	• Daily foot inspection • Routine nail care • Well-fitting protective footwear • Off-loading • Glycemic control
Autoimmune disease	• Anti-inflammatory agents (topical vs. systemic)
Infectious agents (bacterial, fungal, viral)	• Antimicrobial therapy (topical vs. systemic)

BOX 5-1   FACTORS TO CONSIDER IN PROVIDING SYSTEMIC SUPPORT

A. Tissue perfusion and oxygenation
B. Smoking cessation
C. Nutritional support
D. Glycemic control
E. Corticosteroids
F. Age and comorbidities

Tissue Perfusion and Oxygenation

Well-oxygenated blood and the ability to perfuse the tissues are critical to wound healing. Hypoxic cells cannot support tissue repair or defend against bacterial invasion; any condition that affects blood volume, oxygenation, or tissue perfusion compromises wound healing and places the patient at increased risk of infection. This includes such conditions as severe anemia, hypovolemia and hypotension, sepsis, lower extremity arterial disease (LEAD), edema, lower extremity venous disease (LEVD), severe COPD, and radiation damage (Kapetanaki et al., 2013; WOCN, 2014, 2019; Wright et al., 2014). Obesity should also be considered as a high-risk condition since adipose tissue is poorly perfused (Pierpont et al., 2014). In addition, many obese patients suffer from sleep apnea, which can further impact tissue oxygenation. Measures to improve perfusion and oxygenation must be individualized for the patient and the wound. For example, the patient with LEAD should be referred for vascular testing and possible revascularization procedures. General measures to improve tissue oxygenation include use of nasal oxygen for patients who are hypoxic, maintenance of adequate hydration to reduce blood viscosity, and management of edema through elevation and compression. Sleep apnea monitoring would be helpful in patients afflicted with this disorder.

Smoking Cessation

Rice et al. (2017) searched the Cochrane Tobacco Addiction Group Specialized Register and CINAHL in January 2017 to determine the effectiveness of nursing-delivered smoking cessation interventions in adults. Pooling 44 studies (over 20,000 participants) comparing a nursing intervention to a control or to usual care, the authors found that the smoking intervention increased the likelihood of quitting (RR 1.29, 95% CI 1.21 to 1.38). However, statistical heterogeneity was moderate (I^2 = 50%) and not explained by subgroup analysis so the authors concluded that there is moderate quality evidence that behavioral support by nurses to motivate and sustain smoking cessation can lead to a modest increase in the number of people who achieve prolonged smoking abstinence (Rice et al., 2017).

Cahill et al. (2014) summarized the efficacy and side effects of the three commonly used medications for smoking cessation incorporating data from 12 Cochrane reviews of 26 different treatments and using a network meta-analysis to make direct and indirect comparisons of efficacy. The three medications used to help people to quit were nicotine replacement therapy (NRT), bupropion, and varenicline. Combination NRT (using two NRT formulations simultaneously [e.g., patch and inhaler, patch and lozenge]) was associated with higher smoking cessation rates than single NRT formulations. NRT patches were similar in efficacy to NRT gum and other NRTs (e.g., tablets, lozenges, sprays, and inhalers). Varenicline was associated with higher smoking cessation rates compared with single forms of NRT (OR, 1.57 [95% CrI, 1.29–1.91]) and compared with bupropion (OR, 1.59 [95% CrI, 1.29–1.96]). Varenicline and combination NRT were associated with similar smoking cessation rates (OR, 1.06 [95% CrI, 0.75–1.48]). In summary, all three first line medications were associated with higher rates of smoking cessation compared with placebo. Varenicline and combination NRT were associated with higher rates of long-term smoking cessation than bupropion or single formulations of NRT.

There are many forms of tobacco on the market. People often think some forms are safe and do not cause health problems. This is not true. One large cigar can contain as much tobacco as an entire pack of cigarettes.

KEY POINT

There is no safe form of tobacco.

Using electronic or e-cigarettes is often called vaping or JUULing. JUUL is a certain popular brand of e-cigarette. The liquid in these devices is heated and creates an aerosol of tiny particles (sometimes called a "vapor") that is inhaled by users. Although the term "vapor" may sound harmless, the aerosol that comes out of an e-cigarette is not water vapor and can be harmful. E-cigarette vapor can contain nicotine and other substances that are addictive and can cause lung disease, heart disease, and cancer (Siegel et al., 2019). It is important to know that even though e-cigarettes do not contain tobacco, the Food and Drug Administration (FDA) classifies them as "tobacco products." Secondhand smoke (SHS) has the same harmful chemicals that smokers inhale. There is no safe level of exposure for SHS (American Cancer Society, 2019).

KEY POINT

Behavioral support by nurses to motivate and sustain smoking cessation can lead to an increase in the number of people who achieve prolonged smoking cessation.

Cannabis is the most commonly used illicit substance worldwide and the prevalence of users continues to increase with estimates that over 180 million people globally use cannabis for nonmedical, or recreational uses and that approximately 13 million people are dependent on cannabis (Bonomo et al., 2018). Over the past 20 years, there has been significant changes regarding cannabis for recreational and therapeutic use. Delta-9-tetrahydrocannabinol (THC) has been proposed to be beneficial for chronic pain, nausea and vomiting induced by chemotherapy, spasms reduction in multiple sclerosis, and reduction of Parkinsonian symptoms (Bonomo et al., 2018; VanDolah et al., 2019).

Cannabis also has a range of harmful effects and effects vary between products (e.g., smoking, vaporization, oromucosal sprays, sublingual preparations, capsules, oils, transdermal patches). Side effects such as panic attacks, short-term memory loss, tachycardia, or hypertension may occur even in recreational users (Bonomo et al., 2018; Subramaniam et al., 2019).

Cannabis is the most common illicit substance used by youth in the western hemisphere. Evidence indicates that frequent use of cannabis use during adolescence is associated with a range of adverse psychosocial outcomes including other substance use, poorer educational attainment, and mental health issues (Bonomo et al., 2018). Elderly individuals may also be sensitive to the cognitive effects of cannabis. There is growing concern that cannabis use may be associated with dementia. Cannabis has been associated with road traffic accidents and fatalities. The effects of cannabis on motor coordination, reaction time, and judgment are well documented. However, a definition of a threshold serum cannabinoid level that would be expected to impair most people's driving capacity is unknown. It is therefore important for wound care nurses to inform patients that driving is not recommended while taking medicinal cannabinoids (Bonomo et al., 2018).

Nutritional Support

The body requires essential nutrients to synthesize new tissue and fight infection; assessment of the patient's nutritional status and provision of the macronutrients and micronutrients required for repair is a critical aspect of wound management. Chapter 7 details the specific nutrients needed to support wound healing and provides step-by-step guidelines for nutritional assessment and intervention. Any patient with a wound requires adequate calories, additional protein, and sufficient intake of critical vitamins and minerals (e.g., vitamin C, zinc, and iron) (Kaminski & Drinane, 2014). Adding a multivitamin with a mineral supplement is sometimes recommended to ensure adequate intake of these micronutrients.

Allcott et al. (2019) studied the causes of "nutritional inequality" or that low-income neighborhoods are more likely to be "food deserts"—areas with low availability or high prices of healthy foods. The authors reported that exposing low-income households to the same products and prices available to high-income households reduces nutritional inequality by only about 10%, while the remaining 90% is driven by differences in consumer preferences. These findings counter the argument that policies to increase the supply of healthy groceries could play an important role in reducing nutritional inequality.

With any type of injury or infection, there is an increase in the metabolic rate and a resulting increased need for calories. Patients who are trying to heal open wounds should not be on a weight loss diet, as reduced caloric intake may also limit intake of essential nutrients required for wound healing. Caloric restriction should be recommended only in situations where the expertise of a registered dietitian is available.

Patients with chronic wounds should have their nutritional status evaluated. In some settings, such as home care, the nurse may be the person tasked with this assessment. Chapter 7 details the components of a nutritional assessment and provides guidelines the nurse can use to develop nutritional interventions. Strategies for obtaining accurate data regarding current intake include the 24-hour recall method (asking the patient to relay everything they ate or drank in the past 24 hours) and asking the patient to keep a diet journal for 3 days. In addition to assisting the wound care nurse to identify nutritional deficiencies, this journal may provide insight regarding ways to increase protein intake by modifying the foods the patient is already eating. For example, use of powdered milk is an inexpensive way to add protein to many foods, including creamed soups, cereals, puddings, and shakes.

Glycemic Control

Wound healing is frequently impaired in patients with diabetes mellitus (DM). For example, DM may result in vascular compromise that increases the risk for LEAD and impaired healing of lower extremity wounds; this is more common among individuals with long-standing and poorly controlled diabetes and will be discussed further in Chapter 26. The most common complication of diabetes is hyperglycemia, which negatively impacts bacterial balance and all phases of wound healing. Management of wounds in patients with diabetes should include measures to maintain normal blood glucose levels. Goals for glycemic control may be adjusted for life expectancy, comorbidities, and history of severe hypoglycemia. For younger patients with longer life expectancy, fewer complications and comorbid conditions, and no history of severe hypoglycemia, the American Diabetes Association (2019a) recommends the following: A1C 6.5% to 7.0% (mean plasma glucose 140 to 154 mg/dL). Older adults who are otherwise healthy with few coexisting chronic illnesses and intact cognitive function and functional status should have glycemic goals of A1C <7.5%, while those with multiple coexisting chronic illnesses, cognitive impairment, or functional dependence should have less stringent glycemic goals (such as A1C < 8.0% to 8.5%).

Measures for maintaining adherence to established goals include (1) self-monitoring and tracking of blood glucose levels, (2) adherence to the prescribed diet and exercise regimen, and (3) medication management. Effective self-management can slow the progression. Management is complex and requires a collaborative multidisciplinary approach (American Diabetes Association, 2019b). Individuals must assume an active role in their care to be successful. Providing self-management education and support are vital components of diabetes care, and the wound care nurse is in a key position to reinforce that education (Ha Dinh et al., 2016). Depending on the care setting, additional resources such as a dietitian and/or diabetes educator may be needed to assist with comprehensive assessment, teaching, and support. Patients must not only demonstrate the ability to correctly self-monitor their blood glucose but must also be able to use the results to adjust their medication, diet, and exercise therapy. Collaboration with the patient's primary physician is necessary to determine the desired A1C goals and to help the patient develop an algorithm for self-adjustment of insulin based on the results of blood glucose monitoring.

Different practice settings present unique opportunities and challenges. For example, in the acute care setting, diet and activity can be more closely controlled, blood glucose levels can be closely monitored, and medications adjusted. The challenge is to determine the patient's level of understanding and motivation for self-management post discharge. The home care or outpatient setting provides a better opportunity to assess the patient's ability to self-manage their diabetes.

Corticosteroids

Medications that suppress the body's immune response can impair wound healing. The therapeutic effects of these drugs block the normal inflammatory response, which is the first phase of wound healing (Wang et al., 2013). Evidence supports the use of vitamin A supplementation is to counteract the negative effects of steroids on wound healing. When considering supplementation, the potential benefits must be weighed against the risk of harm. Zinder et al. (2019) suggested 15,000 to 20,000 IU/day vitamin A orally for 14 to 21 days for patients on chronic steroids with wounds. The mechanism of action is not fully understood, since vitamin A has no beneficial effects in patients who are not taking steroids. Topical administration of vitamin A has numerous dermatology indications, but application directly on wounds has not been established as a treatment modality, despite some data to suggest it help in diabetic foot ulcer and venous leg ulcer (Zinder et al., 2019).

Patients on long-term steroids often have very thin and fragile epidermis, and striae. Minimizing the use of tapes and adhesive products in wound management reduces the risk of periwound medical adhesive-related skin injury (MARSI) (McNichol et al., 2013; Yates et al., 2017). The use of liquid skin protectants, adhesive remover/releaser products, tape anchors, surgical dressing holders, stretchable netting used as an alternate securement device, and silicone-based adhesives are all useful tools in protection of fragile skin.

Age and Comorbidities

Advanced age and the presence of comorbidities, such as renal or hepatic disease, may adversely affect wound healing. Healthy elderly people retain the ability to heal their wounds but age-related changes and delays occur in all phases of wound healing. In addition, advanced age is associated with a marked increase in the prevalence of comorbidities and use of medications that affect healing (Sgonc & Gruber, 2013). Any acute exacerbation in a systemic condition can cause a wound to stall or deteriorate. It is important to communicate with the patient that wound healing will be delayed. To promote wound healing in a patient of advanced age or with multiple comorbidities, the person's overall health must be optimized by reducing stress, managing pain, assuring adequate sleep, and increasing activity levels.

Evidence-Based Topical Treatment

Another component of a comprehensive plan of care is evidence-based topical treatment. Chapters 9 and 10 provide in-depth discussion and guidelines for wound cleansing, debridement, and dressing selection based on wound characteristics. The optimal dressing at the time of initial assessment may not be the best choice later; topical therapy must change as the wound condition changes. The goal is to manage exudate while maintaining a moist wound bed and to achieve optimal balance. In developing a plan for topical therapy, the wound care nurse should also consider the frequency of dressing change. Wound healing is disrupted whenever the dressing is removed, so reduced frequency of dressing changes may be beneficial to healing. Because the condition of the wound may change rapidly, topical therapy should be reevaluated frequently. Serial assessments are essential and should prompt adjustments in the topical therapy in response to changes in wound depth, exudate, and bioburden.

The importance of comprehensive serial assessments has implications other than modifications in dressing selection. Serial assessments are the basis for prompt recognition of a plateau in wound healing or deterioration in wound status. There is evidence to indicate that absence of progress for 2 to 4 weeks despite appropriate management mandates reassessment of the management plan (WOCN, 2017). Reassessment should include etiologic factors and systemic support as well as topical therapy. Reevaluate topical therapy including exudate management, maintenance of moist wound bed, protection of the healing wound from trauma and bacterial invasion, and control of bacterial burden. For example, in assessing the patient with a nonhealing sacral pressure ulcer, it is important to determine whether or not the wound is being consistently off-loaded, whether the patient has stopped smoking, and whether or not the patient's nutritional intake provides adequate support for healing. Changing the topical dressing will not provide healing if the patient does not adhere to the other elements of the plan of care. Engaging the patient in a meaningful discussion of the factors delaying healing, the patient's role in managing those factors, the barriers to their adherence, and strategies for overcoming those barriers may help the patient achieve their overall goals and promote wound healing.

 CARE TRANSITIONS

The patient with a wound may transition from acute care to home health or outpatient care, and care for the same wound may be delivered by many different practitioners in varied practice settings. The Transitional Care Model (TCM) is an advanced practice nurse (APN) led, team-based, care management model designed to improve outcomes of at risk older adults throughout acute care transitions. In multiple NIH-funded randomized controlled trials and comparative effectiveness studies, the TCM has consistently been demonstrated to enhance older adults' care experiences and improve their health and quality of life while decreasing use of costly health care services (Hirschman et al., 2015; Naylor et al., 2018).

With the aging population increasing, seamless transition of care is crucial to reduce complications and prevent readmissions (Mansukhani et al., 2015). Almost two out of five surgeries are performed on patients over 65 years of age. It has been calculated that about 40% of hospitalized patients over 85 years of age in United States are discharged to a skilled nursing facility. Selecting the appropriate the care setting is important to avoid frequent and preventable readmissions to hospital (Rennke et al., 2013; Zurlo & Zuliani, 2018).

The goal is to make the transition from one care setting and provider to another care setting and provider as seamless as possible. The two processes (planning for discharge and transitional care) constitute a continuum; one (transitional care) cannot be properly conducted without having adequately dealt with the other (discharge planning) (Zurlo & Zuliani, 2018).

To reduce the risk of negative outcomes when discharging patients consider the following:

1. Assessment of the clinical/social/care conditions
2. Expectations of the patient/caregivers
3. Formalization of teams designated to planning and coordination of discharge
4. Knowledge of programs of transitional care, and
5. Good communication/information in patient's transition between facilities (Zurlo & Zuliani, 2018).

The wound care nurse works with the multidisciplinary health care teams across care settings to provide seamless transitions of the wound care plan within the agency and across health care agencies. The wound care nurse provides direct patient care and instructs nonwound care nurses on wound care using procedures, guidelines, and protocols. Agencies who have a wound care nurse are able to provide optimal care, often achieving better patient outcomes. It is estimated that only 10% of all WOC nurses work in home health agencies (WOCN, 2016).

Wound care nurses can help improve continuity of care for patients transitioning to another care setting by considering product availability in the next setting when coordinating discharge plans and discharge wound care orders. If the patients will be purchasing their own supplies, it is important to consider the patient's financial resources (including third-party payer coverage), and any preferred provider for durable medical equipment (DME) and wound care supplies, including dressings. Wound care can take place in a variety of settings which will affect cost of treatment, such as in a hospital, outpatient department, home-care facility, or an ambulatory clinic. For instance, the cost of treatment might be higher in a hospital setting in contrast to an outpatient setting (Al-Gharibi et al., 2018).

A treatment is considered cost-effective only if it is economical in terms of both time and money. The duration of treatment is often directly linked with costs as the shorter the duration of treatment, the less expensive the total costs of treatment. However, apart from increasing the rate of wound healing, a treatment may also be economical in that it reduces the number of wound dressing changes needed or decreases the time required to apply the dressing (Al-Gharibi et al., 2018).

COMMUNITY RESOURCES

If the patient lacks insurance and other financial resources, there may be resources available in the community to assist the patient and product assistance programs. For example, there may be a chapter of the American Cancer Society, hospice, or a church-based lending closet that may have access to dressings and wound care supplies. Local nonprofit organizations may be able to assist with the costs of transportation and wound care supplies. Urban areas may have low or no-cost community health clinics that can offer support.

Advanced wound care products may not be available for every patient. For patients with minimal resources for maintenance wounds, dressings may be simplified to include easily accessible and low cost items, such as disposable diapers or feminine hygiene pads to manage exudate. Clothing items (e.g., socks, compression shorts, sports bras) can be modified to secure dressings.

 CONCLUSION

Effective patient-centered wound care involves establishment of goals (healing vs. maintenance or palliative). When the goal is healing, the wound care nurse must develop a plan of care that includes identification and mitigation of etiologic factors, systemic factors and conditions affecting repair, and provision of evidence-based topical therapy. The wound care nurse contributes to seamless care transitions with good communication and information.

REFERENCES

Al-Gharibi, K. A., Sharstha, S., & Al-Faras, M. A. (2018). Cost-effectiveness of wound care: A concept analysis. *Sultan Qaboos University Medical Journal, 18*(4), e433–e439. doi: 10.18295/squmj.2018.18.04.002.

Allcott, H., Diamond, R., Dubé, J., et al. (2019). Food deserts and the causes of nutritional inequality. *The Quarterly Journal of Economics, 134*(4), 1793–1884.

American Cancer Society. (2019). Is any type of smoking safe? Retrieved from https://www.cancer.org/cancer/cancer-causes/tobacco-and-cancer/is-any-type-of-smoking-safe.html. Accessed on February 15, 2020.

American Diabetes Association. (2019a). Comprehensive medical evaluation and assessment of comorbidities: Standards of medical care in diabetes—2019. *Diabetes Care, 42*(Suppl 1), S34–S45.

American Diabetes Association. (2019b). Standards of Medical Care in Diabetes. Retrieved February 2, 2020, from http://care.diabetesjournals.org/content/42/Supplement_1

Anderson, K., & Hamm, R. L. (2014). Factors that impair wound healing. *The Journal of the American College of Clinical Wound Specialists, 4*(4), 84–91. doi: 10.1016/j.jccw.2014.03.001.

Bonomo, Y., Souza, J., Jackson, A., et al. (2018). Clinical issues in cannabis use. *British Journal of Clinical Pharmacology, 84*(11), 2495–2498. doi: 10.1111/bcp.13703.

Cahill, K., Stevens, S., & Lancaster, T. (2014). Pharmacological treatments for smoking cessation. *JAMA, 311*(2), 193–194. doi: 10.1001/jama.2013.283787.

Demidova-Rice, T. N., Hamblin, M. R., & Herman, I. M. (2012). Acute and impaired wound healing: Pathophysiology and current methods for drug delivery. Part 1: Normal and chronic wounds: Biology, causes and approaches to care. *Advances in Skin & Wound Care, 25*(7), 304–314.

Ha Dinh, T. T., Bonner, A., Clark, R., et al. (2016). The effectiveness of the teach-back method on adherence and self-management in health education for people with chronic disease: A systematic review. *JBI Database of Systematic Reviews and Implementation Reports, 14*(1), 210–247.

Harries, R. L., Bosanquet, D. C., & Harding, K. G. (2016). Wound bed preparation: TIME for an update. *International Wound Journal, 13*(Suppl 3), 8–14. doi: 10.1111/iwj.12662.

Hirschman, K., Shaid, E., McCauley, K., et al. (2015). Continuity of care: The transitional care model. *The Online Journal of Issues in Nursing, 20*(3). Retrieved from http://ojin.nursingworld.org/MainMenuCategories/ANAMarketplace/ANAPeriodicals/OJIN/TableofContents/Vol-20-2015/No3-Sept-2015/Continuity-of-Care-Transitional-Care-Model.html

Kaminski, M. V., & Drinane, J. J. (2014). Learning the oral and cutaneous signs of micronutrient deficiencies. *Journal of Wound Ostomy & Continence Nursing, 41*(2), 127–135.

Kapetanaki, M. G., Mora, A. L., & Rojas, M. (2013). Influence of age on wound healing and fibrosis. *Journal of Pathology, 229*(2), 310–322. Retrieved from http://onlinelibrary.wiley.com/doi/10.1002/path.4122/full

Langemo, D., Haesler, E., Naylor, W., et al. (2015). Evidence-based guidelines for pressure ulcer management at the end of life. *International Journal of Palliative Nursing, 21*(5), 225–232.

Maida, V. (2013). Wound management in patients with advanced illness. *Current Opinion in Supportive and Palliative Care, 7*(1), 73–79.

Mansukhani, R., Bridgeman, M., Candelario, D., et al. (2015). Exploring transitional care: Evidence-based strategies for improving provider communication and reducing readmissions. *Pharmacy and Therapeutics, 40*(10), 690–694.

McNichol, L., Lund, C., Rosen, T., et al. (2013). Medical adhesives and patient safety: state of the science consensus statements for the assessment, prevention, and treatment of adhesive-related skin injuries. *Journal of Wound Ostomy & Continence Nursing, 40*(4), 365–380.

Mold, J. (2017). Goal-directed health care: Redefining health and health care in the era of value-based care. *Cureus, 9*(2), e1043. doi: 10.7759/cureus.1043.

Naylor, M. D., Hirschman, K. B., Toles, M. P., et al. (2018). Adaptations of the evidence-based Transitional Care Model in the U.S. *Social Science & Medicine, 213*, 28–36. doi: 10.1016/j.socscimed.2018.07.023.

Osborn, C. Y., Kripalani, S., Goggins, K. M., et al. (2017). Financial strain is associated with medication nonadherence and worse self-rated health among cardiovascular patients. *Journal of Health Care for the Poor and Underserved, 28*(1), 499–513. doi: 10.1353/hpu.2017.0036.

Pierpont, Y. N., Dinh, T. P., Salas R. E., et al. (2014). Obesity and surgical wound healing: A current review. *International Scholarly Research Network Obesity, 2014*(638936), 1–13. Retrieved from http://www.hindawi.com/journals/isrn/2014/638936/abs

Rennke, S., Nguyen, O., Shoeb, M., et al. (2013). Hospital-initiated transitional care interventions as a patient safety strategy: A systematic review. *Annals of Internal Medicine, 158*(2), 433–440.

Rice, V. H., Heath, L., Livingstone-Banks, J., et al. (2017). Nursing interventions for smoking cessation. *Cochrane Database of Systematic Reviews, 12*(12), CD001188. doi: 10.1002/14651858.CD001188.pub5.

Sgonc, R., & Gruber, J. (2013). Age-related aspects of cutaneous wound healing: A mini review. *Gerontology, 59*(2), 159–164. Retrieved from http://www.karger.com/Article/Fulltext/342344

Siegel, D. A., Jatlaoui, T. C., Koumans, E. H., et al. (2019). Update: Interim guidance for health care providers evaluating and caring for patients with suspected e-cigarette, or vaping, product use associated lung injury—United States, October 2019. *Morbidity and Mortality Weekly Report, 68*(41), 919–927.

Subramaniam, V. N., Menezes, A. R., DeSchutter, A., et al. (2019). The cardiovascular effects of marijuana: Are the potential adverse effects worth the high? *Missouri Medicine, 116*(2), 146–153.

VanDolah, H. J., Bauer, B. A., & Mauck, K. F. (2019). Clinicians' guide to cannabidiol and hemp oils. *Mayo Clinic Proceedings, 94*(9), 1840–1851.

Wang, A. S., Armstrong, E. J., Armstrong, A. W. (2013). Corticosteroids and wound healing: Clinical considerations in the perioperative period. *American Journal of Surgery, 206*(3), 410–417.

Woo, K. (2015). Exploring the effects of pain and stress on wound healing. *Advances in Skin & Wound Care, 25*(1), 38–44.

Wound, Ostomy and Continence Nurses Society (WOCN). (2014). *Guideline for management of wounds in patients with lower extremity arterial disease*. Mt. Laurel, NJ: Author.

Wound, Ostomy and Continence Nurses Society (WOCN). (2016). *WOC Nursing Salary and Productivity Survey*. Mt. Laurel, NJ: Author.

Wound, Ostomy and Continence Nurses Society (WOCN). (2017). Guideline for prevention and management of pressure injuries (ulcers):

An executive summary. *Journal of Wound, Ostomy and Continence Nursing, 44*(3), 241–246. doi: 10.1097/WON.0000000000000321.

Wound, Ostomy and Continence Nurses Society (WOCN). (2019). *Guideline for management of wounds in patients with lower extremity venous disease.* Mt. Laurel, NJ: Author.

Wright, J. A., Richards, T., & Srai, S. K. S. (2014). The role of iron in skin and cutaneous wound healing. *Frontiers in Pharmacology, 5*(156). doi: 10.3389/fphar.2014.00156.

Yates, S., McNichol, L., Heinecke, S. B., et al. (2017). Embracing the concept, defining the practice, and changing the outcome. *Journal of Wound, Ostomy, and Continence Nursing, 44*(1), 13–17.

Zinder, R., Cooley, R., Vlad, L. G., et al. (2019). Vitamin A and Wound Healing. *Nutrition in Clinical Practice, 34*(6), 839–849. doi: 10.1002/ncp.10420.

Zurlo, A., & Zuliani, G. (2018). Management of care transition and hospital discharge. *Aging Clinical and Experimental Research, 30*(3), 263–270. doi: 10.1007/s40520-017-0885-6.

QUESTIONS

1. What should be the focus of wound management for a patient with chronic wounds who has end-stage multiple sclerosis?
 A. Wound healing
 B. Wound maintenance
 C. Palliative
 D. Correction of etiological factors

2. What critical intervention should the wound care nurse recommend to manage chronic wounds of a patient with diabetic neuropathy?
 A. Compression wraps/stockings
 B. Normal glycemic control
 C. Anti-inflammatory agents
 D. Antimicrobial therapy

3. What would a wound care nurse recommend as an intervention to manage a chronic wound for a patient with severe chronic obstructive pulmonary disease (COPD)?
 A. Use of nasal oxygen
 B. Reduction of fluid intake
 C. Weight loss counseling
 D. Use of corticosteroids

4. A wound care nurse is devising a care plan for a patient with a dehisced incision. Which strategy is recommended to promote wound healing?
 A. Use of marijuana
 B. Replacing tobacco cigarettes with e-cigarettes
 C. Use of anticoagulants to improve perfusion
 D. Increasing calories in the diet

5. Which macronutrient would the wound care nurse increase in the diet of a patient to promote wound healing?
 A. Protein
 B. Essential minerals such as zinc
 C. Fat
 D. Vitamins

6. Based on the American Diabetes Association goal for glycemic control, what glucose level would the wound nurse recommend for a young patient with a long life expectancy who has limited complications and no history of severe hypoglycemia?
 A. A1C 5.5% to 6.0%
 B. A1C 6.0% to 6.5%
 C. A1C 6.5% to 7.0%
 D. A1C 7.0% to 7.5%

7. The wound nurse is devising a care plan for a patient with chronic wounds who has been on long-term corticosteroid use for rheumatoid arthritis. What is a recommended strategy to promote wound healing?
 A. Increase the dosage of the corticosteroid.
 B. Use 15,000 to 20,000 IU/day vitamin A orally for 14-21 days for patients on chronic steroids.
 C. Avoid the use of topical antimicrobial ointments and dressings.
 D. Avoid the use of adhesive remover products and silicone-based adhesives.

8. When devising a treatment plan for patients with chronic wounds, the wound nurse should keep in mind that:
 A. Chronic wounds are manifestations of acute conditions.
 B. Dressings heal wounds.
 C. Overall health of the patient must be addressed to promote healing.
 D. Topical therapy should be used as a last resort.

9. What is the priority for the wound care nurse to promote smooth transition of care for a patient moving from an acute care facility to a home care setting?
   A. Clear communication regarding care plan and goals
   B. Ordering wound care products
   C. Assessing the condition of the wound
   D. Providing counseling to the patient

10. Which of the following is an effective strategy for promoting a seamless transition between care settings for patients with chronic wounds?
   A. Use of different wound care protocols and priorities for each facility in the system
   B. Selection of products based on cost considerations alone
   C. Wound care orders that specify trade names/brand of dressing
   D. Generic wound care orders and frequent communication with other providers

ANSWERS AND RATIONALES

1. C. Rationale: There are circumstances for which palliative care is the focus, such as when the chronic disease state is end stage and is no longer deemed responsive to medical treatment, or when the patient is terminally ill.

2. B. Rationale: Wound healing is a systemic process that requires increased calorie, protein, and vitamin/mineral intake, sufficient blood flow and oxygenation to support the repair process, and relatively normal glycemic levels.

3. A. Rationale: General measures to improve tissue oxygenation include use of nasal oxygen for patients who are hypoxic, maintenance of adequate hydration to reduce blood viscosity, and management of edema through elevation and compression.

4. D. Rationale: Wound healing is a systemic process that requires increased calorie, protein, and vitamin/mineral intake, sufficient blood flow and oxygenation to support the repair process, and relatively normal glycemic levels.

5. A. Rationale: Wound healing is a systemic process that requires increased calorie and protein intake for optimal healing.

6. C. Rationale: For younger patients with longer life expectancy, fewer complications and comorbid conditions, and no history of severe hypoglycemia, the American Diabetes Association recommends the following: A1C 6.5% to 7.0% (mean plasma glucose 140 to 154 mg/dL).

7. B. Rationale: Oral administration of Vitamin A is recommended. The recommended dose is 25,000 international units orally per day for up to 10 days to offset the negative effects of corticosteroids.

8. C. Rationale: To promote wound healing in a patient of advanced age or with multiple comorbidities, the person's overall health must be optimized by reducing stress, managing pain, assuring adequate sleep, and increasing activity levels.

9. A. Rationale: Challenges to transitions of care include differences in wound care protocols and products, and lack of communication between care settings and providers.

10. D. Rationale: A specific strategy the wound care nurse can employ to promote seamless transitions includes working with licensed providers to assure that wound care orders are appropriate for the setting, and clear and as simple as possible. Product orders should be written in generic terms.

CHAPTER 6

PATIENT AND CAREGIVER EDUCATION FOR WOUND PREVENTION AND HEALING: TEACHING STRATEGIES FOR LEARNING

Lia van Rijswijk

OBJECTIVES

1. Discuss common challenges in patient and caregiver education.

2. Use the nursing process to develop an appropriate educational intervention and teaching plan for an individual patient and/or caregiver.

3. Identify resources to optimize patient and caregiver education strategies.

TOPIC OUTLINE

INTRODUCTION AND REQUIREMENTS

There will be frequent references to the importance of patient and family education, and the role of the wound care nurse in providing that education in this text. This chapter will provide a framework the wound care nurse may use to assure appropriate and effective instruction regarding wound prevention and wound management.

Education has been a core function of nursing for as long as nursing has been recognized as a unique discipline. The National League of Nursing (previously known as the National League of Nursing Education) observed as early as 1918 that nurses are agents for the promotion of health and the prevention of illness in all settings in which they practice (National League of Nursing Education, 1937). The brochure developed by the American Hospital Association to explain "The Patient Care Partnership: Understanding Expectations, Rights and Responsibilities" (American Hospital Association, 2003) includes several specific patient rights that relate to information and the right to making informed decisions. All State Nurse Practice Acts include teaching within the scope of nursing practice responsibilities, and the American Nurses Association's Scope and Standards of Practice (American Nurses Association [ANA], 2015) includes seven Health Teaching and Health Promotion competencies for Registered Nurses. Similarly, the WOCN Scope and Standards (2018) also references patient education. The latter includes using consumer-appropriate health promotion and health teaching methods as well as feedback and evaluation to determine the effectiveness of the employed strategies. Additional competencies for the Advanced Practice Registered Nurse include synthesis of all relevant behavioral, teaching, and learning theories for designing health education information and programs as well as the evaluation of health information resources (ANA, 2015). In addition to being an effective teacher, the wound care nurse will usually be expected to develop appropriate teaching plans and educational materials for inpatients and outpatients with wounds. The wound care nurse can also be expected to be involved in education of staff members.

Original research examining the effects of patient education on wound prevention and treatment outcomes is limited and generally inconclusive (Dorresteijn et al., 2014; Weller et al., 2016); despite this, guidelines for chronic wound prevention and management currently include patient and caregiver education recommendations, with varying levels of evidence and strength of recommendations (**Table 6-1**). In other words, patient and caregiver education is an integral component of nursing, the wound care nurse's role, and evidence-based care.

GOALS OF CARE AND EDUCATION

The ultimate goal of patient and caregiver education is to assist patients to implement behaviors that help them meet their goals for care. The success of the nurse's efforts at teaching depends not on how much information has been imparted but rather on how much the person has learned (Bastable, 2017). Education involves both teaching and learning with the goal of helping people to achieve optimal independence in their self-care and health. The goals of education change when the goals of care change and can range from recognizing the signs and symptoms of an infection and being able to change a dressing to preventing the development or recurrence of a wound.

KEY POINT

The goal of patient and caregiver education is to achieve optimal independence in self-care and health.

ASSESSMENT

Every nursing process, including teaching and development of instructional content and materials, begins with a complete and thorough assessment of the learner. This includes assessing the values, preferences, expressed and unexpressed needs, and knowledge of the health care situation (ANA, 2015). For assessment (and evaluation) purposes, the Health Belief Model (HBM) (Rosenstock et al., 1988) can provide a useful framework. Originally the HBM was developed to predict and explain health behavior; this model is also useful in explaining the role of culture, values, and beliefs in predicting

outcomes and adherence to the plan of care (Edelman et al., 2014).

Two components of health-related behavior are a desire to avoid illness or to get well and a belief that specific actions will prevent or cure illness (LaMorte, 2019). There are six elements of HBM that are perceived by the individual:

1. Susceptibility of the risk of acquiring an illness or disease.
2. Severity, which refers to feelings on the seriousness of contracting an illness or disease (or leaving the illness or disease untreated). Often a person may consider the medical consequences (e.g., death, disability) and social consequences (e.g., family, social relationships) when evaluating the severity.
3. Benefits, which refer to perception of effectiveness of actions available to reduce the threat of illness or disease (or to cure illness or disease).
4. Barriers, which refer to feelings on the obstacles to performing a recommended health action.
5. Cue to action, which is the stimulus that triggered the decision-making process to accept a recommended health action. These cues can be internal (e.g., non-healing surgical incision, leg wound, etc.) or external (e.g., advice from others, illness of family member, newspaper article, etc.).
6. Self-efficacy, which refers to the confidence in the ability to successfully perform a behavior (LaMorte, 2019).

The model postulates that the likelihood of a person implementing recommended behaviors is affected by a number of factors; these factors are categorized as individual perception variables, modifying variables, and variables determining likelihood of action (**Table 6-2**). Although the predictive value of each factor varies, the effect of perceived benefits and perceived barriers on likelihood of action has consistently been observed in a wide variety of studies (Carpenter, 2010).

Research investigating factors influencing patient adherence with compression stocking use to prevent venous leg ulcer recurrence found only two factors that differed significantly between persons who did and did not wear compression stockings daily: the belief that wearing stockings was worthwhile and the belief that stockings were uncomfortable to wear (Jull et al., 2004; Ratliff et al., 2016; WOCN, 2019). In a study describing skin care behaviors to prevent pressure injuries in persons with spinal cord injury (SCI), King and colleagues (2012) found that turning benefits, turning barriers, perceived susceptibility, and self-efficacy were significant predictors of turning frequency. Similarly, HBM factors that significantly affected daily foot-exam practice among persons with diabetes and peripheral neuropathy included action cues from family, friends, or health professionals; perceived self-efficacy; and perceived barriers to completing a daily foot exam (Chin et al., 2013)

TABLE 6-1 EXAMPLES OF GLOBAL WOUND GUIDELINES WITH PATIENT/FAMILY/CARE PARTNER EDUCATIONAL COMPONENTS

INTERNATIONAL
- National Pressure Ulcer Advisory Panel (NPUAP), European Pressure Ulcer Advisory Panel (EPUAP), and Pan Pacific Pressure Injury Alliance (PPPIA): Prevention and treatment of pressure ulcers/injuries—Clinical practice guideline, 3rd edition (2019)
- International Working Group on the Diabetic Foot (IWGDF): Guidance on the use of interventions to enhance the healing of chronic ulcers of the foot in diabetes (2015)
- Wounds International: Best practice guidelines—Wound management in diabetic foot ulcers (2013)

CANADA
- Wounds Canada: Best practice recommendations for the prevention and management of pressure injuries (2018)
- The Canadian Institute for Health Information (CIHI) and the Canadian Patient Safety Institute (CPSI): Hospital harm improvement resource—Pressure ulcer (2016)

UNITED STATES
- Wound Ostomy and Continence Nurses Society (WOCN): 2016 guideline for prevention and management of pressure injuries (ulcers)—An executive summary (published 2017)
- WOCN: Venous, arterial, and neuropathic lower-extremity wounds—Clinical resource guide (2017)
- Society for Vascular Surgery (SVS), American Podiatric Medical Association (APMA), and the Society for Vascular Medicine (SVM): A clinical practice guideline on the management of diabetic foot (2016)
- WOCN: 2014 guideline for management of wounds in patients with lower-extremity arterial disease (LEAD)—An executive summary (published 2016)
- Wound Healing Society (WHS): Guidelines for arterial ulcers (2016)
- WHS: Guidelines for diabetic foot ulcer treatment, update (2016)
- WHS: Guidelines for pressure ulcers, 2015 update (published 2016)
- WHS: Guidelines for venous ulcers, 2015 update (published 2016)
- American College of Physicians (ACP): A clinical practice guideline for the treatment of pressure ulcers (2015)
- Choosing Wisely: Don't use whirlpools for wound management (2014)
- SVS and American Venous Forum (AVF): Clinical practice guidelines for the management of venous leg ulcers (2014)
- WOCN: Guideline for the management of wounds in patients with lower-extremity neuropathic disease—An executive summary (2013)
- WOCN: Guideline for the management of wounds in patients with lower-extremity venous disease—An executive summary (2020)

EUROPE
- European Dermatology Forum (EDF): S3-Guideline on venous leg ulcer (2016)
- European Society for Vascular Surgery (ESVS): Clinical practice guidelines on management of chronic venous disease (2015)

UNITED KINGDOM
- National Institute for Health and Care Excellence (NICE): Guideline on diabetic foot problems—Prevention and management (2015, updated 2019)
- NICE: Quality standard on pressure ulcers (2015)
- NICE: Clinical guideline on pressure ulcers—Prevention and management (2014)
- Scottish Intercollegiate Guidelines Network (SIGN): A national clinical guideline on the management of chronic venous leg ulcers (2010)

AUSTRALIA
- Australian Wound Management Association (AWMA): Pan Pacific guideline for the prevention and treatment of pressure injury (2012)

JAPAN
- [In English] Japanese Dermatological Association (JDA): The wound/burn guidelines—1. Wounds in general (2016)
- [In English] JDA: The wound/burn guidelines—2. Guidelines for the diagnosis and treatment for pressure ulcers (2016)
- [In English] JDA: The wound/burn guidelines—3. Guidelines for the diagnosis and treatment of diabetic ulcer/gangrene (2016)
- [In English] JDA: The wound/burn guidelines—4. Guidelines for the management of skin ulcers associated with connective tissue disease/vasculitis (2016)
- [In English] JDA: The wound/burn guidelines—5. Guidelines for the management of lower leg ulcers/varicose veins (2016)
- [In English] Japanese Society of Pressure Ulcers (JSPU): Guidelines for the prevention and management of pressure ulcers, 4th edition (2016)

From Armstrong, D. G., & Meyr, A. J. (2020). Basic principles of wound management. In J. F. Eidt, J. L. Mills, Sr, E. Bruera, E. et al. (Eds.), *UpToDate*. Waltham, MA: UpToDate Inc. Retrieved March 3, 2020 from https://www-uptodate-com

KEY POINT

The factors most likely to affect adherence to care recommendations are the individual's perceptions of the *benefits* and *barriers* associated with the recommendation.

The take-home message from these studies is the importance of assessing each individual from the perspective of his or her beliefs and priorities related to the care recommendations. Open-ended questions are more effective than "yes/no" questions when trying to

TABLE 6-2 USING THE HEALTH BELIEF MODEL		
INDIVIDUAL PERCEPTIONS	MODIFYING FACTORS	LIKELIHOOD OF ACTION VARIABLES
• Beliefs about susceptibility to... (e.g., venous ulcer recurrence) *plus* • Beliefs about seriousness of... (e.g., what happens if I get another wound?) *equals* • Perceived threat of... (e.g., what are the risks when I develop another venous ulcer?)	• Demographic variables (e.g., age, race, ethnicity) • Sociopsychological variables (e.g., personality, socioeconomic status, peer and reference group pressure or support) • Structural variables (e.g., knowledge about disease/condition)	• Perceived Benefits of Action (e.g., no wound pain and clinic visits) *minus* • Perceived Barriers to Action (e.g., compression stockings too warm, expensive, difficult to apply) *equals* • *Likelihood of taking action* (e.g., wearing compression stockings daily, repositioning)

Used with permission from Rosenstock, I. M., Strecher, K. J., & Becker, M. H. (1988). The social learning theory and Health Belief Model. *Health Education Quarterly, 15*, 175–183, SAGE Publications.

identify gaps in knowledge and understand a patient's culture (Rankin & Stallings, 2001). Good examples of open-ended questions that address the individual's *beliefs about and understanding* of the disease process, potential *modifying factors*, and perceived ability to *implement care recommendations* include the following:

- What do you think caused your wound? Why do you think it started when it did?
- How severe is it? How does the wound affect you?
- What are you most worried about?
- If you didn't have this wound, what would you be doing right now? What would you like to do when the wound is healed? Do you think it will take a long or short time for the wound to heal?
- Do you know anyone who had a similar problem and what happened to him/her?
- What are your goals for care of this wound?
- What kind of treatment do you think is needed to get the wound to heal?
- How do you feel about the care recommendations that have been made (e.g., smoking cessation, tight glucose control, off-loading)?

Demographic and psychosocial variables are important to assess since they are known to affect outcomes of care. For example, researchers found that leg elevation, use of compression hosiery, social support, and self-efficacy all significantly affected the risk of venous ulcer recurrence (Finlayson et al., 2011). In a study examining risk factors for pressure ulcer development in SCI patients, level of injury and shorter time since injury increased the risk of having a pressure ulcer at the time of the study; however, so did being black, being male, not having a high school diploma, and having a household income <$ 25,000 per year (Saunders et al., 2010). These observations are not surprising since demographic and psychosociologic variables have a profound impact on health literacy.

Health literacy is usually defined as the degree to which individuals have the capacity to obtain, process, and understand basic health information and

services; efforts to improve health literacy have been an area of increased focus in recent years, and are included in the 2010 Affordable Care Act (Koh et al., 2012). Studies suggest that many patients who have or are at risk for a chronic wound have the same demographic characteristics as do persons found to have the highest rates of limited literacy and health illiteracy. Specifically, studies show that one in four adults (25%) has a low level of health literacy, and this number increases to 37.9% for persons >50 years of age (Paasche-Orlow et al., 2005). The percentage of adults with limited health literacy continues to increase with increasing age. These data have profound implications for the wound care nurse. Conservatively, the wound care nurse should expect that at least 40% of her/his wound care patients will have limited ability to obtain, process, and understand information and instructions regarding their care. Low health literacy is associated with a number of adverse health outcomes; these include reduced ability to take medication correctly, reduced ability to interpret labels and health messaging, poorer health outcomes and health status among the elderly, less effective use of health care services, and higher all-cause mortality rates (Berkman et al., 2011).

KEY POINT

Health literacy is defined as an individual's ability to understand and process health-related information ... 40% of individuals >50 years of age have limited health literacy.

Several methods and tools are available to assist the wound care nurse in screening for health literacy (**Table 6-3**). Depending on the care setting and the assessment goals, the wound care nurse may choose either a detailed and extensive assessment tool or a few simple screening questions. For example, in one study involving a random sample of VA patients (average age

TABLE 6-3 HEALTH LITERACY ASSESSMENT AND SCREENING TOOLS

TITLE/NAME	AVAILABILITY
Health Literacy Measurement Tools (SAHL & REALM-SF)	Tool and directions available in English and Spanish at Agency for Healthcare Research and Quality Web site: https://www.ahrq.gov/health-literacy/quality-resources/tools/literacy/index.html
The Newest Vital Sign (health literacy tool)	Available in English and Spanish at: https://www.pfizer.com/health/literacy/public-policy-researchers/nvs-toolkit
Short Test of Functional Health Literacy in Adults (STOFHLA)	https://www.reginfo.gov/public/do/PRAViewIC?ref_nbr=201210-0935-001&icID=204408

61 years) it was found that a single question ("How confident are you filling out medical forms by yourself?") effectively identified individuals with inadequate, though not marginal, health literacy skills (Chew et al., 2008). Preliminary evidence suggests that a conversational health literacy assessment (CHAT) may help supplement existing intake and assessment procedures by asking simple questions about supportive professional relationships, supportive personal relationships, health information access and comprehension ("Where do you get health information that you trust?"), current health behaviors, and health promotion barriers and support ("Thinking about looking after your health, what is difficult for you and what is going well?") (O'Hara et al., 2018). In addition to determining the individual's or caregivers' health literacy, current level of knowledge regarding the disease process, wound treatment plan and goals for care, the nurse must consider all barriers and facilitators for learning and/or providing care. For example, is the patient or caregiver physically capable of applying compression hosiery or changing position to relieve pressure? Is the person with a new SCI emotionally ready to discuss the injury and its impact, let alone pressure injury prevention strategies?

TEACHING GOALS AND OBJECTIVES

Prior to initiating a teaching session or developing an educational program or materials, it is important to consider (1) the teaching goal and objectives based on the goals of care, (2) assessment findings, and (3) the principles of learning across the life span. Principles for teaching pediatric patients should be appropriate to their developmental stage; adult (andragogy) or older adult (geragogy) learning is focused differently. Adults are generally self-directed, have a lifetime of experi-

ence they want to use and share, need to know why they should learn something and how it benefits them, may have difficulty with someone telling them what to do (self-concept), are life, task, and problem centered, and respond more to internal priorities than to external motivators (Knowles et al., 1998). When teaching older adults, the wound care nurse may need to make adaptations to accommodate normal physical and cognitive changes associated with aging: for example, written instructions should be at least 14-point font, good lighting should be provided, hearing aids should be in and on, and information should be shared in shorter teaching sessions with more repetition. At the same time, the wound care nurse should be aware that the vast majority of older adults retain the ability to learn and should avoid assumptions of cognitive decline (ageism) (Bastable, 2017).

Most chronic wound conditions develop as a result of several complex interactions; providing effective education in regard to wound management or wound prevention is not easy. For example, to help an individual patient prevent the development of a pressure injury following discharge (goal of care and education), the patient needs to meet a variety of objectives in the cognitive (knowledge), affective (emotions, feelings), and behavioral or psychomotor domain. Specifically, the patient and/or caregiver needs at least a basic understanding of the role of immobility, shear force damage, moisture, and malnutrition on skin and tissue health, and needs to verbalize and demonstrate the critical measures for prevention: correct positioning, moisture management, and nutritional intake.

A systematic literature review of cancer patient education strategies has shown that, regardless of strategy used, structured, culturally appropriate, and patient-specific teachings are more effective than unstructured ad hoc teaching methods (Friedman et al., 2011). Teaching plans are invaluable to organize the *objectives, content, teaching/learning activities, and evaluation methods,* in part because it requires the wound care nurse to examine the teaching/learning process related to specific areas (Beitz, 2007).

Instructional objectives must be clearly defined and should clearly delineate what it is that the patient/caregiver needs to be able to do, explain, discuss, etc. Verbs used in instructional objectives should be measurable, can be classified based on the behavioral objective domain classifications (cognitive, affective and psychomotor), and can be found in textbooks (Bastable, 2017). The wound care nurse can also use Bloom's Taxonomy verbs, which are available online from a variety of sources (Anderson & Krathwohl, 2001).

An important element in developing a teaching plan is to divide the overall content and skills to be learned into individual "lessons" that are manageable. A sample teaching plan for pressure injury prevention follows:

- Day 1—The patient can explain the relationship between pressure and skin breakdown (cognition/comprehension).
- Day 2—The patient independently shifts weight using appropriate techniques while sitting and lying down (behavioral/psychomotor).
- Day 3—The patient asks questions and discusses the importance of preventing pressure injuries (affective/responding).

An optimal teaching plan also includes evaluation methods, for example, the learner answers questions correctly and demonstrates appropriate off-loading techniques.

The most effective individual teaching plans are based on assessment findings. It is of course important to address identified structural variables (knowledge gaps), but the effect of perceived benefits and perceived barriers (see **Table 6-2**) on likelihood of action is profound (Carpenter, 2010) and must be considered in the teaching objectives and content. For example, if the patient has indicated that his life is very hectic and he sometimes forgets to take his medication, the wound care nurse should assume that remembering to shift weight may be an important barrier to achieving the overall goal of care and strategies that may work for him need to be explored. Similarly, if the patient has stated that her goal is to get the plantar surface wound to heal, but she has also explained that she has to work, cannot take time off, and has a high deductible health insurance plan and financial concerns, an effective management plan must include exploring off-loading devices and strategies that will reduce these barriers to implementing the recommended plan of care.

TEACHING STRATEGIES AND IMPLEMENTATION

Teaching strategies and implementation methods are detailed in the teaching plan. Multiple teaching strategies (e.g., computer technology, audio- and videotapes, written materials, demonstrations) are generally more effective than verbal teaching alone (Friedman et al., 2011). In one study involving the ability of patients at risk for foot ulcers to recall information, videos were found to be more effective than written material only (Gravely et al., 2011). Although every person learns differently, most learn best when exposed to information in more than one mode; for example, a combination of visual, auditory, reading/writing, and kinesthetic (experience and practice) information (Fleming & Mills, 1992). An advantage to one-on-one patient/caregiver teaching strategies is the ability to readily adapt the information to meet individual needs and goals. Immediate responses can be solicited,

learning evaluated, and modifications made. It is important to make sure that the patient does not feel pressured to articulate acquired knowledge. During demonstrations/return demonstrations of psychomotor skills, it is especially important for the learner to know that there is no expectation to perform the task flawlessly—only practice will build competence (Bastable, 2017).

Because one-on-one education is time intensive, other educational materials (videos, printed materials) are widely used in health care to complement face-to-face teaching. It is critical for the wound care nurse to carefully assess all written and audiovisual materials to assure appropriate reading level and comprehension. Population assessments have shown that a large percentage of people have health literacy limitations and they are unable to understand many of the educational materials used today. Including a patient's circle of care in these efforts may help persons with limited health literacy and help address other barriers to optimal health behavior. For example, a meta-analysis of studies examining the effectiveness of strategies for blood pressure control showed that multilevel, multicomponent strategies (including health coaching sessions, team-based care, self-monitoring, audit, and feedback) were significantly more effective in long-term BP control than usual care (office visits and teaching) (Mills et al., 2018).

Written materials can be readily assessed for appropriateness of reading level using one of several reading level analysis tools: for example, the Flesch Reading Ease Formula and Flesch-Kincaid Grade level are included in word processing software tools. Most health education materials are written at a 10th grade reading level; however, among adults 16 to 74 years of age in the United States only 13% have the highest level of proficiency in literacy whereas 19% can read only relatively brief texts to locate a piece of information (low-level literacy) (U.S. Department of Education, 2016). There is obviously a profound "disconnect" between many educational products available today and what we know about health literacy. In a recent analysis of written materials used to teach patients about skin care and pressure ulcer prevention, researchers found that most materials were written at an 8th or 10th grade reading level and none of the materials were appropriate teaching tools for low-literacy patients (Wilson, 2003).

Although reading levels are important, it is only one consideration in developing appropriate health education materials. All educational materials (e.g., videos, printed materials) should be prepared using health literacy universal precautions (Brach et al., 2012; Eigelbach, 2017). *A health literate health care organization simplifies all communication to the greatest extent possible* and verifies comprehension with everyone; they do not make assumptions about who understands or needs extra assistance. Organization-wide health literacy approaches can be very effective in improving the understandability and actionability of patient health information (Mastroianni et al., 2019). Fortunately, there are many resources to help the wound care nurse prepare education materials that meet the needs of patients using scientific principles of health communication that go beyond determining reading levels (**Table 6-4**). Kirkland-Kyhn et al. (2018) describe simple and useful instructions that the wound care nurse could reinforce with patient and family caregivers who perform wound care tasks, including links to instructional videos. An example of an educational sheet for wound care teaching for family caregivers can be found in **Table 6-5**.

KEY POINT

All educational materials should be prepared using health literacy universal precautions (keep it simple!)

EVALUATION

Evaluating the success of educational efforts is determined by the extent to which learning occurred; evaluation of patient/caregiver learning is based on the objectives outlined in the teaching plan and whether or not the goals of care are met. Can the patient safely and correctly shift weight or apply compression stockings (objectives), *and/or* did they implement this practice into their daily life (goals of care/action)? (see **Table 6-2**). In evaluating individual patient/caregiver learning, it is necessary to ask open-ended questions and to observe return demonstrations.

In evaluating an overall educational program, the wound care nurse must determine whether the educational tools that were developed meet the desired objectives. Fortunately, many of the resources available for development of health communication tools also contain strategies for testing and evaluation (see **Table 6-4**) and AHRQ has developed a Patient Education Materials Assessment Tool (PEMAT) and User's Guide (Shoemaker et al., 2013). In general, an educational evaluation can range from a simple formative evaluation of the process used to a more complex impact evaluation (Bastable, 2017). A guiding question for a total program evaluation may be "How well did patient education activities implemented throughout the year meet the goals established for a clinic's patient education program?" (Bastable, 2017). While difficult to use for a specific health care area (e.g., the wound clinic), from a health care systems perspective, the Centers for Medicare and Medicaid Services (CMS) Hospital Consumer Assessment of Healthcare Providers and Systems (HCAHPS) survey outcomes also contain information that may be useful in evaluating teaching strategies. For example, patients are asked to rate how often nurses and doctors listened carefully and explained things in a way they could understand,

TABLE 6-4 RESOURCES TO IMPROVE EDUCATIONAL OUTCOMES AND DEVELOP HEALTH LITERATE EDUCATION COMMUNICATIONS

PUBLISHER AND TITLE	PURPOSE	AVAILABILITY
Centers for Disease Control and Prevention (CDC) Clear Communication Index	Tool for developing and assessing CDC Public Communication Products	http://www.cdc.gov/ccindex/pdf/clear-communication-user-guide.pdf
CDC Clear Communication Index Score Sheet	Helps evaluate appropriateness of communication products	http://www.cdc.gov/healthliteracy/pdf/fillable-form-may-2013.pdf
DHHS office of Disease Prevention and Health Promotion Health Literacy Online Guide	A guide for simplifying health Web sites and digital tools	http://www.health.gov/healthliteracyonline/
Institute for Healthcare Improvement Ask Me 3	Patient education materials to improve communication between health care providers and patients	http://www.ihi.org/resources/Pages/Tools/Ask-Me-3-Good-Questions-for-Your-Good-Health.aspx
AHRQ Health Literacy Universal Precautions Toolkit (second edition)	Toolkit to help improve spoken and written communication, patient self-management, and supportive systems	https://www.ahrq.gov/sites/default/files/wysiwyg/professionals/quality-patient-safety/quality-resources/tools/literacy-toolkit/healthlittoolkit2.pdf
CDC—Simply Put	Guide for creating easy-to-understand teaching materials	http://www.cdc.gov/healthliteracy/pdf/simply_put.pdf
Medline Plus	Patient education materials	https://medlineplus.gov/
National Jewish Health	Patient education materials	https://www.nationaljewish.org/education/patient/print-multimedia/online-materials-2

and are asked how well they understood their care when leaving the hospital (CMS, 2019). *The sheer number of communication questions in the HCAHPS survey serves as yet another reminder that patient/caregiver education affects patient outcomes!*

The entire process of patient/caregiver education, from assessment to evaluation, is cyclical, and evaluation findings should be applied and lead to education improvements wherever they are needed. In this case,

TABLE 6-5 INFORMATION FOR FAMILY CAREGIVERS

WOUND TYPE	ASSESSMENT	PREVENTION AND TREATMENT	WHEN TO CONTACT A HEALTH CARE PROVIDER
Surgical wound	During every dressing change, check for: • Redness • Swelling • A change in drainage (color or amount) • Separation of wound edges • Increased pain	The patient should shower per surgeon's orders. No tub baths until cleared by the surgeon Use prescribed dressings (usually plain or silicone nonstick dressing).	Contact a health care provider if: The patient has chills or a fever of >101°F or 38°C. There is increased amount of pain, swelling, or redness. The wound edges separate. There is a change in wound drainage (color, odor, or amount).
Venous ulcers	During every compression bandage change, check for: • Redness • Swelling • Change in wound drainage (color, odor or amount) • Increased pain	The patient should: Wear compression bandages daily Lose weight if overweight Follow a walking routine Change dressing as prescribed Elevate legs for 30 minutes, 3 times per day	Contact a health care provider if: The patient has chills or a fever of >101°F or 38°C. There is increased amount of pain, swelling or redness. There is a change in wound drainage (color, odor or amount).
Neuropathic (Diabetic) ulcers	Check between toes for any maceration, redness, or breaks in the skin. Monitor the temperature of the feet.	Inspect the patient's feet daily. Practice daily foot hygiene. Practice good skin care, including the use of alcohol-free moisturizers. Control blood sugar levels. Ensure footwear fits properly. Obtain regular toenail care by a professional. Use off-loading techniques to manage wounds. Before putting on shoes, check the inside for irregular, sharp surfaces or foreign objects.	Contact a health care provider if: The patient has chills or a fever of >101°F or 38°C. There is increased amount of pain, swelling or redness. The wound edges separate. There is a change in wound drainage (color, odor, or amount). If calluses develop, they should be removed by a professional.
Arterial ulcers	During every dressing change, check for: • Redness • Change in wound drainage (color, odor, or amount) • Increased pain	Avoid injury. Stop or reduce smoking. Avoid going barefoot. Practice good skin care. Obtain regular toenail care by a professional.	Contact a health care provider if: Patient has chills or a fever >101°F or 38°C. If there is an increased amount of pain, drainage, or redness If there is a change in wound drainage (color, odor, or amount)
Pressure injury	During every dressing change, check for: • Redness • Swelling • A change in wound drainage (color, odor, or amount) • Increased pain	Off-load the affected area. Use dressings as prescribed. Stop or reduce smoking. Eat a healthy diet.	Contact a health care provider If patient has chills or a fever >101°F or 38°C If there is an increased amount of pain, drainage, or redness If there is a change in wound drainage (color, odor, or amount)

Adapted from Kirkland-Kyhn, H., Generao, S. A., Teleten, O., et al. (2018). Teaching wound care to family caregivers. *American Journal of Nursing, 118*(3), 63–67.

we can practice what we preach when teaching psychomotor skills to patients: "Practice makes perfect."

KEY POINT

Learning and teaching improve with practice.

 CONCLUSION

Patient and caregiver education is an integral component of evidence-based practice, nursing, and the wound care nurse role. The goal of education is to influence patient/caregiver behavior, and we have learned over the past few decades that adjustments in behavior require more than delivering information. There are a number of studies that demonstrate a complex and significant relationship between individual perceptions, psychosocial variables, and perceived benefits and barriers of specific actions and interventions; all of these factors must be considered when developing an effective education plan. We have also learned a lot about health literate communications strategies, and providers are encouraged to follow health literacy universal precautions when developing educational materials and approaches because all people have the right to health information that helps them make informed decisions.

Fortunately, patient and caregiver education involves the same basic steps as the nursing process (with which wound care nurses are very familiar), and research examining health behavior can be used to assure that we are asking the right questions and developing appropriate objectives to meet the goals of care. In addition, there are multiple tools available to guide the nurse in designing effective educational programs, including those developed by the Agency for Health Research and Quality (AHRQ) and the Centers for Disease Control and Prevention (CDC).

REFERENCES

American Hospital Association (AHA). (2003). *The patient care partnership: Understanding expectations, rights, and responsibilities*. Atlanta, GA: Author. Retrieved January 31, 2020, from https://www.aha.org/other-resources/patient-care-partnership

American Nurses Association. (2015). *Nursing: Scope and standards of practice* (3rd ed.). Silver Springs, MD: Author.

Anderson, L. W., & Krathwohl, D. R. (2001). *A taxonomy for learning, teaching, and assessing* (Abridged ed.). Boston, MA: Allyn and Bacon.

Armstrong, D. G., & Meyr, A. J. (2020). Basic principles of wound management. In J. F. Eidt, J. L. Mills, Sr, E. Bruera, E. et al. (Eds.), *UpToDate*. Waltham, MA: UpToDate Inc. Accessed March 3, 2020 at https://www-uptodate-com

Association for the Advancement of Wound Care (AAWC). (2010). *Guideline of pressure ulcer guidelines*. Malvern, PA: Association for the Advancement of Wound Care (AAWC). Accessed November 22, 2020 at https://aawconline.memberclicks.net/resources

Bastable, S. B. (Ed.). (2017). *Essentials of patient education* (2nd ed.). Sudbury, MA: Jones & Bartlett.

Beitz, J. (2007). Health promotion and health education. In M. J. Morison, C. J. Moffatt, & P. J. Franks, (Eds.), *Leg ulcers: A problem-based learning approach*. Edinburg, UK: Mosby Elsevier.

Berkman, N. D., Sheridan, S. L., Donahue, K. E., et al. (2011). Low health literacy and health outcomes: An updated systematic review. *Annals of Internal Medicine, 155*(2), 97–107.

Brach, C., Keller, D., Hernandez, L. M., et al. (2012). *Ten attributes of health literate health care organizations*. Washington, DC: Institute of Medicine. Retrieved from http://iom.edu/~/media/Files/Perspectives-Files/2012/Discussion-Papers/BPH_Ten_HLit_Attributes.pdf

Carpenter, C. J. (2010). A meta-analysis of the effectiveness of Health Belief Model variables in predicting behavior. *Health Communication, 25*, 661–669. doi: 10.1080/10410236.2010.521906.

Centers for Medicare and Medicaid Services (CMS). (2019). *Hospital consumer assessment of health care providers and systems. Survey Instruments*. Baltimore, MD: Centers for Medicare and Medicaid Services. Retrieved November 30, 2019, from https://hcahpsonline.org/globalassets/hcahps/survey-instruments/mail/29-item-survey/updated-w-omb-date/2019_survey-instruments_english_mail-updateda.pdf

Chew, L. D., Griffin, J. M., Partin, M. R., et al. (2008). Validation of screening questions for limited health literacy in a large VA outpatient population. *Journal of General Internal Medicine, 23*(5), 561–566. doi: 10.1007/s11606-008-0520-5.

Chin, Y., Huang, T., & Hsu, B. R. (2013). Impact of action cues, self-efficacy and perceived barriers on daily foot exam practice in type 2 diabetes mellitus patients with peripheral neuropathy. *Journal of Clinical Nursing, 22*(1-2), 61–68.

Dorresteijn, J. A., Kriegsman, D. M. W., Assendelft, W. J. J., et al. (2014). Patient education for preventing diabetic foot ulceration. *The Cochrane Database of Systematic Reviews, 2014*(12), CD001488. https://doi.org/10.1002/14651858.CD001488.pub5

Edelman, C. L., Kuzma, E. C., & Mandle, C. L. (2014). *Health promotion throughout the life span* (8th ed.). St. Louis, MO: Elsevier Mosby.

Eigelbach, B. (2017). Ten suggested health literacy attributes of a health care organization. *Journal of Consumer Health on the Internet, 21*(2), 201–208. doi: 10.1080/15398285.2017.1311606.

European Pressure Ulcer Advisory Panel, National Pressure Injury Advisory Panel, and Pan Pacific Pressure Injury Alliance [EPUAP/NPIAP/PPPIA]. (2019). In E. Haesler (Ed.), *Prevention and treatment of pressure ulcers/injuries: Clinical Practice Guideline*. The International Guideline.

Finlayson, K., Edwards, H., & Courtney, M. (2011). Relationships between preventive activities, psychosocial factors and recurrence of venous leg ulcers: A prospective study. *Journal of Advanced Nursing, 67*(10), 2180–2190. doi: 10.1007/s13187-010-0183-x.

Fleming, N. D., & Mills, C. (1992). *Helping students understand how they learn*. The Teaching Professor, 7(4). Madison, WI: Magma Publications.

Friedman, A. J., Cosby, R., Boyko, S., et al. (2011). Effective teaching strategies and methods of delivery for patient education: A systematic review and practice guideline recommendations. *Journal of Cancer Education, 26*, 12–21.

Gravely, S. S., Hensley, B. K., & Hagood-Thompson, C. (2011). Comparison of three types of diabetic foot ulcer education plans to determine patient recall of education. *Journal of Vascular Nursing, 29*(3), 113–119.

Jull, A. B., Mitchell, N., Arroll, J., et al. (2004). Factors influencing concordance with compression stockings after venous leg ulcer healing. *Journal of Wound Care, 13*(3), 90–92.

King, R., Champion, V. L., Chen, D., et al. (2012). Development of a measure of skin care belief scales for persons with spinal cord injury. *Archives of Physical Medicine and Rehabilitation, 9*(10), 1814–1821.

Kirkland-Kyhn, H., Generao, S. A., Teleten, O., et al. (2018). Teaching wound care to family caregivers. *American Journal of Nursing, 118*(3), 63–67. doi: 10.1097/01.NAJ.0000530941.11737.1c.

Knowles, M. S., Holton, E. F., & Swanson, R. A. (1998). *The adult learner*. Houston, TX: Gulf Publishing.

Koh, H. K., Berwic, D. M., Clancy, C. M., et al. (2012). New Federal policy initiatives to boost health literacy can help the nation move beyond the cycle of costly "crisis care." *Health Affairs, 31*(2), 434–443. doi: 10.1377/hlthaff.2011.1169.

LaMorte, W. W. (2019). *Behavioral change models*. Retrieved January 31, 2020, from http://sphweb.bumc.bu.edu/otlt/MPH-Modules/SB/BehavioralChangeTheories/BehavioralChangeTheories2.html#headingtaglink_1

Mastroianni, F., Chen, Y., Vellar, L., et al. (2019). Implementation of an organization-wide health literacy approach to improve the understandability and actionability of patient information and education materials: A pre-post effectiveness study. *Patient Education and Counseling, 102*, 1656–1661. doi: 10.1016/j.pec.2019.03.022.

Mills, K. T., Obst, K. M., Shen, W., et al. (2018). Comparative effectiveness of implementation strategies for blood pressure control in hypertensive patients: A systematic review and meta-analysis. *Annals of Internal Medicine, 168*(2), 110–120.

National League of Nursing Education. (1937). *A curriculum guide for schools of nursing*. New York, NY: Author.

O'Hara, J., Hawkins, M., Batterham, R., et al. (2018). Conceptualisation and development of the conversational health literacy assessment tool (CHAT). *BMS Health Services Research, 18*, 199. doi: 10.1186/s12913-018-3037-6.

Paasche-Orlow, M. K., Parker, R. M., Gazmararian, J. A., et al. (2005). The prevalence of limited health literacy. *Journal of General Internal Medicine, 20*(2), 175–184. doi: 10.1111/j.1525-1497.2005.40245.x.

Rankin, S. H., & Stallings, K. D. (2001). *Patient education: Principles and practices* (4th ed.). Philadelphia, PA: Lippincott Williams & Wilkins.

Ratliff, C. R., Yates, S., McNichol, L., et al. (2016). Compression for primary prevention, treatment, and prevention of recurrence of venous leg ulcers: An evidence- and consensus-based algorithm for care across the continuum. *Journal of Wound, Ostomy, and Continence Nursing, 43*(4), 347–364.

Rosenstock, I. M., Strecher, K. J., & Becker, M. H. (1988). The social learning theory and health belief model. *Health Education Quarterly, 15*, 175–183.

Saunders, L. L., Krause, J. S., Peters, B. A., et al. (2010). The relationship of pressure ulcers, race, and socioeconomic conditions after spinal cord injury. *Journal of Spinal Cord Medicine, 33*(4), 387–395.

Shoemaker, S. J., Wolf, M. S., & Brach, C. (2013). *The Patient Education Materials Assessment Tool (PEMAT) and user's guide*. Rockville, MD: Agency for Health Care Quality and Research. Retrieved December 1, 2019, from https://www.ahrq.gov/ncepcr/tools/self-mgmt/pemat.html

United States Department of Education, National Center for Education Statistics. (2016). *PIAAC 2012/2014 results*. Retrieved from https://nces.ed.gov/surveys/piaac/results/summary.aspx

Weller, C. D., Buckbinder, R., Johnston, R. V. (2016). Interventions for helping people adhere to compression treatments for venous leg ulceration. *Database of Systematic Reviews, 3*(3), CD008378. https://doi.org/10.1002/14651858.CD008378.pub3

Wilson, F. L. (2003). Assessing the readability of skin care and pressure ulcer patient education materials. *Journal of Wound Ostomy & Continence Nursing, 30*(4), 224–230.

Wound, Ostomy and Continence Nurses Society (WOCN). (2016). *Guideline for prevention and management of pressure ulcers (injuries)*. Mount Laurel, NJ: Author.

Wound, Ostomy and Continence Nurses Society (WOCN). (2018). *Scope and standard of practice* (2nd ed.). Mount Laurel, NJ: Author.

Wound, Ostomy, and Continence Nurses Society (WOCN). (2019). *Guideline for management of wounds in patients with lower-extremity venous disease*. WOCN Clinical Practice Guideline. Mount Laurel, NJ: Author.

QUESTIONS

1. What is the ultimate goal of patient and caregiver education?
   A. Imparting as much information as possible to the patient
   B. Helping patients achieve optimal independence in self-care and health
   C. Helping patients recognize signs and symptoms of infection
   D. Teaching patients how to manage the health care system

2. The wound care nurse consults the Health Belief Model when planning teaching strategies to prevent pressure injury development in a patient with spinal cord injury. Which factor should the nurse consider including in the plan?
   A. Belief about susceptibility to pressure injury development
   B. Perceived threat of developing a pressure injury
   C. Perceived benefit of techniques used to prevent pressure injury
   D. Involvement of friends and family

3. The wound care nurse is interviewing a person who has diabetes with a surgical wound that is showing signs of dehiscence. Which interview question best solicits the individual's understanding about glucose control and wound complications?
   A. "What are your goals for care of this wound?"
   B. "How does this wound affect you?"
   C. "What role do you think having diabetes played in this wound condition?"
   D. "Do you feel you are able to follow the treatment plan we discussed?"

4. Which of the following is an example of a psychosociologic variable that may impact health literacy?
   A. Economic status
   B. Individual perceptions of health
   C. Beliefs about the seriousness of the problem
   D. Perceived benefits of action

5. The wound care nurse is developing a patient handout about the use of compression stockings. Which of the following statistics should be considered?
   A. Forty percent of adults over 50 years of age have a low literacy level.
   B. Most adults can read 10th grade level materials.
   C. An estimated 10% of wound care patients have a low level of health literacy.
   D. Sixty percent of patients treated for wounds have incomes <$25,000.

6. Which information about adult learners should the wound care nurse consider when devising a teaching plan for wound care?
   A. Adults are easily motivated to learn a new skill.
   B. Adults may have difficulty with someone telling them what to do.
   C. Adults are not problem centered; rather, they focus on the big picture.
   D. Adults respond more to external motivators than to internal priorities.

7. A wound care nurse is teaching a 70-year-old patient how to care for an arterial ulcer. An evidence-based teaching approach modification would include which of the following?

A. Information should be provided in longer teaching sessions.

B. Written instructions should be 10-point font or higher.

C. Teaching sessions should be short with more repetition.

D. Assume that the vast majority of older adults experience cognitive decline.

8. Meeting a teaching objective based on the psychomotor domain is best achieved using which of the following strategies?

A. The nurse requests a return demonstration of a dressing change.

B. The nurse provides detailed dressing change instructions.

C. The nurse assesses if the patient values his or her health enough to stop smoking.

D. The nurse describes the process of wound healing to a patient.

9. Which teaching strategy should be considered when performing discharge planning for hospitalized patients?

A. Instructional objectives should be broadly defined and applicable to all patients.

B. The teaching plan should be limited to one or two lessons that are manageable.

C. Verbal teaching is generally more effective than using multiple teaching strategies.

D. Individual teaching plans should be based on assessment findings and identify and consider structural variables.

10. Evaluating the success of the teaching plan is based on:

A. Assessing learned psychomotor skills

B. Treatment progress

C. Patient satisfaction scores from HCAPS survey

D. Assessing whether objectives outlined in the teaching plan have been met

ANSWERS AND RATIONALES

1. B. Rationale: The ultimate goal of patient and caregiver education is to assist patients to implement behaviors that help them meet their goals for care. The success of the nurse's efforts at teaching depends not on how much information has been imparted but rather on how much the person has learned.

2. D. Rationale: The only modifiable factor listed is the involvement of the patient's circle of care.

3. C. Rationale: Good examples of open-ended questions that address the individual's beliefs about and understanding of the disease process, potential modifying factors, and perceived ability to implement care recommendations.

4. A. Rationale: Demographic and psychosociologic variables have a profound impact on health literacy.

5. A. Rationale: Health literacy is defined as an individual's ability to understand and process health-related information. Forty percent (40%) of individuals >50 years of age have limited health literacy.

6. B. Rationale: Adults are generally self-directed; have a lifetime of experience they want to use and share; need to know why they should learn something and how it benefits them; may have difficulty with someone telling them what to do (self-concept); are life, task, and problem centered; and respond more to internal priorities than to external motivators.

7. C. Rationale: When teaching older adults, the wound care nurse may need to make adaptations to accommodate normal physical and cognitive changes associated with aging: for example, written instructions should be at least 14-point font, good lighting should be provided, hearing aids should be in and on, and information should be shared in shorter teaching sessions with more repetition.

8. A. Rationale: During demonstrations/return demonstrations of psychomotor skills, it is especially important for the learner to know that there is no expectation to perform the task flawlessly—only practice will build competence.

9. D. Rationale: It is important to address identified structural variables (knowledge gaps), but the effect of perceived benefits and perceived barriers on likelihood of action is profound and must be considered in the teaching objectives and content.

10. D. Rationale: Evaluating the success of educational efforts is determined by the extent to which learning occurred; evaluation of patient/caregiver learning is based on the objectives outlined in the teaching plan and whether or not the goals of care are met.

CHAPTER 7

NUTRITIONAL STRATEGIES FOR WOUND MANAGEMENT

Elizabeth Friedrich, Mary Ellen Posthauer, and Becky Dorner

OBJECTIVES

1. Analyze the relationship between nutrition and wound healing.

2. Differentiate between nutrition screening and nutrition assessment and understand the value of both processes in developing a plan of nutrition care.

3. Demonstrate an understanding of current guidelines for nutrition support for patients with or at risk for skin breakdown.

TOPIC OUTLINE

THE RELATIONSHIP BETWEEN
NUTRITION AND WOUND HEALING

Nutrition plays an important role in both prevention and treatment of wounds. Malnutrition is a major health care problem, and international research studies note the relationship between nutrition and pressure injuries (Banks et al., 2010; Iizaka et al., 2010; Shahin et al., 2010; Verbrugghe et al., 2013). The term "wound" could apply to pressure injuries as well as surgical wounds, lower extremity wounds, or nonhealing skin tears. The majority of studies regarding nutrition and wound care are related to pressure injuries. For that reason, nutrition management for the prevention and treatment of pressure injuries is the major focus of this chapter (Posthauer et al., 2015).

Adequate calories, protein, fluids, vitamins, and minerals are needed by the body to maintain tissue integrity and prevent tissue breakdown; inadequate intake of essential nutrients over time can result in nutritional deficiencies that affect skin integrity. Inadequate intake of protein and calories may result in malnutrition. Malnutrition alters body composition and the normal pathways by which the body uses protein and fat for fuel (Cederholm et al., 2017). As a result, the body breaks down muscle tissue for energy, and there is a loss of lean body mass (Demling, 2009). In addition, inadequate daily intake of calories can result in inadequate intake of vitamins and minerals necessary to support or maintain skin integrity.

Malnutrition is associated with many adverse outcomes, including increased risk of pressure injuries and impaired wound healing (EPUAP/NPIAP/PPPIA, 2019).

KEY POINT

Preventing and/or treating malnutrition is widely recognized as a key to prevention of pressure injuries and promotion of wound healing.

 IDENTIFYING INDIVIDUALS WITH
COMPROMISED NUTRITIONAL STATUS

NUTRITION SCREENING

Nutrition screening is defined as "the process of identifying patients, clients, or groups who may have a nutrition diagnosis and benefit from nutrition assessment and intervention by a registered dietitian nutritionist (RDN)" (Academy of Nutrition and Dietetics, Terms and Definitions, 2019). Evidence indicates that being identified as malnourished or at risk for malnutrition through nutrition screening is associated with increased risk for pressure injury development (EPUAP/NPIAP/PPPIA, 2019). The nutrition screening process is used to identify individuals at nutritional risk, which should prompt referrals to the appropriate health care professionals for more in-depth

assessment. Most nutrition screening tools are composed of a few simple questions that can be asked by a nurse or any qualified health care professional when the patient is admitted to a health care facility or home health care agency. Screening tools should be quick and easy to use, and valid and reliable for the population served. Most screening tools use common parameters to assign risk level including height, weight, appetite, activity level, mobility, and, gastrointestinal issues. A number of screening tools are available, including the Mini-Nutritional Assessment (MNA), the Malnutrition Universal Screening Tool (MUST), the Malnutrition-Screening Tool (MST), and the Subjective Global Assessment (SGA). **Table 7-1** outlines validated screening tools that can be used in a variety of settings and populations.

Once an individual has been identified as at nutritional risk through nutritional screening, a referral to a RDN should be placed. The RDN will complete a comprehensive nutrition assessment and determine a nutrition plan of care. Additional indicators for RDN referral include presence of a pressure injury or chronic wound that is deteriorating or not healing and comorbidities such as diabetes, chronic kidney disease (CKD), heart failure, and chronic obstructive pulmonary disease (COPD). Individuals assessed as being at risk for pressure injury development per the Braden Scale or Norton Scale should also be referred to a RDN for a comprehensive nutrition assessment. Individuals with unique dietary circumstances (such as those following vegan diets) or those with limited economic resources or chewing or swallowing problems are also candidates for nutrition assessment.

Nutrition Assessment

Nutrition assessment is a systematic method for obtaining, verifying, and interpreting the data needed to identity nutrition-related problems and their causes (Academy of Nutrition and Dietetics eNCPT, 2019). Using nutrition assessment data, the RDN determines whether a nutrition diagnosis (problem) exists. The nutrition assessment is grouped into six domains (Academy of Nutrition and Dietetics eNCPT, 2019):

- Food/nutrition-related history (nutrient intake, food behaviors, etc.)
- Anthropometric measurements (height, weight, body composition, body mass index [BMI], weight history)
- Biochemical data, medical tests, and procedures (CBC, CMP, lipid profile, A1C, etc.)
- Nutrition-focused physical findings (overall appearance and any signs and symptoms of nutritional deficiencies or excesses)
- Client history (medical history, weight history, social and socioeconomic history)
- Assessment, monitoring, and evaluation tools (Braden Scale, PUSH tool, and others)

Following assessment, the RDN will determine if there is a nutrition diagnosis that requires intervention. Unintended weight loss, malnutrition, and poor food or fluid intake are all indicators of nutritional deficiencies that increase the risk for pressure injury development and/or impaired healing. Most individuals with pressure injuries will have a nutrition diagnosis and require intervention.

Speech-language pathologists and occupational therapists may recommend interventions that can increase food and nutrient intake, for example, a change in positioning for ease of swallowing or the addition of a self-help feeding device. Frequent monitoring and evaluation are necessary for any patient at nutritional risk, to determine if interventions are having their intended effect.

Mini Nutritional Assessment MNA®

Nestlé NutritionInstitute

Last name: _____   First name: _____

Sex: _____ Age: _____ Weight, kg: _____ Height, cm: _____ Date: _____

Complete the screen by filling in the boxes with the appropriate numbers. Total the numbers for the final screening score.

Screening

A Has food intake declined over the past 3 months due to loss of appetite, digestive problems, chewing or swallowing difficulties?
0 = severe decrease in food intake
1 = moderate decrease in food intake
2 = no decrease in food intake   ☐

B Weight loss during the last 3 months
0 = weight loss greater than 3 kg (6.6 lbs)
1 = does not know
2 = weight loss between 1 and 3 kg (2.2 and 6.6 lbs)
3 = no weight loss   ☐

C Mobility
0 = bed or chair bound
1 = able to get out of bed / chair but does not go out
2 = goes out   ☐

D Has suffered psychological stress or acute disease in the past 3 months?
0 = Yes   2 = no   ☐

E Neuropsychological problems
0 = severe dementia or depression
1 = mild dementia
2 = no psychological problems   ☐

F1 Body Mass Index (BMI) (weight in kg) / (height in m^2)
0 = BMI less than 19
1 = BMI 19 to less than 21
2 = BMI 21 to less than 23
3 = BMI 23 or greater   ☐

IF BMI IS NOT AVAILABLE, REPLACE QUESTION F1 WITH QUESTION F2.
DO NOT ANSWER QUESTION F2 IF QUESTION F1 IS ALREADY COMPLETED.

F2 Calf circumference (CC) in cm
0 = CC less than 31
3 = CC 31 or greater   ☐

Screening score (max. 14 points)

12 - 14 points: Normal nutritional status
8 - 11 points: At risk of malnutrition
0 - 7 points: Malnourished   ☐☐

References
1. Vellas B, Villars H, Abellan G, et al. Overview of the MNA® - Its History and Challenges. *J Nutr Health Aging* 2006;**10**:456-465.
2. Rubenstein LZ, Harker JO, Salva A, Guigoz Y, Vellas B. Screening for Undernutrition in Geriatric Practice: Developing the Short-Form Mini Nutritional Assessment (MNA®-SF). *J Geront* 2001;**56A**: M366–377.
3. Guigoz Y. The Mini-Nutritional Assessment (MNA®) Review of the Literature - What does it tell us? *J Nutr Health Aging* 2006; **10**:466–487.
4. Kaiser MJ, Bauer JM, Ramsch C, et al. Validation of the Mini Nutritional Assessment Short-Form (MNA®-SF): A practical tool for identification of nutritional status. *J Nutr Health Aging* 2009; **13**:782–788.

® Société des Produits Nestlé S.A., Vevey, Switzerland, Trademark Owners. © Nestlé, 1994, Revision 2009. N67200 12/99 10M
For more information: www.mna-elderly.com

TABLE 7-1 SUMMARY OF THE NUTRITION SCREENING TOOL VALIDATION STUDIES

NUTRITION SCREENING TOOL	EVIDENCE FOR IDENTIFYING PI RISK STATUS	EVIDENCE FOR IDENTIFYING FACTORS ASSOCIATED WITH PI RISK	CLINICAL SETTING
Mini Nutritional Assessment full version (MNA®)	Yes	Yes	Older adults in community settings Older adults in long-term care Older adults with PIs and multiple comorbidities Older adults at nutritional risk in long-term care and community settings Older adults in acute care, long-term care and community settings
Malnutrition Universal Screening Tool (MUST)	No	Yes	Older adults in acute care, long-term care and community settings
Nutrition Risk Screening (NRS) 2002	No	No	Adults in acute care Older adults in acute care, long-term care and community settings
Short Nutrition Assessment Questionnaire (SNAQ)	No	No	Adults in acute care Older adults in residential care
Seniors in the Community: Risk Evaluation for Eating and Nutrition (SCREEN©)	No	No	Older adults in community settings

Reference: Adapted with permission from European Pressure Ulcer Advisory Panel, National Pressure Injury Advisory Panel, and Pan Pacific Pressure Injury Alliance [EPUAP/NPIAP/PPPIA]. (2019). In E. Haesler (Ed.), *Prevention and treatment of pressure ulcers/injuries: Clinical Practice Guideline*. The International Guideline.

KEY POINT

The RDN should be routinely consulted for assistance with management of individuals at risk for or demonstrating evidence of undernutrition.

Food/Nutrition-Related History and Client History

Information about an individual's food-related history, medical history, and socioeconomic status can provide important clues to overall nutritional status and potential for implementing effective interventions. For example:

- An individual's ability to perform activities of daily living (ADLs) and instrumental activities of daily living (IADLs) may affect his or her ability to access nutritious food. For community-dwelling individuals who have no mealtime assistance, this can have a significant impact on food consumption.
- Individuals with chewing and/or swallowing problems are at risk for inadequate intake of food and fluids.
- Individuals who have food allergies or intolerances may be unable to consume some nutritious foods. For example, those with lactose intolerance may not be able to consume milk or cheese, which are excellent sources of protein.
- Cognitive impairment can affect the individual's ability to obtain and prepare food and their ability to focus on eating.
- Medications (including prescription, over the counter, and herbal supplements) can impair appetite, cause dry mouth and/or GI distress, or produce other side effects that adversely affect nutrient intake or utilization.
- Socioeconomic status can affect access to food. Referral to appropriate sources for economic assistance or supplemental food may be necessary.
- Comorbidities like diabetes and CKD can necessitate dietary restrictions that affect an individual's food choices.

It is important to remember, particularly when dealing with food habits and access to food, to treat the whole person, not just the pressure injury or wound. This requires sensitivity to individual and cultural preferences, economic issues, and food availability.

Anthropometric Data

Height and weight, including weight history over time, are critical elements of the nutrition assessment for every individual with or at risk for developing pressure injuries. This information is used to estimate daily calorie, protein, and fluid needs and to assess nutritional status over time. One key indicator of undernutrition is unintended weight loss (defined as 5% of body weight in 30 days or 10% of body weight in 180 days) (Thomas, 2008). Slow weight loss over time (sometimes called insidious weight loss) can also indicate a nutritional deficiency. Height and weight are also used to determine BMI; individuals with a low BMI (<22) may be at higher risk for pressure injuries (Horn et al., 2004). For individuals older than 70 years of age, the best health status and lowest risk of mortality has been observed in those with a BMI between 25 and 32 (Dahl et al., 2013). See **Tables 7-2 to 7-4** for classification of weight status based on BMI.

TABLE 7-2 CALCULATION OF BMI

MEASUREMENT UNITS	FORMULA AND CALCULATION
BMI is calculated the same way for both adults and children. The calculation is based on the following formulas:	
Kilograms and meters (or centimeters)	Formula: weight (kg)/[height (m)]^2 With the metric system, the formula for BMI is weight in kilograms divided by height in meters squared. Since height is commonly measured in centimeters, divide height in centimeters by 100 to obtain height in meters. Example: weight = 68 kg, height = 165 cm (1.65 m) Calculation: 68 ÷ (1.65)^2 = 24.98
Pounds and inches	Formula: weight (lb) / [height (in.)]^2 × 703 Calculate BMI by dividing weight in pounds (lbs) by height in inches (in.) squared and multiplying by a conversion factor of 703. Example: weight = 150 pounds, height = 5′5″ (65″) Calculation: [150 ÷ (65)^2] × 703 = 24.96
Interpretation of BMI for adults	
For adults 20 years old and older, BMI is interpreted using standard weight status categories that are the same for all ages and for both men and women. For children and teens, on the other hand, the interpretation of BMI is both age and sex specific.	

Source: Centers for Disease Control and Prevention (2020). Accessed at https://www.cdc.gov/healthyweight/assessing/bmi/adult_bmi/index.html#Interpreted

KEY POINT

Unintended weight loss is a common indicator of malnutrition; thus, ongoing monitoring of patient weight and their response to interventions is a critical element of a nutrition care.

Biochemical Data

Serum albumin and prealbumin have historically been used to determine visceral protein status. However, there is no laboratory test that can provide a stand-alone assessment of an individual's nutritional status (White et al., 2012). It is now recognized that many acute and chronic diseases can contribute to inflammation, resulting in reduced levels of hepatic proteins like albumin and prealbumin. Inflammation exerts a significant effect on serum levels of hepatic proteins by altering metabolism of those proteins and by causing capillaries to become more permeable, permitting proteins to pass through the capillary walls and into surrounding tissues (Furhman et al., 2004). Serum levels of albumin, prealbumin, and transferrin are reduced in conditions causing inflammation, such as infection, injury, or trauma; as the individual recovers from the inflammatory condition, levels of hepatic proteins rise back toward normal (Litchford et al., 2014). In many cases, hepatic protein levels are indicative of inflammation related to acute or chronic disease, as opposed to poor nutritional status (White et al., 2012). Albumin and prealbumin may correlate with overall prognosis, but frequently do not correlate well with nutritional status; their usefulness in nutritional assessment is limited (Covinsky et al., 2002; Johnson & Merlini, 2007; White et al., 2012). While albumin and prealbumin levels are sometimes requested to diagnose malnutrition, these laboratory tests don't correlate well with clinical observations of nutritional status (Covinsky et al., 2002; White et al., 2012).

Identification and classification of anemia is an important element of assessment, because adequate levels of iron are required for collagen formation, oxygen transport, and new cell generation, and low iron stores can adversely affect wound healing. A nutritional anemia profile can help identify and classify anemia.

KEY POINT

Identification of malnutrition should not be based solely on lab values such as albumin and prealbumin, but on a comprehensive evaluation that includes weight history, protein and calorie intake, and overall health status.

TABLE 7-3 BMI CLASSIFICATION FOR ADULTS

BMI	WEIGHT STATUS
Below 18.5	Underweight
18.5–24.9	Normal
25.0–29.9	Overweight
30.0 and above	Obese

Source: Centers for Disease Control and Prevention (2020). Accessed at https://www.cdc.gov/healthyweight/assessing/bmi/adult_bmi/index.html#Interpreted

TABLE 7-4 BMI CLASSIFICATION BASED ON HEIGHT

HEIGHT	WEIGHT RANGE	BMI	WEIGHT STATUS
5′9″	124 pounds or less	Below 18.5	Underweight
	125–168 pounds	18.5–24.9	Normal
	169–202 pounds	25.0–29.9	Overweight
	203 pounds or more	30 or higher	Obese

Source: Centers for Disease Control and Prevention (2020). Accessed at https://www.cdc.gov/healthyweight/assessing/bmi/adult_bmi/index.html#Interpreted

Hydration status is an important indicator of food and fluid intake. An electrolyte and renal profile can be used to help identify overhydration or dehydration (Academy of Nutrition and Dietetics Nutrition Care Manual, 2019a, 2019b). Lab values that are used to evaluate hydration status include serum BUN, sodium, and serum osmolality (Academy of Nutrition and Dietetics Care Manual, 2019a, 2019b).

Nutrition-Focused Physical Examination

Compromised nutritional status can manifest itself in a wide variety of physical symptoms. A component of nutrition assessment is nutrition-focused physical examination (NFPE) (Peterson, 2016). NFPE involves hands-on assessment of an individual with a focus on nutrition-related components of health (Peterson, 2016) and may help the nutrition and dietetics practitioner to identify compromised nutritional status. The International Dietetics and Nutrition Terminology defines nutrition-focused physical findings gathered from a NFPE, interview, or the medical record as muscle and subcutaneous fat, oral health, suck/swallow/breathe ability, appetite, and affect (Academy of Nutrition and Dietetics eNCPT, 2019). **Table 7-5** outlines some common physical signs and symptoms of malnutrition.

TABLE 7-5 NUTRITION-FOCUSED PHYSICAL FINDINGS OF MALNUTRITION

SIGNS	POSSIBLE NUTRITION-RELATED CAUSES
HAIR	
Dull, dry, lack of natural shine, easily plucked	Protein–energy deficiency, malnutrition
	Essential fatty acid (EFA) deficiency
Thin, sparse: alopecia	Zinc, biotin, protein deficiency, iron
Color changes, depigmentation, lack luster	Other nutrient deficiencies: manganese, copper, selenium, protein-calorie malnutrition
Easily plucked with no pain	Protein deficiency
Corkscrew hair; unemerged hair coils	Vitamin C deficiency
EYES	
Xanthoma (small, yellowish nodules around eyes)	Hyperlipidemia
White rings around both eyes	
Angular inflammation of eyelids, "grittiness" under eye lids, superficial vascularization, ulcerations of cornea, photophobia, lacrimation	Riboflavin deficiency
Pale eye and mucous membranes	Vitamin B$_{12}$, folate, and/or iron deficiency
Night blindness, chronic dry eye, dull or soft cornea	Vitamin A, zinc deficiency
Redness and fissures of eyelid corners; red and inflamed conjunctiva, swollen and sticky eyelids	Riboflavin/pyridoxine deficiency
Ring of fine blood vessels around cornea	General poor nutrition
Bitot's spots (white spots in eyes)	Vitamin A deficiency
LIPS	
Stomatitis (redness and swelling of mouth)	Niacin, riboflavin, iron, and/or pyridoxine deficiency
Cheilosis (angular fissures, scars at corner of mouth)	Niacin, riboflavin, iron, and/or pyridoxine deficiency
Soreness, burning lips, pallor	Pyridoxine deficiency
GUMS	
Spongy, swollen, bleed easily, redness (swollen, bleeding gums; retracted gums with teeth)	Vitamin C deficiency
Gingivitis	Vitamin C, niacin deficiency
MOUTH	
Cheilosis, angular scars	Riboflavin, iron, pyridoxine, niacin deficiency
Soreness, burning	Riboflavin deficiency
TONGUE	
Sores, swollen, scarlet, raw, "beef tongue"	Folacin, niacin deficiency
Smooth, beefy red tongue	Vitamin B$_{12}$, niacin deficiency
Soreness, burning tongue, purplish/magenta color	Riboflavin deficiency
Smooth with papillae (small projections)	Riboflavin, vitamin B$_{12}$, pyridoxine, niacin, folate, protein, iron deficiency
Glossitis	Riboflavin, iron, zinc, riboflavin, pyridoxine deficiency
TASTE	
Sense of taste diminished	Zinc deficiency
TEETH	
Gray-brown spots, mottling	Increased fluoride intake
Missing or erupting abnormally	Generally poor nutrition

(Continued)

TABLE 7-5 NUTRITION-FOCUSED PHYSICAL FINDINGS OF MALNUTRITION (*Continued*)

SIGNS	POSSIBLE NUTRITION-RELATED CAUSES
FACE	
Skin color loss, dark cheeks and eyes, enlarged parotid glands, scaling of skin around nostrils	Protein–energy deficiency, specifically niacin, riboflavin, and pyridoxine deficiencies
Pallor	Iron, folacin, vitamin B_{12}, and vitamin C deficiencies
Hyperpigmentation	Niacin deficiency
NECK	
Thyroid enlargement	Iodine deficiency
Symptoms of hypothyroidism	Iodine deficiency
NAILS	
Brittle, banding	Protein deficiency
Spoon shaped	Iron deficiency, protein deficiency
Central line ridges	Folate, iron deficiencies, malnutrition
SKIN	
Slow wound healing	Zinc, vitamin C, protein deficiency; malnutrition
Psoriasis	Biotin deficiency
Eczema, lesions	Riboflavin, zinc deficiency
Scaling of the scalp, dandruff, oiliness of the scalp, lips, and nose	Biotin deficiency, pyridoxine, zinc, riboflavin, essential fatty acids deficiency; vitamin A excess or deficiency
Petechiae (purple or red pinpoint hemorrhages in the skin)	Vitamin C
Dryness, mosaic, sandpaper feel, flakiness	Increased or decreased vitamin A
Follicular hyperkeratosis (gooseflesh)	Vitamin A deficiency
Dark, dry, scaly skin	Niacin deficiency
Lack of fat under skin, cellophane appearance	Protein–energy deficiency, vitamin C deficiency
Bilateral edema	Protein–energy, vitamin C deficiency
Yellow colored	Beta carotene excess, B_{12} deficiency
Cutaneous flushing	niacin
Body edema; round swollen face	Protein, thiamin deficiencies
Pallor, fatigue, depression, apathy	Iron, folate deficiency
GASTROINTESTINAL	
Anorexia, flatulence, diarrhea	Vitamin B_{12}, folate deficiency
MUSCULAR SYSTEM	
Weakness	Phosphorus or potassium deficiency, vitamin C, vitamin D deficiency
Wasted appearance	Protein–energy deficiency
Calf tenderness, absent knee jerks, foot and wrist drops	Thiamin deficiency
Peripheral neuropathy, tingling, "pins and needles"	Folacin, pyridoxine, pantothenic acid, phosphate, thiamine, vitamin B_{12} deficiencies
Muscle twitching, convulsions, tetany	Magnesium or pyridoxine excess or deficiency, calcium, vitamin D deficiencies
Muscle cramps	Chloride decreased, sodium deficiency; calcium, vitamin D, magnesium, potassium deficiencies
Muscle pain	Biotin, vitamin D deficiency
SKELETAL SYSTEM	
Demineralization of bone	Calcium, phosphorus, vitamin D deficiencies
Epiphyseal enlargement of leg and knee, Bowed legs	Vitamin D deficiency
Bone tenderness	Vitamin D deficiency
NERVOUS SYSTEM	
Listlessness	Protein–energy deficiency
Loss of position and vibratory sense, decrease and loss of ankle and knee reflexes, depression, inability to concentrate, defective memory, confabulation, delirium	Thiamin, pyridoxine, vitamin B_{12} deficiencies
Seizures, memory impairment, and behavioral disturbances	Magnesium, zinc deficiencies
Peripheral neuropathy, dementia	Pyridoxine deficiency
Dementia	Niacin, vitamin B_{12} deficiencies

IDENTIFYING MALNUTRITION

Malnutrition is recognized as a complex syndrome that manifests in different ways. In 2012, the Academy of Nutrition and Dietetics (Academy) and the American Society for Parenteral and Enteral Nutrition (ASPEN) published a joint consensus statement on the identification and documentation of adult malnutrition (White et al., 2012). The statement proposed a three-pronged definition of malnutrition based on etiology (White et al., 2012), as follows:

1. **Malnutrition in the context of social or environmental circumstances (starvation-related malnutrition):** This may be pure starvation due to financial or social reasons, or starvation caused by anorexia nervosa.
2. **Malnutrition in the context of acute illness or injury:** This includes malnutrition associated with organ failure, pancreatic cancer, rheumatoid arthritis, or sarcopenic obesity.
3. **Malnutrition in the context of chronic illness:** This includes malnutrition associated with major infections, burns, trauma, or closed head injury.

The Academy/ASPEN consensus statement, in addition to providing a definition of malnutrition, suggests the following criteria for diagnosis:

- Insufficient energy intake
- Weight loss
- Loss of muscle mass
- Loss of subcutaneous fat
- Localized or generalized fluid accumulation that may sometimes mask weight loss
- Diminished functional status as measured by hand-grip strength

If an individual has two or more of these criteria, they meet the proposed guidelines for malnutrition. Using specific parameters related to each of these six criteria, malnutrition can be classified as nonsevere or severe.

The basic characteristics used to make a malnutrition diagnosis are detailed in **Box 7-1.** These characteristics and criteria rely on medical history, physical examination/clinical signs, anthropometric data, assessment of food and nutrient intake, and functional assessment (White et al., 2012). Laboratory markers of inflammation (C-reactive protein [CRP], white blood cell count, and blood glucose levels) may also be used to help determine if the condition is starvation related, chronic disease related, or acute disease or injury related. The Academy and ASPEN criteria are a work in progress and may change over time.

The European Society for Parenteral and Enteral Nutrition (ESPEN) recognizes that malnutrition is a state resulting from lack of intake or uptake of nutrition that leads to altered body composition (decreased fat-free mass) and body cell mass leading to diminished physical and mental function and impaired clinical outcome from disease (Cederholm et al., 2017). The Global Leadership Initiative on Malnutrition (GLIM) developed the most current definition of malnutrition. Prior

| BOX 7-1 | PROPOSED CLINICAL CHARACTERISTICS USED TO IDENTIFY AND CATEGORIZE MALNUTRITION* |

1. **Energy intake:** Malnutrition is the result of inadequate food and nutrient intake or assimilation; thus, recent intake compared to estimated requirements is a primary criterion for defining malnutrition. The clinician may obtain or review the food and nutrition history, estimate optimum energy needs, compare needs to estimates of energy consumed. Inadequate intake should be reported as a percentage of estimated energy requirements over time.
2. **Interpretation of weight loss:** The clinician may evaluate weight in light of other clinical findings including the presence of underhydration or overhydration. The clinician may assess weight change over time reported as a percentage of weight loss from baseline.
3. **Body fat:** Loss of subcutaneous fat (e.g., orbital, triceps, fat overlying the ribs)
4. **Muscle mass:** Muscle loss (e.g., wasting of the temples [temporalis muscle], clavicles [pectoralis and deltoids], shoulders [deltoids], interosseous muscles, scapula [latissimus dorsi, trapezius, deltoids], thigh [quadriceps], and calf [gastrocnemius])
5. **Fluid accumulation:** The clinician may evaluate generalized or localized fluid accumulation evident on examination (extremities, vulvar/scrotal edema, or ascites). Weight loss is often masked by generalized fluid retention (edema), and weight gain may be observed.
6. **Reduced grip strength:** Use standards supplied by the manufacturer of the measurement device (dynamometer).

*A minimum of two characteristics are required for a diagnosis of malnutrition. Based on criteria proposed by the Academy/A.S.P.E.N, malnutrition can be identified into one of three categories (malnutrition in the context of acute illness or injury, malnutrition in the context of chronic illness, and malnutrition in the context of environmental circumstances) and can be classified as severe or nonsevere within each category. Refer to source below for more information. Source: White et al. (2012).

to diagnosing malnutrition, the GLIM committee recommends nutrition screening using a validated screening tool to determine nutrition risk. This consensus diagnostic criteria, based on previous ASPEN and ESPEN criteria, helps to identify malnutrition in adults in clinical settings on a global scale. The criteria consist of three phenotype characteristics (weight loss, low BMI, decreased muscle mass) and two etiologic characteristics (decreased food intake or assimilation and disease burden/inflammation). The presence of one phenotype and one etiologic characteristic meets the GLIM criteria for malnutrition (Cederholm et al., 2018).

A comprehensive assessment to identify malnutrition requires more time than a simple blood draw but provides helpful information as to the etiology of malnutrition, which provides guidance as to best approach to intervention. An RDN should be routinely consulted for assistance in management of individuals at risk for or demonstrating evidence of malnutrition.

It is important to share the data and planned interventions with other members of the interdisciplinary team. The plan should include strategies to monitor the individual's nutritional status as they move from one care setting to another.

 NUTRIENTS THAT PLAY A ROLE IN WOUND HEALING

For overall good health, it is important to consume all essential nutrients in the quantities recommended by the Dietary Reference Intakes. A diet that contains good sources of protein, low-fat dairy foods, fruits, vegetables, and grains (especially whole grains) can provide the essential nutrients in adequate amounts to maintain good health (U.S. Department of Agriculture, 2015). Nutrients are generally broken down into macronutrients (those needed in large amounts) and micronutrients (those needed in small amounts). Protein, carbohydrate, fat, and fluid are known as macronutrients. Vitamins and minerals are considered micronutrients. Each nutrient plays a different role in the body, with some having more of an influence on wound healing than others. **Table 7-6**

TABLE 7-6 NUTRIENTS AND THEIR THERAPEUTIC PROPERTIES

NUTRIENT	FUNCTION	SOURCE
Calories	Supply energy, prevent weight loss, preserve lean body mass.	Carbohydrate, protein, and fat, with carbohydrate and fat the preferred sources
Carbohydrates	Deliver energy. Energy needs must be met to spare protein from being used for energy. Glucose supports cell growth, fibroblasts, and leukocytes.	Grains, fruits, and vegetables, with complex carbohydrate the preferred source
Protein	Contains nitrogen, which is essential for wound healing. Is a component of the immune system. Supplies the binding material of skin, cartilage, and muscle. Note: Arginine becomes a conditionally indispensable amino acid during times of physiological stress.	Meats, fish, poultry, eggs, legumes, milk, and dairy products; favor lean meat and reduced-fat or low-fat dairy products
Fat	Most concentrated energy source, carries the fat-soluble vitamins, provides insulation under the skin and padding of bony prominences, helps modulate inflammation and the immune response.	Meats, eggs, dairy products, and vegetable oils
Fluids	Solvent for minerals and vitamins, amino acids and glucose; help maintain body temperature; transport materials to cells and waste products from cells; maintain skin integrity.	Water, juices, beverages; fruits and vegetables contain ~95% water. Most supplements are 75% water
Vitamin A	Important for protein synthesis, collagen formation, maintenance of epithelium, immune function. May also delay healing in older adults on corticosteroids. UL is 3,000 µg; DRI females older than 70 years is 700 µg, males older than 70 years is 900 µg.	Beef liver, milk, dark green and yellow vegetables, especially carrots, sweet potatoes, broccoli, spinach, apricots
Vitamin C	Water-soluble, noncaloric organic nutrient essential for collagen formation; enhances activation of leukocytes and macrophages to the wound site; improves tensile strength; aids in absorption of iron.	Citrus fruits and juices, tomatoes, potatoes, broccoli
Vitamin E	Antioxidant important in metabolism of fat, collagen synthesis, stabilization of cell membranes.	Vegetable oils, sweet potatoes
Copper	Inorganic, noncaloric nutrient; assists in the formation of red blood cells; responsible for collagen cross-linking and erythropoiesis. UL is 10,000 µg. DRI females and males 70 years and older is 900 µg.	Nuts, dried fruit, organ meats, dried beans, whole grain cereal
Iron	Transports oxygen to the cells as a component of hemoglobin, important in collagen formation, creates energy from cells.	Heme iron: meats, poultry, and fish. Nonheme iron: vegetables, grains, eggs, meat, fish
Zinc	Inorganic, noncaloric nutrient; cofactor for collagen formation; metabolizes protein; assists in immune function; liberates vitamin A from the liver; interacts with platelets in blood clotting. Mega doses of zinc may inhibit healing and cause copper deficiency. UL is 40 mg. DRI females 70 years and older is 8 mg, males 70 years and older is 11 mg.	Meats, liver, eggs, and seafood

DRI, dietary reference intake; UL, tolerable upper intake level.
Reference: Posthauer, M. E. (2020). Nutritional implications of wound healing. In M. Bernstein & N. Munoz (Eds.), *Nutrition for the older adult* (3rd ed., pp. 418–419). Burlington, MA: Jones and Bartlett Learning. Reprinted with permission.

outlines the key nutrients that play a role in wound healing and their specific functions.

 ## NUTRITIONAL NEEDS OF INDIVIDUALS AT RISK FOR OR WITH PRESSURE INJURIES

Each individual has unique nutritional needs that are based on their body weight, activity level, and comorbidities. A comprehensive nutrition assessment assists the RDN to identify areas of concern and to develop an individualized plan of care. The 2019 International Guideline, *Prevention and Treatment of Pressure Ulcers/Injuries Clinical Practice Guideline,* which was developed by three organizations and 14 associate organizations, provides information on specific nutritional needs for prevention and treatment of pressure injuries in adults and children (EPUAP/NPIAP/PPPIA, 2019). These guidelines were developed following a systematic, comprehensive review of peer-based research on pressure injury prevention and treatment. All studies meeting the inclusion criteria were reviewed for quality, summarized in evidence tables, and classified according to their level of evidence using an established classification system (EPUAP/NPIAP/PPPIA, 2019). The goal of the international collaboration was to provide a comprehensive review of the current research and develop recommendations based on recent evidence. The intention is for health professionals throughout the world to apply the recommendations in clinical practice.

The 2019 EPUAP/NPIAP/PPPIA guideline provides ratings for recommendations according to the strength of cumulative evidence supporting the recommendation plus the strength of recommendation. A summary of the 2019 Clinical Practice Guideline (CPG) on nutrition and wounds is outlined in **Box 7-2**.

Food sources of nutrients are preferred over supplements. Supplements are prescribed if an individual cannot or will not consume adequate nutrients through food alone. Major food sources for each of the macronutrients and micronutrients are listed in **Table 7-6**. Energy, measured in the form of kilocalories, is provided in the diet by the macronutrients, protein, carbohydrates, and fats. Providing adequate energy promotes anabolism (tissue building), nitrogen and collagen synthesis, and wound healing and acts to spare protein by providing alternative sources of energy (Quain & Khardon, 2015). Any condition that increases the metabolic rate (e.g., infection, trauma, stress, pressure injury, etc.) creates a hypermetabolic state that increases energy (caloric) needs.

KEY POINT

The *Clinical Practice Guideline for Prevention and Treatment of Pressure Ulcers/Injuries* provides recommendations for intake of calories, protein and amino acids, fluid, and vitamins and minerals (EPUAP/NPIAP/PPPIA, 2019).

BOX 7-2   NUTRITION GUIDELINES FOR PRESSURE INJURY PREVENTION AND MANAGEMENT

Nutrition Screening
- Conduct nutritional screening for individuals at risk for pressure ulcer/injury.

Nutrition Assessment
- Conduct a comprehensive nutrition assessment for adults at risk of a pressure ulcer/injury who are screened to be at risk of malnutrition and for all adults with a pressure ulcer/injury.

Nutrition Care Planning
- Develop and implement an individualized nutrition care plan for individuals with, or at risk of, a pressure ulcer/injury who are malnourished or who are at risk of malnutrition.

Energy and Protein Intake for Individuals at Risk of Pressure Injuries
- Optimize energy intake for individuals at risk of pressure ulcer/injuries who are malnourished or at risk of malnutrition.
- Adjust protein intake for individuals at risk of pressure ulcer/injuries who are malnourished or at risk of malnutrition.

Energy and Protein Intake for Individuals with Pressure Injuries
- Provide 30 to 35 kcal/kg body weight/day body weight for adults with a pressure injury who are malnourished or at risk of malnutrition.
- Provide 1.25 to 1.5 g/kg body weight/day for adults with a pressure ulcer/injury who are malnourished or at risk of malnutrition.

Nutritional Supplementation
- Offer high calorie, high protein fortified foods and/or nutritional supplements in addition to the usual diet for adults who are at risk of developing a pressure ulcer/injury and who are also malnourished or at risk of malnutrition, if nutritional requirements cannot be achieved by normal dietary intake.
- Offer high calorie, high protein nutritional supplements in addition to the usual diet for adults with a pressure ulcer/injury who are malnourished or at risk for malnutrition, if nutritional requirements cannot be achieved by normal dietary intake.
- Provide high-calorie, high-protein, arginine, zinc and antioxidant oral nutritional supplements, or enteral formula for adults with a Category/Stage 2 or greater pressure ulcer/injury who are malnourished or at risk for malnutrition.

Artificial Nutrition: Enteral and Parenteral Feeding
- Discuss the benefits and harms of enteral or parenteral feeding to support overall health in light of preferences and goals of care with individuals at risk of pressure ulcer/injury who cannot meet their nutritional requirements through oral intake despite nutritional interventions.
- Discuss the benefits and harms of enteral or parenteral feeding to support pressure injury treatment in light of preferences and goals of care for individuals with pressure ulcer/injury who cannot meet their nutritional requirements through oral intake despite nutritional interventions.

Hydration
- Provide and encourage adequate water intake for hydration for an individual with or at risk of a pressure ulcer/injury, when compatible with goals of care and clinical condition.

ENERGY (KILOCALORIES)

The 2019 EPUAP/NPIAP/PPPIA guideline recommends optimizing energy intake for individuals at risk of pressure ulcer/injuries who are malnourished or at risk of malnutrition, specifically, to provide 30 to 35 kcal/kg of body weight for adults with a pressure injury who are malnourished or at risk of malnutrition. In contrast, a severely obese individual may require a caloric range below the recommended level. Using the 2019 EPUAP/NPIAP/PPPIA guideline as a resource, the RDN should calculate the appropriate caloric intake based on the individual's nutrition assessment.

Food before supplements is the general rule; when supplements are required, they should be offered between meals rather than with meals to maximize meal consumption. The 2019 EPUAP/NPIAP/PPPIA guideline recommends (and research supports) measures to liberalize dietary choices, especially when meals are refused due to the type of food served (Dorner & Friedrich, 2017). For example, if a person with heart failure and pressure injuries is refusing to eat a 2-g sodium therapeutic diet as ordered, then moving to a less restrictive diet is appropriate.

PROTEIN

Sufficient protein should be provided to maintain positive nitrogen balance for any individual who has a pressure injury or is assessed at risk for a pressure injury. Clinical judgment should be used when determining the appropriate level of protein for each person, based on overall nutritional status, comorbidities, and tolerance to the interventions. Renal function is of concern, as high levels of protein intake may be contraindicated in some patients with CKD (Harvey, 2013). The 2019 EPUAP/NPIAP/PPPIA guideline provides the following recommendations:

- Adjust protein intake for individuals at risk of pressure ulcer/injuries who are malnourished or at risk of malnutrition.
- Provide 1.25 to 1.5 g/kg body weight/day for adults with a pressure ulcer/injury who are malnourished or at risk of malnutrition.

AMINO ACIDS

Amino acids are the building blocks of protein. Specialized protein supplements with selected amino acids are often recommended to promote wound healing when standard care has proven unsuccessful. Some amino acids must be provided through dietary intake (essential or indispensable amino acids), while others can be synthesized by the body (nonessential or dispensable amino acids). Three amino acids (arginine, glutamine, and cysteine) are commonly linked to wound healing because they are indispensable, meaning they become essential in situations causing physiologic stress, such as trauma, chronic disease, or poor dietary intake.

According to the 2019 EPUAP/NPIAP/PPPIA guideline, growing evidence supports nutritional supplementation with additional protein, arginine, and micronutrients for adults with a Stage 2 or greater pressure injury who are malnourished or at risk for malnutrition to promote pressure injury healing. One study showed more than three times greater likelihood of a pressure injury healing when a high calories high-protein oral nutritional supplement containing arginine, zinc, and antioxidants is provided for more than 4 weeks (Cereda et al., 2015). Other studies provide evidence for improvements in wound healing measures using this type of supplement (EPUAP/NPIAP/PPPIA, 2019).

FLUIDS

Adequate fluids should be provided to prevent dehydration. Individuals with draining wounds, emesis, diarrhea, or increased insensible losses due to fever, excessive perspiration, or air-fluidized beds may need additional fluids daily. Recommended fluid intake for healthy adults is 2.4 L/day for women and 3.7 L/day for men (IOM, 2004). Hydration needs are met by consuming liquids as well as from fluids found in foods.

Fluid needs can be estimated using a number of methods including 1.0 mL/kcal consumed or body weight in kg × 30 mL/kg (EPUAP/NPIAP/PPPIA, 2019). Fluid needs may vary based on comorbidities and/or acute illnesses or heavily draining wounds. Inadequate fluid intake is a common problem, especially among older adults; strategies that have been proven effective are listed in **Box 7-3**.

BOX 7-3   STRATEGIES TO ENHANCE FLUID INTAKE

- Identify and offer the individual's favorite beverages.
- Offer a beverage following wound care treatment.
- Offer extra fluids with each medication pass.
- Keep water at the bedside and within reach.
- Offer a variety of beverages with meals.
- Offer beverages before or after physical therapy sessions.
- Monitor all individuals for signs and symptoms of dehydration.

VITAMINS AND MINERALS

Adequate vitamins and minerals are needed for overall good health and to promote skin integrity and wound healing. No research has demonstrated a positive effect on wound healing when large doses of a supplement were offered, such as vitamin C or zinc. Vitamin C is a cofactor, along with iron, that contributes to the oxidation of lysine and proline, which is required for the production of collagen. A deficiency of vitamin C could delay wound healing, but mega doses of ascorbic acid have not resulted in accelerated healing (ter Riet et al., 1995). Zinc is a cofactor for collagen formation and is also necessary for protein metabolism; mega doses of elemental zinc above the upper limit (UL) of 40 mg/day is not recommended unless a deficiency is confirmed (IOM, 2006). Zinc status is difficult to measure since it is widely distributed throughout the body. Plasma and serum zinc levels are the most widely used methods of zinc assessment, but they do not necessarily reflect cellular zinc status. A serum zinc level is not recommended to determine status.

If an individual with wounds is consistently consuming a diet that is low in vitamins and minerals, a daily multivitamin with minerals may be beneficial. Health professionals should use clinical judgment and evaluate nutrient intake from food, beverages, and oral nutritional supplements (ONS). Because of the lack of evidence-based research on the validity of recommending mega doses of specific vitamin or minerals, the 2019 EPUAP/NPIAP/PPPIA guideline small working group did not study the issue. The guideline does recommend that when dietary intake is inadequate, or deficiencies are suspected or confirmed, a multivitamin and mineral supplement should be provided. See **Table 7-6** for additional sources of nutrients and their specific functions.

KEY POINT

A multivitamin–mineral supplement should be recommended when inadequate intake is known or suspected.

CARE PLANNING: DEVELOPING NUTRITION INTERVENTIONS TO PREVENT AND/OR TREAT PRESSURE INJURIES

An individualized/interdisciplinary plan for nutrition should be developed in conjunction with the individual and/or caregivers and should include a discussion of the risks and benefits of recommended interventions. Interventions to help improve nutritional status might include but are not limited to the following:

- Individualized diets: Those individuals who are on therapeutic diets might benefit from a more liberal, less restrictive diet, especially if intake is poor (Dorner & Friedrich, 2017).

- Texture modifications: If chewing or swallowing problems are preventing food intake, food textures or fluid consistencies might need to be modified to maximize meal intake.
- Assistance with food preparation and/or eating, as needed.
- Improved access to food (including transportation) if financial limitations affect nutritional status.
- Targeted nutrition interventions, including fortified foods, ONS, or enteral nutrition.
- Offering six small meals daily to ensure increased caloric intake.
- Rotating the type of high-calorie/high-protein snacks offered between meals to avoid flavor fatigue.

Oral Nutritional Supplements

When an individual cannot meet their nutritional needs through consumption of meals and snacks, then other strategies are necessary. Options include adding fortified foods to meals or snacks or offering high-calorie, high-protein supplements (such as those made with milk and ice cream) between meals.

Fortified or enhanced foods can be made by adding ingredients to regular foods consumed that increase the calories and/or protein provided. Examples include oatmeal made with whole milk or half and half, powdered milk and brown sugar, or cream soup made with whole milk or half and half.

ONS are commercial products that supply nutrients such as protein, carbohydrates, fat, vitamins, minerals, and/or amino acids. Several studies conducted in a variety of settings have demonstrated significant improvements in pressure injury healing in individuals using high calorie, high protein ONS (EPUAP/NPIAP/PPPIA, 2019). A wide variety of commercial supplements are available, and many can be purchased over the counter by community-dwelling individuals.

Appetite Enhancers

Appetite stimulants and anabolic steroids may contribute to improved food intake and/or to treatment of unintended weight loss. A number of different medications are available that can enhance appetite; however, more research is needed to determine their effectiveness in promoting pressure injury healing (Levine, 2017). In the long-term care setting, there is insufficient evidence to support the use of most appetite enhancers (Rudolph, 2009). Some evidence suggests that megestrol acetate may be of benefit in this setting; however, there are risks associated with its use, and there are no studies addressing benefits and risks if used for long periods of time (Rudolph, 2009). Use of appetite enhancers should be considered on an individual basis.

Oxandrin is an anabolic steroid sometimes used to promote anabolism and weight gain in patients with significant unintended weight loss. Animal studies have shown promise for improvements in collagen synthesis and other parameters associated with wound healing, but evidence in humans has not shown a positive effect (Levine, 2017).

Enteral Nutrition

When oral intake is inadequate, enteral or parenteral feeding may be recommended if consistent with an individual's wishes. Enteral feeding is preferred over parenteral nutrition as long as the gut is functioning. One of the potential benefits of enteral nutrition is reduced risk of pressure injury development and/or improved wound healing. Research on the benefits of enteral nutrition in prevention and/or treatment of pressure injuries is limited. Studies have not shown benefits to the incidence of pressure injuries (EPUAP/NPIAP/PPPIA, 2019). Two small studies do support a link between high protein nutrition support and a decrease in the incidence of pressure injuries in older adults (Cereda et al., 2009; Ohura et al., 2011). Specific adverse effects associated with enteral feedings include GI complications (diarrhea, nausea, and vomiting), aspiration pneumonia, metabolic complications, and mechanical complications with tube placement (Chernoff & Seres, 2014; Malone et al., 2019). Given the mixed data regarding benefits, each individual should be evaluated for the risks versus benefits of tube placement. If an individual is catabolic and the source of the catabolism is untreatable, such as chronic or critical illness, enteral feeding is less likely to positively affect outcome (Chernoff & Seres, 2014).

KEY POINT

The decision to initiate enteral feedings must be individualized and made with caution after analyzing the risks versus benefits.

Nutrition Care and the Wound Care Center

Patients at risk for or with pressure injuries that reside in acute or post-acute care settings typically have access to a RDN. Wound care centers (WCC) provide treatment to individuals living in the community and those referred from a health care setting. They may not have an RDN on staff but should have a system in place for referral to an RDN for individualized counseling. Medicare and some private insurance carriers provide coverage for nutrition services for management of diabetes and renal disease when specific criteria are met.

Screening individuals to determine malnutrition risk using a validated nutrition screening tool could be the initial step in the referral process. A research study in Ohio resulted in the development of a nutrition screening tool for an outpatient wound center called The MEAL Scale for Malnutrition in Chronic Wound Patients (Fulton et al., 2016). The MEAL scale includes questions about wounds, food intake, appetite, and activity.

It is recommended that MEAL be completed by the wound care nurse or RDN at their initial visit and again in 6 months. Individuals with a 2 or greater score are referred to an RDN for a complete assessment and those who score a 1 or at risk should have a discussion with the nurse or physician about the value of consuming an adequate diet.

Individuals who receive services at a WCC may have language or literacy difficulties, which hamper their ability to understand the value of consuming good sources of protein and adequate calories. Providing pamphlets with colorful pictures of high protein foods and discussing the importance of eating a balanced diet and linking their diet to wound healing reinforces the concept of "food as medicine." See Chapter 6 Patient and Caregiver Education for suggestions for addressing this concern.

Some individuals face limited resources to purchase food due to lack of transportation. Hospitals in some communities have a Fresh Food Pharmacy that offers food including high calories supplements to individuals who have limited access to affordable food. The physician writes an order for food just as they would for medicine that can be used at the food pharmacy.

CASE STUDY

DIAGNOSING MALNUTRITION

A 70-year-old woman admitted to the hospital with a hip fracture after a fall. She lives alone and her son found her on the floor 10 hours after her fall. Lying 10 hours in one position increased her risk of PI. Additional diagnoses: obesity, hypertension, and diabetes mellitus (DM).

History: Typical meals include breakfast of sweet roll and coffee, noon: Meals on Wheels 5 days a week, sandwiches and chips, cookies, ice cream, overall poor diet

Admission weight: 325 pounds, height 60 inches (152.4 cm), BMI 63.6 (obese)

Medications: oral hypoglycemic, diuretic, beta blocker, and NSAID

Intake: past 6 days is 50% of her estimated energy requirement

Current weight: 315 pounds (a 7 pound loss due to diuresis)

Biochemical data: HgbA1C, 8%; fasting glucose (FG) 195 mg/dL; serum albumin, 2.6 g/dL; hemoglobin, 10 g/dL; hematocrit, 32%.; C-reactive protein, 18 mg/L

Nutrition Focused Physical Assessment: handgrip dynamometer notes reduced handgrip strength for age and gender

Physical Therapy: Poor endurance, difficulty walking

Activity Preference: Watching TV in recliner, refuses to reposition or elevate heels

Clinical Malnutrition Diagnosis: Acute injury-associated malnutrition (hip surgery) and chronic

disease-associated malnutrition as evidenced by less than optimal intake and reduced handgrip strength. Factors contributing to the diagnosis include:

- Hip surgery linked to acute inflammatory response compounded by comorbidities
- Elevated C-reactive protein typical of inflammation noted with surgery
- Anthropometric data: BMI consistent with obesity
- Laboratory data: Elevated FG and HgbA1C consistent with poor control of DM
- Low hemoglobin and hematocrit characteristic of blood loss from surgery

SPECIFIC POPULATIONS

Neonates and Children

Neonates and children are at risk for developing pressure injuries. Multicenter studies report most pressure injuries in this population are facility acquired with the highest prevalence rates occurring in intensive care units (ICUs) (Schlüer et al., 2012, 2014). Medical devices account for the majority of pressure injuries in neonates and young children (Curley et al., 2018; Schlüer et al., 2014).

Pediatric malnutrition or undernutrition in developed countries occurs as a result of an acute or chronic illness (Grover & Ee, 2009). Pediatric malnutrition related to complications of an underlying disease and conditions such as slow wound healing leads to longer complex hospital stays, which increase hospital costs (Hecht et al., 2015).

ASPEN defines pediatric malnutrition (undernutrition) as an imbalance between nutrient requirement and intake, resulting in cumulative deficits of energy, protein or micronutrients that may negatively affect growth, development, and other relevant outcomes (Mehta et al., 2013). Children at risk for pressure injuries and those with pressure injuries usually have other comorbidities that compromise their ability to consume adequate nutrients to promote healing (Mehta et al., 2009). Early nutrition screening and assessment are important to identify malnutrition risk and implement a nutrition care plan. The 2019 EPUAP/NPIAP/PPPIA guideline recommends conducting an age-appropriate nutritional screen and assessment for neonates and children at risk of pressure injuries as a Good Practice Statement (EPUAP/NPIAP/PPPIA, 2019). Validated nutrition screening tools for this population include the Subjective Global Nutritional Assessment for Children, Pediatric Nutritional Risk Score (PMRS), Screening Tool for the Assessment of Malnutrition in Pediatrics (STAMP), the Paediatric Yorkhill

Malnutrition Score (PYMA), and the Screening Tool for the Risk of Impaired Nutritional Status and Growth (STRONG-kids) (EPUAP/NPIAP/PPPIA, 2019).

Studies recommend that an RDN should complete a nutrition assessment weekly for critically ill children. The individualized care plan designed by the interdisciplinary team for children should include the method of feeding, frequent monitoring of intake, and growth status. The need for oral supplements, nutrition support, and feeding strategies for parents and caregivers to promote adequate intake of nutrients should also be considered (Ranade & Collins, 2011; Skillman & Wischmeyer, 2008). The 2019 EPUAP/NPIAP/PPPIA guideline recommends for neonates and children with or at risk of pressure ulcer/injury who have inadequate oral intake, consider fortified foods, age appropriate nutritional supplements, or enteral or parenteral nutritional support as a good practice statement (EPUAP/NPIAP/PPPIA, 2019). If enteral feeding is needed, pediatric enteral formulas designed for children from age 1 to 13 years of age meet the Dietary Reference Intakes (DRI) for children ages 1 to 8 in 1,000 mL/day and 1,500 mL/day for children ages 9 to 14 (Malone et al., 2019).

Older Adults

The aging process leads to multiple changes in the skin. Dermal thickness decreases by 20%, leading to a paper-thin appearance on the legs and forearms. Fatty layers decrease, leaving bony prominences less protected, and reduced collagen deposition could lead to slow wound healing (Baranoski et al., 2016). Older adults have a decrease in pain sensation making them susceptible to environmental insults such as stepping on objects or hitting their legs on furniture that can result in bruising or skin tears. Aging skin retains less moisture because of a reduction in dermal proteins leading to diminished fluid homeostasis, placing older adults at risk for dehydration. Water content of the skin is usually 10% to 15%; and when below 10%, the skin becomes dry and more vulnerable to damage (Dealey, 2009). Studies suggest that age is a factor and an indicator of likely deficits risk for pressure injury development (EPUAP/NPIAP/PPPIA, 2019). The 10-year International Prevalence Survey (2006–2015) noted the prevalence of pressure injuries in long-term at 25.2% and 11.8% in long-term care (VanGilder et al., 2017). The majority of the residents in these settings are older adults.

Sarcopenia and frailty are conditions that impact the older adult's nutritional status, increase risk for pressure injury, and affect the healing process. The European Working Group on Sarcopenia in Older People (EWGSOP) published a definition of sarcopenia; sarcopenia, that is muscle failure, is a muscle disease rooted in adverse muscle changes that accrue across a lifetime; sarcopenia is common among adults of older age but can also occur earlier in life. Sarcopenia is defined by low levels of measures for three parameters: (1) muscle strength, (2) muscle quantity/quality, and (3) physical performance as an indicator of severity (Cruz-Jentoft et al., 2019). Sarcopenia increases the risk of falls and fractures, decreases the ability of older adults to perform ADLs, may lead to mobility disorders, which decreases their quality of life and is associated with cardiac disease, respiratory failure, and loss of independence. According to the EWGSOP, sarcopenia may be acute or chronic.

The sarcopenia phenotype associated with malnutrition is irrespective of whether the condition is caused by undernutrition or malabsorption, medication-caused anorexia, overnutrition/obesity, or high nutrient requirement caused by an inflammatory disease or condition, such as pressure injury. Low fat mass is associated with malnutrition, which is also present in sarcopenia, and low muscle mass has also been proposed as part of the GLIM malnutrition definition (Cederholm et al., 2018).

Frailty is a geriatric syndrome also characterized by a decline in multiple body systems leading to poor outcomes including disability and increased hospital stays (Langiois et al., 2012). Weight loss is common in frail older adults and physical changes such as low grip strength and slow gait speed is distinctive of frailty and sarcopenia. Treatment for physical frailty and for sarcopenia includes provision of optimal protein intake, supplementation of vitamin D, and physical exercise (Dodds & Sayer, 2015).

Spinal Cord Injuries

Spinal cord injury (SCI) can result in permanent physical deficits (Bigford & Nash, 2017) including paraplegia or quadriplegia. SCI also results in metabolic abnormalities including increased risk for all-cause cardiovascular disease, central obesity, dyslipidemia, hypertension, insulin resistance, and long-term declines in muscle mass

(Bigford & Nash, 2017). Individuals with limited mobility following SCI are at increased risk for pressure injuries (EPUAP/NPIAP/PPPIA, 2019) but information on nutrition recommendations to prevent and treat pressure injury in individuals with SCI is limited. Clinical judgment is necessary to determine nutritional needs of each individual with SCI to prevent or treat comorbidities, maintain muscle mass, and prevent and/or treat pressure injuries.

Muscle energy expenditure in SCI patients in the acute and rehabilitation phases is at least 10% below predicted (Academy of Nutrition and Dietetics Evidence Analysis Library, SCI, 2009). The Academy of Nutrition and Dietetics Evidence Analysis Library recommends providing 22.7 kcal/kg for individuals with tetraplegia and 27.9 kcal/kg for individual with quadriplegia (Academy of Nutrition and Dietetics Evidence Analysis Library, SCI, 2009). During the acute phase of SCI, as much as 2.0 g protein/kg body weight may be needed (Academy of Nutrition and Dietetics Evidence Analysis Library, SCI, 2009). Specific guidelines for protein needs following the acute phase are not available (Bigford & Nash, 2017) but estimating needs at 0.8 to 1.0 g/kg body weight (with changes as needed based on comorbidities) is recommended (Academy of Nutrition and Dietetics Evidence Analysis Library, SCI, 2009). SCI patients with pressure injuries may need as much as 30 to 40 kcal/kg of body weight and 1.2 to 1.5 g protein (Stage 2) and 1.5 to 2.0 g/kg protein (Stage 3 and 4) (Academy of Nutrition and Dietetics Evidence Analysis Library, SCI, 2009). See Chapter 16 for additional information specific to SCI patients.

 ISSUES THAT AFFECT NUTRITION ASSESSMENT AND INTERVENTIONS FOR PRESSURE INJURIES AND WOUNDS

OVERWEIGHT AND OBESITY

Overweight and obesity are defined based on BMI. **Tables 7-2 to 7-4** outline BMI definitions. The subject of nutritional management of overweight and obese individuals with pressure injuries raises more questions than it provides answers. Research is needed to better define appropriate caloric intake for overweight and obese individuals with pressure injuries.

According to the Academy of Nutrition and Dietetics Evidence Analysis Library, caloric needs for healthy obese individuals are most accurately estimated by the Mifflin St. Jeor formula using *actual* body weight (Academy of Nutrition and Dietetics Evidence Analysis Library, Adult Weight Management, 2014). The American Society of Parenteral and Enteral Nutrition/Society of Critical Care Medicine recommends using 11 to 14 kcal/kg actual weight or 22 to 25 kcal/kg ideal body weight for critically ill obese adults (Malone & Russell, 2016). It is unclear if any guidelines provide appropriate recommendations for the obese individual who presents with wounds or pressure injuries in the absence of critical illness. Practitioners may choose to use the 2019 EPUAP/NPIAP/PPPIA guideline recommendation of 30 to 35 kcal/kg body weight, recognizing that the resulting estimates may be unrealistically high. Clinical judgment should be used to adjust caloric intake goals based on the individualized nutrition assessment.

Standard estimates of protein and fluid needs for underweight or normal weight individuals with pressure injuries may not apply to those who are overweight or obese. Protein needs of critically ill obese patients can be estimated at 1.2 g/kg actual weight or 2.0 to 2.5 g/kg ideal body weight, with adjustment of goals based on nutrition balance (Malone & Russell, 2016). There is little evidence-based guidance available for practitioners on how to estimate protein needs for overweight or obese individuals in the absence of critical illness.

When applying the 2019 EPUAP/NPIAP/PPPIA guideline recommendations for protein and fluids, estimates may be unrealistically high, so clinical judgment is required to make adjustments based on the individualized nutrition assessment.

Because estimating the nutritional needs of overweight and obese individuals is problematic, ongoing monitoring of calorie, protein, and fluid intake; weight; and progress in wound healing is important and may be the best way to determine whether nutritional needs are being met.

When caring for patients who are overweight or obese, wound-healing goals usually take priority overweight loss goals. Although weight loss is usually recommended for obese individuals, weight loss efforts may need to be postponed temporarily, or at least modified, to assure provision of sufficient nutrients for wound healing (Posthauer et al., 2015). An obese individual with wounds should consume a diet adequate in protein and calories to meet wound-healing needs instead of a low-calorie diet designed for weight reduction (Posthauer & Thomas, 2012). Because the wound-healing process depends on an adequate flow of nutrients, reducing caloric and/or protein intake could compromise wound healing by resulting in a breakdown of lean body mass (Demling, 2009).

VEGAN DIETS

Vegetarian-based diets are growing in popularity as Americans focus on healthy eating; approximately 4% of U.S. adults, follow a vegetarian diet. Approximately 2.0% of those are vegans, who consume no animal products (The VRG, 2019). Planned vegetarian or vegan diets are healthful and nutritionally adequate for most people, including older adults (Melina et al., 2016). Vegans and some other vegetarians tend to have lower intake of selected nutrients, including zinc, which is thought to have a role in wound healing. Other nutrients that may not be provided in sufficient amounts in a vegan diet include vitamin B_{12} and iron. Dry beans, nuts, peas, lentils, and tofu are all protein sources that should be encouraged for vegans. Meat analogs made of soy, microproteins, or seitan are also good sources of protein. The diet of a vegan with wounds or pressure injuries should be evaluated for adequacy of intake related to key nutrients, with supplements ordered if a deficiency is confirmed or suspected.

Oral Nutritional Supplements for Vegans

If meal intake is poor, ONS may be necessary to help meet calorie, protein, and nutrient needs. Supplements for vegans should contain no dairy, meat, or egg products. Milk protein is commonly used as a base for commercial nutritional supplements available through medical supply companies and pharmacies. It may be necessary to find alternate sources for vegan supplements.

DIABETES MELLITUS

Individuals with diabetes are at increased risk for non-healing wounds and wound infections. Poorly managed blood glucose levels can affect the ability of a wound to heal. Glycemic control is a key issue for individuals with both wounds and diabetes (Litchford, 2010).

Effective blood glucose control requires an interdisciplinary approach that addresses diet, physical activity, and medication management. There is no conclusive evidence regarding the ideal amount of carbohydrate intake for people with diabetes (Standards of Diabetes Care-Lifestyle, 2019) and no "one size fits all" eating pattern for individuals with diabetes. Goals of nutrition therapy for adults with diabetes include to promote and support healthful eating patterns, emphasizing a variety of nutrient-dense foods in appropriate portion sizes, to improve overall health and (1) achieve and maintain body weight goals, (2) attain individualized glycemic, blood pressure, and lipids goals, and (3) delay or prevent the complications of diabetes. Ideally an individualized diet that takes into account preferences, cultural norms, and lifestyle is recommended.

Older adults who are functional, are cognitively intact, and have significant life expectancy should receive diabetes care similar to younger individuals (Standards of Medical Care in Diabetes-Older adults, 2019); in these individuals, the glycemic goal is usually 90 to 130 mg/dL. Glycemic control may be less important in those with life-limiting illness or substantial cognitive or functional impairment (Standards of Medical Care in Diabetes-Older adults, 2019). Those with poorly controlled diabetes may be subject to complications such as dehydration, impaired wound healing, or wound infection, so glycemic goals should be established with the goal of preventing these consequences (Standards of Medical Care in Diabetes-Older adults, 2019).

CHRONIC KIDNEY DISEASE

Individuals with CKD often have comorbidities that affect their nutrition care. An individual with CKD, diabetes, and wounds or pressure injuries has complicated and conflicting nutritional needs. The diet often suggested for management of stage 3 or 4 CKD that is limited in calories, protein, potassium, phosphorus, sodium, and fluid may not meet the protein or nutrient needs required for wound healing. Clinical consultation with an RDN is important when treating individuals with CKD and wounds. The RDN is prepared to provide in-depth assessment of the risks versus the benefits of therapeutic diets, especially for older adults (Dorner & Friedrich, 2017).

END OF LIFE/PALLIATIVE CARE/ HOSPICE CARE

Nutrition care for end of life and/or hospice care should focus on comfort, quality of life, and minimizing symptoms (Dorner & Friedrich, 2017; EPUAP/NPIAP/PPPIA, 2019). The individual and/or their family or surrogate should be at the center of decision-making regarding the use of supplemental nutrition to prevent and/or treat pressure injuries and other types of wounds near the end of life (EPUAP/NPIAP/PPPIA, 2019). An individual receiving palliative or end of life care that does not have pressure injury healing as a goal should be allowed to consume foods and fluids as desired and tolerated (EPUAP/NPIAP/PPPIA, 2019). Supplemental nutrition is appropriate for palliative and/or end of life wound care (EPUAP/NPIAP/PPPIA, 2019). The plan of nutrition care should reflect an individual's choices and preferences and include foods and fluids that they can safely consume (Dorner & Friedrich, 2017). Individuals have the right to refuse nutrition and hydration, including food, beverages, supplements, and enteral or parenteral nutrition as medical treatment (Academy Nutrition Care Manual: End of Life, 2019), and that right should be respected as part of the plan of care. See Chapter 35 for additional information about palliative wound care.

CONCLUSION

Nutrition plays a key role in the prevention and treatment of wounds and pressure injuries. Early identification of individuals at risk for malnutrition and/or pressure injuries as well as identification of malnutrition and/or pressure injury is critical and should prompt a referral to a RDN. Comprehensive assessment by an RDN can identify medical, nutritional, and situational problems that can contribute to poor nutritional status and increase the risk for further complications.

Nutrition interventions to prevent or treat pressure injuries should be individualized and designed to improve each individual's health status and contribute to their quality of life. Regular monitoring and evaluation are needed to assess the effects of nutrition interventions.

REFERENCES

Academy of Nutrition and Dietetics. (2019). Terms and definitions. Retrieved December 9, 2019, from https://www.eatrightpro.org/-/media/eatrightpro-files/practice/scope-standards-of-practice/20190910-academy-definition-of-terms-list.pdf

Academy of Nutrition and Dietetics Electronic Nutrition Care Process Terminology. (2019). Nutrition assessment. Retrieved November 14, 2019, from https://www.ncpro.org/pubs/encpt-en/category-1

Academy of Nutrition and Dietetics Evidence Analysis Library. (2009). Spinal cord injury (SCI) guideline. Retrieved November 27, 2019, from https://www.andeal.org/topic.cfm?menu=5292&cat=3485

Academy of Nutrition and Dietetics Evidence Analysis Library. (2014). Adult weight management guideline. Retrieved December 10, 2019, from https://www.andeal.org/template.cfm?template=guide_summary&key=4341

Academy of Nutrition and Dietetics Nutrition Care Manual. (2019a). End-of-life nutrition. Retrieved November 14, 2019, from https://www.nutritioncaremanual.org/topic.cfm?ncm_category_id=31&lv1=255663&lv2=270395&ncm_toc_id=270395&ncm_heading=Older%20Adult%20Nutrition

Academy of Nutrition and Dietetics Nutrition Care Manual. (2019b). Hydration: Biochemical data, medical tests, and procedures. Retrieved November 14, 2019, from https://www.nutritioncaremanual.org/topic.cfm?ncm_category_id=1&lv1=272918&lv2=272925&ncm_toc_id=272925&ncm_heading=Nutrition%20Care

Banks, M., Bauer, J., Graves, N., et al. (2010). Malnutrition and pressure ulcer risk in adults in Australian health care facilities. *Nutrition in Clinical Practice, 26*(9), 896–901. doi: 10.1016/j.clnu.2012.09.008.

Baranoski, S., Ayello, E. A., Levine, J., et al. (2016). Skin: An essential organ. In S. Baronski & E. A. Ayello (Eds.), *Wound care essentials: Practice principles* (4th ed., pp. 52–62). Ambler, PA: Lippincott Williams & Wilkins.

Bigford, G., & Nash, M. (2017). Nutritional health considerations for persons with spinal cord injury. *Topics in Spinal Cord Injury Rehabilitation, 23*(3), 188–206. doi: 10.1310/sci2303-188.

Cederholm, T., Barazzoni, R., Austin, P., et al. (2017). ESPEN guidelines on definitions and terminology of clinical nutrition. *Clinical Nutrition, 36*, 49–64. Retrieved November 25, 2019, from https://www.espen.org/files/ESPEN-guidelines-on-definitions-and-terminology-of-clinical-nutrition.pdf

Cederholm, T., Jensen, G. L., Correia, M. I. T. D., et al. (2018). GLIM criteria for the diagnosis of malnutrition—A consensus report from the global clinical nutrition community. *Clinical Nutrition, 38*(1), 1–9. Retrieved November 25, 2019, from https://ntvd.media/wp-content/uploads/2018/09/GLIM-criteria-ondervoeding-2018.pdf

Centers for Disease Control and Prevention (2010). About BMI for adults. Retrieved December 10, 2019, from http://www.cdc.gov/healthyweight/assessing/bmi/adult_bmi/index.html#Interpreted. Web site. Reviewed September 17, 2020.

Cereda, E., Gini, A., Pedrolli, C., et al. (2009). Disease-specific, versus standard, nutritional support for the treatment of pressure ulcers in institutionalized older adults: A randomized controlled trial. *Journal of the American Geriatrics Society, 57*(8), 1395–1402.

Cereda, E., Kiersy, C., Serioli, M., et al. (2015). A nutritional formula enriched with arginine, zinc and antioxidants for the healing of pressure ulcers: A randomized trial. *Annuals of Internal Medicine, 162*(3), 167–174. doi: 10.7326/M14-0696.

Chernoff, R., & Seres, D. (2014). Nutritional support for the older adult. In R. Chernoff (Ed.), *Geriatric nutrition* (4th ed., pp. 465–485). Burlington, MA: Jones and Bartlett Learning.

Covinsky, K. E., Covinsky, M. H., & Palmer, R. M. (2002). Serum albumin concentration and clinical assessments of nutrition status in hospitalized older people; different sides of different coins? *Journal of the American Geriatric Society, 50*, 631–637.

Cruz-Jentoft, A. J., Bahat, G., Bauer, J., et al. (2019). Sarcopenia: Revised European consensus on definition and diagnosis. *Age and Aging, 48*(4), 601. doi: 10.1093/ageing/afy169.

Curley, M. A. Q., Hasbari, N. R., Quigley, S. M., et al. (2018). Predicting pressure injury risk in pediatric patients: The Barden QD scale. *Journal of Pediatrics, 192*, 168–195.e2. doi: 10.1016/j.jpeds.2017.09.045.

Dahl, A. K., Fauth, E. R., Ernest-Bravell, M., et al. (2013). Body mass index change in body mass index, and survival in old and very old persons. *Journal of the American Geriatrics Society, 61*(4), 512–518. doi: 10.1111/jgs.12158.

Dealey, C. (2009). Skin care and pressure ulcers. *Advances in Skin and Wound Care, 22*(9), 421–430.

Demling, R. H. (2009). Nutrition, anabolism, and the wound healing process: An overview. *Eplasty, 9*, e9. Retrieved July 11, 2014, from http://www.ncbi.nlm.nih.gov/pmc/articles/PMC2642618/

Dodds, R., & Sayer, A. A. (2015). Sarcopenia and frailty: New challenges for clinical practice. *Clinical Medicine, 15*(Suppl 6), S88–S91. doi: 10.7861/clinmedicine.15-6-s88.

Dorner, B., & Friedrich, E. (2017). Position of the Academy of Nutrition and Dietetics: Individualized nutrition approaches for older adults: Long-term care, post-acute care, and other settings. *Journal of the Academy of Nutrition and Dietetics, 118*, 724–735. doi: 10.1016/j.jand.2018.01.022.

European Pressure Ulcer Advisory Panel, National Pressure Injury Advisory Panel, and Pan Pacific Pressure Injury Alliance [EPUAP/NPIAP/PPPIA]. (2019). In E. Haesler (Ed.), *Prevention and treatment of pressure ulcers/injuries: Clinical Practice Guideline*. The International Guideline.

Fulton, J., Evans, B., Miller, S., et al. (2016). Development of a nutrition screening tool for an outpatient wound center. *Advances in Skin and Wound Care, 29*(3), 136–141.

Furhman, M. P., Charney, P., & Mueller, C. (2004). Hepatic proteins and nutrition assessment. *Journal of the American Dietetic Association, 104*, 1258–1264.

Grover, Z., & Ee, L. C. (2009). Protein energy malnutrition. *Pediatric Clinics of North America, 56*(5), 1055–1068. doi: 10.1016/j.pcl.2009.07.001.

Harvey, K. S. (2013). Nutrition management in chronic kidney disease stages 1 through 4. In L. Byham-Gray, J. Stover, & K. Wiesen (Eds.), *A clinical guide to nutrition care in chronic kidney disease* (2nd ed., pp. 25–37). Chicago, IL: Academy of Nutrition and Dietetics.

Hecht, C., Weber, M., Grote, V., et al. (2015). Disease associated malnutrition correlates with length of hospital stay in children. *Clinical Nutrition, 34*(1), 53–59. doi: 10.1016/j.clnu.2014.01.003.

Horn, S. D., Bender, S. A., Ferguson, M. L., et al. (2004). The National Pressure Ulcer Long-Term Care Study: Pressure injury development in long-term care residents. *Journal of the American Geriatrics Society, 52*(3), 359–367.

Iizaka, S., Okuwa, M., Sugama, J., et al. (2010). The impact of malnutrition and nutrition-related factors on the development and severity of pressure ulcers in older patients receiving home care. *Clinical Nutrition, 29*(1), 47–53. doi: 10.1016/j.clnu.2009.05.018.

Institute of Medicine. (2004). *Dietary reference intakes for water, potassium, sodium, chloride, and sulfate*. Washington, DC: National Academy of Sciences. Retrieved December 10, 2019, from https://www.nap.edu/download/10925

Institute of Medicine. (2006). *Dietary reference intakes: The essential guide to nutrient requirements*. Washington, DC: National Academy of Sciences. Retrieved December 10, 2019, from https://www.nap.edu/catalog/11537/dietary-reference-intakes-the-essential-guide-to-nutrient-requirements

Johnson, A. M., & Merlini, G. (2007). Clinical indications for plasma protein assays: Transthyretin (prealbumin) in inflammation and malnutrition. *Clinical Chemistry and Laboratory Medicine, 45*(3), 419–426.

Langiois, F., Vu, T. T., Kergoat, M. J., et al. (2012). The multiple dimensions of frailty: Physical capacity, cognition, and quality of life. *International Psychogeriatrics, 24*, 1429–1436. doi: 10.1017/S1041610212000634.

Levine, J. (2017). The effect of oral medication on wound healing. *Advances in Skin and Wound Care, 30*, 136–142.

Litchford, M. D. (2010). *The advanced practitioner's guide to nutrition and wounds*. Greensboro, NC: Case Software and Books.

Litchford, M. D., Dorner, B., & Posthauer, M. E. (2014). Malnutrition as a precursor of pressure ulcers. *Advances in Wound Care, 3*(1), 54–63.

Malone, A., Carney, I. N., Mays, A., et al. (Eds.) (2019). *ASPEN enteral nutrition handbook* (2nd ed., pp. 354–401). Silver Springs, MD: American Society for Parenteral and Enteral Nutrition.

Malone, A., & Russell, M. K. (2016). Nutrient requirements. In P. Charney & A. Malone (Eds.), *Academy of Nutrition and Dietetics pocket guide to nutrition assessment* (3rd ed., pp. 213–236). Chicago, IL: Academy of Nutrition and Dietetics.

Mehta, N. M., Compher, C., & ASPEN Board of Directors. (2009). A.S.P.E.N. clinical guidelines: Nutrition support of the critically ill child. *JPEN Journal of Parenteral and Enteral Nutrition, 33*(3), 260–276. doi: 10.1177/0148607109333114.

Mehta, N. M., Corkins, M. R., Lyman, B., et al. (2013). Defining pediatric malnutrition: A paradigm shift towards etiology-related definitions. *Journal of Parenteral and Enteral Nutrition, 37*(4), 460–481. doi: 10.1177/0148607113479972.

Melina, V., Craig, W., & Levin, S. (2016). Position of the academy of nutrition and dietetics: Vegetarian diets. *Journal of the Academy of Nutrition and Dietetics, 116*, 1970–1890. doi: 10.1016/j.jand.2016.09.025.

Ohura, T., Nakajo, T., Okada, S., et al. (2011). Evaluation of the effects of nutrition intervention on healing of pressure ulcers and nutritional states. *Wound Repair and Regeneration, 19*(3), 330–336.

Peterson, S. (2016). Nutrition-focused physical assessment. In P. Charney & A. Malone (Eds.), *Academy of Nutrition and Dietetics pocket guide to nutrition assessment* (3rd ed., pp. 76–102). Chicago, IL: Academy of Nutrition and Dietetics.

Posthauer, M. E. (2020). Nutritional implications of wound healing. In M. Bernstein & N. Munoz (Eds.), *Nutrition for the older adult* (3rd ed., pp. 418–419). Burlington, MA: Jones and Bartlett Learning.

Posthauer, M. E., Banks, M., Dorner, B., et al. (2015). The role of nutrition for pressure ulcer management: National Pressure Ulcer Advisory Panel, European Pressure Ulcer Management, Pan Pacific Pressure Injury Alliance White Paper. *Advances in Skin and Wound Care, 28*(4), 175–188.

Posthauer, M. E., & Thomas, D. R. (2012). Nutrition and wound care. In S. Baronski & E. A. Ayello (Eds.), *Wound care essentials* (3rd ed., pp. 240–264). Ambler, PA: Lippincott Williams & Wilkins.

Quain, A. M., & Khardon, N. M. (2015). Nutrition in wound care management: A comprehensive review. *Wounds, 27*(12), 327–335.

Ranade, D., & Collins, N. (2011). Children with wounds: The importance of nutrition. *Ostomy Wound Management, 57*(10), 14–24.

Rudolph, D. (2009). Appetite stimulants in long term care: A literature review. *The Internet Journal of Advanced Nursing Practice, 11*(1). Retrieved November 25, 2019, from http://ispub.com/IJANP/11/1/9279

Schüler, A. B., Halfens, R. J., & Schols, J. M. G. A. (2012). Pediatric pressure ulcer prevalence: A multicenter, cross-sectional, point-prevalence study in Switzerland. *Journal of Ostomy Wound Management, 58*(7), 18–31.

Schlüer, A. B., Schols, J. M. G. A., & Halfens, R. J. (2014). Risk associated factors of pressure ulcers in hospitalized children over one year of age. *Journal for Specialists in Pediatric Nursing, 1*, 80–89. doi: 10.1111/jspn.12055.

Shahin, E. S., Meijers, J. M. M., Schols, J. M. G. A., et al. (2010). The relationship between malnutrition parameters and pressure ulcers in hospitals and nursing homes. *Nutrition, 26*(9), 886–889. doi: 10.1016/j.nut.2010.01.016.

Skillman, J., & Wischmeyer, P. (2008). Nutrition therapy in critically ill infants and children. *Journal of Parenteral and Enteral Nutrition, 32*(5), 520–534. doi: 10.1177/0148607108322398.

Standards of Medical Care in Diabetes-2019. (2019a). Lifestyle management. *Diabetes Care, 42*(Suppl 1), SA46–SA60. doi: 10.2337/dc19-S005.

Standards of Medical Care in Diabetes-2019. (2019b). Older adults. *Diabetes Care, 42*(Suppl 1), S139–S147. doi: 10.2337/dc19-S012.

ter Riet, G., Kessels, A. G., & Knipschild, P. G. (1995). Randomized clinical trial of ascorbic acid in the treatment of pressure ulcers. *Journal of Clinical Epidemiology, 48*(12), 1453–1460.

The Vegetarian Resource Group (VRG). (2019). How many people are vegan? How many eat vegetarian when eating out? Retrieved November 18, 2019, from https://www.vrg.org/nutshell/Polls/2019_adults_veg.htmOUT?

Thomas, D. R. (2008). Unintended weight loss in older adults. *Ageing Health, 4*(2), 191–200.

United States Department of Agriculture and United States Department of Health and Human Services. (2015). *Dietary guidelines for Americans–2020.* (HHS Publication No. HHS-ODPHP-2015-2020-DGA0-A). Retrieved November 15, 2019, from https://health.gov/dietaryguidelines/2015/

VanGilder, C., Lachenbruch, C., Algrim-Boyle, C., et al. (2017). The International Pressure Ulcer Prevalence Survey: 2006–2015: A 10-year pressure injury prevalence and demographic trend analysis by care setting. *Journal of Wound, Ostomy and Continence Nursing, 44*(1), 20–28. doi: 10.1097/WON.0000000000000292.

Verbrugghe, M., Beeckman, D., Van Hecke, A., et al. (2013). Malnutrition and associated factors in nursing home residents: A cross-sectional, multi-centre study. *Clinical Nutrition, 32*(3), 438–443.

White, J. V., Guenter, P., Jensen, G., et al. (2012). Consensus statement of the Academy of Nutrition and Dietetics/American Society for Parenteral and Enteral Nutrition: Characteristics recommended for the identification and documentation of adult malnutrition (undernutrition). *Journal of the Academy of Nutrition and Dietetics, 112,* 730–738. doi: 10.1177/0148607112440285.

QUESTIONS

1. A nutritional assessment is performed on a patient to determine if he is undernourished. Which of the following is a key indicator of undernutrition?
   A. Loss of 5% of body weight in 30 days
   B. Loss of 10% of body weight in 30 days
   C. Loss of 25% of body weight in 180 days
   D. Loss of 30% of body weight in 90 days

2. Which patient would the RDN consider at high risk for the development of pressure injury?
   A. A patient with BMI > 25
   B. A patient who has increased levels of hepatic proteins
   C. A patient who has a BMI < 18
   D. A patient who runs marathons

3. Which patient criteria support a diagnosis of malnutrition using the Academy of Nutrition and Dietetics/ASPEN Criteria?
   A. Insufficient energy intake and increased subcutaneous fat
   B. Loss of muscle mass and loss of subcutaneous fat
   C. Fluid accumulation and weight gain
   D. Diminished functional status and increased muscle mass

4. What is the primary reason for taking the time to perform a comprehensive assessment to identify malnutrition, as opposed to ordering a simple blood draw to formulate a diagnosis?
   A. Blood tests do not provide a definitive diagnosis.
   B. Blood tests for malnutrition are expensive and unreliable.
   C. There are no blood tests available.
   D. There is a high incidence of false-positive results with blood tests.

5. An RDN is preparing a nutrition plan of care for a patient diagnosed with malnutrition with a stage 4 pressure injury. Which of the following might be included in the plan of care?
   A. Vitamin C and zinc sulfate daily for a duration of 2 to 3 weeks
   B. Vitamin C daily for a duration of 2 to 3 weeks
   C. Zinc sulfate daily until wound is healed
   D. Multivitamin with mineral supplement daily

6. An RDN is explaining the role of energy in the diet to a patient diagnosed with starvation-related malnutrition. Which statement accurately describes the effect of energy on the body?
   A. "Energy is provided in the diet by micronutrients."
   B. "Providing adequate energy prevents anabolism."
   C. "Energy acts to spare protein by providing alternative sources of energy."
   D. "Conditions increasing the metabolic rate decrease energy needs."

7. An RDN is determining energy needs for a patient who has a Stage 3 pressure injury and weights 70 kg. According to the *2019 Prevention and Treatment of Pressure Ulcers/ Injuries Clinical Practice Guidelines*, how many kilocalories would the nurse recommend?
   A. 1,500 to 1,800
   B. 2,100 to 2,450
   C. 2,500 to 2,750
   D. 3,200 to 3,500

8. How many grams of protein are recommended for an adult patient with a Stage 3 pressure injury and malnutrition, who weighs 50 kg?
   A. 62.5 to 75
   B. 75 to 90
   C. 90.5 to 12.5
   D. 112.5 to 127

9. Based on the GLIM diagnostic characteristics for malnutrition, which of the following is considered a phenotype characteristic?
   A. Disease burden
   B. Low food intake
   C. Low BMI
   D. Risk per validated screening tool

10. Which of the following statements is most accurate regarding the nutritional management of special populations?
   A. An obese individual with wounds should consume a low-calorie diet designed for weight reduction.
   B. Nutritional supplements for vegans should contain dairy, meat, or egg products.
   C. The American Diabetes Association endorses the "ADA diet" plan for individuals with diabetes.
   D. The diet for stage 3 or 4 CKD may not meet the protein or nutrient needs required for wound healing.

ANSWERS AND RATIONALES

1. A. Rationale: One key indicator of undernutrition is unintended weight loss (defined as 5% of body weight in 30 days or 10% of body weight in 180 days).

2. C. Rationale: Height and weight are also used to determine body mass index (BMI); individuals with a low BMI (<22) may be at higher risk for pressure injuries.

3. B. Rationale: The Academy/ASPEN consensus statement, in addition to providing a definition of malnutrition, suggests the following criteria for diagnosis: insufficient energy intake, weight loss, loss of muscle mass, loss of subcutaneous fat, localized or generalized fluid accumulation that may sometimes mask weight loss, diminished functional status as measured by handgrip strength. If an individual has two or more of these criteria, they meet the proposed guidelines for malnutrition.

4. A. Rationale: While albumin and prealbumin levels are sometimes requested to diagnose malnutrition, these laboratory tests don't correlate well with clinical observations of nutritional status.

5. D. Rationale: When dietary intake is inadequate, or deficiencies are suspected or confirmed, a multivitamin and mineral supplement should be provided.

6. C. Rationale: Malnutrition alters body composition and the normal pathways by which the body uses protein and fat for fuel. As a result, the body breaks down muscle tissue for energy, and there is a loss of lean body mass.

7. B. Rationale: The 2019 EPUAP/NPIAP/PPPIA guideline recommends optimizing energy intake to provide 30 to 35 kcal/kg of body weight for adults with a pressure injury who are malnourished or at risk of malnutrition. (30 x 70 = 2100 – 35 x 70 = 2450)

8. A. Rationale: The 2019 EPUAP/NPIAP/PPPIA guideline provides the following recommendations: adjust protein intake for individuals and provide 1.25 to 1.5 g/kg body weight/day for adults with a pressure ulcer/injury who are malnourished or at risk of malnutrition. (1.25 x 50 = 62.5 – 1.5 x 50 =75)

9. C. Rationale: The criteria consist of three phenotype characteristics (weight loss, low BMI, and decreased muscle mass) and two etiologic characteristics (decreased food intake or assimilation and disease burden/inflammation). The presence of one phenotype and one etiologic characteristic meets the GLIM criteria for malnutrition.

10. D. Rationale: The diet often suggested for management of stage 3 or 4 CKD that is limited in calories, protein, potassium, phosphorus, sodium, and fluid may not meet the protein or nutrient needs required for wound healing.

CHAPTER 8

GENERAL PRINCIPLES OF TOPICAL THERAPY

JoAnn M. Ermer-Seltun and Bonnie Sue Rolstad

OBJECTIVES

1. Describe the principles of moist wound healing and wound bed preparation.
2. Explain the impact of wound care goals on wound care management and topical therapy.
3. Develop an individualized plan of care based on assessment data and current evidence-based guidelines that addresses each of the following factors:
   a. Correction or amelioration of etiologic factors
   b. Attention to systemic factors affecting repair process
   c. Evidence-based topical therapy
   d. Pain management
   e. Patient and caregiver education

4. Recommend or provide topical therapy based on best available evidence, to include
   a. Debridement of necrotic tissue when indicated
   b. Identification and management of wound-related infections
   c. Management of epibole and hypertrophic granulation tissue
   d. Selection of dressings to maintain a physiologic environment
   e. Judicious utilization of advance therapies for the refractory wound
   f. Identification of social and patient-related factors that may negatively impact wound healing
5. Describe indications and procedure for chemical cauterization of closed wound edges and/or hypertrophic granulation tissue.

TOPIC OUTLINE

● INTRODUCTION

People with chronic wounds are considered to be a global health care challenge, and chronic wounds now occur in epidemic proportions (Sen, 2019). Wound care nurses are challenged to utilize resources to promote wounds to close quickly while avoiding long-term complications. In addition to the impact on morbidity and potential mortality, chronic wound care costs to Medicare only in 2014 in a retrospective study of Medicare beneficiaries for all wound types ranged from $28.1 to $98.6 billion dollars, with the average spending for wound care alone estimated to be $35.3 billion dollars with the highest costs seen in the outpatient setting (Nussbaum et al., 2018). Factors contributing to the persistence and cost of chronic wounds include a delay in identification and correction of etiologic factors and impediments to healing, wound care inconsistencies among practitioners and clinics, and a lack of evidence-based wound management (Gupta et al., 2017). There is a need for an evidence-based approach to chronic wound management that can be implemented by wound care nurses in a variety of settings (Atkin et al., 2019; Gupta et al., 2017). Chronic wound management must have a holistic, patient-centered focus where the etiology of the wound is identified and comorbidities and cofactors are corrected, and local wound care is implemented that reestablishes physiologic wound environment. This chapter focuses on wound bed preparation as it relates to providing an optimal physiologic environment. The wound care nurse must remember that effective therapy requires attention to all three principles: correction of causative factors, optimization of systemic factors affecting healing, and enhancement of the physiologic wound environment through evidence-based topical therapy (Atkin et al., 2019; Gupta et al., 2017). A holistic approach to chronic wound management requires a multidisciplinary team and an individualized plan of care that addresses patient/family-centered concerns and preferences.

KEY POINT

Effective wound management must include correction of etiologic factors, systemic support for healing, and evidence-based topical therapy that provides a local physiologic environment that supports repair.

● PRIORITIES IN WOUND MANAGEMENT

An effective wound management plan must be consistent with the goals of care, individualized for the patient, and based on current evidence and scientific principles.

ESTABLISHMENT APPROPRIATE WOUND CARE GOALS

Following a comprehensive and focused assessment of the patient and problem, the next step in developing an effective and individualized plan of care is to determine the cause of the wound and determine whether it is healable, maintenance, or nonhealable (Gupta et al., 2017). Determining the goal for the wound will in turn direct treatment priorities and modalities that are individualized and realistic. Chapter 5 provides a thorough discussion regarding goal setting and patient-centered support.

Healing Goal

Individuals with healable wounds have the resources (physical, psychosocial, and health system support) to successfully heal the wound in a reasonable time frame (and within their lifespan). In order to determine the wound is healable, it must meet the following criteria: (1) causative factors have been identified and can be corrected or ameliorated and (2) there is sufficient systemic support (perfusion, nutritional support, glycemic control, etc.) to promote healing. Treatment goals for healable wounds should focus upon wound bed preparation as described later in the chapter using the TIME acronym as a framework.

Maintenance Goal

Maintenance wounds are wounds that might be healable, but the potential for healing is delayed or negated either by the individual's concurrent treatments (i.e., chemotherapy), choice (nonadherence in edema management, poor glycemic control, lack of self-care efforts), or by insufficient health care resources to correct the causative factors and provide sufficient systemic support and topical therapy to optimize healing. For these wounds, care is focused on wound maintenance (stabilization) and prevention of complications.

Comfort Goal

The nonhealable wound cannot proceed through the wound healing phases due to decreased tissue perfusion, inability to effectively correct etiologic factors, or end-of-life status. For these patients, comfort and symptom management are the primary focus of care.

For patients at end of life and patients in palliative care, comfort is the primary goal. Palliative care is a complex care model that is patient and family centered (Emmons & Lachman, 2010; Letizia et al., 2010). The aim in palliative wound care is to improve the quality of life for those with life-threatening or debilitating disorders through symptom control and improvement of psychosocial well-being by a multidisciplinary team approach (Emmons & Lachman, 2010). Patients receiving palliative wound care often have nonhealable (comfort) or maintenance wounds. However, some have wounds that are healable from the ability to correct etiologic and systemic factors that support wound healing (Atkin et al., 2019; Gupta et al., 2017). Wounds may heal during comfort care. The care is conservative and focused on comfort, but the wound may heal as the patient is dying. Chapter 35 describes the concept of palliative care and the primary goals in palliative wound management.

KEY POINT

Identifying a wound in terms of ability to heal determines whether the goal is wound healing, maintenance, or comfort.

ESTABLISHMENT OF INDIVIDUALIZED WOUND CARE PLAN

Once the ability of the wound to heal is determined, the next priority is to assure that the plan of care is patient centered and individualized. The plan must address the patient's unique risk factors, comorbidities, and quality of life issues; must include consideration of their circle of care or support system and their ability to access care; and must address personal concerns such as pain control, activities of daily living, psychosocial well-being, and financial constraints (Atkin et al., 2019; Gupta et al., 2017). Specific dressing selection is based upon the characteristics of the wound (type of tissue, depth of tissue destruction, amount of drainage, presence of odor or pain, evidence of infection) but must be consistent with the principles of wound bed preparation. The plan of care should be written and a permanent part of the health care record, reevaluated at least every 30 days or more frequently depending on the care setting and updated/modified whenever there is no measurable progress for 2 to 3 weeks or when there is a significant change in the patient's health care status (Gupta et al., 2017). The wound care nurse must be cognizant of common barriers to effective wound care and develop strategies to eliminate these barriers. Examples may include inappropriate goals, complicated treatment modalities, impaired cognition or dexterity, financial barriers, and

lack of resources and lack of knowledge due to inadequate or ineffective patient education (Nix et al., 2016).

EVIDENCE-BASED WOUND CARE

A model for evidence-based medicine was proposed by Sackett et al. (2000) that involves clinical decision-making based on the following essential elements: best available clinical evidence, clinical expertise, and patient preferences. These three elements must drive the wound plan of care. The use of evidence-based clinical practice guidelines (WOCN, 2012, 2014, 2016, 2019) and best practice documents to guide care for various types of chronic wounds may be mandated and linked to reimbursement (Nussbaum et al., 2018). Wound care nurses should seek to improve population-based wound outcomes, the patient care experience, and fiscal outcomes through improved delivery systems (Flattau et al., 2013).

● EVIDENCE-BASED WOUND CARE: MOIST WOUND HEALING

Evidence supports that moist wound healing promotes key characteristics in reestablishing a wound's normal physiologic environment. The purpose of this section is to provide the wound care nurse with high-level evidence that includes randomized controlled trials (RCTs), bench research, and sentinel references related to the science of moist wound healing, the ability of moist wound healing to foster a physiologic wound environment and to provide examples of how that research is translated into clinical practice. Most wounds healing in a moist environment heal two to three times faster than dry wounds with fewer infections from autolytic debridement. There is also less pain and scarring and care is more cost-effective than those dressed with dry or saline impregnated gauze (Bolton et al., 1996; Hesketh et al., 2017; Ovington, 2002; van Rijswijk, 2004).

KEY POINT

Wounds managed in a moist environment heal faster, with fewer infections, less pain and scarring, and more cost-effectively than wounds managed in a dry environment.

Moist wound healing maintains body surface temperature so cellular activities, chemical reactions, and processes within the wound are optimized. Moist wound healing promotes fibroblast proliferation while maintaining a neutral pH (7.4), which inhibits bacterial growth, optimizes WBC phagocytosis, and creates a physical barrier to the entrance of pathogens (Kruse et al., 2017; Lawrence, 1994; MacFie et al., 2005; McGuinness et al., 2004; Ovington, 2002; Schneider et al., 2007). The original research supporting many of these statements was

---

BOX 8-1   ADVANTAGES OF MOIST WOUND HEALING

Prevents wound desiccation
Enhances cell migration
Promotes angiogenesis
Promotes autolysis
Reduces risk for wound infection
Improves thermoregulation
May alter biological factors
Diminishes fibrosis
Reduces dressing frequency
Enhances patient comfort
Reduces scar formation

---

published (Winter, 1962) and continues to be validated (Brölmann et al., 2013; Vloemans et al., 2014) (see **Box 8-1**). Moist wound healing has not been fully integrated into clinical practice. The wound care nurse should educate patients and care providers about the importance of moist wound healing.

KEY POINT

Moist wound healing promotes the reestablishment of a physiologic wound environment: appropriate moisture levels, neutral pH, local thermoregulation, bacterial balance, and protection from external contamination.

MOIST WOUND HEALING: THE EVIDENCE

Knowledge of the repair process for both partial-thickness and full-thickness wounds leads to an understanding of the importance of hydration for all living tissue. Cells living within a fluid environment are actively involved in the destruction of any debris. They are also observed to migrate freely, to reproduce, and to contribute actively to tissue repair and proliferation. These functions are critical to the repair process. When a wound occurs, the protective barrier of the skin is compromised. Since one of the primary functions of the skin is protection, skin injury and skin loss result in exposure of the underlying tissues to the external environment where dehydration occurs. Without intervention to restore and maintain the protective barrier, the dehydration results in cell death and tissue desiccation. Monitoring and maintenance of moisture in the wound is a primary goal for the wound care nurse.

The seminal publication on the benefits of moist wound healing in soft tissue injuries is credited to George Winter in 1962. Winter demonstrated that porcine partial-thickness wounds covered with a polyethylene film epithelialized twice as fast as those exposed to the air. He also reported an increased rate of regeneration in the underlying connective tissue, indicating

that a moist wound environment positively affected the deeper structures as well. Hinman and Maibach (1963) reported on a study of partial-thickness wounds created on human volunteers where they found faster epithelialization among wounds that were occluded. De Coninck et al. (1996) repeated Winter's work with full-thickness wounds utilizing a semipermeable polyurethane film dressing. They also reported a shorter time to healing among wounds managed with the moisture-retentive dressing.

In addition to proving there is reduced time to wound closure, Winter (1962), and later Rogers (2000), demonstrated that moist wound healing prevented trauma to the wound bed. They demonstrated that allowing gauze to dry onto the surface of the wound causes trauma to the healing tissue with removal. They found that the new blood vessels and newly formed tissue became attached to the dry gauze and were removed during dressing changes, reinjuring the wound and delaying closure. Ovington (2002) later reported that gauze (wet or dry) is not an effective barrier to bacteria.

KEY POINT

The wound care nurse should realize that gauze remains a mainstay of wound care because of its availability and familiarity as opposed to clinical outcomes or cost-effectiveness.

Winter's research indicated that epithelial cellular migration (i.e., wound resurfacing) and extracellular matrix (ECM) formation (i.e., wound filling) occurs optimally in a moist environment. Wounds dressed with gauze or exposed to the air require twice the time to heal because of tissue desiccation and development of a scab. The presence of a scab inhibits epithelial cell migration and requires that the cells migrate downward (i.e., under the scab) in order to complete wound resurfacing. Healing in this manner increases the time required to heal the wound (**Fig. 8-1A and B**).

MOISTURE BALANCE

A moist wound healing environment is defined as one that maintains moisture balance at the interface between the wound and the dressing by use of therapies that maintain, absorb, or donate moisture. Wounds may be dry, moist, or heavily exudating. Topical therapies are selected to manage exudate with the goal of maintaining a moist surface, while avoiding the accumulation and pooling of exudate. The moisture in the wound is exudate from the interstitial tissues. Exudate has been defined as fluid composed of serum, fibrin, and white blood cells that escapes into a superficial lesion or area of inflammation. See Chapter 9 for specifics on dressing properties and selection.

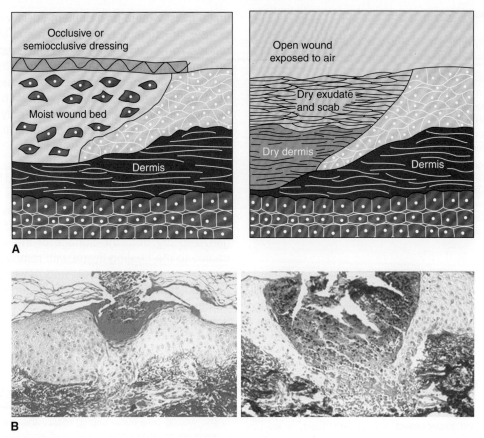

FIGURE 8-1. A. Wound healing in moist versus dry environment. **B.** Histology of a human incision covered with a moisture-retentive dressing and another of identical depth protected, but air exposed. (From Bryant, R., & Nix, D. (Eds.) (2016). *Acute and chronic wounds, current management concepts* (5th ed.). New York, NY: Elsevier, reprinted with permission.)

KEY POINT

Moisture is critical to wound healing and requires a balancing act between absorption of exudate and prevention of desiccation.

MOISTURE-RETENTIVE DRESSINGS

The dressings and advanced therapies used to maintain moisture balance at the wound surface are most accurately termed moisture retentive, meaning they are designed to maintain continuous moisture at the wound–dressing interface and to prevent desiccation of the wound surface. Another frequently used term is semiocclusive dressing in that they permit limited moisture vapor transfer rate (MVTR). Moisture-retentive dressings are appropriately used for infected as well as noninfected wounds. They allow evaporation of some moisture from the skin and wound. Dressings with limited moisture vapor transmission (<35 g/m²/h) have been reported to optimize healing of a wide variety of acute and chronic animal and human wounds (Bolton, 2007; Bolton & van Rijswijk, 1991; Powers et al., 2016). In addition to maintaining an optimally moist wound surface, some moisture-retentive dressings are impermeable

to viruses and bacteria, providing high-level protection against infection (Bowler et al., 1993).

KEY POINT

Occlusive dressing is an outdated term, which has been replaced with moisture-retentive dressings. They permit evaporation of moisture from the skin and wound; they are not occlusive.

EXUDATE MANAGEMENT

Appropriate moisture balance at the wound surface includes management of wound exudate as well as prevention of dehydration. Wound exudate derived from blood is composed primarily of water, but electrolytes, nutrients, protein digesting enzymes (matrix metalloproteinases [MMPs]), growth factors, neutrophils, macrophages, platelets, and microorganisms are also present (Romanelli et al., 2010). All open wounds contain microorganisms, as does wound exudate, but the presence of microorganisms does not necessarily signal infection; infection occurs when the bacterial loads overwhelm host defenses and is manifest by additional findings such as wound deterioration and periwound erythema and induration.

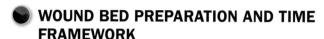

The fluid produced by an acute wound typically contains large amounts of growth factors and other substances supporting ECM production. In contrast, the fluid produced by a chronic wound is typically proinflammatory and contains large concentrations of cytokines and proteases that tend to maintain the wound in an inflammatory state.

CLINICAL APPLICATION

1. **Maintain a moist wound base**

   Wound healing is enhanced in a moist environment, and moisture-retentive dressings are designed with this goal in mind. They protect the wound from external contaminants while maintaining balanced moisture at the wound base via absorption, moisture donation, and/or moisture retention.

   Caution: Maintain stable, dry eschar in the patient with a poorly vascularized noninfected wound of the lower extremity (see Chapter 10).

2. **Protect the periwound skin**

   In a wound with well-controlled moisture balance and less frequent dressing changes, periwound skin may not require additional skin protection. However, in most situations, routine protection of the periwound skin, with either a liquid skin protectant or a moisture barrier ointment, is indicated. Wounds on the trunk are typically managed with adhesive dressings; in this situation, a liquid skin protectant is the best option for periwound skin protection to prevent medical adhesive–related skin injury (MARSI). In contrast, moisture barrier ointments are a good choice for protection of the skin surrounding extremity wounds being managed with wrap dressings to prevent moisture-associated skin damage (MASD). See Chapter 18 for more information about MARSI and MASD.

3. **Manage exudate**

   Wound exudate may be affected by many factors, and the volume of exudate changes throughout the healing process and in response to changes in bacterial loads. Exudate may be higher during the early inflammatory phase of healing and may increase when there is wound infection, either local or invasive (Golinko et al., 2009; IWII, 2016; WUWHS, 2019). An aspect of topical wound care is effective management of exudate while maintaining a moist wound surface; this requires careful matching of the dressing (and its absorptive qualities) with the wound (and volume of exudate). The type of dressing may change depending on wound characteristics.

4. **Educate patient, family, and health care team**

   Teach the importance of moist wound healing to dispel the myth that drying wounds promotes healing (Jones et al., 2014).

WOUND BED PREPARATION AND TIME FRAMEWORK

Wound bed preparation summarized by the TIME mnemonic (Tissue, Inflammation/infection, Moisture imbalance, Epithelial edge advancement) is a systematic approach for assessing chronic wounds. Each of these components must be addressed and optimized to improve the chances of successful wound closure (Atkin et al., 2019; Schultz et al., 2003; Sibbald et al., 2011). TIME provides a framework for wound care nurses and other clinicians to address the challenges of hard-to-heal wounds in a—systematic way. In 2003, research highlighted the key differences between healing and hard-to-heal wounds, with particular emphasis placed on understanding the biological imbalances present in wounds that are hard to heal.

The fluid from hard-to-heal wounds was found to differ substantially from that of healing wounds, showing an imbalance between the production of proteases and their inhibitors. This imbalance causes an excess production of proteases, such as matrix metalloproteinases (MMPs), which negatively impact the functionality of growth factors and extracellular matrix (ECM). This inhibits the proliferation of the essential cells required for wound healing. From a cellular perspective, the requirement for a focused approach to correction of the imbalance within hard-to-heal wounds was seen as being of distinct importance (Brambilla et al., 2016; Moore et al., 2019).

In 2005, the "E" character of the TIME mnemonic was changed from epidermis to edge of wound. The rationale for this change was to ensure that the focus was not just on a failure of the epidermis but also on the potential for problems within the ECM, or with the cells at the wound edge itself. The TIME framework has been widely adopted into practice and research. The developments in wound management have helped reinforce the clinical relevance of TIME (Moore et al., 2019) (**Table 8-1**).

KEY POINT

Wound bed preparation utilizing the TIME framework is an excellent example of a simple, structured approach to assessing chronic wounds.

The TIME concept is dynamic, not a static nor linear process; as the wound stalls or progresses through the phases of wound healing, different aspects of the framework will necessitate attention. For example, a necrotic wound that has been debrided and is now free of devitalized tissue but begins to drain excessively as a result of inflammation caused by biofilm formation requires attention to both the underlying local infection and the resulting problem with moisture balance. The TIME framework also enables clinicians to evaluate the therapeutic value

TABLE 8-1 TIME FRAMEWORK FOR CHRONIC WOUND MANAGEMENT

CLINICAL OBSERVATIONS	PROPOSED PATHOPHYSIOLOGY	WBP CLINICAL ACTIONS	EFFECT OF WBP ACTIONS	CLINICAL OUTCOME
Tissue nonviable or deficient	Defective matrix and cell debris	Debridement (episodic or continuous): Autolytic, enzymatic/chemical/surfactant, biosurgical/larval, mechanical, sharp	Restoration of wound base and functional extracellular matrix proteins	Viable wound base
Infection or inflammation	High bacterial counts or prolonged inflammation ↑Inflammatory cytokines ↑Protease activity ↓Growth factor activity	Remove infected foci topical/systemic: Antimicrobials Anti-inflammatories Protease inhibition	Low bacterial counts or controlled inflammation: ↓Inflammatory cytokines ↓Protease activity ↑Growth factor activity	Bacterial balance and reduced inflammation
Moisture imbalance	Desiccation slows epithelial cell migration	Apply moisture-retentive dressings	Restored epithelial cell migration, desiccation avoided	Moisture balance
	Excessive fluid causes maceration of wound margin	Compression, negative pressure, or other methods of removing fluid	Edema, excessive fluid controlled, maceration avoided	
Edge of wound—nonadvancing or undermining	Nonmigration of keratinocytes Nonresponsive wound cells and abnormalities in extracellular matrix or abnormal protease activity	Reassess cause or consider corrective therapies: Debridement Skin grafts Biological agents Adjunctive therapies	Migration of keratinocytes and responsive wound cells Restoration of appropriate protease profile	Advancing edge of wound

Used with permission from Moore, Z., Dowsett, C., Smith, G., et al. (2019). TIME CDST: An updated tool to address the current challenges in wound care. *Journal of Wound Care, 28*(3), 154-161.

of a specific intervention; for example, sharp debridement may result in establishment of a viable wound bed (T) and reduced bioburden (I) as evidenced by diminished volumes of exudate to prepare for an advanced adjunctive therapy. Wound cleansing with a microfilament pad may reduce nonviable tissue (T), bacteria, and surface containments, thereby impacting tissue quality and lessening of proinflammatory processes (I). These examples demonstrate a single intervention can impact several components of the framework simultaneously (Atkin et al., 2019; Leaper et al., 2012; McCallon et al., 2015).

T = TISSUE MANAGEMENT

The concept of tissue management is removal of nonviable and unhealthy tissue from the wound bed to promote transition from the inflammatory phase into the proliferative phase. The goal is to move the chronic wound to an acute wound to promote healing. Tissue management addresses the removal of senescent cells, cellular debris, biofilm, callus, foreign material, and exudate that may negatively impact the extracellular matrix (ECM). Types of tissue to be addressed in wound management include nonviable tissue and debris, hypergranulation tissue, and hypertrophic scar. Methods for removal include varying techniques of debridement, wound cleansing, and selective forms of negative pressure wound therapy (NPWT) (Atkin et al., 2019; Manna & Morrison, 2019).

Nonviable Tissue

It is well accepted by wound care nurses that the removal of nonviable tissue such as slough, eschar, fibrin, or callus promotes wound healing. The importance of debridement in wound healing was not fully appreciated until landmark randomized clinical trials demonstrated higher rates of wound closure in patients with diabetic foot ulcers (Cardinal et al., 2009) and venous ulcers (Cardinal et al., 2009). Necrotic and nonviable tissues are excellent culture medium for bacterial growth. The presence of necrotic tissue prolongs the inflammatory phase by recruiting macrophages and neutrophils. Inflammatory proteases and cytokines are produced, which degrade the ECM and retard wound healing (Bjarnsholt et al., 2017; Roy et al., 2018). Devitalized tissue prevents visualization of the extent of the wound, impedes angiogenesis, granulation formation, and re-epithelialization. Debridement through various methods is recognized as a component in wound bed preparation (Atkin et al., 2019). See Chapter 10 for additional information on debridement.

Biofilm Removal

Evidence suggests that the majority of chronic wounds (approximately 60% to 100%) contain bacteria embedded in an extracellular polymeric substance (EPS) matrix known as a biofilm (Malone et al., 2017a), which are not detected with wound cultures (Keast et al., 2014; Malone et al., 2017b). Biofilms are detrimental to wound healing. They prolong inflammation through increasing levels of proinflammatory cytokines, which lead to elevated proteases, matrix metallopeptidases (MMP), neutrophil elastases (NE), and reactive oxygen species (ROS) that degrade the ECM and growth factors (Bjarnsholt et al., 2017; Malone et al., 2017a; Ulrich et al., 2011); sharp debridement removes the biofilm and helps to control the associated inflammation and tissue damage (Bianchi et al., 2016; Wolcott et al., 2010). The International Wound Infection Institute (IWII) (2016) provides several tips for prevention and control of biofilms: (1) irrigate the wound with body temperature solution at 4 to 15 psi (cold fluid reduces mitotic activity) to remove surface contaminants, bacteria, exudate, and residual dressing; (2) debride the wound of nonviable, poor-quality tissue frequently; and (3) apply an antimicrobial dressing between debridements since biofilms can reform quickly but are more susceptible to antimicrobial agents in the 24 to 48 hours following debridement (Serena et al., 2016a, 2016b; Serra et al., 2017). Silver and cadexomer iodine have shown bactericidal effectiveness with weakened biofilms (Snyder et al., 2017). Other antimicrobial agents (e.g., polyhexamethylene biguanide [PHMB], medical grade honey) have been linked to slowing the formation of biofilms following debridement (Bianchi et al., 2016; Snyder et al., 2017). Another method to control biofilm formation is to prevent excessive wound moisture using absorptive products and manage underlying conditions that cause edema (e.g., venous insufficiency, chronic heart, renal and/or liver failure).

KEY POINT

The first goal of topical therapy for most wounds is elimination of nonviable, inflammatory, and unhealthy tissue from the wound bed via debridement, cleansing, and appropriate use of antimicrobial agents.

Hypergranulation

Hypergranulation tissue may be referred to as overgranulation, proud flesh, exuberant granulation, hypertrophic granulation, hyperplasia of granulation, or granulation hypertrophy. It may be defined as an excess of granulation tissue that fills the wound bed to a greater extent than what is required and goes beyond the height of the surface of the wound resulting in a raised tissue mass. Clinically, it is identified as a red friable, shiny tissue with a soft appearance above the level of the surrounding skin. Hypergranulation occurs in an array of wounds including burns and venous and pressure ulcers. This tissue prevents migration of epithelial cells across the surface of the wound bed and impedes wound healing. The etiology behind the development of hypergranulation

tissue is not well understood. Predisposing factors that have been suggested include healing by secondary intention, excessive moisture, prolonged inflammation related to infection or residue dressing fibers, external friction, and the repeated use of occlusive dressings. A prolonged stimulation of fibroplasia and angiogenesis may result in the formation of hypergranulation tissue that impairs wound healing. Treatment of hypergranulation tissue includes dressings that are less occlusive or more absorbent with or without antimicrobials, surgical excision, chemical cautery with silver nitrate, hypertonic saline, timolol maleate ophthalmic gel, and laser ablation. These treatments may not be successful (Hawkins-Bradley & Walden, 2002; Jaeger et al., 2016; Lain & Carrington, 2005; Vuolu, 2010; Waldman et al., 2019). (For chemical cauterization procedure, see Chapter 10.)

The use of topical steroids to treat hypergranulation tissue has been reported. Topical steroids demonstrate improved wound healing rates by reducing the inflammatory process (Ae et al., 2016; Borkowski, 2005). One retrospective review was conducted of all patients being treated with a topical preparation containing a steroid (clobetasone butyrate 0.05%) at a tertiary wound healing center over a 10-year period. Healing rates were calculated before and during this treatment period for each patient. Changes in symptom burden (pain, odor, and exudate levels) following topical application were also calculated. Overall, 34 wounds were identified from 25 individual patients (mean age: 65 years, range: 37 to 97 years) and 331 clinic visits were analyzed, spanning a total time of 14,670 days (7,721 days "before treatment" time, 6,949 days "during treatment" time). Following treatment, 24 wounds demonstrated faster rates of healing, 3 wounds showed no significant change in healing rates, and 7 were healing more slowly ($p = 0.0006$). Treatment generally reduced the burden of pain and exudate, without affecting odor (Bosanquet et al., 2013). In summary, research is needed to clearly identify the etiologic factors, clinical characteristics, and management of hypergranulation tissue.

KEY POINT

There is limited research on the etiology and management of hypergranulation tissue. Empiric approaches to management include dressings that are less occlusive or more absorbent with or without antimicrobials, surgical excision, chemical cautery with silver nitrate, hypertonic saline, and laser ablation.

Hypertrophic Scar Tissue

Hypertrophic scars and keloids represent an excessive tissue response to dermal injury characterized by local fibroblast proliferation and overproduction of collagen. Hypertrophic scars and keloids may have a similar clinical appearance. Hypertrophic scars are confined within the boundaries of the wound area and tend to regress spontaneously over time. Keloids are fibrous growths that extend beyond the original area of injury to involve the adjacent normal skin (Berman & Elston, 2018; Goldstein et al., 2020).

The incidence and prevalence of keloids and hypertrophic scars are unknown. Keloids have been reported in 5% to 16% of individuals of Hispanic and African ancestry. An annual incidence of 15 per 10,000 has been reported in Taiwan. Keloids affect men and women equally and are more common in younger individuals. There is a familial tendency to develop keloids (Goldstein et al., 2020).

The pathogenesis of abnormal scarring is poorly understood. The last phase of normal wound healing, maturation or remodeling, involves degradation of the immature ECM (type 3 collagen) produced during the proliferative phase, and replacement with type 1 collagen, which provides tensile strength to the wound (see Chapter 3). Fibroblast proliferation and collagen synthesis are greatly increased in hypertrophic scars and keloids. Overexpression of growth factors, such as transforming growth factor-beta (TGF-beta), vascular endothelial growth factor (VEGF), and connective tissue growth factor (CTGF), appear to play a role in the formation of these lesions (Goldstein et al., 2020; Luo et al., 2017).

Hypertrophic scars and keloids are conditions that may require treatment if symptomatic such as pain, pruritus, functional impairment, and cosmetic disfigurement. Although multiple medical and surgical therapies have been used for the treatment of hypertrophic scars and keloids, there is no universally accepted treatment approach.

For hypertrophic scars, the wound care nurse may initiate first-line therapies including silicone gel sheeting and pressure therapy. Silicone gel sheets should be cut to fit the size of the keloid. The sheet is placed on top of the scar, taped into place, and left on for 12 to 24 hours per day for 2 to 6 months. The sheet may be washed daily and replaced every 10 to 14 days. Pressure therapy with pressure garments, bandages, or devices for special locations, if feasible and tolerated by the patient, may be an alternative to silicone sheeting. Pressure between 20 to 30 mm Hg should be maintained for 12 to 24 hours per day for 6 to 12 months (Goldstein et al., 2020).

For keloids, the wound care nurse may consider referral to dermatology or plastic surgery for intralesional corticosteroid injections as first-line therapy for the treatment of minor keloids (<0.5 cm). Triamcinolone acetonide 10 to 40 mg/mL can be injected. Injections can be repeated at 4-week intervals. Silicone gel sheeting or pressure dressings may be used as adjunctive treatment (Goldstein et al., 2020).

I = INFLAMMATION AND INFECTION CONTROL

The inflammatory phase of repair may be prolonged by a number of local and systemic factors: presence of nonviable tissue, high bacterial loads, impaired leukocyte function (as seen in diabetes), and other conditions resulting in reduced ability to control bacterial loads (e.g., ischemia, hypoxia, anti-inflammatory medications such as steroids, and immunosuppression) (Zhao et al., 2016). Research has identified high protease levels as the mediator for prolonged inflammation. MMPs are enzymes that act on proteins to physically degrade them (Jones et al., 2019). They play an important role in wound healing by eliminating damaged ECM and bacteria, by promoting cell migration, and by assisting with the degradation of type 3 collagen required for normal remodeling of the ECM. MMPs are produced by host wound cells (keratinocytes, fibroblasts, and endothelial cells), and activated inflammatory cells (macrophages and neutrophils) secrete large numbers of MMPs and ROS into the wound bed to control microbial loads and inhibit biofilm formation (Keast et al., 2014). As long as there are high microbial loads and/or biofilm present in the wound bed, the high levels of MMPs and inflammatory process will persist. The MMPs and ROS are damaging to normal tissue, and they degrade growth factors, interfering with repair (Jones et al., 2019). The best biochemical marker for predicting poor wound healing is high protease levels especially MM-9 in diabetic foot ulcers (Cowan et al., 2018; Jones et al., 2019). There is currently a point of care test designed to measure MMP levels in wound fluid, which will allow detection of high protease levels in nonhealing wounds.

KEY POINT

Management of inflammation requires management of microbial loads, correction of wound etiologic factors, and use of dressings that reduce MMP (protease) levels.

Regardless of the specific factors resulting in prolonged inflammation, nonhealing wounds exhibit similar biochemical traits: high levels of inflammatory cytokines and MMPs, reduced growth factor activity, and diminished quantities and response of proliferative cells (Gupta et al., 2017; Zhao et al., 2016). These traits create a hostile wound microenvironment resulting in inflammation that can persist for months or even years if not addressed. In order to break the cycle, the wound care nurse must correct wound etiology, eliminate factors contributing to persistent inflammation (nonviable tissue and high microbial loads), and reduce MMP levels through use of MMP inhibiting and antimicrobial dressings.

The importance of correcting wound etiology cannot be overemphasized (Atkin et al., 2019; Gupta et al., 2017; Jones et al., 2017). For example, studies indicate that nonhealing venous ulcers are characterized by excessive inflammation and high bacterial loads. When compression therapy is initiated and edema resolves, the heavy bioburden decreases without antimicrobial interventions (Harris et al., 1995). Failure to correct etiologic factors results in persistent tissue damage; bacteria thrive in this environment resulting in persistent inflammation.

Wound infection (either localized or spreading) is a major cause of persistent inflammation, and infectious wound complications are addressed in detail in Chapter 11. All chronic wounds are colonized with bacterial and/or fungal organisms, and colonization does not typically result in prolonged inflammation or impaired healing. It is only when the numbers and virulence of the colonizing organisms rise to a level that interferes with repair (subtle signs of local infection) that intervention is required (IWII, 2016). Indicators of subtle signs of local wound infection are reflected by the mnemonic NERDS (*n*onhealing wound, increased *e*xudate, dusky *r*ed or bright red and friable tissue, *d*ebris or necrotic tissue, and odor (*s*mell) (Sibbald et al., 2011; Woo & Sibbald, 2009). The wound care nurse should be alert to indicators of subtle signs of infection and should intervene appropriately (e.g., with antimicrobial dressings). The wound care nurse must closely monitor the wound to assure desired response to therapy and must modify or discontinue the therapy when it is ineffective or no longer indicated (Atkin et al., 2019; IWII, 2016).

KEY POINT

All wounds are colonized, but this does not interfere with healing; intervention is required only for evidence of local (subtle or "classic" signs) or spreading infection. NERDS and STONEES mnemonics may be used to assess for local and spreading infection requiring treatment (see **Box 8-2**).

BOX 8-2   CRITERIA FOR COLONIZATION AND INFECTION

Local Infection (NERDS)
   N = Nonhealing wound
   E = Exudative wound
   R = Red and bleeding wound
   D = Debris
   S = Smell from the wound
Spreading Infection (STONEES)
   S = Size is bigger
   T = Temperature increased
   O = Os (probes to or exposed bone)
   N = New area of breakdown
   E = Erythema/edema
   E = Exudate
   S = Smell

Adapted from Sibbald, R. G., Goodman, L., Woo, K. Y., et al. (2011). Special considerations in wound bed preparation 2011: An update©. *Advances in Skin & Wound Care, 24*(9), 415–436.

The wound care nurse must assess for indicators of spreading infection, which require prompt initiation of systemic antimicrobial therapy. The mnemonic STONEES represents the signs and symptoms of spreading tissue infection: increasing *s*ize of wound, elevated *t*emperature (local or systemic), development of *o*pening that probes to underlying tissue and possibly bone, *n*ew area of breakdown, *e*rythema and *e*dema, increased levels of *e*xudate, and development of odor (*s*mell) (Sibbald, Woo, & Ayello, 2006; Sibbald et al., 2011). Indicators of spreading infection require notification of the provider so that appropriate systemic antimicrobial therapy may be initiated. A wound culture may be obtained from an area of clean viable wound tissue prior to initiation of therapy to assure that the antimicrobial agent prescribed is effective against the infecting organism. Wound cultures must be obtained according to evidence-based protocols; see Chapter 11 for proper wound culturing techniques.

KEY POINT

A critical aspect of effective wound management is prompt identification and treatment of wound-related infection and inflammation. Infectious complications range from surface infection (subtle local signs and biofilm formation) to invasive infection (cellulitis) to osteomyelitis and sepsis.

M = MOISTURE BALANCE

A wound surface that is too wet or too dry is a major impediment to repair; a critical element of effective wound management is maintenance of a wound surface that is moist but not wet. Establishing and maintaining this balance may be one of the most challenging aspects of the TIME wound bed preparation model. The amount of wound exudate may change over a short period of time, which negatively impacts the repair process (Bianchi et al., 2016; WUWHS, 2019). Accurate assessment and description of exudate levels is important to determine the etiology of the change in exudate level and to select the appropriate dressing for exudate management.

Chronic wound fluid has different properties than acute wound fluid. Acute wound fluid tends to promote healing; it contains high levels of proliferative cytokines and growth factors, which promote fibroblast, endothelial cell, and keratinocyte activity. Chronic wound fluid contains high levels of inflammatory cytokines and proteolytic MMPs, which promote persistent inflammation and ECM degradation (Falanga, 2004; Smeets et al., 2008; WUWHS, 2019). It is thought that inflammation increases interstitial fluid levels by increasing capillary permeability, elevating exudation levels. The wound care nurse should select topical products that effectively absorb the wound fluid to avoid pooling of exudate or an excessively dry wound bed while maintaining a moist wound bed that promotes cell migration and healing.

Chapter 9 provides an in-depth discussion of types of moisture-retentive dressings and the process of dressing selection.

E = EPITHELIAL (EDGE) ADVANCEMENT

In order for epithelialization to occur in full-thickness wounds, there must be an open epithelial edge that permits the keratinocytes (epidermal cells) to migrate from the wound edge onto the granulating wound base (Atkin et al., 2019; Schlutz et al., 2003). The ideal wound edge is attached to and flush with the wound bed, moist, and open (**Fig. 8-2A–D**). If the wound edges heal prematurely (as evidenced by a dry closed edge), epithelial migration cannot occur. It is important for the wound care nurse to assess the wound margin or edge for color, thickness, and degree of attachment. The optimal epithelial rim is thin and pale pink to translucent. Wound edge abnormalities include closed edges that appear rolled (epibole) and may be thickened, wound edges that are unattached (as seen in undermining), and wound edges that are not advancing (as seen in hyperkeratotic or calloused edges).

Epibole is the term used to describe wound edges that have rolled down and under until the advancing epithelial wound edge meets the inside edge impeding cellular migration (contact inhibition) (**Fig. 8-2B–D**). Factors thought to contribute to closed wound edges include premature keratinization, calloused edges, too little moisture in the wound bed, and an unhealthy wound bed that does not support epithelial resurfacing (e.g., absence of granulation tissue or hypergranulation tissue). Inadequate absorption of wound exudate may result in periwound maceration, which inhibits cellular migration. See Chapter 9 for additional information on dressings to manage exudate. Wound margins that are unattached are those with a space or undermining between the intact skin and the underlying wound bed. Wound resurfacing is delayed until the wound bed fills with granulation tissue. Factors contributing to edge failure are the same as those for delayed wound healing, such as hypoxia, infection, desiccation, repetitive trauma, elevated blood glucose levels, and high MMPs (Atkin et al., 2019; Falanga, 2004; Harries et al., 2016).

Treatment involves reestablishment of an open and proliferative wound edge. This may be accomplished by chemical cauterization or surgical excision. Wounds with significant undermining require comprehensive evidence-based management to establish and maintain a

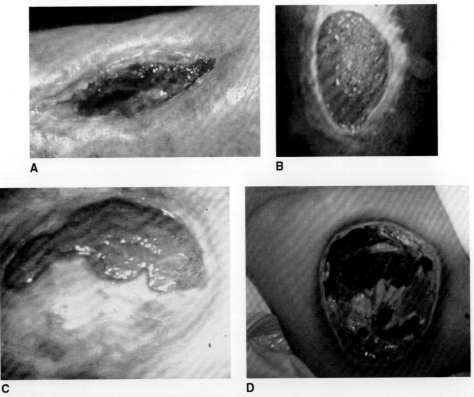

FIGURE 8-2. A. Advancing epithelium: Note greater epithelial advancement from superior edge as compared to inferior edge; this is because the wound bed at the superior aspect is much healthier and more able to support cellular migration and attachment. **B.** Epibole: Wound has granulated to surface but is not epithelializing due to closed wound edges. **C.** Closed versus open wound edges: Note all epithelial resurfacing has occurred from "bottom up" because there is open wound edge at the inferior aspect of the wound while the edges at the superior aspect of the wound are closed. **D.** Closed wound edges: All wound edges closed and will have to be opened once the wound has granulated to surface. (From Ermer-Seltun & Rolstad, 2016.)

moist wound surface that supports granulation tissue until the wound edge approximates the wound bed.

Wounds with closed wound edges that do not respond to conservative therapies require surgical removal of the nonadvancing edge (saucerization); this involves removal of any callus, senescent cells, and dried exudate and establishes an open edge that promotes epithelial cell advancement (Falanga, 2004).

 ## EVOLUTION OF TIME FRAMEWORK

The general TIME framework addresses standardization of wound bed preparation. The framework has been expanded to TIMERS to provide more comprehensive guidance with the integration of repair/regeneration (R) and social factors (S) (Atkin et al., 2019).

R = REGENERATION OR REPAIR OF TISSUE

The "R" in TIMERS emphasizes the consideration of regenerative/repair therapies to expedite wound closure (Atkin et al., 2019). The use of advanced therapies may be expensive, but in a refractory wound may be cost effective. For instance, many cellular and tissue-based products (CTP) may move a wound from a chronic stalled state to wound healing. Advanced therapies should only be considered if the wound care nurse has addressed the cause of the wound, optimized systemic support and patient-related factors that may affect wound healing. Regenerative or repair modalities promote wound closure by enhancement of growth factors, angiogenesis, and improve oxygen to deprived tissues. Chapter 12 reviews guidelines for use of advanced regenerative or repair therapies for the refractory wound.

S = SOCIAL OR PATIENT-RELATED FACTORS

The "S" of TIMERS envelops the entire framework and recognizes the importance of patient engagement in increasing the likelihood of healing (Atkin et al., 2019). The plan of care must be holistic, realistic, patient centered with mutually agreed upon goals. Patients should understand the risk and benefits of treatment modalities as well as the right to refuse treatment. Potential social or patient-related barriers must be identified and addressed, for example, psychosocial, physical, and factors that affect adherence. Use of medical jargon should be avoided (Atkin et al., 2019). Chapters 5 and 6 provide additional information about goal setting and patient education.

A criticism of the TIME concept was that it was wound focused and not patient centered. Another update of the TIME framework included holistic patient assessment and involving a multidisciplinary team (MDT) (Moore et al., 2019). The TIME clinical decision support tool (CDST) offers an A, B, C, D, and E approach as follows:

- **A**ssessment, measurement, and diagnosis of the patient and their wound

- **B**ring in the MDT to promote holistic care
- **C**ontrol and treat systemic causes
- **D**ecide appropriate treatment
- **E**valuate treatment and wound management goals

The TIME framework will continue to evolve as wound care nurses use expanded versions and determine the applicability in clinical practice.

 ## MANAGEMENT OF WOUND-RELATED PAIN

Pain is a very personal and subjective phenomenon, a sensory and emotional experience that affects one's physical, psychological, and spiritual well-being and social functioning. Pain is what the person says it is and strikes whenever the person says it does (McCaffery & Pasero, 1999). The phenomenon of pain is often influenced by one's ethnicity, culture, level of support, past medical history, and previous pain experiences. Unmanaged or poorly managed pain can dramatically and negatively affect one's quality of life (Fiala et al., 2018; Krasner, 2014; Newbern, 2018; Woo et al., 2013). Research has linked pain to poor wound healing due to initiation of the stress response, which activates sympathetic activity and vasoconstriction; this contributes to tissue ischemia (Woo, 2008) and altered immune function/increased risk of infection (Braden, 1998; Kiecolt-Glaser et al., 1995) due to the production of cortisol and catecholamines. Any patient with a wound is at risk for acute or chronic pain of varying severity (Shukla et al., 2005). Pain is too often not addressed or undertreated (Hollinworth, 1995; Serena et al., 2016a; Woo et al., 2008b). A wound care nurse should always assume someone with a wound has some level of discomfort. Performing an assessment is the first step in developing successful management strategies to reduce or eliminate pain. Chapter 4 provides a discussion on systematic pain assessment; the discussion in this chapter will focus on pain prevention and management in acute and chronic wounds.

NOCICEPTIVE VERSUS NEUROPATHIC PAIN

Wound associated pain may be nociceptive, neuropathic, or both, occurring persistently or episodically. Nociceptive pain is caused by an injury or inflammation in tissue that stimulates somatic (skin, fascia, muscles, ligaments, joints, or bones) or visceral (internal organs or linings of body cavities) pain receptors. Nociceptive pain is considered a normal physiological response to a known painful stimulus. It is described as dull, sharp, aching, or throbbing. It may be acute, in surgical or traumatic wounds, or chronic, as in venous leg ulcers, arterial ulcers, or pressure injuries. Persistent inflammation associated with chronic wounds may result in increased sensitivity. Primary hyperalgesia describes pain in the wound itself while secondary hyperalgesia describes pain in the periwound tissue (WUWHS, 2007). In contrast, neuropathic pain is a physiological response that develops when pain pathways are damaged by trauma, infection, metabolic or neurologic disorders, or malignancies affecting the central or peripheral nervous system. Neuropathic pain is often described as burning, shooting, pins and needles, prickling, tingling, or like an electric shock. A stimulus such as a light touch of the skin may elicit an exaggerated painful response called allodynia. One example is pain from the bedsheet resting on the foot.

Krasner (1995) developed a conceptual framework to describe the patient's chronic wound experience, in which she classified wound-related pain as episodic (cyclic or noncyclic) or persistent (as seen in chronic wound pain) (**Fig. 8-3**). Acute pain that is cyclic occurs at regular or predictable intervals (e.g., with dressing removal, wound cleansing, or scheduled turning/positional changes) while acute noncyclic pain is less predictable and associated with procedures and factors such as excisional debridement, biopsy, drain removal, coughing, dressing slippage, and/or friction. Persistent or chronic wound pain is usually related to the underlying cause of the wound (i.e., pressure, arterial insufficiency, venous congestion, neuropathy, vasculitis), aggravating factors (i.e., maceration, inflammation, edema, infection), or other

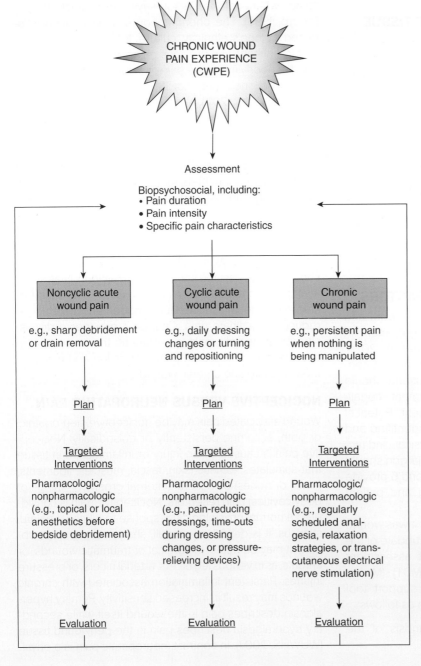

FIGURE 8-3. Chronic Wound Pain Model. (From Woo, K.Y., Krasner, D. L., Sibbald, R. C. (2014). Pain in people with chronic wounds: Clinical strategies for decreasing pain and improving quality of life. In D. L. Krasner. (Ed.), *Chronic wound care: The essentials. A clinical source book for healthcare professionals* (pp. 111–122). Malvern, PA: HMP Communications.)

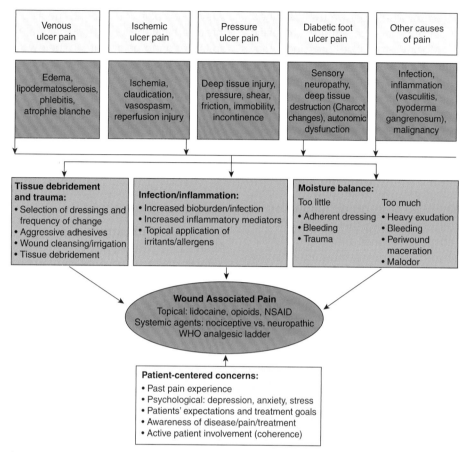

FIGURE 8-4. Wound-associated Pain Model. (Copyright K. Y. Woo and R. Gary Sibbald, 2007.)

pathologies (i.e., malignancy, dermatological conditions, rheumatoid arthritis). Often persistent or chronic wound pain is described as background pain. Background pain is noted at rest and is usually persistent, with potential periodic exacerbations due to care procedures or other factors. Woo and Sibbald (2008) provide an additional model of the complexity of chronic wound pain that includes causative factors, wound-related factors, and patient-centered concerns and guides the clinician in development of an individualized, strategic plan for managing chronic wound pain (**Fig. 8-4**).

KEY POINT

Wound-related pain is a major concern for most patients and may be nociceptive, neuropathic, or both and either persistent or episodic in nature.

MANAGEMENT OPTIONS

Wound-associated pain management must be individualized, patient centered, and multifaceted to address both background pain and cyclic and noncyclic triggers. The goal is to prevent pain or its exacerbation when

possible, relieve or limit pain and discomfort, enhance function, and ultimately restore quality of life. A stepwise approach is necessary along with proper utilization of pharmacotherapy as mainstay therapy. Pain management begins with a comprehensive pain assessment that starts with patients' own words to describe their pain and includes location, type, quality, and intensity, if any aggravating or relieving factors, and impact on daily life, including sleep (see Chapter 4) (**Figs. 8-3 and 8-4**).

KEY POINT

Effective management of wound-related pain involves a multimodal treatment approach, including appropriate use of analgesic and adjuvant medications, use of nonadherent dressings and atraumatic wound care, and adjunctive non-pharmacologic therapies, including the option to call time out during wound care.

Atraumatic Dressings and Other Topical Measures

The application of atraumatic dressings to minimize pain and pruritus during dressing changes is recommended (EPUAP/NPIAP/PPPIA, 2019; WUWHS, 2007). Moisture-retentive dressings may reduce the number of dressing changes as compared to wet-to-dry gauze dressings. Dressings may dry out and become adherent, causing pain with removal. Moisture-retentive dressings may provide painless autolytic debridement, minimizing the need for sharp debridement. Low-adhesive or nonadhesive dressings (e.g., silicone or gel adhesive dressings) do not adhere to moist wound beds and significantly reduce pain related to dressing removal (Woo et al., 2008a; WUWHS, 2007). For wounds with moderate to large amounts of exudate, hydrofibers and alginates minimize trauma and dressing frequency as compared to gauze-type dressings (dry, wet to dry, or wet to damp), which adhere to the wound base, disrupt granulation tissue, and require frequent dressing changes, all of which promote pain. In contrast, wounds that are dry/desiccated benefit from hydrogels or other moisture-retentive dressing to minimize dressing adherence. The application of antimicrobial dressings may also help to reduce pain, due to reduction in bacterial loads and inflammation (Fiala et al., 2018).

Protection of the periwound skin should be a routine consideration in topical therapy; liquid skin protectants and moisture barrier ointments can be used to protect the skin from maceration (moisture associated skin damage [MASD]) and medical adhesive–related skin injury (MARSI). It is important to select dressings for effective exudate management and that do not allow exudate to pool on the skin (Woo et al., 2018). Gentle cleansing with use of noncytotoxic agents such as surfactant wound cleanser, saline, or water is recommended as opposed to abrasive techniques or harsh cleansers (Chan et al., 2016; Rodeheaver & Ratliff, 2018; Woo et al., 2018). See Chapter 9 for additional information about dressing selection and wound cleansing.

Adjunctive Therapies

Other patient-oriented nonpharmacologic approaches such as diversional activities (relaxation, touch, slow rhythmic breathing, imagery, aromatherapy, music, hypnosis, stress reduction, and relaxation activities) can be used to reduce wound-related pain. The individual should be given the option to call a time out during wound-related procedures (Fiala et al., 2018). Additional complementary and integrative health modalities listed in the "Pain Management Best Practices Report" include TENS (transcutaneous electrical nerve stimulation), massage, manipulative therapy, spirituality, mindfulness-based stress reduction, art therapy, yoga, and Tai Chi (USDHHS, 2019). Patient education regarding wound care, dressings, and pain management is also essential for reduction of anxiety (which increases pain), adherence to moist wound care principles, and appropriate use of analgesics. Patients must be assured that the prescribed analgesics will not lead to addiction. They should be educated regarding prevention and management of side effects related to analgesics, as well as the negative

effects of pain on wound healing. Building rapport through active listening and mutual respect as well as an invitation to participate in their wound care (timing of dressing changes, removing the dressing themselves, choice of diversional activities, etc.) are effective patient empowerment methods.

In summary, pain is a complex, subjective, biopsychosocial experience that greatly impacts the quality of life in patients with wounds. It is vital for wound care nurses to collaborate with the primary care provider or pain specialist to properly assess and manage cyclic, noncyclic, and persistent pain in order to promote wound healing and improved quality of life.

Analgesic Medications

Pharmacological agents are selected based upon the type of pain and severity and in collaboration with the patient's primary care provider. The World Health Organization (2014) provides an analgesic three-step ladder (www.who.int/cancer/palliative/painladder/en) that was designed for management of cancer pain but is also suitable for nociceptive cyclic and chronic wound (background) pain (Carlson, 2016; Woo et al., 2018; WUWHS, 2007) (see **Fig. 8-5**). The ladder guides the prescriber to begin with pharmacological interventions at the lowest level based upon the intensity of pain. If pain control is inadequate, then the ladder guides the clinician to add medication with greater potency alone or in combination with other drugs until adequate pain control is reported. Step 1 on the ladder involves nonopioid analgesics such as acetaminophen, acetylsalicylic acid, or nonsteroidal

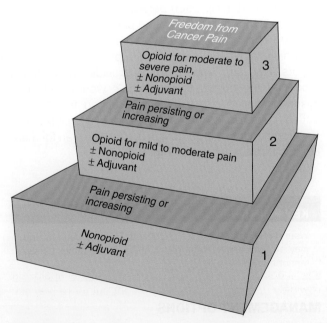

FIGURE 8-5. WHO Analgesic Ladder. (From World Health Organization. (1996). *Cancer pain relief: With a guide to opioid availability* (2nd ed., p. 15). Geneva, Switzerland: Author, with permission. Copyright © World Health Organization. All rights reserved.)

anti-inflammatory drugs (NSAIDs) for mild pain (1 to 4 out of 10) to moderate pain (5 to 6 out of 10) plus or minus adjuvant therapy to help manage anxiety, depression, or neuropathic pain. Step 2 agents are recommended for pain that is moderate to severe (5 to 10 out of 10) and for less severe pain that is refractory to step 1 interventions; agents at this level include weak opioids such as hydrocodone for those who have limited opioid exposure, with or without a nonopioid and adjuvant therapy. Step 3 agents are required for severe pain (8 to 10 out of 10) and involve stronger opioids such as morphine, oxycodone, or hydromorphone in possible conjunction with nonopioid and adjuvant therapy. Selection of pharmacologic agents is impacted by the patient's age, comorbidities (e.g., renal/liver status), and possible drug-to-drug interactions with concurrent medications including over the counter and herbal remedies. In general, prescribers need to start with the least invasive route (i.e., oral, patches, creams). The medication should be prescribed at the lowest dose and titrated slowly, especially in the elderly, to avoid adverse effects such as dizziness, drowsiness, delirium, nausea, or vomiting (AGS, 2012; USDHHS, 2019). Side effects are common with analgesics. It is critical to provide ongoing monitoring and education of patients and caregivers regarding their occurrence. Patients with chronic wound-related pain benefit from long-acting formulations supplemented with short-acting formulations as needed for painful procedures while those with more acute or procedural-type pain benefit from regular dosing of short-acting formulations (Dowell et al., 2016).

Adjuvant Medications

Adjuvant medications are often utilized in combination with analgesics for neuropathic pain or for management of other symptoms such as anxiety or depression. Tricyclic antidepressants such as amitriptyline, nortriptyline, or doxepin are often recommended for milder neuropathic pain (burning/stinging pain) while antiepileptics such as gabapentin, pregabalin, and carbamazepine are used for more severe nerve damage (shooting/stabbing pain). Antispasmodics may be helpful as many chronic pain conditions can be accompanied by muscle spasms. Topical lidocaine patches 5% have also proven to be beneficial for neuropathic pain (USDHHS, 2019; Woo et al., 2018).

Topical anesthetics and dressings with nonadherent/atraumatic interfaces are crucial in managing procedural (cyclic and noncyclic nociceptive) pain. Topical analgesia is widely utilized prior to debridement but there is a lack of evidence for its safe use. In an animal study by Kesici et al. (2018), topical lidocaine and prilocaine did not exhibit any deleterious effects on wound healing.

Topical analgesics come in multiple forms: jelly, cream, ointment, liquid, and patches. Lidocaine (2% to 4% jelly) is the most commonly used agent. It should be used with caution, particularly in large wounds, because systemic absorption could cause adverse neurologic or cardiovascular side effects. The agent with the strongest evidence is EMLA® cream (lidocaine/prilocaine). The EMLA® cream must be in contact with the wound for a minimum of 20 minutes under occlusion (plastic wrap over the top); in some cases, 60 minutes is required for effective prevention of pain related to sharp debridement (Briggs & Nelson, 2010; Woo et al., 2018).

Lidocaine, an amide anesthetic, has been used as a topical anesthetic to control pain in chronic wound pain for many years. Pain relief with most of the commercially available topical lidocaine preparations lasts a few hours (3 to 8 hours) requiring multiple daily applications. In an attempt to improve the management of chronic wound pain, a gel containing 4% lidocaine in TRI-726 matrix (lidocaine gel) was evaluated in 33 patients with chronic painful wounds. The study gel was applied once on day 0. Patients recorded their perceived pain level for the next 7 days. Mean reported pain scores and pain intensity difference (PID) were statistically significantly lower on days 1 to 4 compared to day 0 and days 5 to 7. The study gel was effective in reducing the pain in the majority of patients for multiple days after one application (Treadwell et al., 2019).

Topical uses of morphine, NSAIDs, aspirin, clonidine, tricyclic antidepressants, and capsaicin have all been reported in the literature. All lack pharmacokinetic, safety, and efficacy evidence; at present these agents are not routinely used in the clinical setting (Woo et al., 2018).

In response to the epidemic of opioid abuse, patients and clinicians continue to look for alternative options in managing chronic pain and wound-related pain as seen in the increase interest and use of medical cannabis and cannabidiol (CBD) oil (Grinspoon, 2018; Kroenke et al., 2019; Suzuke, 2019). Anecdotal reports from patients show a significant reduction in pain, discomfort, anxiety, insomnia, and the improvement in function and mobility for multiple health ailments such as chronic pain, inflammation associated with osteoarthritis, rheumatoid arthritis, fibromyalgia, cancer, and neuropathic pain (Joshi, 2018). Delta-9-tetrahydrocannabinol (THC) has been proposed to be beneficial for chronic pain, nausea and vomiting induced by chemotherapy, spasms reduction in multiple sclerosis, and reduction of parkinsonian symptoms (Bonomo et al., 2018; VanDolah et al., 2019).

Another alternative to manage a variety of symptoms is cannabidiol or CBD oil. CBD oil is used to manage seizure disorders especially in children unresponsive to antiseizure medications, anxiety, pain, neuropathy, arthritis, and cancer. Patients experiencing severe pain have reported premedicating with CBD oil sublingual or applied topically prior to procedures (i.e., dressing changes, sharp debridement) (Suzuke, 2019). Side effects of CBD oil include nausea, fatigue, irritability, and drug interactions with warfarin and any medications that are affected by grapefruit juice. CBD oil is obtained over the counter without FDA regulation; purity, amount of actual active ingredients listed on label, and presence of other foreign elements are unknown. Research is needed to determine the dosage as well as which diseases or health issues benefit from CBD or medical cannabis (Grinspoon, 2018).

● CONCLUSION

Wound management begins with identification of wound-related goals. When the goal is comfort or maintenance, the focus in topical therapy is symptom management and complication prevention. When the goal is healing, management must involve correction of etiologic and contributing factors, systemic support for healing, and evidence-based topical therapy. Evidence-based topical therapy should adhere to the concepts outlined in the TIME framework for wound management. For patients with wounds, effective pain management is an important aspect of care and involves use of both pharmacologic and nonpharmacologic interventions.

REFERENCES

Ae, R., Kosami, K., & Yahata, S. (2016). Topical corticosteroid for the treatment of hypergranulation tissue at the gastrostomy tube insertion site: A case study. *Ostomy & Wound Management, 62*(9), 52–55.

Atkin, L., Bućko, Z., Montero, E. C., et al. (2019). Implementing TIMERS: The race against hard-to-heal wounds. *Journal of Wound Care, 28*(Suppl 3a), S1-S50.

American Geriatrics Society (AGS). (2012). AGS Panel on the pharmacological management of persistent pain in older persons. *Journal of the American Geriatrics Society, 57*, 1331–1346.

Berman, B., & Elston, D. M. (2018). Keloid and hypertrophic scar. Retrieved November 9, 2019, from https://emedicine.medscape.com/article/1057599-overview

Bianchi, T., Wolcott, R. D., Peghetti, A., et al. (2016). Recommendations for the management of biofilm: A consensus document. *Journal of Wound Care, 25*(6), 305–317.

Bjarnsholt, T., Eberlein, T., Malone, M., et al. (2017). Management of wound biofilm Made Easy. *Wounds International, 8*(2). Retrieved from https://www.woundsinternational.com/resources/details/management-of-wound-biofilm-made-easy

Bolton, L. L. (2007). Evidence-based report card: Operational definition of moist wound healing. *Journal of Wound, Ostomy, and Continence Nursing, 34*(1), 23–29.

Bolton, L., & van Rijswijk, L. (1991). Wound dressings: Meeting clinical and biological needs. *Dermatology Nursing, 3*, 146–161.

Bolton, L., van Rijswijk, L., & Shaffer, F. (1996). Quality wound care equals cost effective wound care: A clinical model. *Nursing Management, 27*(7), 30–33, 37.

Bonomo, Y., Souza, J. D. S., Jackson, A., et al. (2018). Clinical issues in cannabis use. *British Journal of Clinical Pharmacology, 84*(11), 2495–2498.

Borkowski, S. (2005). G tube care: Managing hypergranulation tissue. *Nursing, 25*(8), 24.

Bosanquet, D. C., Rangaraj, A., Richards, A. J., et al. (2013). Topical steroids for chronic wounds displaying abnormal inflammation. *Annals of the Royal College of Surgeons of England, 95*(4), 291–296. doi.org/10.1308/003588413X13629960045634.

Bowler, P. G., Delargy, H., Prince, D., et al. (1993). The viral barrier properties of some occlusive dressings and their role in infection control. *Wounds, 5*(1), 1–8.

Braden, B. J. (1998). The relationship between stress and pressure sore formation. *Ostomy and Wound Management, 44*(3A Suppl), 26S–36S.

Brambilla, R., Hurlow, J., Landis, S., et al. (2016). WUWHS clinical report: Innovations in hard-to-heal wounds. *Wounds International*. Retrieved November 2, 2019, from https://www.woundsinternational.com/resources/details/clinical-report-innovations-hard-heal-wounds

Briggs, M., & Nelson, E. A. (2010). Topical agents or dressings for pain in venous leg ulcers. *Cochrane Database of Systematic Reviews* (4), CD001177.

Brölmann, F. E., Eskes, A. M., Goslings, J. C., et al., & REMBRANDT study group. (2013). Randomized clinical trial of donor-site wound dressings after split-skin grafting. *British Journal of Surgery, 100*(5), 619–627.

Cardinal, M., Eisenbud, D. E., Armstrong, D. G., et al. (2009). Serial surgical debridement: A retrospective study on clinical outcomes in chronic lower extremity wounds. *Wound Repair and Regeneration, 17*(3), 306–311.

Carlson, C. L. (2016). Effectiveness of the World Health Organization cancer relief guidelines: An integrative review. *Journal of Pain Research, 9*, 515–534. doi: 10.2147/JPR.S97759.

Chan, M. C., Cheung, K., & Leung, P. (2016). Tap water versus sterile normal saline in wound swabbing. *Journal of Wound, Ostomy and Continence Nursing, 43*(2), 140–147. doi.org/10.1097/WON.0000000000000213.

Cowan, L., Stechmiller, J., Phillips, P., et al. (2018). Science of wound healing: Translation of bench science into advances for chronic wound care. In D. L. Krasner & L. van Rijswijk (Eds.), *Chronic wound care: The essentials e-book*. Malvern, PA: HMP.

De Coninck, A., Draye, J. P., Van Strubarq, A., et al. (1996). Healing of full-thickness wounds in pigs: Effects of occlusive and non-occlusive dressings associated with gel vehicle. *Journal of Dermatological Science, 13*(3), 202–211.

Dowell, D., Haegerich, T. M., Chou, R. (2016). CDC guideline for prescribing opioids for chronic pain—United States, 2016. *MMWR Recommendations and Reports, 65*(No. RR-1), 1–49. doi: http://dx.doi.org/10.15585/mmwr.rr6501e1.

Emmons, K. R., & Lachman, V. D. (2010). Palliative wound care: A concept analysis. *Journal of Wound Ostomy Continence Nursing, 37*(6), 639–646.

European Pressure Ulcer Advisory Panel, National Pressure Injury Advisory Panel, and Pan Pacific Pressure Injury Alliance [EPUAP/NPIAP/PPPIA]. (2019). In E. Haesler (Ed.), *Prevention and treatment of pressure ulcers/injuries: Clinical Practice Guideline*. The International Guideline.

Falanga, V. (2004). The chronic wound: Impaired healing and solutions in the context of wound bed preparation. *Blood Cells Molecules & Diseases, 32*(1), 88–94.

Fiala, C. A., Abbott, L. I., Carter, C. D., et al. (2018). Severe pain during wound care procedures: A cross-sectional study protocol. *Journal of Advanced Nursing, 74*(8), 1964–1974.

Flattau, A., Thompson, M., & Meara, A. (2013). Developing and integrating a practice model for health finance reform into wound healing programs: An examination of the triple aim approach. *Ostomy & Wound Management, 59*(10), 42–51.

Goldstein, B. G., Goldstein, A. O., & Hong, A. M. (2020). Keloids and hypertrophic scars. In R. P. Dellavalle & M. L. Levy (Eds.), *UpToDate*. Waltham, MA: UpToDate Inc. Retrieved February 15, 2020, from https://www.uptodate-com.proxy.lib.duke.edu

Golinko, M. S., Clark, S., Rennert, R., et al. (2009). Wound emergencies: The importance of assessment, documentation, and early treatment using a wound electronic medical record. *Ostomy & Wound Management, 55*(5), 54–61.

Grinspoon, P. (2018). *Cannabidiol (CBD)—What we know and what we don't*. Retrieved on November 28, 2019, from https://www.health.harvard.edu/blog

Gupta, S., Andersen, C., Black, J., et al. (2017). Management of chronic wounds: Diagnosis, preparation, treatment, and follow-up. *Wounds, 29*(9), S19–S36.

Harries, R. L., Bosanquet, D. C., Harding, K. G. (2016). Wound bed preparation: TIME for an update. *International Wound Journal, 13*(S3), 8–14.

Harris, I. R., Yee, K. C., Walters, C. E., et al. (1995). Cytokine and protease levels in healing and non-healing chronic venous leg ulcers. *Experimental dermatology, 4*(6), 342–349. https://doi.org/10.1111/j.1600-0625.1995.tb00058.x

Hawkins-Bradley, B., & Walden, M. (2002). Treatment of a non-healing wound with hypergranulation tissue and rolled edges. *Journal of Wound, Ostomy, and Continence Nursing, 29*(6), 320–324.

Hesketh, M., Sahin, K. B., West, Z. E., et al. (2017). Macrophage phenotypes regulate scar formation and chronic wound healing. *International Journal of Molecular Sciences, 18*(7), 1545. Retrieved November 11, 2019, from https://doi.org/10.3390/ijms18071545

Hinman, C. D., & Maibach, H. (1963). Effect of air exposure and occlusion on experimental human skin wounds. *Nature, 200*, 377–379.

Hollinworth, H. (1995). Nurses' assessment and management of pain at wound dressing changes. *Journal of Wound Care, 4*(2), 77–83.

International Wound Infection Institute (IWII). (2016). Wound infection in clinical practice. *Wounds International*. Retrieved March 27, 2020, from https://www.woundsinternational.com/resources/details/iwii-wound-infection-clinical-practice

Jaeger, M., Harats, M., Kornhaber, R., et al. (2016). Treatment of hypergranulation tissue in burn wounds with topical steroid dressings: A case series. *International Medical Case Reports Journal, 9*, 241–245. doi.org/10.2147/IMCRJ.S113182.

Jones, C. J., Smith, H., & Llewellyn, C. (2014). Evaluating the effectiveness of health belief model interventions in improving adherence: A systematic review. *Health Psychology Review, 8*(3), 253–269.

Jones, C. M., Rothermel, A. T., & Mackay, D. R. (2017). Evidence-based medicine: Wound Management. *Plastics and Reconstructive Surgery, 140*, 201e–216e.

Jones, J. I., Nguyen, T. T., Peng, Z., et al. (2019). Targeting MMP-9 in diabetic foot ulcers. *Pharmaceuticals, 12*(2), 79. doi: 10.3390/ph12020079.

Joshi, J. (2018). 5 trends in pain management for Today's wound care clinicians. *Today's Wound Clinic, 12*(6). Retrieved March 27, 2020, from https://www.todayswoundclinic.com/articles/5-trends-pain-management-todays-wound-care-clinicians

Keast, D., Swanson, T., & Carville, K. (2014). Ten top tips: Understanding and managing wound biofilm. *Wounds International, 5*(2), 20–24.

Kesici, S., Kesici, U., Ulusoy, H., et al. (2018). Effects of local anesthetics on wound healing. *Brazilian Journal of Anesthesiology, 68*(4), 375–382.

Kiecolt-Glaser, J. K., Marucha, P. T., Malarkey, W. B., et al. (1995). Slowing of wound healing by psychological stress. *Lancet, 346* (8984), 1194–1196.

Kroenke, K., Alford, D. P., Argoff, C., et al. (2019). Challenges with implementing the CDC prevention opioid guideline: A consensus panel report. *Pain Medicine, 20*(4), 724–735.

Krasner, D. (1995). The chronic wound pain experience: A conceptual model. *Ostomy & Wound Management, 41*(3), 20–25.

Krasner, D. (2014). *Chronic wound care: The essentials*. Malvern, PA: HMP Publications.

Kruse, C. R., Singh, M., Targosinski, S., et al. (2017). The effect of pH on cell viability, cell migration, cell proliferation, wound closure, and wound reepithelialization: In vitro and in vivo study. *Wound Repair and Regeneration, 25*(2), 260–269.

Lain, E. L., & Carrington, P. R. (2005). Imiquimod treatment of exuberant granulation tissue in a nonhealing diabetic ulcer. *Archives of Dermatology, 141*(11), 1368–1370.

Lawrence, C. L. (1994). Dressings and wound infection. *American Journal Surgery, 167*(1A), S21–S24.

Leaper, D. J., Schultz, G., Carville, K., et al. (2012). Extending the TIME concept: What have learned in the past 10 years? *International Wound Journal, 9*(Suppl 2), 1–19.

Letizia, M., Uebelhor, J., & Paddack, E. (2010). Providing palliative care to seriously ill patients with nonhealing wounds. *Journal of Wound Ostomy Continence Nursing, 37*(3), 277–282.

Luo, L., Li, J., Liu, H., et al. (2017). Adiponectin is involved in connective tissue growth factor-induced proliferation, migration and overproduction of the extracellular matrix in keloid fibroblasts. *International Journal of Molecular Sciences, 18*(5), 1044. doi.org/10.3390/ijms18051044.

MacFie, C. C., Melling, A. C., & Leaper, D. J. (2005). Effects of warming on healing. *Journal Wound Care, 14*(3), 133–136.

Malone, M., Bjarnsholt, T., McBain, A. J., et al. (2017a). The prevalence of biofilms in chronic wounds: A systematic review and meta-analysis of published data. *Journal of Wound Care, 26*(1), 20–25.

Malone, M., Goeres, D. M., Gosbell, I., et al. (2017b). Approaches to biofilm-associated infections: The need for standardized and relevant biofilm methods for clinical applications. *Expert Review of Anti-infective Therapy, 15*(2), 147–156. doi: 10.1080/14787210.2017.1262257.

Manna, B., & Morrison, C.A. (2019). Wound debridement. In *StatPearls [Internet]*. Treasure Island, FL StatPearls Publishing. Retrieved September 26, 2019, from https://www.ncbi.nlm.nih.gov/books/NBK507882

McCaffery, M., & Pasero, C. (1999). How can we improve the way we perform our pain assessments to meet the needs of patients from diverse cultures? *American Journal of Nursing, 99*(8), 18.

McCallon, S. K., Weir, D., & Lantis, J. C. (2015). Optimizing wound bed preparation with collagenase enzymatic debridement. *Journal American College of Clinical Wounds Specialists, 6*, 14-23.

McGuinness, W., Vella, E & Harrison, D. (2004). Influence of dressing changes on wound temperature. *Journal of Wound Care, 13*(9), 383–385.

Moore, Z., Dowsett, C., Smith, G., et al. (2019). TIME CDST: An updated tool to address the current challenges in wound care. *Journal of Wound Care, 28*(3), 154–161.

Newbern, S. (2018). Identifying pain and effects on quality of life from chronic wounds secondary to lower-extremity vascular disease: An integrative review. *Advances in Skin & Wound Care, 31*(3), 102–108.

Nix, D. P., Peirce, B., & Haugen, V. (2016). Eliminating noncompliance. In R. A. Bryant & D. P. Nix (Eds.), *Acute and chronic wounds: Current management concepts* (5th ed.). St. Louis, MO: Elsevier Inc.

Nussbaum, S. R., Carter, M. J., Fife, C. E., et al. (2018). An economic evaluation of the impact, cost, and medicare policy implications of chronic nonhealing wounds. *Value in Health, 21*(1), 27–32.

Ovington, L. (2002). Hanging wet to-dry dressings out to dry. *Journal of Prevention and Healing, 15*(2), 79–84.

Powers, J. G., Higham, C., Broussard, K., et al. (2016). Wound healing and treating wounds: Chronic wound care and management. *Journal of the American Academy of Dermatology, 74*(4), 607–626. doi.org/10.1016/j.jaad.2015.08.070

Rodeheaver, G. T., & Ratliff, C. R. (2018). Wound cleansing, wound irrigation, wound disinfection. In: D. L. Krasner & L. van Rijswijk (Eds.), *Chronic wound care: The essentials e-book*. Malvern, PA: HMP.

Rogers, M. (2002). Treatment of angiomas: A modern commentary. *Australasian Journal of Dermatology, 41* (suppl) S89–S91.

Romanelli, M., Vowden, K., & Weir, D. (2010). Exudate management made easy. *Wounds International, 1*(2), 1–6.

Roy, R., Tiwari, M., Donelli, G., et al. (2018). Strategies for combating bacterial biofilms: A focus on anti-biofilm agents and their mechanisms olfaction. *Virulence, 9*(1), 522–554. doi: 10.1080/21505594.2017.1313372.

Sackett, D. L., Strauss, S. E., Richardson, W. S., et al. (2000). Evidenced-based medicine: How to practice and teach. *Evidenced based medicine* (2nd ed.). *Edinburgh, NY*: Churchill Livingstone.

Schneider, A. K., Korber, A., Grabbe, S., et al. (2007). Influence of pH on wound healing: A new perspective for wound therapy? *Archives of Dermatological Research, 298*(9), 413–420.

Schultz, G. S., Sibblad, R. G., Falanga, V., et al. (2003). Wound bed preparation: A systematic approach to wound management. *Wound Repair and Regeneration, 11*(Suppl 1), S1–S28.

Sen, C. K. (2019). Human wounds and its burden: An updated compendium of estimates. *Advances in Wound Care, 8*(2), 39–49.

Serena T. E., Cullen, B. M., Bayliff, S. W., et al. (2016a). Defining a new diagnostic assessment parameter for wound care: Elevated protease activity, an indicator of nonhealing, for targeted protease-modulating treatment. *Wound Repair and Regeneration, 24*(3), 589–595.

Serena, T. E., Yaakov, R. A., Aslam, S., et al. (2016b). Preventing, minimizing, and managing patients with chronic wounds: Challenges and solutions. *Chronic Wound Care Management and Research, 3*, 85–90.

Serra, M. B., Barroso, W. A., Silva, N. N. D., et al. (2017). From inflammation to current and alternative therapies involved in wound healing. *International Journal of Inflammation, 2017*, 3406215. Retrieved November 11, 2019, from https://doi.org/10.1155/2017/3406215

Shukla, D., Tripathi, A. K., Agrawal, S., et al. (2005). Pain in acute and chronic wounds: A descriptive study. *Ostomy & Wound Management, 51*(11), 47–51.

Sibbald, R. G., Goodman, L., Woo, K. Y., et al. (2011). Special considerations in wound bed preparation 2011: An update©. *Advances in Skin & Wound Care, 24*(9), 415–436.

Sibbald, R. G., Woo, K. Y., & Ayello, E. (2006). Increased bacterial burden and infection: The story of NERDS and STONEES. *Advances in Skin and Wound Care, 19*(8), 447–463.

Smeets, R., Ulrich, D., Unglaub, F., et al. (2008). Effect of oxidized regenerated cellulose/collagen matrix on proteases in wound exudate of patients with chronic venous ulceration. *International Wound Journal, 5*(2), 195–203.

Snyder, R. J., Bohn, G., Hanft, J., et al. (2017). Wound biofilm: Current perspectives and strategies on biofilm disruption and treatments. *Wounds, 29*(6), S1–S17.

Suzuke, K. (2019). Emerging insights on wound care and pain management. *Podiatry Today, 32*(7), 24–26.

Treadwell, T., Walker, D., Nicholson, B. J., et al. (2019). Treatment of pain in wounds with a topical long acting lidocaine gel. *Chronic Wound Care Management and Research, 6*, 117–121. doi.org/10.2147/CWCMR.S224092.

Ulrich, D., Smeets, R., Unglaub, F., et al. (2011). Effect of oxidized regenerated cellulose/collagen matrix on proteases in wound exudate of patients with diabetic foot ulcers. *Journal of Wound Ostomy & Continence Nursing, 38*(5), 522–528.

U.S. Department of Health and Human Services (USDHHS). (2019). Pain Management Best Practices Inter-Agency Task Force Report: Updates, Gaps, Inconsistencies, and Recommendations. Retrieved March 27, 2020, from U.S. Department of Health and Human Services website: https://www.hhs.gov/sites/default/files/pmtf-final-report-2019-05-23.pdf

VanDolah, H. J., Bauer, B. A., & Mauck, K. F. (2019). Clinicians' guide to cannabidiol and hemp oils. *Mayo Clinic proceedings, 94*(9), 1840–1851. https://doi.org/10.1016/j.mayocp.2019.01.003

Van Rijswijk, L. (2004). Bridging the gap between research and practice. *American Journal of Nursing, 104*(2), 28–30.

Vloemans, A. F., Hermans, M. H., van der Wal, M. B., et al. (2014). Optimal treatment of partial thickness burns in children: A systematic review. *Burns, 40*(2), 177–190.

Vuolu, J. (2010). Hypergranulation: Exploring possible management options. *British Journal of Nursing, 19*(6), S4, S6–S8.

Waldman, R. A., Lin, G., & Sloan, B. (2019). Clinical pearl: Topical timolol for refractory hypergranulation. *Cutis, 104*(2), 118–119.

Winter, G. D. (1962). Formation of the scab and the rate of epithelialization of superficial wounds in the skin of the young domestic pig. *Nature, 193*, 293–294.

Wolcott, R. D., Rumbaugh, K. P., James, G. M., et al. (2010). Biofilm maturity studies indicate sharp debridement opens a time-dependent therapeutic window. *Journal of Wound Care, 19*(8), 320–328.

Woo, K. Y. (2008). Meeting the challenges of wound-associated pain: Anticipatory pain, anxiety, stress, and wound healing. *Ostomy & Wound Management, 54*(9), 10–12.

Woo, K. Y., Abbott, L. K., & Librach, L. (2013). Evidence-based approach to manage persistent wound-related pain. *Current Opinion in Supportive and Palliative Care, 7*(1), 86–94. https://doi.org/10.1097/SPC.0b013e32835d7ed2

Woo, K. Y., Harding, K., Price, P., et al. (2008a). Minimizing wound-related pain at dressing change: Evidence-informed practice. *International Wound Journal, 5*(2), 144–157.

Woo, K. Y., Krasner, D. L., & Sibbald, R. G. (2018). Pain in people with chronic wounds: Clinical strategies for decreasing pain and improving quality of life. In D. L. Krasner, L. van Rijswijk (Eds.), *Chronic wound care: the essentials e-book* (pp. 111–122). Malvern, PA: HMP.

Woo, K. Y., & Sibbald, R. G. (2008). Chronic wound pain: A conceptual model. *Advances in Skin and Wound Care, 21*(4), 175–190.

Woo, K. Y., & Sibbald, R. G. (2009). A cross-sectional validation study of using NERDS and STONEES to assess bacterial burden. *Ostomy & Wound Management, 55*(8), 40–48.

Woo, K. Y., Sibbald, R. G., Fogh, K., et al. (2008b). Assessment and management of persistent (chronic) and total wound pain. *International Wound Journal, 5*(2), 205–215.

World Health Organization (WHO). (2014). WHO's pain ladder. Retrieved October 25, 2014, from http://www.who.int/cancer/palliative/pain-ladder/en/

World Union of Wound Healing Societies (WUWHS). (2007). *Principles of best practice: Minimizing pain at wound dressing-related procedures. A Consensus Document.* London: MEP Ltd.

World Union of Wound Healing Societies (WUWHS) Consensus Document. (2019). Wound exudate: Effective assessment and management. *Wounds International.* Retrieved March 27, 2019, from https://www.woundsinternational.com/resources/details/wuwhs-consensus-document-wound-exudate-effective-assessment-and-management

Wound, Ostomy & Continence Nurses Society (WOCN). (2016). *Guidelines for the prevention and management of pressure ulcers, WOCN clinical practice guideline series #2.* Mount Laurel, NJ: Author.

Wound, Ostomy & Continence Nurses Society (WOCN). (2019). *Guideline for management of wounds in patients with lower extremity venous disease (LEVD), WOCN clinical practice guideline series #4.* Mount Laurel, NJ: Author.

Wound, Ostomy & Continence Nurses Society (WOCN). (2012). *Guidelines for Management of Wounds in Patients with Lower Extremity Neuropathic Disease (LEND). WOCN clinical practice guideline series #3.* Mount Laurel, NJ: Author.

Wound, Ostomy & Continence Nurses Society (WOCN). (2014). *Guideline for Management of Patients with Lower Extremity Arterial Disease (LEAD). WOCN clinical practice guideline series #1.* Mount Laurel, NJ: Author.

Zhao, R., Liang, H., Clarke, E., et al. (2016). Inflammation in chronic wounds. *International Journal of Molecular Sciences, 17*(12), 2085.

QUESTIONS

1. A wound care nurse is caring for a patient with a wound determined to be healable. What is the focus of treatment for this type of wound?
   A. Proper wound bed preparation
   B. Consistent use of debridement
   C. Wound stabilization
   D. Prevention of complication

2. The wound care nurse is managing hypergranulation tissue. Which of the following is the best option?
   A. Continue to use occlusive dressing
   B. Change to a less absorbent dressing
   C. Change to a more absorbent dressing
   D. Leave wound open to air

3. Which of the following is an outcome of moist wound healing?
   A. Increased pain
   B. Increased fibroblast proliferation
   C. Increased nonviable tissue
   D. Increased risk of infection

4. What is a primary intervention when treating wounds?
   A. Packing the wound with plain gauze to absorb excess exudate
   B. Maintaining moisture balance in the wound
   C. Exposing the wound to air to allow a protective scab to form
   D. Avoiding the use of moisture-retentive dressings

5. What is one effect of managing a wound in a moist environment?
   A. Revascularization occurs at a slower rate.
   B. Wounds heal in disorganized manner.
   C. The breakdown of avascular tissue and fibrin is slowed.
   D. Collagen production is increased.

6. The wound care nurse is following the TIME framework to promote wound healing in an efficient manner. Which statement accurately describes an aspect of healing measures based on the tissue management step of this framework?
   A. The removal of nonviable tissue prolongs wound healing time.
   B. Biofilms are beneficial to wound healing as they degrade the ECM.

   C. Hypergranulation tissue slows wound healing by preventing epithelialization.
   D. Keloids will resolve on their own when the incision heals.

7. The wound care nurse is reassessing a patient's venous leg ulcer and notes subtle signs of wound infection. Which of the following may indicate local wound infection?
   A. The wound size is increasing.
   B. Temperature is elevated.
   C. Tissue is more friable than at last assessment.
   D. The wound probes to underlying tissue or bone.

8. The wound care nurse notes wound edges that are closed and rolled despite conservative therapies. What would be the best next step in addressing the closed edges?
   A. Refer for surgical intervention.
   B. Apply an antimicrobial foam dressing.
   C. Wait and see if improves over time.
   D. Add a compression dressing.

9. Which of the following accurately describes the occurrence of nociceptive pain?
   A. It is an abnormal physiological response that develops when pain pathways affecting the central or peripheral nervous system are damaged.
   B. It is caused by a disruption or inflammation in tissue that stimulates somatic or visceral pain receptors.
   C. It is frequently described as burning, shooting, electric shock like, pins and needles, prickling, or tingling.
   D. It is considered to be an abnormal physiological response to a known painful stimulus.

10. The nurse assessing the pain of a patient with chronic leg ulcers documents a pain level of 5 on a scale of 0 to 10. What patient-orientated, nonpharmacologic modality would be appropriate to reduce this level of pain?
   A. Acetaminophen
   B. Apply heating pad
   C. Perform dressing change rapidly
   D. Diversional activities

ANSWERS AND RATIONALES

1. A: Treatment goals for healable wounds should focus upon proper wound bed preparation using the TIME framework.

2. C: Excess moisture may be a contributing factor to hypergranulation tissue formation requiring a more absorptive type of dressing.

3. B: Moist wound healing promotes fibroblast proliferation while maintaining a neutral pH, which inhibits bacterial growth, optimizes WBC phagocytosis, and creates a physical barrier to the entrance of pathogens.

4. B: Monitoring and maintenance of moisture in the wound is a primary goal for the wound care nurse.

5. D: There is increased production of collagen in the wound in a moist environment.

6. C: A prolonged stimulation of fibroplasia and angiogenesis may result in the formation of hypergranulation tissue that impairs wound healing.

7. C: Indicators of subtle signs of local wound infection are reflected by the mnemonic NERDS (nonhealing wound, increased exudate, dusky red or bright red and friable tissue, debris or necrotic tissue, and odor [smell]).

8. A: Wounds with closed wound edges that do not respond to conservative therapies require sharp (surgical) debridement to open edges.

9. B: Nociceptive pain is caused by an injury or inflammation in tissue that stimulates somatic (skin, fascia, muscles, ligaments, joints, or bones) or visceral (internal organs or linings of body cavities) pain receptors. Nociceptive pain is considered to be a normal physiological response to a known painful stimulus.

10. D: Other patient-oriented nonpharmacologic approaches such as diversional activities (relaxation, touch, slow rhythmic breathing, imagery, aromatherapy, music, hypnosis, stress reduction, and relaxation activities) can be used to reduce wound-related pain.

CHAPTER 9

WOUND CLEANSING AND DRESSING SELECTION

Kelly Jaszarowski and Rose W. Murphree

OBJECTIVES

1. Discuss the rationale for wound cleansing and dressing application based upon wound characteristics.

2. Recommend or apply topical wound therapy, based on best available evidence, including the following:

   a. Selection of dressings to manage exudate and maintain moist wound bed

   b. Selection of dressings to facilitate autolytic debridement

   c. Selection of dressings to address bioburden

3. Develop an individualized plan of care based on assessment data and current evidence-based guidelines that addresses each of the following factors:

   a. Wound cleansing

   b. Dressing selection

TOPIC OUTLINE

● INTRODUCTION

Wound healing requires comprehensive and holistic management. Considerations include etiology and systemic factors as well as provision of evidence-based topical therapy. Topical therapy selection considerations include factors needed to interrupt the cycle of injury, perfusion, nutritional status, glycemic control, antiproliferative medications, and comorbidities.

Material selection is important to design an ideal wound dressing. Naturally occurring polymers may make excellent wound dressing components because they are biocompatible and biodegradable, making them environmentally friendly. Chitin, starch, cellulose, and β-glucan are just some of the products being studied for wound dressings (Naseri-Nosar & Ziora, 2018).

The goal of topical therapy is to create a local environment that supports healing, through appropriate cleansing and dressing selection. Promoting an environment that fosters healing may involve evaluating the need for debridement, management of infection, exudate management, and management of wound depth and undermining (Cox, 2019). This chapter provides clear guidelines for wound cleansing and dressing selection based on the phase of healing and the specific characteristics of the wound.

● WOUND CLEANSING

Wound bed preparation begins with cleansing and requires attention to both the cleansing agent and the technique. Wound assessment guides the approach to cleansing and the identification of the appropriate agent. Wounds in the inflammatory phase of repair are characterized by the presence of devitalized tissue (eschar and/or slough) and/or by high bacterial loads and large amounts of exudate, which can frequently be malodorous. The goal in cleansing wounds is to remove as much of the devitalized tissue, bacterial burden, and exudate as possible without damaging the viable tissue within the wound bed.

CLEAN WOUNDS

Wounds in the proliferative phase of repair are characterized by healthy tissue within the wound bed (granulation tissue and/or new epithelium), relatively low levels of bacteria, and lower volumes of exudate. The goal in cleansing of these wounds is to flush away exudate without damaging the proliferative cells and newly formed tissue. Appropriate solutions include saline, commercial wound cleansers, and potable tap water. A bulb syringe can effectively deliver a gentler flush pressure (0.5 psi) for the proliferative phase wound (Atiyeh et al., 2009; Edlich et al., 2010; Rodeheaver & Ratliff, 2016).

NECROTIC OR INFECTED WOUNDS

Cleansing of infected or dirty wounds requires irrigation and may involve the use of a cytotoxic cleansing agent. These wounds require irrigation rather than gentle flushing to effectively reduce bacterial loads and loosen and remove avascular tissue and debris. Irrigation should be done with low pressure (4 to 15 psi) that may be obtained with a 35-mL syringe and 19-gauge catheter (7 psi) (Atiyeh et al., 2009; Edlich et al., 2010; Rodeheaver & Ratliff, 2016) or a commercial cleanser packaged in a pressurized container that delivers the desired irrigation force. Low pressure should be utilized for three reasons: (1) to prevent splash back and contamination of other areas/surfaces/persons, (2) to prevent invasion of the bacteria into healthy tissue or bloodstream, and (3) to prevent damage to any healthy tissue present in the wound bed.

Another option for irrigating a wound is pulsatile lavage. Pulsatile lavage irrigation involves delivery of an irrigating solution under pressure, from an electrically powered device, with or without suction. A key consideration in the use of pulsatile lavage is the level of irrigation force. Low pulsatile lavage delivers 5 to 10 psi, while high-pressure lavage pulsations can reach >20 psi (Mundy et al., 2017). Studies examining this approach report increased risk of bacterial invasion into the soft tissues if the irrigating force is excessive (>15 psi).

Consequently, companies are currently working to perfect the delivery system to assure safe levels of irrigation force (Fry, 2017; Hughes et al., 2012). Another consideration is the potential for aerosolization of bacteria (Angobaldo et al., 2015). The wound care nurse must follow all   manufacturer's guidelines to assure safe use.

Agents used for cleansing dirty wounds may be either noncytotoxic (saline, potable/tap water, or commercial cleansing solutions) or cytotoxic (antiseptics such as sodium hypochlorite or acetic acid solution). Antiseptic solutions are generally preferred if the goal is to kill bacteria (e.g., a heavily necrotic and infected wound). However, the wound care nurse must be aware that use of these agents can potentially damage viable wound tissue. In determining the best cleansing agent for a specific wound, the wound care nurse should consider the goals of care and the status of the wound bed. When the goal is swift cleansing of the wound and >50% of the wound bed is covered with devitalized tissue or there is a large amount of malodorous exudate indicating active wound infection, most wound experts believe an antiseptic solution is the best choice. Use of an antiseptic for cleansing should be a short-term intervention. Once the bacterial loads have been controlled and the volume of necrotic tissue has been reduced to >40% of the wound bed, the antiseptic should be discontinued.

ANTISEPTIC SOLUTIONS

The discussion of antiseptic agents that follows is not considered all-encompassing. It is important to consider the cytotoxicity of the solution along with its impact on healthy tissues and wound healing. Studies report varying outcomes regarding these solutions. Chlorhexidine is not discussed here because it is primarily utilized for surgical skin cleansing and not for wound cleansing (Edlich et al., 2010). Instead, a discussion of commonly utilized antiseptic agents follows.

When using the following agents, a thorough wound assessment is imperative. The wound care nurse should monitor for evidence of effectiveness and needs to change the wound plan of care if there is a poor response. The nurse also needs to monitor for any adverse or allergic reaction. The product in use should be accurately labeled to avoid accidental misuse. Finally, the wound care nurse should collaborate with the staff to provide ongoing monitoring of wound status and assure the use of the antiseptic solution is discontinued once the wound bed is clean.

Acetic Acid (e.g., Vinegar Solution)

Acetic acid can be used as a cleansing/irrigating agent alone or as a wound packing agent. It is sometimes used because of its bactericidal effectiveness against *Pseudomonas aeruginosa*. This common wound pathogen produces a classic "green" hue to both the wound bed and wound exudate, as well as has a very distinct odor. The most commonly used concentration is ¼ (0.25%) strength. While these typically come premixed, they can also be formulated by mixing one cup of vinegar and three cups of distilled water.

Clinical Considerations

Cytotoxicity to fibroblasts is a concern when applying acetic acid solutions, so attention to concentration and length of use is essential. Periwound skin can be damaged if acetic acid remains in contact for a prolonged period. The periwound skin should be protected with a liquid barrier film or a moisture barrier ointment. Application may cause a stinging/burning sensation or even pain. If this occurs, the acetic acid may require further dilution.

Hydrogen Peroxide

Hydrogen peroxide has been utilized primarily as a first-line wound cleanser by many disciplines including the lay person. Studies document the negative effects of hydrogen peroxide, particularly the cytotoxicity to wound healing cells (De Luna et al., 2017; Thomas et al., 2009; Zhu et al., 2017). The bubbling effect noted with its use produces a misconception of a positive action occurring on the cellular level. Hydrogen peroxide has been noted to kill fibroblasts. In a classic study by Lineaweaver et al. (1985), a 0.03% hydrogen peroxide solution was utilized to clean a wound. Their results demonstrated that 60% to 70% of the wound's fibroblasts were killed. In another study evaluating the cytotoxic effect of commercially available cleansers, 17 cleansers and 3 liquid bath soaps were evaluated for their effect on infant dermal fibroblasts and epidermal keratinocytes. Hydrogen peroxide was found to be one of the most toxic cleansers (Wilson et al., 2005).

Clinical Considerations

Hydrogen peroxide solution is readily available and inexpensive. It can be used in initial cleansing of a superficial traumatic wound when gross contamination is present. If utilized, it should be discontinued once the wound bed is clean, and a noncytotoxic solution should be utilized instead.

Povidone–Iodine

Data regarding use of povidone–iodine are mixed, with results depending on form and concentration. This product is supplied in several formulations. The scrub form is intended for presurgical use on intact skin and contraindicated for use as a wound cleanser. Povidone–iodine is considered as a broad-spectrum antimicrobial, which is effective against many organisms. Advancements in wound healing research have demonstrated that povidone–iodine, even in low concentrations, has been found to interfere with granulation tissue development and delay wound healing (De Luna et al., 2017; Ruder & Springer, 2017).

Clinical Considerations

Povidone–iodine solution is readily available and inexpensive. Dilute povidone–iodine solution, 1% concentration, may be beneficial as an initial treatment for infected wounds. It should be discontinued once the wound bed is clean, and a noncytotoxic solution should be utilized instead. Application may cause a stinging/burning sensation or even pain. If this occurs, the povidone–iodine may require further dilution.

Silver

Silver has been utilized in wound dressings and is most recently being introduced into wound cleansers. It is believed to be bactericidal and effective against a number of pathogens. More research needs to be conducted to determine its effectiveness and benefits as a wound cleanser.

Sodium Hypochlorite Solution (e.g., Dakin's Solution®, Clorpactin®, Di-Dak-Sol®, Anasept®)

The active ingredient in these products is dilute bleach; sodium bicarbonate may be added as a buffering agent. As a wound cleanser, this solution has demonstrated bactericidal effectiveness against most of the bacteria in chronic wounds and significantly reduces wound odor. Studies have shown sodium hypochlorite to be an effective bactericidal agent even at low concentrations. Some investigators recommend 0.025% or 0.0125% as the optimal concentration for killing bacteria (e.g., *MRSA*, *MSSA*, *Escherichia coli*) while preserving fibroblasts (Agostinho et al., 2011; Bradley & Cunningham, 2013). Some studies indicate reduced toxicity with quarter strength concentration while retaining bactericidal effects (Fonder et al., 2008; Heggers et al., 1991). While available in retail stores, it may also be formulated by the pharmacy to adhere to specific dilution requirements. It can also be mixed at home. Anecdotally, sodium hypochlorite solutions are sometimes used to promote debridement when used as a wound dressing. When used in this way, sodium hypochlorite solution–moistened gauze is placed into the wound bed and changed every 12 hours. Some studies suggest that it may also be effective in reducing biofilm formation (Agostinho et al., 2011; Bradley & Cunningham, 2013). The solution should be discontinued once the wound bed is clean, and a noncytotoxic solution should be utilized instead.

Clinical Considerations

Sodium hypochlorite solutions can be easily formulated utilizing common household products. For example, the formula for half strength Dakin's Solution® (0.25%) is three tablespoons + half teaspoon of regular strength household bleach (48 mL) and half teaspoon baking soda added to 32 ounces of sterile water (or water that has been boiled). The formula for quarter strength (0.125%) Dakin's Solution® is one tablespoon + two teaspoons bleach (24 mL) + half teaspoon baking soda added to 32 ounces of water. The wound care nurse should be aware full strength Dakin's Solution® is a 0.5% concentration. It must be stored in the refrigerator and replaced every 48 hours. Unopened jars can be stored for up to 1 month after preparation. It should be stored away from sunlight, kept out of the reach of children, and clearly marked as poisonous to prevent accidental oral ingestion. Clorpactin® and other hypochlorite solutions are readily available without prescription at many retailers and Web sites.

NONCYTOTOXIC SOLUTIONS

Cleansing of noninfected wounds in the proliferative phase of repair involves gentle flushing with noncytotoxic solutions, saline, tap water, or commercial wound cleansers. Normal saline (0.9%) is widely available, especially in health care facilities. Commercially prepared saline is available in most retail and pharmacy stores, either in spray cans or in bottles. It can also safely be prepared at home (Fellows & Crestodina, 2006).

Commercial wound cleansers may also be used. Borges et al. (2018) investigated the effect of polyhexamethylene biguanide (PHMB) (Prontosan®) solution as a wound cleanser on bacterial load and bacterial biofilm in patients with venous leg ulcers. Forty-four patients were divided into two groups: the intervention group had their wounds cleansed with PHMB, and the control group had their wound cleansed with a 0.9% saline solution. The bacterial load was reduced in both groups compared to baseline values; no significant difference was found when groups were compared. When considering use of a commercial wound cleanser, the wound care nurse should verify that the agent is noncytotoxic. Hypochlorous acid solution (Vashe®) is naturally produced in the body, so it may be less cytotoxic compared with other wound cleansers. Day et al. (2017) studied the antimicrobial effects of Vashe® compared with those of other common wound cleansers (1% and 10% povidone–iodine [PI], 0.05% chlorhexidine wound solution [CWS], or normal saline) in vitro using biofilms of two common wound pathogens: the gram-positive *Staphylococcus aureus* and the gram-negative *P. aeruginosa*. All agents tested significantly neutralized methicillin-resistant *S. aureus* and *P. aeruginosa* biofilms compared with saline control. Vashe® was as effective as CWS at disrupting MRSA biofilms and *P. aeruginosa* biofilms but demonstrated less cytotoxicity being comparable to normal saline.

In some situations, tap water is an acceptable cleanser. Fernandez and Griffiths (2012) performed a Cochrane review, which found very few studies on the use of tap water for wound cleansing. The data available indicated that tap water is a safe agent provided it is potable (Resende et al., 2016). The use of a gentle shower may be the most effective approach to cleanse wounds (Fernandez & Griffiths, 2012).

Clinical Considerations

Saline is inexpensive, widely available, and easy to use. A simple formula for 0.9% concentration is two teaspoons of salt added to 1,000 mL or 1 quart of distilled or boiled water. Studies have shown effective shelf life without contamination when stored in the refrigerator up to 1 month (Fellows & Crestodina, 2006). In the hospital, open bottles of saline should be discarded after 24 hours. Saline does not provide any antimicrobial effect. The wound care nurse should monitor for appropriate use of saline or commercial cleansing agents and modify the care protocol if signs of infection or poor wound healing develop.

 ## DRESSING SELECTION

Selection of the most appropriate dressing(s) for a specific wound represents another challenge for the wound care nurse. A clear understanding of the principles of topical therapy (see Chapter 8) coupled with knowledge of dressing functions and characteristics will guide the nurse in effectively matching the dressing to the wound. The remainder of this chapter addresses the products currently available and provides guidance in selection of appropriate products based on wound characteristics.

Wound dressings can be divided into two general categories: those that provide passive support for wound healing and those that actively impact the processes involved in wound repair. The majority of the products on the market are passive, meaning that they promote wound healing by providing exudate control, maintaining a moist wound surface, reducing bacterial loads, as well as protecting the wound against trauma and pathogenic invasion This chapter focuses on these types of dressings. Active therapy dressings and products will be discussed in the chapter on refractory wounds (Chapter 12).

Passive dressings can be classified in several different ways. One approach is based on the form of the dressing in relationship to the contours of the wound. From this perspective, dressings can be classified as wicking agents, filler dressings, or cover dressings. Another approach to classification is based on the dressing's role in maintaining moisture balance within the wound bed. Dressings are hydrating, absorbent, or moisture retentive. All dressings can be classified as either having antimicrobial properties or not (plain), and many products are available in both forms. Additionally, dressings can be classified based on the primary materials from which they are constructed, for example, gauze, hydrogels, alginates, foams, etc. In this chapter, we discuss dressings primarily from the perspective of their form (wick, filler, cover) and function (absorb, hydrate, and/or retain moisture). Specific dressing materials are discussed within the functional categories.

WICK VERSUS FILLER VERSUS COVER DRESSING

Wicking agents are ribbon or rope dressings that are placed into tunneled and undermined areas to evacuate fluid. They are available in plain and antimicrobial form and in a variety of materials (alginate, hydrofiber, foam, textile, nonwoven gauze). They may also be impregnated with a solution or dry. There are two clinical considerations in selecting an appropriate wicking agent: width of the tunnel and volume of exudate. When placing a wick into a narrow tunnel, the wound care nurse should select a wick that will not leave any residual dressing material. For example, nonwoven gauze strips would be appropriate, but woven gauze would not be appropriate. When selecting a wick for a tunnel in a highly exudative and/or infected wound, the wound care nurse should consider selection of an antimicrobial wicking product or a nonwoven gauze strip impregnated with hypertonic saline, which provides "active" wicking through osmotic effects.

Filler dressings are dressings that are designed to go into the wound and conform to the contours of the wound. Cover dressings are solid "sheet-type" dressings that are designed to cover the wound. Wounds with depth require both a filler dressing and a cover dressing, whereas surface wounds require only a cover dressing. Filler dressings and cover dressings are available in both absorbent and hydrating forms, and in plain and antimicrobial forms.

The wound with tunnels and depth will require a wick, a filler, and a cover (**Fig. 9-1**); the wound with depth but

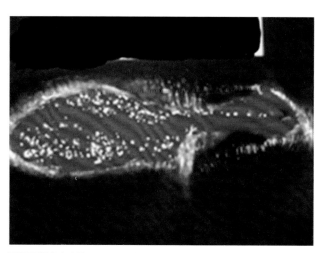

FIGURE 9-1. Wound with Depth and Tunnel (at 3 o'clock): Needs Wick, Filler, Secondary Dressing.

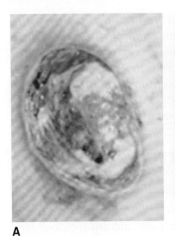 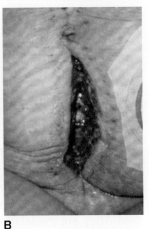

A   B

FIGURE 9-2. A, B. Wounds with Depth: Need Filler and Secondary Dressing.

no tunnels will require a filler and a cover (**Fig. 9-2**); and the wound with no tunnels and no depth will require only a cover dressing (**Fig. 9-3**).

KEY POINT

The wound care nurse must assess the contours of the wound to determine the appropriate dressing. Is a wick required? Is a filler required? Is only a cover dressing needed?

ABSORBENT VERSUS HYDRATING VERSUS MOISTURE-RETENTIVE DRESSING

Maintenance of moisture balance at the wound surface is a key element of evidence-based topical therapy. The goal is to absorb any excess exudate and to maintain a continually moist wound surface. The wide array of dressings currently available allows the wound care nurse to effectively match absorptive/hydrating capacity of the

dressing to the volume of exudate produced by the wound. In selecting an appropriately absorptive dressing, the nurse must also consider frequency of dressing change. Very wet or very dry wounds may require more frequent dressing changes to maintain optimal moisture balance at the wound surface. Dressings classified as absorptive include alginates, hydrofibers, foams, fabric/textiles, and gauze. Dressings classified as moisture retentive include contact layer/nonadherent dressings, hydrocolloids, and transparent adhesive dressings. Dressings classified as hydrating include hydrogel dressings and wet gauze dressings. These specific categories are discussed in more detail later in this chapter.

KEY POINT

The wound care nurse must select addressing based on the amount of wound exudate and the absorptive capacity of available dressings.

ANTIMICROBIAL VERSUS PLAIN DRESSINGS

Antimicrobial dressings may be needed for wounds at high risk of infection and wounds with evidence of colonization or biofilm (Haesler et al., 2019). Antimicrobial dressings include those that incorporate silver, cadexomer iodine, polyhexamethylene biguanide (PHMB), and polyvinyl alcohol (PVA) with crystal violet and methylene blue, those with medicinal honey, and those that attract and remove bacteria. All antimicrobial dressings affect a broad spectrum of organisms including essentially all known wound pathogens. Antimicrobial agents are available in various forms including creams, ointments, powder, sprays, and all forms of dressings. Each antimicrobial dressing varies in physical properties including amount and release properties of the antimicrobial, duration of antimicrobial effectiveness, absorptive capacity,

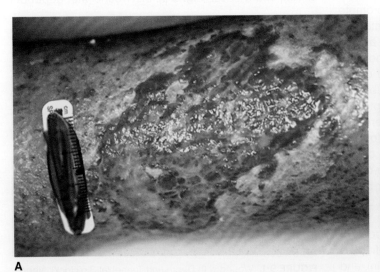 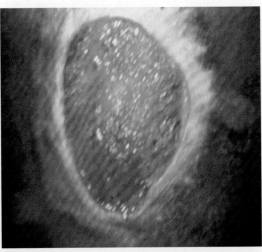

A   B

FIGURE 9-3. A, B. Superficial/Shallow Wounds: Need Single Dressing Only.

management of odor, and management of pain (Vowden et al., 2011). These properties, along with wound status and treatment goals, that should be considered when choosing a specific dressing.

As with any therapy, length of use is determined by the wound and its progression or other negative response to treatment and manufacturer's guidelines. A lack of progress or a deterioration in wound status suggests the need for reassessment and change in treatment. In contrast, significant improvement in wound status usually indicates control of bacterial loads, which may signify the ability to transition away from an antimicrobial dressing. Antimicrobial dressings are available without a prescription and are effective against essentially all wound pathogens. Therefore, a wound culture is not required, and antimicrobial dressings can be used in lieu of antibiotics to treat local wound infection. The risk of resistance to antimicrobial dressings is low. (A more detailed examination of these dressings can be found in Chapter 11.)

KEY POINT

Antimicrobial dressings provide broad-spectrum control of bacterial bioburden at the wound surface, and therefore, when using these dressings, wound culture is not recommended.

 ## DRESSING CATEGORIES

ALGINATES

Description and Characteristics

Alginate dressings are nonwoven dressings composed of polysaccharide fibers or xerogel, which is derived from brown seaweed. These dressings are available in a variety of forms, including sheets and ropes. Some alginates are impregnated with antimicrobial agents such as silver. Alginate dressings absorb moderate amounts of exudate. Some form a gel as the result of an ion exchange that occurs during exudate absorption, while others absorb the exudate into the dressing so that the dressing becomes soft and moist. The frequency of dressing change is dependent upon the amount of exudate and the secondary dressing utilized but typically ranges from daily to every 3 days. These dressings are indicated for wounds with moderate to heavy exudate. If the wound is highly exudative, the absorptive capacity of the alginate should be supplemented by an absorbent cover dressing. The wound care nurse should follow the manufacturer's recommendations for use of the specific dressing.

Alginates are conformable to irregular wound beds, easily filling dead space in deep wounds. The formation of a gel or a soft moist dressing permits easy and atraumatic dressing removal with wound irrigation, resulting with less pain with dressing changes. The gel formation of these dressings also facilitates autolytic debridement.

These advantages, coupled with less frequent dressing changes, may result in cost savings in supplies and labor, especially in postacute care.

Clinical Considerations

The wound should be thoroughly irrigated to remove all dressing residue. The rope form of alginate dressing may be used in narrow tunnels. Alginate dressings should not be layered; if the wound is deep and highly exudative, apply the alginate as a base (primary) dressing and use another absorptive dressing as a secondary filler. Intended for exudating wounds, alginate dressings are inappropriate for use in relatively dry wounds. Alginates are generally considered an inappropriate choice as the primary dressing for wounds with exposed tendons, joint capsules, or bone due to the risk of tissue desiccation.

COLLAGENS

Collagen is the most common protein in the body and is essential for wound healing. Collagen enhances the deposition of organized collagen fibers and granulation tissue to promote wound healing (Hess, 2020). Collagen makes up a large portion of the extracellular matrix, which acts as a structural scaffold in the tissues. There are many types of collagen, but the types most often used in collagen dressings are type 1 or a combination of type 1 and denatured collagen. Most collagen dressings contain bovine, ovine, or porcine collagen that has been treated; making it nonantigenic (Wu et al., 2017). Matrix metalloproteinases (MMPs) found in the extracellular fluid of wounds break down collagen. Wound dressings containing collagen give MMPs an alternative collagen source, allowing the body's collagen available for wound healing.

Description and Characteristics

Collagen dressings can be used in a variety of wounds as a primary dressing for partial- or full-thickness wounds. These dressings may be used on minimal to heavily exudating wounds, which may or may not be infected. They are absorbent and promote a moist wound healing environment, requiring a secondary dressing, and can be used with other topical agents. Collagen dressings are not recommended for use on third-degree burns or necrotic wounds (Hess, 2020).

COMPOSITES

Description and Characteristics

Composite dressings are available in a variety of sizes and combinations, with varying degrees of absorptive capacity. These dressings contain two or more physically distinct products manufactured as a single dressing, serving several functions. The layers may include a contact layer, an absorptive layer, a cover layer, and an adhesive border. The outer covering provides a physical bacterial barrier to the wound. Available with or without impregnated antimicrobial agents, they are frequently used as secondary dressings but are also appropriate as primary dressings for surface wounds.

The frequency of dressing change is dependent upon the specific components of the dressing and whether it is being used as a primary or secondary dressing. Composite dressings are intended for use as a primary dressing for partial-thickness or shallow full-thickness wounds with minimal exudate. They are convenient, easy to apply, and readily available regardless of setting.

Clinical Considerations

Composite dressings are selected based on amount of wound exudate, quality of wound bed tissue, and need for waterproof outer layer, depending on wound location. These dressings should not be cut since the structure of the dressing design will be compromised. Sizing should allow for a 1 to 2.5 cm (1/2 to 1 inch) border of intact skin surrounding the wound. Composite dressings may be used on full-thickness wounds to facilitate autolytic debridement. In order to appropriately use these dressings, the wound care nurse should be familiar with the product types included in the layers of the dressing. Wear time or dressing changes are dependent upon the combination of products being utilized (Hess, 2020).

CONTACT LAYERS

Description and Characteristics

Contact layer dressings are placed in direct contact with the wound bed. These dressings help to maintain a moist and protected wound surface. While they are minimally adherent, contact layer dressings are porous, permitting exudate to pass through the contact layer to a secondary dressing that provides absorption. These dressings are usually single layer, nonadherent, and contain perforations of varying size. Some dressings are designed so that one surface wicks fluid away from the wound (hydrophilic) and the other retains fluid (hydrophobic). They are available in sheets, rolls, and strip forms. These dressings may also contain an antimicrobial agent. Commonly used contact layer dressings include woven polyamide net and silicone-based material.

Clinical Considerations

These dressings are used for wounds with depth, applying the contact layer followed by a secondary filler dressing and secured with a cover dressing. They are not recommended for stage 1 pressure injuries, wounds with viscous exudate, shallow or desiccated wounds, or wounds covered with eschar. Contact layer dressings are not intended to be changed at each dressing change; follow manufacturer's recommendations for specific product use. Topical medications may also be used with these dressings.

FOAM DRESSINGS

Description and Characteristics

Foam dressings are available in a variety of shapes and sizes. They may also contain antimicrobial agents and have adhesive borders. Foam dressings are most commonly made of polyurethane and contain small, open cells for absorbing wound exudate. The absorptive capacity varies depending on the specific components of the dressing. Foam dressings can be used effectively as both primary and secondary dressings. They are appropriate for wounds with low, moderate, or heavy exudate. Because foam dressings maintain a moist wound surface while absorbing excess exudate, they also promote autolytic debridement of moist avascular tissue or slough (Avent, 2010). It should be noted that foams are absorbent dressings and are inappropriate for use on dry wounds or wounds with minimal exudate. Foam dressings would not be effective in promoting autolysis of dry eschar because they do not donate moisture and cannot create a fluid environment. Frequency of dressing change is dependent upon the volume of exudate and absorptive capacity of the dressing. If used under a compression wrap, the foam would be changed only at the time wrap is changed. Manufacturers often classify a foam by absorptive capacity using descriptors such as "light" or "extra."

Clinical Considerations

Foam dressings may macerate periwound skin and should be changed before they become overly saturated with exudate. Macerated skin increases the risk of bacterial invasion. Foam dressing use should be avoided on minimally draining wounds and are contraindicated for third-degree burns or ischemic wounds with dry eschar.

In the absence of a wound, foam dressings have been utilized as preventative dressings for patients with fragile skin at risk for friction injury. International guidelines also suggested their use in pressure injury, particularly in the sacral and heel areas (EPUAP/NPIAP/PPIA, 2019; Truong et al., 2016; WOCN, 2016).

GAUZE DRESSINGS (IMPREGNATED/ NONIMPREGNATED)

Description and Characteristics

Gauze can be used for wound cleansing and as a wick, filler, or cover dressing. It can be moistened with various products to address the wound environment need. Gauze comes in various forms, including pads, precut to fit around tubes, rolled, and narrow strips. Gauze is available with or without antimicrobial properties. The primary characteristic to consider when selecting gauze for wound care is whether it is woven or nonwoven. Woven gauze is composed of cotton fibers, which can be classified as fine or coarse. Loosely woven gauze allows for wound exudate absorption. Loose fibers can become embedded in the wound bed and act as foreign bodies (Ovington, 2001). Gauze is generally considered a less than optimal choice for a primary dressing. It is more appropriately used for a secondary dressing.

Nonwoven gauze is typically composed of synthetic material: rayon, polyester, or a combination of these. This material provides for better wicking and absorbency and is less likely to leave fibers in the wound. Nonwoven gauze is also believed to provide some protection from bacterial invasion (Dhivya et al., 2015). This type of gauze dressing is also considered more optimal as a primary dressing and can be appropriately utilized as a secondary dressing.

KEY POINT

Gauze may be used as a primary or secondary dressing. Nonwoven gauze is preferred as a primary dressing.

Clinical Considerations

Consideration should be given to the type of gauze dressing and its intended use. As a wound filler, gauze is often moistened with saline or other noncytotoxic solution. Wet-to-moist gauze dressings are used to maintain a moist wound base and must be changed frequently to avoid drying. Gauze is used to fill the deeper space in the wound in order to avoid premature closure. Care should be taken to avoid overfilling as packing tightly puts internal pressure on the wound and will interfere with perfusion and compromise fibroblast activity and granulation tissue development. Packing strips should be used in tunnels with a portion protruding into the wound to assure easy and complete removal.

Highly exudating wounds may indicate the need for dry gauze. If the gauze is dry and adherent at time of removal, it will need to be moistened to avoid trauma to the wound bed. The exception to this is the use of gauze for debridement. This form of nonselective mechanical debridement can become painful as the percentage of healthy tissue increases. (See Chapter 10 for more information about wound debridement.)

A comparison of gauze to advanced wound dressings (e.g., those that control moisture level and/or control microbial level) demonstrates gauze to be an inexpensive dressing until the total cost of care is calculated. When factoring in the time and frequency of change and cost of the person performing multiple dressing changes, the result is a higher cost with gauze.

IMPREGNATED GAUZE

Impregnated gauze dressings may be woven or nonwoven and are saturated with a variety of products such as iodinated agents, petroleum, zinc compounds, crystalline sodium chloride, chlorhexidine gluconate, bismuth tribromophenate, hydrogel, and aqueous saline (Hess, 2020). Impregnated gauze dressings are often nonadherent to the wound bed and may provide additional moisture to the wound, absorb exudate, and have antimicrobial properties. They are used on a variety of wounds from partial thickness to full thickness, skin tears, skin grafts, burns, as well as chronic wounds.

HYDROCOLLOIDS

Description and Characteristics

Hydrocolloids are occlusive or semiocclusive sheet, powder, and paste dressings made of gelatin, pectin, and carboxymethylcellulose. The sheet dressing is available in varying thicknesses. These dressings are also available in varying sizes and shapes with many designed for specific body locations. Some sheet hydrocolloids have tapered borders to prevent loosening at the edge. Sheet dressings tend to be totally occlusive. This occlusive nature promotes a moist wound environment, promotes autolytic debridement, insulates the wound from temperature changes, and serves as a barrier to other contaminants. These dressings are appropriate for shallow wounds with low to moderate exudate.

Components of the dressing interact with wound exudate to form a gel, which decreases trauma to the wound bed. This gel has a characteristic odor and appearance that should not be confused with signs of wound infection. The adhesive may be aggressive to fragile skin and care should be taken on removal.

These dressings are contraindicated for wounds that are infected; have heavy exudate, sinus tracts, or exposed tendons and bone; or are with fragile periwound skin. Wear time varies from 3 to 7 days, depending on the volume of exudate. If wear time is <3 days, an alternative dressing should be considered.

Clinical Considerations

Correct size of a hydrocolloid should allow about 1 inch of intact periwound skin. After dressing removal, wound assessment should be performed only after thoroughly cleansing the wound. Some anatomical locations are challenging to achieve and maintain a seal, without lifting of the edges. Gentle warming hand pressure after application may help the dressing conform and adhere. Recommended removal technique for hydrocolloids is pushing away the skin while gently lifting the dressing away to prevent medical adhesive–related skin injury (MARSI) (Yates et al., 2017).

HYDROFIBERS

Description and Characteristics

Hydrofibers are similar to alginate dressings. Hydrofibers are composed of carboxymethylcellulose, which makes them highly absorbent. These dressings are indicated for use in a variety of wounds with moderate to heavy exudate. The carboxymethylcellulose interacts with wound exudate to form a gel, much like the alginate dressings. Hydrofibers are available in both plain and antimicrobial forms. They are also available in sheet and rope form. They are nonadherent resulting in the need for a secondary dressing. Frequency of dressing change is dependent upon the dressing saturation and manufacturer's recommendation. This could range from daily to every 3 days.

Clinical Considerations

Given the gelling nature of these dressings, the wound should be thoroughly cleansed to remove all remnants. The wound should be regularly assessed for moisture level to determine ongoing need. Hydrofiber dressings are contraindicated in dry wounds, wounds with dry eschar, and third-degree burns.

HYDROGELS

Description and Characteristics

Hydrogels dressings are designed to hydrate the wound through the donation of water. They are available in solid gel sheets, viscous liquids (also known as amorphous), and gel-impregnated dressings. These dressings may be used in wounds with depth or tunnels or in shallow wounds with minimal exudate or in minor burns or tissue damaged by radiation. They have also been used to promote autolytic debridement. Some hydrogels have antimicrobial agents added.

Solid gel sheet dressings can be either water or glycerin based. They are available with and without adhesive borders. The sheets can absorb varying amounts of drainage depending upon their composition and promote autolysis. These sheets offer a cooling effect, which may be beneficial for pain management. Hydrogel dressings are ideal for any wound with minimal or no exudate and should be considered for management of minor burns and radio dermatitis. The frequency of dressing changes is dependent upon the type of hydrogel, volume of exudate, and characteristics of the secondary dressing but in general ranges from every 1 to 3 days.

Clinical Considerations

Sheet hydrogel dressings are easy to apply. The sheets with adhesive may allow visualization of the wound bed, reducing the need for premature removal. In addition, hydrogel dressings can be safely utilized during radiation therapy, and no allergies have been associated with this dressing.

Caution should be taken to avoid over filling the wound bed when using gel-impregnated gauze. Placement of hydrogel directly to the wound bed should be done per manufacturer's recommendations and should cover the wound bed. Periwound skin should be protected from maceration. The wound should be assessed for excess moisture and dryness with the plan of care altered as indicated.

OTHER PRODUCTS

InterDry®

Description and Characteristics

InterDry® is a polyurethane-coated polyester fabric impregnated with an antimicrobial silver, which reduces odor. It is used between skin folds and other skin-to-skin contact areas to manage moisture by wicking it away. Its low-friction surface reduces skin-to-skin trauma. It reduces colonization of bacteria and yeast. Use and frequency of dressing change is dependent upon manufacturer's recommendations (Hess, 2020).

Clinical Considerations

Position the textile appropriately based upon the dressing characteristics. When placed in a body fold, a portion of the dressing should be easily visible during assessment. The dressing should be placed flat against the skin. It is not a wound dressing and so should not be used with open wounds (Hess, 2020).

Plurogel® Burn and Wound Dressing

Descriptions and Characteristics

Plurogel® Burn and Wound Dressing is a translucent water-soluble dressing that provides moisture to the wound to prevent wound desiccation. It contains a non-cytotoxic surfactant that provides softening and loosening of wound debris with the added advantage of breaking up biofilm or preventing biofilm formation to aid in wound healing (in vitro) (Yang et al., 2017).

Clinical Considerations

Plurogel® Burn and Wound Dressing may be used on partial- to full-thickness wounds with minimal to moderately draining wounds. Plurogel® Burn and Wound Dressing is contraindicated for use on third- and fourth-degree burns. It may be applied directly to the wound or onto a sterile dressing using a sterile applicator. For wounds with minimal drainage, a thickness of 3 mm is recommended; for wounds with moderate drainage, a thickness of 5 mm is recommended. A secondary dressing is required. The dressing should be changed every 1 to 3 days (Hess, 2020).

A case series of 18 patients with lower extremity wounds were treated with Plurogel® Burn and Wound Dressing. On follow-up clinic visits, the wound was assessed, measurements were obtained, and Pressure Ulcer Scale for Healing (PUSH) Tool scores were completed. The mean Total PUSH score before the concentrated surfactant dressing (CSD) dressing was applied was 10.7 (range from 5 to 15) (standard deviation [SD] 3.09) and posttreatment was 8.3 (range from 0 to 14) (SD 4). All 18 patients had a decrease in their pretreatment score from the first clinic visit compared with the posttreatment PUSH Tool score, indicating that Plurogel® Burn and Wound Dressing may be an effective dressing in the management of lower extremity arterial and venous wounds (Ratliff, 2018b). Groin wounds are difficult to keep clean and maintain dressing integrity because of their location and complex topography. Ratliff (2018a) described the use of Plurogel® Burn and Wound Dressing to promote healing of an infected groin wound from a vascular graft infection.

TRANSPARENT FILMS

Description and Characteristics

Transparent films are thin sheets of polyurethane with a layer of acrylic hypoallergenic adhesive on one side. The adhesive is inactivated by moisture and will not adhere to a moist surface. The technology involved in production of the film renders these dressings semiocclusive or semipermeable. They allow for moisture vapor transfer and atmospheric gas exchange while remaining impermeable to liquids, solids, and bacteria.

Semiocclusive dressings keep a wound moist by retaining moisture lost by the wound. Their ability to maintain tissue hydration can be described using a measurement of moisture vapor transmission rate (MVTR). Traditional films have a low MVTR, ranging from 400 to 800 $g/m^2/d$. High-permeability film dressings have an MVTR of 3,000 $g/m^2/d$ or higher and are designed for use on intravenous (IV) sites (Bryant & Nix, 2016; Sussman, 2010).

KEY POINT

The wound care nurse should be knowledgeable about the MVTR of the transparent films available when recommending topical care for wounds versus IV site care.

Transparent films retain moisture at the wound surface but have no absorptive capacity. Transparent films are widely utilized as both primary and secondary dressings. They may be used as primary dressings for superficial wounds that are dry or have minimal exudate. They can serve as a secondary or securement for other products when a moisture-retentive cover dressing is needed as well as when wounds are at risk for contamination from urine and stool. Wear time is variable and is dependent upon wound depth, exudate, and location. When used as a primary dressing for a minimally exudating wound, a wear time of 3 to 7 days is appropriate.

Transparent films can promote autolytic debridement of eschar if indicated. They are available in a variety of sizes and shapes that conform to various anatomical locations. This conformability also allows the dressing to stay in place with body movement.

Clinical Considerations

When used to promote autolysis, the liquifying of the necrotic tissue results in increased volume of fluid, which can loosen the film adhesive requiring more frequent dressing changes. Because the film is minimally absorbent, excess fluid can cause maceration of the periwound skin. The liquefied nonviable tissue can be incorrectly assessed as purulent drainage. The wound should be thoroughly cleansed prior to assessment to determine the presence of an infectious process. Dressing size

should accommodate a perimeter of 2.5 cm (1 inch) of intact skin. In vulnerable populations, care should be taken with removal to avoid trauma. Transparent film dressings should not be pulled back across themselves as this action may result in skin stripping. Instead, the dressing should be gently stretched parallel with skin level allowing for adhesive release and then lifted (Bryant & Nix, 2016). In addition to the technique described, it is sometimes necessary to use a liquid skin protectant prior to application and adhesive remover/releaser products to prevent MARSI and pain with dressing removal (McNichol et al., 2013; Yates et al., 2017).

KEY POINT

Transparent film dressings should be gently stretched parallel to skin level allowing for adhesive release.

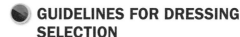

GUIDELINES FOR DRESSING SELECTION

Dressing selection for wound care is multifactorial. Decision-making guidelines and a simple decision table can be used to facilitate product selection (**Box 9-1; Table 9-1**). The key is to match wound characteristics with dressing attributes. The most important wound characteristics are amount of wound exudate and wound depth. One approach is to identify all available dressings and place them in a decision table based on those two characteristics (**Table 9-1**). This approach may identify areas of duplication and/or gaps in an agency's wound care formulary. Streamlining the wound care formulary and simplifying the decision-making process will aide in appropriate dressing selection.

Ongoing wound assessment per agency protocol requires reevaluation of the dressings in use. As a wound evolves, progressing, regressing, or plateauing, adjustments in dressing selection will be needed. Not all dressings are appropriate for continuous use until the wound is healed. Failure to change to different dressings can result in complications of wound healing. The wound care nurse is responsible for following manufacturer's

BOX 9-1   GUIDELINES FOR WOUND CLASSIFICATION

- Wounds with depth, tunnels, or undermining and moderate–large amounts of exudate: *deep/wet*
- Wounds with depth, tunnels, or undermining and minimal or no exudate: *deep/dry*
- Wounds that are shallow/superficial with no tunnels or undermining and moderate-to-large amounts of exudate: *shallow/wet*
- Wounds that are shallow/superficial with no tunnels or undermining and minimal or no exudate: *shallow/dry*

TABLE 9-1 SELECT DRESSING OPTION FROM THE APPROPRIATE GRID

DEEP WET WOUNDS	DEEP DRY WOUNDS
Need: Absorbent filler + secondary dressing to manage drainage	*Need: Moisture-retentive filler + secondary dressing to donate moisture to the wound*
Filler Dressing Options: • Alginate (sheet or rope) • Hydrofiber (sheet or rope) • Gauze and specialty gauze (nonwoven, moistened, loosely fluffed) • If tunnel, use "wick"	**Filler Dressing** Options: • Viscous gel to wound bed + lightly fluffed damp saline gauze • Gel-soaked gauze fluffed into wound bed • If tunnel, use "wick"
Secondary Dressing Options: • Gauze/tape (if wound exposed to contaminants, use transparent film instead of tape) • Waterproof adhesive foam dressing (good choice when bacterial barrier needed)	**Secondary Dressing** Options: • Gauze + transparent film dressing • Waterproof adhesive foam dressing

SHALLOW WET WOUNDS	SHALLOW DRY WOUNDS
Options *(may require both a primary and secondary)*: • Foam dressing with adhesive border • Sheet alginate + adhesive foam or roll gauze • Hydrofiber + adhesive foam or hydrofiber + roll gauze • Nonadherent contact layer (e.g., silicone perforated dressing) + gauze secondary • Textile dressing + roll gauze	Options: • Sheet hydrogels • Hydrocolloids • Transparent film dressings • Nonadherent contact layer + gauze secondary • Ointments

recommendations for dressing use and should avoid combining products without consideration for product compatibility.

 ## CONCLUSION

The wound care nurse should have a thorough understanding of wounds, wound healing, and dressings to provide evidence-based care to each patient with a wound (Hamdan et al., 2017). Dressing selection should be based on wound characteristics including depth, amount of exudate, tunnels or undermined areas, presence of infection, and location. Wound care should be individualized and based on goals of care.

REFERENCES

Agostinho, A. M., Hartman, A., Lipp, C., et al. (2011). An in vitro model for the growth and analysis of chronic wound MRSA biofilms. *Journal of Applied Microbiology, 111*(5), 1275–1282. doi: 10.1111/j.1365-2672.2011.05138.x.

Angobaldo, J., Sanger, D. O., & Marks, M. (2015). Prevention of projectile and aerosol contamination during pulsatile lavage irrigation using a wound irrigation bag. *Wounds, 20*(6), 167–170.

Atiyeh, B. S., Dibo, S. A., & Hayek, S. N. (2009). Wound cleansing, topical antiseptics and wound healing. *International Wound Journal, 6*, 420–430.

Avent, Y. (2010). Wound wise: Keep wounds moist with foam dressings. *Nursing Made Incredibly Easy!, 8*(1), 17–19.

Borges, E. L., Frison, S. S., Honorato-Sampaio, K., et al. (2018). Effect of polyhexamethylene biguanide solution on bacterial load and biofilm in venous leg ulcers: A randomized controlled trial. *Journal of Wound Ostomy & Continence Nursing, 45*(5), 425–431. doi: 10.1097/WON.0000000000000455.

Bradley, B. H., & Cunningham, M. (2013). Biofilms in chronic wounds and the potential role of negative pressure wound therapy: An integrative review. *Journal of Wound, Ostomy, and Continence Nursing, 40*(2), 143–149. doi: 10.1097/WON.0b013e31827e8481.

Bryant, R. A., & Nix, D. P. (2016). Principles of wound healing and topical management. In R. A. Bryant, & D. P. Nix (Eds.), *Acute & chronic wounds: Current management concepts* (5th ed.). St. Louis, MO: Elsevier.

Cox, J. (2019). Wound care 101. *Nursing2019, 49*(10), 32–39. doi: 10.1097/01.NURSE.0000580632.58318.08.

Day, A., Alkhalil, A., Carney, B.C., et al. (2017). Disruption of biofilms and neutralization of bacteria using hypochlorous acid solution: An in vivo and in vitro evaluation. *Advances in Skin & Wound Care, 30*(12), 543–551.

De Luna, V., Mancini, F., Maio, F. D., et al. (2017). Intraoperative disinfection by pulse irrigation with povidone-iodine solution in spine surgery. *Advances in Orthopedics*, Article ID 7218918, 1–8. doi: 10.1155/2017/7218918.

Dhivya, S., Padma, V. V., & Santhini, E. (2015). Wound dressings—A review. *BioMedicine, 5*(4), 22. doi: 10.7603/s40681-015-0022-9.

Edlich, R. F., Rodeheaver, G. T., Thacker, J. G., et al. (2010). Revolutionary advances in the management of traumatic wounds in the emergency department during the past 40 years: Part I. *Journal of Emergency Medicine, 38*(1), 40–50. doi: 10.1016/j.jemermed.2008.09.029.

European Pressure Ulcer Advisory Panel, National Pressure Injury Advisory Panel, and Pan Pacific Pressure Injury Alliance [EPUAP/NPIAP/PPPIA]. (2019). In E. Haesler (Ed.), *Prevention and treatment of pressure ulcers/injuries: Clinical Practice Guideline*. The International Guideline.

Fellows, J., & Crestodina, L. (2006). Home prepared saline: A safe, cost-effective alternative for wound cleansing in home care. *Journal of Wound, Ostomy, and Continence Nursing, 33*(6), 606–609. doi: 10193-03_WJ3306-Fellows.qxd.

Fernandez, R., & Griffiths, R. (2012). Water for wound cleansing: Review/Update of Cochrane database systematic review 2008. *Cochrane Database Systematic Reviews*, (2), CD003861. doi: 10.1002/14651858.CD003861.pub3.

Fonder, M. A., Lazarus, G. S., Cowan, D. A., et al. (2008). Treating the chronic wound: A practical approach to the care of nonhealing wounds and wound care dressings. *Journal of the American Academy of Dermatology, 58*(2), 185–206. doi: 10.1016/j.jaad.2007.08.048.

Fry, D. E. (2017). Pressure irrigation of surgical incisions and traumatic wounds. *Surgical Infections, 18*(4), 424–430. doi: 10.1089/sur.2016.252.

Haesler, E., Swanson, T., Ousey, K., et al. (2019). Clinical indicators of wound infection and biofilm: Reaching international consensus. *Journal of Wound Care, 28*(Sup3b), s4–s12. doi: 10.12968/jowc.2019.28.Sup3b.S4.

Hamdan, S., Pastar, I., Drakulich, S., et al. (2017). Nanotechnology-driven therapeutic interventions in wound healing: Potential uses and applications. *ACS Central Science, 3*(3), 163–175. doi: 10.1021/acscentsci.6b00371.

Heggers, J. P., Sazy, J. A., Stenberg, B. D., et al. (1991). Bactericidal and wound-healing properties of sodium-hypochlorite solutions: The

1991 Lindberg Award. *The Journal of Burn Care & Rehabilitation, 12*(5), 420–424.

Hess, C. T. (2020). *Product guide to skin and wound care* (8th ed.). Philadelphia, PA: Wolters Kluwer.

Hughes, M. S., Moghadamian, E. S., Yin, L. I., et al. (2012). Comparison of bulb syringe, pressurized pulsatile, and hydrosurgery debridement methods for removing bacteria from fracture implants. *Orthopedics, 35*(7), e1046–e1050. doi: 10.3928/01477447-20120621-19.

Lineaweaver, W., Howard, R., Soucy, D., et al. (1985). Topical antimicrobial toxicity. *Archives of Surgery, 120*(3), 267–270.

McNichol, L., Lund, C., Rosen, T., et al. (2013). Medical adhesives and patient safety: State of the science consensus statements for the assessment, prevention, and treatment of adhesive-related skin injuries. *Journal of Wound, Ostomy, and Continence Nursing, 40*(4), 365–380.

Mundy, L. R., Cage, M. J. Yoon, R. S., et al. (2017). Comparing the speed of irrigation between pulsatile lavage versus gravity irrigation: An ex-vivo experimental investigation. *Patient Safety in Surgery, 11*(7). doi: 10.1186/s13037-017-0124-2.

Naseri-Nosar, M., & Ziora, Z. M. (2018). Wound dressings from naturally-occurring polymers: A review on homopolysaccharide-based composites. *Carbohydrate Polymers, 189*, 379–398. doi: 10.1016/j.carbpol.2018.02.003.

Ovington, L. G. (2001). Hanging wet-to-dry dressings out to dry. *Home Healthcare Nurse, 19*(8), 477–483.

Ratliff, C. R. (2018a). Management of a groin wound using a concentrated surfactant-based gel dressing. *Journal of Wound, Ostomy, and Continence Nursing, 45*(5), 465–467.

Ratliff, C. R. (2018b). Case series of 18 patients with lower extremity wounds treated with a concentrated surfactant–based gel dressing. *Journal of Vascular Nursing, 36*(1), 3–7.

Resende, M. M., Rocha, C. A., Corrêa, N. F., et al. (2016). Tap water versus sterile saline solution in the colonisation of skin wounds: Tap water in wound cleansing. *International Wound Journal, 13*(4), 526–530. doi: 10.1111/iwj.12470.

Rodeheaver, G. T., & Ratliff, C. R. (2016). Wound cleansing, wound irrigation, wound disinfection. In D. L. Krasner (Ed.), *Chronic wound care: The essentials*. Malvern, PA: HMP Publications.

Ruder, J. A., & Springer, B. D. (2017). Treatment of periprosthetic joint infection using antimicrobials: Dilute povidone-iodine lavage. *Journal of Bone and Joint Infection, 2*(1), 10–14. doi: 10.7150/jbji.16448.

Sussman, G. (2010). Technology update: Understanding film dressings. *Wounds International, 1*(4), 23–25.

Thomas, G. W., Rael, L. T., Bar-Or, R., et al. (2009). Mechanisms of delayed wound healing by commonly used antiseptics. *Journal of Trauma and Acute Care Surgery, 66*(1), 82–91. doi: 10.1097.TA.0b013e31818b146d.

Truong, B., Grigson, E., Patel, M., et al. (2016). Pressure ulcer prevention in the hospital setting using silicone foam dressings. *Cureus, 8*(8). doi: 10.7759/cureus.730.

Vowden, P., Vowden, K., & Carville, K. (2011). Antimicrobial dressings made easy. *Wounds International, 2*(1). www.woundsinternational.com.

Wilson, J. R., Mills, J. G., Prather, I. D., et al. (2005). A toxicity index of skin and wound cleansers used on in vitro fibroblasts and keratinocytes. *Advances in Skin & Wound Care, 18*(7), 373–378.

Wound, Ostomy and Continence Nurses Society (WOCN). (2016). *Guideline for prevention and management of pressure ulcers (Injuries). WOCN clinical practice guideline series 2*. Mount Laurel, NJ: Author.

Wu, S., Applewhite, A. J., Niezgoda, J., et al. (2017). Oxidized regenerated cellulose/collagen dressings: Review of evidence and recommendations. *Advances in Skin & Wound Care, 30*(11S Suppl 1), S1–S18.

Yang, Q., Larose, C., Della Porta, A. C., et al. (2017). A surfactant-based wound dressing can reduce bacterial biofilms in a porcine skin explant model. *International Wound Journal, 14*(2), 408–413.

Yates, S., McNichol, L., Heinecke, S. B., et al. (2017). Embracing the concept, defining the practice, and changing the outcome: Setting the standard for medical adhesive-related skin injury interventions in WOC nursing practice. *Journal of Wound Ostomy & Continence Nursing, 44*(1), 13–17. doi: 10.1097/WON.0000000000000290.

Zhu, G., Wang, Q., Lu, S., et al. (2017). Hydrogen peroxide: A potential wound therapeutic target. *Medical Principles and Practice, 26*(4), 301–308. doi: 10.1159/000475501.

QUESTIONS

1. The wound nurse is assessing a patient's wound and documents: "wound is in the inflammatory stage with visible eschar and slough and large amounts of exudate." What is the goal in cleansing this wound?

A. Flush away exudate without damaging the proliferative cells and newly formed tissues.

B. Gradually scrape away dead tissue and slough without damaging healthy tissue.

C. Remove as much devitalized tissue, bacteria, and exudate as possible without damaging viable tissue.

D. Use a cytotoxic cleansing agent to irrigate the wound without disturbing granulation tissue.

2. A patient has a gunshot wound infected with *Pseudomonas aeruginosa*. What would be the best cleansing solution for this patient?

A. Acetic acid

B. Sodium hypochlorite

C. Bleach

D. Normal saline

3. For what adverse wound condition would the wound care nurse monitor when using saline-moistened gauze as a wound dressing?

A. Dehiscence of the wound

B. Tissue hypoxia

C. Desiccation of the wound bed

D. Hernia

4. A wound care nurse recommends a hydrating dressing for the wound. What would be the best choice?
A. Adhesive foam
B. Alginate
C. Hydrofiber
D. Hydrogel

5. The wound care nurse is choosing a dressing for a dehisced incision that measures 6 × 3 × 2 cm with areas of tunneling. What dressing would be an appropriate choice?
A. Wick, filler, and secondary dressing.
B. Filler dressing + secondary dressing.
C. Secondary (cover) dressing only.
D. Dressings are contraindicated for this type of wound.

6. Which type of dressing protects a wound from trauma and permits drainage to pass through to a secondary dressing?
A. Contact layer dressing
B. Alginate dressing
C. Hydrofiber dressing
D. Composite dressing

7. The wound nurse is choosing a dressing for a wound that is a deep, dry wound. What would be an appropriate choice?
A. Amorphous hydrogel to wound bed
B. Sheet hydrocolloid
C. Transparent film
D. Hydrofiber

8. A shallow wound is being treated with a transparent film dressing. To avoid skin stripping, the dressing removal technique includes
A. Always using a skin adhesive remover while lifting straight up on the dressing
B. Stretching the dressing at skin level, then lifting up
C. Lifting up on the dressing
D. Moistening the dressing with saline, then lifting up

9. The by-product of a hydrocolloid dressing is a gel with a characteristic odor. This gel and odor formation
A. Is normal and the wound should be cleansed
B. Indicates an infection and the wound should be cultured
C. Indicates an infection and the dressing should be changed to an antimicrobial
D. Is normal, but a different dressing should be chosen

10. Key wound characteristics to be considered in dressing selection include
A. Wound type, presence of odor, and wound location
B. Goals of treatment, wound location, and use of an antimicrobial dressing
C. Depth of the wound and the amount of exudate
D. Using an antimicrobial dressing, wound depth, and wound location

ANSWERS AND RATIONALES

1. C. Rationale: The goal is to cleanse the wound and remove as much of the devitalized tissue to reduce bacterial burden without damaging the viable tissue within the wound bed.

2. A. Rationale: Acetic acid can be used as a cleansing/irrigating agent alone or as a wound packing agent. It is sometimes used because of its bactericidal effectiveness against *Pseudomonas aeruginosa*.

3. C. Rationale: Wet-to-moist gauze dressings are used to maintain a moist wound base and

must be changed frequently to avoid drying (desiccation).

4. D. Rationale: Hydrogels dressings are designed to hydrate the wound through the donation of water.

5. A. Rationale: The wound with tunnels and depth will require a wick, a filler, and a secondary dressing to fill the open (dead) space in the wound.

6. A. Rationale: While they are minimally adherent, contact layer dressings are porous, permitting exudate to pass through the contact layer to a secondary dressing that provides absorption.

7. A. Rationale: Hydrogels may be used in wounds with depth or tunnels or in shallow wounds with minimal exudate or in minor burns or tissue damaged by radiation.

8. B. Rationale: Transparent film dressings should not be "pulled back" across themselves as this action may result in skin injury, specifically medical adhesive–related skin injury (MARSI). Instead, the dressing should be gently stretched at skin level allowing for adhesive release and then lifted.

9. A. Rationale: Components of the dressing interact with wound exudate to form a gel, which decreases trauma to the wound bed. This gel has a characteristic odor and appearance that should not be confused with signs of wound infection.

10. C. Rationale: Key wound characteristics to be considered in dressing selection include the following: depth of the wound and amount of exudate because these factors determine the need for a wick, filler, and/or secondary dressing.

CHAPTER 10

PRINCIPLES AND GUIDELINES FOR WOUND DEBRIDEMENT

Janet Ramundo

OBJECTIVES

1. Recommend or provide topical therapy based on best available evidence, to include

   a. Debridement of necrotic tissue when indicated

   b. Identification and management of wound-related infections

2. Demonstrate correct procedure for each of the following:

   a. Conservative sharp wound debridement (CSWD)

   b. Use of chemical cautery with silver nitrate applicators

3. Identify indications and contraindications to debridement.

4. Identify advantages, disadvantages, and guidelines for each of the following: CSWD, autolytic debridement, enzymatic debridement, chemical debridement, surfactant debridement, biosurgical/larval debridement therapy, mechanical (wet-to-dry) debridement, ultrasonic debridement, and surgical debridement.

TOPIC OUTLINE

INTRODUCTION

Debridement is the removal of necrotic tissue from a wound. Necrotic tissue is an impediment to healing, particularly in the chronic wound; removal of this tissue is essential to wound healing (Percival & Suleman, 2015; Ramundo, 2016). Debridement is also used for removal of biofilm and bioburden along with senescent cells (Manna & Morrison, 2020). As explained in other chapters, elimination of necrotic tissue is a critical element of wound bed preparation when the goal is healing; this chapter addresses indications, contraindications, options, and guidelines for debridement.

KEY POINT

Necrotic tissue interferes with healing and supports bacterial growth.

Necrotic tissue presents in two forms: eschar (the hard, leathery form) and slough (the soft yellow form) (**Figs. 10-1 and 10-2**). The components of necrotic tissue include avascular tissue, fibrinous exudate, and bacteria; these substances support bacterial growth and interfere with repair. Debridement (removal of eschar and slough) is an essential component of wound bed preparation. A wound containing necrotic material remains in the inflammatory phase of wound healing and is at increased risk of infection. Debridement allows visualization of the wound base, reduces the chance for infection, reduces odor, and allows the wound healing process to continue.

Many factors must be considered when determining the best approach to debridement, including the type of necrotic material in the wound base. Wounds containing slough may respond to autolytic, enzymatic, chemical, surfactant debridement methods, biosurgical/larval

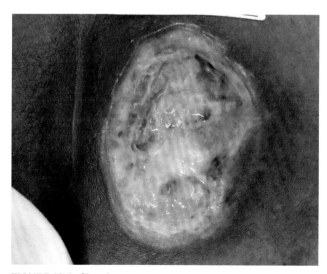

FIGURE 10-1. Slough.

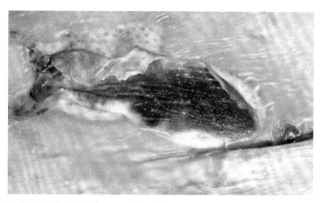

FIGURE 10-2. Eschar and Slough.

therapy, and conservative sharp wound debridement (CSWD). Eschar can be removed by autolytic, enzymatic (following crosshatching of the eschar), and instrumental debridement, either CSWD or surgical debridement. Infected wounds require rapid debridement that does not cause further harm to the surrounding tissue. Surgical debridement is often indicated (along with antibiotic therapy); if surgical intervention is contraindicated, more conservative approaches to debridement can be utilized (e.g., enzymatic, biosurgical/larval, chemical, surfactant, and CSWD) so long as infection is controlled with concomitant antibiotic therapy. These methods are discussed in further detail later in this chapter.

DECISION-MAKING REGARDING DEBRIDEMENT

CONTRAINDICATIONS TO DEBRIDEMENT

The wound care nurse must be aware that there are situations in which debridement is actually contraindicated. The most important contraindication is the poorly perfused wound, such as an uninfected foot ulcer in a patient with severe lower extremity arterial disease (LEAD). In this situation, removal of the eschar would convert the wound from closed to open and would significantly increase the risk of infection. In addition, removal of the eschar would provide no benefit, because a poorly perfused wound often does not progress to healing. Current guidelines state that this wound should be left closed and monitored for any signs of infection (WOCN, 2012, 2014). Development of infection usually mandates removal of the necrotic tissue, since necrotic tissue supports bacterial growth. Another situation in which debridement is usually contraindicated is a heel wound with dry eschar in a nonambulatory patient; the eschar is left intact as long as there are no signs of infection. Occasionally, intact eschar is left on a trunk wound as well when there are no signs of infection and other care priorities take precedence. If the eschar begins to separate or the wound shows signs of infection, then proceeding with debridement is recommended.

SELECTING THE BEST APPROACH TO DEBRIDEMENT

Other factors will guide the clinician in selecting the most appropriate method for removal of necrotic tissue. Foremost should be a consideration of the individual goals of care for the patient. In end-of-life care, the decision may be to forego removal of necrotic tissue and a focus on healing and to focus instead on comfort measures.

Clinician level and skill will also factor into the debridement method selection process. CSWD and surgical debridement require specialized training, whereas the application of enzymes to the wound or application of dressings to enhance autolytic debridement may be safely taught to nurses, nursing assistants, and caregivers. The care setting is another important consideration. A wound care nurse considering debridement options in home care might elect a more conservative approach to debridement than the wound care nurse practicing in acute care, due to the difference in access to support personnel and supplies. Autolytic debridement and enzymatic debridement are typical choices in the home setting, whereas surgical debridement or serial CSWD is frequently used in the acute care setting.

Decision-making about the method of debridement is often a challenge for clinicians as there is limited guidance regarding the best methods and many factors to consider. The few studies that have been done have different end points (healing vs. amount of debridement), are limited in scope, or are in vitro (lab) studies; thus, they fail to provide any definitive evidence as to the best approach for an individual patient. **Table 10-1** provides a brief summary of various methods of debridement.

TABLE 10-1 METHODS OF DEBRIDEMENT

TYPE OF DEBRIDEMENT	METHOD	EFFECT ON BIOFILM
Surgical	Performed in the operating room using scalpel and scissors	Disrupts biofilm and removes foci of infection
Conservative/sharp	Performed using aseptic technique with sterile curette, scalpel, and scissors	Removes and disrupts biofilm
Autolytic	Selective, slow debridement that occurs naturally and can be aided by using topical agents and moisture retentive wound dressings, including • Cadexomer iodine • Manuka honey • Alginate/hydrofiber wound dressing • Polyhexamethylene biguanide (PHMB) • Hydrogel	Varying efficacy on biofilm depending on the product and the phase of the biofilm cycle in which it is applied
Mechanical	Nonselective debridement performed using • Therapeutic irrigation • Monofilament fiber pads • Low-frequency ultrasound • Hydrosurgery	Some levels of disruption and removal of biofilm
Enzymatic/chemical/surfactant	Application of exogenous enzymes or chemicals to the wound surface, including • Alginogel • Enzymatic debriders • Wound cleansers and gels with high or low concentrations of surfactant	Some levels of disruption and removal of biofilm
Biosurgical/larval therapy	Sterile fly larvae that produce a mixture of proteolytic enzymes	Good evidence of removal of biofilm in vitro

From Swanson, T., Angel, D., Sussman, G., et al. (2016). *Wound infection in clinical practice: Principles of best practice*. International Wound Infection Institute (IWII). Wounds International. Retrieved from http://eprints.hud.ac.uk/id/eprint/30637/

See **Box 10-1** for critical questions to be addressed when considering debridement.

PROGRESSION AND MAINTENANCE DEBRIDEMENT

The wound must be closely monitored during the debridement process. The wound nurse should monitor for the removal of necrotic tissue, and this should be documented at each assessment. Necrotic tissue in the wound bed is typically expressed as a percentage of the total wound bed. It should be noted that the wound dimensions typically increase as the necrotic tissue is removed from the wound. Early in the debridement process, the wound is commonly exudative; the amount of exudate typically decreases as the necrotic tissue is removed. As debridement progresses, there should be increasing exposure of healthy viable tissue in the wound base. Regardless of the type of debridement utilized, a gradual transition in the type of necrotic tissue present in the wound is typically observed. Eschar gradually softens, and densely adherent slough loosens and becomes moister in appearance (**Fig. 10-3**). Post-

debridement, there should also be a reduction in signs of infection (e.g., periwound erythema and induration) in an infected wound, especially when the patient is also being treated with systemic antibiotics. Typically, wound debridement is discontinued when all necrotic tissue is removed from the wound base; the wound nurse will then select appropriate topical therapy based on the characteristics of the clean wound bed.

Some clinical experts propose continuing debridement even when the wound bed is visibly free of necrotic tissue, particularly in recalcitrant wounds (those that fail to respond to moist wound healing) (Falanga et al., 2008; Snyder et al., 2017). Maintenance debridement or repeated debridement may be recommended at each dressing change to delay biofilm re-formation especially if wound healing has stalled. It may be accomplished using a scalpel and scissors or a ring curette (Schultz et al., 2017; Snyder et al., 2017).

TYPES OF DEBRIDEMENT

Debridement is often categorized as selective or nonselective or instrumental versus noninstrumental. Selective debridement methods remove only necrotic material from the wound bed and leave healthy tissue intact. Examples of selective debridement include autolytic, enzymatic/chemical/surfactant, biosurgical/larval therapy, and CSWD. Nonselective debridement methods, such as surgical debridement, remove both viable and nonviable tissue from the wound bed. The indications for surgical debridement include (1) removal of the source of sepsis in the presence of infection; (2) decrease bacterial burden; (3) obtain accurate cultures taken after debridement for systemic antibiotic treatment; and (4) stimulation of the wound bed to promote healing with the release of platelet-derived growth factors (Yamakawa & Hayashida, 2019). Other examples of nonselective debridement include mechanical debridement such as wet-to-dry dressings, hydrosurgery, therapeutic irrigation (4 to 15 psi), and low-frequency ultrasound debridement. Instrumental debridement includes surgical and CSWD; noninstrumental methods include autolytic, enzymatic/chemical/surfactant, biosurgical/larval therapy, and mechanical (e.g., hydrotherapy, ultrasonic) debridement. Each method of debridement has a unique mechanism of action and indications and considerations for selection and use.

KEY POINT

Surgical debridement to the point of bleeding may stimulate healing via the release of platelet-derived growth factors.

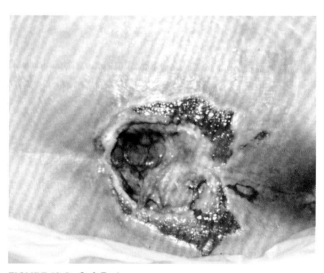

FIGURE 10-3. Soft Eschar.

NONINSTRUMENTAL METHODS OF DEBRIDEMENT

Noninstrumental methods of debridement are widely used due to their safety and availability. The various types of noninstrumental debridement are discussed individually.

Autolytic Debridement

Autolytic debridement involves the removal of necrotic tissue by the body's own white blood cells and natural enzymes, which migrate to the wound site during the normal inflammatory process. The body's proteolytic, fibrinolytic, and collagenolytic enzymes are released to digest the devitalized tissue present in the wound while leaving the healthy tissue intact (Rodeheaver et al., 1994; WOCN, 2015). Autolysis occurs naturally when the wound is kept in a moist, vascular environment with adequate leukocyte function. Because autolysis relies on white blood cells in the wound, there must be perfusion to the area and an adequate white blood cell count. Autolytic debridement is indicated for noninfected wounds or as an adjunct in infected wounds. It can be used with other debridement techniques such as mechanical debridement in the case of infected wounds (Manna & Morrison, 2020).

KEY POINT

Autolytic debridement is generally considered a safe though slow method of debridement. It is most effective on slough, and, because it is slow, it is generally considered more appropriate for noninfected wounds.

The use of moisture retentive dressings can enhance autolysis. Examples of dressings that support autolysis include transparent films, Manuka honey, hydrogels (amorphous and sheet), and any topical agent that adds and/or maintains a moist wound bed. Studies comparing autolytic to other methods of debridement are difficult to interpret as they use different end points as outcome measures; many studies focus on healing rather than the effectiveness of debridement (Jull et al., 2013). Konig et al. (2005) report that autolysis compares favorably to other methods of debridement in terms of effectiveness; however, autolytic debridement is slower than some alternative methods, such as mechanical and sharp. A multicenter randomized trial conducted by Burgos et al. (2000) showed no significant difference in healing of stage 3 pressure ulcers managed with a hydrocolloid for autolytic debridement and those managed with a commercially prepared topical enzyme. In contrast, another randomized study comparing the same products (hydrocolloid and enzyme) in management of stage 4 pressure ulcers on the heel following surgical debridement found that the enzyme provided faster results (Müller et al., 2001). Milne et al. (2010) also compared autolytic debridement (using hydrogel) to enzymatic debridement in 27 patients with pressure ulcers and also reported faster results with the enzyme.

Other dressings that promote autolysis include Manuka honey (Al-Waili et al., 2011; Jull et al., 2013) and polyacrylate dressings containing Ringer's solution (Paustian & Stegman, 2003; Skórkowska-Telichowska et al., 2013). Large-scale studies regarding the effectiveness of these products are lacking.

Gethin et al. (2015) conducted a systematic review of 10 RCTs (N = 715) to determine the effects of various debridement methods or debridement compared to no debridement on the rate of debridement and VLU healing. Seven RCTs focused on various methods of autolytic debridement; two RCTs compared enzymatic debridement to autolytic debridement; and one RCT compared biodebridement (larval) to autolytic debridement. There were no RCTs that evaluated sharp, surgical, or mechanical methods or that compared debridement to no debridement. Gethin et al. (2015) concluded that due to the small number of studies, small sample sizes, high risk of bias in most of the trials, and lack of meta-analysis due to heterogeneity of the trials, there was only limited evidence that debriding VLUs had a significant clinical impact on healing, and it was not possible to determine if any of the methods performed better than the others (WOCN, 2019).

KEY POINT

Autolytic debridement involves breakdown of necrotic tissue via the body's own WBCs and enzymes; it requires a moist wound surface and normal WBC counts.

Guidelines for Autolytic Debridement

Typically, the wound is cleansed with normal saline or wound cleanser; a moisture retentive dressing is then applied and monitored for excessive drainage. There is typically a significant amount of drainage during the early phases of autolytic debridement, due to liquefaction of the slough and other debris. The periwound area usually needs to be protected from maceration by the application of a liquid skin protectant. Frequency of dressing changes will be determined by the amount of drainage, in accordance with the manufacturer's guidelines for the particular dressing selected. For example, although Manuka honey dressings may generally be left in place for up to 7 days; the drainage and potential for maceration may necessitate more frequent changes.

Education is essential so that the patient, family, and other caregivers will know to expect the increased drainage and to alleviate concerns that the drainage is indicative of infection. The wound should be assessed at each dressing change for reduction in the amount of necrotic tissue, amount of exudate, and any signs of infection. The time frame for results with autolysis varies depending on the size of the wound and the amount and type of necrotic tissue. This type of debridement induces softening of the necrotic tissue and eventual separation from the wound bed. The effectiveness of this type of debridement is mandated by the amount of devitalized tissue to be removed as well as the actual wound size. Autolytic debridement will take a few days. If a significant decrease in necrotic tissue is not seen in 1 or 2 days, a different method of debridement should be considered (Manna & Morrison, 2020).

Enzymatic Debridement

Topical application of enzymes is another selective method of debridement. The only enzymatic debriding agent currently available in the United States is collagenase, which is derived from *Clostridium* bacteria. Collagenase digests the denatured collagen in necrotic tissue by dissolving the collagen anchors that secure the necrotic tissue to the underlying wound bed (Howes et al., 1959; Manna & Morrison, 2020).

Indications for enzymatic debridement include patients who are poor surgical debridement candidates, as an adjunct to surgical debridement and those who do not have access to a wound care nurse to provide sharp debridement (WOCN, 2015). Enzymatic debridement is a safe choice with infected wounds, especially when the patient is also receiving antibiotic therapy. Collagenase can also be effectively used with selected topical antibiotics and antibacterial dressings. Studies have demonstrated compatibility between collagenase and topical antibiotics, such as polymyxin B/bacitracin and mupirocin, and with selected antibacterial dressings (e.g., polyvinyl alcohol [PVA] dressings containing gentian violet and methylene blue). A relative contraindication of enzymatic debridement is its use in heavily infected wounds. The enzyme may cause mild and transient burning pain or slight erythema if it contacts the periwound. However, the wound care nurse must be aware that collagenase is *not* compatible with iodine products, silver-based products, and Dakin® solution (Jovanovic et al., 2012; Konig et al., 2005; Manna & Morrison, 2020; Ramundo & Gray, 2009). The length of time required to achieve debridement may range from several days to weeks. Early studies have shown collagenase to be an effective debriding agent for peripheral arterial ulcers and pressure ulcers (Boxer et al., 1969), and recent studies indicate that collagenase may provide faster debridement when compared to autolysis (Milne et al., 2010, 2012). A limited case series observed efficacy and safety when collagenase was used for debridement of necrotic wounds in the infant and neonate patient (Huett et al., 2017).

Collagenase is applied to the necrotic tissue in the wound bed every 24 hours. The secondary dressing should be one that it is practical to change within this timeframe. Certain cleansers will also deactivate the enzymatic activity; products should be selected carefully, and the manufacturer's guidelines should be followed (Jovanovic et al., 2012).

The current manufacturer recommends a 2-mm thick application of the enzyme, covered with a moist normal saline dressing or a moisture-retentive dressing. The product is most effective at a wound bed pH of 6.0 to 8.0 but has been demonstrated to be effective in a pH range up to 9.5 (Shi et al., 2010). There is currently no practical way to measure pH in the wound bed; however, pH issues must be considered if the product does not appear to be effective.

KEY POINT

Enzymatic debridement requires a 2-mm thick application of the enzyme, a moist wound environment, and avoidance of antiseptics that inactivate the enzyme, such as iodine and many silver dressings.

The enzyme should be continued as long as there is necrotic tissue visible in the wound bed; the product is generally discontinued once the wound bed is clean. Collagenase works most effectively on slough; when used on eschar, the wound care nurse must first crosshatch the eschar to permit the collagenase to penetrate to the collagen anchoring strands (**Fig. 10-4**). Another option is to apply the enzyme to the periphery of the eschar (if it has begun to lift from the wound bed); this will promote further lifting of the eschar, which then allows for CSWD. If prescribed for a home care patient, the patient or family member is taught the application of the product with application of secondary dressing. Enzymes are often used in conjunction with serial conservative wound debridement. Enzymes are a prescription item, so the

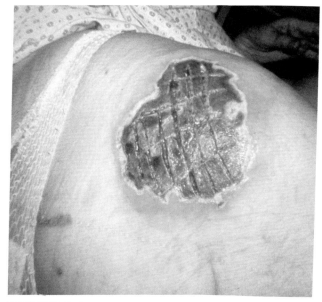

FIGURE 10-4. Eschar that Has Been Crosshatched Prior to Application of Enzyme.

Cost is another consideration; however, there are studies that show enzymatic debridement to be a cost-effective treatment (Waycaster & Milne, 2013; Woo et al., 2015).

Biosurgical/Larval Therapy

Biosurgical/larval therapy is a method of debridement that involves the application of sterile larvae of the *Lucilia sericata* (green bottle fly) to a wound with necrotic tissue. The larvae secrete enzymes that digest the necrotic tissue without harming the viable tissue in the wound bed. It is often used with infected necrotic wounds, particularly if surgical debridement is not an option (Gray, 2008; WOCN, 2015). This therapy is often referred to as MDT (maggot debridement therapy), LDT (larval debridement therapy), or biosurgical debridement. Biosurgical/larval therapy has been described in historical literature; its use in debridement was documented during the Civil War and in WWI. With the advent of antibiotics in the 1940s, the use of biosurgical/larval debridement declined. There is renewed interest due to the rise in antibiotic-resistant bacteria (Courtenay et al., 2000).

Some studies have noted successful removal of biofilm with biosurgical/larval debridement (Cowan, 2012). A randomized controlled trial noted a significant reduction in *Staphylococcus aureus* and *Pseudomonas aeruginosa* in the treatment of diabetic foot ulcers when treated with maggot therapy (Malekiam et al., 2019). A large-scale study of venous ulcers (VenUS II) concluded that there was no difference in healing rates between MDT and hydrogel despite more rapid debridement in the MDT group (Dumville et al., 2009). Another study compared MDT to hydrogel (autolytic) in lower extremity wounds (VLU and mixed) and found improved healing rates with MDT, along with less frequent dressing changes that may factor into decision-making. However, larger ulcers did not heal as well as smaller ones regardless of the choice of therapy (Mudge et al., 2014; Zarachi & Gergor, 2012).

Davies et al. (2015) conducted an RCT to assess the effectiveness of larval debridement of VLUs under compression bandages and the effect on healing. Patients (N = 40) were randomized to treatment with a four-layer compression bandage (n = 20) or to a four-layer compression bandage plus larval therapy (n = 20) for 4 days. Patients were seen on day 4 after the initial application of the bandages, with follow-up every 2 weeks for up to 12 weeks, to assess the slough and surface area of the wound. The investigators concluded that larval therapy demonstrated a significant reduction in the amount of slough in the wound, but there was no additional impact on healing over that of compression (WOCN, 2019).

Gethin et al. (2015), one RCT of patients with VLUs (N = 12), compared biodebridement (n = 6) to autolytic debridement (n = 6) of the ulcers. One-hundred percent (n = 6) of VLUs treated with biodebridement achieved a clean wound bed within a month, compared to 33%

(n = 2) of VLUs treated with autolytic debridement using a hydrogel (RR = 2.6, 95% CI [0.94, 7.17], p = 0.065), which was a nonsignificant difference. The authors of the RCT reported that the time to complete debridement was significantly quicker with biodebridement than with autolytic debridement (3 days vs. 22, p = 0.003). The participants in the biodebridement group required only one application of larvae. Healing rates were not reported by the investigators in the RCT (WOCN, 2019).

Guidelines for Biosurgical/Larval Debridement

Biosurgical/larval therapy can be used in acute or chronic wounds. It is contraindicated in the presence of active bleeding or those at high risk of bleeding, copious wound exudate that may flush the maggots out of the wound, and wounds with deep cavities or sinus tracts. Pain and bleeding have been reported with the use of biosurgical/larval debridement (Mudge et al., 2014; Shih et al., 2018; Steenvorde et al., 2005; Steenvorde & van Doorn, 2008), so careful assessment is essential for the duration of therapy, particularly in patients on anticoagulation therapy. Biosurgical/larval therapy is also contraindicated in wounds in close proximity to blood vessels, devitalized bone or tendon, with inadequate circulation or if patient is allergic or sensitive to larval proteins or the nutrient media (WOCN, 2015). A major concern about use of biosurgical/larval debridement is the possible aversion to this therapy by the patient and caregivers.

Medical grade, sterilized maggots are applied directly to the wound and covered with a containment dressing; the recommended "dose" is approximately 5 to 8 larvae per cm^2. There are commercially available containment dressings from the distributor of the larvae, or dressings may be designed for this purpose. Typically, the periwound skin is protected with a hydrocolloid-type dressing, and a small aperture (fine) mesh dressing is applied over the wound (and the larvae) and secured to the hydrocolloid border. It is critical to assure that the secondary dressing permits oxygen delivery to the wound bed, to prevent death of the larvae. Amount of drainage will be moderate to large as the necrotic tissue is liquefied.

Chemical Debridement

Sodium hypochlorite (Dakin® solution) has been theorized to promote debridement. Sodium hypochlorite has mostly been studied for cleansing properties rather than debridement but may be a viable option for use in an infected necrotic wound. It is thought that Dakin® solution will loosen the anchoring strands holding eschar on the wound and allow for easier removal. In addition, it is effective against most bacteria, yeast, and viruses, reduces odor, and is relatively inexpensive to use. The most common concentration is 0.25%, but this strength should not be used in a clean wound as it will destroy fibroblasts. Heggers et al. (1991) noted that at 0.0125%, the solution provides effective antimicrobial action without destroying fibroblasts. Other studies have challenged the debridement qualities of sodium hypochlorite (Thomas, 1991), and some authors state that the concentration and frequency needed to facilitate removal of necrotic tissue is impractical and possibly harmful to the wound. In clinical practice, Dakin® solution is typically used in heavily necrotic wounds particularly when infection and odor are a concern. Dakin® solution should be applied to gauze until it is moderately wet, packed lightly into the wound with a cover dressing, and changed every 12 hours. Care should be taken to protect the periwound skin and confine the solution-moistened gauze to the wound bed. The solution should be contained in a colored bottle away from light as it breaks down easily. Commercial solutions are available now with stabilizers, which eliminate concerns about stability. Dakin® solution dressings should be considered short term while the wound is treated for infection and debrided; once concerns about infection are eliminated, another method of debridement should be considered.

KEY POINT

Chemical debridement using sodium hypochlorite and similar agents is typically reserved for wounds that are necrotic, infected, and malodorous; use remains controversial.

Surfactants

Surfactants cleanse and remove slough and most types of necrotic tissue. Surfactants are considered a form of debridement because of their ability to prevent and breakdown biofilms. Plurogel® Burn and Wound Dressing is a translucent water-soluble dressing that provides moisture to the wound to prevent wound desiccation. It contains a noncytotoxic surfactant that provides softening and loosening of wound debris with the added advantage of breaking up biofilm or preventing biofilm formation to aid in wound healing. Yang et al. (2017) tested the concentrated surfactant dressing (CSD) on porcine skin infected with a biofilm. They found that daily application and removal of the CSD reduced the biofilm to undetectable levels within 3 days in the pig model.

A case series of 18 patients with lower extremity wounds were treated with Plurogel® Burn and Wound Dressing. On follow-up clinic visits, the wound was assessed, measurements were obtained, and Pressure Ulcer Scale for Healing (PUSH) Tool scores completed. The mean total PUSH score before the CSD dressing was applied was 10.7 (range from 5 to 15) (standard deviation [SD] 3.09) and posttreatment was 8.3 (range from 0 to 14) (SD 4). All 18 patients had a decrease in their pretreatment score from the first clinic visit compared with the posttreatment PUSH Tool score, indicating that

Plurogel® Burn and Wound Dressing may be an effective dressing in the management of lower extremity arterial and venous wounds (Ratliff, 2018a). Groin wounds are difficult to keep clean and maintain dressing integrity because of their location and complex topography. Ratliff (2018b) describes the use of Plurogel® Burn and Wound Dressing to promote healing of an infected groin wound from a vascular graft infection.

Hydrotherapy

Hydrotherapy involves the use of water or other fluid to cleanse and possibly loosen necrotic tissue in an attempt to remove it from the wound bed. There are few studies that look at irrigation or hydrotherapy as a method of debridement; most focus on the cleansing properties of the fluid. Historically, whirlpool has been used as a mechanical method of debridement. However, contemporary guidelines do not mention whirlpool as a recommended option for debridement (EPUAP/NPIAP/PPPIA, 2019; Robson et al., 2006; Steed et al., 2006; WOCN, 2016, 2019). Concerns about cross-contamination as well as the development of alternate methods have largely eliminated whirlpool as a method of cleaning or debriding a wound.

Therapeutic wound irrigation and pulsatile lavage involve debridement of necrotic tissue with fluid and between 4 and 15 pounds per square inch (psi) of pressure, which is adequate to remove debris from the wound bed without damaging healthy tissue or inoculating the underlying tissue with bacteria (Federman et al., 2016; Robson et al., 2006; Steed et al., 2006; WOCN, 2016). The wound care nurse should be aware that delivery of fluid under pressure can cause aerosolization and dissemination of wound bacteria over a wide area, exposing the patient and care provider to potential contamination. Consequently, the care provider should wear personal protective equipment (mask, gloves, gown, goggles) while performing irrigation. Therapeutic wound irrigation may be accomplished using a 19-gauge angiocatheter and a 35-mL syringe, or with prepackaged canisters of pressurized saline or products that attach to saline bags for continuous low-pressure irrigation (EPUAP/NPIAP/PPPIA, 2019; WOCN, 2016).

A pulsatile lavage device combines intermittent high-pressure lavage with suction to loosen necrotic tissue and facilitate its removal (Morgan & Hoelscher, 2000). Pulsatile lavage is effective for removing larger amounts of debris and should be discontinued once the wound is clean. Pulsatile lavage should be used with caution to prevent damage to blood vessels, graft sites, and exposed muscle, tendon, and bone. Patients on anticoagulant therapy should be observed carefully for any bleeding, and treatment should be discontinued immediately if bleeding occurs. Disadvantages of debridement with pulsatile lavage include cost and time. The irrigators are designed for one-time use, and large necrotic wounds may require daily treatments. Pulsatile lavage treatment should be delivered in an enclosed area separate from any other patients to prevent contamination (Maragakis et al., 2004). Once the wound bed is clean, pulsed lavage is usually discontinued, and the wound is assessed for topical therapy that will support the goals of healing. Pulsed lavage is often combined with other methods of debridement such as CSWD, enzyme application, or selection of a dressing that supports autolytic debridement. It is typically utilized three to seven times per week and is often performed by physical therapists who are certified in wound care.

Wet-to-Dry Gauze

Wet-to-dry debridement is a mechanical, nonselective method of debridement. This method can be painful and may damage newly formed viable tissue; it is therefore generally considered suboptimal therapy (Hopf et al., 2006; Ovington, 2001; Robson et al., 2006; Steed et al., 2006). If wet-to-dry debridement must be used, it is most appropriate with heavily necrotic and infected wounds without visible granulation tissue. Correct technique consists of lightly packing moistened woven cotton gauze in the wound bed, and allowing it to dry on the wound, to trap debris and necrotic tissue. Once dry, usually 4 to 6 hours after application, the dressing is pulled off the wound along with the trapped debris and necrotic tissue. The gauze should not be moistened prior to removal. The wound is then cleansed, and the process is repeated. Wet-to-dry gauze debridement requires dressing changes several times per day until all necrotic tissue is removed. The perception that wet–dry debridement is cost-effective may not be accurate once caregiver time is factored into the equation. Woo et al. (2015) compared the cost of various methods of debridement and noted mechanical wet-to-dry debridement as one of the most costly methods.

> **KEY POINT**
>
> Mechanical debridement using wet-to-dry gauze is nonselective and painful; it is generally considered contraindicated.

Moist to damp is often the method employed when gauze dressings are used and may promote autolysis. This approach is also not cost-effective when the time to add fluid to the dressing is factored in. In addition, there are no studies to support moist to damp gauze dressings as a method of autolytic debridement.

A newer method of mechanical debridement using a monofilament debridement pad has been shown to be effective with the removal of slough and biofilm (Schultz et al., 2018). The pad is moistened and rubbed over the wound surface to loosen and remove necrotic tissue.

One review noted that this is a cost-effective treatment in comparison with other methods of debridement (Mead et al., 2015).

Ultrasound

Ultrasound uses acoustic energy to remove necrotic tissue from the wound bed and promote healing. Contact ultrasound used for debridement may be either high or low frequency and uses saline coupled with the acoustic wave to produce mechanical and thermal effects (**Fig. 10-5**). For example, low-frequency ultrasound with high intensity produces cavitation, which may cause breakdown of fibrin (Madhok et al., 2013; Stanisic et al., 2005). This debridement effect is not seen when there is no contact with the wound, as in low-frequency, low-intensity, noncontact ultrasound. A review of the literature on the use of ultrasound revealed insufficient evidence to determine its effectiveness in debridement (Cullum et al., 2010; Ramundo & Gray, 2008), although a positive impact on healing has been noted (Carville et al., 2018; Kavros et al., 2008; Kavros & Coronado, 2018; Messa et al., 2018). Most of the studies use healing as the endpoint, so the exact impact on efficacy of debridement is difficult to determine.

INSTRUMENTAL METHODS OF DEBRIDEMENT

Instrumental methods of debridement have the advantage of providing faster elimination of necrotic tissue. Instrumental methods include surgical approaches and conservative sharp debridement at the bedside; surgical debridement is typically a one-step approach to debridement, while conservative sharp debridement is usually used in conjunction with noninstrumental approaches.

Surgical Debridement

Surgical debridement is the nonselective removal of large amounts of necrotic tissue with a scalpel, laser, or water (hydrosurgery). It typically is performed in the operating room or special procedures area, and the patient is frequently anesthetized. It is the debridement method

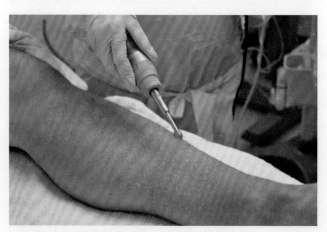

FIGURE 10-5. Contact Ultrasound Debridement.

recommended for wounds with advancing cellulitis, wound-related sepsis, large amounts of necrotic tissue, and/or infected bone or hardware that must be removed (EPUAP/NPIAP/PPPIA, 2019). It is the most rapid way to remove large amounts of necrotic tissue.

Risk must be considered as the patient will likely need to have anesthesia, and there is the potential for bleeding and infection. Surgical debridement requires a high skill level and should be performed by a surgeon or advanced practice nurse with training in surgical debridement.

In additional to traditional debridement with a scalpel, new surgical methods of debridement are available. *Laser debridement,* a form of surgical debridement, uses focused beams of light to slice through tissue. Advantages of laser debridement are that the wound bed is sterilized and instantly cauterized (Flemming et al., 1986). Animal studies using a laser to debride partial-thickness burns have demonstrated results similar to those of sharp debridement but with hemostasis and no disturbance of periwound skin (Graham et al., 2002; Lam et al., 2002). Disadvantages of laser debridement include risk of injury to adjacent healthy tissue; however, newer pulsed lasers have reduced that risk (Glatter et al., 1998; Smith et al., 1997).

The *hydrosurgical water knife* is a method of surgical debridement that dispenses normal saline at high power, which provides debridement and cleansing of the wound base. This water jet device is regulated so that the clinician is able to precisely control the depth of debridement; debris from the wound is removed at the same time. The main advantage to hydrosurgery over traditional surgery is the shorter time required with similar outcomes; the shorter time contributes to the cost-effectiveness of the method (Caputo et al., 2008; Gravante et al., 2007).

Conservative Sharp Wound Debridement

CSWD is a method for the removal of loosely adherent necrotic tissue using sterile instruments such as scalpel, forceps, and scissors (see **Box 10-2**).

CSWD involves the removal of nonviable tissue, so no blood loss is anticipated. If minor bleeding occurs, apply direct pressure with a gauze dressing or use chemical cautery via silver nitrate applicator (see **Box 10-3**). CSWD is typically used with other methods of debridement and done serially. For example, a wound care nurse might remove necrotic slough from a wound bed, then apply an enzyme to the wound bed along with a dressing that will support autolytic debridement. CSWD would be performed at each professional visit, usually one to three times per week. CSWD is more rapid than non-instrumental methods but slower than surgical removal. Since only necrotic tissue is removed, it is considered selective.

BOX 10-2   CSWD PROCEDURE

Conservative Sharp Wound Debridement Procedure
1. Review medical record to assure licensed provider order.
2. Review medications that would increase the risk for bleeding.
3. Rule out contraindications such as ischemia or active cellulitis.
4. Obtain informed consent and complete time out process (if required).
5. Wash hands; apply clean gloves.
6. Set up clean field with sterile scalpel and sterile forceps/pickups or hemostats.
7. Position the patient for comfort; drape appropriately.
8. Prep wound with povidone–iodine solution or alternative antiseptic; allow to dry.
9. Remove gloves. Sanitize the hands and apply clean gloves.
10. Grasp loose necrotic tissue and hold tautly so that line of dissection is clearly visualized. Use scalpel or scissors to establish plane of dissection and to cut away loose necrotic tissue.
11. Flush wound with saline following procedure and apply appropriate dressing.

Throughout Procedure
1. Avoid all vascular structures and any structures/tissues not clearly identified.
2. Monitor patient tolerance and discontinue procedure if evidence of pain or discomfort.
3. Control minor bleeding with direct pressure and/or silver nitrate.

Documentation
1. Wound status at the beginning and end of the procedure.
2. Procedure performed.
3. Patient tolerance and any adverse effects (bleeding or pain).

From Wound, Ostomy and Continence Nurses Society (WOCN). (2005). *Conservative sharp wound debridement: Best practice for clinicians.* Mt. Laurel, NJ: Author.

CSWD may be used in conjunction with noninstrumental forms of debridement to facilitate wound cleanup; the wound care nurse must assure that she or he is covered to do CSWD by the state nurse practice act and facility policy. The wound care nurse must rule out any conditions that would be contraindications prior to performing CSWD.

CSWD has several advantages. It removes the necrotic tissue more quickly than the previously discussed methods, and it can be accomplished in a serial manner. This method of debridement can be combined with other debridement techniques (autolytic or enzymatic) to shorten this phase of wound care. Theoretically, a more rapid approach to debridement decreases the body's expenditure of energy during a time of high resource use.

Because of the low risk involved, CSWD in many states is a delegated medical function that can be performed in a variety of settings by a clinician who is competent and credentialed in the technique. Therefore, conservative sharp debridement is a viable option for patients residing in nonacute care settings without the need for transfer to a hospital. A variety of requirements may need to be satisfied, depending on the nurse practice act specific to the state and the employer's requirements.

A disadvantage of CSWD is that, depending on the size of the wound and the amount of necrotic tissue involved, it could conceivably take weeks to remove all of the nonviable tissue. The procedure may be uncomfortable for the patient, so the need for analgesia should be considered. Blood loss is not expected during conservative sharp debridement but remains a possibility. As a result, the patient should be assessed for factors that place him or her at risk for clotting problems if a small vessel is accidentally severed. Factors to consider include medications (e.g., anticoagulants, high-dose nonsteroidal anti-inflammatory drugs) and pathologic conditions (e.g., thrombocytopenia, impaired hepatic function, vitamin K deficiency, malnutrition). When any of these factors are present, the wound care nurse should confer with the provider before proceeding with CSWD. Another consideration prior to CSWD is the presence of active wound infection; in this case, severing of a small vessel could cause a bacteremia. Most wound care nurses either delay CSWD until the periwound cellulitis is under control or are very cautious when debriding these wounds to eliminate the risk of unintentional injury.

PROFESSIONAL PRACTICE CONSIDERATIONS

Although debridement methods such as autolysis, wound irrigation, wet-to-dry dressings, and enzymes ideally are initiated under the direction of the provider or wound care nurse, they are procedures that can be performed by nurses, physical therapists, the patient, and caregivers. However, the more aggressive methods of debridement, specifically sharp debridement, require a greater level of skill and competence. CSWD should be performed only by a wound care nurse or provider with demonstrated and documented competence. Although there is currently no certification for debridement, most institutions will require evidence of didactic and clinical education. In addition, many will require demonstration of competency at designated intervals. Most state boards of nursing do not address this function specifically. The wound care nurse should ensure that there is a policy in place that states who is able to perform CSWD and a written procedure that is approved by the institution.

CONCLUSION

Debridement is a critical component of topical therapy for necrotic wounds. The wound care nurse should be knowledgeable about the various methods available for debridement and should consider options based on goals of care, wound assessment, and skill level of involved clinicians. Debridement methods are often combined and modified as the wound conditions change. Continual, accurate wound assessments during the debridement phase are essential to ensure an outcome consistent with the stated wound goals.

REFERENCES

Al-Waili, N., Salom, K., & Al-Ghamdi, A. A. (2011). Honey for wound healing, ulcers and burns; data supporting its use in clinical practice. *The Scientific World Journal, 11*, 766–787.

Boxer, A. M., Gottesman, N., Bernstein, H., et al. (1969). Debridement of dermal ulcers and decubiti with collagenase. *Geriatrics, 24*(7), 75–86.

Burgos, A., Gimenez, J., Moreno, E., et al. (2000). Cost, efficacy, efficiency and tolerability of collagenase ointment versus hydrocolloid occlusive dressing in the treatment of pressure ulcers: A comparative, randomised, multicenter study. *Clinical Drug Investigation, 19*(5), 357–365. Retrieved May 10, 2014, from http://link.springer.com/article/10.2165/00044011-200019050-00006

Caputo, W. J., Beggs, D. J., DeFede, J. L., et al. (2008). A prospective randomised controlled clinical trial comparing hydrosurgery debridement with conventional surgical debridement in lower extremity ulcers. *International Wound Journal, 5*(2), 288–294.

Carville, K., Howse, L., Edmondson, M., et al. (2018). Nurse practitioners and their use of low-frequency ultrasound debridement in the management of chronic wounds. *Journal of the Australian Wound Management Association, 26*(3), 122–126.

Courtenay, M., Church, J., & Ryan, T. (2000). Larva therapy in wound management. *Journal of Royal Society of Medicine, 93*, 72–74.

Cowan, T. (2012). Visible biofilms: A controversial issue! *Journal of Wound Care, 21*(3), 106.

Cullum, N., Al-Kurdi, D., & Bell-Syer, S. E. M. (2010). Therapeutic ultrasound for venous leg ulcers. *Cochrane Database of Systematic Reviews*, (6), CD001180. doi: 10.1002/14651858.CD001180.pub3.

Davies, C. E., Woolfrey, G., Hogg, N., et al. (2015). Maggots as a wound debridement agent for chronic venous leg ulcers under graduated compression bandages: A randomised controlled trial. *Phlebology*, *30*(10), 693–699. doi: 10.1177/0268355514555386.

Dumville, J., Worthy, G., Soares, M., et al. (2009). VenUS II: A randomized controlled trial of larval therapy in the management of leg ulcers. *Health Technology Assessment, 13*(55), 1–182.

European Pressure Ulcer Advisory Panel, National Pressure Injury Advisory Panel, and Pan Pacific Pressure Injury Alliance [EPUAP/NPIAP/PPPIA]. (2019). In E. Haesler (Ed.), *Prevention and treatment of pressure ulcers/injuries: Clinical Practice Guideline*. The International Guideline.

Evans, K., & Kim, P. J. (2019). Overview of treatment of chronic wounds. In C. E. Butler, R. S. Berman, & E. Bruera (Eds.), *UpToDate*. Waltham, MA: UpToDate Inc. Accessed online on January 31, 2020. https://www.uptodate.com/contents/overview-of-treatment-of-chronic-wounds

Falanga, V., Brem, H., Ennis, W. J., et al. (2008). Maintenance debridement in the treatment of difficult to heal wounds, recommendations of an expert panel. *Ostomy Wound Management*, (Suppl), 2–13.

Federman, D. G., Ladiiznski, B., Dardik, A., et al. (2016). Wound healing society 2014 update on guidelines for arterial ulcers. *Wound Repair and Regeneration, 24*(1), 127–135.

Flemming, A., Frame, J. D., & Dhillon, R. (1986). Skin edge necrosis in irradiated tissue after carbon dioxide laser excision of tumor. *Lasers in Medical Sciences, 1*, 263–265.

Gethin, G., Cowman, S., & Kolbach, D. N. (2015). Debridement for venous leg ulcers. *Cochrane Database of Systematic Reviews*, (9), CD008599. doi: 10.1002/14651858.CD008599.pub2.

Glatter, D., Goldberg, J. S., Schomacker, K. T., et al. (1998). Carbon dioxide laser ablation with immediate auto-grafting in a full-thickness porcine burn model. *Annals of Surgery, 228*(2), 257.

Graham, J. S., Schomacker, K. T., Glatter, R. D., et al. (2002). Efficacy of laser debridement with autologous split-thickness skin grafting in promoting improved healing of deep cutaneous sulfur mustard burns. *Burns, 28*, 719.

Gravante, G., Delogu, D., Esposito, G., et al. (2007). Versajet hydrosurgery versus classic escharectomy for burn débridement: A prospective randomized trial. *Journal of Burn Care & Research, 28*(5), 720–724.

Gray, M. (2008). Is larval (maggot) debridement effective for removal of necrotic tissue from chronic wounds? *Journal of Wound Ostomy & Continence Nursing, 35*(4), 378.

Heggers, J., Sazy, J. A., Stenberg, B. D., et al. (1991). Bactericidal and wound-healing properties of sodium hypochlorite solutions: The 1991 Lindberg award. *Journal of Burn Care & Rehabilitation, 12*, 420–424.

Hopf, H. W., Ueno, C., Aslam, R., et al. (2006). Guidelines for the treatment of arterial insufficiency ulcers. *Wound Repair and Regeneration, 14*(6), 693–710.

Howes, E. L., Mandl, I., Zaffuto, S., et al. (1959). The use of *Clostridium histolyticum* enzymes in the treatment of experimental third degree burns. *Surgery Gynecology & Obstetrics, 109*, 177.

Huett, E., Bartley, W. Morris, D., et al. (2017). Collagenase for wound debridement in the neonatal intensive care unit: A retrospective case series. *Pediatric Dermatology, 34*(3), 277–281.

Jovanovic, A., Ermis, R., Mewaldt, R., et al. (2012). The influence of metal salts, surfactants, and wound care products on enzymatic activity of collagenase, the wound debriding enzyme. *Wounds, 24*(9), 242–253.

Jull, A. B., Cullum, N., Dumville, J. C., et al. (2013). Honey as a topical treatment for wounds. *Cochrane Database of Systematic Reviews*, (2), CD005083.

Kavros, S. J., & Coronado, R. (2018). Diagnostic and therapeutic ultrasound on venous and arterial ulcers: A focused review. *Advances in Skin and Wound Care, 31*(2), 55–65.

Kavros, S. J., Liedl, D. A., Boon, A. J., et al. (2008). Expedited wound healing with noncontact low frequency ultrasound in chronic wounds: A retrospective analysis. *Advances in Skin & Wound Care, 21*, 416–423.

Konig, M., Vanscheidt, W., Augustin, M., et al. (2005). Enzymatic versus autolytic debridement of chronic leg ulcers: A prospective randomized trial. *Journal of Wound Care, 14*(7), 320–323.

Lam, D., Rice, P., & Brown, R. (2002). The treatment of Lewisite burns with laser debridement—"Lasablation". *Burns, 28*(1), 19–25.

Madhok, B. M., Vowden, K., & Vowden, P. (2013). New techniques for wound debridement. *International Wound Journal, 10*, 247–251.

Malekiam, A., Djavid, G. E., Akbarzadeh, K., et al. (2019). Efficacy of maggot therapy on *Staphylococcus aureus* and *Pseudomonas aeruginosa* in diabetic foot ulcers. *Journal of Wound Ostomy and Continence Nursing, 46*(1), 25–29.

Manna, B., & Morrison, C. A. (2020). Wound debridement [Updated November 23, 2019]. In *StatPearls* [Internet]. Treasure Island, FL: StatPearls Publishing. Retrieved from https://www.ncbi.nlm.nih.gov/books/NBK507882

Maragakis, L. L., Cosgrove, S. E., Song, X., et al. (2004). An outbreak of multidrug-resistant *Acinetobacter baumannii* associated with pulsatile lavage wound treatment. *Journal of American Medical Association, 292*(24), 3006–3011.

Mead, C., Lovato, E., & Longworth, L. (2015). The Debrisoft® monofilament pad for use in acute or chronic wounds: A NICE medical technology guidance. *Applied Health Economics and Health Policy, 13*(6), 583–594.

Messa, C. A., Rhemtulla, I. A., Mauch, J. T., et al. (2018). Institutional experience with ultrasound debridement for the treatment of complex wounds. *Plastic and Reconstructive Surgery, 6*(8S), 189–190.

Milne, C. T., Ciccarelli, A. O., & Lassy, M. (2010). A comparison of collagenase to hydrogel dressings in wound debridement. *Wounds, 22*, 270–274.

Milne, C. T., Ciccarelli, A. O., & Lassy, M. (2012). A comparison of collagenase to hydrogel dressings in maintenance debridement and wound closure. *Wounds, 24*(11), 317–322.

Morgan, D., & Hoelscher, J. (2000). Pulsed lavage: Promoting comfort and healing in home care. *Ostomy Wound Management, 46*(4), 44–49.

Mudge, E., Price, P., Neal, W., et al. (2014). A randomized controlled trial of larval therapy for the debridement of leg ulcers: Results of a multicenter, randomized, controlled, open, observer-blind, parallel group study. *Wound Repair & Regeneration, 22*(1), 43–51.

Müller, E., van Leen, M. W., & Bergemann, R. (2001). Economic evaluation of collagenase-containing ointment and hydrocolloid dressing in the treatment of pressure ulcers. *Pharmacoeconomics, 19*(12), 1209–1216.

Ovington, L. (2001). Hanging wet-to-dry dressings out to dry. *Home Healthcare Nurse, 19*(8), 477–483.

Paustian, C., & Stegman, M. R. (2003). Preparing the wound for healing: The effect of activated polyacrylate dressing on debridement. *Ostomy Wound Management, 49*(9), 34–42.

Percival, S. L., & Suleman, L. (2015). Slough and biofilm: Removal of barriers to wound healing by desloughing. *Journal of Wound Care, 24*(11), 498–510.

Ramundo, J. (2016). Wound debridement. In R. A. Bryant & D. P. Nix (Eds.), *Acute and chronic wounds: Current management* (5th ed.). St. Louis, MO: Mosby.

Ramundo, J., & Gray, M. (2008). Is ultrasonic mist therapy effective for debriding chronic wounds? *Journal of Wound Ostomy & Continence Nursing, 35*(6), 579.

Ramundo, J., & Gray, M. (2009). Collagenase for enzymatic debridement: A systematic review. *Journal of Wound Ostomy & Continence Nursing, 36*(6S), S4–S11.

Ratliff, C. R. (2018a). Case series of 18 patients with lower extremity wounds treated with a concentrated surfactant-based gel dressing. *Journal of Vascular Nursing, 36*(1), 3–7.

Ratliff, C. R. (2018b). Management of a groin wound using a concentrated surfactant-based gel dressing. *Journal of Wound Ostomy Continence Nursing, 45*(5), 465–467.

Robson, M. C., Cooper, D. M., Aslam, R., et al. (2006). Guidelines for the treatment of venous ulcers. *Wound Repair and Regeneration, 14*(6), 649–662.

Rodeheaver, G. T., Baharestani, M. M., Brabec, M. E., et al. (1994). Wound healing and wound management: Focus on debridement. *Advances in Wound Care, 7*(1), 22–24.

Schultz, G., Bjarnsholt, T., James, G. A., et al., & Global Wound Biofilm Expert Panel. (2017). Consensus guidelines for the identification and treatment of biofilms in chronic nonhealing wounds. *Wound Repair and Regeneration, 25*(5), 744–757.

Schultz, G., Woo, K., Weir, D., et al. (2018). Effectiveness of a monofilament wound debridement pad at removing biofilm and slough: *Ex vivo* and clinical performance. *Journal of Wound Care, 27*(2), 80–90.

Shi, L., Ermis, R., Kiedaisch, B., et al. (2010). The effect of various wound dressings on the activity of debriding enzymes. *Advances in Skin & Wound Care, 23*(10), 456–462.

Shih, A. F., Little, A. J., Panse, G., et al. (2018). Maggot therapy for calciphylaxis wound debridement complicated by bleeding. *Journal of the American Academy of Dermatology, 4*(4), 396–398.

Skórkowska-Telichowska, K., Czemplik, M., Kulma, A., et al. (2013). The local treatment and available dressings designed for chronic wounds. *Journal of the American Academy of Dermatology, 68*(4), e117–e126. doi: 10.1016/j.jaad.2011.06.028.

Smith, K., Skelton, H. G., Graham, J. S., et al. (1997). Depth of morphologic skin damage and viability after one, two, and three passes of a high-energy, short pulse CO_2 laser (Tru-Pulse) in pig skin. *Journal of the American Academy of Dermatology, 37*(2), 204.

Snyder, R. J., Bohn, G., Hanft, J., et al. (2017). Wound biofilm: Current perspectives and strategies on biofilm disruption and treatments. *Wounds, 29*(6), S1–S17.

Stanisic, M. C., Provo, B. J., Larson, D. L., et al. (2005). Wound debridement with 25 kHz ultrasound. *Advances in Skin & Wound Care, 18*(9), 484.

Steed, D. L., Attinger, C., Colaizzi, T., et al. (2006). Guidelines for the treatment of diabetic ulcers. *Wound Repair and Regeneration, 14*(6), 680–692.

Steenvorde, P., Budding, T., & Oskam, J. (2005). Determining pain levels in patients treated with maggot debridement therapy. *Journal of Wound Care, 14*(10), 485.

Steenvorde, P., & van Doorn, L. P. (2008). Maggot debridement therapy: Serious bleeding can occur. Report of a case. *Journal of Wound Ostomy & Continence Nursing, 35*(4), 412.

Swanson, T., Angel, D., Sussman, G., et al. (2016). *Wound infection in clinical practice: Principles of best practice*. International Wound Infection Institute (IWII). Wounds International. Retrieved from http://eprints.hud.ac.uk/id/eprint/30637/

Thomas, S. (1991). Evidence fails to justify use of hypochlorite. *Journal of Tissue Viability, 1*(1), 9–10.

Waycaster, C., & Milne, C. T. (2013). Clinical and economic benefit of enzymatic debridement of pressure ulcers compared to autolytic debridement with a hydrogel dressing. *Journal of Medical Economics, 16*(7), 976–986.

Woo, K. Y., Keast, D., Parsons, N., et al. (2015). The cost of wound debridement: A Canadian perspective. *International Wound Journal, 12*(4), 402–407. doi: 10.1111/iwj.12122.

Wound, Ostomy and Continence Nurses Society (WOCN). (2012). *Guideline for management of patients with lower extremity neuropathic disease*. WOCN Society clinical practice guideline series #1. Mt. Laurel, NJ: Author.

Wound, Ostomy and Continence Nurses Society (WOCN). (2014). *Guideline for management of patients with lower extremity arterial disease*. WOCN Society clinical practice guideline series #1. Mt. Laurel, NJ: Author.

Wound, Ostomy and Continence Nurses Society (WOCN). (2015). *Methods of wound debridement: Best practices for clinicians*. Mt. Laurel, NJ: Author.

Wound, Ostomy and Continence Nurses Society (WOCN). (2016). *Guideline for prevention and management of pressure ulcers (injuries)*. Mt. Laurel, NJ: Author.

Wound, Ostomy and Continence Nurses Society (WOCN). (2019). *Guideline for management of wounds in patients with lower-extremity venous disease*. Mt. Laurel, NJ: Author.

Yamakawa, S., & Hayashida, K. (2019). Advances in surgical applications of growth factors for wound healing. *Burns & Trauma, 7*, 10. doi: 10.1186/s41038-019-0148-1.

Yang, Q., Larose, C., Della Porta, A. C., et al. (2017). A surfactant-based wound dressing can reduce bacterial biofilms in a porcine skin explant model. *International Wound Journal, 14*(2), 408–413. doi: 10.1111/iwj.12619.

Zarachi, K., & Gergor, J. (2012). The efficacy of maggot debridement therapy—A review of comparative clinical trials. *International Wound Journal, 9*(5), 469–477.

QUESTIONS

1. The wound care nurse is explaining to a patient why debridement was ordered to clean his pressure injury. Which statement by the nurse accurately explains an aspect of this process?

A. "Debridement obscures visualization of the wound base."

B. "Debridement increases the chance for infection."

C. "Debridement replaces necrotic tissue with eschar."

D. "Debridement allows the wound healing process to continue."

2. The wound care nurse is recommending use of an enzymatic ointment for debridement. Which of the following is the best approach?

A. Apply thick layer and cover with dry gauze.

B. Crosshatch eschar before application.

C. Cover with silver dressing to prevent infection.

D. Protect any viable tissue with petrolatum.

3. A patient with an infected wound is scheduled for conservative sharp wound debridement. Which statement accurately describes a step in this process?
   A. Wash hands and apply sterile gloves.
   B. Prep wound with a normal saline wash.
   C. Peel off loose necrotic tissue using a scalpel.
   D. Avoid all vascular structures throughout the procedure.

4. For which patient would the wound care nurse recommend a wound remain closed and monitored for signs of infection rather than ordering debridement?
   A. A patient with advanced LEAD and closed heel ulcer
   B. A patient with advanced Parkinson disease
   C. A patient with a wound with loose eschar over the malleolus
   D. A patient with a wound that develops infection

5. Which assessment question would the nurse ask to determine the method and safety of the debridement process?
   A. What are the goals of care for this patient?
   B. What is the care setting of the patient?
   C. Where is the wound?
   D. What type of necrotic tissue is involved?

6. The wound care nurse is assessing the results of debridement for a patient with a sacral pressure injury. Which statement accurately describes a characteristic of this progressive process?
   A. Necrotic tissue is typically expressed as centimeters in length.
   B. Wound dimensions typically decrease as the necrotic tissue is removed.
   C. Amount of exudate typically decreases as the necrotic tissue is removed.
   D. After debridement, eschar gradually hardens.

7. Which of the following methods of debridement is considered nonselective and should be chosen in very select circumstances?
   A. Autolytic
   B. Enzymatic
   C. Biosurgical/larval therapy
   D. Wet-to-dry mechanical

8. Which type of debridement is appropriate only for noninfected wounds?
   A. Autolytic
   B. Enzymes
   C. Chemical debridement
   D. Hydrotherapy

9. The wound care nurse is choosing a debridement method for a home care patient who is also on anticoagulant therapy due to atrial fibrillation. Which method would be most appropriate for this patient?
   A. Hydrotherapy
   B. Conservative sharp wound debridement
   C. Enzymes
   D. Biosurgical/larval therapy

10. A wound care nurse recommends chemical debridement for a patient with an infected stage 4 pressure injury. What is a disadvantage of this procedure?
   A. There is a risk for bacteremia with an infected wound.
   B. It is readily available and requires weekly dressing changes.
   C. A greater length of time is needed to remove nonviable tissue.
   D. Possible loss of blood may occur.

ANSWERS AND RATIONALES

1. D: Necrotic tissue is an impediment to healing, particularly in the chronic wound; removal of this tissue is essential to wound healing.

2. B: Collagenase works most effectively on slough; when used on eschar, the wound care nurse must first crosshatch the eschar to permit the collagenase to penetrate to the collagen anchoring strands.

3. D: A consideration prior to CSWD is the presence of active wound infection; in this case, severing of a small vessel could cause a bacteremia.

4. A: Debridement is usually contraindicated as a heel wound with dry eschar in a nonambulatory patient; the eschar is left intact as long as there are no signs of infection.

5. B: The care setting must be considered when selecting a debridement method. A wound care nurse in home care might select a more conservative approach to debridement than the wound care nurse practicing in acute care, due to differences in access to support personnel and supplies.

6. C: Wound dimensions typically increase as the necrotic tissue is removed from the wound. Early in the debridement process, the wound is commonly exudative; the amount of exudate typically decreases as the necrotic tissue is removed.

7. D: Wet-to-dry debridement is a mechanical, nonselective method of debridement.

8. A: Autolytic debridement is generally considered a safe though slow method of debridement. It is most effective on slough, and, because it is slow, it is generally considered more appropriate for noninfected wounds.

9. C: Hydrotherapy is not available in home care setting. Anticoagulants increase the risk of bleeding in CSWD and biosurgical/larval therapy is not readily available in home care.

10. C: Infected wounds require rapid debridement that does not cause further harm to the surrounding tissue. Surgical debridement is often indicated (along with antibiotic therapy).

CHAPTER 11

ASSESSMENT AND MANAGEMENT OF WOUND-RELATED INFECTIONS

Dorothy Weir and Gregory Schultz

OBJECTIVES

1. Explain how an open wound places the individual at risk for infection.

2. Differentiate among contamination, colonization, local infection, spreading infection, and systemic infection, to include implications for wound healing and wound management.

3. Identify indications, options, and guidelines for wound culture.

4. Describe guidelines for diagnosis and management of local and spreading infection.

5. Describe guidelines for diagnosis and management of osteomyelitis.

6. Discuss current guidelines for appropriate use of topical antimicrobial agents and dressings.

TOPIC OUTLINE

INTRODUCTION

A key function of the skin is to maintain a boundary between the individual and the outside environment, providing an effective barrier to bacterial invasion into the deeper tissues. As discussed in Chapter 2, specific ways in which the skin protects against bacterial invasion include the following: (1) the dry keratinized cells on the surface create a physical barrier to penetration by microorganisms; (2) the constant shedding of the keratinocytes causes shedding of any attached organisms (Wysocki, 2016); (3) the normally acidic pH (4 to 6.5) produced by the production of sebum by the sebaceous glands creates a hostile environment to microbial growth (Maliyar et al., 2020; McNichol et al., 2018); (4) the breakdown of skin lipids produces toxic by-products that inhibit the growth of potential pathogens; (5) sweat inhibits microorganism growth through its low pH and high sodium concentration; and (6) resident bacteria (e.g., *Staphylococcus epidermidis* and skin diphtheroids) inhibit colonization by more pathogenic organisms (such as *Staphylococcus aureus*) (Mufti et al., 2016; Sussman & Bates-Jensen, 2012).

Any wound involves a break in the skin that permits access of both normal flora and pathogenic organisms. The warmth, moisture, reduced oxygen, and nutrient-rich environment of the subepidermal tissues promotes bacterial survival and multiplication. Infection is a constant risk and common complication for all types of wounds, and prevention, prompt detection, and effective management of wound-related infection is a key responsibility for the wound care nurse, which is the focus of this chapter.

KEY POINT

An open wound permits access of pathogenic organisms, and the warmth, moisture, reduced oxygen, and nutrient-rich environment of the subepidermal tissues promotes bacterial survival and multiplication—infection is a constant risk and common complication for all types of wounds.

MICROBES AND WOUND HEALING

Bioburden is the degree or load of microorganisms (e.g., bacteria, virus, fungi) that create contamination in a wound. It is influenced by the quantity of colony-forming units (CFUs) per gram of tissue or per cm^2 and the virulence of microbes (IWII, 2016). In clinical practice, the term bioburden is often used to reflect the presence of bacteria on the wound surface and to justify the use of antimicrobial dressings.

Wound healing is generally not impaired simply due to the presence of microbes on the wound surface. The impact of the microorganisms is determined by their number, their virulence, the microbial "mix" (numbers and types of bacteria, viruses, and fungi), and the host's resistance (Bowler, 2003; IWII, 2016).

BACTERIAL CHARACTERISTICS

Bacteria may be defined as prokaryotic unicellular organisms that may range from benign to invasive pathogens. They may be aerobic or anaerobic, motile or immotile. They typically have a cell wall and membrane, which become the targets of many antibacterial compounds. Bacteria are identified and described based on shape, results of Gram stain, need or lack of need for oxygen, and mode of growth (IWII, 2016).

Shape

While there is great variation in the shape, size, and arrangement of bacteria, they are most basically described by one of the three most common shapes: round or ball shaped, described as a coccus (or cocci); cylindrical in shape, described as a rod or bacillus; and a spiral-shaped cylinder, known as a spirillum or spirochete, depending on the thickness and regularity of the spirals or coils. The description is broadened when there is a combination of two shapes, such as a rod that is short and rounded (coccobacillus), when the bacteria are found in chains or clusters, are paired together, or are curved or twisted (Yang et al., 2016) (**Fig. 11-1**).

Gram Positive versus Gram Negative

Gram staining has been used for over a century as a method for identifying and classifying bacteria as either gram positive or gram negative. Gram staining provides rapid information for the wound care nurse that facilitates empirical management while awaiting the outcome of a culture.

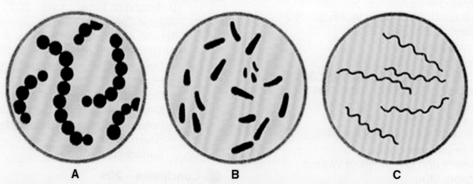

FIGURE 11-1. Shapes of Bacteria. **A.** Coccus. **B.** Bacillus or rod shaped. **C.** Spirillum or spirochete.

Gram staining is named for Hans Christian Gram, the Danish scientist who developed the technique in 1884. It is still widely used in hospital and community laboratories and is based on a differentiation between two major cell wall types. A basic description of the methodology is that a sample of the bacterial culture is smeared onto a slide and dried. The sample is heated. Once cooled, the sample is flooded with the stain crystal or gentian violet, washed off, further stained with an iodine solution (Gram's iodine), and then again washed with a decolorizing agent such as alcohol or acetone. The slide is then again stained with a red dye (safranin or fuchsin) and rinsed a final time. After a final drying, the slide is examined under a microscope to identify whether the bacterial cell wall has retained the purple dye (gram positive), lost the purple color (gram negative), or retained a mix of the purple and red dyes (gram variable). Common gram-positive bacteria include various species of the genera *Streptococcus*, *Staphylococcus*, *Enterococcus*, *Corynebacterium*, and *Listeria*. Common gram-negative bacteria include various species of the genera *Pseudomonas*, *Proteus*, *Escherichia coli*, *Klebsiella*, *Enterobacter*, *Serratia*, *Salmonella*, *Shigella*, and others (American Society of Microbiology, 2019; Cowan & Talaro, 2006) (**Fig. 11-2**).

KEY POINT

Bacteria are commonly identified and described based on their shape, response to Gram staining, need for oxygen, and mode of growth. Gram staining can be used to provide rapid general information to the wound care nurse that guides initial antibiotic therapy while awaiting definitive culture results.

Aerobic versus Anaerobic

Bacteria are further differentiated by those that survive and grow in an oxygenated environment (aerobes), those that do not require oxygen to grow and may even die in the presence of oxygen (anaerobes), and those that can use oxygen but also have anaerobic methods of energy production (facultative anaerobes). **Figure 11-3** graphically illustrates the relative distribution of these functional categories among a variety of wound types.

Planktonic versus Biofilm

Discussions about bacterial growth in wounds, culture results, antibiotic therapy, and bactericidal efficacy of topical dressings and agents are referring to free-floating or planktonic bacteria. Planktonic bacteria are free-living bacteria, that is, the bacteria that grow out in the laboratory flask or dish. They have been recognized for centuries, are relatively hydrophilic, and are characterized by cell walls that can be eradicated by the host's immune system and/or targeted antimicrobials. Most of the current knowledge about antibiotics is based on studies and experiments involving planktonic bacteria. The opposite mode of growth is the adherent, or sessile, mode of growth, known as biofilm (**Fig. 11-4**).

Description of Biofilms

Biofilms are complex microbial communities. They are usually polymicrobial, containing multiple species of bacteria and fungi (Dowd et al., 2008a; IWII, 2016; Trengove et al., 1996). In contrast to single, planktonic bacteria, which are not attached (or are only weakly attached) to the wound surface (see **Fig. 11-4**), the microorganisms in a biofilm community synthesize and secrete a matrix that firmly attaches the biofilm to either a living or nonliving surface (Stoodley et al., 2002). The matrix secreted by the organisms in the biofilm consists mainly of polysaccharide chains but also typically contains substantial amounts of bacterial DNA entwined within the polysaccharide chains (see **Fig. 11-4**). Biofilms are dynamic heterogenous communities that are continuously changing in response to factors in the immediate environment (Hall-Stoodley & Stoodley, 2009).

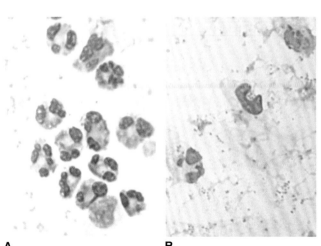
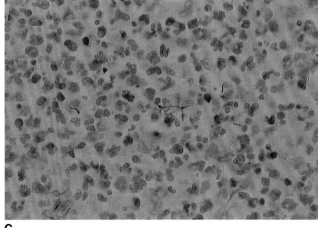

A   B   C

FIGURE 11-2. Gram Staining. **A.** Gram positive. **B.** Gram negative. **C.** Gram variable. (Reprinted with permission from McClatchey, K. D. (2002). *Clinical laboratory medicine* (2nd ed). Philadelphia, PA: Lippincott Williams & Wilkins.)

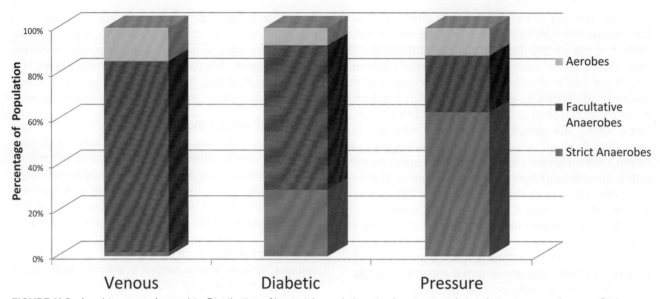

FIGURE 11-3. Aerobic versus Anaerobic. Distribution of bacterial populations in chronic wounds in relation to aerotolerance. Diabetic, venous, or pressure injury types were analyzed separately using pyrosequencing and the resulting populations grouped into three categories based upon their suggested aerotolerance. This figure graphically illustrates the relative distribution of these functional categories among the wound types. (Used with permission from Dowd, S. E., Sun, Y., Secor, P. R., et al. (2008). Survey of bacterial diversity in chronic wounds using Pyrosequencing, DGGE, and full ribosome shotgun sequencing. *BioMed Central Microbiology, 8*, 43. © 2008 Dowd et al.; licensee BioMed Central Ltd.)

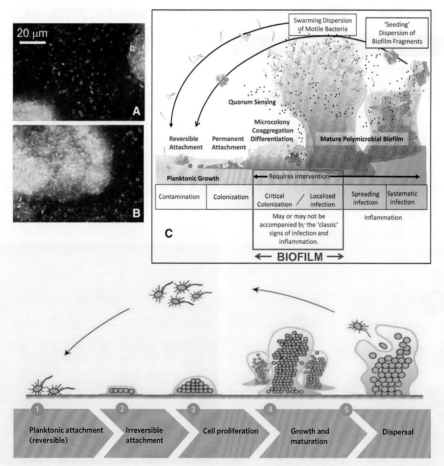

FIGURE 11-4. Biofilm. Confocal laser scanning microscopy (top view) of planktonic *Pseudomonas aeruginosa* (**A**), biofilm community (**B**). **C.** Schematic representation of biofilm cycle (IWII, 2016). (Courtesy Priscilla Phillips, PhD, Assistant Professor, Kirksville College of Osteopathic Medicine.)

Formation of Biofilms

Biofilms begin with reversible attachment of free-floating, planktonic bacteria to a surface. As the bacteria multiply, they become more firmly attached (sessile). These multiplying planktonic bacteria produce specific molecules known as quorum molecules. When the concentration of quorum molecules reaches a sufficient threshold, it triggers a change in gene expression patterns. This change in gene expression patterns causes the bacteria to begin synthesizing and secreting components of the protective exopolymeric matrix (IWII, 2016). It is this protective matrix (or slime) that distinguishes planktonic bacteria from biofilm bacteria (see **Fig. 11.4**).

Purpose of Biofilms

Bacteria living in polymicrobial communities that are typical of biofilms are afforded protective advantages, which allow them to share their individual strengths in ways that benefit the group and increase resistance to environmental stresses (Hibbing et al., 2010; Xavier & Foster, 2007). For example, formation of the protective polymeric matrix encases the biofilm bacteria and provides an evolutionary defense against natural predators: bacterial viruses, amoebae, and microbicides. The tightly attached exopolymeric matrix also protects bacteria against phagocytosis by neutrophils and macrophages, reduces penetration by antibodies, and can neutralize natural reactive oxygen species (ROS) and many chemically reactive antiseptics and disinfectants, such as sodium hypochlorite (bleach) solutions. Many bacteria in the center of large, mature biofilm communities become metabolically inactive, or quiescent. Since all antibiotics kill bacteria by interfering with essential bacterial processes including energy metabolism, membrane/cell wall synthesis, and synthesis of proteins, RNA and DNA, the metabolically quiescent bacteria in biofilms become highly tolerant to antibiotics that efficiently kill rapidly proliferating bacteria. These quiescent biofilm bacteria are often termed persister bacteria because they can survive much higher levels of antibiotics than rapidly dividing planktonic bacteria. Formation of polymicrobial biofilms enables bacteria to survive in conditions that rapidly and efficiently kill planktonic bacteria (IWII, 2016) (**Fig. 11-5**).

Another clinically important feature of bacterial biofilms is that bacterial biofilms can form both on and under the surface of a chronic wound bed. As shown in **Figure 11.6**, panel B, scanning electron microscopy (SEM) reveals a classical image of a bacterial biofilm community on the surface of punch biopsies taken from chronic wound beds. As shown in panel A, bacterial biofilm structures can also form beneath the surface of chronic wound beds. Measurements of biopsies show that biofilm aggregates of *Pseudomonas aeruginosa* form at an average 50 to 60 μm and *S. aureus* aggregate biofilms form at an average of 20 to 30 μm beneath the surface of wound beds. Also, biofilms are not uniformly distributed across a wound bed (**Fig. 11-6, panel D**). Effective removal of biofilms from chronic wound beds must involve procedures that include both surface and subsurface biofilm aggregates (Sauer et al., 2002).

Step-Down-Then-Step-Up Paradigm

The step-down-then-step-up paradigm, shown in **Figure 11-7**, summarizes the current state of knowledge regarding management of wound bioburden (Schultz et al., 2017). When a chronic wound presents after weeks

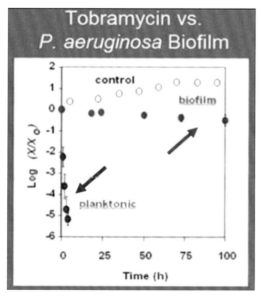

FIGURE 11-5. Antibiotics versus Biofilm on Inert Surfaces. Tobramycin rapidly kills planktonic *Pseudomonas aeruginosa* (*blue*) very effectively but is not effective against biofilm *Pseudomonas* (*red*).

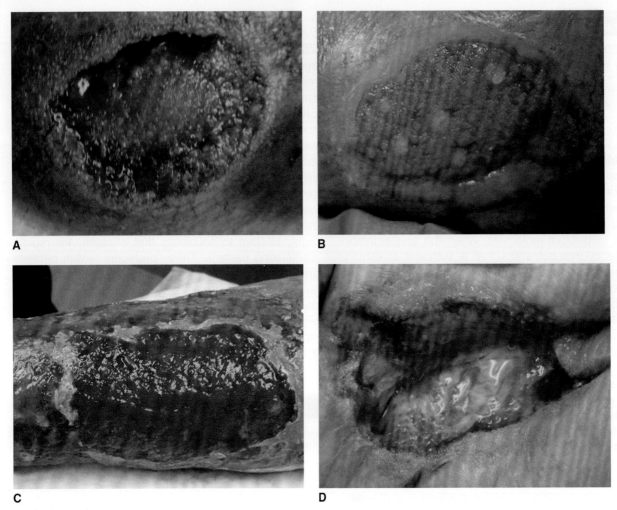

FIGURE 11-6. Bacterial Loads in Wounds. **A.** Contamination: The presence of bacteria on wound surfaces with no replication or multiplication of the bacteria and no clinical host response. **B.** Colonization: The act or process of establishing a colony or colonies; the spreading of species into a new habitat. Bacteria replicating; no host response. **C.** Local Infection: The point at which the bacteria multiplying on the surface begin to interfere with wound healing, resulting in a mild host response. **D.** Spreading Infection: Invasion by and multiplication of pathogenic microorganisms in tissue, which may produce subsequent tissue injury and progress to overt disease through a variety of cellular or toxic mechanisms.

of failing to heal with standard care, it should be assumed that the wound contains a major bacterial bioburden that includes biofilm aggregates. The first step in correcting this problem is to perform aggressive debridement of the wound bed by whatever methods are available and appropriate for each patient's wound. Optimally, this would be some form of sharp debridement that would remove both planktonic and biofilm bacteria. It is important to combine debridement with a topical treatment that effectively kills any remaining biofilm (and planktonic) bacteria and prevents reformation of biofilm aggregate. Biofilm can occur in 3 days in chronic wounds that are not treated with antimicrobial dressings (Wolcott et al., 2016). As the bioburden of planktonic and biofilm bacteria decreases, the frequency and aggressiveness of debridement can "step-down" and a variety of topical antimicrobial treatments that prevent biofilm reformation can be used. The wound bed then re-enters an initial

healing phase, which may be adequate to progress to full healing. However, if a patient's wound is not healing at an acceptable rate, treatments can be "step(ped)-up." Advanced wound care products such as cellular- and tissue-based products, growth factors, or skin grafts enhance healing because the wound bed has been prepared by correcting the bioburden and molecular barriers preventing healing.

BACTERIAL LOADS IN CHRONIC WOUNDS

Contamination

There is wide agreement in the literature that all open wounds are contaminated, regardless of the age of the wound. Contamination is defined as the presence of non-replicating bacteria on the wound surface with no clinical host response (Browne et al., 2001; Landis et al., 2007;

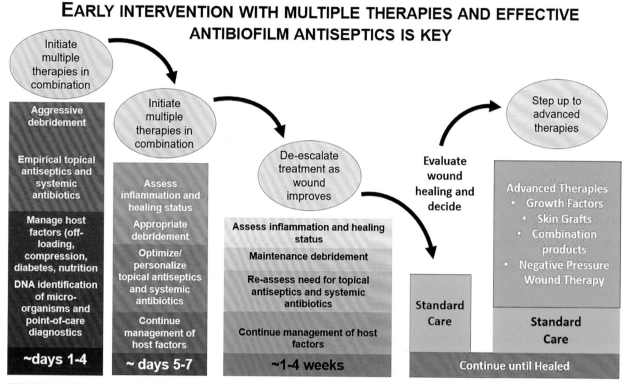

FIGURE 11-7. Step-Down-Then-Step-Up Paradigm.

Stotts, 2016). The presence of some level of bacteria is thought to be beneficial, in that the bacteria help to stimulate the inflammatory response needed to initiate the normal cascade of events resulting in wound repair. Chronic wounds may become contaminated from endogenous sources (i.e., natural flora) and peri-wound skin, and exogenous sources such as an outdoor environment or the hands and contaminated gloves of health care workers. As time progresses, it is the number and activity of the bacteria and the host's ability to balance the bacteria that determines the impact on wound healing.

Colonization

Bacterial replication on the wound surface begins the change in the dynamics between the host and the bacterial organisms. The environment on the wound surface offers an ideal milieu for bacterial growth and replication. It provides warmth, moisture, oxygen, and nutrients. Once the bacteria begin to multiply and attach to the wound surface, the wound is considered to be colonized. Low levels of colonization do not incite a significant host response and do not generally interfere with wound healing.

Local Infection

The point at which the bacteria multiplying on the surface begin to interfere with wound healing had been termed critical colonization, a term that was coined by Davis in 1996 (White & Cutting, 2006b). This concept represented a significant advancement in our understanding of the relationship between bacteria and wound healing. For decades, wounds were considered to be either infected or not infected. Infected wounds were typically defined as those with bacterial loads >10^5 (>100,000 CFU/g of tissue) and displaying the classic host response (e.g., erythema, induration, edema, increased exudate, warmth, and pain) (Robson et al., 2006). The concept of critical colonization fell under scrutiny in the past decade with questions raised about the identification of wound infection through clinical observation rather than microbial confirmation. In 2016, the International Wound Infection Institute (IWII) convened a meeting of wound specialists to reach consensus on wound infection issues with minimal or lacking evidence. The newer term replacing critical colonization is local infection. It is generally accepted that a wound is influenced by an imbalance of microbes exhibits subtle differences that can be observed by experienced clinicians (EPUAP/NPIAP/PPPIA, 2019; IWII, 2016). The awareness that pathogens can interfere with wound healing without evoking a host response is fundamental to understanding the concept of local infection. The concept of local infection has enabled wound care nurses to make treatment decisions by determining the point where the bacteria had reached a critical level and management with an antimicrobial dressing was warranted. If treatment with the antimicrobial dressing results in an improvement in the healing trajectory, then the treatment is justified.

Clinical Indicators of Local Infection

An obvious sign of local infection is a plateau in the wound's healing trajectory, evidenced by minimal or no reduction in wound dimensions or by a sudden unexplained increase in wound size. Additional subtle signs and symptoms include hypergranulation, bleeding, friable granulation, epithelial bridging and pocketing in granulation tissue, wound breakdown and enlargement, delayed wound healing, and new or increasing pain and odor. Overt or classic signs of local infection include erythema, local warmth, swelling, purulent drainage, delayed wound healing, and new or increasing pain and odor (EPUAP/NPIAP/PPPIA, 2019; IWII, 2016) (**Figs. 11-8 to 11-10**).

Pathology of Local Infection

Suggested causative factors for the negative effects of local infection include the effects of proteases produced by the bacteria, the competition between wound healing cells and bacteria for oxygen and nutrients, the effects of exotoxins released by bacterial and fungal organisms, and the release of endotoxins caused by breakdown of the cell walls of gram-negative organisms. Increasing bacterial loads stimulate white blood cell activity, and the proteases produced by the neutrophils and macrophages (especially the matrix metalloproteases, MMPs) can degrade proteins that are essential for healing (Lindsay et al., 2017; WUWHS, 2016). Bacterial loads also increase production of proinflammatory mediators including tumor necrosis factor alpha (TNFα) and interleukins such as IL-1β. Bacteria can also stimulate angiogenesis and contribute to the production of a deficient matrix.

Spreading Wound Infection

The IWII defines spreading wound infection as the presence of microbes in sufficient numbers or virulence to cause a host response locally and/or systemically. Depending on the location of the wound and the

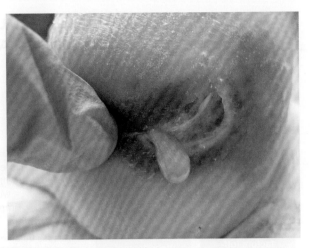

FIGURE 11-9. Purulent Exudate.

condition of the host, the presenting signs may be subtle or profound. They include extending induration with or without erythema, lymphangitis, crepitus, wound breakdown or dehiscence with or without satellite lesions, malaise or lethargy, loss of appetite, inflammation, and swelling of lymph glands (EPUAP/NPIAP/PPPIA, 2019; IWII, 2016).

Systemic Infection

Systemic infection from a wound affects the whole body as microorganisms are spread via the vascular or lymphatic systems, which can result in severe sepsis, septic shock, organ failure, and death (EPUAP/NPIAP/PPPIA, 2019; IWII, 2016). See **Table 11-1** for a comparative list of the signs and symptoms associated with the wound infection continuum. **Figure 11-11** illustrates the stages in the wound infection continuum.

Bacterial Loads and Characteristics

A quantitative threshold of $>10^5$ CFU/g of tissue biopsied has been used to define burn wound infection (Bamberg et al., 2002) and to predict skin graft failure.

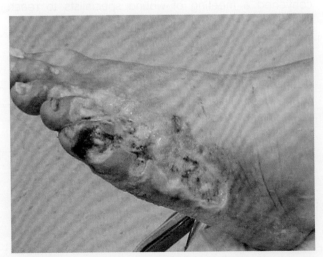

FIGURE 11-8. Infected Foot.

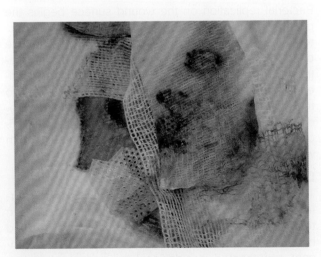

FIGURE 11-10. Exudate Color Change.

TABLE 11-1 SIGNS AND SYMPTOMS ASSOCIATED WITH STAGES OF THE WOUND INFECTION CONTINUUM

CONTAMINATION	COLONISATION	LOCAL INFECTION		SPREADING INFECTION	SYSTEMIC INFECTION
All wounds may acquire micro-organisms. If suitable nutritive and physical conditions are not available for each microbial species, or they are not able to successfully evade host defences, they will not multiply or persist; their presence is therefore only transient and wound healing is not delayed	Microbial species successfully grow and divide but do not cause damage to the host or initiate wound infection	Covert (subtle) signs of local infection: • Hypergranulation (excessive "vascular" tissue) • Bleeding, friable granulation • Epithelial bridging and pocketing in granulation tissue • Wound breakdown and enlargement • Delayed wound healing beyond expectations • New or increasing pain • Increasing malodour	Overt (classic) signs of local infection: • Erythema • Local warmth • Swelling • Purulent discharge • Delayed wound healing beyond expectations • New or increasing pain • Increasing malodour	• Extending in duration +/– erythema • Lymphangitis • Crepitus • Wound breakdown/ dehiscence with or without satellite lesions • Malaise/lethargy or nonspecific general deterioration • Loss of appetite • Inflammation, swelling of lymph glands	• Severe sepsis • Septic shock • Organ failure • Death

Chronic wounds have been reported to progress to closure despite levels of microorganisms as great as 10^8 CFU/g of tissue (Bamberg et al., 2002). Wound infection has also been defined in terms of bacterial load and virulence relative to the patient's level of resistance.

KEY POINT

A quantitative threshold of $>10^5$ CFU of bacteria per gram of tissue has been used as the cutoff for laboratory diagnosis of infection, based on burn wound infection and skin graft failure. Chronic wounds have been reported to progress to closure despite levels as high as 10^8.

The majority of chronic wounds are polymicrobial. Certain pathogens (e.g., *S. aureus*, *P. aeruginosa*, and beta-hemolytic *Streptococci*) have been cited as the most common cause of wound infection and delayed healing (Martin & Drosou, 2005). Stacey and colleagues (2019) evaluated whether any of a panel of biomarkers can determine the healing status of chronic venous leg ulcers. Forty-two patients with chronic venous leg ulcers had their wound measured and wound fluid collected at weekly time points for 13 weeks. Wound fluid was analyzed using multiplex enzyme-linked immunosorbent assay to determine the concentration of biomarkers in the wound fluid at each weekly time point. Healing status

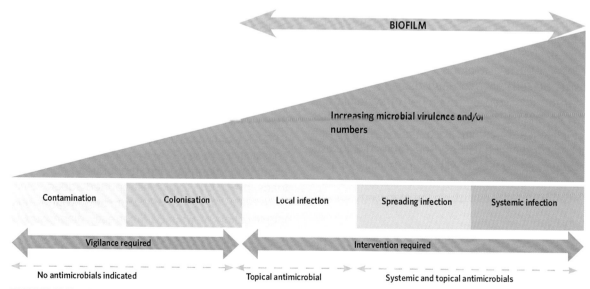

FIGURE 11-11. Wound Infection Continuum (IWII, 2016).

was determined by examining the change in wound size at the previous and subsequent weeks. They found that two biomarkers from wound fluid can predict healing status in chronic venous leg ulcer. Granulocyte macrophage-colony stimulating factor ($p < 0.001$) and matrix metalloprotease-13 ($p = 0.004$) were the best predictors of wound healing (Stacey et al., 2019). These data provide further support for the impact of microbial interactions on overall pathogenicity. It is not just the presence of bacteria but the type and virulence of the organism(s), the interaction with other microbial agents, and the interaction with the host that determine the influence on healing of chronic wounds.

While the presence of bacteria is not believed to increase the risk of infection, beta-hemolytic *Streptococcus* is an important exception to the rule. The presence of one virulent beta-hemolytic *Streptococcus* should be considered significant and appropriate treatment initiated. Some bacterial combinations may develop synergy with each other. This can result in a previously nonvirulent organism becoming virulent and causing damage to the host. Antimicrobial therapy may eliminate selected organisms, allowing overgrowth of other organisms that may impair healing and result in infection. Collaboration with an infectious disease specialist is recommended if a lack of healing is thought to be due to bacterial influence in spite of appropriate measures to reduce microbes and address biofilm.

KEY POINT

The presence of bacteria is not believed to increase the risk of infection. Beta-hemolytic *Streptococcus* is the notable exception to this rule.

Host Resistance

Bacterial quantity and virulence are important determining factors in development of wound infection. Host resistance is also significant. Host resistance is defined as the ability of the host to produce an immune response that resists bacterial invasion and damage. This resistance can be impacted by a number of systemic and local factors, and the ability to mitigate these factors has a direct influence on the impact of the bacteria on the wound and surrounding tissues. See **Table 11-2** for lists of local and systemic factors with the potential to impact host resistance. Clinical interventions to minimize factors that affect host resistance include the following:

- Wound debridement
- Interventions to control comorbid conditions such as diabetes
- Measures to enhance tissue perfusion and oxygenation (e.g., revascularization)
- Nutritional support

TABLE 11-2 LOCAL AND SYSTEMIC FACTORS AFFECTING HOST RESISTANCE TO BACTERIA

LOCAL	SYSTEMIC
Size, location, and age of the wound	Poorly controlled diabetes
Necrotic tissue or foreign bodies	Inadequate vascular perfusion
Presence of scar	Edema
Previous radiation	Immunosuppressive drugs
Inadequate or improper topical treatments	Malnutrition Alcohol and/or tobacco abuse
	Neutrophil disorders

- Counseling related to lifestyle changes (e.g., weight loss, smoking cessation)
- Compression therapy to eliminate interstitial edema
- Advanced wound management therapies to promote wound healing (e.g., topical biologic therapies; negative pressure wound therapy [NPWT]; hyperbaric oxygen therapy [HBOT])

KEY POINT

Host resistance to infection is affected by systemic and local factors such as tissue necrosis and edema. Comprehensive care is required for prevention and management of infection.

ASSESSMENT AND DIAGNOSIS OF WOUND INFECTION

Determining the presence of wound infection begins with the clinical examination and observance for the signs and symptoms. Microbiological tests can be used to determine the specific offending organism(s) and to assure that the prescribed antimicrobial agents appropriately target those organisms. Studies indicate that reliance on clinical evaluation alone may lead to false assumptions as to the infectious status of a wound. Serena et al. (2019) examined 17 venous leg ulcers and 2 diabetic foot ulcers to compare clinical signs and symptoms (CCS) alone, use of bacterial fluorescence imaging in combination with CCS. Use of fluorescence images significantly improved sensitivity (22% vs. 72%) and accuracy (26% vs. 74%) for identifying wounds with moderate-to-heavy bacterial loads, $p = 0.002$. Clinicians reported added value of fluorescence images in >90% of study wounds, including identification of wounds incorrectly diagnosed by CCS (47% of study wounds) and treatment plan modifications guided by fluorescence (73% of study wounds). Modifications to care included image-guided cleaning, treatment selection, debridement, and antimicrobial stewardship (Serena et al., 2019).

Research suggests that clinical examination alone underestimates the incidence of wound infection.

In guidelines published by the Wound Healing Society, the following recommendation is made: if infection is suspected in a debrided ulcer, or if epithelialization from the margin of a wound is not progressing within 2 weeks, despite appropriate therapy, the presence of infection should be determined by tissue biopsy or quantitative swab technique (EPUAP/NPIAP/PPPIA, 2019; Gould et al., 2016; Lavery et al., 2016; Marston et al., 2016).

WOUND CULTURES

Wound cultures are used to confirm or modify the plan for treatment when antibiotic therapy is indicated. The culture results should be compared to the clinical assessment. The patient presenting with clinical signs and symptoms of infection requires prompt response. Treatment is initiated with antibiotics to which pathogens most commonly involved in a particular type of wound are usually sensitive. If previous cultures from the specific wound are available, the data regarding bacterial type and sensitivity can be used to guide initial treatment. The antibiotic can be changed if indicated when culture results are obtained. Collaboration with an infectious disease specialist is recommended for wounds that culture positive for multiple types of bacteria. Treatment decisions should be based upon current trends of known bacterial synergies and/or resistance in a particular hospital or community.

KEY POINT

Wound cultures are used to confirm or modify the plan for treatment when antibiotic therapy is indicated.

Data comparing the accuracy and usability of culture results obtained by various techniques have been widely published (EPUAP/NPIAP/PPPIA, 2019; Drosou et al., 2003; Fernandez et al., 2008). The quantitative information generated by a tissue biopsy remains the gold standard; while it is the methodology most commonly used in research and clinical trials, it is least used in clinical practice.

General Guidelines for Wound Cultures

Regardless of the procedure used, there are two aspects that assure accurate information from the culture. The first is adherence to the time frame for transport of the specimen to the lab. Use of culture specimen containers and tubes that stabilize and fix the bacteria reduces the risk of bacterial replication or death and allows for a reasonable time frame for transport. This is particularly important for cultures obtained in the home or in an institution without a lab on the premises, such as an outpatient wound care center or skilled nursing facility. Aerobic specimens maintained in appropriate transport media will survive, and the media will not promote continued growth. Specimens obtained specifically for anaerobic culture should be placed into anaerobically sterilized transport media (Landis et al., 2007). Secondly, the specimen must be carefully and accurately obtained.

KEY POINT

Regardless of the specific procedure used to obtain a wound culture, it is important to adhere to guidelines regarding transport to the lab and to obtain the specimen from viable tissue using meticulous technique.

Specimens are obtained by three methods: tissue removal, aspiration, and swab.

Tissue Removal Technique

Tissue removal methods include standard punch biopsy and use of instruments such as a scalpel or curette to obtain tissue (**Figs. 11-12 and 11-13**). When obtaining tissue specimens for quantitative culture, it is important to determine the individual laboratory requirements for the size of the specimen. A 3-mm sample is required by most labs.

Another consideration when obtaining a tissue specimen for bacterial culture is the potential impact of topical and injectable anesthetic agents, which are commonly used prior to tissue removal. Some of these agents have antimicrobial properties that influence bacterial survival (Berg et al., 2006; Johnson et al., 2008). Preservative-free lidocaine 1% solution as an injectable infiltrate was found to be safe for a wound biopsy performed within 2 hours.

The advantage of tissue cultures is the ability to identify organisms that have invaded the tissues beyond the wound surface, which optimizes antibiotic

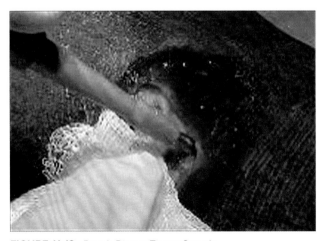

FIGURE 11-12. Punch Biopsy Tissue Sample.

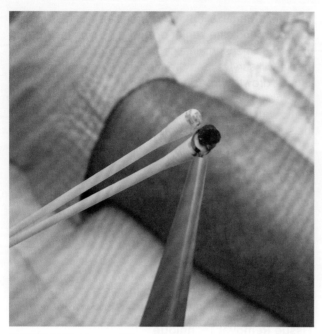

FIGURE 11-13. Curetted Tissue Sample.

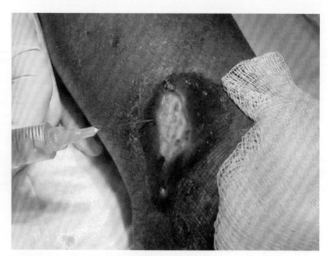

FIGURE 11-14. Aspiration.

therapy. Disadvantages are that the technique is invasive, painful, and must be performed by a trained health care provider. Tissue biopsy is not practical in many clinical sites.

Aspiration Technique

The goal of aspiration culture is to obtain fluid from the tissue below the wound bed to avoid surface contaminants. In clinical practice, this method is more commonly used to obtain a specimen from an abscess or loculated fluid collection. The skin over or adjacent to the area to be aspirated is disinfected and allowed to dry for 60 seconds. Fanning the area to speed drying is not recommended because organisms may be dispersed in the environment and settle on the aspiration site. A 10-mL syringe with a 22-g needle should be prefilled with 0.5 mL of air and inserted through the skin toward the area to be aspirated. Suction is achieved by withdrawing the plunger the length of the syringe to the 10-mL mark. The needle is then moved backward and forward through the tissue in the area at different angles for 2 to 4 explorations. The plunger is then released back to the 0.5-mL mark, the needle is withdrawn, excess air is removed from the syringe, and the syringe is capped and sent to the laboratory. This technique requires understanding of the underlying structures to avoid inadvertent damage (Lee et al., 1985; Stotts, 2016). The challenge in obtaining a culture utilizing aspiration is that it is an invasive procedure not likely to be performed by the bedside care provider. Compared to tissue biopsy, this technique tends to underestimate the number of organisms. Overall, it is a technique rarely used in general practice (**Fig. 11-14**).

Swab Technique

Swab cultures have historically been considered the least appropriate method for obtaining a culture due to the potential for contamination by surface debris and skin contaminants.

Swab cultures continue to be the primary method of culture used and clinicians should utilize specific technique when obtaining the specimen. Swab cultures should not be taken of the accumulated exudate under moisture retentive dressings. The results will likely show high numbers of microbes that may not reflect actual bacterial status of the wound. Current guidelines recommend wound cleansing prior to obtaining a swab culture. Specifically, the wound surface should be cleansed with normal saline to remove surface debris, residual dressing material, and any coagulum easily removed from the surface. Wound debridement should be carried out to remove necrotic and devitalized tissue. The wound should be cleansed again after debridement and the swab should be taken from the clean healthy appearing tissue (Gardner et al., 2006; Stotts, 2016).

The two swab techniques most often described in the literature are the Z-stroke and Levine's technique. The Z-stroke method involves swabbing the wound by gently rotating a sterile calcium alginate or rayon swab. Swab the wound from margin to margin in a 10-point zig-zag fashion from top to bottom. Use enough pressure to express fluid from within the wound tissue. The inherent challenge of this technique is the probability of contamination of the swab(s) with resident bacteria from the skin as well as from any devitalized tissue remaining on the wound surface. This can lead to overtreatment with antibiotics (Rushing, 2007).

Levine et al. (1976) described a method for obtaining a viable sample of aerobic bacteria on the surface of wounds. This method involves thoroughly cleansing the wound surface with saline and identifying a 1-cm

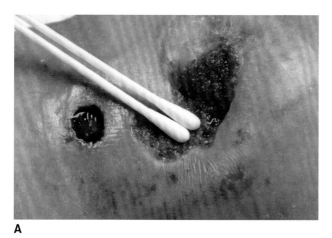 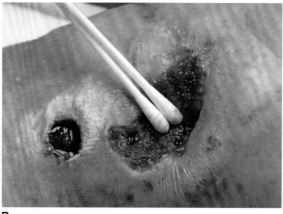

A   **B**

FIGURE 11-15. A, B. Levine Technique. Thoroughly cleanse the wound surface and identify a 1-cm area of the wound that is free from necrotic tissue. Rotate the swab while applying pressure sufficient to express fluid from the wound tissue.

area of the wound that is free from necrotic tissue. The swab is rotated while applying pressure sufficient to express fluid from the wound tissue (see Box 11-1). Comparison of these 2 swab techniques to tissue biopsy showed the Levine technique had a 91% sensitivity and 57% specificity compared with the Z-stroke technique which had a 63% sensitivity and 53% specificity. The Levine technique is recommended for obtaining a swab culture (EPUAP/NPIAP/PPPIA, 2019; Levine et al., 1976) (**Fig. 11-15A and B**).

Stallard (2018) reviewed seven studies to determine best evidence related to cultures, looking at when cultures should be performed and by what method. The results revealed that quantitative cultures are still the gold standard but that the swab technique is an acceptable alternative, and that the Levine technique is more reliable than the Z-stroke technique to determine the microbial load in the wound (Stallard, 2018).

Additionally, Haalboom et al. (2018) evaluated Levine swab and biopsy cultures taken from the same site from 180 wounds of different types. Skin flora was found to be contaminated more of the swabs, but swabs and biopsies tend to identify the same microorganisms when taken from the same locations. Agreement ranged from 78% to 97%. They reported that there seems to be no need for invasive biopsy in clinical practice (Haalboom et al., 2018) (see **Box 11-1**).

KEY POINT

Swab cultures should be obtained using Levine technique, which includes thorough irrigation of the wound bed with a noncytotoxic solution and rotating the swab in a 1 cm² area of viable tissue with enough force to express fluid.

ASSESSMENT OF CULTURE RESULTS

Final wound culture results take up to 72 hours to be reported. If Gram staining is provided, these preliminary

results are available within hours and provide information that can be used to guide initial therapy. Determining whether the organism(s) is/are gram negative or gram positive provides general direction in terms of appropriate antibiotic agents.

Qualitative versus Quantitative Reports

Culture results may be classified as qualitative, semiquantitative, or quantitative, depending on the methodology used to obtain and process the specimen.

A qualitative culture is obtained by plating the specimen on solid media and identifying the organisms grown. Semiquantitative cultures are plated on solid media and then serially streaked into four quadrants. Results are reported as 1+ to 4+, identifying the number of quadrants where there was bacterial growth. Quantitative cultures are generally performed on tissue specimens, though swab specimens can be utilized. Tissue specimens are homogenized and plated, whereas the swab specimens are serially diluted and plated. This technique allows for quantification of the number of CFU of the bacteria identified and is reported as CFU per gram of tissue for wound biopsies and CFU per cm² for swab cultures.

BOX 11-1   PROCEDURE FOR LEVINE SWAB CULTURE

The Levine Quantitative Swab Technique:
1. Cleanse wound with normal saline.
2. Pat dry wound bed with sterile gauze.
3. Culture the healthiest looking tissue, excluding exudate, purulent, devitalized tissue.
4. Roll the end of the sterile applicator over a 1 cm × 1 cm area for at least 5 seconds.
5. Apply sufficient pressure to swab, causing tissue fluid to be expressed.

Bill and colleagues (2001) quantitated the level of bacteria in 38 clean, nonhealing, chronic wounds that showed no classical clinical signs of infection. Tissue biopsies showed that 74% of these nonhealing, clean wounds contained >10^5 organisms/g of tissue. The quantitative swab technique detected 79% of these infected wounds (Bill et al., 2001). Ratliff & Rodeheaver (2002) examined a total of 124 wounds that were swabbed using alginate swabs and processed using both the semiquantitative and quantitative techniques. Alginate swabs were chosen over cotton-tipped swabs because the cotton-tipped swabs may be bacteriostatic secondary to the oxidative sterilization procedure. Processing quantitative swabs requires several steps, and many routine microbiology services may not want to deal with a process that complex. In contrast, the procedures for processing a semiquantitative swab are routine in most laboratories. Fifty-three quantitative swabs contained 10^5 or more bacteria/cm^2. These wounds were defined as infected. For the semiquantitative swabs, this correlated with 42 swabs that had growth in quadrant III or quadrants III and IV for a sensitivity of 79% (42/53). Linear regression analysis demonstrated a statistically significant correlation between the 2 techniques with a coefficient of $r = 0.84$ with a $p < 0.001$ (Ratliff & Rodeheaver, 2002).

Bacterial Sensitivity Data

In addition to identification of the specific bacteria, culture results provide information regarding sensitivity of the bacterial strain to antibiotics common to the setting, laboratory, or hospital. The final culture report will identify the organism(s) grown, the sensitivity (S) or resistance (R) to the antibiotics tested, and the minimum inhibitory concentration (MIC) relative to those antibiotics. The MIC identifies the lowest concentration of the antibiotic tested, which resulted in inhibition or reduction of the inoculums. Minimum bactericidal concentrations (MBCs) are the lowest concentration of antimicrobial that will prevent the growth of an organism after culture onto antibiotic-free media. MICs are used by diagnostic laboratories mainly to confirm resistance. As a rule, the lower the MIC, the more effective the antibiotic. This information must be considered in relation to the species of the bacteria, other species identified, and possible synergies that may exist. Consultation with an infectious disease specialist may be warranted in the presence of multiple organisms, significant resistance, and in the patient experiencing persistent or recurring infections.

KEY POINT

The minimum inhibitory concentration (MIC) identifies the lowest concentration of antibiotics tested that produce inhibition or reduction of bacterial growth. The lower the MIC, the more effective the antibiotic.

Limitations and Considerations

There are several concepts the clinician should understand about standard clinical microbiology laboratory culture methods:

- Only planktonic bacteria are typically detected by standard culture techniques. Detecting bacteria in biofilm communities requires additional processing of wound samples. Biofilm communities that are tightly attached to tissue samples must be dislodged and dispersed into single cells using ultrasonic energy and extensive vortexing prior to plating on agar culture dishes. A recent review and meta-analysis of published papers indicated structures that are consistent with biofilm aggregates were present in approximately 80% of biopsies from chronic wounds (Malone et al., 2017).

- Only a small fraction (perhaps approximately 20%) of all the bacterial species that are present in a chronic wound bed are typically detected by standard aerobic agar plating techniques. For example, identification of all bacterial species present in a series of pressure injuries using DNA-sequencing techniques found that approximately 60% were strict anaerobic bacteria, which are very difficult to grow under standard culturing conditions (Dowd et al., 2008a, 2008b, 2011).

- The polymerase chain reaction (PCR) is a molecular technique utilized to target and amplify bacterial DNA. This technique generates thousands to millions of copies of a particular DNA sequence, which allows them to be detected. The method relies on thermal cycling, cycles of repeated heating and cooling for melting, and then enzymatic replication of the DNA. Bacteria are identified by amplifying a tiny sample of their DNA, without actually having to grow bacterial cultures in the microbiology laboratory. This technology is sensitive, specific, and can be completed in hours.

KEY POINT

Only planktonic bacteria are recovered and identified by wound culture. We currently lack the technology to identify biofilm bacteria, and only a small percentage of the bacterial species present in a chronic wound are detected by standard culture techniques.

Standard clinical microbiology laboratory results obtained by traditional aerobic plating of wound samples provide only partial information about the actual spectrum of bacteria in the wound bed. The results of standard clinical microbiology laboratory assays may be helpful to clinicians in developing a therapy plan. Wound cultures should be done whenever clinical signs and symptoms indicate invasive infection requiring systemic therapy, or when a wound has failed to respond adequately to current antimicrobial therapy (either systemic or topical). However, as identification of bacteria species by DNA-sequencing techniques becomes more widely available, it is very likely that new patterns of bacterial species will be identified that correlate with, and predict, poor wound healing (Dowd et al., 2011).

OSTEOMYELITIS

Infection of the bone, or osteomyelitis, should be considered separately, as cultures taken of soft tissue may not accurately reflect bacterial penetration into bone. The absolute diagnosis of osteomyelitis is a difficult one, often requiring imaging or bone biopsies. Lavery et al. (2007) sought to assess the accuracy of the probe to bone (PTB) test in diagnosing foot osteomyelitis. The investigators enrolled 1,666 consecutive diabetic individuals. Over a mean of 27.2 months, 247 patients developed a foot wound and 151 developed 199 foot infections. Osteomyelitis was found in 30 patients (in 12% with a foot wound and in 20% with a foot infection). The PTB test was found to be highly sensitive (0.87%) and specific (0.91%). The authors concluded that a negative PTB test could be used to exclude the diagnosis (Lavery et al., 2007).

Dinh et al. (2008) performed a meta-analysis of diagnostic tests for osteomyelitis in diabetic foot wounds summarizing sensitivity and specificity. They concluded that exposed bone or positive probe-to-bone test was moderately predictive of osteomyelitis. MRI was the most accurate imaging test for diagnosis. The Infectious Disease Society of America (IDSA) recommends performing a PTB test for any diabetic foot infection (DFI) with an open wound to help diagnose or exclude diabetic foot osteomyelitis (DFO). They also recommend plain radiographs (x-rays) of the foot initially, and serial plain radiographs to monitor for suspected DFO. For diagnostic imaging for DFO, they recommend use of MRI (Lipsky et al., 2012) (**Figs. 11-16 to 11-18**).

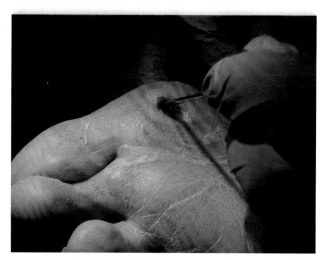

FIGURE 11-16. Probe to Bone.

osteomyelitis. Neither clinical evaluation nor radiologic examinations correlate well with the histopathologic diagnosis of bone infection. Bone scans in deep non-healing stage 4 pressure injuries often yield confusing results. While a bone scan is highly sensitive (almost 100%), it is poorly specific (<33%), meaning that overdiagnosis is a common problem. This is due to the tendency of the nuclear molecules to concentrate in areas of bone that are affected by pressure-induced changes and in foci of heterotopic bone ossification. A bone scan should be used to rule out osteomyelitis. An accurate positive diagnosis of osteomyelitis underlying a pressure

---

KEY POINT

The probe to bone (PTB) test has high negative predictive value for osteomyelitis in foot wounds. This test can be used to rule out osteomyelitis. MRI is usually required to confirm the diagnosis of osteomyelitis in patients with foot ulcers.

The diagnosis of osteomyelitis in the bone beneath pressure injuries is problematic. In patients with deep nonhealing pressure injuries, clinical evaluation does not accurately detect or predict the existence of underlying

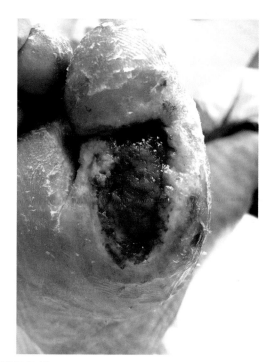

FIGURE 11-17. Plantar First Met Head DFU that Probed Deeply.

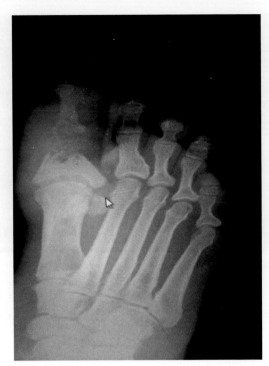

FIGURE 11-18. Correlating Plain Film X-ray Showing Bone Destruction.

injury usually requires examination of bone. This is best obtained intraoperatively, because osteomyelitis is likely to be a focal process, and percutaneous biopsy may fail to sample the infected bone (Steinberg & Warren, 2007) (**Fig. 11-19**).

KEY POINT

An accurate diagnosis of osteomyelitis in the bone underlying a pressure ulcer usually requires examination of bone obtained intraoperatively.

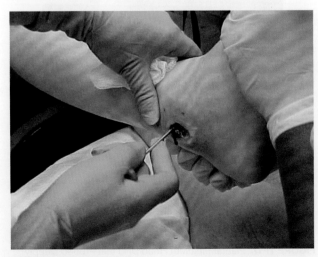

FIGURE 11-19. Bone Biopsy.

CONTROLLING AND MANAGING BIOBURDEN

Bioburden management begins with correction of the factors that can impair resistance to infection. These factors are frequently overlooked components of the plan to control infection. Evaluation and management of nutritional status, glycemic control, blood flow, edema, and exposure to trauma and pressure must be incorporated into the overall management plan and serial assessments of the patient.

The concept of wound bed preparation implies comprehensive care that prepares a wound to heal and involves the foundational elements of wound care at every wound encounter as follows: cleansing, debridement of necrotic or nonviable tissue with attention to wound edges, and management and prevention of infection (Moore et al., 2019). Wound cleansing and debridement are covered in depth in Chapters 9 and 10. Necrotic tissue provides a medium for bacterial growth and must be debrided (Schultz et al., 2003). Wounds in which debridement is not indicated (e.g., an eschar on an ischemic heel) should be monitored frequently for signs of infection (e.g., separation and/or drainage at wound edges, erythema, induration, or fluctuance).

DEFINITION OF TERMS USED

The wound care nurse must understand terms and definitions related to the wound infection continuum. Terminology related to cleansing and topical agents is often misunderstood and misused (WOCN, 2019). The overall evidence on the efficacy of topical antimicrobials in the management of wounds is confusing. Recommendations for use of antimicrobials are based on laboratory studies rather than clinical research. Common definitions of topical agents include

- Antibacterial: An agent that inhibits the growth of bacteria (Doughty & McNichol, 2016).
- Antibiotic: A natural or synthetic agent with the capacity to destroy or inhibit bacterial growth (IWII, 2016).
- Antimicrobial: An agent that acts directly on a microbe to either kill the organism or hinder the development of new colonies (IWII, 2016).
- Antiseptic: A nonselective, topical agent that inhibits multiplication of microorganism, or it may kill microorganisms (IWII, 2016).

WOUND CLEANSING

All wounds should be cleansed at each dressing change, before and after debridement, and in the event of contamination using a neutral, nonirritating, nontoxic solution. Routine cleansing should minimize chemical and mechanical trauma (Gould et al., 2016; Lavery et al., 2016; Marston et al., 2016). An exception to the requirement for routine cleansing may be the recent application of a skin graft or cellular tissue product that should be left undisturbed. In this case, the surrounding skin should be cleansed.

The choice of solution used as well as the method of delivery is driven by the condition of the wound and local factors in the wound. Evidence suggests use of a nontoxic cleaning solution in combination with a delivery device that will create sufficient mechanical force to remove the surface debris without injury to healthy tissue (EPUAP/NPIAP/PPPIA, 2019).

The perceived risks of cytotoxicity with the use of antiseptics and the potential for tissue and cellular trauma associated their use have been debated. The data against the use of antiseptics such as hydrogen peroxide, acetic acid, Dakin solution, and povidone–iodine are based primarily on in vitro models demonstrating the toxicity of these agents to the viability of cells important to wound healing, such as fibroblasts, keratinocytes, and leukocytes. In clinical practice, the choice of solution used for wound cleansing should be made based on the presence of necrotic tissue and exudate on the wound surface, the location of the wound, and the potential for environmental or other contamination such as incontinence.

In choosing the appropriate wound cleanser, the wound care nurse should consider whether cleansing or disinfection is the desired outcome. This decision will depend on the characteristics of the wound and the properties of the agent. The wound care nurse should weigh the risks and benefits of a specific cleanser to the wound. Antiseptic agents such as superoxide water solutions with hypochlorous acid and dilute sodium hypochlorite can be advantageous in management of wounds with high bacterial loads because they are able to reduce microbes on the surface of the wound without causing injury to the wound cells.

KEY POINT

In determining the most appropriate wound cleanser, the wound care nurse must decide whether the goal is wound cleansing or wound disinfection.

Commercially available wound cleansers contain surface active agents (surfactants) that break the bonds attaching contaminants and debris to the wound surface, allowing them to be rinsed away mechanically when the solution is sprayed or poured over the wound. A concentrated, noncytotoxic, nonionic surfactant product that forms a stable gel at body temperature (Plurogel®) improves cleansing and debridement of burns and chronic wounds (Mayer et al., 2018; Percival et al., 2017). The wound care nurse should consider use of cleansing solutions with surfactants or antimicrobials

for wounds with debris, confirmed infection, suspected infection, or suspected high levels of bacterial colonization (EPUAP/NPIAP/PPPIA, 2019). Any potential toxicity of these cleansers should be weighed against the need for removal of surface debris and contaminants based on the assessment of the wound. Normal saline is an effective agent for wound cleansing when delivered with enough pressure to ensure adequate removal of surface debris. Pressures below 4 pounds per square inch (psi) are not sufficient to remove debris, and pressures exceeding 15 psi increase the risk that bacteria will be driven into the tissues (Gabriel, 2017; Wolcott & Fletcher, 2014).

The use of potable water (tap water) for cleansing chronic wounds has been questioned many times. A Cochrane Review published in 2008 concluded that, based on the randomized trials available at that time, tap water is unlikely to be harmful if used for wound cleansing. The decision to use tap water to cleanse wounds should take into account the quality of water, nature of wounds, and the patient's general condition, including the presence of comorbid conditions (Fernandez et al., 2008). Recent guidelines suggest that most pressure injuries can be cleansed with potable water (i.e., water suitable for drinking) or normal saline (EPUAP/NPIAP/PPPIA, 2019; Huang & Choong, 2019). If the wound is going to be cleansed as part of the patient's personal shower, the decision should also take into account the location of the wound, water conditions in a geographic area, the patient's physical condition and immune system, and the overall hygienic advantage (Watret & McLean, 2014). Patients should be advised not to immerse an open wound into a tub.

Skin cleansers designed for use in care of the incontinent patient should not be used as a wound cleanser. The surface-active agents in these preparations are of a concentration sufficient to emulsify and lift adherent fecal matter from the skin and are damaging to the cells of an open wound.

TOPICAL ANTIMICROBIALS

Topical antimicrobials include both antibiotics and antiseptics. The use of topical antibiotics, which contain a low-dose form of antibiotic, may induce resistance. Controversy surrounds the use topical antibiotics and the debate is compounded by extensive work on the microbiota of the individual wound. Given the global concern regarding antibiotic resistance, use of topical antibiotics for wound management should only be considered in infected wounds under very specific circumstances by experienced clinicians. Examples include the use of

- Topical metronidazole for the treatment of odor in fungating wounds
- Silver sulfadiazine for the treatment of burns and wounds

- Mupirocin for the treatment of bacterial skin infections from *S. aureus* (particularly methicillin-resistant *Staphylococcus aureus* [MRSA]), beta-hemolytic *Streptococcus* and *Streptococcus pyogenes*.

While the specific mechanism of action varies from one antibiotic to another, the antibiotic has a single defined microbial target, which limits their effectiveness against multiple pathogens (International Consensus, 2012). Some topical antibiotics may cause hypersensitivity reactions in certain patients and should be avoided (Lipsky & Hoey, 2009).

Topical antimicrobials should be reserved for local clinical infection and in conjunction with culture-based systemic antibiotic therapy for spreading and systemic infections. When a topical antimicrobial is being considered for use in management of an infected wound, the wound care nurse must select the specific agent based on the infecting organism and the topical agent's spectrum of bactericidal activity. If the infecting organism is unknown, it is best to obtain a culture (IWII, 2016).

ANTIMICROBIAL WOUND DRESSINGS

The wound care nurse should assure prompt recognition of changes in the wound that indicate either local, spreading or systemic infection. When changes in the previously healing wound are noted, the wound care nurse may initiate topical measures to reduce the bacterial load, preventing continued replication and potential invasion into the deeper tissues. See Chapter 8 for additional information on the identification of colonization and infection.

There has been an increase in the number of antimicrobial dressings that address the wound infection continuum. Each antimicrobial dressing option provides unique mechanisms of action. The development of resistant organisms with use of these dressings is not yet known (Hess, 2020). Advantages of antimicrobial dressing include the following:

- Provides a broad range of sustained antimicrobial or antibacterial activity
- Provides a moist wound healing environment
- Prevents or reduces infection
- May alter metalloproteinases (MMPs) within wound

The primary differentiating factor for the various dressings is the particular antimicrobial agent incorporated into the dressing. Antimicrobial agents are bound into or coated onto the dressing materials. They act as a barrier to outside contaminants in addition to interacting with wound exudate to further enhance the barrier effects and to reduce bacterial loads on the surface of the wound. Commonly used agents include dialkylcarbamoylchloride (DACC), honey, iodine, methylene blue and gentian violet, polyhexamethylene biguanide (PHMB), silver, and surfactants.

Dialkylcarbomoyl chloride

Dialkylcarbomoyl chloride (DACC)-coated dressings irreversibly bind bacteria at the wound surface that are then removed when the dressing is changed. While the bacteria are not killed, they are unable to disassociate from the surface of the dressing, which means they are rendered inactive and are then physically removed when the dressing is changed. Totty et al. (2017) identified 17 studies with a total of 3,408 patients, which were included in the systematic review. The DACC-coating was suggested to reduce postoperative surgical site infection (SSI) rates and result in chronic wounds that subjectively looked cleaner and had less bacterial load on microbiological assessments. The authors concluded that existing evidence for DACC-coated dressings in managing chronic wounds or as a SSI prophylaxis is limited but encouraging with evidence in support of DACC-coated dressings preventing and treating infection without adverse effects (Totty et al., 2017) (**Fig. 11-20**).

If DACC dressings are to be used effectively for wound care, appropriate levels of moisture are important. Adequate moisture at the surface of the wound is essential for optimal attachment of the bacteria to the dressing. Common antiseptics and analgesics may interfere with hydrophobic attachment, including eutectic mixture of local anesthetic (EMLA) and the use of any products or topical treatments that are petrolatum based. For a wound that is dry and nonexudative, a hydrogel or moisture retentive cover dressing should be used in conjunction with the DACC dressing to provide the moisture needed for effective use (Hamptson, 2007).

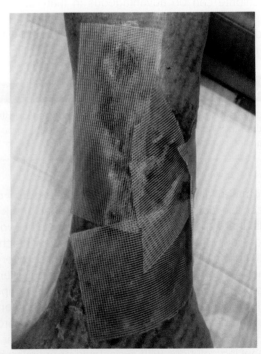

FIGURE 11-20. Dialkylcarbamoylchloride.

Another consideration in the use of DACC is the frequency of dressing changes. As the dressings remove bacteria with each change, wounds with clinical signs of spreading infection may require dressing changes every 12 to 24 hours to achieve the needed reduction in wound bioburden (Gentili et al., 2012). An appropriately absorptive secondary dressing should be used to manage exudate (Bruce, 2012; von Hallern & Lang, 2005). In cases of prophylaxis when there are no clinical signs of infection, dressing change frequency may be decreased (Bua et al., 2017).

Honey

The form of medical grade honey used today differs greatly from that of the natural or culinary versions. Medical grade honey has two general sources: *Leptospermum scoparium* (manuka), which is derived from tea plants, and *Leptospermum polygalifolium*, jelly bush honey. These forms have specific qualities related to processing that affect the end product's bacterial count, pH, enzyme activity, and overall benefit in wound care. Culinary honey uses heat to prepare the product for consumption, which invariably reduces the enzyme responsible for hydrogen peroxide production, whereas medical grade honey's gamma radiation sterilization process allows it to retain biologic activity (Pieper, 2009) **(Fig. 11-21)**.

Honey has demonstrated antimicrobial effects on a broad spectrum of viruses, fungi, protozoa, and over 50 species of bacteria, including clinically relevant organisms such as *P. aeruginosa*, *S. aureus*, MRSA, and vancomycin-resistant *enterococcus* (VRE) (Gethin & Cowman, 2008; Lipsky & Hoey, 2009). The antimicrobial activity of honey has been attributed to its high sugar content (87%) and low water activity, which creates an osmotic effect that dehydrates the bacteria (Hess, 2020). This effect, along with the acidic pH of 3.2 to 4.5, inhibits bacterial growth. Honey inhibits biofilm growth and

reduces biofilm colony formation (EPUAP/NPIAP/PPPIA, 2019). The reduction in wound pH leads to increased oxygen release, reduced toxicity of bacterial end products, enhanced removal of abnormal wound collagen, decreased protease activity, promotion of angiogenesis, increased macrophage and fibroblast activity, and regulation of enzyme activity. The fluid shift produced by the osmotic effect helps to create a moist wound healing environment, promoting autolytic debridement (Grothier & Cooper, 2011). One study found that honey was more effective at desloughing wounds with >50% necrotic tissue than standard hydrogel, leading to statistically significant reduction in healing rates and time to epithelialization (Gethin & Cowman, 2008).

KEY POINT

Medical grade honey has unique properties that provide demonstrated antimicrobial effects, most likely as a result of osmotic activity that dehydrates the organism, and high acidity, which is generally toxic to bacteria.

Honey dressings are available in an alginate, hydrocolloid, and paste form. Dressings can be left in place for up to 7 days, but the actual wear time is determined by the volume of exudate, patient response, and soiling of secondary dressings. Stinging or burning pain has been reported after initial application of the dressing to the wound bed, most likely because of the osmotic effects and the acidic pH of the dressing. Often, these symptoms are transient. A change in therapy is warranted if these symptoms persist. Contraindications to the use of honey include know sensitivity to honey and use in third-degree burns. A common fear is that sensitivity to bee venom would be a contraindication. While most clinicians will not use honey dressings for the patient with a known bee allergy, no reports of anaphylaxis have been described to date with medical grade honey wound care products (Hess, 2020; Pieper, 2009).

Iodine (Povidone and Cadexomer)

Many iodine preparations exist but not all are appropriate for wound care secondary to the cytotoxicity that may occur relative to overall concentration, release, and solubility of the iodine. Iodine has a broad spectrum of activity and works in many ways, for example, by disrupting cell walls and nuclei and by facilitating oxidative killing of microorganisms and neutrophils (Cooper et al., 1991). In vitro and in vivo studies have demonstrated iodine toxicity at the cellular level (Lineaweaver et al., 1985a, 1985b), and iodine has traditionally been perceived as an inhibitor of wound healing. More recent studies suggest that different iodine compounds have different levels of toxicity and that the difference in toxicity associated with povidone–iodine compounds and cadexomer iodine may lie

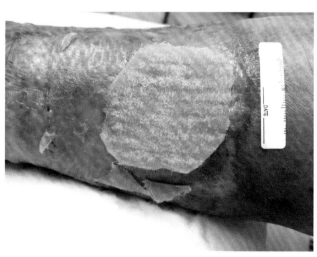

FIGURE 11-21. Honey.

in the components of iodine delivery (Mertz et al., 1999). A clinically beneficial iodine compound would control the speed and amount of iodine released into the wound bed, maintaining bactericidal effects while avoiding cytotoxicity, and would be incorporated into a dressing that permitted decreased frequency of dressing changes for the patient. Povidone–iodine may be used topically over eschar to decrease the bacterial count and to desiccate a maintenance wound (Bigliardi et al., 2017).

The term cadexomer iodine actually describes a delivery system rather than an antimicrobial agent. In this novel delivery system, the iodine is contained within a cadexomer starch bead. As wound exudate is absorbed, it enters the cadexomer bead, causing the openings to swell and allowing a slow, sustained release of the iodine molecule (**Fig. 11-22**). This maintains a steady-state 0.9% concentration at the wound bed, which is nontoxic to healing wounds (Leaper & Durani, 2008). Iodine (I_2) is a potent microbicide, and the uncharged iodine molecule can penetrate the exopolymeric matrix of most biofilms, which partially explains the ability of cadexomer iodine dressings to kill biofilm bacteria in laboratory experiments (Phillips et al., 2015). The microbicidal form of the iodine is brown, and iodide (I^-), which is the inactive form of iodine, is colorless. The dressing progresses from brown to colorless, which signals depletion of the iodine and acts as a signal to change the dressing. The dressing lasts for an average of 72 hours, depending on the amount of exudate, the size of the wound, and the amount of the dressing/gel used.

Contraindications to use of cadexomer iodine are known allergy to iodine, contrast dyes, or shellfish and in those with thyroid or renal disorders. It is also contraindicated in extensive burns (EPUAP/NPIAP/PPPIA, 2019). The structure of the cadexomer starch requires an adequate amount of exudate or moisture to allow for breakdown and release of the iodine. Dry wounds without exudate may not properly activate the dressing. Iodine reduces the activity of topically applied collagenase ointment, so these products should not be used simultaneously (Jovanovic et al., 2012).

Methylene Blue and Gentian Violet

Methylene blue and gentian violet have been used in medicine for over 50 years as laboratory stains and have demonstrated antibacterial activity against a broad spectrum of yeast and bacteria commonly found in wounds, including MRSA and *P. aeruginosa* (Woo & Heil, 2017) (**Fig. 11-23**). The methylene blue and gentian violet dye molecules are bound to a polyvinyl alcohol (PVA) foam. When hydrated, the foam becomes a soft, conformable wound filler and contact dressing. Methylene blue and gentian violet are available bound to polyurethane foams that do not require hydration. In vitro, PVA foam absorbs up to 12 times its weight in exudate (Hess, 2020; Woo & Heil, 2017). Coupled with its absorptive capacity, the methylene blue/gentian violet–bound foam absorbs and retains bacteria-laden exudate. In clinical use, the foam also has been noted to reduce hypergranulation tissue and to flatten rolled wound edges (epibole) (Hess, 2020). One advantage of gentian violet and methylene blue dressings is compatibility with collagenase (Jovanovic et al., 2012). Color change may occur in the dressing, from deep blue to a lighter blue or white caused by bacterial inhibition and depletion of the methylene blue and gentian violet components, providing an important visual

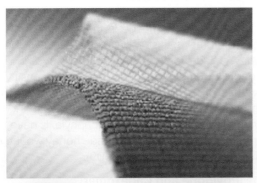
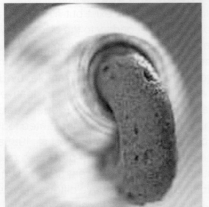

FIGURE 11-22. Cadexomer Iodine.

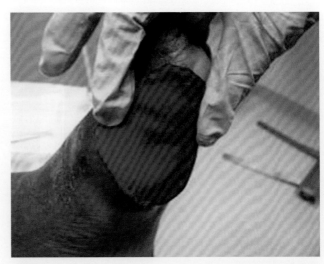

FIGURE 11-23. Methylene Blue and Gentian Violet Foam.

indicator to guide dressing change. Dressing change frequency is dependent on the level of exudate, and the polyurethane foam may be left in place 3 to 7 days. If the dressing completely dries out, it may be rehydrated with normal saline or water. Contraindications include third-degree burns and with hypersensitivity to the ingredients of the dressing.

Polyhexamethylene Biguanide

Polyhexamethylene biguanide (PHMB) is a bactericidal that has been used for many years with no known resistance. It is used in a variety of products, including wound care dressings, contact lens cleaning solutions, perioperative cleansing products, and swimming pool cleaners (Gray et al., 2010; Moore & Gray, 2007; Mullder et al., 2007) (**Fig. 11-24**). PHMB is a synthetic compound similar in structure to naturally occurring molecules that are produced by inflammatory cells to protect against infection. By attaching itself to the bacterial cell membrane, PHMB causes structural changes that kill the bacteria. The incorporation of PHMB into dressings, including gauze, nonadherent dressings, foams, and cellulose wound dressings, has been shown to provide an effective barrier to outside contamination in addition to bactericidal activity against bacteria absorbed into the dressing material. One study found that PHMB-impregnated foam showed a significant log reduction of *P. aeruginosa* within the wound compared to standard gauze and did not allow *Pseudomonas* to colonize the PHMB-impregnated foam nor change the normal wound milieu. These results support one of the most common uses of PHMB by the wound care nurse, which is to prevent infection in high-risk individuals (Cazzaniga et al., 2010). PHMB must come into direct contact with the bacterial organism. Once bound to a dressing material such as gauze, foam, or alginate, it can only affect bacteria that have been absorbed into the dressing (Butcher, 2012). PHMB is also available as a wound irrigation solution. Time of

exposure is the key determinant of effectiveness, with 10 to 20 minutes of exposure required to provide optimal antimicrobial effects (Hess, 2020). Wound care nurses utilizing PHMB in solution form should allow the solution to dwell in the wound bed when using NPWT devices that instill and allow dwell time (NPWTi-d) (Gupta et al., 2016; Hess, 2020; Kim et al., 2015).

Contraindications to the use of PHMB include known adverse reactions to PHMB or chlorhexidine. Care should be taken to avoid saturation of PHMB-impregnated gauzes with solutions other than normal saline, sterile water, or potable water, as certain antiseptic solutions such as sodium hypochlorite may result in a chemical reaction that inactivates these agents and produces a nontoxic yellow stain. PHMB has been shown in vitro to significantly reduce the activity of exogenously applied collagenase (Jovanovic et al., 2012). The frequency of dressing change is dependent upon the dressing into which the PHMB is impregnated.

Silver

Silver has been used for centuries originally in vessels used to preserve water and has had medicinal uses documented from AD 750. The use of ionic silver in topical antimicrobial dressings has resulted in multiple studies to assess its ability to reduce bacterial growth and the risk of wound infection, to manage active infection, and to reduce the risk of hospital-acquired wound infections. This interest is attributed to silver's bactericidal efficacy at low concentrations and its relatively limited toxicity to human cells. Silver has proven antimicrobial activity at a low concentration, which includes antibiotic-resistant bacteria such as MRSA and vancomycin-resistant enterococci (VRE). Silver used in clinical practice in topical dressings has displayed limited toxicity to human cells. Advances in impregnation techniques and polymer technologies, resulting in numerous delivery systems in the form of dressing materials, have supported its use (White & Cutting, 2006a). Silver is now available in amorphous hydrogels, sheet hydrogels, alginates, hydrofibers, foams, silicones, contact layers, wound powders, ointments, and nanocrystalline sheets (**Fig. 11-25**).

Silver dressings work via one of two delivery systems: the silver may be donated to the wound bed and may kill organisms on the wound surface or the silver may be retained in the dressing and work by destroying bacteria contained in the exudate and absorbed into the carrier dressing. For silver to realize its full bactericidal potential, there must be controlled and sustained release of silver over time at sufficient levels to cause bacterial death but within a range that prevents tissue toxicity (Cutting et al., 2009). A scoping review was conducted to examine the extent, range, and nature of research activity surrounding chronic wound care that employed silver-impregnated dressings. In comparative analyses of the 26 studies that investigated wound healing, 15 revealed significantly

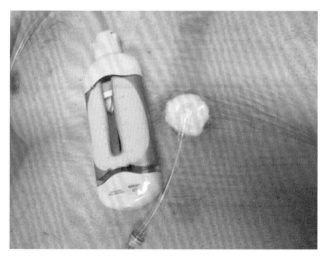

FIGURE 11-24. PHMB Gauze Under Nonpowered NPWT Device.

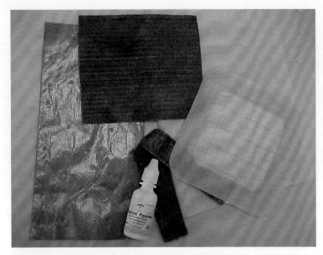

FIGURE 11-25. Examples of Silver Dressings.

positive wound healing outcomes with silver treatments versus 9 that did not. Of 17 studies that presented data on microbiology, 3 reported significant microbial load improvement for silver dressings, 9 noted nonsignificant findings, and 4 provided no statistical values. They noted that the heterogeneous evidence regarding the impact of silver dressings on clinical outcomes may be related to differences in the silver treatments themselves, study designs, outcomes, and measures used (Rodriguez-Arguello et al., 2018). The ability of the dressing to conform, remain in place, and provide consistent coverage of the wound bed also contributes to antimicrobial effectiveness. The quantity, chemical form, delivery, release, and ability to conform influence the clinical outcomes associated with silver dressings (Hamm, 2010; International Consensus, 2012; Jones et al., 2005).

KEY POINT

Silver dressings work through one of two mechanisms: (1) donation of silver to wound surface, with direct bactericidal activity at the wound surface or (2) destruction of bacteria within the dressing itself.

Silver sulfadiazine is a broad-spectrum antimicrobial that has been available for over 40 years, with extensive use in management of burn wounds. Silver sulfadiazine cream has a relatively short period of action, its penetration of burn eschar is poor, and it forms a pseudo-eschar with repeated applications. As a result, frequent dressing changes are required with thorough cleaning at each change. Silver sulfadiazine is not water soluble, making it difficult to remove. It may be contraindicated in patients who are allergic to sulfa. Alternative methods of silver delivery may provide equally effective bacterial control with a more patient-friendly delivery system. For example, a study involving partial-thickness burns

showed no statistically significant difference in the rate of infection or time required for reepithelialization between burns managed with silver sulfadiazine and those managed with a silver hydrogel; however, the author reported less pain and increased patient satisfaction in the hydrogel group (Glat et al., 2009).

Silver has a potent antimicrobial effect that destroys microorganisms immediately by blocking cellular respiration and disrupting bacterial cell membranes. Specifically, silver cations bind to tissue proteins, causing structural changes in the bacterial cell membranes that cause cell death. Silver also binds and denatures bacterial DNA and RNA, inhibiting cell replication (Fong & Wood, 2006). Further, silver may increase the sensitivity of a biofilm to antibiotics and may also reduce its adhesion to the wound bed (Kostenko et al., 2010).

Concerns related to the use of silver dressings relate to the potential for development of bacterial resistance, potential for cellular toxicity, and assuring appropriate use of the right amount of silver at the right time. The toxicity of silver to normal cells and tissues has also been assessed. Silver dressings with demonstrated toxicity at 1 day in "in vitro" studies demonstrated no cytotoxicity at 1 week in "in vivo" studies; these results suggest that in vitro cytotoxicity is greater than in vivo because the silver in "in vitro" studies is not diluted by wound fluid, perfusion effects, and/or effects of the tissue reservoir or metabolism (White & Cutting, 2006a).

Considerations and contraindications related to the use of silver fall into two primary areas. Of lesser concern is the use of silver in conjunction with exogenously applied collagenase. The use of dressings with heavy metal ions is discouraged due to their impact on activity of the enzyme (Jovanovic et al., 2012). Wound care nurses should avoid the use of silver in combination with collagenase. Silver should not be used close to any oil-based products (e.g., petrolatum, zinc oxide) where the oil molecules may interfere with the ionization of the silver. Products that produce a continuous supply of ionized silver are likely to be more efficacious, and higher levels of silver release are often necessary to treat microorganisms such as pseudomonas in a complete environment, such as a wound (Sibbald, et al., 2011).

The use of silver in the pediatric population should be limited (Barrett & Rutter, 1994). While there have been reports in the literature of safe use of silver in this population, those studies utilized traditional end points in wound healing trials (e.g., time to healing, pain, and length of stay), rather than risk of harm (Jester et al., 2008). The in vitro toxicity data need to be considered when considering use of silver-based products for the pediatric population (Poon & Burd, 2004). For example, silver toxicity was a reported concern in the assessment of pediatric burn patients managed with nanocrystalline silver dressings. Specifically, serum silver levels were elevated, and the elevation was closely proportional to the surface area of the wounds treated. When considering the use of a silver dressing for a pediatric patient, the age of the patient, size of the wound, level of silver, and delivery system should be taken into consideration. Wound care nurses should avoid silver dressings in neonates and should limit the use of such products in the pediatric population to no more than 2 weeks (International Consensus, 2012).

Surfactant

Surfactants are widely used as detergents, emulsifiers, wetting, and foaming agents. Many wound cleansers contain surfactants (surface active agents). Surfactants are defined as amphiphilic agents, which means that they contain both water soluble (hydrophilic) and water insoluble (hydrophobic structures). They reduce the surface tension between two liquids or a liquid and solid, which allows for greater penetration of fluids (Percival et al., 2017). The use of surfactants to manage biofilms is a new treatment. Surfactants are now included as a method of debridement (IWII, 2016).

Poloxamer 188 (Pluronic F68) is a nonionic surfactant, which was approved by the FDA over 50 years ago to reduce viscosity of blood before transfusions (**Fig. 11-26**). Yang et al. (2017) conducted an ex vivo study on porcine skin using a concentrated surfactant dressing (CSD) to treat biofilm infections (**Fig. 11-24**). They found that daily application and removal of this dressing reduced the biofilm to undetectable levels within 3 days in the pig model. Percival et al. (2017) conducted an in vivo study that demonstrated the effectiveness of CSD in breaking down biofilms. Zölß & Cech (2016) conducted

a cohort design study at a European outpatient tertiary wound center using the CSD with the addition of 1% silver sulfadiazine on 226 chronic wound patients. Eighty-eight patients had been undergoing standard of care treatment while the remainder (*n* = 138) began treatment with the CSD. Seventy-three percent of patients in the first group healed or showed improvement, with 60% healing by a median of 17 weeks. Eighty-six percent of the group of new enrollees healed or showed improvement with 73% healing within a median of 12 weeks of beginning treatment with the CSD (Zölß & Cech, 2016).

Ratliff (2018a) conducted a case series of 18 patients with lower extremity wounds that were treated with CSD. On follow-up clinic visits, the wound was assessed, measurements were obtained, and Pressure Ulcer Scale for Healing (PUSH) Tool scores completed. The mean total PUSH score before the CSD dressing was applied was 10.7 (range from 5 to 15) (standard deviation [SD] 3.09) and posttreatment was 8.3 (range from 0 to 14) (SD 4). All 18 patients had a decrease in their pretreatment score from the first clinic visit compared with the posttreatment PUSH Tool score, indicating that it may be an effective dressing in the management of lower extremity arterial and venous wounds (Ratliff, 2018a). Ratliff (2018b) also describes a clinical case of using the dressing to promote healing of an infected groin wound from a vascular graft infection.

⬤ CONCLUSION

Management of bioburden in the chronic wound requires an assessment that includes systemic and local risk factors, wound status, and monitoring of the progress in healing. While avoidance of unnecessary systemic antibiotics is ideal, judicious use is warranted. Although wound care nurses rely on the appearance of the wound to drive decisions regarding culture and treatment, the fact that a wound is not progressing should alert the wound care nurse that excessive bioburden is present. Consultation with colleagues in infectious disease should be considered when management of bacterial bioburden is beyond the scope of the wound care nurse.

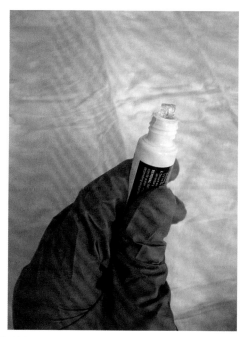

FIGURE 11-26. Surfactant (Pluronic F68).

REFERENCES

American Society of Microbiology. (2019). Gram Stain Protocols. Retrieved from https://www.asm.org/Protocols/Gram-Stain-Protocols. Accessed on March 23, 2020.

Bamberg, R., Sullivan, P. K., & Conner-Kerr T. (2002). Diagnosis of wound infections: Current culturing practices of US wound care professionals. *Wounds, 14*, 314–321.

Barrett, D. A., & Rutter, N. (1994). Transdermal delivery and the premature neonate. *Critical Reviews in Therapeutic Drug Carrier Systems, 11*(1), 1–30.

Berg, J. O., Mossner, B. K., Skov, M. N., et al. (2006). Antibacterial properties of EMLA and lidocaine in wound tissue biopsies for culturing. *Wound Repair and Regeneration, 14*(5), 581–585.

Bigliardi, P. L., Alsagoff, S. A. L., El-Kafrawi, H. Y., et al. (2017). Povidone iodine in wound healing: A review of current concepts and practices. *International Journal of Surgery, 44*, 260–268.

Bill, T., Ratliff, C., Donovan, A., et al. (2001). Quantitative swab culture versus tissue biopsy: A prospective comparison in chronic wounds. *Ostomy/Wound Management, 47*(1), 34–37.

Bowler, P. G. (2003). The 10^5 bacterial growth guideline: Reassessing its clinical relevance in wound healing. *Ostomy/Wound Management, 49*(1), 44–53.

Browne, A., Dow, G., & Sibbald, R. G. (2001). Infected wounds: Definitions and controversies. In V Falanga (ed.), *Cutaneous Wound Healing* (pp. 203–219). London, UK: Martin Dunitz.

Bruce, Z. (2012). Using Cutimed Sorbact Hydroactive on chronic infected wounds. *Wounds UK, 8*(1), 119–129.

Bua, N., Smith, G. E., Totty, J. P., et al. (2017). Dialkylcarbamoyl chloride dressings in the prevention of surgical site infections after nonimplant vascular surgery. *Annals of Vascular Surgery, 44*, 387–392.

Butcher, M. (2012). PHMB: An effective antimicrobial in wound bioburden management. *British Journal of Nursing, 21*, s16–s21.

Cazzaniga, A., Serralta, V., Davis, S. C., et al. (2010). The effect of an antimicrobial gauze dressing impregnated with 0.2-percent polyhexamethylene biguanide as a barrier to prevent *Pseudomonas aeruginosa* wound invasion. *Wounds, 14*, 169–176.

Cooper M. L., Laxer J. A., & Hansbrough J. F. (1991). The cytotoxic effects of commonly used topical antimicrobial agents on human fibroblasts and keratinocytes. *Journal of Trauma, 31*(6), 775–782.

Cowan, D. K., & Talaro, K. P. (2006). Infectious diseases affecting the skin and eyes. In M. K. Cowan & K. P. Talaro (Eds.), *Microbiology: A Systems Approach* (pp. 540–576). New York, NY: McGraw-Hill.

Cutting, K., White, R., & Hoekstra, H. (2009). Topical silver-impregnated dressings and the importance of the dressing technology. *International Wound Journal, 6*(5), 396–402.

Dinh, M. T., Abad, C. L., & Safdar, N. (2008). Diagnostic accuracy of the physical examination and imaging tests for osteomyelitis underlying diabetic foot ulcers: meta-analysis. *Clinical Infectious Diseases, 47*(4), 519–527.

Doughty, D. B., & McNichol, L. L. (Eds.) (2016). *WOCN core curriculum: Wound management.* Philadelphia, PA: Wolters Kluwer.

Dowd, S. E., Sun, Y., Secor, P. R., et al. (2008a). Survey of bacterial diversity in chronic wounds using Pyrosequencing, DGGE, and full ribosome shotgun sequencing. *BMC Microbiology, 8*(1), 43.

Dowd, S. E., Wolcott, R. D., Kennedy, J., et al. (2011). Molecular diagnostics and personalized medicine in wound care: Assessment of outcomes. *Journal of Wound Care, 20*(5), 234–239.

Dowd, S. E., Wolcott, R. D., Sun, Y., et al. (2008b). Polymicrobial nature of chronic diabetic foot ulcer biofilm infections determined using bacterial tag encoded FLX amplicon pyrosequencing (bTEFAP). *PLoS One, 3*(10), e3326.

Drosou, A., Falabella, A., & Kirsner, R. S. (2003). Antiseptics on wounds: An area of controversy. *Wounds, 15*, 149–166.

European Pressure Ulcer Advisory Panel, National Pressure Injury Advisory Panel, and Pan Pacific Pressure Injury Alliance [EPUAP/NPIAP/PPPIA]. (2019). In E. Haesler (Ed.), *Prevention and treatment of pressure ulcers/injuries: Clinical Practice Guideline*. The International Guideline.

Fernandez, R., Griffiths, R., & Ussia, C. (2008). Water for wound cleansing. *Cochrane Database of Systematic Reviews*, (2), CD003861.

Fong, J., & Wood, F. (2006). Nanocrystalline silver dressings in wound management: A review. *International Journal of Nanomedicine, 1*(4), 441–449.

Gabriel, A. (2017). Wound Irrigation. *Medscape*. Retrieved from https://emedicine.medscape.com/article/1895071-overview. Accessed on December 15, 2019.

Gardner, S. E., Frantz, R. A., Saltzman, C. L., et al. (2006). Diagnostic validity of three swab techniques for identifying chronic wound infection. *Wound Repair and Regeneration, 14*(5), 548–557. https://doi.org/10.1111/j.1743-6109.2006.00162.x

Gentili, V., Gianesini, S., Balboni, P. G., et al. (2012). Panbacterial real-time PCR to evaluate bacterial burden in chronic wounds treated with Cutimed Sorbact. *European Journal of Clinical Microbiology and Infectious Diseases, 31*(7), 1523–1529.

Gethin, G., & Cowman, S. (2008). Bacteriological changes in sloughy venous leg ulcers treated with manuka honey or hydrogel: An RCT. *Journal of Wound Care, 17*(6), 241–247.

Glat, P. M., Kubat, W. D., Hsu, J. F., et al. (2009). Randomized clinical study of SilvaSorb® gel in comparison to Silvadene® silver sulfadiazine cream in the management of partial-thickness burns. *Journal of Burn Care & Research, 30*(2), 262–267.

Gould, L., Stuntz, M., Giovannelli, M., et al. (2016). Wound Healing Society 2015 update on guidelines for pressure ulcers. *Wound Repair and Regeneration, 24*(1), 145–162.

Gray, D., Barrett, S., Battacharya, M., et al. (2010). PHMB and its potential contribution to wound management. *Wounds UK, 6*(2), 40–46.

Grothier, L., & Cooper, R. (2011). Medihoney dressings made easy. *Wounds UK, 6*(2), 1–6.

Gupta, S., Gabriel, A., Lantis, J., et al. (2016). Clinical recommendations and practical guide for negative pressure wound therapy with instillation. *International Wound Journal, 13*(2), 159–174.

Haalboom, M., Blokhuis-Arkes, M. H., Beuk, R. J., et al. (2018). Wound swab and wound biopsy yield similar culture results. *Wound Repair and Regeneration, 26*, 192–199. doi:10.1111/wrr.12629

Hall-Stoodley, L., & Stoodley, P. (2009). Evolving concepts in biofilm infections. *Cellular Microbiology, 11*(7), 1034–1043.

Hamm, R. (2010). Antibacterial dressings. In C Sen (Ed.), *Advances in wound care* (pp. 148–154). New Rochelle, NY: Mary Ann Liebert, Inc.

Hamptson, S. (2007). An evaluation of the efficacy of Cutimed Sorbact in different types of non-healing wounds. *Wounds UK, 3*, 1–6.

Hess, K. T. (2020). *Product Guide to Skin & Wound Care* (8th ed.). Philadelphia, PA: Wolters Kluwer.

Hibbing, M. E., Fuqua, C., Parsek, M. R., et al. (2010). Bacterial competition: Surviving and thriving in the microbial jungle. *Nature Reviews Microbiology, 8*(1), 15–25.

Huang, C. Y., & Choong, M. Y. (2019). Comparison of wounds' infection rate between tap water and normal saline cleansing: A meta-analysis of randomised control trials. *International Wound Journal, 16*(1), 300–301.

International Consensus. (2012). *Appropriate use of silver dressings in wounds. An expert working group consensus*. London: Wounds International. Retrieved from http://www.woundsinternational.com. Accessed on March 22, 2020.

International Wound Infection Institute (IWII). (2016). *Wound Infection in Clinical Practice*. London, England: Wounds International.

Jester, I., Bohn, I., Hannmann, T., et al. (2008). Comparison of two silver dressings for wound management in pediatric burns. *Wounds, 20*, 303–308.

Johnson, S. M., Saint John, B. E., & Dine, A. P. (2008). Local anesthetics as antimicrobial agents: A review. *Surgical Infections, 9*(2), 205–213.

Jones, S., Bowler, P. G., & Walker, M. (2005). Antimicrobial activity of silver-containing dressings is influenced by dressing conformability with a wound surface. *Wounds, 17*, 263–270.

Jovanovic, A., Ermis, R., Mewaldt, R., et al. (2012). The influence of metal salts, surfactants, and wound care products on enzymatic activity of collagenase, the wound debriding enzyme. *Wounds, 24*, 242–253.

Kim, P. J., Attinger, C. E., Olawoye, O., et al. (2015). Negative pressure wound therapy with instillation: review of evidence and recommendations. *Wounds, 27*(12), S2–S19.

Kostenko, V., Lyczak, J., Turner, K., et al. (2010). Impact of silver-containing wound dressings on bacterial biofilm viability and susceptibility to antibiotics during prolonged treatment. *Antimicrobial Agents and Chemotherapy, 54*(12), 5120–5131.

Landis, S., Ryan, S., & Woo, K. (2007). Infections in chronic wounds. In D Krasner, G. T. Rodeheaver, & R. G. Sibbald (Eds.), *Chronic wound care: A clinical source book for healthcare professionals* (pp. 299–321). Malvern, PA: HMP Communications.

Lavery, L. A., Armstrong, D. G., Peters, E. J., et al. (2007). Probe-to-bone test for diagnosing diabetic foot osteomyelitis: Reliable or relic? *Diabetes Care, 30*(2), 270–274.

Lavery, L. A., Davis, K. E., Berriman, S. J., et al. (2016). WHS guidelines update: Diabetic foot ulcer treatment guidelines. *Wound Repair and Regeneration, 24*(1), 112–126.

Leaper, D. J., & Durani, P. (2008). Topical antimicrobial therapy of chronic wounds healing by secondary intention using iodine products. *International Wound Journal, 5*(2), 361–368.

Lee, P. C., Turnidge, J., & McDonald, P. J. (1985). Fine-needle aspiration biopsy in diagnosis of soft tissue infections. *Journal of Clinical Microbiology, 22*(1), 80–83.

Levine, N. S., Lindberg, R. B., Mason, A. D. Jr, et al. (1976). The quantitative swab culture and smear: A quick, simple method for determining the number of viable aerobic bacteria on open wounds. *Journal of Trauma, 16*(2), 89–94.

Lindsay, S., Oates, A., & Bourdillon, K. (2017). The detrimental impact of extracellular bacterial proteases on wound healing. *International Wound Journal, 14*(6), 1237–1247.

Lineaweaver, W., Howard, R., Soucy, D., et al. (1985a). Topical antimicrobial toxicity. *Archives of Surgery, 120*(3), 267–270.

Lineaweaver, W., McMorris, S., Soucy, D., et al. (1985b). Cellular and bacterial toxicities of topical antimicrobials. *Plastic and Reconstructive Surgery, 75*(3), 394–396.

Lipsky, B. A., & Hoey, C. (2009). Topical antimicrobial therapy for treating chronic wounds. *Clinical Infectious Diseases, 49*(10), 1541–1549.

Lipsky, B. A., Berendt, A. R., Cornia, P. B., et al. (2012). 2012 Infectious Diseases Society of America clinical practice guideline for the diagnosis and treatment of diabetic foot infections. *Clinical Infectious Diseases, 54*(12), e132–e173. https://doi.org/10.1093/cid/cis346

Maliyar, K., Persaud-Jaimangal, R., & Sibbald, R. G. (2020). Associations among skin surface pH, temperature, and bacterial burden in wounds. *Advances in Skin & Wound Care, 33*(4), 180–185. doi: 10.1097/01.ASW.0000655488.33274.d0.

Malone, M., Bjarnsholt, T., McBain, A. J., et al. (2017). The prevalence of biofilms in chronic wounds: A systematic review and meta-analysis of published data. *Journal of Wound Care, 26*(1), 20–25.

Marston, W., Tang, J., Kirsner, R. S., et al. (2016). Wound healing society 2015 update on guidelines for venous ulcers. *Wound Repair and Regeneration, 24*, 136–144.

Martin, L. K., & Drosou, A. (2005). Wound microbiology and the use of antibacterial agents. In A. F. Falabella & R. S. Krisner (Eds.), *Wound healing* (pp. 83–101). Boca Raton, FL: Taylor & Francis Group.

Mayer, D., Armstrong, D., Schultz, G., et al. (2018). Cell salvage in acute and chronic wounds: A potential treatment strategy. Experimental data and early clinical results. *Journal of Wound Care, 27*(9), 594–605.

McNichol, L. L., Ayello, E. A., Phearman, L. A., et al. (2018). Incontinence-associated dermatitis: State of the science and knowledge translation. *Advances in Skin & Wound Care, 31*(11), 502–513.

Mertz, P. M., Oliveira-Gandia, M. F., & Davis, S. C. (1999). The evaluation of a cadexomer iodine wound dressing on methicillin resistant *Staphylococcus aureus* (MRSA) in acute wounds. *Dermatologic Surgery, 25*(2), 89–93.

Moore, K., & Gray, D. (2007). Using PHMB antimicrobial to prevent wound infection. *Wounds UK, 3*, 96–102.

Moore, Z., Dowsett, C., Smith, G., et al. (2019). TIME CDST: an updated tool to address the current challenges in wound care. *Journal of Wound Care, 28*(3), 154–161.

Mufti, A., Ayello, E. A., & Sibbald, R. G. (2016). Anatomy and Physiology of the Skin. In D. B. Doughty & L. L. McNichol (Eds.). *WOCN Core Curriculum: Wound Management.* Philadelphia, PA: Wolters Kluwer.

Mullder, G. D., Cavorsi, J. P., & Lee, D. K. (2007). Polyhexamethylene biguanide (PHMB): An addendum to current topical antimicrobials. *Wounds, 19*, 173–182.

Percival, S. L., Mayer, D., & Salisbury, A. M. (2017). Efficacy of a surfactant-based wound dressing on biofilm control. *Wound Repair and Regeneration, 25*(5), 767–773.

Phillips, P. L., Yang, Q., Davis, S., et al. (2015). Antimicrobial dressing efficacy against mature *Pseudomonas aeruginosa* biofilm on porcine skin explants. *International Wound Journal, 12*(4), 469–483. doi: 10.1111/iwj.12142.

Pieper, B. (2009). Honey-based dressings and wound care: An option for care in the United States. *Journal of Wound, Ostomy, and Continence Nursing, 36*(1), 60–66.

Poon, V. K., & Burd, A. (2004). In vitro cytotoxicity of silver: Implication for clinical wound care. *Burns, 30*(2), 140–147.

Ratliff, C. R. (2018a). Case series of 18 patients with lower extremity wounds treated with a Concentrated Surfactant–Based Gel Dressing. *Journal of Vascular Nursing, 36*(1), 3–7.

Ratliff, C. R. (2018b). Management of a groin wound using a concentrated surfactant-based gel dressing. *Journal of Wound, Ostomy, and Continence Nursing, 45*(5), 465–467.

Ratliff, C. R., & Rodeheaver, G. T. (2002). Correlation of semi-quantitative swab cultures to quantitative swab cultures from chronic wounds. *Wounds, 14*(9), 329–333.

Robson, M. C., Cooper, D. M., Aslam, R., et al. (2006). Guidelines for the treatment of venous ulcers. *Wound Repair and Regeneration, 14*(6), 649–662.

Rodriguez-Arguello, J., Lienhard, K., Patel, P., et al. (2018). A scoping review of the use of silver-impregnated dressings for the treatment of chronic wounds. *Ostomy/Wound Management, 64*(3), 14–31.

Rushing, J. (2007). Obtaining a wound culture specimen. *Nursing, 37*(11), 18.

Sauer, K., Camper, A. K., Ehrlich, G. D., et al. (2002). *Pseudomonas aeruginosa* displays multiple phenotypes during development as a biofilm. *Journal of Bacteriology, 184*(4), 1140–1154.

Schultz, G. T., Bjarnsholt, G. A., James, D. J., et al. (2017). Consensus guidelines for the identification and treatment of biofilms in chronic non-healing wounds. *Wound Repair and Regeneration, 25*(5), 744–757.

Schultz, G. S., Sibbald, R. G., Falanga, V., et al. (2003). Wound bed preparation: A systematic approach to wound management. *Wound Repair and Regeneration, 11*(Suppl 1), S1–S28.

Serena, T. E., Harrell, K., Serena, L., et al. (2019). Real-time bacterial fluorescence imaging accurately identifies wounds with moderate-to-heavy bacterial burden. *Journal of Wound Care, 28*(6), 346–357.

Sibbald, R. G., Goodman, L., Woo, K. Y., et al. (2011). Special considerations in wound bed preparation 2011: an update©. *Advances in Skin & Wound Care, 24*(9), 415–436.

Stacey, M. C., Phillips, S. A., Farrokhyar, F., et al. (2019). Evaluation of wound fluid biomarkers to determine healing in adults with venous leg ulcers: A prospective study. *Wound Repair and Regeneration, 27*, 509–518. doi: 10.1111/wrr.12723

Stallard, Y. (2018). When and How to Perform Cultures on Chronic Wounds? *Journal of Wound, Ostomy, and Continence Nursing, 45*(2), 179–186. doi: 10.1097/WON.0000000000000414

Steinberg, J. S., & Warren, J. S. (2007). Point-counter point: Probe to bone: Is it the best test for osteomyelitis? *Podiatry Today, 20*, 50–54.

Stoodley, P., Sauer, K., Davies, D. G., et al. (2002). Biofilms as complex differentiated communities. *Annual Review of Microbiology, 56*, 187–209.

Stotts, N. A. (2016). Wound infection: Diagnosis and management. In R. A. Bryant & D. P. Nix (Eds.). *Acute and Chronic Wounds: Current Management Concepts* (5th ed.). St. Louis, MO: Elsevier, Inc.

Sussman, C., & Bates-Jensen, B. M. (2012). Skin and soft tissue anatomy and wound healing physiology. In C. Sussman & B. M. Bates-Jensen (eds.), *Wound Care: A Collaborative Practice Manual for Health Professionals.* Philadelphia, PA: Lippincott Williams & Wilkins.

Totty, J. P., Bua, N., Smith, G. E., et al. (2017). Dialkylcarbamoyl chloride (DACC)-coated dressings in the management and prevention of wound infection: A systematic review. *Journal of Wound Care, 26*(3), 107–114.

Trengove, N. J., Stacey M. C., McGechie D. F., et al. (1996). Qualitative bacteriology and leg ulcer healing. *Journal of Wound Care, 5*(6), 277–280.

Von Hallern, B., & Lang, F. (2005). Has Cutimed® Sorbact® proved its practical value as an antimicrobial dressing? *Medizin & Praxis Spezial*, 2–7.

Watret, L., & McLean, A. (2014). Cleansing diabetic foot wounds: Tap water or saline? *Wounds International, 5*, 1–5.

White, R. J., & Cutting, K. (2006a). Exploring the effects of silver in wound management—What is optimal? *Wounds, 18*, 307–314.

White, R. J., & Cutting, K. F. (2006b). Critical colonization—The concept under scrutiny. *Ostomy/Wound Management, 52*, 50–56.

Wolcott, R., & Fletcher, J. (2014). The role of wound cleansing in the management of wounds. Retrieved from https://www.woundsinternational.com/resources/details/the-role-of-wound-cleansing-in-the-management-of-wounds. Accessed on March 23, 2020.

Wolcott, R., Sanford, N., Gabrilska, R., et al. (2016). Microbiota is a primary cause of pathogenesis of chronic wounds. *Journal of Wound Care, 25*(Suppl 10), S33–S43.

Woo, K. Y., & Heil, J. (2017). A prospective evaluation of methylene blue and gentian violet dressing for management of chronic wounds with local infection. *International Wound Journal, 14*(6), 1029–1035.

World Union of Wound Healing Societies (WUWHS). (2016). Florence Conference, *Position Document: Management of Biofilm*. England: Wound International.

Wound, Ostomy and Continence Nurses Society (WOCN). (2019). *Guideline for management of wounds in patients with lower extremity venous disease (LEVD)*. Mount Laurel, NJ: Author.

Wysocki, A. B. (2016). Anatomy and physiology of the skin and soft tissue. In R. A. Bryant & D. P. Nix (eds.), *Acute and Chronic Wounds: Current Management Concepts* (5th ed.). St Louis, MO: Elsevier.

Xavier, J. B., & Foster, K. R. (2007). Cooperation and conflict in microbial biofilms. *Proceedings of the National Academy of Sciences of the United States of America, 104*(3), 876–881.

Yang, D. C., Blair, K. M., & Salama, N. R. (2016). Staying in shape: the impact of cell shape on bacterial survival in diverse environments. *Microbiology and Molecular Biology Reviews, 80*(1), 187–203.

Yang, Q., Larose, C., Della Porta, A. C., et al. (2017). A surfactant-based wound dressing can reduce bacterial biofilms in a porcine skin explant model. *International Wound Journal, 14*(2), 408–413.

Zölß, C., & Cech, J. D. (2016). Efficacy of a new multifunctional surfactant-based biomaterial dressing with 1% silver sulfadiazine in chronic wounds. *International Wound Journal, 13*(5), 738–743.

QUESTIONS

1. Which statement accurately describes the relationship between skin and microorganisms?
A. The dry keratinized cells on the surface create a physical barrier to penetration by microorganisms.
B. The keratinocytes bind and inactivate pathogens.
C. The normally alkalinic pH produced by the production of sebum by the sebaceous glands creates a hostile environment to microbial growth.
D. Sweat promotes microorganism growth due to its low pH and high sodium concentrations.

2. The wound care nurse assesses a patient for factors that may delay wound healing. Which of the following is a local factor to consider?
A. Poorly controlled diabetes
B. Immunosuppressive drugs
C. Alcohol and/or tobacco use
D. Necrotic tissue or foreign bodies

3. The wound care nurse assessing a patient's wound determines that the wound is infected. What is a clinical indicator of this adverse condition?
A. Reduction of wound dimensions
B. A plateau in the wound's healing trajectory
C. Decreasing wound exudate
D. The continued development of granulation tissue

4. The wound care nurse is reviewing results from a wound culture on an infected pressure injury. Which of the following requires immediate initiation of antibiotic therapy?
A. *Pseudomonas aeruginosa*
B. Beta-hemolytic *Streptococcus*
C. *S. aureus*
D. *Escherichia coli*

5. For which of the following reasons would a wound culture be performed?
A. Determine the stage of healing.
B. Refer the patient for surgical debridement.
C. Determine the type of antibiotic to be used.
D. Determine the wound dressing to be used.

6. The wound care nurse is obtaining a wound culture using the swab technique. When performing this technique, the practitioner would:
A. Saturate the swab with purulent fluid
B. Cleanse the wound with antimicrobial cleanser prior to obtaining the culture.
C. Move the swab in a circular pattern around the perimeter of the wound.
D. Identify a 1-square cm area of wound free from necrotic tissue to obtain swab specimen.

7. The wound care nurse is assessing wound culture results. Which statement accurately describes a possible finding and its relevancy?
A. Only biofilm communities are typically detected by standard culture techniques; detection of planktonic bacterial requires additional samples.
B. A high percentage of all the bacterial species that are present in a chronic wound bed are typically detected by standard aerobic agar plating techniques.
C. Bacteria are identified by growing bacterial cultures in the lab using the DNA from the bacteria itself.
D. The MIC identifies the lowest concentration of an antibiotic that inhibits or reduces bacterial growth.

8. For which condition does the probe to bone test have a high negative predictive value for osteomyelitis?
A. Deep nonhealing pressure injuries
B. Diabetic foot ulcers
C. Brain tumors
D. Cancer of the long bones in children

9. The wound care nurse is planning care for a patient with a stage 2 pressure injury. What principle of wound cleansing would the nurse incorporate into the plan?
A. Wounds should be cleansed before debridement but not after debridement.
B. Wounds should be cleansed with antimicrobial cleanser if the wound is accidentally contaminated.
C. Wounds should be cleansed at each dressing change with a nonirritating, nontoxic solution.
D. For most clinical situations, wound cleansing has been replaced by wound disinfection.

10. The wound care nurse is using methylene blue/gentian violet–impregnated foam as a wound filler. What is the *unique* advantage of this line of products?
A. Compatibility with enzymatic agents containing collagenase
B. Antimicrobial effects
C. Increased inflammatory response due to released toxins in wound bed
D. Physically binding and removing bacteria as opposed to killing them

ANSWERS AND RATIONALES

1. A. Rationale: Specific ways in which the skin protects against bacterial invasion include the dry keratinized cells on the surface create a physical barrier to penetration by microorganisms.

2. D. Rationale: Necrotic tissue provides a medium for bacterial growth and must be debrided.

3. B. Rationale: An obvious sign of local infection is a plateau in the wound's healing trajectory, evidenced by minimal or no reduction in wound dimensions or by a sudden unexplained increase in wound size.

4. B. Rationale: The presence of one virulent beta-hemolytic *Streptococcus* should be considered significant and appropriate treatment initiated.

5. C. Rationale: Wound cultures are used to confirm or modify the plan for treatment when antibiotic therapy is indicated.

6. D. Rationale: The Levine technique involves thoroughly cleansing the wound surface with saline and identifying a 1-cm area of the wound that is free from necrotic tissue. The swab is rotated while applying pressure sufficient to express fluid from the wound tissue.

7. D. Rationale: The MIC identifies the lowest concentration of the antibiotic tested, which resulted in inhibition or reduction of the inoculums. As a general rule, the lower the MIC, the more effective the antibiotic.

8. B. Rationale: The probe to bone test (PTB) has high negative predictive value for osteomyelitis in foot wounds. This test can be used to rule out osteomyelitis.

9. C. Rationale: All wounds should be cleansed at each dressing change, before and after debridement, and in the event of contamination using a neutral, nonirritating, nontoxic solution.

10. A. Rationale: One advantage of gentian violet and methylene blue dressings is compatibility with collagenase.

CHAPTER 12

REFRACTORY WOUNDS: ASSESSMENT AND MANAGEMENT

Debra Netsch

OBJECTIVES

1. Use data from serial wound assessments to identify wound deterioration or failure to progress.

2. Discuss potential causes for failure to heal and implications for assessment and management.

3. Identify indications and guidelines for use of adjunctive therapies, referrals for further evaluation, or medical–surgical intervention.

4. Describe mechanism of action, indications and contraindications, and guidelines for use of each of the following: MMP inhibitors; matrix dressings; growth factors; bioengineered/biologic dressings; negative pressure wound therapy (NPWT); and flaps and grafts.

TOPIC OUTLINE

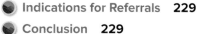 **Indications for Referrals   229**

Conclusion   229

INTRODUCTION

Throughout this text, the following pathway has been described for effective wound management: (1) identification and correction of etiologic factors; (2) systemic support for healing; and (3) evidence-based and individualized topical therapy. The majority of wounds heal when this pathway is followed consistently. A significant minority will plateau. This chapter will cover the assessment and management of these refractory wounds, with a focus on active wound therapies.

REFRACTORY WOUNDS

Wound healing is a complex interactive process with an anticipated sequence of events. Acute wounds in healthy individuals heal in a timely predictable manner, and healing results in durable closure. Chronic wounds occur when this predictable sequence of events is interrupted. The term refractory or recalcitrant wound describes a chronic nonhealing or difficult-to-manage wound that does not progress toward healing or is stagnant (Moore et al., 2006; Rolstad & Nix, 2007; Zhao et al., 2016). Chronic or refractory wound terminology also applies to a frequently recurrent wound. The wound fails to heal in a timely manner or recurs despite appropriate management (Fonder et al., 2008; Gray & Ratliff, 2006; Lazarus et al., 1994). The Wound Healing Society (WHS) defines a recalcitrant wound as one that fails to proceed through an orderly and timely process to produce anatomical and functional integrity or proceeded through the repair process without establishing a sustained anatomic and functional result (WHS, 2006). The term refractory or nonhealing

wound will be used throughout this chapter to avoid confusion.

> **KEY POINT**
>
> Acute wounds in healthy individuals heal in a timely predictable manner, with durable closure—chronic wounds occur when this predictable sequence of events is interrupted.

DEFINITION OF REFRACTORY WOUND

A significant minority of chronic wounds do not respond normally to treatment. A wound is considered refractory if there has not been improvement within 2 to 4 weeks of comprehensive evidence-based therapy or there is no expected and predicted reduction in size of the wound in an established period of time, for example, 50% reduction in size of diabetic neuropathic ulcers in 4 weeks; 40% reduction in size of venous ulcers in 3 weeks (Doughty & Sparks, 2016; Li et al., 2007; WOCN, 2019). Wound size and duration are predictive factors for wound healing outcomes and wound healing time. Data indicate that the percentage of healing at 3 to 4 weeks is a good predictor of healing outcomes (Rolstad & Nix, 2007; Sussman & Bates-Jensen, 2012)

> **KEY POINT**
>
> A wound is considered refractory if there has not been improvement within 2 to 4 weeks of comprehensive evidence-based therapy, or there is not the expected and predicted reduction in wound size within an established period of time.

Refractory wounds represent a significant worldwide health problem, afflicting approximately 5 to 7 million per year in the United States (U.S.) alone. The physical and psychological burden is substantial. Individuals with non-healing wounds experience significant morbidity and even mortality related to wound infections and amputations and have a negative effect on quality of life (Asadi et al., 2014). There is substantial financial impact. The estimated annual cost of care is $20 billion, with additional costs related to treatment of complications, missed work, and assisted living and long-term care (Asadi et al., 2014; Samson et al., 2004).

Refractory wounds are most commonly those that develop as a result of a chronic condition. Ninety percent of all nonhealing wounds are classified as venous ulcers, arterial ulcers, diabetic neuropathic ulcers, or pressure injuries. Refractory wounds are often multifactorial in nature.

FACTORS RESULTING IN NONHEALING WOUNDS

Effective management of a nonhealing wound begins with identification and correction of the factors impairing or delaying repair. These factors fall into four broad categories: inability or failure to correct etiologic factors, imbalance in one or more of the multiple systemic factors affecting repair, local factors delaying or preventing repair, and imbalance in the molecular environment governing the repair process. Patient adherence factors can adversely affect all aspects of management. Patient adherence is important for correction or amelioration of causative factors (e.g., offloading), to systemic support for wound healing (e.g., tight glycemic control or smoking cessation), and to topical wound care. Etiologic factors have been controlled, both systemic and local wound conditions have been established that support repair, but the wound fails to heal. The reason for failure to heal is thought to be an imbalance in the molecular environment and structures controlling the repair process.

> **KEY POINT**
>
> Ninety percent of all nonhealing wounds are classified as venous ulcers, arterial ulcers, diabetic neuropathic ulcers, or pressure injuries.

Inability or Failure to Correct Etiologic Factors

Chronic wounds can be examined by contrasting normal healing and the inflammatory response created by chronic wounds such as hypoxia, ischemia-reperfusion injury, and bacterial colonization (Zhao et al., 2016). The wound fails to heal because the cycle of injury has not been effectively interrupted. Examples include inconsistent offloading of a plantar surface neuropathic ulcer or pressure injury, or nonadherence to compression and elevation for a venous ulcer. The wound care nurse must reevaluate the wound and the management plan to assure accurate identification and treatment of the causative factors. A biopsy should be done whenever the wound is nonhealing and the reason for failure to heal is not clear (IWII, 2016).

> **KEY POINT**
>
> A biopsy should be obtained when a wound is nonhealing and the reasons for failure to heal are not clear.

Imbalance in Systemic Factors Affecting Repair

Systemic factors affecting repair can be divided into intrinsic and extrinsic factors. Each of the common factors will be briefly discussed here and is addressed in greater depth in other chapters (**Fig. 12-1**).

Intrinsic Factors

Intrinsic (systemic) factors are the patient's comorbidities and physiologic conditions impacting wound healing. These include advanced age, poor nutritional status,

---

Intrinsic	Extrinsic	Latrogenic	Adherence
• Age • Chronic disease • Perfusion & oxygenation • Immunosuppression • Neurologically impaired skin	• Medications • Nutrition • Irradiation & chemotherapy • Psychophysiologic stress • Wound bioburden & infection	• Local ischemia • Inappropriate wound care • Trauma • Wound extent & duration	• Psychosocial issues • Financial impact • Life commitments • Comprehension • Accessibility • Differing goals

FIGURE 12-1. Cofactors Impacting Nonhealing. (Modified from Sussman, C., & Bates-Jensen, B. (2012). Wound healing physiology: Acute and chronic. In C. Sussman, & B. Bates-Jensen (Eds.), *Wound care: A collaborative practice manual for health professionals* (4th ed.). Baltimore, MD: Lippincott Williams & Wilkins, Table 2-5, p. 43; Additional information: Nix, D., & Peirce, B. (2012). Noncompliance, nonadherence, or barriers to a sustainable plan? In R. Bryant & D. Nix (Eds.), *Acute & chronic wounds: Current management concepts* (4th ed., pp. 408–415). St Louis, MO: Elsevier-Mosby; Rolstad, B., & Nix, D. (2007). Management of wound recalcitrance and deterioration. In D. L. Krasner, G. T. Rodeheaver, & R. G. Sibbald (Eds.). *Chronic wound care: A clinical source book for healthcare professionals* (4th ed., pp. 743–750). Malvern, PA: HMP Communications.)

chronic diseases (such as diabetes and renal disease), immunosuppression, reduced perfusion and oxygenation, and neurologically impaired skin.

Age

The elderly are at increased risk of skin injury due to thinning of the epidermis, reduced barrier function, and dermal atrophy. The elderly are also at risk for impaired healing. The negative effects of aging are compounded by the comorbidities that are seen in the elderly. The diminished proliferative process includes a delayed cellular response to injury, delayed collagen deposition, and reduced tensile strength. The aging process implies physiological changes in tissues and systems. The pathological changes in blood vessels have an effect on refractory wounds. Mechanisms proposed as underlying causes of the age-related impairment of angiogenesis, such as the production of growth factors (GFs) and nitric oxide reduction, the number and function of endothelial or progenitor cells decrease, changes in microenvironment (extracellular matrix [ECM], pH, etc.), and cellular senescence (Cheng & Fu, 2018). Exercise has been shown to enhance impaired angiogenesis in the elderly through a variety of mechanisms (Cheng & Fu, 2018).

The increased prevalence of chronic disease among the elderly contributes to recognition of age as a cofactor for impaired healing. For additional information on geriatric population, see Chapter 14.

Chronic Disease

Chronic diseases involving the cardiopulmonary system adversely affect the oxygen transport pathway, reducing delivery of oxygen to the tissues and removal of carbon dioxide, both of which are required for healing. Diabetic ulcers, pressure injuries, and arterial ulcers are an impairment of angiogenic processes, and the subsequent pathological remodeling of the microcirculation contributes to compromised tissue perfusion (Cheng & Fu, 2018).

Persons with diabetes are also at risk for impaired healing. Biochemical abnormalities may accelerate neuropathy and vascular foot changes, including hyperglycemia that inhibits the production and activation of endothelial nitric oxide synthase and the reaction of protein with sugars (Malllard reaction) that is linked to diabetic complications. Diabetic foot ulcers (DFUs) are caused by neuropathy, ischemia, or both. The pathophysiology of DFUs requires an appreciation of the role of contributory factors, including peripheral neuropathy, vascular disease, and inflammatory cytokines and the susceptibility to infection (Alavi et al., 2014).

High glucose levels impair leukocyte function, increasing the risk of infection, and have a negative impact on collagen synthesis, tensile strength, and keratinocyte migration. Growth factors and growth factor receptor sites appear to be reduced. Microvascular and neuropathic disease are common, and both negatively impact healing.

Perfusion and Oxygenation

Adequate perfusion and oxygenation are essential for wound healing. Inadequate perfusion results in failure to heal, and perfusion and oxygenation are compromised by many chronic disease processes, including cardiovascular, pulmonary, and renal diseases. Any condition causing hypovolemia reduces transportation of oxygen and nutrients to the tissues and removal of waste products, and prolonged hypovolemia impairs collagen production and compromises leukocyte function. Overcorrection of hypovolemia can lead to cardiac overload, which further reduces perfusion and oxygenation (Doughty & Sparks, 2016; Stotts et al., 2014; Sussman & Bates-Jensen, 2012).

Immunosuppression

Patients with immunosuppressive conditions (e.g., patients with cancer, human immunodeficiency virus [HIV] infection, and diabetes and those undergoing corticosteroid therapy or chemotherapy) are at risk for poor wound healing due to impairment of the initial inflammatory response required for healing (Doughty & Sparks, 2016; Sussman & Bates-Jensen, 2012).

Neurological Impairment

Patients with spinal cord injuries are known to have delayed healing below the level of the injury, due to changes in perfusion and persistent inflammation, among other factors (see Chapter 16). These individuals are high risk for pressure injury development due to sensory loss, immobility, and altered weight bearing (Doughty & Sparks, 2016; Sussman & Bates-Jensen, 2012). Other types of neurological impairment also place individuals at high risk of ulcer development with peripheral neuropathy contributing to development of 70% of all foot ulcers and 78% of DFUs (WOCN, 2012).

Extrinsic Factors

Extrinsic factors include external or environmental sources that disrupt the wound healing process. These extrinsic factors include medications, malnutrition, radiation and chemotherapy, psychophysiologic stress, and wound bioburden and infection.

Medications

Many individuals with chronic wounds take multiple medications to treat chronic conditions. Some of these medications negatively impact wound healing. For example, platelet activation is a critical first step along the wound healing pathway and can be disrupted by anticoagulant medications (warfarin, heparin, etc.), antiplatelet medications (clopidogrel, salicylates, aspirin, etc.), and nonsteroidal anti-inflammatory medications (cyclooxygenase-2 [COX-2] inhibitors, ibuprofen, naproxen, etc.). Steroids are another class of medications that adversely affect all phases of wound healing. Many other medication classes also disrupt wound healing including immunosuppressive agents, antiprostaglandins, and opioids including morphine (Karukonda et al., 2000; Martin et al., 2010)..

KEY POINT

Many medications have the unintended effect of impairing wound healing. Medications with an adverse effect on repair include anticoagulants, antiplatelets, anti-inflammatory agents, steroids, chemotherapeutic agents, antiprostaglandins, and opioids.

Nutrition

Malnutrition, especially protein and calorie malnutrition, is well known to alter wound healing. Micronutrient deficiencies can also adversely affect repair. Nutritional management must include attention to both macronutrient and micronutrient intake along with adequate calories for wound repair. (See Chapter 7.)

Radiation Therapy and Chemotherapy

Radiation therapy interferes with wound healing for years after treatment, due to persistent damage to the vessels and the proliferative cells (fibroblasts) in the treatment area. The end result of radiation therapy is tissue ischemia and compromised proliferative processes in the irradiated field. Chemotherapy interrupts the cell cycle for proliferative cells, profoundly and adversely affecting the tissue repair process. The severity and duration of the negative impact of chemotherapy depends on the dose and duration of therapy. The wound care goal for a patient receiving radiation or chemotherapy is maintenance until therapy is complete. (See Chapter 31.)

Psychophysiologic Stress

Stress and depression release hormones that negatively affect immune function. Cortisol levels are increased during times of stress, and cortisol is known to adversely affect cytokine production and fibroblast proliferation. Cortisol is also associated with increased matrix degradation. Cortisol can disrupt the growth hormone–somatomedin system, contributing to poor healing outcomes. Stress management strategies such as biofeedback, sleep, positive imagery, hypnosis, and exercise have all been associated with improved healing outcomes (Doughty & Sparks, 2016; Stotts et al., 2014; Sussman & Bates-Jensen, 2012).

Wound Bioburden and Infection

Bioburden is the degree or load of microorganisms (e.g., bacteria, virus, fungi) that create contamination in a wound. The degree of bioburden is influenced by the quantity and virulence of microbes (IWII, 2016). Wound infection is the invasion of proliferating microorganisms in a wound to a level that causes a local or systemic response in the host (IWII, 2016). Biofilms are complex microbial communities. They are usually polymicrobial, containing multiple species of bacteria and fungi (IWII, 2016).

Bacteria in the wound compete with fibroblasts for the nutrients and oxygen essential to ECM formation. Bioburden can result in biofilm formation, which further impairs healing and increases the risk for infection. Osteomyelitis is another infection-related cause of refractory wounds. Effective wound management must include ongoing assessment and management of bioburden, and antimicrobial dressings are often used as a first step intervention for a poorly healing or plateaued wound and referral for MRI and bone biopsy may be necessary when bone is probed or visible in the wound (Gray & Ratliff, 2006; IWII, 2016; Stotts et al., 2014; Sussman & Bates-Jensen, 2012). (See Chapters 8 and 11 for wound healing principles and infection.)

KEY POINT

Antimicrobial dressings are often used as a first step intervention for a poorly healing or plateaued wound.

IATROGENIC FACTORS PREVENTING REPAIR

Iatrogenic factors are treatment-related factors that compromise wound healing, such as inappropriate wound care and trauma to the wound bed.

Local Ischemia

Local ischemia occurs inadvertently with inappropriate application of compression wraps, total contact casts and failure to identify offloading equipment used inappropriately.

Inappropriate Wound Care

Appropriate wound management and topical therapy requires appropriate wound etiology with clear understanding of the wound healing process and available products and appropriate utilization of dressings and therapies to promote repair. The goal is to establish and maintain a clean moist wound bed. Products that are appropriate for highly exudative wounds would be very inappropriate for minimally exudative wounds. Inappropriate topical therapy can lead to disruption of the wound healing trajectory. Misuse of topical antiseptics can lead to cytotoxicity, and either overhydration or desiccation of the wound bed compromises function of the cells essential to repair.

Trauma

Trauma to the wound bed and periwound area occurs frequently due to inappropriate approaches to wound debridement, improper removal of dressings, or excessively high-pressure irrigation. Trauma impedes wound healing and leads to increased susceptibility for wound infection.

ADHERENCE FACTORS

Factors affecting patient adherence to the wound treatment plan include more than the presence or lack of motivation. Many aspects of living with a chronic wound impact the patient's ability to actively and effectively contribute to the management plan, including psychosocial issues, financial impact, life commitments, comprehension, accessibility to care, and ability to carry out critical aspects of care. Effective wound outcomes require a patient-centered approach and the ability to collaborate with the patient and caregivers to establish and modify the wound management plan based on wound status and patient concerns and priorities. Adherence is related to the ability of the person with the wound to participate in and carry out the treatment plan (Miller, 2016). Adherence can be achieved only when the individual is an active participant in formulating the plan of care in a safe open environment.

KEY POINT

Effective wound outcomes require a patient-centered approach and the ability to collaborate with the patient and caregivers to establish and modify the wound management plan based on wound status and patient concerns and priorities.

Financial Impact

Management of refractory wounds has a negative financial impact that is both societal and personal. Missed work, product costs, medication costs, and the impact of underinsurance or lack of insurance all impact the ability to provide or obtain proper wound management.

Life Commitments

Life commitments such as caring for family members, household chores, attending family functions, and providing for the family may result in competing priorities that disrupt the treatment plan.

Comprehension

Comprehension of the treatment plan, including causative and corrective factors and the consequences of adherence or nonadherence on healing, is one of the factors most critical to adherence. The wound care nurse must consistently work with the patient and family to assure that they understand treatment options and the impact of adherence or nonadherence on outcomes. Factors impacting comprehension include the patient's and family's ability to learn and comprehend and the wound nurse's ability to explain at a level the patient and family can understand (DiMatteo, 2004). Patient adherence is primarily determined by their perception

of the benefits and disadvantages of the behaviors they are being asked to adopt. The level of comprehension needs to be reassessed at each visit.

Psychosocial Aspects

Psychosocial aspects including beliefs, attitudes, expectations, and cultural issues are factors that affect adherence and that may necessitate adjustments to the management plan.

Accessibility and Ability

The availability and accessibility of wound care products and wound care expertise have an impact on adherence. The wound care nurse must be holistic in the approach to wound care and assist the patient to obtain the necessary supplies and access to care.

Differing Goals

Goal setting is important to adherence. Healing is not always the appropriate goal. When healing is the goal, it is important to clearly identify interventions that are the responsibility of the health care team (e.g., selection of appropriate wound therapies) and interventions that are the responsibility of the patient and caregivers (e.g., pressure relief/offloading and tight glycemic control). Once an appropriate goal has been established and agreed upon, guidelines can be established. The establishment of the goal and care plan related to wound care is important to patient and caregiver adherence (Nix et al., 2016; Rolstad & Nix, 2007).

Imbalance in Molecular Microenvironment

There are significant differences in the molecular environment of healing wounds as opposed to nonhealing wounds. Normal wound healing is characterized by a balanced interaction among inflammatory and proliferative factors and by steady progression of the wound through the repair process, whereas chronic wounds are characterized by a proinflammatory environment and failure of the wound to progress normally. Chronic wounds exhibit a high level of matrix metalloproteases (MMPs), which degrade the matrix proteins and growth factors necessary for healing (**Table 12-1**). Nonhealing wounds frequently have high numbers of proliferative cells such as fibroblasts that are senescent. These cells are unable to reproduce and less able to contribute to repair (Doughty & Sparks, 2016; Harding et al., 2005; Lobmann et al., 2005).

KEY POINT

Chronic wounds are characterized by a proinflammatory environment that contributes to failure to heal.

With normal repair, the ECM provides a scaffold for migrating cells and stores the growth factors controlling

TABLE 12-1 CHARACTERISTICS OF ACUTE VERSUS CHRONIC WOUNDS

CHARACTERISTICS	HEALING WOUNDS	CHRONIC WOUNDS
Proliferative cellular activity	High	Low
Inflammatory cytokines	Low	High
Protease levels	Low	High
Growth factors	High	Low
Cell response to growth factors	Mitotically competent	Senescent

Compiled from Doughty, D., & Sparks-DeFriese, B. (2012). Wound-healing physiology. In R. Bryant & D. Nix (Eds.), *Acute & chronic wounds: Current management concepts* (5th ed., pp. 63–82). St Louis, MO: Elsevier-Mosby; Lobmann, R., Schultz, G., & Lehnert, H. (2005). Proteases and the diabetic foot syndrome: Mechanisms & therapeutic implications. *Diabetes Care, 28*(2), 462–471.

the repair process. An ECM is required for cell attachment and migration and for neoangiogenesis and collagen synthesis and epithelial resurfacing. The high concentrations of proteases (MMPs) to tissue inhibitors of matrix metalloproteases (TIMPs) in chronic wounds may contribute to ECM destruction and to degradation of growth factors and growth factor receptors (Caley et al., 2015). While the high levels of proteases are a characteristic of chronic wounds, it is unknown whether the imbalance in inflammatory and proliferative factors is the causative factor for wound chronicity or the result of chronicity (Vowden, 2011).

KEY POINT

While the high levels of proteases are a characteristic of chronic wounds, it is unknown whether the imbalance in inflammatory and proliferative factors is the causative factor for wound chronicity or the result of chronicity.

 ASSESSMENT OF THE NONHEALING WOUND

To manage a nonhealing wound, the wound care nurse provides serial wound assessments to detect a plateau or deterioration in the wound. A wound that deteriorates or fails to demonstrate measurable progress in 2 to 4 weeks despite appropriate care is considered to be refractory. Deterioration is typically identified faster, while failure to progress (a plateau) is more insidious and may be overlooked. Iatrogenic factors such as lack of follow-up, multiple different providers, inconsistent documentation, or insufficient understanding of wound healing, and wound care may contribute to delayed recognition of a refractory wound (Bryant & Nix, 2016; Rolstad & Nix, 2007).

Lack of progress or deterioration should prompt a reassessment of the patient, wound, and management plan to assure that there is no undiagnosed pathology or inappropriately managed or new cofactors. These wounds may have been previously evaluated and treated with a narrow focus on the wound alone. A thorough history and physical assessment are key in

distinguishing whether the wound deterioration or plateau is the result of (1) misdiagnosis, (2) uncontrolled associated cofactors, (3) inappropriate wound management, or (4) any combination of these (Han & Ceilley, 2017; Harding, 2000; Rolstad & Nix, 2007). Any gaps in the management plan should be promptly corrected.

KEY POINT

Failure of a wound to progress or sudden deterioration should prompt a reassessment of the patient, wound, and management plan to rule out undiagnosed pathology, inadequately managed cofactors, or inappropriate wound management.

 MANAGEMENT OF THE NONHEALING WOUND

Correction of all known etiologic and contributing factors may be insufficient to correct a negative healing trajectory for a chronic wound. The wound may remain refractory despite best efforts due to changes in the microenvironment that create chronicity and prevent repair. In this case, the focus of topical therapy will need to shift from passive support for wound healing to active management of the stalled repair process.

PATHWAY FOR MANAGEMENT

Refractory wound management presents a clinical challenge. The three principles of wound care are to: (1) control or eliminate causative factors, (2) support the host to reduce existing and potential cofactors, and (3) optimize the microwound environment or physiologic wound environment (Rolstad et al., 2012).

Control or Elimination of Causative Factors

A first step in effective wound management is accurate identification and correction of the causative factors. For example, a venous ulcer requires compression and/or elevation to control the underlying venous insufficiency in addition to topical therapy to provide moisture balance; topical therapy alone will not promote healing. Management of etiologic factors requires accurate diagnosis on the part of the provider and patient adherence to the prescribed management plan.

Identification and correction of etiologic factors is not easy, and misdiagnosis of primary etiology or contributing cofactors may occur. A systematic approach to wound care is promoted by the use of evidence-based guidelines and algorithms such as those created by the Wound Ostomy Continence Nurses Society (WOCN). These guidelines are specific to the type of wound. The wound care nurse must determine wound etiology, contributing comorbid conditions, and topical wound care using evidence-based guidelines. If a wound is diagnosed as a venous ulcer, then the guidelines pertaining to venous ulcers are instituted. When the ulcer is not responding according to anticipated time frames or normal sequence of healing, then the wound care nurse should reassess the cause or etiology and cofactors. Even if the primary etiology has been accurately identified, a wound care nurse may miss significant confounding factors such as medications. There are case studies where failure to heal a venous ulcer was due to medication (hydroxyurea) prescribed for treatment of polycythemia vera. Once the hematologist discontinued or changed the medication, the wound healed quickly. The first step in management of a refractory wound is reassessment of etiologic and contributing factors by a multidisciplinary team (Rolstad & Nix, 2007; Stotts et al., 2014).

Biopsy

A biopsy is indicated when a wound fails to heal and the reasons are unclear. A Marjolin's ulcer is a rare, aggressive skin cancer developing in scar tissue, chronic ulcers, and areas affected by inflammation. Its incidence is estimated to range from 1% to 2% of all burn scars. It frequently takes the form of squamous cell carcinoma (Bazaliński et al., 2017). A Marjolin ulcer exemplifies transformation from a chronic wound to a malignancy. Malignant transformation occurs in 1.7% of chronic wounds, and refractory wounds are at high risk for transformation to malignancy. Any suspicion of malignant transformation necessitates biopsy at multiple sites and depths of the wound. Re-biopsy is warranted if the wound does not respond to appropriate treatment (Bryant, 2016). The WOCN Pressure Ulcer/Injury guideline recommends a biopsy for histology if the injury fails to heal and the wound base has changes inconsistent with the patient's overall condition (WOCN, 2016).

KEY POINT

Chronic wounds can transform into a malignant wound. A biopsy should always be obtained when a wound fails to progress despite appropriate management.

Goal Verification/Adherence Factors

Mutual goal setting requires open communication with the patient as the center of the care plan. An exemplar of mutual goal setting would be a paraplegic patient with an ischial pressure injury. The wound care nurse may be focused on wound healing, while the patient's primary goal may be to remain active, up in the wheelchair, and enjoying life. The goals are misaligned. Many providers would consider this nonadherence, but the issue is failure to communicate and to come to agree upon goals with the patient (Nix et al., 2016).

Systemic Support for Healing

Wound healing involves all of the body's major systems. Support of the host is important to optimize treatment outcomes. Dressings alone will not heal the wound without support of the host and management of cofactors. Glycemic control, nutritional management, adequate hydration, edema reduction, adequate perfusion, and control of comorbidities are aspects of systemic support that are critical to positive outcomes. Support for the host seems logical but is difficult if cofactors are not identified or if management of comorbid conditions conflicts with goals of wound care. For example, wound healing requires adequate protein intake, but low-protein diets are a key management factor for patients in renal failure, requiring referral to a registered dietitian nutritionist (RDN) to optimize systemic support for healing. Another common situation is the need for chronic systemic steroid use. While the steroid is necessary to control the comorbidity impacting healing, the steroid interferes with the inflammatory response and decreases proliferation of keratinocytes and fibroblasts with some reversal of these factors by use of topical vitamin A (Doughty & Sparks, 2016).

Optimal Local Wound Care

Topical management or wound bed preparation is achieved through topical therapy (wound cleansing and dressing selection), with the goal of establishing a physiologic wound environment that supports healing. The key characteristics of the physiologic wound environment are adequate moisture balance, temperature control, pH regulation, and control of bioburden. The acronym of TIME (Tissue management, Inflammation and infection control, Moisture balance, Epithelial [edge] advancement) provides a quick reference to the key principles of wound bed preparation and a guideline for assessment of wound management and wound status (Atkin et al., 2019; Leaper et al., 2012; Schultz et al., 2003; Sibbald et al., 2011).

ACTIVE WOUND THERAPIES

Approaches to refractory wound management have been and continue to be developed (active wound therapies) to improve treatment outcomes. Active wound therapies are designed to correct the molecular imbalances characteristic of the refractory wound and to actively stimulate the repair process (Asadi et al., 2014).

Active wound therapies are indicated for refractory wounds and are not indicated for routine management of an appropriately healing wound. The criteria for implementation of active wound therapies have not been well defined. Their use is well established in wounds that have plateaued or deteriorated despite appropriate comprehensive therapy when the goal is healing. Selected therapies may also be utilized for wounds that are very unlikely to heal in a timely manner with routine care (**Fig. 12-2**) (Houghton & Campbell, 2012; Trovato et al., 2012).

Appropriate use of active wound therapies requires the wound care nurse to understand the mechanisms of action, indications, and contraindications for each of the therapies. Additional issues to be addressed include reimbursement guidelines, qualifications of the provider providing the active wound therapy, and availability of the product or therapy (Houghton & Campbell, 2012).

Each of the currently available active wound therapies will be briefly discussed in terms of mechanism of action, guidelines for use, and current evidence base.

MMP Inhibitors

There are several dressings available that act to reduce the levels of MMPs in the wound bed.

Mechanism of Action

MMPs are essential in all phases of normal wound healing and comprise a large and diverse group of molecules, some of which are proinflammatory and some of which support proliferation and oppose inflammation. The proinflammatory MMPs are particularly important during the inflammatory and remodeling phases of repair because they act as natural enzymes to support the breakdown of necrotic tissue. Normal wound healing is characterized by high levels of these proinflammatory MMPs during early inflammation with a marked reduction in levels as the wound transitions out of the inflammatory phase and into the proliferative phase. Chronic wounds are characterized by persistent high levels of MMPs and persistent inflammation despite the absence of necrotic tissue or infection. Elevated levels of MMP proteases and reduced levels of MMP inhibitors create or contribute to the imbalance found in chronic wounds. The topical application of dressings that provide MMP inhibitors in high concentrations has been shown to reduce the levels of MMPs in the wound bed. The MMPs are attracted to and bound by the ORC (oxidized regenerated cellulose). There are also dressings available that act to down-regulate production of MMPs (Klein, 2020). Once point-of-care testing for elevated protease levels becomes available, the wound care nurse will be able to make better informed decisions regarding use of these dressings. Use of dressings that modulate MMP activity

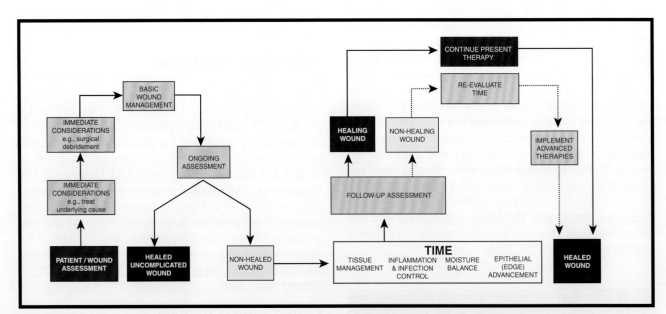

FIGURE 12-2. Decision Tree for Wound Management and Implementation of Advanced Therapies. (Reprinted with permission from European Wound Management Association (EWMA). (2004). *Position Document: Wound bed preparation in practice* (p. 4). London, United Kingdom: MEP Ltd. http://ewma.org/fileadmin/user_upload/EWMA/pdf/Position_Documents/2004/pos_doc_English_final_04.pdf. Copyright © Medical Education Partnership Ltd., 2004. All rights reserved.)

is a reasonable first step in the management of a non-healing wound.

KEY POINT

Once point-of-care testing for elevated protease levels becomes available, the wound care nurse will be able to make better informed decisions regarding use of these dressings. Until then, use of dressings that modulate MMP activity is a very reasonable first step in the management of a non-healing wound

Guidelines for Use

The wound should be cleansed, and the dressing should then be applied to the viable wound bed. If the wound bed is dry, the dressing should be moistened with a small amount of saline. An appropriate secondary dressing should then be applied. Dressing change frequency is based on volume of exudate but is typically every 2 to 3 days (Klein, 2020).

Current Evidence

Klein (2020) reported that treatment with a protease inhibitor dressing significantly reduced elastase and plasmin activity in the wound bed. Lobmann and colleagues (2005) found that use of these dressings was associated with increased numbers of healed ulcers and reduced time to healing in patients with DFUs and venous ulcers (Lobmann et al., 2005). Many randomized controlled trials (RCTs) have been done that show significant improvement in healing rates with use of these dressings for venous ulcers, diabetic ulcers, and pressure injuries (Klein, 2020; Westby et al., 2018).

Cost Considerations

These dressings are more expensive than standard moisture retentive dressings, but much less costly than other active wound therapies. For many patients, the cost of the dressing may be covered by insurance. Consideration should be given to the benefit versus cost, but the wound care nurse should remember that, when the goal is healing, it is much more cost-effective to use a more expensive therapy that promotes repair than to use a less expensive therapy that does not promote healing.

Matrix Dressings (Acellular Scaffold Dressings)

Acellular products (ECM scaffolds) are nonliving products derived from allogeneic, xenographic, biosynthetic, or synthetic materials. Because there are no living cells, these products do not cause an antigen–antibody response.

Mechanism of Action

A healthy wound bed is required for healing because the cells responsible for repair (e.g., fibroblasts and keratinocytes) must be able to attach to the wound bed in order to migrate and carry out repair processes. When the existing wound bed does not support attachment and migration, wound healing does not occur. Use of ECM dressings is postulated to provide a scaffold for attachment and migration of host cells (keratinocytes, fibroblasts, and endothelial cells), supporting neoangiogenesis, collagen synthesis, and reepithelialization. As the new ECM is developed, the matrix dressing undergoes controlled degradation (Capito et al., 2012; Cazzell et al., 2017).

KEY POINT

Matrix dressings provide a scaffold for migration and attachment of fibroblasts, endothelial cells, and keratinocytes, supporting granulation tissue formation and epithelial resurfacing.

Guidelines for Use

All measures to address etiologic factors must be continued as well as measures for systemic support of wound healing. Matrix dressings should be applied to clean, noninfected, debrided wounds. The dressing should be sized slightly larger than the wound and anchored to the wound bed, followed by an appropriate secondary dressing. Matrix dressings can be used for a wide variety of chronic wounds, including pressure injuries, nonhealing surgical wounds, venous leg ulcers, and DFUs (International Consensus, 2010).

Current Evidence

There are multiple ECM dressings available. There is little evidence for use of some of the dressings and RCT evidence supporting the use of others. An RCT of one of the most widely available products showed 55% of 120 patients with venous ulcers healed at 12 weeks compared to 34% in the control group (Cazzell et al., 2017; Mostow et al., 2005).

Cost Consideration

These dressings are more costly than standard moist wound healing products and MMP inhibitors, but less expensive than cellular skin substitutes. There is an application procedure fee that may be covered by insurance. Prior authorization is recommended (Saim et al., 2016; Snyder et al., 2020). The wound care nurse should collaborate with the reimbursement experts in the agency to assure that all documentation and coverage guidelines are being followed.

Cellular- and Tissue-based Products

Cellular skin substitutes contain living cells embedded in a bioabsorbable matrix; selected products may use autologous cells (cells donated by the individual) but most involve allogeneic cells obtained from neonatal foreskin or amniotic membrane, which have limited antigenicity (Sheikh et al., 2014). These skin substitutes can be epidermal, dermal, or bilayer (both the epidermal and dermal layers).

Mechanism of Action

Allogeneic skin substitutes deliver healthy living cells to the chronic wound where they secrete growth factors and ECM proteins to stimulate wound repair because the cells are embedded in a bioabsorbable matrix, and these products also provide a scaffold for migration and attachment of host cells. Dermal skin substitutes can be used on wounds with depth. The bilayered skin substitutes function as a nonsurgical skin graft and are appropriate for use only on shallow or superficial wounds that are well vascularized and free of necrotic tissue and infection (Saim et al., 2016).

KEY POINT

Bioengineered cellular and tissue-based products provide both a scaffold for cell migration and healthy cells to support repair. Cells are typically harvested from neonatal foreskin or amniotic membrane, so there is limited antigenic activity.

Guidelines for Use

These products are intended as adjunct therapy and must be used as one component of a comprehensive wound management program, in conjunction with measures to address wound etiology and systemic support. The specific product must be prepared and applied in strict adherence to the manufacturer's recommendations. Dermal substitutes require thawing according to very specific protocols, with immediate application to the wound bed following thawing. Bilayered tissue-based products may be meshed prior to application to permit drainage of exudate, and it is important to apply the product dermal side down. The tissue-based product is anchored and covered with an appropriate secondary dressing. Frequency of secondary dressing change is based on volume of exudate, frequency of reapplication of the cellular dressing is based on wound status and response, but must be consistent with the manufacturer's recommendation, evidence-based protocols, and third-party reimbursement.

KEY POINT

Bioengineered cellular and tissue-based products are expensive. They must be used according to manufacturers' guidelines to a wound bed that is viable, free of infection, and well perfused.

Current Evidence

Numerous studies are available that address the efficacy of specific skin substitutes in the management of particular wounds. The AHRQ Technology Assessment Program reviewed the evidence behind the 76 commercially available skin substitutes and categorized them based on the Davison-Kotler classification system. Sixty-eight (89%) were categorized as acellular dermal substitutes, mostly replacements from human placental membranes and animal tissue sources. Three systematic reviews and 22 RCTs examined use of 16 distinct skin substitutes, including acellular dermal substitutes, cellular dermal substitutes, and cellular epidermal and dermal substitutes in DFUs, pressure injuries, and venous leg ulcers. All of the skin substitutes evaluated in the RCTs were associated with improved healing outcomes as compared to control groups, which were managed with saline-moistened dressings and petrolatum-impregnated dressings. The strength of the evidence for these studies was reported as low to medium, and most lacked assessment of efficacy. The report suggested that studies need to be better designed (Snyder et al., 2020).

Cost Considerations

Cellular and tissue-based products are expensive, and there may be significant product wasted with each application. It is important to assure that the product selected has demonstrated effectiveness with the type of wound for which it is being used (Samsell et al., 2019). The wound care nurse must assure that the wound bed is ready for the advanced therapy product such as free of necrotic tissue, and infection, and well vascularized. It is important to assure that the patient has the ability to heal from a systemic and etiologic perspective. Guidelines for who can apply the product, treatment time, and response to treatment must be followed. Insurance prior authorization for skin substitutes is recommended (Saim et al., 2016; Snyder et al., 2020).

Growth Factors

Chronic wound fluid has low concentrations of several growth factors, and normal concentrations and combinations of growth factors are known to be essential to repair. It has been postulated that topical application of exogenous growth factors might rectify the growth factor deficiency and promote healing. Initial experience with autologous growth factors obtained by drawing the patient's blood, treating the platelets to cause release of growth factors, and then applying the growth factors to the wound did show promise. There is a commercially available gel with exogenous growth factors produced by recombinant DNA technology; specifically, the B chain of the platelet-derived growth factor (PDGF) gene has been inserted into yeast to produce the growth factor, which is incorporated into a gel. There is a therapy that involves production of platelet-rich plasma gel by drawing and treating the patient's blood to generate the plasma gel. In the future, different combinations and concentrations of growth factors may be applied to different types of chronic wounds at different phases of healing.

Mechanism of Action

The recombinant PDGF has the same mechanisms of action as endogenous PDGF or PDGF in platelet-rich plasma gel. It has the ability to control migration of cells needed for repair through chemoattraction, to promote proliferation of the cells needed for repair, and to stimulate cellular activities required for granulation tissue formation and epithelial migration. The limitation of current growth factor therapy is the fact that it provides only one type of growth factor, when a healing wound is characterized by a constantly changing mix of growth factors and concentrations. The use of recombinant PDGF or platelet-rich plasma gel replicates the growth factors released during the initial phase of healing in an acute wound.

Guidelines for Use

The commercially available growth factor (becaplermin gel) is approved for use only with nonhealing DFUs that are free of necrotic tissue and infection and effectively offloaded. A layer of gel should be applied to the wound base and covered with a saline-moistened gauze. The manufacturer recommends removing the gel after 12 hours and replacing with moist saline gauze. If the wound fails to show measurable progress within 2 weeks or if wound size does not decrease by 30% in 10 weeks, therapy should be discontinued. Platelet-rich plasma gel has been used with a variety of nonhealing wounds, and studies are ongoing to determine wounds most likely to respond to this therapy and best protocols for use.

KEY POINT

The growth factor that is currently available commercially (becaplermin gel) is approved for use only with diabetic foot ulcers that are viable, uninfected, and effectively offloaded.

Precautions and Contraindications

Becaplermin gel is contraindicated in patients with known hypersensitivity to any product components or known neoplasms at the application site. A rash at the application site occurs in 2% of patients treated. Safety in pregnancy has not been determined.

Current Evidence

Multiple clinical studies of DFUs treated with recombinant PDGF showed improved healing rates and reduced time to healing. Smiell and colleagues (1999) reported full healing of wounds treated with PDGF at a rate of 39% higher than those treated with placebo (Lobmann et al., 2005; Smiell et al., 1999; Trovato et al., 2012). A meta-analysis of 21 studies comparing chronic or acute wounds treated with platelet-rich plasma (PRP) to those treated with saline-moistened gauze, Bacitracin, or Vaseline gauze revealed significant reduction in wound area and volume or complete wound closure and reduced incidence of complications such as infection among the wounds treated with PRP (Carter et al., 2011).

Cost Considerations

The recombinant DNA gel product is costly but frequently covered by third-party payers. Significant differences in cost can exist between pharmacies. The platelet-rich plasma therapy is also covered by some third-party payers.

Negative Pressure Wound Therapy

NPWT is one of the most commonly used active wound therapies. It involves filling the wound defect and any tunnels or undermined areas with gauze or foam and then applying subatmospheric negative pressure to the wound through suction at controlled levels. There are a number of different NPWT systems, some of which are gauze based and some of which are foam based. Some are designed for acute care settings, with multiple therapy options including intermittent wound irrigation (NPWTi-d), while others are simple peel and stick systems designed for closed surgical incisions (ciNPWT).

Mechanism of Action

Controlled subatmospheric pressure is utilized to enhance moist wound healing. Primary effects demonstrated in multiple in vivo studies include the following: (1) elimination of chronic wound exudate, which is known to impair healing; (2) maintenance of a moist wound surface; (3) reduction in edema, with resultant improvement in perfusion; (4) macrodeformation described as traction on the sides of the wound, which promotes wound contraction; and (5) microdeformation and mechanical stretch on the cells in the wound bed, which changes cell shape and activates intracellular processes that promote healing. Clinically, these cellular effects are manifested as increased angiogenesis and granulation tissue formation and reduction in bacterial bioburden.

KEY POINT

NPWT works by eliminating edema that improves perfusion and removing exudate while maintaining a moist wound surface, and activating intracellular processes that promote healing through deformation, or stretch.

Guidelines for Use

NPWT is indicated when the goal is wound healing, the wound bed has minimal or no necrotic tissue, and bacterial loads are under control. The NPWTi-d can be used with soft slough in the wound bed. Kim et al. (2014) compared NPWTi-d with standard NPWT and found higher closure rates with NPWTi-d 6 minute or 20-minute dwell time compared with standard NPWT. It must be noted that only specific fluids are approved for instillation. All other elements of care must be continued (control of etiologic factors and systemic support for healing) despite the type of NPWT utilized. Each type of NPWT system has its own nuances and use and application must be consistent with manufacturers' guidelines. The application process usually involves the following: wound cleansing; protection of the periwound skin with a liquid skin protectant and transparent adhesive drape; application of appropriate gauze or foam to the wound bed; application of the transparent adhesive dressing to cover the wound; and application of negative pressure via suction catheters or a negative pressure control pad applied to a cutout area of the cover drape. The negative pressure settings should be individualized for the patient and goals of therapy. Options include intermittent versus continuous suction and varied levels of negative pressure. Faster granulation has been demonstrated when intermittent suction is used as opposed to continuous. Continuous suction may be needed for exudate control and pain management and is the standard of care when negative pressure is used to promote fistula closure. The guidelines for levels of negative suction vary based on the manufacturer. Additional considerations include type of foam to be used (when using a foam-based system) and the potential need for a contact layer to reduce tissue trauma, bleeding, and pain with dressing changes (Rhee et al., 2014). For example, manufacturers providing foam-based systems frequently provide both an open cell reticulated foam (standard care product) and a soft white hydrophilic foam. The open cell foam has been associated not only with faster formation of granulation tissue but also with increased risk of tissue trauma, bleeding, and pain with removal, due to the fact that the tissue becomes adherent to the open cell foam. A contact layer (impregnated porous gauze or silicone adhesive contact layer) can be placed in the wound bed prior to application of the open cell foam. This protects the structures in the wound bed by preventing adherence, without interfering with the negative pressure therapy. Dressings are typically changed every 48 to 72 hours.

KEY POINT

Standard NPWT is indicated when the goal is wound healing, the wound bed is viable (or there is minimal necrotic tissue), and any infection, including osteomyelitis, is being treated.

The wound care nurse must educate staff on the appropriate use of NPWT, troubleshooting guidelines, and the importance of removing the dressing any time therapy cannot be reestablished within a 2-hour time period. The staff must understand that, when suction is lost, there is no mechanism for exudate control. Allowing the dressing to remain in place without suction for exudate control significantly increases the risk of wound infection.

NPWT is intended for short-term use to establish a healthy bed of granulation tissue. Once this goal has been met, most patients can be transitioned to moist wound healing. NPWT should be discontinued when there is a plateau in response or any deterioration.

The most common complications of NPWT are bleeding, pain, tissue trauma and retained foam dressing. The risk of complications can be significantly reduced through use of the hydrophilic foam or a nonadherent contact layer dressing in the base of the wound to prevent tissue adherence.

Contraindications

There are many contraindications to negative pressure therapy, including untreated osteomyelitis, necrotic tissue, exposed blood vessels, exposed organs, nonenteric or unexplored fistulas, and malignancy in the wound. The NPWTi-d has additional contraindications of not being used for sternal or open compartment abdominal wounds. NPWT is also usually contraindicated for use in wounds where the goal of care is comfort or maintenance. The wound care nurse should review manufacturers' guidelines for the system used in their setting and should develop protocols that assure adherence to those guidelines.

Current Evidence

The evidence base for use of NPWT supports efficacy. More research is needed to support the use of NPWTi-d. Many best practice clinical guidelines recommend use of NPWT.

KEY POINT

NPWT should be discontinued when there is a plateau in response or deterioration.

Cost Considerations

NPWT may be cost-effective when considering decreased frequency of dressing changes and enhanced wound healing. Prior authorization from third-party payers is recommended (Gupta et al., 2016; Netsch et al., 2016; Rhee et al., 2014; Smith et al., 2014).

Hyperbaric Oxygen Therapy

Hyperbaric oxygen therapy (HBOT) is the systemic administration of oxygen delivered under pressure (atmospheric pressure >1 atmosphere absolute). The patient is placed in a pressurized chamber and is then administered 100% oxygen.

Mechanism of Action

Normally, almost all oxygen delivered to the tissues is attached to the hemoglobin molecule on the red blood cell. Tissue oxygenation is normally totally dependent on normal perfusion and blood vessels of sufficient patency to permit unimpeded passage of RBCs. Breathing oxygen under pressure significantly increases the amount of oxygen dissolved in the plasma, which provides increased delivery of oxygen to the tissues. Adequate oxygen levels are essential for all phases of healing and for control of bacterial burden. The ability to increase oxygen delivery to the tissues is of potential benefit to patients with compromised perfusion due to vascular disease or prior radiation and to those with complex infections (Gray & Ratliff, 2006).

Guidelines for Use

HBOT should be considered when wound healing is compromised by severe infection or impaired tissue perfusion. The wound care nurse should be aware that HBOT is likely to be of benefit when a wound is ischemic but viable, for example, the patient with peripheral arterial disease and low ABI but a pale viable wound bed. HBOT is not of benefit when the wound is already necrotic, for example, with dry gangrene because it works by delivering oxygenated plasma and necrotic wounds have no plasma flow. HBOT should be considered as adjunct therapy for soft tissue radionecrosis and limb-threatening wounds caused by diabetes and/or vascular insufficiency. HBOT reduces edema by meeting the tissues' oxygen needs, inducing vasoconstriction. This further improves tissue oxygenation. HBOT may contribute to resolution of osteomyelitis by providing increased oxygen to the bone, thus improving leukocyte activity. HBOT may also promote healing of compromised grafts and flaps by reducing edema and improving oxygenation.

KEY POINT

HBOT should be considered when wound healing is compromised by inadequate tissue perfusion or by severe infection.

The wound care nurse should refer patients who may benefit from HBO for evaluation. The HBOT center will evaluate the patient to rule out contraindications and can also conduct preliminary testing to determine probability that the patient will benefit. There are a number of absolute or relative contraindications to HBOT, including advanced lung disease, ear disorders that place the patient at risk for barotrauma, selected medications, malignancy, and severe claustrophobia. Testing to determine likelihood of effectiveness includes an oxygen challenge test; baseline $TcPO_2$ levels are obtained and then repeated following administration of oxygen via nasal cannula or mask, and significant improvement in tissue oxygen levels suggests that HBOT will be of benefit.

Current Evidence

Boykin and Baylis (2007) reported enhanced nitric oxide levels in DFUs following treatment with HBOT, and a systematic review of RCTs involving HBOT revealed improved healing in DFUs in the short term and reduced rates of major amputations for DFUs (Kranke et al., 2015).

In a review by Gray and Ratliff (2006), HBOT was associated with demonstrated benefit in treatment of DFUs; in contrast, HBOT was of no benefit in treatment of pressure injuries and venous ulcers.

Cost Considerations

HBO therapy is covered by insurance for specific conditions. Insurance prior authorization is recommended (Broussard, 2016).

Electrical Stimulation (E-stim)

Electrical stimulation has been used in a variety of settings and for a variety of wounds and has in general been found to support healing.

Mechanism of Action

Various types of electrical current can be delivered to the wound and periwound tissues to support wound healing. The most commonly used type is high-voltage pulsed current (HVPC). E-stim is thought to work by reducing edema, increasing perfusion, and promoting migration of the cells critical to repair.

Guidelines for Use

E-stim is a nonspecific stimulus for repair that can be used for multiple types of chronic wounds. Wounds are typically treated 3 to 7 times a week for 8 to 12 weeks. If there is no evidence of progress within 10 to 14 days, therapy should be reevaluated. While best practice guidelines recommend consideration of electrical stimulation for nonhealing wounds (EPUAP/NPIAP/PPPIA, 2019; WOCN, 2016), the therapy is not yet FDA approved for use in wound care although it is approved for pain and edema management (Frantz, 2016; Isseroff & Dahle, 2012). Electrical stimulation is best provided in conjunction with a physical therapist, as they have the expertise to assure optimal use of this modality.

KEY POINT

Electrical stimulation is best provided in conjunction with a physical therapist, as they have the expertise to assure optimal use of this treatment modality.

Current Evidence

Studies indicate improved blood flow and enhanced resistance to infection in refractory wounds treated with electrical stimulation. Wolcott and colleagues (1969) evaluated the use of E-stim with ischemic nonhealing wounds and found that wounds treated with standard care and electrical stimulation demonstrated a healing rate of 30%, as compared to 14.7% for wounds managed with standard care alone. Carley and Wainapel (1985) evaluated the effects of E-stim on sacral and lower extremity wounds of varying etiology and found that wounds treated with electrical stimulation healed at a rate of

1.5 to 2.5 times that of the control (no E-stim) group. Lala and colleagues (2016) conducted a systematic review and meta-analysis regarding E-stim. They found that e-stimulation is an effective adjunctive therapy for treating pressure ulcers in individuals with SCI. The results of the meta-analysis showed that electrical stimulation decreases pressure ulcer size at a rate of 1.32% per day and increases pressure ulcer closure by 1.55 times more than with standard wound care alone or sham electrical stimulation. Study parameters varied, and no one protocol or treatment plan could be recommended (EPUAP/NPIAP/PPPIA, 2019; Lala et al., 2016).

Cost Considerations

Cost is typically covered by insurance through physical therapy application; prior authorization of insurance coverage is recommended (Frantz, 2016; Unger, 2007).

Ultrasound (Low-Frequency Noncontact, Nonthermal Ultrasound)

Low-frequency noncontact ultrasound has been used as a method of debridement and as a nonspecific stimulus to repair.

Low-frequency noncontact, nonthermal ultrasound utilizes acoustic/sound energy to deliver ultrasound energy through saline mist or open air to the wound bed and periwound tissue. Evidence suggests that this therapy may augment wound healing through a combination of the following: enhanced debridement of necrotic tissue through enzymatic and fibrinolytic activity, reduced bacterial counts and biofilm production, increased fibroblast migration, and improved blood flow.

KEY POINT

Low-frequency noncontact, nonthermal ultrasound may promote healing through enhanced fibrinolytic activity, reduced bacterial counts, and improved blood flow.

Guidelines for Use

This therapy is indicated as an adjunctive therapy for refractory wounds and burns, with ongoing monitoring to assure effectiveness.

Current Evidence

A retrospective observational study comparing 163 patients with vascular wounds treated with ultrasound + standard care to 47 patients treated with standard care alone revealed significantly higher healing rates among the ultrasound group (Kavros et al., 2008). Driver and colleagues (2011) conducted a meta-analysis of eight studies involving 444 patients with a variety of chronic wounds with similar findings. They found higher healing rates among the patients treated with low-frequency noncontact, nonthermal ultrasound. Anecdotal reports also note reduced pain and exudate, and this therapy

has been reported to be of benefit in the management of patients with deep tissue pressure injury (DTPI). A prospective randomized, double-blind, sham control, single-center study compared noncontact low frequency airborne ultrasound to sham in Wagner 2 and 3 ulcers. Rastogi and colleagues (2019) found >50% wound area reduction in 97.1% and 73.1% subjects in ultrasound and sham groups, respectively. Wound contraction during the first 2 weeks occurred faster with ultrasound therapy, compared with sham treatment. Overall, faster wound area reduction was found in the ultrasound group.

Cost Considerations

In the outpatient setting, this therapy may be covered under a debridement code (Unger, 2007).

Flaps and Grafts

In selected refractory wounds, surgical closure may be required. This usually involves either a split-thickness skin graft or a myocutaneous flap procedure. Split-thickness skin grafts are appropriate for burn care and for shallow wounds with a healthy well-vascularized wound bed. The principles of management include post-op immobilization of the graft site, use of a bolster dressing or NPWT to maintain close contact between the graft and the underlying wound bed, and prevention of infection. Myocutaneous flaps are generally reserved for large defects overlying bony prominences in nonambulatory patients with good potential for healing, such as a wheelchair-bound spinal cord–injured patient with an ischial ulcer. Management priorities include establishment of a healthy granulating wound bed prior to surgery, assurance of adequate nutritional status and systemic support for healing, and protection and close monitoring of the flap to prevent complications due to ischemia, venous congestion, or exposure to pressure and shear (Kane, 2014).

KEY POINT

Split-thickness skin grafts are appropriate for management of burns and well-vascularized superficial wounds. Post-op management should be focused on maintenance of close adherence between the graft and the underlying wound bed.

NOVEL TECHNOLOGIES

Nanotechnology

Despite efforts to create dressings that regenerate tissue quickly, reduce bacterial bioburden, and heal without scarring, approximately 40% of chronic wounds never heal. This continues to advance research in medical and wound healing technology. Nanotechnology is an area that is gaining in interest and research. Scientifically nanotechnology provides a new platform for the next generation of advanced wound healing.

Nanotechnology involves the study of manipulating matter at the nanometric particle size (maximum diameter of 100 nm) and their synthesis, structure and the dynamics of atoms, molecules, and supramolecular particles. The nanometric size increases a particle's surface exponentially as the volume decreases. The size and shape of the nanoparticles determine their biological efficiency.

The size and shape of the different types of nanoparticles are properties that determine their biological efficiency, through influencing active substance delivery, penetrability, and cellular receptor recognition. Wound treatment research involves the nanomaterial types of nanoparticles, nanocomposites, coatings, and scaffolds. Theoretically the size and shape of the nanoparticles allow active compounds, surfactants, therapeutic agents, and antibacterial agents to demonstrate increased biocompatibility, efficacy, and their eventual use in clinical practice. Metal nanoparticles such as silver, gold, and zinc are ideal to incorporate into wound dressings due to their antibacterial properties and low toxicity. Research incorporating stem cells into nanomaterials is currently under development.

Nanoparticles are anticipated to be efficiently incorporated in countless medical treatments including new wound treatment modalities, with further study (Hamdan et al., 2017; Mariappan, 2019; Mihai et al., 2019).

Low Level Laser (Light) Therapy

Low level laser (light) therapy (LLLT) has shown promise as an adjunctive treatment in lower extremity venous ulcers. It has not shown the same response in pressure injuries. Low-dose laser (light) affects enzymatic chain reactions, immune cell activation, and cellular proliferation.

Laser is appropriate for medical therapy by the dissemination of the laser beam absorption by tissue. Because of the broadness of the absorption bands a spectrally narrow laser is not essential and the LLLT provides a nonthermal energy application without accumulative thermal energy or temperature elevation. This stimulation of various biological events using light energy without significant temperature change is referred to as photo-bioactivation and is a common term for LLLT.

The low-level laser–tissue interaction physiological and cellular effects are many key to wound healing. These effects are modulation of cell proliferation, phagocyte and macrophage activation, fibroblast proliferation, alteration of cell membrane potentials, and stimulation of angiogenesis. Essentially, LLLT has been found to have analgesic, vasodilating, and anti-inflammatory properties.

Use of laser therapy in the clinical setting has been significantly limited by the lack of studies reporting in the same global dose units, as different laser machines utilize different measurements of energy density. Thus, the dose calculations are not universal nor consistent between the different studies. Treatment outcomes are influenced by the different parameters of LLLT (wavelength, power, energy, pulse frequency, pulse duration, etc.) and conditions like exposure time, frequency, and

duration. The mechanisms of laser-tissue interaction, crucial parameters, therapeutic outcomes, and efficacy of LLLT as adjunctive treatment for different chronic wounds are the main issues needing further study in large-scale unbiased RCTs (Rashidi et al., 2015; Wang et al., 2017).

Fluorescence Light Device

Diagnostics providing accurate wound measurements and level of bacterial burden facilitate evidence-based treatment decisions to facilitate wound healing. A hand-held device providing wound measurements was found in pilot studies to immediately document wound area, length and width with an accuracy >95% when these measurements were overlaid on an image of the wound. In addition, bacterial fluorescence was assessed across diverse wound types and compared with microbiological cultures confirming bacterial status approximately 3 days later. In the clinical trial, swab culture was found to underreport bacterial loads relative to fluorescence-guided cultures. Pilot studies suggest that bacteria fluorescence-targeted debridement may improve healing rates, but larger controlled studies are necessary.

Visualization of bacteria in and around a wound does not mean infection is present, though delayed healing has been shown when bacteria levels reach the detection threshold. Limitations of this device include inability to detect bacteria deeper than 1.5 mm from the wound surface due to inherent limitations of the device's optical imaging. The device does not identify the bacterial species present nor does it provide antibiotic sensitivities. Microbiological cultures are still required if this information is necessary. Fluorescence imaging must be performed in dark conditions, and a disposable drape attachment can be used to achieve sufficient darkness.

Routine future incorporation of bacterial fluorescence imaging in wound care may reduce wound size through more aggressive debridement and decreasing bacterial loads (Raizman et al., 2019).

 ## INDICATIONS FOR REFERRALS

A team approach is necessary for refractory wound management. Referrals are essential whenever the etiology is unclear or specific therapies are required to correct the etiologic factors such as revascularization or offloading with a boot, medical, or nutritional intervention is needed to assure potential for healing, or medical or surgical intervention is needed for wound closure. The wound care nurse needs to assure optimal outcomes for their patients and needs to appreciate the knowledge and skills of other disciplines.

 ## CONCLUSION

Refractory wounds are complex and require comprehensive assessment to determine probable cause for failure to heal. Interventions are based on assessment data. Key interventions include reassessment of causative and contributing factors and biopsy whenever the etiology is unclear or there is any suspicion of malignant deterioration, evaluation of all systemic factors, and comorbid conditions affecting repair. Topical therapy must be reevaluated to assure appropriate moisture management and control of bacterial loads. Implementation of active wound therapies for wounds determined to be nonhealing despite appropriate comprehensive wound care should be considered. While active wound therapies continue to evolve, there are a number of options available, including protease-inhibiting dressings, matrix dressings, bioengineered skin substitutes, NPWT, and HBOT. The wound care nurse must align the features of the available technology to the specific wound characteristics.

REFERENCES

Alavi, A., Sibbald, R. G., Mayer, D., et al. (2014). Diabetic foot ulcers: Part I. Pathophysiology and prevention. *Journal of the American Academy of Dermatology, 70*(1), 1.e1–1.e20. doi: 10.1016/j.jaad.2013.06.055.

Asadi, M., Alamdari, D. H., Rahimi, H. R., et al. (2014). Treatment of life-threatening wounds with a combination of allogeneic platelet-rich plasma, fibrin glue and collagen matrix, and a literature review. *Experimental and Therapeutic Medicine, 8*, 423–429.

Atkin, L., Bućko, Z., Montero, E. C., et al. (2019). Implementing TIMERS: The race against hard-to-heal wounds. *Journal of Wound Care, 28*(Sup3a), S1–S50.

Bazaliński, D., Przybek-Mita, J., Barańska, B., et al. (2017). Marjolin's ulcer in chronic wounds—review of available literature. *Contemporary Oncology (Poznan, Poland), 21*(3), 197–202. doi: 10.5114/wo.2017.70109.

Boykin, J. V., Jr., & Baylis, C. (2007). Hyperbaric oxygen therapy mediates increased nitric oxide production associated with wound healing: A preliminary study. *Advances in Skin & Wound Care, 20*(7), 382–388.

Broussard, C. (2016). Hyperbaric oxygenation. In R. Bryant, & D. Nix (Eds.), *Acute & chronic wounds: Current management concepts* (5th ed., pp. 361–368). St. Louis, MO: Elsevier Inc.

Bryant, R. (2016). Uncommon wounds and manifestations of intrinsic diseases. In R. Bryant, & D. Nix (Eds.), *Acute & chronic wounds: Current management concepts* (5th ed., pp. 441–461). St Louis, MO: Elsevier Inc.

Bryant, R., & Nix, D. (2016). Principles of wound healing and topical management. In R. Bryant, & D. Nix (Eds.), *Acute & chronic wounds: Current management concepts* (5th ed., pp. 306–324). St Louis, MO: Elsevier Inc.

Caley, M. P., Martins, V. L., & O'Toole, E. A. (2015). Metalloproteinases and wound healing. *Advances in Wound Care, 4*(4), 225–234.

Capito, A. E., Tholpady, S. S., Agrawal, H., et al. (2012). Evaluation of host tissue integration, revascularization, and cellular infiltration within various dermal substrates. *Annals of Plastic Surgery, 68*(5), 495–500.

Carley, P. J., & Wainapel, S. F. (1985). Electrotherapy for acceleration of wound healing: Low intensity direct current. *Archives of Physical Medicine and Rehabilitation, 66*(7), 443–446.

Carter, M. J., Fylling, C. P., & Parnell, L. K. (2011). Use of platelet rich plasma gel on wound healing: A systematic review and meta-analysis. *Eplasty, 11*, e38.

Cazzell, S., Vayser, D., Pham, H., et al. (2017). A randomized clinical trial of a human acellular dermal matrix demonstrated superior healing rates for chronic diabetic foot ulcers over conventional care and an active acellular dermal matrix comparator. *Wound Repair and Regeneration, 25*(3), 483–497.

Cheng, B., & Fu, X. (2018). The focus and target: Angiogenesis in refractory wound healing. *The International Journal of Lower Extremity Wounds, 17*(4), 301–303.

DiMatteo, M. R. (2004). Social support and patient adherence to medical treatment: A meta-analysis. *Health Psychology, 23*(2), 207.

Doughty, D., & Sparks, B. (2016). Wound healing physiology and factors that affect the repair process. In R. Bryant, & D. Nix (Eds.), *Acute & chronic wounds: Current management concepts* (5th ed., pp. 63–81). St. Louis, MO: Elsevier Inc.

Driver, V. R., Yao, M., & Miller, C. J. (2011). Noncontact low-frequency ultrasound therapy in the treatment of chronic wounds: A meta-analysis. *Wound Repair and Regeneration, 19*(4), 475–480.

European Pressure Ulcer Advisory Panel, National Pressure Injury Advisory Panel, and Pan Pacific Pressure Injury Alliance [EPUAP/NPIAP/PPPIA]. (2019). In E. Haesler (Ed.), *Prevention and treatment of pressure ulcers/injuries: Clinical Practice Guideline*. The International Guideline.

European Wound Management Association (EWMA). (2004). *Position Document: Wound bed preparation in practice*. London, United Kingdom: MEP Ltd.

Fonder, M. A., Lazarus, G. S., Cowan, D. A., et al. (2008). Treating the chronic wound: A practical approach to the care of nonhealing wounds and wound care dressings. *Journal of the American Academy of Dermatology, 58*(2), 185–206.

Frantz, R. (2016). Electrical stimulation. In R. Bryant, & D. Nix (Eds.), *Acute & chronic wounds: Current Management Concepts* (5th ed., pp. 369–376). St Louis, MO: Elsevier Inc.

Gray, M., & Ratliff, C. (2006). Is HBO therapy effective for the management of chronic wounds? *Journal of Wound, Ostomy, and Continence Nursing, 33*, 21–25.

Gupta, S., Gabriel, A., Lantis, J., et al. (2016). Clinical recommendations and practical guide for negative pressure wound therapy with instillation. *International Wound Journal, 13*, 159–174.

Hamdan, S., Pastar, I., Drakulich, S., et al. (2017). Nanotechnology-driven therapeutic interventions in wound healing: Potential uses and applications. *ACS Central Science, 3*, 163–175

Han, G., & Ceilley, R. (2017). Chronic wound healing: A review of current management and treatments. *Advances in Therapy, 34*(3), 599–610.

Harding, K. (2000). Nonhealing wounds: Recalcitrant, chronic, or not understood? *Ostomy/wound management, 46*(1A Suppl), 4S–7S.

Harding, K., Moore, K. & Phillips, T. (2005). Wound chronicity and fibroblast senescence—Implications for treatment. *International Wound Journal, 2*, 364–368.

Houghton, P., & Campbell, K. (2012). Therapeutic modalities in the treatment of chronic recalcitrant wounds. In D. L. Krasner, G. T. Rodeheaver, & R. G. Sibbald (Eds.), *Chronic wound care: A clinical source book for healthcare professionals* (5th ed.). Malvern, PA: HMP.

International Consensus. (2010). *Acellular matrices for the treatment of wounds. An expert working group review*. London, United Kingdom: Wounds International.

International Wound Infection Institute (IWII). (2016). *Wound infection in clinical practice*. London, United Kingdom: Wounds International. Retrieved April 25, 2020 from http://www.wound-infection-institute.com/wp-content/uploads/2017/07/IWII-Consensus_Final-2017.pdf

Isseroff, R. R., & Dahle, S. E. (2012). Electrostimulation therapy and wound healing: Where are we now? *Advances in Wound Care, 1*(6), 238–243.

Kane, D. P. (2014). Surgical repair in advanced wound caring. In D. L. Krasner (Ed.), *Chronic wound care: The Essentials* (pp. 279–291). Malvern, PA: HMP Communications.

Karukonda, S. R., Flynn, T. C., Boh, E. E., et al. (2000). The effects of drugs on wound healing—Part II. Specific classes of drugs and their effect on healing wounds. *International Journal of Dermatology, 39*, 321–333.

Kavros, S. J., Liedl, D. A., Boon, A. J., et al. (2008). Expedited wound healing with noncontact, low-frequency ultrasound therapy in chronic wounds: A retrospective analysis. *Advances in Skin & Wound Care, 21*(9), 416–423.

Kim, P. J., Attinger, C. E., Steinberg, J. S., et al. (2014). The impact of negative-pressure wound therapy with instillation compared with standard negative-pressure wound therapy: A retrospective, historical, cohort, controlled study. *Plastic and Reconstructive Surgery, 133*(3), 709–716.

Klein, R. J. (2020). Use of oxidized regenerated cellulose (ORC)/collagen/silver-ORC dressings alone or subsequent to advanced wound therapies in complex wounds. *Wounds, 32*(2), 37–43.

Kranke, P., Bennett, M. H., Martyn-St James, M., et al. (2015). Hyperbaric oxygen therapy for chronic wounds. *Cochrane Database of Systematic Reviews,* (6), CD004123.

Lala, D., Spaulding, S., Burke, S., et al. (2016). Electrical stimulation therapy for the treatment of pressure ulcers in individuals with spinal cord injury: A systematic review and meta-analysis. *International Wound Journal, 13*, 1214–1226.

Lazarus, G. S., Cooper, D. M., Knighton, D. R., et al. (1994). Definitions and guidelines for assessment of wounds and evaluation of healing. *Wound Repair and Regeneration, 2*(3), 165–170.

Leaper, D. J., Schultz, G., Carville, K., et al. (2012). Extending the TIME concept: What have we learned in the past 10 years? *International Wound Journal, 9*, 1–19.

Li, J., Chen, J., & Kirsner, R. (2007). Pathophysiology of acute wound healing. *Clinics in Dermatology, 25*(1), 9–18.

Lobmann, R., Schultz, G., & Lehnert, H. (2005). Proteases and the diabetic foot syndrome: Mechanisms & therapeutic implications. *Diabetes Care, 28*(2), 462–471.

Mariappan, N. (2019). Recent trends in nanotechnology applications in surgical specialties and orthopedic surgery. *Biomedical and Pharmacology Journal, 12*(3), 1095–1127.

Martin, J. L., Koodie, L., Krishnan, A. G., et al. (2010). Immunopathy and infectious diseases: Chronic morphine administration delays wound healing by inhibiting immune cell recruitment to the wound site. *American Journal of Pathology, 176*(2), 786–799.

Mihai, M., Dima, M., Dima, B., et al. (2019). Review nanomaterials for wound healing and infection control. *Materials, 12*(2176), 1–16.

Miller, T. A. (2016). Health literacy and adherence to medical treatment in chronic and acute illness: A meta-analysis. *Patient Education and Counseling, 99*(7), 1079–1086.

Moore, K., McCallion, R., Searle, R. J., et al. (2006). Prediction and monitoring the therapeutic response of chronic dermal wounds. *International Wound Journal, 3*, 89–96.

Mostow, E. N., Haraway, G. D., Dalsing, M., et al.; OASIS Venus Ulcer Study Group. (2005). Effectiveness of an extracellular matrix graft (Oasis wound matrix) in the treatment of chronic leg ulcers: A randomized clinical trial. *Journal of Vascular Surgery, 41*(5), 837–843.

Netsch, D. S., Nix, D. P., & Haugan, V. (2016). Negative pressure wound therapy. In R. Bryant, & D. Nix (Eds.), *Acute & chronic wounds: Current management concepts* (5th ed., pp. 350–360). St Louis, MO: Elsevier Inc.

Nix, D., Peirce, B., & Haugen, V. (2016). Eliminating noncompliance. In R. Bryant, & D. Nix (Eds.), *Acute & chronic wounds: Current management concepts* (5th ed., pp. 428–440). St Louis, MO: Elsevier Inc.

Raizman, R., Dunham, D., Lindvere-Teene, L., et al. (2019). Use of a bacterial fluorescence imaging device: Wound measurement, bacterial detection and targeted debridement. *Journal of Wound Care, 28*(12), 824–834.

Rashidi, S., Yadollahpour, A., & Mirzaiyan, M. (2015). Low level laser therapy for the treatment of chronic wound: Clinical considerations. *Biomedical and Pharmacology Journal, 8*(2), 1121–1127.

Rastogi, A., Bhansali, A., & Ramachandran, S. (2019). Efficacy and safety of low-frequency, noncontact airborne ultrasound therapy (glybetac) for neuropathic diabetic foot ulcers: A randomized, double-blind, sham-control study, *The International Journal of Lower Extremity Wounds, 18*(1), 81–88.

Rhee, S. M., Valle, M. F., Wilson, L. M., et al. (2014). *Technology assessment: Negative pressure wound therapy technologies for chronic wound care in the home setting* [Internet]. Rockville, MD: Agency for Healthcare Research and Quality (US). Retrieved April 25, 2020 from https://www.ncbi.nlm.nih.gov/books/NBK285361/

Rolstad, B., Bryant, R., Nix, D. (2012). Topical management. In R. Bryant & D. Nix (Eds.), *Acute & chronic wounds: Current management concepts* (4th ed., pp. 289–306). St. Louis, MO: Elsevier-Mosby.

Rolstad, B., & Nix, D. (2007). Management of wound recalcitrance and deterioration. In D. L. Krasner, G. T. Rodeheaver, & R. G. Sibbald (Eds.), *Chronic wound care: A clinical source book for healthcare professionals* (4th ed., pp. 743–750). Malvern, PA: HMP Communications.

Saim, S., Heintzelman, A. B., & Bryant, R. A. (2016). Cellular- and tissue-based products for wounds. In R. Bryant, & D. Nix (Eds.), *Acute & chronic wounds: Current management concepts* (5th ed., pp. 308–323). St Louis, MO: Elsevier Inc.

Samsell, B., McLean, J., Cazzell, S., et al. (2019). Health economics for treatment of diabetic foot ulcers: A cost-effectiveness analysis of eight skin substitutes. *Journal of Wound Care, 28*(Sup9), S14–S26.

Samson, D., Lefevre, F., & Aronson, N. (2004). 111 Wound-healing technologies: Low-level laser and vacuum-assisted closure: Summary. In *AHRQ Evidence Report Summaries* (pp. 1998–2005). Rockville, MD: Agency for Healthcare Research and Quality (US). Retrieved from https://www.ncbi.nlm.nih.gov/sites/books/NBK11882/

Schultz, G. S., Sibblad, R. G., Falanga, V., et al. (2003). Wound bed preparation: A systematic approach to wound management. *Wound Repair and Regeneration, 11*(Suppl 1), S1–S28.

Sheikh, S. S., Sheikh, S. S., & Fetterolf, D. E. (2014). Use of dehydrated human amniotic membrane allografts to promote healing in patients with refractory non healing wounds. *International Wound Journal, 11*(6), 711–717. doi: 10.1111/iwj.12035.

Sibbald, R. G., Goodman, L., Woo, K. Y., et al. (2011). Special considerations in wound bed preparation 2011: An update©. *Advances in Skin & Wound Care, 24*(9), 415–436.

Smiell, J. M., Wieman, T. J., Steed, D. L., et al. (1999). Efficacy and safety of becaplermin (recombinant human platelet-derived growth factor-BB) in patients with non-healing, lower extremity diabetic ulcers: A combined analysis of four randomized studies. *Wound Repair and Regeneration, 7*, 335–346.

Smith, A., Whittington, K., Frykberg, R., et al. (2014). Negative pressure wound therapy. In: D. L. Krasner (Ed.), *Chronic wound care: The essentials* (pp. 195–223). Malvern, PA: HMP Communications.

Snyder, D., Sullivan, N., Margolis, D., et al. (2020). *Technology assessment: Skin substitutes for treating chronic wounds* [Internet]. Rockville, MD: Agency for Healthcare Research and Quality (US). Retrieved April 25, 2020 from: https://www.ncbi.nlm.nih.gov/books/NBK554220/

Stotts, N. A., Wipke-Tevis, D. D., & Hopf, H. W. (2014). Cofactors in impaired wound healing. In D. L. Krasner (Ed.), *Chronic wound care: The essentials* (pp. 79–86). Malvern, PA: HMP Communications.

Sussman, C., & Bates-Jensen, B. (2012). Wound healing physiology: Acute and chronic. In C. Sussman, & B. Bates-Jensen (Eds.), *Wound care: A collaborative practice manual for health professionals* (4th ed.). Baltimore, MD: Lippincott Williams & Wilkins.

Trovato, M., Granick, M., Tomaselli, N., et al. (2012). Management of the wound environment with advanced therapies. In C. Sussman, & B. Bates-Jensen (Eds.), *Wound care: A collaborative practice manual for health professionals* (4th ed.). Baltimore, MD: Lippincott Williams & Wilkins.

Unger, P. (2007). The physical therapist's role in wound management. In D. L. Krasner, G. T. Rodeheaver, R. G. Sibbald (Eds.), *Chronic wound care: A clinical source book for healthcare professionals* (4th ed., pp. 381–388). Malvern, PA: HMP Communications.

Vowden, P. (2011). Hard-to-heal wounds: Made easy. *Wounds International, 2*(4), 1–6.

Wang, H. T., Yuan, J. Q., Zhang, B., et al. (2017). Phototherapy for treating foot ulcers in people with diabetes. *Cochrane Database of Systematic Reviews, 6*(6), CD011979.

Westby, M. J., Dumville, J. C., Stubbs, N., et al. (2018). Protease activity as a prognostic factor for wound healing in venous leg ulcers. *Cochrane Database of Systematic Reviews, 9*(9), CD012841.

Wolcott, L. E., Wheeler, P. C., Hardwicke, H. M., et al. (1969). Accelerated healing of skin ulcer by electrotherapy: Preliminary clinical results. *Southern Medical Journal, 62*(7), 795–801.

Wound Healing Society (WHS). (2006). Guidelines for the treatment of venous ulcers. *Wound Repair and Regeneration, 14*, 649–662.

Wound Ostomy & Continence Nurses Society (WOCN). (2012). *Guideline for management of wounds in patients with lower extremity neuropathic disease (LEND), WOCN clinical practice guideline series #2*. Mount Laurel, NJ: Author.

Wound Ostomy & Continence Nurses Society (WOCN). (2016). *Guideline for prevention and management of pressure ulcers/injuries, WOCN clinical practice guideline series #2*. Mount Laurel, NJ: Author.

Wound Ostomy & Continence Nurses Society (WOCN). (2019). *Guideline for management of wounds in patients with lower extremity venous disease (LEVD), WOCN clinical practice guideline series #4*. Mount Laurel, NJ: Author.

Zhao, R., Liang, H., Clarke, E., et al. (2016). Inflammation in Chronic Wounds. *International Journal of Molecular Sciences*, 17(12), 2085. doi: 10.3390/ijms17122085.

QUESTIONS

1. The wound care nurse is assessing a patient with a neuropathic ulcer. What criteria must exist for the wound to be considered refractory?
  A. There is no improvement in the wound in 1 week.
  B. There is no reduction in the size of the wound in 2 to 4 weeks despite appropriate management.
  C. The wound becomes infected after 1 week of management.
  D. The wound heals in a timely predictable manner with durable closure.

2. Which of the following is an extrinsic factor affecting wound repair?
  A. Patient comorbidities
  B. Patient age
  C. Medications
  D. Perfusion and oxygenation

3. Which medication places a patient at greater risk for delayed wound healing?
  A. Antiplatelet medication
  B. Insulin
  C. Antidepressants
  D. Human growth factor

4. What is the wound care goal for a patient who is receiving radiation to treat cancer?
  A. Maintenance
  B. Topical therapy
  C. Pharmacological therapy
  D. Identification of etiologic factors

5. What is one effect of psychophysiologic stress on wound healing?
  A. Bacteria form that release by-products deleterious to the wound repair process.
  B. Stress causes persistent damage to the proliferative cells in the wound.
  C. Increased cortisol levels adversely affect cytokine production.
  D. Biofilm formation occurs, impairing wound healing.

6. Which characteristic of nonhealing wounds is responsible for degrading the matrix proteins and growth factors essential for healing?
  A. Low ratio of matrix metalloproteases (MMPs) to tissue inhibitors of matrix metalloproteases (TIMPs)
  B. High levels of matrix metalloproteases (MMPs), which degrade the matrix proteins and growth factors essential for healing
  C. A balanced interaction among inflammatory and proliferative factors and slowing progression of the wound through the repair process
  D. Excessive bioburden (critical colonization) resulting in biofilm formation, increasing the risk for infection

7. The wound care nurse recommends active wound therapy to treat a refractory wound. What is the goal of this therapy?
  A. Correct the molecular imbalances in the wound.
  B. Increase the levels of MMPs in the wound bed.
  C. Reduce the levels of MMP inhibitors.
  D. Increase elastase and plasmin activity in the wound bed.

8. The wound care nurse recommends a bioengineered skin substitute to treat a venous ulcer that has progressed to refractory wound stage. What is a therapeutic effect of this type of cellular dressing?
  A. Provides a scaffold for cell migration
  B. Reduces the level of biofilms in the wound
  C. Promotes an antigen–antibody response
  D. Reduces elastase and plasmin activity in the wound bed

9. What is one of the criteria that must be met to consider negative pressure wound therapy (NPWT)?

A. The goal of wound healing is maintenance.

B. The wound bed has a high level of necrotic tissue.

C. Any infection in the wound bed is being treated.

D. There is a malignancy in the wound.

10. For which patient would the wound care nurse most likely recommend hyperbaric oxygen therapy (HBOT)?

A. A patient who has a comorbid malignancy

B. A patient whose wound healing is compromised by inadequate tissue perfusion

C. A patient who has a viable wound bed not responding to NPWT

D. A wheelchair-bound patient with an ischial ulcer

ANSWERS AND RATIONALES

1. B: A wound is considered refractory if there has not been improvement within 2 to 4 weeks of comprehensive evidence-based therapy or there is no expected and predicted reduction in size of the wound in an established period of time.

2. C: Extrinsic factors include medications, malnutrition, radiation and chemotherapy, psychophysiologic stress, and wound bioburden and infection.

3. A: Platelet activation is a critical first step along the wound healing pathway and can be disrupted by anticoagulant medications, antiplatelet medications, and nonsteroidal anti-inflammatory medications.

4. A: The wound care goal for a patient receiving radiation or chemotherapy is maintenance until therapy is complete.

5. C: Cortisol levels are increased during times of stress, and cortisol is known to adversely affect cytokine production and fibroblast proliferation.

6. B: Chronic wounds exhibit a high level of proteases (matrix metalloproteases, or MMPs), which degrade the matrix proteins and growth factors essential for healing.

7. A: The reason for failure to heal is thought to be an imbalance in the molecular environment and structures controlling the repair process.

8. A: Use of ECM dressings is postulated to provide a scaffold for attachment and migration of host cells, supporting neoangiogenesis, collagen synthesis, and reepithelialization.

9. C: NPWT is indicated when the goal is wound healing, the wound bed has minimal or no necrotic tissue, and bacterial loads are under control.

10. B: HBOT should be considered when wound healing is compromised by severe infection or impaired tissue perfusion.

CHAPTER 13

SKIN AND WOUND CARE FOR NEONATAL AND PEDIATRIC POPULATIONS

Carolyn Lund and Charleen Singh

OBJECTIVES

1. Describe the anatomy and physiology of the skin and soft tissue, changes across the life span, and implications for maintenance of skin health.

2. Describe the pathology, assessment, and management of wounds unique to the neonatal and pediatric populations.

TOPIC OUTLINE

INTRODUCTION

Skin and wound care for neonates, infants, and children requires an understanding of skin characteristics unique to these populations. The skin is one of the most important organs at birth, with the following functions: barrier protection against water loss and absorption control of substances; temperature regulation; acid-mantle formation and infection control; water and electrolyte regulation; and tactile sensory function (AWHONN, 2018). Daily skin care practices such as antimicrobial skin disinfection and adhesive removal place these newborns at risk for skin trauma and loss of normal skin barrier function. Premature infants in the NICU who are critically ill or require surgery are at high risk for alterations in skin integrity. Other causes of skin damage include intravenous extravasation, diaper dermatitis, and pressure injuries. An understanding of the unique anatomic and physiologic differences in premature, full-term newborn, and young infant skin is fundamental to providing effective care to these populations.

CHARACTERISTICS OF NEWBORN, INFANT, AND PREMATURE INFANT SKIN

Each year, an estimated 15 million babies are born preterm (before 37 weeks of pregnancy) and the number is increasing (WHO, 2018). Preterm birth complications are the leading cause of death among children under 5 years of age. Preterm is defined as babies born before 37 weeks of pregnancy are completed. There are subcategories of preterm birth, based on gestational age: extremely preterm (<28 weeks), very preterm (28 to 32 weeks), and moderate to late preterm (32 to 37 weeks). Preterm birth and being small for gestational age are the reasons for low birth weight (LBW), which are also indirect causes of neonatal deaths (WHO, 2018). Examples of health risks associated with prematurity include increased risk for infections, thermoregulation issues, enhanced percutaneous drug absorption due to thinner skin, and higher ratio of total body surface area to body mass. There are also health risks associated with post maturity of pregnancy >42 weeks of gestation. These infants have a decrease in amniotic fluid with dry, peeling skin present at birth (Kline-Tilford & Haut, 2016).

Newborn skin undergoes an adaptation process during the transition from the aquatic environment of the uterus to the aerobic environment after birth. The skin assists in thermoregulation, serves as a barrier against toxins and microorganisms, is a reservoir for fat storage and insulation, and is a primary interface for tactile sensation and communication.

STRATUM CORNEUM AND EPIDERMIS

The stratum corneum (SC) which is the outermost layer of the epidermis provides the most important barrier function of the skin. It contains 10 to 20 cell layers in the adult and in the full-term newborn. Full-term newborns have been shown to have skin barrier function comparable to that of adult skin as indicated by transepidermal water loss (TEWL), the rate at which water vapor from respiration passes through the skin layers into the environment. TEWL is accepted as an indicator of epidermal barrier function and skin integrity (Vongsa et al., 2019; Yosipovitch et al., 2000). Normal TEWL is 4 to 8 $g/m^2/h$. with lower values generally indicating an effective SC barrier. High values mean the barrier is damaged, not well formed, or has fewer than the normal 16 layers. Evidence from age-related TEWL studies support the view that infant skin barrier function at birth or within 2 to 4 weeks of birth is in the same range as that of healthy adults (Visscher et al., 2015; Vongsa et al., 2019).

The skin of the full-term newborn is coated with vernix caseosa, which is predominantly composed of water (80.5%). The vernix caseosa contains proteins, lipids, and antimicrobial peptides (Oranges et al., 2015). Vernix begins to form as early as 17 to 20 weeks gestation with the thickest coating noted between 36 and 38 weeks. By 40 weeks, it is found primarily in the skin folds. Vernix protects the fetus from water exposure, preventing maceration from amniotic fluid, and facilitates development of the SC. Babies born prematurely (i.e., <28 weeks) do not have the covering of vernix (Visscher et al., 2015). Vernix caseosa assists in the development of the acid mantle of the skin surface which inhibits the growth of microorganisms and provides immunologic properties to the skin (AWHONN, 2018; Coughlin & Taïeb, 2014; Visscher et al., 2015).

The SC does not function as well as adult skin during the first year of life and is approximately 30% thinner than that of adult skin (AWHONN, 2018; Nikolovski et al., 2008). The SC is thinner, the microvasculature of the skin is not as organized, and there is a lower concentration of melanin than in adults. Infant skin pH levels range from 6.34 to 7.5, which is higher than adult skin but the skin pH decreases within 96 hours of birth (McNichol et al., 2018; Visscher et al., 2015). The basal layer of the epidermis is 20% thinner than of the adult, and the keratinocytes in this layer have a high cell turnover rate, which may account for the faster wound healing observed in neonates (AWHONN, 2018; Stamatas et al., 2011).

At <30 weeks of gestation, there may be as few as two or three layers, and the extremely premature infant (23 to 24 weeks of gestation) has almost no SC and negligible barrier function (Agren et al., 1998; McNichol et al., 2018; Visscher et al., 2015). The deficient SC results in excessive fluid and evaporative heat losses during the first weeks of life, leading to increased risk of dehydration and significant alterations in electrolyte levels, such as hypernatremia (AWHONN, 2018; Bhatia, 2006). Premature infants are at risk of increased TEWL, increased absorption of topical agents, and increased susceptibility to chemical and mechanical injury. Careful attention must be paid to the type of product used with this population (McNichol et al., 2018). Maturation of the skin barrier, particularly for infants of 23 to 25 weeks of gestation, occurs over time (Agren et al., 1998; Sedin et al., 1985), with evidence of mature barrier function delayed until about 30 to 32 weeks of postconceptional age (Kalia et al., 1998). The structure of epidermal and dermal layers also differs according to the body site with some areas of the body thicker and less at risk than other sites. Over the palm, sole, and along the joints, the epidermal layer is thicker, whereas between scapulae, the dermal layer is thicker (de-Souza et al., 2019).

DERMIS

The dermis of the full-term newborn is thinner, and not as well developed as the adult dermis. The collagen and elastin fibers are shorter and less dense, and the reticular layer of the dermis is absent, which makes the skin feel very soft. There are reduced total lipid levels and fewer sebaceous glands in the dermal layer in infancy (Stamatas et al., 2011).

Premature and newborn infants exhibit decreased cohesion between the epidermis and dermis, which places them at risk for skin injury from removal of medical adhesives. When extremely aggressive adhesives are used, the bond between the adhesive and epidermis may be stronger than that between the epidermis and dermis, resulting in stripping of the epidermal layer (medical adhesive–related skin injuries [MARSI]) with loss of significantly diminished skin barrier function (AWHONN, 2018; Lund et al., 1997; Visscher et al., 2015).

SKIN pH

Skin normally has an acidic pH due to chemical and biologic processes involving the SC. This acid mantle of the skin (pH < 5) has been documented extensively in children and adults. The acidic skin surface contributes to the immune function of the SC by inhibiting the growth of pathogenic microorganisms and supporting the proliferation of commensal, or healthy, bacteria on the skin (Larson & Dinulos, 2005; Visscher et al., 2015).

Full-term newborns are born with an alkaline skin surface (pH > 6.0), but within the first 4 days after birth, the pH falls to <5.0 (Behrendt & Green, 1971). A study comparing full-term newborns to adults, the mean pH of the newborn skin measured 7.08 on the first day of life, as compared to 5.7 for adult skin pH (AWHONN, 2018; Yosipovitch et al., 2000). Another study reported that full-term newborns had a mean skin pH of 6.0 for the first 15 days of life and that the pH dropped to 5.1 by 5 to 6 weeks of life. Skin surface pH in premature infants of varying gestational ages has been reported to be >6 on the first day of life. It decreases to 5.5 by the end of the first week and 5.1 by the end of the first month (Fox et al., 1998; McNichol et al., 2018). Bathing and other topical treatments transiently alter skin pH (Gfatter et al., 1997), and diapered skin has a higher pH due to the combined effects of urine contact and occlusion (Visscher et al., 2002; Vongsa et al., 2019). The higher pH of diapered skin reduces the barrier function of the SC, rendering it more susceptible to mechanical damage from friction (Visscher et al., 2011; Vongsa et al., 2019).

RISK OF TOXICITY FROM TOPICAL AGENTS

Toxicity from topically applied substances has been reported in numerous case reports due to the increased permeability of both preterm and full-term newborn skin. This is due to a number of factors including the fact that newborn skin is 20% to 40% thinner than adult skin, and the ratio of body surface to weight is nearly five times greater in newborns than in older children and adults, which places newborns at increased risk for percutaneous absorption and toxicity. Examples of toxicity from percutaneous absorption include encephalopathy and death among premature infants bathed with hexachlorophene (Anderson et al., 1981; Kline-Tilford & Haut, 2016; Lund, 2014), and alterations in iodine levels and thyroid function related to routine use of povidone–iodine in intensive care nurseries (Aitken & Williams, 2014; Lund, 2014; Siegfried, 2008).

KEY POINT

The skin of premature infants and neonates is very permeable. The wound care nurse must assure that topical agents are approved for use in this population.

 ## SKIN ASSESSMENT AND RISK FACTORS FOR SKIN BREAKDOWN

In the NICU, a thorough examination of all skin surfaces should be done once or twice daily to monitor skin integrity. Early signs such as skin abrasions or small excoriations may call for either diagnostic or treatment procedures. A scoring tool can be used to objectively document skin status. The Neonatal Skin Condition Score (NSCS) is a valid and reliable tool (Lund & Osborne, 2004) that has demonstrated effectiveness as an outcome measure for evaluation of interventions (Morris et al., 2015). The three domains on the NSCS are dryness, erythema, and breakdown. The scale is used to assess all skin surfaces. Scores range from 1 to 3 on each domain with cumulative scores ranging from 3 to 9. A score of 3 equates to normal skin with no dryness, erythema, or breakdown. A score of 9 equates to very dry, cracked skin with visible erythema and extensive skin breakdown (AWHONN, 2018; Schardosim et al., 2014).

This scoring system may be integrated into skin care protocols to identify neonates with excessive dryness, erythema, or skin breakdown.

PRESSURE INJURY PREVENTION

The Braden Q scale was adapted from the adult Braden Scale for Predicting Pressure Sore Risk©. Curley and colleagues (2003) published their reexamination of the Braden Q Scale's predictive validity and critical cutoff point for classifying risk of pressure injuries in the pediatric population. The Braden Q Scale has the same six subscales as the Braden Scale with an additional seventh subscale: tissue perfusion and oxygenation (Curley et al., 2003).

The Braden QD Scale is a pediatric-specific, risk assessment instrument that reliably predicts both immobility-related and medical device–related pressure injuries (MDRPIs) in the pediatric acute care environment. A revision of the Braden Q Scale, the Braden QD Scale can be used to assess risk among the wide range of infants, children, and adolescents commonly treated in acute care environments. Braden QD Scale examines the five subscales of the Braden Q with the addition of the number of medical devices and repositionability/skin protection. A total score of 13 or higher indicates that the patient is at risk (Curley et al., 2018) (**Fig. 13-1**).

Curley et al. (2018) conducted a multicenter, prospective cohort study enrolling 652 hospitalized patients,

Braden QD Scale				
Intensity and Duration of Pressure				**Score**
Mobility The ability to independently change & control body position	**0. No Limitation** Makes major and frequent changes in body or extremity position independently.	**1. Limited** Makes slight and infrequent changes in body or extremity position OR <u>unable</u> to reposition self independently (includes infants too young to roll over).	**2. Completely Immobile** Does not make even slight changes in body or extremity position independently.	
Sensory Perception The ability to respond meaningfully, in a <u>developmentally</u> appropriate way, to pressure-related discomfort	**0. No Impairment** Responsive **and** has no sensory deficits which limit ability to feel or communicate discomfort.	**1. Limited** Cannot always communicate pressure-related discomfort **OR** has some sensory deficits that limit ability to feel pressure-related discomfort.	**2. Completely Limited** Unresponsive due to diminished level of consciousness or sedation **OR** sensory deficits limit ability to feel pressure-related discomfort over most of body surface.	
Tolerance of the Skin and Supporting Structure				
Friction & Shear *Friction:* occurs when skin moves against support surfaces *Shear:* occurs when skin & adjacent bony surface slide across one another	**0. No Problem** Has sufficient strength to completely lift self up during a move. Maintains good body position in bed/chair at all times. Able to completely lift patient during a position change.	**1. Potential Problem** Requires **some** assistance in moving. Occasionally slides down in bed/chair, requiring repositioning. During repositioning, skin often slides against surface.	**2. Problem** Requires **full** assistance in moving. Frequently slides down and requires repositioning. Complete lifting without skin sliding against surface is impossible **OR** spasticity, contractures, itching or agitation leads to almost constant friction.	
Nutrition *Usual* diet for age – assess pattern over the most recent 3 consecutive days	**0. Adequate** Diet for age providing **adequate** calories & protein to support metabolism and growth.	**1. Limited** Diet for age providing **inadequate** calories **OR inadequate** protein to support metabolism and growth **OR** receiving supplemental nutrition any part of the day.	**2. Poor** Diet for age providing **inadequate** calories **and** protein to support metabolism and growth.	
Tissue Perfusion & Oxygenation	**0. Adequate** Normotensive for age, & oxygen saturation ≥ 95%, & normal hemoglobin, & capillary refill ≤ 2 seconds.	**1. Potential Problem** Normotensive for age **with** oxygen saturation <95%, **OR** hemoglobin <10 g/dl, **OR** capillary refill > 2 seconds.	**2. Compromised** Hypotensive for age **OR** hemodynamically unstable with position changes.	
Medical Devices				
Number of Medical Devices	**Score 1 point for each medical device* up to 8 (Score 8 points maximum)** **Any diagnostic or therapeutic device that is currently attached to or traverses the patient's skin or mucous membrane.*			
Repositionability/ Skin Protection	**0. No Medical Devices**	**1. Potential Problem** All medical devices can be repositioned **OR** the skin under each device is protected.	**2. Problem** Any one or more medical device(s) can<u>not</u> be repositioned **OR** the skin under each device is not protected.	
			Total **(≥ 13 considered at risk)**	

© Curley MAQ; Adapted with permission from B. Braden and N. Bergstrom, Braden Scale for Predicting Pressure Sore Risk, (1987)

FIGURE 13-1. Braden QD Scale.

preterm to 21 years of age, on bed rest for at least 24 hours with a medical device in place. They found that Braden QD Scale reliably predicts both immobility-related and MDRPIs in the pediatric acute care environment. Common sites for immobility-related pressure injuries included the anterior rib, sacrum, buttock, and head. External monitoring, oxygen delivery, and airway maintenance devices caused the most MDRPIs (Curley et al., 2018).

Many factors have been identified as contributing to skin breakdown in the pediatric population. Suggested risk factors for skin breakdown may be intrinsic, such as duration and amount of pressure, friction, shear, and moisture, or extrinsic, such as perfusion, malnutrition, infection, anemia, and immobility. The sacrum, the largest bony area, is the most common location for pressure injuries in adults. In the pediatric population, the occiput of the infant's head is the most common location of pressure injuries, as the head is larger in a newborn or young infant compared to the rest of their body. Hair braids may also be a potential risk factor for occipital pressure injuries. Dixon and Ratliff (2011) describe a case study of a 7-year-old boy admitted to the pediatric intensive care unit (PICU) with severe sepsis. Hair braids that were placed before admission were taken down, revealing five full-thickness occipital lesions. Measures to prevent occipital pressure injuries include the use of gel pillows or mattresses, and frequent repositioning. Older children are likely to develop a PI in the same areas as an adult (sacrum, heels, etc.).

On admission, all neonates and children should have a documented comprehensive examination, including a skin assessment and a risk assessment for pressure injuries. Pressure injury risk assessment should be performed at least daily with a documented head-to-toe skin assessment. Thorough examination of high-risk areas, such as under splints, braces, cervical collars, tracheostomy sites, tubing devices, intravenous catheters, and arm boards, is important. Patients receiving continuous positive airway pressure (CPAP) also need close assessment and monitoring of the nares and septum.

According to the National Pressure Injury Advisory Panel (NPIAP), MDRPIs result from the use of devices designed and applied for diagnostic or therapeutic purposes. The resultant pressure injury generally conforms to the pattern or shape of the device. The injury should be staged using the NPIAP staging system.

The leading cause of PIs in pediatrics is MDRPIs (Baharestani & Ratliff, 2007; Delmore & Ayello, 2017). Visscher and Taylor (2014) conducted a 2-year prospective study and found that nearly 80% of all PIs and 90% of PIs in premature infants were associated with MDRPIs.

Pressure injuries from medical devices are more common than those caused by immobility. A device that causes pressure injuries with increased frequency is due

to nasal continuous positive airway pressure (NCPAP). Thin silicone foam dressings may provide some protection for the skin under nasal prongs and mask of the NCPAP device.

Dai et al. (2020) conducted a study to examine nasal pressure injuries due to NCPAP treatment in newborns over a 1-year period. Nasal pressure injuries were observed in 149 (34.7%). The risk was significantly higher when gestational age was <32 weeks and in those who received NCPAP treatment for more than 6 days.

Boyar (2020) studied the incidence of PI in premature infant receiving CPAP. A polyvinyl chloride foam dressing was used to pad the CPAP device in two arms of the study. There were fewer PIs that developed when using the foam padding and the PIs were less severe compared to use of the device with no padding. This reflected a sixfold decrease in nasal injuries when a protective foam dressing was used.

Every newborn and infant in the NICU is at risk for skin damage, including chemical burns from skin disinfectants, MARSIs, diaper dermatitis, and intravenous extravasations. Evidence-based recommendations for preventing and treating skin breakdown, maintaining barrier function of the immature skin, and promoting skin integrity are integrated into a skin care guideline for neonatal nurses, which is available through the Association of Women's Health, Obstetric and Neonatal Nursing (AWHONN, 2018).

 ## PREVENTION AND TREATMENT OF COMMON CAUSES OF SKIN BREAKDOWN IN NEONATES AND INFANTS

DAMAGE DUE TO SKIN DISINFECTANTS

Decontamination of the skin prior to invasive procedures such as venipuncture and placement of umbilical catheters and chest tubes is common practice in NICUs. Case reports of skin injury describe blisters, burns, and sloughing after the use of disinfectants with chlorhexidine gluconate (CHG) of varying concentrations in both aqueous forms or combined with isopropyl alcohol (IA) (Kutsch & Ottinger, 2014; Sardesai et al., 2011). Most occur in premature infants <26 weeks gestation and <1,000 g during the first week of life (Beresford, 2015).

Janssen et al. (2018) reported that a 0.2% CHG solution in acetate (0.2% CHG-acetate) was introduced as skin disinfectant for extremely preterm infants in the NICU. The main finding of this study was that the introduction of a skin disinfectant with a lower percentage of CHG in a nonalcoholic solution resulted in a reduced incidence of skin lesions as compared with alcohol-based skin disinfectants, but without increasing the risk for infection (Janssen et al., 2018).

A number of studies support the efficacy of chlorhexidine-containing solutions in preventing colonization and infection of peripheral intravenous (PIV) catheters in neonates (Chaiyakunapruk et al., 2002; Garland et al., 1995). A randomized controlled trial (RCT) compared 2% CHG/IA to 10% povidone–iodine for skin disinfection prior to placement of central venous catheters in premature infants and found no difference in bloodstream infections between the two groups (Kieran et al., 2018). Chapman et al. (2013) conducted a study to assess chlorhexidine absorption and skin tolerability in premature infants following skin antisepsis with 2% aqueous CHG prior to peripherally inserted central catheter (PICC) placement. No CHG-related skin irritation occurred in any infant. CHG was detected in the blood of preterm infants receiving CHG skin antisepsis for PICC insertion. Highest serum concentrations occurred 2 to 3 days after exposure. Further investigation is needed to determine the clinical relevance of CHG absorption in preterm infants (Chapman et al., 2013).

Lai and colleagues (2016) found that it is not clear whether cleaning the skin around CVC insertion sites with antiseptic reduces catheter–related blood stream infection compared with no skin cleansing. Skin cleansing with chlorhexidine solution may reduce rates of CLABSI and catheter colonization compared with cleaning with povidone–iodine. These results may be influenced by the nature of the antiseptic solution (i.e., aqueous or alcohol-based) (Lai et al., 2016).

KEY POINT

The wound care nurse must be aware that the combination (CHG and isopropyl alcohol) has a significant potential for skin injury in very-low-birth-weight (VLBW) infants and cannot be recommended for use in these patients (**Fig. 13-2**).

CHG products are commonly used for daily bathing in critical care units and have been shown to decrease infections in PICU patients >2 months of age (Milstone et al., 2013). CHG bathing was studied in a NICU population using an algorithm based on gestational and postnatal age. They report a decrease in bloodstream infections although the cohort used for comparison had an extremely high infection rate. They excluded infants <1,000 g and <28 days of age (Quach et al., 2014). Further study is needed regarding the antimicrobial benefits, the duration of effect, and the potential risks, especially in the NICU population. Concerns have also been raised about the potentially negative effect of CHG on normal skin colonization.

MEDICAL ADHESIVE–RELATED SKIN INJURY

One of the most common practices in the NICU is the application and removal of adhesives that secure ET tubes, IV devices, and monitoring probes and electrodes. MARSI results when the skin to adhesive attachment is stronger than skin cell to skin cell attachment. As a result, the epidermal layers separate or the epidermis separates completely from the dermis. Adhesive removal itself results in detachment of varying amounts of superficial epidermal cell layers even in adult skin, and repeated application and removal result in changes in skin barrier function (Lund, 2014).

Medical adhesives are pressure sensitive. Firm pressure applied to the surface of the medical tape/dressing/device will activate the adhesive by increasing the surface area contact. Over time, the adhesive will warm and flow to fill in the gaps between the adhesive and the irregularities in the skin surface, increasing the strength of the bond. The length of time for this process differs among different types of adhesive products. Some softer adhesives, such as silicone, have a lower surface tension and fill in these gaps quickly and maintain the same

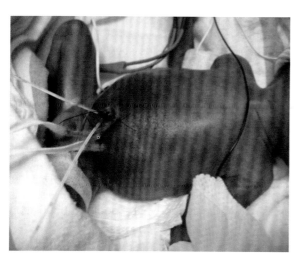 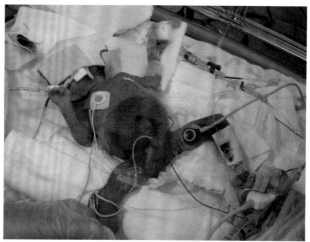

FIGURE 13-2 Chemical Burns in a Very-Low-Birth-Weight Infants from Disinfectant Containing 2% Chlorhexidine Gluconate and 70% Isopropyl Alcohol.

level of adherence over time. Other adhesives, such as the acrylates, act more slowly, and adherence increases over time to a state of maximal adherence, and then gradually the bond weakens. This is why, whenever possible, leaving an adhesive in place even when not in use, can assist in the removal process when the adhesive bond starts to lessen (Lund, 2014). See Chapter 18 for more information about MARSI.

An evidence-based practice project involving 2,820 premature and term newborns found that adhesives were the primary cause of skin breakdown among NICU patients (Lund et al., 2001). Changes in TEWL and skin barrier function are seen in adults after 10 consecutive removals of adhesive tape. However, these changes occur after only one removal of plastic perforated tape in neonates (Lund et al., 1997). MARSI includes epidermal stripping, tearing, maceration, tension blisters, contact and irritant dermatitis, and folliculitis (Lund, 2014; McNichol et al., 2013).

Kim et al. (2019) conducted a prospective observational study to identify the purpose, type, and site of medical adhesives (MAs) used for patient care to measure the incidence of MARSI among patients in a PICU. The number of MARSI occurrences was 35 cases in 23 patients. Skin stripping was the most common form of MARSI (26/35) (Kim et al., 2019).

Wang et al. (2019) investigated the prevalence of MARSI and associated risk factors in a PICU. A total of 232 patients were enrolled. Tracheal intubation (transoral or nasal, 37.58%), vascular access (22.67%), and ECG monitor (13.35%) accounted for most MARSIs. Tracheal intubation was the most common cause of MARSI. Skin stripping was the most common type of MARSI, followed by skin tears, tension injury/blisters, contact dermatitis, and maceration. Mild skin stripping was usually caused by electrode pads on the trunk. Extended use of electrode pads could also cause moderate skin tears attributable to increased adhesion. Severe skin tears were usually caused by acrylate tapes with soft elastic cloth or nonstretching cloth, and it was almost always documented on the face as a result of fixation of tracheal intubation (Wang et al., 2019) **(Fig. 13-3)**.

Medical Adhesive Removers

Adhesive removers are sometimes used to prevent discomfort and skin disruption from adhesive removal. There are three categories of adhesive removers: alcohol/organic-based solvents, oil-based solvents, and silicone-based removers (Black, 2007; Lund, 2014). The alcohol/organic-based removers contain hydrocarbon derivatives or petroleum distillates that have potential or proven toxicities. This is of particular concern with premature infants, due to their underdeveloped SC, increased skin permeability, larger surface area/body weight ratio, and immature hepatic and renal function. Mineral oil, petrolatum, and citrus-based products may be helpful

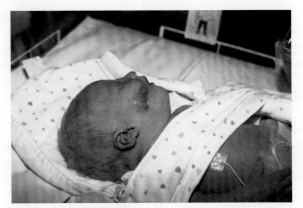

FIGURE 13-3. Example of Epidermal Stripping (MARSI) in Premature Infant.

in removing adhesives, and the area must be cleansed following removal. Silicone-based removers form an interposing layer between adhesive and skin, evaporate readily after application, and do not leave a residue (Black, 2007; Cooper et al., 2011; Lund, 2014). They have been recommended for patients with extremely fragile skin, such as infants with epidermolysis bullosa (EB) (Cooper et al., 2011; Denyer, 2011, Lund, 2014). Removing adhesives with water-soaked cotton balls sometimes helps, and gently pulling the adhesive parallel to the skin surface rather than straight up at a 90 degrees angle may facilitate removal with less skin trauma (Lund, 2014).

Despite using an adhesive remover prior to removal of adhesive dressings, epidermal stripping continues to be seen in neonates and pediatric patients with compromised skin integrity. Use of products with soft silicone adhesive technology may be better tolerated by neonates and children with skin fragility or impaired epidermal barrier. The use of dressings with soft silicone adhesive technology has also been associated with significantly reduced pain during dressing changes and minimizing TEWL (King et al., 2014).

Tackifiers

Substances that increase the stickiness or tack of adhesives, called bonding agents or tackifiers, are used to increase the cohesive strength of adhesives such as to promote adherence of wound closure tapes to surgical incisions. Examples of these products include tincture of benzoin (Compound Benzoin Tincture®) and gum mastic (Mastisol®). They may create a bond between the adhesive and epidermis that is stronger than the fragile cohesion of the epidermis to the dermis. When the adhesive is removed, epidermal stripping may result. Use of tackifiers is not recommended in the pediatric population.

Barrier Products

Liquid skin protectants that are silicone based and alcohol free are reported to reduce skin trauma from repeated adhesive removal (Black, 2007; Lund, 2014).

The use of a skin protectant underneath the tape used to secure intravenous lines in newborns provided skin protection (Irving, 2001) and reduced TEWL (Brandon et al., 2010).

Hydrocolloid skin barriers are sometimes used in the NICU as a platform between the skin and adhesive. This practice is based on the reduction in visible evidence of skin trauma with removal of the hydrocolloid as opposed to tape removal (Dollison & Beckstrand, 1995). Hydrocolloid adhesive products continue to be used in the NICU because they mold well to curved surfaces and adhere even with moisture.

Morris et al. (2015) conducted a retrospective two-group longitudinal comparative study to determine if a double hydrocolloid barrier prevents skin breakdown in very-low-birth-weight (VLBW) infants weighing <1,500 g who received oxygen via heated humidified high-flow nasal cannula (HHHFNC) when compared with a matched cohort who did not have the hydrocolloid dressing. Nurses evaluated the infants' skin for signs of trauma using the NSCS instrument. The authors found no differences in skin scores between the two groups. The use of HHHFNC, which exerts less pressure on the delicate nares tissues, is becoming increasingly common in the NICU, and fewer infants are receiving NCPAP, a device with a higher incidence of skin trauma. They concluded that a double-barrier hydrocolloid dressing between the HHHFNC cannula and infant's skin in addition to vigilant nursing care may help prevent nares breakdown (Morris et al., 2015).

Preventive Measures

Prevention of skin trauma from adhesive removal includes minimizing tape use when possible by using smaller pieces, backing the adhesive with cotton, and delaying tape removal until adherence is reduced. The use of soft wraps to secure pulse oximeter probes and hydrogel electrocardiogram electrodes is one strategy when feasible. Silicone-based adhesive products have been shown to improve adherence to wounds and to reduce discomfort with removal (Dykes et al., 2001; Gotschall et al., 1998; King et al., 2014). Silicone tapes are gentle to the skin but do not adhere well to plastic materials and cannot be used to secure critical tubes and appliances (McNichol et al., 2013; Yates et al., 2017). Higher performing acrylate adhesive tapes designed to withstand moisture may be beneficial to secure critical tubes and lines in NICU patients and may prevent the need for frequent retaping.

INTRAVENOUS EXTRAVASATIONS

Extravasation injuries can be serious in the neonatal population. Every effort must be made to prevent extravasation, and any injury that does occur must be promptly detected and treated.

Prevention

Prevention of tissue injury from IV extravasations includes securing IV devices with transparent dressings or plastic tape so that the insertion site is clearly visible, and observing the site with appropriate documentation every hour. If the IV device is placed in a limb, the tape securing the arm or leg to the rigid board should be placed loosely over the joint (such as the elbow or knee) and not over the skin directly above the insertion site. This allows any extravasated fluid and medications to diffuse over a larger surface rather than being concentrated and confined to a small, constricted area, which may result in greater tissue injury. An alternative approach that is being used by some NICUs with success is to eliminate use of the rigid board. Using central venous lines (such as peripherally inserted central venous catheters) to infuse highly irritating solutions and medications is also recommended. Many nurseries limit the glucose concentrations in peripheral lines to 12.5% and the amino acid concentrations to 2%. Use of peripheral veins for infusion of calcium-containing intravenous fluids is debatable as calcium is extremely irritating to the intima of the vein. When used, the concentration of calcium gluconate should be limited to 200 mg/100 mL (Thigpen, 2007; Treadwell, 2012).

The majority of infants in the NICU receive PIV therapy for administration of fluids, nutrition, medications, and blood products. The potential complications of infiltration and extravasation are common in this population. Extravasation is estimated to occur in 11% of NICU patients at <27 weeks' gestation (Thigpen, 2007). The terms "infiltration" and "extravasation" are defined by the Infusion Nurses Society (INS) based on the type of medication or fluid that inadvertently enters the tissues (infiltration). Vesicants are agents known to cause blistering, tissue sloughing, or necrosis. When this type of medication or fluid is involved, the infiltration is further described as an extravasation (Vizcarra et al., 2014).

Prevention strategies may include the following: avoid areas difficult to immobilize or secure (e.g., elbows, wrists, knees), tape loosely to promote circulation and venous return, do not tape proximal to the IV site to prevent tourniquet effect, stabilize the insertion site with a sterile, transparent adhesive dressing to allow visualization of the insertion site, peripheral dextrose solution should never exceed 12.5%, dilute medications according to pharmacologic recommendations, avoid peripheral infusion of calcium preparations, if possible, assess catheter site, compare both extremities (e.g., distal site, fingers, toes) and touch for coolness every hour, and do not use how easily the IV flushes as the only means of assessment (Desarno et al., 2018).

Management

If IV fluid has extravasated into surrounding tissue, the IV device should be removed and the extremity elevated (**Fig. 13-4**). Use of moisture, heat, or cold is not recommended because the tissue is vulnerable at this point to further injury. Hyaluronidase (Amphadase®, Vitrase®) can be helpful if administered shortly after the extravasation is identified. This medication is an enzyme that breaks down the interstitial barrier and allows the extravasated fluid to diffuse over a larger area, thus preventing or limiting tissue necrosis (Beaulieu, 2012; Doellman et al., 2009; Gorski et al., 2017; Treadwell, 2012). Extravasations for which hyaluronidase may be helpful include those with evidence of blanching, discoloration, or blistering and extravasations involving hypertonic or calcium-containing solutions, even if the site appears relatively undisturbed. The use of an extravasation scale for treatment of IV extravasations may improve communication and consistency in providing appropriate immediate care (Amjad et al., 2011; Gorski et al., 2017; Simona, 2012).

Calcium-containing solutions may cause deep tissue damage even when the epidermal tissues are not involved. In addition to hyaluronidase administration, creating multiple puncture holes over the area of swelling and gently palpating the involved area, or allowing the extravasated fluid to leak out, can promote removal of the infiltrate and reduce the risk of tissue necrosis (Chandavasu et al., 1986; Sawatzky-Dicksson & Bodnaryk, 2006). Saline washout is another technique described to facilitate the removal of extravasated irritants from tissues surrounding an IV site (Casanova et al.,

2001; Davies et al., 1994). Hyaluronidase is not recommended in the extravasation of vasoconstrictive medications such as dopamine, because it may extend the area of vasoconstriction. Phentolamine (Regitine®) is used in this case because it directly counteracts the action of dopamine (Thigpen, 2007).

Signs that alert the nurse to a possible extravasation include blanching extending more than ¼ inch past the insertion site or ½ inch in diameter and spreading, and skin cool and/or firm to touch (Desarno et al., 2018). Amjad and associates (2011) presented a revised grading scale proposed to represent the degree of severity relative to the size of the patient. By referring to the number of joints involved, and not a set number of inches, this scale represents the degree of severity relative to the size of the patient. A reference distance of 2 cm is included to ensure that infiltrations can be detected before involvement of any joints. A grade 1 is swelling <2 cm from the site or <1 joint involved. A grade 2 is swelling >2 cm from the site or blanched skin or involvement of 1 to 2 joints. A grade 3 is swelling involving >2 joints or any localized tissue damage.

Management of extravasation should include: stop the infusion, remove the catheter, elevate affected extremity, apply saline-soaked gauze to draw out the infiltrated fluid, and notify physician or nurse practitioner. One should not apply warm or cold compresses. Warm compresses may help reabsorb the infiltrating fluid, or it may cause further tissue damage by increasing metabolic rate. Cold compresses may limit further dispersion of the infusate into the surrounding tissue (Desarno et al., 2018).

Wound Care

When tissue injury occurs after extravasation, moist wound-healing principles are utilized to promote healing without scarring. In most cases, major tissue loss and the need for skin grafts can be prevented by the wound

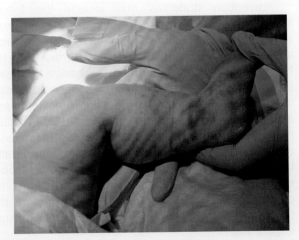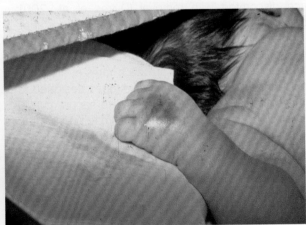

FIGURE 13-4. Intravenous Extravasation that Will Require Immediate Intervention to Prevent Wound.

care nurse. In the most severe cases involving compartment syndrome to the extremity or deep-tissue necrosis, a plastic surgery consultation may be necessary.

Wound care products include transparent film dressings that utilize silicone adhesive technology. These dressings adhere only to intact dry skin, not the surface of moist wounds, thereby avoiding damage to fragile new tissue upon removal. Silicone dressings may be left in place for several days, permitting observation of the site, yet allowing healing as the wound bed remains undisturbed. Amorphous hydrogels donate moisture to dry wounds to help maintain a moist healing environment. The high moisture content serves to rehydrate wound tissue, facilitating debridement or sloughing of necrotic tissue (Desarno et al., 2018).

DIAPER DERMATITIS

A common skin disruption that occurs in neonates and infants is diaper dermatitis. Diaper dermatitis is an irritant contact dermatitis (ICD) seen in the diaper area in neonates and infants (Tüzün et al., 2015). It predominantly occurs in infants and children aged <2 years with the highest incidence found in infants at the age of 7 to 12 months (Yuan et al., 2018). Diaper dermatitis is reported to account for approximately 20% of all pediatric office visits (Yuan et al., 2018). Diaper dermatitis may also be referred to as incontinence-associated dermatitis (IAD). IAD may affect the perineum, groin, thighs, buttocks, and anal region. Signs of IAD may include erythema, edema, blistering, skin erosion, weeping, and pain. Over time, the skin may even look sunburned and involve the skin folds between the buttocks and the inner thighs (Ratliff & Dixon, 2007).

The pathogenesis of IAD involves maceration, compounded by friction injury and/or damage from microbial invasion or enzymatic activity. Skin that is moist and macerated becomes more permeable and susceptible to injury because wetness increases friction. Moisture-laden skin is associated with higher levels of microorganisms as compared to dry skin. Another contributing factor to skin injury is the effect of an alkaline skin pH. The normal skin pH is acidic, ranging between 4.0 and 5.5; however, occluded and macerated skin is typically alkaline (McNichol et al., 2018; Visscher et al., 2015). When the skin pH is more alkaline, there is increased vulnerability to injury and penetration by microorganisms. An alkaline pH stimulates fecal enzyme activity. Stool contains both proteases and lipases, which, when activated, can cause significant damage to the protein and fat components of the skin. This enzymatic damage is responsible for much of the contact irritant diaper dermatitis commonly seen in clinical practice. Stools from breastfed infants have been shown to have a lower pH and may be less irritating to the skin, and so infants that are breastfed are less likely to develop severe IAD (Wesner et al., 2019).

Prevention

Strategies for preventing diaper dermatitis include maintaining a dry and acidic skin surface. Frequent diaper changes are recommended, especially in the newborn period. Superabsorbent gelling diapers with breathable covers have been shown to keep the skin surface drier by wicking the moisture away from the skin and separating urine from feces (Kosemund et al., 2009; Lin et al., 2005; Nield & Kamat, 2007; Rai et al., 2009; Scheinfeld, 2005). The routine use of petrolatum-based ointments may prevent the progression to diaper dermatitis in neonates and infants at risk, such as those with watery stools from opiate withdrawal or malabsorption. Use of powders is discouraged because of the risk of inhalation of particles into the respiratory tract. Liquid silicone-based and alcohol-free barrier films, which are designed to repel moisture and protect the skin from irritants (Heimall et al., 2012), can be used as barriers to prevent diaper dermatitis. These products are FDA approved for use in infants >28 days of age but are frequently used off-label and have been beneficial when used on neonatal ostomy patients.

Burdall et al. (2019) conducted a literature search to review different practices in neonatal care to maintain skin barrier function to prevent diaper dermatitis. They concluded from the search that super-absorbent diapers reduce moisture at skin level to reduce diaper dermatitis. Barrier creams may be beneficial both in prevention and treatment but do not provide a substitute for frequent diaper changes. Also they found that the literature does not demonstrate superiority of one cleansing method over another, but neither the use of wipes nor water increases diaper dermatitis prevalence.

Vongsa et al. (2019) reviewed the clinical evidence comparing the use of baby wipes to water and cloth wipes. They found that clinical studies over the past 15 years have demonstrated the safety and efficacy of using formulated baby wipes on diapered infant skin. Baby wipes were found to be superior to water and cloth in 4 out of 5 published studies comparing cleaning with water and cloth to cleaning with formulated baby wipes. None of the studies found baby wipes to be inferior to water and cloth. There were no studies with preterm infants and the use of baby wipes. One major concern associated with using any skincare products on very preterm infants is the potential percutaneous absorption of ingredients found in the products. Special consideration must be taken when cleaning the skin of very premature infants, especially during the first 2 weeks of life while the skin is undergoing rapid maturation (Vongsa et al., 2019).

Diaper wipes should be free of alcohol (benzyl alcohol is mild and considered safe), perfumes, or preservatives, such as methylisothiazolinone, that may contribute to skin irritation and increase risk for allergic contact dermatitis (ACD) (Visscher et al., 2015).

Treatment

Once skin injury from diaper dermatitis has occurred, protecting the damaged skin to prevent reinjury is the primary goal of treatment (**Fig. 13-5**). Topical treatment for diaper dermatitis involves ointments and creams containing a variety of ingredients such as zinc oxide and petrolatum (Heimall et al., 2012). Generous application of protective skin barriers that contain zinc oxide may prevent further injury while allowing the skin to heal. Once denudation occurs, keeping the skin open to air is not an effective strategy. The damaged tissue requires a moist surface for healing, and leaving the damaged surface open to air provides no protection against exposure to stool during recurrent diarrheal episodes. All caregivers must be taught that it is not necessary or desirable to completely remove the skin barrier ointment with each diaper change, because this causes additional trauma that disrupts healing tissue. The caregiver should remove the layers of ointment soiled with stool and should reapply the barrier generously to the affected areas with each diaper change.

The skin should be cleansed with water and/or gentle cleansers. Products with a more acidic pH similar to the skin (pH of 5 to 5.5) may help combat alkalization from fecal enzymes. Barrier creams that contain zinc oxide and/or petroleum provide a protective layer over the skin to reduce contact with urine and stool and allow the underlying skin to heal. These creams can also be used to prevent or treat IAD. A thick coat should be applied at each diaper change after gently removing stool or other contaminants. Noncontaminated residual barrier cream does not have to be completely removed at each change. Cornstarch may be used to reduce moisture and friction in the diaper area but should be used with caution to prevent inhalation. Baby powders that contain talcum should be avoided due to concerns of asbestos contamination and increased risk of ovarian cancer (Wesner et al., 2019).

Candidiasis

Candida albicans can be a contributing factor to diaper dermatitis. The yeast rash presents as a bright erythematous, sharply demarcated dermatitis that involves the inguinal folds as well as the buttocks, thighs, and genitalia, typically with characteristic satellite lesions (**Fig. 13-6**). Treatment with an antifungal ointment or cream is necessary. Antifungal preparations include nystatin, miconazole, clotrimazole, and ketoconazole in ointment or cream forms; ointments are preferable to coat the skin and repel moisture (AWHONN, 2018). If the dermatitis involves both a fungal rash and denudation due to contact irritant dermatitis, it may be necessary to layer the ointment with the antifungal preparation. In this case, nystatin or miconazole powder can be dusted onto the area, followed by application of an alcohol-free liquid skin protectant to seal the powder onto the skin surface, followed by a generous application of a skin barrier cream such as zinc oxide or pectin paste (AWHONN, 2018; Heimall et al., 2012).

When *Candida* is present, treatment and the application of a barrier for the prevention of skin breakdown or further skin breakdown are the goals (AWHON, 2018). Low concentrations of antifungal agents in a zinc–petrolatum base have shown to be well tolerated and effective in treating mild to severe diaper dermatitis complicated by *Candida* (AWHONN, 2018).

Occasionally, infants may experience extremely severe diaper dermatitis from intestinal malabsorption syndromes, opiate withdrawal, or constant dribbling of stool due to compromised sphincter function (e.g., infants with myelomeningocele or those undergoing a pull-through procedure for Hirschsprung disease or anorectal atresia). In the case of malabsorption, there is rapid transit through the small intestine. This results in a complex clinical situation that includes abnormally alkaline stool, increased stool volume, higher levels of activated enzymes, and undigested carbohydrates and

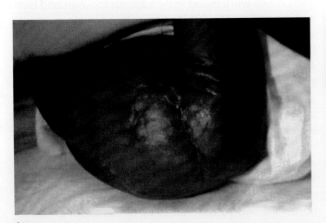
A

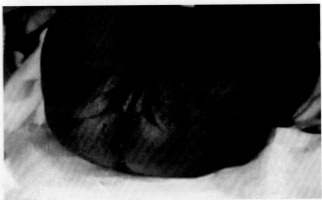
B

FIGURE 13-5. A. Contact Irritant Dermatitis (IAD). **B.** IAD Improved with Treatment. (Used with permission from Ratliff, C., & Dixon, M. (2007). Treatment of incontinence-associated dermatitis (diaper rash) in a neonatal unit. *Journal of Wound, Ostomy and Continence Nursing, 34*(2):158–161.)

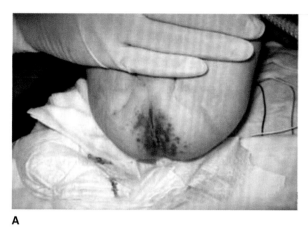
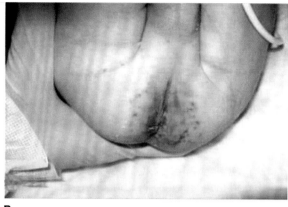

A   **B**

FIGURE 13-6. A. Diaper Dermatitis (IAD) Caused by *Candida albicans*. **B.** IAD Improved with Treatment. (Used with permission from Ratliff, C., & Dixon, M. (2007). Treatment of incontinence-associated dermatitis (diaper rash) in a neonatal unit. *Journal of Wound, Ostomy and Continence Nursing, 34*(2):158–161.)

fats. Infants with malabsorption syndromes are at risk for nutritional deficiencies and dehydration in addition to severe diaper dermatitis and require thorough medical evaluation.

While optimal nutritional therapy is being addressed with special diets or parenteral nutrition, skin protection from injury should be initiated. Products that contain carboxymethylcellulose, petrolatum, and zinc oxide without alcohol may provide a sturdier barrier for these infants than zinc oxide alone. The skin should be thoroughly but gently cleansed followed by a very thick application of the barrier paste. The barrier paste is then covered by a greasy ointment such as petrolatum to prevent adherence of the barrier paste to the diaper. When the infant has a stool, it is not necessary to completely remove the barrier paste. The stool can be gently wiped away before reapplying the thick paste barrier. The skin will heal under this protective covering as long as it is protected from reinjury. Another approach described is the crusting technique. Pectin-based powder is dusted onto the skin followed by application of an alcohol-free liquid skin protectant (AWHONN, 2018; Gray, 2007; Heimall et al., 2012). Products that contain cyanoacrylates adhere well to excoriated skin and provide an excellent barrier which lasts up to 5 to 7 days (Brennan et al., 2017).

🌑 UNIQUE CHALLENGES IN PEDIATRIC SKIN AND WOUND CARE

In neonatal and pediatric clinical settings, wound care concepts are generalizable from the adult literature. Knowledge of pediatric nursing should be applied to wound care practice to meet the needs of this population.

Coupled with the age range and developmental stages is the range of both congenital and acquired diagnoses in the pediatric population. It is important for the pediatric wound care nurse to serve as a liaison between various disciplines, the child and family, and develop a plan of care that reflects the goals of the child, family, and care team. Communication and collaboration skills are important in meeting the needs of the pediatric population. The pediatric wound care nurse must realize that, in many situations, the wound is a complication of a primary diagnosis, surgical procedure, or trauma, which means the child and family have multiple competing issues and challenges in addition to the wound. As in any complex situation, the tolerance for discussion of multiple ideas and plans of care is limited. To avoid overwhelming children and families or adding confusion, wound care management plans should be presented within the context of the overall plan of care. This approach avoids conflicting information as well as promoting the team approach. It is the responsibility of the pediatric wound care nurse to explain to the parents the common principles underlying all recommendations and to work with the entire team to develop a plan that works for the parents and the child. It is important to acknowledge that wound care is challenging and to use available resources and strategies (such as the child life specialist and premedication) to facilitate dressing changes and wound management at home. These approaches support family centered care. More than family-centered care, the wound care plan of care should be centered on the needs of the child.

KEY POINT

Most wound care principles are generalizable to a variety of populations in all care settings. Products used in premature and neonatal patients should be evaluated for skin toxicity.

KEY POINT

Wound care for the pediatric patient must be evidence-based and feasible for the child and parent.

PHYSIOLOGY PEDIATRIC SKIN AND WOUND HEALING

Throughout childhood, the skin continues to change as the child grows. These changes involve general appearance of the skin, its texture and elasticity, and the time frame for healing. During early childhood, wounds that are appropriately managed heal quickly and with minimal scarring. Moving a wound rapidly through the inflammatory phase, eliminating necrotic tissue and controlling bacterial loads, is an important strategy for minimizing scarring (Occleston et al., 2010). Scars acquired in early childhood fade, stretch, and become less obvious in later years (Occleston et al., 2010). The wound care nurse must be able to explain the basic healing process in simple terms and must also address concerns regarding both short-term and long-term outcomes and expectations, for example, wound healing and wound management short term and scar appearance long term.

Scar Appearance

A concern for all parents is impact of the wound and eventual scar on the child's body image and the appearance of the healed wound and scar. The wound care nurse should be prepared to discuss wound-healing outcomes and options for scar management. They should provide the family with future management strategies including a referral to plastic surgery if there is a history of keloid formation. Prevention of scar formation and keloid formation includes early intervention with silicone-based dressings. After an incision or wound is well healed, scar formation is further prevented with the use of a thin silicone dressing. The silicone dressing when worn for 23 hours out of the day for several weeks after wound healing minimizes scar formation.

Impact of Developmental Stage

Pediatric skin and wound care is provided within the framework of overall growth and development. The plan of care includes attention to differences in skin condition, activity levels, and perspiration. Dressing options may vary based on the age and development of a child. For example, a toddler who has soft supple skin will benefit from a silicone-based dressing or a dressing that has a 5-day wear time, whereas a teenager who is prone to sweating may need a dressing with greater adhesion and more resistance to moisture and activity.

The generalized knowledge of skin conditions or pediatric conditions combined with the specialty body of knowledge around wounds places the pediatric wound care nurse in a unique position to provide comprehensive care. The pediatric wound care nurse shares responsibility for facilitating, coordinating, and providing input on care transitions. The pediatric wound care nurse is frequently asked to provide recommendations for wound management.

SKIN DISORDERS COMMONLY SEEN IN THE PEDIATRIC POPULATION

ATOPIC DERMATITIS

Over the last 5 decades, the prevalence of atopic dermatitis (AD) has increased dramatically. If one parent is affected, there is a 20% risk of a child developing the disease. If both parents have AD, there is up to a 50% chance of a child developing it. Close to 60% of people diagnosed with eczema are diagnosed between 3 and 6 months of age. Along with genetic factors, this rise in cases seems to be related to environmental exposure of infants to agents that break down the skin barrier, such as washing with soaps and detergents (Kuller, 2016).

Atopic dermatitis is commonly known as eczema, is a chronic inflammatory disease (Janmohamed et al., 2014) that occurs in children, but persists into adulthood. The classic symptoms include skin dryness, erythema, intense pruritus, weeping, and crusting, all of which impact quality of life (Janmohamed et al., 2014). The lichenification process can also cause disfigurement, which impacts body image. The goal of treatment is not cure but elimination of triggers and symptom management (Janmohamed et al., 2014).

Management

Eczema is a challenging disease that requires a multidimensional approach. The five main principles underlying topical therapy include maintaining the pH balance of the skin, restoring and maintaining skin hydration through use of humectant and emollients, minimizing exacerbating factors, providing patient education, and assuring appropriate pharmacological treatment (Visser, 2014).

Skin cleansers are primarily made up of surfactants, which act by decreasing the surface tension between water and air, and create lather, allowing the fat-soluble impurities to be removed from the skin surface. Surfactants in cleansers can potentially weaken the skin barrier, increase TEWL, and lower hydration, leading to skin dryness, irritation, and redness when the product is not designed to be mild and infant skin compatible. Ideal cleansers should be a mild liquid, remove unwanted material, interact minimally with the skin, have a skin-compatible pH value below 7.0, have minimal dyes and fragrance, and have been tested on infants so that the infant's acid mantle and skin barrier are not disrupted (Kuller, 2016).

Emollients can be applied after a bath if the skin shows any signs of dryness or cracking. Because emollients provide a temporary artificial repair of the SC, they must be applied frequently. One of the safest and most effective emollients available for newborns is white petrolatum ointment (Aquaphor ointment) (Kuller, 2016).

The formulation of diaper wipes are free of alcohol, with a mild surfactant to lower surface tension. They also include a preservative, an ingredient that enhances glide across the skin to minimize frictional damage (e.g., dimethicone), and have a pH of approximately 5.5.

Talcum powder is not recommended for use in an infant's diaper area because inhaled particles can lead to respiratory complications. Also, these products may promote the growth of bacteria and *Candida* sp. and can worsen diaper dermatitis (Kuller, 2016).

The pediatric wound care nurse comanages the child with a dermatologist or can manage the child independently within scope of practice and knowledge level. Open eczematous lesions are at risk for bacterial, viral, and dermatophyte infections, which manifest intense erythema, tenderness to touch, increased drainage, or odor. A punched out appearance and hemorrhagic vesicles are indicative of a secondary herpes simplex infection that requires systemic treatment. Initial treatment should include a systemic antiviral, a broad-spectrum antibacterial, an antimicrobial dressing, and close monitoring.

Initial treatment with a broad-spectrum antibacterial in addition to the antiviral ensures that a staph infection which may be masked is not left untreated. Identification of exacerbating factors is crucial for minimizing flares. Triggering factors commonly include food allergies, heat, and humidity. Given the correlation between food allergies and eczema, consultation with an allergist is extremely helpful for most children to identify which food or items in the environment are triggers.

The pediatric wound care nurse should develop a therapeutic relationship with the child and family. Education should emphasize skin hygiene, identification and avoidance of irritants, and the routine use of emollients and humectants to maintain soft supple skin. The wound care nurse is in a unique position to provide ongoing education and support for the child and family.

Description of Clinical Scenario

Wound care nurse was consulted for care of 4-year-old girl with extensive eczema involving her face, neck, and arms. The patient was admitted to rule out bacterial, viral, and/or dermatophyte infection secondary to lesions from eczema; transported from outside facility with wet dressings over her arms and neck that are to be kept moist at all times. The child is bothered by the dressings, and her day care facility is questioning her ability to participate in activities.

Plans for Wound Care

The wound care nurse established the following goals: (1) establish a trusting relationship with the child and family; (2) obtain a history of previously used products and current skin care routine; (3) identify a dressing that meets the goals of care and allows the child to return to preschool; and (4) educate the child and family regarding eczema management.

The wound care nurse talked with the patient and family regarding low-profile dressings that are easy to

conceal and showed them samples of a medical-grade honey alginate dressing that could be applied directly to the open wounds and covered with a light silicone adhesive foam or wicking fabric secured with stretch net. These dressings could be changed daily with minimal or no discomfort, could be easily concealed under long sleeve clothing, and would keep her clothing dry. The wound care nurse also emphasized the importance of maintaining skin pH using a pH-balanced cleanser with an antimicrobial agent followed by daily use of a dimethicone 6% moisturizer. **Figures 13-7 to 13-10** show progression of healing.

CONTACT DERMATITIS

Contact dermatitis is a category of diseases whose common denominator is an external inciting factor. Included in this group are ICD, contact urticaria (CU), protein contact dermatitis (PCD), and ACD (Admani & Jacob, 2014).

Contact dermatitis is inflammation of the dermis and epidermis, which has been triggered by a substance that came in contact with the skin surface. There are two broad categories of contact dermatitis: irritant dermatitis and allergic dermatitis. ICD involves either diaper dermatitis or dermatitis involving intact dry skin. Diaper dermatitis is common in children of all ages who require diapering (even short term) for incontinence. During an acute illness requiring antibiotics, stool pH frequently changes, which makes it highly irritating to the skin. Prevention

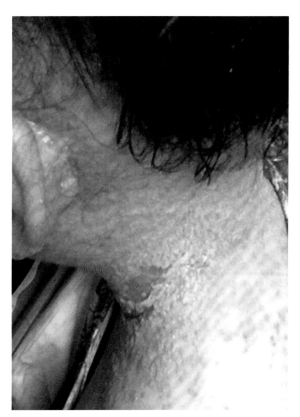

FIGURE 13-7. A Young Girl with Severe Eczema on Initial Presentation.

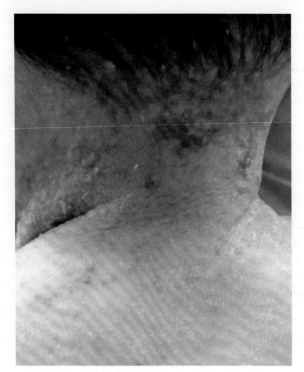

FIGURE 13-8. Response to Treatment that Included Antivirals, Antibiotics, Medical-Grade Honey to Open Lesions; Daily Cleansing with pH-balanced Cleanser; and Moisturizing with 6% Dimethicone.

includes application of a thin clear skin barrier with all diapered children during an acute illness, either a petrolatum-based ointment or a liquid barrier film. If the diaper dermatitis involves a fungal infection, the child should be

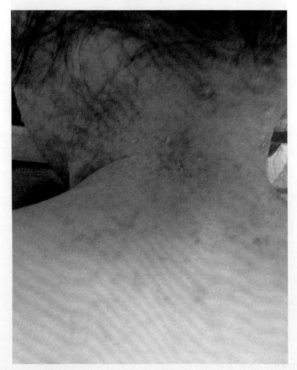

FIGURE 13-9. Skin at the Time of Discharge.

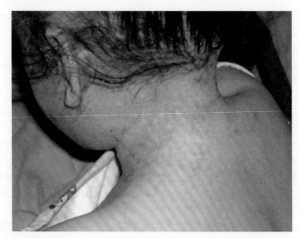

FIGURE 13-10. Skin Showing Progressive Healing.

treated with an antifungal agent, as discussed earlier in this chapter. The wound care nurse should be aware that there are multiple strands of *C. albicans* and not all are responsive to nystatin; if the child with a fungal rash fails to respond to nystatin, she or he should be treated with a broad-spectrum antifungal such as miconazole (Fridkin & Jarvis, 1996).

The wound care nurse should realize that fungal rashes that develop following broad spectrum antibiotic therapy are more likely to be resistant to nystatin than those developing following milder oral agents (Fridkin & Jarvis, 1996). There is ongoing research into treatment for resistant fungal infections (Vandeputte et al., 2012). The wound care nurse should always query patients in regard to recent antibiotic therapy and continence status. In the interest of avoiding polypharmacy at the bedside and simplifying skin care routines, a combined barrier and antifungal ointment is recommended for children who are incontinent and who present with a fungal rash. Prompt treatment of diaper dermatitis is important in order to prevent denudation, which increases the risk for *Candida* invasion of the skin, soft tissue, and even blood (Fridkin & Jarvis, 1996).

KEY POINT

Algorithms are effective tools for improving standards of care and outcomes.

See **Figure 13-11** for a sample algorithm addressing prevention and management of diaper dermatitis.

EPIDERMOLYSIS BULLOSA

Epidermolysis bullosa (EB) is a rare skin condition affecting the junction between the epidermis and dermis, with an incidence of 1/50,000 live births or 50 in 1 million live births. There are three main types of EB: EB simplex, junctional EB, and dystrophic EB. EB simplex accounts for

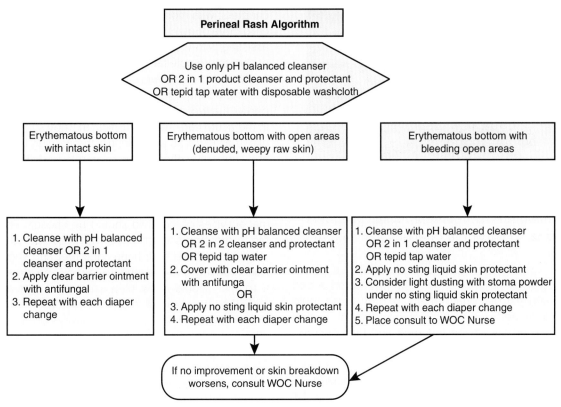

FIGURE 13-11. Sample Perineal Rash Algorithm.

92% of all cases and is autosomal dominant; junctional is autosomal recessive and rare, accounting for only 1% to 2% of the cases. Dystrophic EB can be either dominant or recessive and accounts for approximately 5% to 6% of cases. EB simplex typically affects the hands and feet and is the simplest form of EB. During the first year of life, the infant may experience blistering over the arms and legs. Toward the end of the first year of life, the blistering becomes limited to the hands and feet. Autosomal recessive EB is the severest form. These infants have blisters present at birth caused by the friction experienced during delivery. The mucous membranes and lining of the gastrointestinal tract are also involved, which makes feeding difficult. The child often suffers from calorie deficiencies due to the combined problems of impaired intake and increased caloric demands related to wound healing (Singer et al., 2018; Thompson et al., 2014).

Management

EB is diagnosed in infancy, often within the first few weeks of life. EB is initially managed in the neonatal intensive care unit. The NICU must have a policy for management of these infants and their lesions. The child is managed by dermatology and the neonatologist. The pediatric wound care nurse can assist with initiation of treatment, education of the parents, and case management (e.g., ordering supplies).

The pediatric wound care nurse supports the families during adjustment to the unexpected and devastating diagnosis by connecting them to the Debra foundation (debra.org, 2014). The families are not expecting a diagnosis of EB and need support in adjusting to the diagnosis and in preparing to bring the baby home (debra. org, 2014). The baby diagnosed with EB needs to be protected from friction. Even light pressure and friction caused by hugging and kissing can result in blisters. Adjustment to the diagnosis includes changing perceptions regarding good parenting behaviors and how to include the extended family (debra.org, 2014). Providing ongoing support prior to and following discharge home is a team approach that includes social work, case management, dermatology, and wound care (debra.org, 2014). Research in wound healing for children with EB is ongoing. Evolving treatment strategies include gene therapy and advanced topical therapy (Cutlar et al., 2014).

Older children who have lived their entire lives with EB have an established routine for dressing changes and preferences regarding dressings (debra.org, 2014). Children with EB easily verbalize what they can and cannot do. The pediatric wound care nurse needs to involve the child and follow their lead in dressing changes and activity.

Topical Therapy

Only nonadhesive dressings or those with gentle adhesive technology comes in direct contact with the child. Moisturizers should be used in generous amounts to prevent friction and blister formation. Low-friction

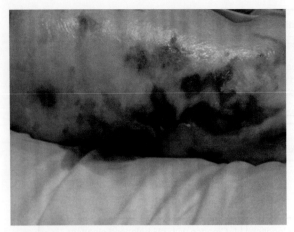

FIGURE 13-12. A Child with EB: Open blisters on the lower back.

antimicrobial linens should be strongly recommended for routine use (Coladonato et al., 2012). Blisters should be drained immediately to prevent enlargement. Central lines if needed should be tunneled and then secured with a single stitch. Special considerations in the OR include avoiding use of tapes directly on the skin. ET tubes should be secured with a mask placed behind the child's head with the ties then secured around the ET tube (**Fig. 13-12**).

The dressing regimen for an individual child is created in conjunction with dermatology and modified over time to reflect the child's growth and changes in activity. The child is continually monitored for sepsis, and the parents are given instructions as to signs of wound infection and proper response, as well as daily skin and wound care and blister management.

REPERFUSION INJURY

Reperfusion injury is seen after periods of extreme ischemia. Irreversible tissue damage can occur within 3 hours of extreme ischemia (Blaisdell, 2002). The thrombotic and inflammatory responses associated with reperfusion injury begin after the ischemia has been corrected. The tissue damage associated with reperfusion injury may be uniform (as if a tourniquet was applied) or may be patchy (Blaisdell, 2002). The injury often involves the tips of the ears, fingers, nose, or toes. The extent of reperfusion injury will depend on the duration of the ischemia and level of damage to collateral vessels (Blaisdell, 2002). Once the blood flow and blood pressure are normalized and stabilized, the reperfusion injury becomes evident. Reperfusion injury is a complicated pathologic process with the potential for devastating consequences including amputation. Smaller areas of ischemic damage may be managed with advanced wound care (Mohr et al., 2014).

⬤ WOUND CARE FOR THE PEDIATRIC POPULATION

Pediatric wound care is based on the principles of wound care and topical therapy addressed in previous chapters, with modifications based on issues related to child development. Families and caregivers providing or assisting with wound care must be involved in the plan of care to promote family-centered care and compliance. Families and caregivers need to be encouraged to practice the wound care and dressing change with the support of the wound care nurse as often as possible while in the acute care setting. Topical therapy should be simplified as much as possible, nonthreatening to the child, and supportive of concerns related to body image.

DRESSING SELECTION

Low-profile dressings that do not interfere with the normal activities of the child should be chosen. For example, a dressing should, whenever possible, allow older infants to explore their hands and feet and should support crawling and learning to stand. The dressing for a toddler should allow play activities. The older child should be encouraged to discuss what they want from a dressing. Topical therapy should always be designed to minimize pain and discomfort. Key strategies include use of dressings with gentle adhesives, such as silicone, and advanced wound dressings that reduce dressing change frequency. Options for advanced dressings that do not require daily dressing changes include foam dressings, silver-impregnated dressings, alginate dressings (plain, silver impregnated, or impregnated with leptospermum honey), hydrofiber dressings (plain or silver impregnated), gel dressings, and silicone-based contact layer dressings. Using appropriate primary and secondary dressings can reduce dressing changes to every few days or weekly (Mohr et al., 2014; Weissenstein et al., 2014).

Advanced dressings should be considered as first-line dressings in pediatrics to promote healing while minimizing pain and trauma. Creating a chart for dressing selection that includes a picture of the product, indications for use, directions for use, and special considerations can assure appropriate selection and utilization of dressings by staff throughout the facility. As value-based purchasing progresses, it is important that wound care follow evidence-based practice that includes advanced dressings.

NEGATIVE PRESSURE WOUND THERAPY

NPWT has been commonly used to treat pediatric patients, including neonates and premature infants, and its use includes the traditional indications established for adults and congenital or age-specific diseases. Neonates and small infants are the most common pediatric surgery patients treated with NPWT, due to abdominal complications, especially necrotizing enterocolitis and bowel necrosis, and complicated abdominal wall malformations in this population (de Jesus et al., 2018).

NPWT is commonly recommended for nonhealing wounds, and pediatric wound care nurses are frequently asked about safety of use in this population (Rentea et al., 2013). Small studies have demonstrated safe use in children >1 year of age, and a larger retrospective study demonstrated safe use in 290 pediatric cases (Boyar, 2018; Copeland et al., 2018; Rentea et al., 2013). There are increasing data that support the use of NPWT in infants younger than 1 year of age. Stoffan et al. (2012) reported safe use of NPWT in neonates and infants. They reviewed cases over a 10-year period of time in which NPWT was used in infants. Most authors recommend beginning NPWT at low levels of pressure for small infants (e.g., −50 to −75 mm Hg) and gradually increasing for older infants and toddlers (Rentea et al., 2013; Stoffan et al., 2012). Anecdotally, pediatric surgeons have reported good outcomes when the pressure was kept close to the child's mean arterial pressure. Pressure limits of −50 to −75 mm Hg are recommended for hemodynamically unstable children. For all children, the NPWT should be managed by an interdisciplinary team, which should include members from the surgical service, the wound care nurse, and child life therapy. Principles underlying effective use of NPWT in the pediatric population are the same as those for adults, with a few additional considerations related to pain management such as use of a nonadhesive layer under the wound vacuum sponge.

KEY POINT

NPWT can be safely used in neonatal and pediatric populations with modifications and careful monitoring.

To reduce trauma, bleeding, and pain during dressing changes, the pediatric wound care nurse implements measures to prevent tissue adherence and growth into the wound vacuum sponge. Use of a contact layer between the wound bed and the sponge is a simple and effective way to prevent adherence and ingrowth. Options for contact layer include a silicone fenestrated dressing, emollient-impregnated dressing, and ionic silver fenestrated dressing. Use of a contact layer minimizes the effort required to remove the sponge from the wound bed and reduces the overall dressing change time while minimizing pain.

Measures to prevent sponge adherence to organs is an important element of care when NPWT is used for wounds with exposed organs in the wound bed. Organ adherence to the sponge may result in organ perforation, fistula formation, or massive bleeding with sponge removal. The hydrophobic white sponge used in conjunction with a contact layer effectively prevents adherence and ingrowth of organ tissue into the sponge. The wound care nurse collaborates with the physician groups to educate all involved staff regarding safe use of NPWT in the pediatric population. A NPWT policy and procedure should be in place.

The hydrophobic dressing is used when there is uneven healing and differing rates of granulation within the wound bed. Areas of more exuberant granulation tissue can be covered with the hydrophobic dressing to provide slower granulation, and the areas where granulation is less active can be covered with a contact layer and black foam to optimize granulation. The wound care nurse should assess the wound at each dressing change. When the rate of granulation throughout the wound bed is equal, the entire wound can be managed with a contact layer and black foam.

Another measure to reduce pain associated with NPWT is to utilize the continuous setting as opposed to intermittent setting on the vacuum pump. When the pump is in intermittent mode, the cyclical contraction and relaxation of the foam is likely to be perceived as pain. Use of the continuous setting reduces the need for pain medication during therapy. Typically, analgesics are limited to premedication just prior to dressing changes. For younger children and children with very difficult and painful wounds, it may be necessary to do the NPWT dressing changes in an ambulatory procedure unit with sedation managed by anesthesiology.

The time frame for NPWT ranges from 1 week to several weeks, depending on the size and location of the wound. If therapy is prolonged for more than 2 weeks, the plan of care should be discussed with the child and family to ensure minimal disruption of school and related activities.

All caregivers should be taught to monitor the drainage collected in the NPWT canister. The volume of drainage varies based on the wound type and stage of healing. Normally there is a progressive reduction in the volume of drainage as the wound progresses. If the volume of drainage suddenly increases or remains unexpectedly high, further evaluation is needed to rule out complications. Surgical evaluation may be needed. Sanguineous drainage or a change from serous to sanguineous drainage is monitored. Sanguineous drainage exceeding 5% of the child's blood volume should be reported immediately (Rentea et al., 2013).

A sudden increase in volume of drainage accompanied by a change in character of the drainage requires evaluation to ensure no fistula has developed between the wound bed and underlying organs or the lymphatic system. Pale yellow thin exudate usually requires radiologic evaluation to ensure that no communication to the lymphatic system or the bladder depending on the location of the NPWT. There is a higher risk of fistula development when NPWT is used inappropriately and with poor technique.

NPWT is a valuable adjunctive therapy in wound management but requires appropriate and cautious use to prevent complications. The pediatric wound care nurse provides support to the surgical service and nursing staff in decision-making regarding indications and contraindications to use, appropriate settings, and use of appropriate contact layers. The wound care nurse should establish policies and procedures and ensure that education is provided to all caregivers regarding problem solving and monitoring of patients receiving NPWT.

BIOLOGIC DRESSINGS

Biologic dressings may be used in pediatric wound care as an option for challenging wounds or wounds in patients with complicated systemic disease processes. The pediatric wound care nurse may recommend them in situations where there is delayed healing. It is important to assure that the wound bed is ready for a biologic dressing, and all systemic factors have been addressed to eliminate impediments to healing.

 PREVENTION OF SKIN BREAKDOWN

Maintaining skin integrity is another responsibility of the pediatric wound care nurse. Products used in skin and wound care should be approved for use in children. Silicone- or gel-based adhesive products are best practice in pediatric care to minimize skin trauma and pain from adhesives. Any medical device requires care to minimize the risk of skin damage. Thin adhesive foam or hydrocolloid dressings may be used under a device to provide padding and absorb moisture (e.g., silicone or gel based). When use of a protective dressing is not feasible, the device requires routine repositioning at least every 8 hours and skin integrity assessed every 4 hours. All dressing and adhesive products should be removed with silicone-based adhesive remover to promote skin integrity and reduce the risk of adhesive trauma.

Support surfaces in the pediatric care setting should redistribute pressure. They may be foam based, gel based, or air based. Positioners should be utilized for off-loading and to support natural alignment. Techniques to protect and float at risk areas, for example, ears, elbows, heels, and occiput, should be used. There are options to have customized mattresses built for any size crib or isolette.

The pediatric wound care nurse collaborates with staff and leadership to ensure an evidence-based pressure injury prevention program is maintained. At-risk patients should be identified through use of a pressure injury risk assessment tool. A prevention protocol should include appropriate support surfaces and repositioning devices as well as guidelines for routine turning and positioning, moisture management, and nutrition (Singh et al., 2018). Most pediatric hospitals participate in initiatives to collect data on outcomes and risk assessments, which allow each facility to compare their outcomes with comparable facilities (Singh et al., 2018). The white paper by the NPIAP recommends a bundled approach to pressure injury prevention (Delmore et al., 2019).

Responsibilities of the wound care nurse in pressure injury prevention include maintenance of current evidence-based protocols for risk assessment and prevention and collaboration with purchasing and value analysis committee to assure appropriate support surfaces, positioners, and skin care products are available (Delmore et al., 2019). Collaboration with clinical educators and staff is important for educational strategies to keep staff current in risk assessment and pressure injury prevention. Implementation of prevention programs, education, and engagement of parents in pressure injury prevention are all part of the pediatric wound care nurse role.

 CONCLUSION

The pediatric wound care nurse plays an important role in skin protection and wound care for the neonatal and pediatric population. Major responsibilities include selection of quality products that promote skin integrity and wound healing, maintenance of evidence-based protocols and staff education regarding prevention of pressure injuries, MDRPIs, MARSI, skin tears, and extravasation injuries. Individualized wound care that is both evidence based and family oriented is the desired outcome. The ultimate responsibility is to advocate for the children and their families.

REFERENCES

Admani, S., & Jacob, S. E. (2014). Allergic contact dermatitis in children: Review of the past decade. *Current Allergy and Asthma Reports*, *14*(4), 421.

Agren, J., Sjors, G., & Sedin, G. (1998). Transepidermal water loss in infants born at 24 and 25 weeks of gestation. *Acta Paediatrica*, *87*, 1185–1190.

Aitken, J., & Williams, F. L. R. (2014). A systematic review of thyroid dysfunction in preterm neonates exposed to topical iodine. *Archives of Disease in Childhood-Fetal and Neonatal Edition*, *99*(1), F21–F28.

Amjad, I., Murphy, T., Nylander-Housholder, L., et al. (2011). A new approach to management of intravenous infiltration in pediatric patients: Pathophysiology, classification, and treatment. *Journal of Infusion Nursing, 34*(4), 242–249.

Anderson, J. M., Cockburn, F., Forfar, J. O., et al. (1981). Neonatal spongioform myelinopathy after restricted application of hexachlorophane skin disinfectant. *Journal of Clinical Pathology, 34*(1), 25–29.

Association of Women's Health, Obstetric and Neonatal Nurses (AWHONN). (2018). *Evidence-based clinical practice guideline: Neonatal skin care* (4th ed.). Washington, DC: Association of Women's Health, Obstetric and Neonatal Nurses.

Baharestani, M. M., & Ratliff, C. R. (2007). Pressure ulcers in neonates and children: An NPUAP white paper. *Advances in Skin & Wound Care, 20*(4), 208–220.

Beaulieu, M. J. (2012). Hyaluronidase for extravasation management. *Neonatal Network, 31*(6), 413–418.

Behrendt, H., & Green, M. (1971). *Patterns of Skin PH from Birth Through Adolescence: With a Synopsis on Skin Growth*. Springfield, IL: Charles C. Thomas.

Beresford, D. (2015). MHRA report chlorhexidine solutions: Risk of chemical burn injury to skin in premature infants. *Journal of Neonatal Nursing, 21*, 47–49.

Bhatia, J. (2006). Fluid and electrolyte management in the very low birth weight neonate. *Journal of Perinatology, 26*(Suppl 1), S19–S21.

Black, P. (2007). Peristomal skin care: An overview of available products. *British Journal of Nursing*, *16*(17), 1048, 1050, 1052–1054 passim.

Blaisdell, F. W. (2002). The pathophysiology of skeletal muscle ischemia and the reperfusion syndrome: A review. *Vascular*, *10*(6), 620–630.

Boyar, V. (2018). Treatment of dehisced, thoracic neonatal wounds with single-use negative pressure wound therapy device and medical-grade honey. *Journal of Wound, Ostomy, and Continence Nursing*, *45*(2), 117–122.

Boyar, V. (2020). Pressure injuries of the nose and columella in preterm neonates receiving noninvasive ventilation via a specialized nasal cannula: A retrospective comparison cohort study. *Journal of Wound, Ostomy, and Continence Nursing*, *47*(2), 111–116.

Brandon, D. H., Coe, K., Hudson-Barr, D., et al. (2010). Effectiveness of No-Sting skin protectant and Aquaphor® on water loss and skin integrity in premature infants. *Journal of Perinatology*, *30*(6), 414–419.

Brennan, M. R., Milne, C. T., Agrell-Kann, M., et al. (2017). Clinical evaluation of a skin protectant for management of incontinence associated dermatitis (IAD) in an open label, non-randomized prospective study. *Journal of Wound Ostomy & Continence Nursing*, *44*, 172–180.

Burdall, O., Willgress, L., & Goad, N. (2019). Neonatal skin care: Developments in care to maintain neonatal barrier function and prevention of diaper dermatitis. *Pediatric Dermatology*, *36*(1), 31–35. doi: 10.1111/pde.13714.

Casanova, D., Bardot, J., & Magalon, G. (2001). Emergency treatment of accidental infusion leakage in the newborn: Report of 14 cases. *British journal of plastic surgery*, *54*(5), 396–399.

Chaiyakunapruk, N., Veenstra, D. L., Lipsky, B. A., et al. (2002). Chlorhexidine compared with povidone-iodine solution for vascular catheter-site care: A meta-analysis. *Annals of Internal Medicine*, *136*, 792–801.

Chandavasu, O., Garrow, E., Valsa, V., et al. (1986). A new method for the prevention of skin sloughs and necrosis secondary to intravenous infiltration. *American Journal of Perinatology*, *3*, 4–5.

Chapman, A. K., Aucott, S. W., Gilmore, M. M., et al. (2013). Absorption and tolerability of aqueous chlorhexidine gluconate used for skin antisepsis prior to catheter insertion in preterm neonates. *Journal of Perinatology*, *33*(10), 768–771.

Coladonato, J., Smith, A., Watson, N., et al. (2012). Prospective, nonrandomized controlled trials to compare the effect of a silk-like fabric to standard hospital linens on the rate of hospital-acquired pressure ulcers. *Ostomy Wound Management*, *58*(10), 14.

Cooper, P., Russell, F., Stringfellow, S., et al. (2011). The use of Appeel® Sterile sachet to treat a very old and a very young patient. *Wounds UK*, *7*, 124–127.

Copeland, H., Newcombe, J., Yamin, F., et al. (2018). Role of negative pressure wound care and hyperbaric oxygen therapy for sternal wound infections after pediatric cardiac surgery. *World Journal for Pediatric and Congenital Heart Surgery*, *9*(4), 440–445.

Coughlin, C. C., & Taïeb, A. (2014). Evolving concepts of neonatal skin. *Pediatric Dermatology*, *31*, 5–8.

Curley, M. A., Hasbani, N. R., Quigley, S. M., et al. (2018). Predicting pressure injury risk in pediatric patients: The Braden QD Scale. *The Journal of Pediatrics*, *192*, 189–195.

Curley, M. A., Razmus, I. S., Roberts, K. E., et al. (2003). Predicting pressure ulcer risk in pediatric patients: The Braden Q Scale. *Nursing Research*, *52*(1), 22–33.

Cutlar, L., Greiser, U., & Wang, W. (2014). Gene therapy: Pursuing restoration of dermal adhesion in recessive dystrophic epidermolysis bullosa. *Experimental Dermatology*, *23*(1), 1–6.

Dai, T., Lv, L., Liu, X., et al. (2020). Nasal pressure injuries due to nasal continuous positive airway pressure treatment in newborns: A prospective observational study. *Journal of Wound, Ostomy, and Continence Nursing*, *47*(1), 26–31.

Davies, J., Gault, D., & Buchdahl, R. (1994). Preventing the scars of neonatal intensive care. *Archives of Disease in Childhood—Fetal and Neonatal Edition*, *70*, F50–F51.

de Jesus, L. E., Martins, A. B., Oliveira, P. B., et al. (2018). Negative pressure wound therapy in pediatric surgery: How and when to use. *Journal of Pediatric Surgery*, *53*(4), 585–591.

Debra: The Dystrophic Epidermolysis Bullosa Research and Association of America. (2014). Retrieved from http://www.debra.org/

Delmore, B. A., & Ayello, E. A. (2017). Pressure injuries caused by medical devices and other objects: A clinical update. *The American Journal of Nursing*, *117*(12), 36–45. doi: 10.1097/01.NAJ.0000527460.93222.31.

Delmore, B., Deppisch, M., Sylvia, C., et al. (2019). Pressure injuries in the pediatric population: A national pressure ulcer advisory panel white paper. *Advances in Skin & Wound Care*, *32*(9), 394–408.

Denyer, J. (2011). Reducing pain during the removal of adhesive and adherent products. *British Journal of Nursing*, *20*, S28, S30–S35.

Desarno, J., Sandate, I., Green, K., et al. (2018). When in doubt, pull the catheter out: Implementation of an evidence-based protocol in the prevention and management of peripheral intravenous infiltration/extravasation in neonates. *Neonatal Network*, *37*(6), 372–377.

de-Souza, I., Vitral, G., & Reis, Z. (2019). Skin thickness dimensions in histological section measurement during late-fetal and neonatal developmental period: A systematic review. *Skin Research and Technology*, *25*(6), 793–800. doi: 10.1111/srt.12719.

Dixon, M., & Ratliff, C. (2011). Hair braids as a risk factor for occipital pressure ulcer development: A case study. *Ostomy Wound Management*, *57*(9), 48–53.

Doellman, D., Hadaway, L., Bowe-Geddes, L. A., et al. (2009). Infiltration and extravasation: Update on prevention and management. *Journal of Infusion Nursing*, *32*(4), 203–211.

Dollison, E., & Beckstrand, J. (1995). Adhesive tape vs. pectin-based barrier use in preterm infants. *Neonatal Network*, *14*, 35–39.

Dykes, P. J., Heggie, R., & Hill, S. A. (2001). Effects of adhesive dressings on the stratum corneum of the skin. *Journal of Wound Care*, *10*, 7–10.

Fox, C., Nelson, O., & Wareham, J. (1998). The timing of skin acidification in very low birth weight infants. *Journal of Perinatology*, *18*(4), 272–275.

Fridkin, S. K., & Jarvis, W. R. (1996). Epidemiology of nosocomial fungal infections. *Clinical Microbiology Reviews*, *9*(4), 499–511.

Garland, J., Buck, R., & Maloney, P. (1995). Comparison of 10% povidone-iodine and 0.5% chlorhexidine gluconate for the prevention of peripheral intravenous catheter colonization in neonates: A prospective trial. *Pediatric Infectious Disease Journal*, *14*, 510–516.

Gfatter, R., Hack, P., & Braun, F. (1997). Effects of soap and detergents on skin surface pH, stratum corneum hydration and fat content in infants. *Dermatology*, *195*, 258–262.

Gorski, L. A., Stranz, M., Cook, L. S., et al. (2017). Development of an evidence-based list of noncytotoxic vesicant medications and solutions. *Journal of Infusion Nursing*, *40*(1), 26–40.

Gotschall, C. S., Morrison, M., & Eichelberger, M. (1998). Prospective, randomized study of the efficacy of Mepitel on children with partial-thickness scalds. *Journal of Burn Care and Rehabilitation*, *19*, 279–283.

Gray, M. (2007). Incontinence-related skin damage: Essential knowledge. *Ostomy Wound Management*, *53*, 28–32.

Heimall, L. M., Storey, B., Stellar, J. J., et al. (2012). Beginning at the bottom: Evidence-based care of diaper dermatitis. *MCN: The American Journal of Maternal Child Nursing*, *37*(1), 10–16.

Irving, V. (2001). Reducing the risk of epidermal stripping in the neonatal population: An evaluation of an alcohol-free barrier film. *Journal of Neonatal Nursing*, *7*, 5–8.

Janmohamed, S. R., Oranje, A. P., Devillers, A. C., et al. (2014). The proactive wet-wrap method with diluted corticosteroids versus emollients in children with atopic dermatitis: A prospective, randomized, double-blind, placebo-controlled trial. *Journal of the American Academy of Dermatology*, *70*(6), 1076–1082.

Janssen, L. M., Tostmann, A., Hopman, J., & Liem, K. D. (2018). 0.2% chlorhexidine acetate as skin disinfectant prevents skin lesions in extremely preterm infants: A preliminary report. *Archives of Disease in Childhood-Fetal and Neonatal Edition, 103*(2), F97–F100.

Kalia, Y. N., Nonato, L. B., Lund, C. H., et al. (1998). Development of skin barrier function in premature infants. *Journal of Investigative Dermatology, 111*(2), 320–326.

Kieran, E. A., O'Sullivan, A., Miletin, J., et al. (2018). 2% chlorhexidine–70% isopropyl alcohol versus 10% povidone–iodine for insertion site cleaning before central line insertion in preterm infants: A randomised trial. *Archives of Disease in Childhood-Fetal and Neonatal Edition, 103*(2), F101–F106.

Kim, M. J., Jang, J. M., Kim, H. K., et al. (2019). Medical adhesives-related skin injury in a pediatric intensive care unit: A single-center observational study. *Journal of Wound, Ostomy, and Continence Nursing, 46*(6), 491–496.

King, A., Stellar, J. J., Blevins, A., & Shah, K. N. (2014). Dressings and products in pediatric wound care. *Advances in Wound Care, 3*(4), 324–334.

Kline-Tilford, A. M., & Haut, C. (2016). *Lippincott certification review: Pediatric acute care nurse practitioner.* Philadelphia, PA: Wolters Kluwer.

Kosemund, K., Schlatter, H., Ochsenhirt, J., et al. (2009). Safety evaluation of superabsorbent baby diapers. *Regulatory Toxicology and Pharmacology, 53*(2), 81–89.

Kuller, J. M. (2016). Infant skin care products: What are the issues? *Advances in Neonatal Care, 16*, S3–S12.

Kutsch, J., & Ottinger, D. (2014). Neonatal skin and chlorhexidine: A burning experience. *Neonatal Network, 33*, 19–23.

Lai, N. M., Lai, N. A., O'Riordan, E., et al. (2016). Skin antisepsis for reducing central venous catheter-related infections. *The Cochrane Database of Systematic Reviews, 7*(7), CD010140. doi: 10.1002/14651858.CD010140.pub2.

Larson, A. A., & Dinulos, J. G. (2005). Cutaneous bacterial infections in the newborn. *Current Opinion in Pediatrics, 17*, 481–485.

Lin, R., Tinkle, L., & Janniger, C. (2005). Skin care of the healthy newborn. *Cutis, 75*, 25–30.

Lund, C. (2014). Medical adhesives in the NICU. *Newborn and Infant Nursing Reviews, 14*(4), 160–165.

Lund, C., Nonato, L., Kuller, J., et al. (1997). Disruption of barrier function in neonatal skin associated with adhesive removal. *Journal of Pediatrics, 131*, 367–372.

Lund, C. H., & Osborne, J. W. (2004). Validity and reliability of the neonatal skin condition score. *Journal of Obstetric, Gynecologic, and Neonatal Nursing, 33*, 320–327.

Lund, C., Osborne, J., Kuller, J., et al. (2001). Neonatal skin care: Clinical outcomes of the AWHONN/NANN evidence-based clinical practice guideline. *Journal of Obstetric, Gynecologic, and Neonatal Nursing, 30*, 41–51.

McNichol, L. L., Ayello, E. A., Phearman, L. A., et al. (2018). Incontinence-associated dermatitis: State of the science and knowledge translation. *Advances in Skin & Wound Care, 31*(11), 502–513.

McNichol, L., Lund, C., Rosen, T., et al. (2013). Medical adhesives and patient safety: State of the science. *Journal of Wound, Ostomy, and Continence Nursing, 40*, 365–380.

Milstone, A. M., Elward, A., Song, X., et al.; Pediatric SCRUB Trial Study Group. (2013). Daily chlorhexidine bathing to reduce bacteraemia in critically ill children: A multicenter, cluster-randomised, crossover trial. *Lancet, 381*, 1099–1106.

Mohr, L. D., Reyna, R., & Amaya, R. (2014). Neonatal case studies using active leptospermum honey. *Journal of Wound, Ostomy, and Continence Nursing, 41*(3), 213–218.

Morris, L. D., Behr, J. H., & Smith, S. L. (2015). Hydrocolloid to prevent breakdown of nares in preterm infants. *MCN: The American Journal of Maternal/Child Nursing, 40*(1), 39–43.

Nield, L., & Kamat, D. (2007). Prevention, diagnosis, and management of diaper dermatitis. *Clinical Pediatrics, 46*, 480–486.

Nikolovski, J., Stamatas, G. N., Kollias, N., et al. (2008). Barrier function and water-holding and transport properties of infant stratum corneum are different from adult and continue to develop through the first year of life. *Journal of Investigative Dermatology, 128*, 1728–1736.

Occleston, N. L., Metcalfe, A. D., Boanas, A., et al. (2010). Therapeutic improvement of scarring: Mechanisms of scarless and scar-forming healing and approaches to the discovery of new treatments. *Dermatology Research and Practice, 2010*, 405262.

Oranges, T., Dini, V., & Romanelli, M. (2015). Skin physiology of the neonate and infant: Clinical implications. *Advances in Wound Care, 4*(10), 587–595. doi: 10.1089/wound.2015.0642.

Quach, C., Milstone, A. M., Perpête, C., et al. (2014). Chlorhexidine bathing in a tertiary care neonatal intensive care unit: Impact on central line–associated bloodstream infections. *Infection Control & Hospital Epidemiology, 35*(2), 158–163.

Rai, P., Lee, B. M., Liu, T. Y., et al. (2009). Safety evaluation of disposable baby diapers using principles of quantitative risk assessment. *Journal of Toxicology and Environmental Health, Part A, 72*(21–22), 1262–1271.

Ratliff, C., & Dixon, M. (2007). Treatment of incontinence-associated dermatitis (diaper rash) in a neonatal unit. *Journal of Wound Ostomy & Continence Nursing, 34*(2), 158–161.

Rentea, R. M., Somers, K. K., Cassidy, L., et al. (2013). Negative pressure wound therapy in infants and children: A single-institution experience. *Journal of Surgical Research, 184*(1), 658–664.

Sardesai, S. R., Kornacka, M. K., Walas, W., et al. (2011). Iatrogenic skin injury in the neonatal intensive care unit. *The Journal of Maternal-Fetal & Neonatal Medicine, 24*(2), 197–203.

Sawatzky-Dicksson, D., & Bodnaryk, K. (2006). Neonatal intravenous extravasation injuries: Evaluation of a wound care protocol. *Neonatal Network, 25*, 13–19.

Schardosim, J. M., Ruschel, L. M., Motta, G. D. C. P. D., et al. (2014). Cross-cultural adaptation and clinical validation of the Neonatal Skin Condition Score to Brazilian Portuguese. *Revista Latino-Americana de Enfermagem, 22*(5), 834–841.

Scheinfeld, N. (2005). Diaper dermatitis. A review and brief survey of eruptions of the diaper area. *American Journal of Clinical Dermatology, 6*, 273–281.

Sedin, G., Hammarlund, K., Nilsson, G., et al. (1985). Measurements of transepidermal water loss in newborn infants. *Clinics in Perinatology, 12*, 79–99.

Siegfried, E. (2008). Neonatal skin care and toxicology (chapter 5). In L. Eichenfield, I. Frieden, & N. Esterly (Eds.), *Textbook of neonatal dermatology.* Philadelphia, PA: W. B. Saunders Co.

Simona, R. (2012). A pediatric peripheral intravenous infiltration assessment tool. *Journal of Infusion Nursing, 35*, 243–248.

Singer, H. M., Levin, L. E., Garzon, M. C., et al. (2018). Wound culture isolated antibiograms and caregiver-reported skin care practices in children with epidermolysis bullosa. *Pediatric Dermatology, 35*(1), 92–96.

Singh, C. D., Anderson, C., White, E., et al. (2018). The impact of pediatric pressure injury prevention bundle on pediatric pressure injury rates. *Journal of Wound, Ostomy, and Continence Nursing, 45*(3), 209–212.

Stamatas, G. N., Nikolovski, J., Mack, M., et al. (2011). Infant skin physiology and development during the first years of life: A review of recent findings based on in vivo studies. *International Journal of Cosmetic Science, 33*(1), 17–24.

Stoffan, A. P., Ricca, R., Lien, C., et al. (2012). Use of negative pressure wound therapy for abdominal wounds in neonates and infants. *Journal of Pediatric Surgery, 47*(8), 1555–1559.

Thigpen, J. (2007). Peripheral intravenous extravasation: Nursing procedure for initial treatment. *Neonatal Network, 26*, 379–384.

Thompson, K. L., Leu, M. G., Drummond, K. L., et al. (2014). Nutrition interventions to optimize pediatric wound healing an evidence-based clinical pathway. *Nutrition in Clinical Practice, 29*, 473.

Treadwell, T. (2012). The management of intravenous infiltration injuries in infants and children. *Ostomy Wound Management, 58*, 40–44.

Tüzün, Y., Wolf, R., Bağlam, S., et al. (2015). Diaper (napkin) dermatitis: A fold (intertriginous) dermatosis. *Clinics in Dermatology, 33*(4), 477–482. doi: 10.1016/j.clindermatol.2015.04.012.

Vandeputte, P., Ferrari, S., & Coste, T. (2012). Antifungal resistance and new strategies to control fungal infections. *International Journal of Microbiology, 2012*. doi: 10.1155/2012/713687.

Visscher, M., & Taylor, T. (2014). Pressure ulcers in the hospitalized neonate: rates and risk factors. *Scientific Reports, 4*(1), 1–6.

Visscher, M. O., Adam, R., Brink, S., et al. (2015). Newborn infant skin: Physiology, development, and care. *Clinics in Dermatology, 33*(3), 271–280.

Visscher, M. O., Chatterjee, R., Ebel, J. P., et al. (2002). Biomedical assessment and instrumental evaluation of healthy infant skin. *Pediatric Dermatology, 19*(6), 473–481.

Visscher, M. O., Utturkar, R., Pickens, W. L., et al. (2011). Neonatal skin maturation—vernix caseosa and free amino acids. *Pediatric Dermatology, 28*, 122–132.

Visser, W. I. (2014). Non-pharmacological management of atopic dermatitis, including emollients. *Current Allergy & Clinical Immunology, 27*(2), 88.

Vizcarra, C., Cassutt, C., Corbitt, N., et al. (2014). Recommendations for improving safety practices with short peripheral catheters. *Journal of Infusion Nursing, 37*(2), 121–124.

Vongsa, R., Rodriguez, K., Koenig, D., et al. (2019). Benefits of using an appropriately formulated wipe to clean diapered skin of preterm infants. *Global Pediatric Health, 6*, 2333794X19829186. doi: 10.1177/2333794X19829186.

Wang, D., Xu, H., Chen, S., et al. (2019). Medical adhesive-related skin injuries and associated risk factors in a pediatric intensive care unit. *Advances in Skin & Wound Care, 32*(4), 176–182.

Weissenstein, A., Luchter, E., & Bittmann, S. (2014). Medical honey and its role in paediatric patients. *British Journal of Nursing, 23*(6 Suppl), S30–S34.

Wesner, E., Vassantachart, J. M., & Jacob, S. E. (2019). Art of prevention: The importance of proper diapering practices. *International Journal of Women's Dermatology, 5*(4), 233–234. doi: 10.1016/j.ijwd.2019.02.005.

World Health Organization (WHO). (2018). Preterm birth. Retrieved from https://www.who.int/news-room/fact-sheets/detail/preterm-birth

Yates, S., McNichol, L., Heinecke, S. B., et al. (2017). Embracing the concept, defining the practice, and changing the outcome. *Journal of Wound, Ostomy, and Continence Nursing, 44*(1), 13–17.

Yosipovitch, G., Maayan-Metzger, A., Merlob, P. P., et al. (2000). Skin barrier properties in different body areas in neonates. *Pediatrics, 106*, 105.

Yuan, C., Takagi, R., Yao, X. Q., et al. (2018). Comparison of the effectiveness of new material diapers versus standard diapers for the prevention of diaper rash in Chinese babies: A double-blinded, randomized, controlled, cross-over study. *BioMed Research International, 2018*, 5874184. doi: 10.1155/2018/5874184.

QUESTIONS

1. The wound care nurse must pay special attention to the skin of a neonate. What is a characteristic of a newborn's skin that makes it more fragile?

A. The stratum corneum of full-term newborns functions as well as adult skin.

B. The basement layer of the epidermis has not yet formed.

C. The keratinocytes in the basal layer have a slower turnover rate.

D. The dermis of a neonate is thicker than an adult.

2. Neonates in the NICU are at greatest risk for pressure injury development related to

A. Shear forces

B. Devices used

C. Adhesive use

D. Ischemia

3. The wound care nurse is managing the care of neonates in the NICU. Which intervention is a recommended prevention/treatment measure for this population?

A. Neonates in the NICU should be bathed daily with a chlorhexidine gluconate product.

B. Silicone-based adhesive removers should be used for neonates.

C. IV devices should be secured with transparent dressings and checked every 3 hours.

D. If IV extravasation occurs, the device should be removed and cold compress applied.

4. The wound care nurse is caring for a neonate whose IV fluid has extravasated into the surrounding tissue. Treatment to the site should include

A. Administration of hyaluronidase for all types of extravasated fluids

B. Application of warm compresses

C. Removal of the device and elevating the extremity

D. Application of gentle compression to the extremity

5. The wound care nurse is teaching the parents of a 1-year-old child how to treat severe diaper rash (IAD) following infectious diarrhea. Which teaching point is a recommended intervention?

A. Avoid use of topical treatments containing zinc oxide and petrolatum.

B. Once skin is "raw," leave the area open to air.

C. Do not remove the skin barrier ointment completely with each diaper change.

D. Use baby powder on damaged skin to keep the area dry.

6. In which age group would the Braden Q+D Scale be used to predict pressure injury risk?

A. Birth—5 years

B. Birth—8 years

C. Birth—12 years

D. Birth—21 years

7. The wound care nurse is caring for an adolescent with atopic dermatitis. What should be the emphasis of education for this patient?
A. Skin hygiene and use of emollients
B. Exfoliating hair from the area
C. Frequent dressing changes
D. Nutritional counseling

8. The wound care nurse is planning care for patients on a pediatric unit. Which intervention does not follow recommended guidelines for pediatric wound care?
A. Use low profile dressings to protect wounds from childhood activities.
B. Use dressings that require daily changes whenever possible.
C. Use advanced dressings as first-line treatment.
D. Include caregivers assisting or providing wound care in plan of care.

9. The wound care nurse is recommending use of negative pressure wound therapy (NPWT) for a 6-year-old pediatric patient with a pressure injury. Which of the following adjustments should be made for a pediatric patient?
A. Use black foam as contact layer in wound base.
B. Use suction setting of 125 mm Hg.
C. Use intermittent setting for suction.
D. Use white foam or contact layer in wound base.

10. A key responsibility of the pediatric wound care nurse is to maintain skin integrity for children. What intervention is recommended to prevent skin damage for this population?
A. Use aggressive adhesive products to reduce device dislodgement.
B. Place thin foam under any medical device used.
C. Remove all adhesive products with an alcohol-based adhesive remover.
D. Use circular donut device to offload the occipital area.

ANSWERS AND RATIONALES

1. A. Rationale: The stratum corneum contains 10 to 20 cell layers in the adult and in the full-term newborn. Full-term newborns have been shown to have skin barrier function comparable to that of adult skin as indicated by transepidermal water loss (TEWL), the rate at which water vapor from respiration passes through the skin layers into the environment.

2. B. Rationale: Pressure injuries from medical devices are more common than those caused by immobility.

3. B. Rationale: All dressing and adhesive products should be removed with silicone-based adhesive remover to promote skin integrity and reduce the risk of adhesive trauma, especially in the NICU.

4. C. Rationale: If IV fluid has extravasated into surrounding tissue, the IV device should be removed and the extremity elevated. Use of moisture, heat, or cold is not recommended because the tissue is vulnerable to further injury.

5. C. Rationale: All caregivers must be taught that it is not necessary or desirable to completely remove the skin barrier ointment with each diaper change, because this causes additional trauma that disrupts healing tissue.

6. D. Rationale: A multicenter, prospective cohort study of the Braden QD on patients preterm to 21 years of age, on bed rest for at least 24 hours with a medical device in place demonstrated its effectiveness.

7. A. Rationale: Principles underlying topical therapy include maintaining the pH balance of the skin and restoring and maintaining skin hydration through use of humectants and emollients among others.

8. B. Rationale: Key considerations for dressing selection include use of dressings with gentle adhesives, such as silicone, and advanced wound dressings that reduce dressing change frequency.

9. D. Rationale: The hydrophobic white sponge used in conjunction with a contact layer effectively prevents adherence and ingrowth of tissue into the sponge.

10. B. Rationale: Thin adhesive foam or hydrocolloid dressings may be used under a medical device to provide padding and absorb moisture.

CHAPTER 14

SKIN AND WOUND CARE FOR THE GERIATRIC POPULATION

Leanne Richbourg

OBJECTIVES

1. Describe the anatomy and physiology of the skin and soft tissue, changes across the lifespan, and implications for management of skin health.

2. Describe skin conditions and lesions that are common among the elderly and implications for the skin and wound care nurse.

3. Discuss the role of the skin and wound care nurse in prevention and management of the following: delirium, elder abuse, malnutrition, polypharmacy, and pain.

TOPIC OUTLINE

INTRODUCTION

Longer lifespans and aging baby boomers will combine to double the population of Americans aged 65 years or older in the next 40 years (to about 98 million). By 2060, older adults will constitute about 24% of the U.S. population (Mather et al., 2015). As a result of our aging population, the leading causes of death have shifted over the last 100 years from acute illness and infection to degenerative illness and chronic conditions, many of which contribute to skin and wound conditions (CDC, 2013). The leading causes of death for those over age 65 are heart disease, cancer, chronic lower respiratory diseases, stroke, and Alzheimer disease (Heron, 2018).

This chapter will cover the cellular changes that affect wound healing in the elderly person, common skin conditions experienced by the aged, and geriatric syndromes encountered by the wound care nurse when caring for this population. The overarching term geriatric syndrome has been used to highlight common conditions experienced by elders, especially frail ones.

> **KEY POINT**
>
> By 2060, older adults will constitute 24% of the U.S. population.

 AGE-RELATED CHANGES IN SKIN AND WOUND HEALING

Changes in the skin associated with aging are due to a combination of intrinsic and extrinsic factors. Intrinsic factors are typically unalterable and include the normal aging process and related changes in the DNA of skin cells. Extrinsic factors include lifestyle, environment, pollution, exposure to nicotine, exposure to ultraviolet (UV) light, diet, and hydration. Medications may also affect the skin. For example, drugs to lower cholesterol may cause abnormal desquamation of the skin (Farage et al., 2008, 2009). The normal function of proliferative cells (epithelial cells, fibroblasts, and endothelial cells) plays a vital role in maintenance of skin integrity throughout life. Unfortunately, endogenous and exogenous changes associated with aging cause a reduction in the proliferative ability of these cells, with eventual progression to senescence.

CELLULAR SENESCENCE AND APOPTOSIS

Senescence is a term used interchangeably with aging and describes cells that remain viable but no longer continue the process of mitosis (reproduction). The hallmark of senescent cells is their inability to initiate DNA replication and subsequent cell division. They have lost the ability to progress through the cell cycle. Senescence is different than apoptosis, which signifies cell death programmed within the cell's DNA (cell self-destruction). One example of apoptosis is the normal cell cycle for keratinocytes, in which the migrating keratinocyte loses its DNA and becomes filled with keratin, and the mature keratinocyte is shed from the skin surface as new keratinocytes arrive to take its place. This normal apoptosis maintains the structural integrity and homeostatic function of the epidermis. Extreme physiologic stress can cause premature senescence or apoptosis of normally proliferating cells. Research indicates that proliferating cells respond to extreme stress in one of three ways: (1) complete recovery with the ability to continue subsequent cell cycles; (2) senescence; or (3) apoptosis (Bonte et al., 2019; Campisi & d'Adda di Fagagna, 2007).

> **KEY POINT**
>
> Senescence refers to cells that no longer have the ability to reproduce. Apoptosis refers to programmed cell death.

Clinical manifestations of aging are the result of cumulative cellular damage and mutations in cellular DNA. It is well documented that DNA damage and mutations increase with age while the cells' capacity to repair such damage decreases every year. Cells seem to have a genetically determined reproductive lifespan involving the number of telomeres. Telomeres are lengths of duplicate DNA pairs located at the end of chromosomes, and with each DNA replication, one base pair of telomeric DNA is lost. The loss of telomeres results in cellular senescence (the inability to reproduce) or in spontaneous cellular death (apoptosis).

CHANGES TO PARTIAL-THICKNESS WOUND HEALING

Elderly skin is in a progressive state of decline and is more susceptible to damage from friction, medical adhesive–related skin injury (MARSI), and moisture-associated skin damage (MASD). See Chapter 18 for further discussion of common skin injuries.

In addition to increased risk for partial-thickness skin loss, the time required for healing is frequently prolonged, even when the wound is relatively superficial. This is because aging keratinocytes have reduced proliferative capacity and reduced ability to produce cytokines and other molecules critical to cell-to-cell communication. This compromise in keratinocyte function may be due in part to the marked reduction in Langerhans cells. There is considerable evidence that Langerhans cells regulate the function, differentiation, and proliferation of epidermal keratinocytes.

KEY POINT

Partial-thickness wound healing is frequently prolonged in the elderly, due to reduced keratinocyte proliferative capacity and reduced cell-to-cell communication.

There are also marked changes in the basement membrane (junction between the epidermis and dermis) that contribute to the elderly individual's risk for skin tears and for delayed partial-thickness healing. The basement membrane is not a true membrane; it is composed of thin layers of specialized extracellular matrix that become less organized with aging. This area is normally characterized by the interlocking dermal papillae and epidermal rete pegs. With age, the matrix dermal papillae flatten and the interlocking configuration is lost, resulting in reduced epidermal tensile strength and increased risk for skin tears and MARSI.

While there are changes in the epidermis and basement membrane associated with aging, it is the dermis that sustains the greatest structural and atrophic changes. These changes include a loss of fibroblasts and a doubling of replication time for the remaining fibroblasts. This causes reduced production of dermal collagen, elastin, and proteoglycans and an increase in the time required for repair of dermal damage (Farage et al., 2009).

Reduced blood flow is another characteristic of aging skin that negatively impacts healing. There is a 30% decrease in the cross-sectional area of dermal venules in older skin and a 60% decrease in basal and peak cutaneous blood flow (Archer, 2012). These vascular changes render the elderly more susceptible to pressure injuries and vascular ulcers and compromise their ability to effect skin repair. Despite the vulnerability of the older patient's skin, partial-thickness wounds will heal by epithelialization as long as the cause can be eliminated, and the wound surface is kept clean and moist.

KEY POINT

Despite changes in proliferative capacity, partial-thickness wounds in the elderly will heal so long as causative factors are eliminated and the wound surface is kept clean and moist.

 CHANGES TO FULL-THICKNESS WOUND HEALING

Chapter 3 provides foundational information regarding the pathology of full-thickness injury and the processes involved in full-thickness wound healing. This section addresses aspects of healing unique to the elderly.

The primary processes involved in full-thickness repair include hemostasis (acute wounds), inflammation, proliferation of new tissue (granulation tissue formation), contraction (in open wounds), and epithelial resurfacing. There are changes unique to aging that affect each of these processes.

HEMOSTASIS (ACUTE WOUNDS ONLY)

Platelet aggregation and adherence to the endothelium is enhanced in aged subjects. In addition, there is increased degranulation of platelets and release of growth factors (TGF-β, TGF-α, and PDGF) (Gosain & DiPietro, 2004).

INFLAMMATION

The inflammatory phase is critical to repair and is dependent on normal numbers and function of neutrophils and macrophages, with macrophages playing the more important role. Aging is associated with reduced numbers of macrophages, which partially explains the diminished inflammatory response that is typically seen. The reduced numbers of mast cells, B lymphocytes, and T cells compromises the ability to manage bacterial loads. Reduced immune responsiveness in older age is known as immunosenescence. Changes in capillary permeability limit neutrophil migration into the wound bed. The result is a prolonged inflammatory phase and increased risk of infection. The wound care nurse must supplement the reduced inflammatory response through debridement and use of antimicrobial agents.

A study by Jiang et al. (2012) provides additional insight into the ways in which the normal inflammatory response may be altered in the elderly. They measured the levels of two different proteins in full-thickness (stage 3) pressure injuries. The first protein (Bax protein) is known to induce suicide (apoptosis) in T cells, impairing the normal inflammatory response. The second protein (Bcl 2) is found in healthy skin and inhibits cell death (apoptosis). Samples were taken from the surrounding skin, the wound edge, and the necrotic center. The investigators found that the number of Bax cells progressively increased from the wound edge to the necrotic center of the wound, while the Bcl-2 cells were significantly lower in the center with increasingly higher numbers at the skin edge. They concluded that an imbalance between apoptotic and proliferative cells contributed to impaired healing (Jiang et al., 2012). This is important because the percentages of senescent and apoptotic cells is higher in the elderly.

PROLIFERATION

All aspects of the proliferative phase are compromised to some extent in the elderly, including angiogenesis, collagen synthesis, contraction, and epithelial resurfacing. The two factors that have the greatest negative impact on angiogenesis and collagen synthesis (granulation tissue formation) are impaired perfusion and diminished fibroblast function. Adequate perfusion is critical to all phases of healing and aging is associated with a reduction in blood flow to the soft tissues. At best, the rate of granulation tissue formation will be reduced in the elderly. If the individual with the wound also suffers from macrovascular and/or microvascular disease, the delay may be significant or healing may be impossible. Assessment of perfusion status is important. The wound care nurse must optimize perfusion in the elderly.

Fibroblasts are the cells responsible for synthesis of collagen and other connective tissue proteins, but the cellular senescence associated with aging reduces the number of proliferative fibroblasts and their response to growth factors. This results in a prolonged time frame for collagen synthesis and the collagen may be of poor quality (Chang et al., 2013a).

Contraction of newly formed extracellular matrix proteins can significantly reduce the time to healing by reducing the size of the defect. Contraction is impaired in the elderly, possibly due to reduced numbers of myofibroblasts, which are derived from fibroblasts and are essential for wound contraction.

The proliferative phase ends with epithelial resurfacing, which can be impaired by a number of factors. The rate of keratinocyte proliferation is reduced in the elderly. Keratinocytes require a healthy wound bed to migrate and attach. If collagen synthesis is impaired, the defective new tissue inhibits epithelial migration and resurfacing. Macrophages normally produce substances that promote keratinocyte proliferation (such as ceramides), and macrophage numbers are diminished in the elderly (Seyfarth et al., 2011). Age-related stress can result in increased production of cortisol, glucocorticoids, and epinephrine, and epidermal cells can serve as an extra-adrenal source of both epinephrine and cortisol. This has been linked to impaired healing in experimental models (Stojadinovic et al., 2012).

REMODELING

During the maturation phase, the early provisional (type III) collagen that lacks tensile strength is replaced with mature (type I) collagen, which is essential to development of tensile strength. This involves the dual processes of breakdown of the early collagen and synthesis of the mature collagen. The elderly are at risk for defective remodeling that results in failure to develop tensile strength. This may be due in part to compromised fibroblast function and also to comorbidities affecting tissue oxygenation and nutritional status. In some situations, the rate of collagen breakdown exceeds the rate of collagen synthesis, creating increased risk for breakdown of the newly closed wound. The wound care nurse needs to be aware that full-thickness wounds are at risk even after they have closed. Since full-thickness wounds heal by replacing the lost tissue with scar tissue, they never return to the original state of health or tensile strength. At best, closed full-thickness wound attains 80% of original tensile strength. They are always at risk for breakdown (Armstrong & Meyr, 2020).

> **KEY POINT**
>
> Multiple factors increase the risk for impaired full-thickness wound healing in the elderly, including reduced proliferation and activity of endothelial cells, fibroblasts, and keratinocytes, reduced perfusion, and any comorbidities. Most elderly retain the capacity to heal with comprehensive and appropriate management.

 ## ADDITIONAL INTRINSIC CHANGES

ALTERED MELANOCYTE FUNCTION

There is a change in the distribution and number of melanocytes, those cells that produce melanin, an ultraviolet protective pigment, and transfer it to adjacent keratinocytes. There is a 10% to 40% reduction in number of melanocytes per decade of life. This explains the lightening of skin in some ethnic groups with aging and results in reduced photoprotection. The remaining melanocytes may deteriorate or lose the normal contact and interaction with keratinocytes. The most obvious effect of melanocyte dysfunction in aging is the graying of hair. A more significant effect is interference with the Langerhans cells' ability to eradicate carcinogenic cells (Bonte et al., 2019; Eckhart et al., 2019; Farage et al., 2008).

REDUCED VITAMIN D PRODUCTION

Another change that may affect the individual's health is a decline in vitamin D production and vitamin D receptors. Vitamin D deficiency is linked to many conditions experienced by elders: cognitive decline, depression, osteoporosis, hypertension and cardiovascular disease, diabetes, and cancer. Studies suggest that the prevalence of vitamin D deficiency in U.S. elders varies from 20% to 100% (Meehan & Penckofer, 2014). Vitamin D is involved in regulation of T-cell differentiation and expression of cathelicidin, a peptide lethal to many infectious organisms (Eckhart et al., 2019).

REDUCED SENSORY FUNCTION

In addition to changes in the skin that render the individual more vulnerable to cutaneous infections and malignancies, there are changes in the skin's nervous system that adversely affect the person's ability to recognize and respond appropriately to warning signs of impending damage. The reduction in nerve receptors in the skin and in the production of neurotransmitters means that an elderly patient is less aware of pain, pressure, and exposure to heat and cold, even if they are alert and oriented. This is one reason the elderly are at increased risk for pressure injuries, burns, and frostbite (Bonte et al., 2019).

KEY POINT

The elderly have reduced sensory function, which means they may not sense impending damage from unrelieved pressure or thermal trauma, even if they are alert and oriented.

THINNING OF ADIPOSE LAYER

While this discussion has focused on the layers and structures of the skin itself, it should be noted that the subcutaneous adipose tissue also undergoes changes with aging. This tissue provides cushioning, insulation, and long-term storage of energy. With aging, lipids are redistributed from the subcutaneous to the abdominal visceral compartment (Mancuso & Bouchard, 2019).

IMPACT OF ETHNICITY

Wound care nurses provide care for individuals of all ethnicities and need to be knowledgeable regarding the impact of ethnicity on skin structure and function. The obvious differences relate to the melanin cells and ceramides in the epidermis. While our understanding of ethnic skin differences remains incomplete, it is known that darkly pigmented skin retains a younger appearance with less visible signs of aging than lightly pigmented skin. This may be due to greater protection against photoaging afforded by the increased activity of skin melanocytes. However, skin of all ethnicities is eventually affected by photoaging. Darker skin demonstrates greater intercellular cohesion and higher ceramide levels, which helps to explain their lower incidence of skin tears. Considering that people of darker skin tones constitute most of the world's population, it is evident that we need more research into ethnic skin differences and the implications for skin care (Rawlings, 2006).

REDUCTION OF SEX HORMONES

Estrogen and testosterone are the hormones commonly associated with the development of secondary sexual characteristics. They also play a role in the condition of the skin and wound healing. Both of these hormones are found in males and females.

Estrogen

Estrogen, produced by the ovaries, the adrenal glands, and adipose tissue, influences the function of all major organ systems within the body. Estrogen receptors are found in fibroblasts, keratinocytes, and endothelial cells, all critical to the synthesis of new tissue. Estrogen stimulates the expression of PDGF by monocytes and macrophages, which contributes to the overall regulation of wound-healing processes (Gilliver et al., 2007). Estrogen precursors are converted within the skin to 17β-estradiol (E2), promoting skin thickness, collagen content, and moisture. E2 is known to inhibit keratinocyte apoptosis and a reduction of E2 correlates to a reduction in skin thickness (Wend et al., 2012). Prolonged inflammatory response, up-regulated protease activity, and reduced matrix deposition in age-related impaired healing, and high neutrophil counts have been demonstrated in the wounds of elderly patients (Gilliver et al., 2007). Estrogen has been shown to decrease neutrophil chemotaxis and adhesion, reducing the inflammatory response and allowing for improved matrix formation (Ashcroft et al., 1999; Shu & Maibach, 2011).

Collagen loss per postmenopausal year is estimated to be 2.1%, independent of a woman's age. This is accompanied by a 1.1% decline in skin thickness per postmenopausal year (Archer, 2012). The combined effects of skin aging and loss of estrogen can result in loss of as much as 30% of the dermal collagen in the first 5 years after menopause. Estrogen may reduce the rate of collagen loss, because estrogen has been shown to increase fibroblast proliferation and collagen production. Estrogen can reduce the levels of tissue-degrading matrix metalloproteinases (MMPs) in the connective tissue (Shu & Maibach, 2011).

KEY POINT

Estrogen to known to affect skin health and skin softness, and evidence suggests that estrogen may also significantly impact wound healing.

Testosterone

Testosterone, an androgen, is produced by the Leydig cells in the testes of men and the ovaries and adrenal glands in women. It acts on androgenic receptors found in the skin and is responsible for the differences in skin thickness and texture between the sexes (Demling, 2005). The epidermis is 20% thicker in males as compared to females (Kopera, 2015). Aging skin is characterized by a progressive decline in skin thickness, due primarily to atrophic changes affecting the dermis. These changes include a reduction in fibroblasts, which results in reduced production of dermal collagen, elastin, and proteoglycans (Archer, 2012). Androgens stimulate the production of sebum from the sebaceous glands, a mixture of lipids (glycerides, free fatty acids, wax esters, squalene, cholesterol esters, and cholesterol) that provide photoprotection, plus antimicrobial, antioxidant, and pro- and anti-inflammatory activity (Picardo et al., 2009). Skin oils have a major impact both on skin texture and softness and on the barrier function of the skin. Skin oils are responsible for filling the gap between skin cells to create an intact barrier that prevents water loss and prevents penetration by irritants and pathogens (Pappas, 2009). The effects of decreased testosterone production with aging include thinner, weaker skin, loss of muscle mass, and impaired wound healing (Demling, 2005).

IMPACT OF PH

For nearly 100 years, an acid mantle has been considered a characteristic of healthy skin. Specifically, pH has been shown to be a key factor in maintenance of an intact barrier, the integrity and hydration of the stratum corneum (SC), and added protection against microbes (Ali & Yosipovitch, 2013). The optimal skin pH is approximately 5.4, with a range of 4 to 6. Aging can adversely affect skin pH, due in part to reduced numbers and activity of the sebaceous and sweat glands. This results in reduced production of the skin lipids and sweat that help to maintain acidic pH. It is well documented that skin pH rises with aging, beginning as early as age 50 and rising significantly by age 70 and beyond. The rising pH reduces the integrity of the skin barrier and supports the growth of pathogens. Normal skin flora appears to thrive in an acidic environment, while pathogens grow best in a neutral or alkaline environment. An acidic pH seems to promote attachment of the resident bacteria to the skin, while an alkaline pH promotes shedding of the good bacteria from the skin (Ansari, 2014). For more information on skin pH, see Chapter 2.

KEY POINT

Skin pH rises with aging, compromising skin health and barrier function. This is due in part to reduced activity of the sebaceous and sweat glands.

EXTRINSIC FACTORS

PHOTOAGING

The most damaging extrinsic factors affecting skin health is photodamage caused by exposure to UV light. It is estimated that up to 90% of visible skin aging is the effect of sunlight. It was once thought that sun only affected the epidermis, but it is now known that both UVA and UVB rays penetrate to the dermis and contribute to the chronic skin damage associated with photoaging (Tobin, 2017). The changes in the dermis include degradation of collagen and impaired deposition of elastin. With severe damage, the dermis becomes a mess of tangled elastic fibers and tightly packed collagen. The damaged dermal tissue is unable to maintain normal vasculature, and photoaged skin demonstrates reduced perfusion. Sun-damaged skin is also less able to mount a normal inflammatory response to injury. In addition to causing significant damage to both the epidermis and dermis and accelerating the visible signs of aging, photodamage

also increases the risk of cutaneous neoplasms. This is because UV light damages genetic material through replication errors and the creation of free radicals. UV light interferes with enzymatic activities required for repair of damaged DNA and compromises the function of Langerhans cells, which are responsible for the eradication of carcinogenic cells (Farage et al., 2008). The wound care nurse should be alert to patient history and physical findings consistent with high levels of UV exposure and should be cognizant of the increased risk for all forms of skin cancer in these individuals. The wound care nurse should educate the patient regarding the importance of routine dermatologic checkups and prompt reporting of any lesion that is increasing in size or atypical in appearance. All elderly individuals should be encouraged to use sunscreen routinely and to wear light long-sleeved clothing and broad-brimmed hats when outside. Elderly individuals should be counseled to wear sunglasses on a routine basis for protection against cataract formation as well as protection of the eyelids against skin malignancy (**Fig. 14-1**).

SMOKING

Another extrinsic factor with severe negative effects on skin health is smoking. Tobacco usage has many deleterious effects on the skin. Nicotine is absorbed through the mouth, lungs, gastrointestinal tract, bladder, and the epidermis. Cigarette smoke creates a mild inflammatory reaction and reduces moisture levels in the SC. **Box 14-1** describes the effects that smoking has on skin components. Tobacco smoke contains many mutagens and carcinogens. It is an independent risk factor for developing cutaneous squamous cell carcinoma. There is also a connection between smoking and psoriasis, a condition common to elders (Ortiz & Grando, 2012).

KEY POINT

Sun exposure and cigarette smoking are the most significant extrinsic factors contributing to skin aging and skin damage.

The aging process is responsible for a number of changes in cellular DNA that influence cellular activity and the capacity for reproduction as well as the ability to self-protect. These changes lead to deviant cellular responses that may adversely affect maintenance of normal skin and the ability to heal (Yaar, 2006). While it is the visible signs of aging that sometimes create the most concern, it is the underlying histological changes that are most likely to interfere with normal healing.

MAINTAINING SKIN HEALTH

In a study of 223 elderly nursing home residents, dermatologists found that nearly every resident had at least one dermatological diagnosis. Among the most common

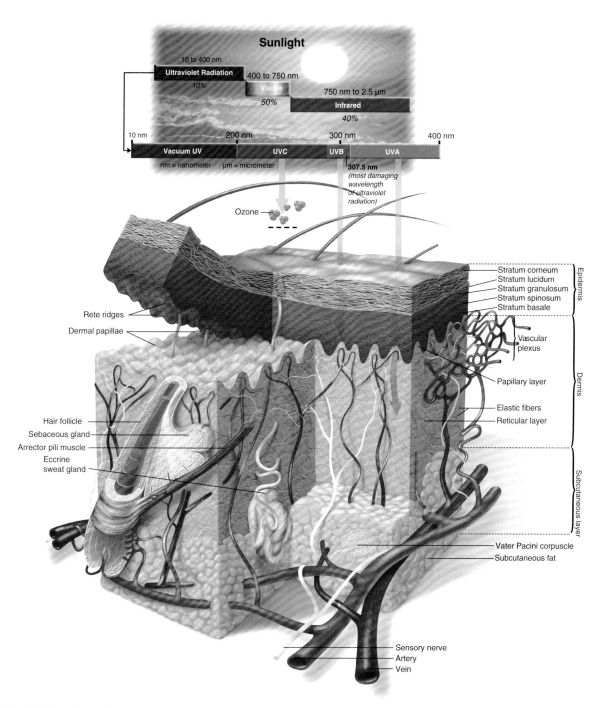

FIGURE 14-1. Skin Cross Section with UV Rays Labeled.

BOX 14-1   DELETERIOUS EFFECTS OF SMOKING ON SKIN CELLS

- Alters extracellular matrix turnover
- Down-regulates collagen synthesis
- Increases collagen degradation
- Up-regulates expression of matrix metalloproteinases (MMPs)
- Decreases tissue inhibitor of metalloproteinases (TIMP-1)

conditions identified were xerosis cutis, incontinence-associated dermatitis (IAD), and tinea pedis (Hahnel et al., 2017). A study of hospitalized elders found the most common skin disorders were solar lentigines (84%), senile angiomas (60%), xerosis (59%), seborrheic warts (54%), and pruritus (35%) (Reszke et al., 2015). One priority in management of the elderly individual is maintenance of skin health. The wound care nurse must carefully evaluate both skin care products and skin care practices in their setting. Attention should be given to agents used for general cleansing and for perineal cleansing following incontinent episodes (McNichol et al., 2018). Products should be selected that promote and maintain an acidic pH and that do not require rinsing. Unnecessary use of antimicrobial agents should be avoided, since normal skin flora help to maintain skin health and acidity. The wound care nurse should also consider the type of bathing cloth used. Soft disposable wipes are preferable, and abrasive cloths and scrubbing technique should be avoided. Routine use of emollients helps to maintain skin softness and an intact barrier (Kottner et al., 2013; White-Chu & Reddy, 2011).

Other factors affecting overall skin health include temperature, humidity, and overall hydration. High temperatures increase evaporative loss, as does an environment with low humidity, and systemic hydration affects hydration of the skin. The wound care nurse should promote adequate fluid intake for any elderly patient and should recommend bathing with water that is warm but not hot.

The EPUAP/NPIAP/PPPIA Prevention and Treatment of Pressure Ulcers/Injuries: Clinical Practice Guideline (2019) recommends the following when caring for vulnerable aged skin:

1. Protect aged skin from pressure and shear forces.
2. Use a barrier product to protect aged skin from exposure to excessive moisture.
3. Select atraumatic wound dressings to reduce further injury to frail older skin.
4. Develop and implement an individualized continence management plan.
5. Assure that elders are regularly repositioned, including the head, as medical condition allows.

XEROSIS AND PRURITUS

Xerosis is a broad term used to denote abnormal dryness of mucous membranes, skin, and eyes. Xerosis cutis is a specific term for abnormally dry skin. In clinical practice, the term xerosis is typically used to indicate very dry skin. Xerosis is found in 52% of home care patients, 58% of nursing home residents, and 85% of individuals >70 years of age (Chang et al., 2013a; Lichterfeld-Kottner et al., 2018). Xerosis accompanied by intense itching and repetitive scratching can result in secondary lesions with a cracked porcelain pattern or linear fissures, particularly on the lower legs. In some cases, fissures penetrate into the dermis, disrupting capillaries and causing bleeding (Farage et al., 2009) (**Fig. 14-2**).

Pruritus or itch is the unpleasant skin sensation that provokes the urge to scratch. Pruritus in the elderly is caused by xerosis, immunosenescence, and neuropathic/neural changes. Conditions associated with pruritus include seborrheic and stasis dermatitis, psoriasis, renal and liver disease, diabetes, HIV, malignancies, depression, anxiety, and dementia (Shevchenko et al., 2018). Medications common to the elderly and associated

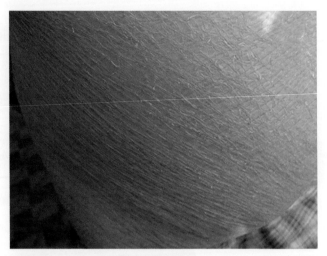

FIGURE 14-2. Xerosis. Minimal dryness, manifested by the slightest fine scaling.

with pruritus (without rash or only transient rash) include angiotensin-converting enzyme inhibitors (ACEIs), salicylates, chloroquine, and calcium channel blockers (Berger et al., 2013). Elders can also suffer from senile pruritus, a condition of chronic itch with no clear etiology.

PATHOLOGY OF XEROSIS

Xerosis is due in part to reduced production of sebaceous lipids (sebum) and epidermal skin lipids produced by the keratinocytes (ceramides, cholesterol, free fatty acids). The end result is increased dryness and scaling of the skin and compromised barrier function. Both external humidity and water in the SC are needed to produce natural moisturizing factor (NMF), a component that binds water in the skin (Toncic et al., 2018; White-Chu & Reddy, 2011). Other age-related causes include defective desquamation, changed function of proteases, changes in skin pH, and decreased estrogen levels (Shevchenko et al., 2018).

Medications can also play a role in xerosis. Systemic as well as topical agents should be reviewed, as polypharmacy is prevalent in the elderly and there are numerous medications that could cause or contribute to xerosis. These include antibacterials, diuretics, NSAIDs, calcium channel antagonists (Farage et al., 2009), hypercholesterolemic agents, antiandrogens, cimetidine, opioids, and ACEI (White-Chu & Reddy, 2011).

KEY POINT

Xerosis (dry skin) and pruritus (itching) are common in the elderly due to reduced production of sebum and skin lipids. Routine use of moisturizers is an important element of care.

MANAGEMENT

The first steps in managing xerosis in the aging patient are rehydration of the skin followed by application of an agent to seal in the hydration. Common recommendations for treatment of dry skin include the following:

reduce frequency of bathing and use of lukewarm (not hot) water; limit showering or bathing to <5 minutes; minimize use of nonirritating, moisturizing soap (apply only to hair-bearing or soiled areas); and apply cream or ointment-type moisturizer of choice to the skin while still damp (Brooks et al., 2017; Chang et al., 2013b; Kottner et al., 2013; LeBlanc & Baranoski, 2009; White-Chu & Reddy, 2011). Although traditional recommendations include restricted bathing, some authors point out that immersion in water is actually needed to rehydrate the SC and suggest that the best approach is to provide at least 10 minutes of immersion in tepid water. These authors agree with minimal use of soaps and stipulate that a better approach is use of a gentle nonirritating cleanser (e.g., a moisturizing foam cleanser or shower gel). They also emphasize the need for generous application of moisturizers immediately following the bath. The moisturizer provides lipids to fill the gaps between the keratinocytes, helping to maintain an intact barrier and reduce flaking (Farage et al., 2009; White-Chu & Reddy, 2011).

Moisturizers are a critical aspect of treatment for xerosis and pruritus and should be applied at least twice a day. Moisturizers have four basic actions; they can act as a humectant, occlusive, emollient, or protein rejuvenator, as shown in **Table 14-1** (Purnamawati et al., 2017; Shevchenko et al., 2018).

Most moisturizing products combine emollients, occlusives, and humectants. They also come in varying formulations: lotions, creams, ointments, and gels. Lotions are appropriate when the moisturizer is to be distributed across a large surface area and no occlusive property is required. Creams have more moisturizing effect than lotions but again offer no occlusion. Ointments provide occlusion and are particularly helpful in low humidity environments. Gels are easily absorbed, often designed for the face (Purnamawati et al., 2017). Products should be rubbed gently over the skin, avoiding excessive friction.

Hyperkeratotic skin will benefit from a humectant, designed to attract and hold water within the SC and to promote desloughing of thick dry skin. Common ingredients are urea compounds and alpha-hydroxy acids (AHAs). One potential advantage of humectants containing lactic acid or AHAs, for example, ammonium lactate 12% lotion is the acidic pH, which can help restore normal skin pH. If the skin is fissured or cracked, stinging and irritation might limit AHA usage (Chang et al., 2013a). Humectants are not appropriate for use on overhydrated or thin fragile skin because humectants attract water and promote desloughing.

KEY POINT

Humectants are designed to attract water and to deslough dry rough skin. These agents are inappropriate for overhydrated or thin fragile skin.

While the ideal moisturizer would be acidic, information regarding the pH of available moisturizers is not readily accessible (Shi et al., 2012). In a recent study, investigators measured the pH of several moisturizers commonly used in the United States and found that some had quite alkaline pH levels. While there are guidelines for appropriate use of emollients versus humectants, there is little evidence that any one emollient or any one humectant is better than another (Young & Chakravarthy, 2014). Decisions at present should be based at least in part on the patient's preference and the cost involved.

One potential problem with use of moisturizing products is the potential for contact dermatitis. Moisturizing products can include a number of common skin sensitizers, for example, balsam of Peru, lanolin, propylene glycol, parabens, formaldehyde, fragrance, vitamin E, aloe vera, and antibiotics, and contact dermatitis is common in the elderly. An irritant or allergen in the topical agent should be considered whenever symptoms worsen with

TABLE 14-1 ACTIONS OF MOISTURIZERS

	HUMECTANT	OCCLUSIVE	EMOLLIENT	PROTEIN REJUVENATORS
Mechanism of Action	Attract water/lipids into the stratum corneum Increase movement of water from dermis to epidermis	Block transepidermal water loss (TEWL)	TEWL prevention Stimulation of epidermal repair	Replenish skin proteins
Substances	Urea Hyaluronic acid Sorbitol Honey Panthenol Glycerol/glycerin Propylene glycol Alpha hydroxy acids	Mineral oil Petrolatum Beeswax Dimethicone Zinc oxide Lanolin	Petrolatum Vegetable oil Dimethicone Propylene glycol Castor oil Jojoba oil Balsam of Peru	Collagen Elastin Keratin

therapy. Patch testing or switching to another moisturizer with different ingredients may be helpful (Bains et al., 2019; White-Chu & Reddy, 2011).

AGE-RELATED SKIN LESIONS

Many health care providers do not differentiate between skin changes caused by intrinsic and extrinsic factors; they simply attribute any skin changes to old age. The effects of one are superimposed on the other. Older individuals who have also been exposed to UV light are at increased risk for the skin changes typically attributed to aging, and the lesions may occur at an earlier age in these individuals.

Eczema is a skin condition characterized by xerosis, pruritus, erythema, lichenification, blistering, cracking, and weeping. Eczema has several distinct types; this chapter will discuss three that are common to the senior population: atopic dermatitis, allergic contact dermatitis, and seborrheic dermatitis.

ATOPIC DERMATITIS

Atopic dermatitis (AD) is a multifactorial inflammatory disease involving an impaired skin barrier function and abnormal immune response with a genetic component. While there are limited studies that characterize the features of IgE-mediated allergy specifically in older age groups, there is a growing trend to consider the elderly as a distinct subgroup of patients with distinct manifestations. Lichenification at the antecubital and popliteal fossae is common, rather than lesions localized to skin folds as found in adult-type AD. Williamson et al. (2019) consolidated this evidence in their review, finding that the age-related changes to the physical skin barrier and to the immune system play a key role. There is a 2% to 3% prevalence of AD in the elderly. Sixty to eighty percent of elderly patients experiencing AD will have IgE-allergic type (extrinsic) and 20% to 30% will have a non-IgE allergic type (intrinsic).

Common environmental extrinsic factors that most affect elders are dust mites, pollens, Balsam of Peru, nickel, and cobalt. Less common agents include milk, eggs, wheat, animal dander, and grasses. The mainstay treatments for AD are emollients and topical drugs such as gluco-corticosteroids and calcineurin inhibitors (Ratliff et al., 2016; WOCN, 2019). AD can have a profound effect on a person's quality of life and lead to depression and anxiety, psychological illnesses common with advanced age (Bieber et al., 2013).

ALLERGIC CONTACT DERMATITIS

Allergic contact dermatitis occurs in as many as 11% of the older population. It is more common in women (Balato et al., 2011; Farage et al., 2009). The allergic reaction is specific to the offending antigen, requires a sensitizing interaction, and only occurs if the person is genetically

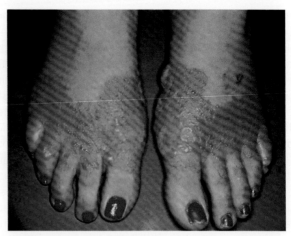

FIGURE 14-3. Allergic Contact Dermatitis. (Used with permission from Nicol, N. (2016). *Dermatology Nursing Essentials* (3rd ed). Philadelphia, PA: Wolters Kluwer.)

capable of sensitization to that antigen. This contrasts with irritant dermatitis, which does not require prior sensitization and can occur in anyone. The higher incidence may be due in part to the fact that the elderly have had years of exposure and sensitization to potential allergens. The sensitivity reaction may be delayed in the older individual due to a reduction in Langerhans cells and vascular response. It typically manifests within 24 hours of exposure. Common offenders include topical antibiotics (neomycin), nickel, latex, lanolin, Balsam of Peru, formaldehyde, adhesives, and sunscreens. Like atopic dermatitis, the topical treatments for allergic contact dermatitis are emollients, which can provide a barrier function, and topical glucocorticosteroids and nonsteroidal calcineurin inhibitors (Prakash & David, 2010) (**Fig. 14-3**).

Up to 81% of patients treated for chronic leg ulcers exhibit allergic reactions to topical products (Farage et al., 2009). The clinician should limit use of topical products to those that are essential, should be alert to products containing common sensitizing agents, and should consider patch testing high-risk patients such as those with ulcers or dermatitis involving the lower extremities (Rzepecki & Blasiak, 2018).

SEBORRHEIC DERMATITIS

Seborrheic dermatitis (SD) is a chronic inflammation involving lipid-rich areas of the body, which affects approximately 31% of the geriatric population. Common sites of involvement are areas with numerous sebaceous glands, such as the eyebrows, paranasal area, scalp, axillae, trunk, and groin. While the cause is not known, limited studies have implicated lipid-dependent fungi of the genus *Malassezia*, normally found on the skin (Saunders et al., 2012). The lesions typically present as areas of greasy-looking yellow or white scales. The underlying skin may be erythematous (**Fig. 14-4**). Treatment is usually topical, and therapies include anti-inflammatory

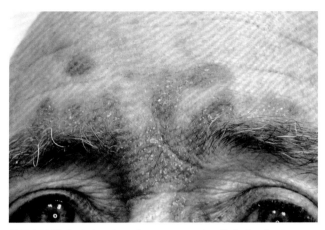

FIGURE 14-4. Seborrheic Dermatitis on the Glabellar Region.

preparations, for example, low-potency topical corticosteroids to the face or intertriginous areas, medium-potency corticosteroids to the chest and back, or calcineurin inhibitors, antifungal medications, for example, ketoconazole, zinc pyrithione, selenium sulfide, and keratolytic agents, for example, coal tar, salicylic acid.

SD of the scalp is typically treated with a medicated shampoo, left on for 5 minutes, twice weekly, for 4 weeks. Ongoing use once a week may prevent relapse. A cream is typically recommended for SD of the face, applied once or twice a day, depending on the medication (Farage et al., 2009; Sasseville, 2018).

BULLOUS PEMPHIGOID

This autoimmune blistering disease is primarily found in the elderly and the incidence has dramatically increased in recent decades. U.S. prevalence of this condition was 38 cases/100,000 adults over age 60, increasing to 124 cases/10,000 adults age 90 and above. Women are affected slightly more than men, and there is no difference in prevalence between the black and white races (Wertenteil et al., 2018). An epidemiologic study conducted in the United Kingdom found a 5-fold increase (17% per year) in incidence of bullous pemphigoid over 11 years (1996–2006) (Langan et al., 2008). Refer to Chapter 30 for information on assessment and care.

INFECTIONS

Skin and soft tissue infections (SSTIs) have become the second most common type of infection among persons residing in long-term care facilities (Kish et al., 2010; McHugh & Gil, 2018). This may be due in part to cellular senescence, which leads to thinning of the epidermis and a compromised epidermal barrier. Defects in the barrier may permit penetration by pathogens. There is a 40% reduction in mast cells and an almost 50% reduction in intradermal macrophages and Langerhans cells, the cells responsible for cellular immunity and for identifica-

tion and destruction of pathogens. There is a reduction in the number and activity of the sweat glands. Sweat normally provides antimicrobial activity against a variety of pathogenic microorganisms (White-Chu & Reddy, 2011). The dry skin commonly found in the elderly is associated with itching and scratching, and the subsequent microabrasions allow invasion by pathogens.

> **KEY POINT**
>
> SSTIs are the second most common type of infection among individuals living in long-term care facilities.

Candidiasis

Cutaneous fungal infection is one of the most common skin diseases in the elderly, due to alterations in barrier function of the skin (**Fig. 14-5**) (Chang et al., 2013a). Risk is further increased by exposure to moisture as occurs with diaphoresis and incontinence, and antibiotic administration, as well as poorly controlled diabetes (Ali & Yosipovitch, 2013; Chang et al., 2013a). Fungal infections caused by yeast organisms (such as *Candida albicans*) typically present as a tender and pruritic maculopapular rash that is confluent in the center with distinct border lesions. Infections caused by tinea organisms are characterized by a rash that is most intense at the periphery, with central clearing (Chang et al., 2013a). Diagnosis is usually made on the basis of clinical presentation but can be confirmed by skin scrapings examined under a microscope. Treatment involves an antifungal agent. The

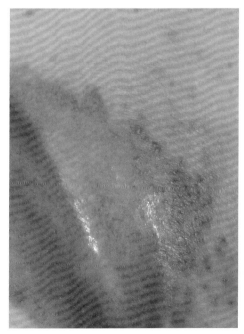

FIGURE 14-5. Cutaneous Candidiasis Classically Produces Red Plaques with Peripheral Pustules and Satellite Lesions.

specific treatment depends on the location and severity of infection. Nonpharmacologic treatment of fungal rashes in moist skin folds includes measures to keep the area dry. This may be achieved with the use of a wicking fabric (Interdry®) containing silver, an antimicrobial component. It is effective against bacterial pathogens in the skin folds (Hess, 2020). Additional interventions include utilizing fans or air conditioning, wearing loose lightweight clothing, and changing clothing when it becomes wet from perspiration. Fungal skin infections usually respond to medicated powders or creams. Medicated suppositories may be used to treat vaginal yeast infections. Thrush may be treated with a medicated mouthwash or lozenges that dissolve in the mouth. Severe infections or infections in a patient with a compromised immune system may be treated with oral antifungal medications. Refer to Chapters 18 and 19 for additional information on intertrigo and candidiasis.

Onychomycosis

Fungal infections of the nail are also very common in older adults, possibly due to vascular insufficiency, diabetes, trauma, immunosuppression, poor hygiene, and inactivity. Ninety percent of infections are due to the dermatophyte tinea unguium (Pierwola et al., 2017). See Chapter 28 for information on assessment and care.

Tinea Pedis

Tinea pedis, a dermatophyte infection, is seen regularly in the elder population (Hahnel et al., 2017). The wound care nurse should assess for this infection whenever caring for elders. The resulting breaks in the skin can serve as portals for bacterial infections with potentially serious consequences (**Fig. 14-6**). Refer to Chapter 28 for assessment and treatment information.

Herpes Zoster

Aging also increases the risk for herpes zoster (shingles), which is caused by reactivation of the varicella virus. Varicella zoster virus (VZV) lies dormant in the major

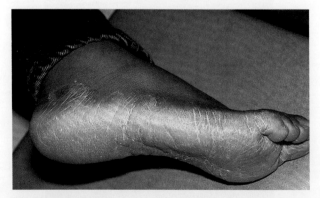

FIGURE 14-6. Tinea Pedis, Moccasin Distribution. (Used with permission from Goodheart, H., Gonzalez, M. (2015). *Goodheart's Photoguide to Common Pediatric and Adult Skin Disorders.* Philadelphia, PA: Wolters Kluwer.)

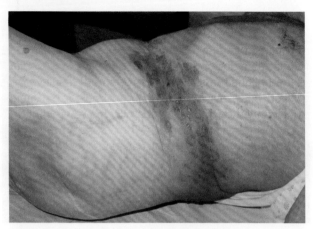

FIGURE 14-7. Herpes Zoster: Cutaneous Findings that Typically Appear Unilaterally, Stopping Abruptly at the Midline of the Limit of Sensory Coverage of the Involved Dermatome.

sensory ganglia following primary infection earlier in life (**Fig. 14-7**). One factor that increases the risk for herpes zoster in the elderly is the substantial reduction in the number of Langerhans cells in all layers of the epidermis. Langerhans cells are equipped to destroy incoming viruses. VZV often presents with prodromal pain, itching or burning, or a sharp stabbing pain that occurs before the onset of rash. Depending on the affected dermatome, prodromal pain may be misdiagnosed as myocardial infarction, appendicitis, or a gallbladder or kidney stone attack. Acute herpes zoster typically manifests as acute pain accompanied by a vesicular rash that follows the path of the involved dermatome. The pain persists until the rash subsides and sometimes past that point. Disseminated zoster is the term used when more than 20 vesicles occur outside the primary dermatome. Zoster is diagnosed by a Tzanck smear of scraped sample from the base of an intact vesicle (Chang et al., 2013a; Pierwola et al., 2017).

Management of herpes zoster requires administration of systemic antiviral agents within 72 hours of onset. These medications reduce viral replication and thereby reduce nerve damage, inflammation, and duration and severity of pain (Pierwola et al., 2017). Early and consistent pain management is an essential part of the care plan.

Complications can include pain, lasting for months or even years after the disappearance of the rash. This is known as postherpetic neuralgia (PHN). Approximately half of all zoster patients will experience PHN persisting at least 120 days after rash onset (Chang et al., 2013a). The Food and Drug Administration (FDA) has approved usage of the lidocaine 5% patch for PHN, but superior pain relief may be received from systemic gabapentin or tricyclic antidepressants. The patch is contraindicated in patients with advanced liver failure (American Geriatric Society [AGS], 2009; Bruckenthal & Barkin, 2013).

Another very serious complication involves the eye, which can occur if the involved dermatome involves the ophthalmic division of the trigeminal nerve. The appearance and location of the rash on the face does not predict eye involvement. Rash on the tip of the nose can be associated with eye involvement. Ramifications can include corneal ulceration, glaucoma, optic neuritis, eyelid scarring, visual impairment, and blindness (Schmader, 2016). Any patient with facial lesions requires prompt referral to ophthalmology.

Further complications of herpes zoster in older persons include secondary bacterial infection of the rash, stroke, focal motor paresis, disordered balance, hearing loss, facial paresis, and meningoencephalitis (Schmader, 2016). Varicella zoster virus is also discussed in Chapter 29.

The Center for Disease Control and Prevention recommends that people 60 years of age and older receive the shingles vaccine, regardless of whether or not they recall having chicken pox. Even those who have already had shingles can receive the vaccine, to prevent a reoccurrence. The vaccine is contraindicated for those with a weakened immune system. More information is available at https://www.cdc.gov/vaccines/vpd/shingles/.

Scabies

Scabies is common among residents in nursing homes and extended care facilities in the United States (**Fig. 14-8**). It is caused by a mite with a lifespan of about 1 month. The mite burrows under the skin to lay eggs. The eggs, saliva, feces, and the mite itself cause a delayed hypersensitivity reaction 2 to 6 weeks after contact (or in 1 to 4 days in those previously infected). Superficial burrows, papules, nodules, or pustules are typically seen on the hands (particularly the finger webs), wrists, waistline, axilla, buttocks, and external genitalia (the face and scalp are usually spared). Intense itching develops, especially

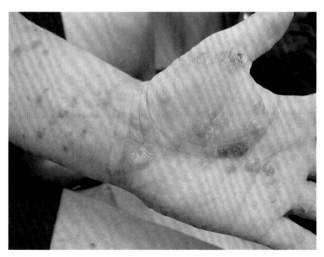

FIGURE 14-8. Scabies: Caused by a Burrowing Mite, which Produces Severe, Intensely Itching Lesions in the Area of its Burrows.

at night, resulting in scratching and excoriations that make it difficult to distinguish from other pruritic skin conditions. Scabies can be problematic among residents in nursing home facilities, spreading rapidly and persistently by cross transmission. It is spread by direct skin contact and is exceptionally contagious, being passed easily from patient to patient and patient to staff. Scabies should always be included in the differential assessment of any acutely pruritic skin condition. Accurate diagnosis can be difficult because it requires visualization of the mites or eggs from a skin scraping. Sometimes the decision is made to treat empirically with topical or systemic scabicidal agents (e.g., permethrin). Treatment must include meticulous attention to laundering of clothing and bedding (Kish et al., 2010; Pierwola et al., 2017).

KEY POINT

Scabies is common in long-term care facilities and is extremely contagious. It should be included in the differential assessment of any pruritic rash.

BENIGN AND MALIGNANT LESIONS

In addition to inflammatory and infectious lesions, the elderly are at risk for a number of benign skin conditions and a range of skin malignancies (**Table 14-2**). See Chapters 2, 27, and 31 for more information about benign and malignant lesions.

GERIATRIC SYNDROMES

Medical and nursing literature identify several conditions as geriatric syndromes. A comprehensive list includes delirium, dementia, falls, frailty, incontinence, pressure injuries (Chapter 20), functional decline, depression, vertigo, bone fractures, neglect, abuse, polypharmacy, osteoporosis, malnutrition (Chapter 7), and pain. The wound care nurse will encounter many of these issues when providing care to an older adult population and should include assessment for and attention to these comorbid conditions (Brown-O'Hara, 2013; Cesari et al., 2017; Inouye et al., 2007). The Hartford Institute for Geriatric Nursing Web site offers many practical nursing resources to assist with management of the full complement of geriatric syndromes (www.consultgeri.org or www.hartfordign.org).

ELDER ABUSE

The prevalence of elder abuse is estimated to be 10% (Lachs & Pillemer, 2015). A literature review performed by the U.S. Government National Center on Elder Abuse (https://ncea.acl.gov/What-We-Do/Research/Statistics-and-Data.aspx) found the most common forms are financial, emotional, physical, and neglect. Statistics also

TABLE 14-2 BENIGN AND MALIGNANT LESIONS COMMON IN THE ELDERLY

TYPE OF LESION	FEATURES	PHOTOAGING	LOCATION	EXAMPLE	TREATMENT
Acrochordon (skin tag)	Papilloma; soft, pedunculated papilloma is typical of a fibroepithelial polyp	No	Neck, axilla, trunk		Electrocautery scalpel or scissors Cryotherapy Ligation
Solar lentigines (age spots, liver spots)	Macule with various colors, from light tan to black. Round or oval; flat or slightly elevated	Yes	Anywhere on the body		Prescription-strength retinol and hydroquinone (HC) cream, microdermabrasion, chemical peels, chemical spot treatments, laser treatments, and light therapy to lighten
Senile angiomas (cherry angiomas, Campbell de Morgan spots)	Firm, smooth, red papules, range in size from 0.5 to 5 mm	No	Anywhere on the body		Electrocautery or laser coagulation
Solar elastosis (dermatoheliosis)	Abnormal accumulation of elastin within the dermis; appears as thickened, dry, wrinkled skin	Yes	Sun-exposed skin		Treatment usually ineffective; minimize sun exposure; sunscreen
Seborrheic keratosis	Elevated sharply defined edge; color varies from light brown to black; warty scale that crumbles; can sometimes be scratched away but looks attached	No	Face, arms, back, and trunk Can be irritated or traumatized depending on the location		Cryotherapy Electrocautery Curettage Trichloroacetic acid Laser surgery Usually not precancerous but needs to be evaluated to determine if precancerous
Actinic keratosis	Small, rough, poorly demarcated lesion. Seldom larger than 1 cm. May develop a white rough surface scale	Yes; cumulative long-term sun exposure	Head, neck, forearms, and hands. Difficult to see on the lips		Benign lesions that may give rise to squamous cell carcinoma (if unsure, biopsy)

TABLE 14-2 BENIGN AND MALIGNANT LESIONS COMMON IN THE ELDERLY (*Continued*)

TYPE OF LESION	FEATURES	PHOTOAGING	LOCATION	EXAMPLE	TREATMENT
Squamous cell carcinoma	Opaque nodule or red nodule; rough, scaly, sometimes ulcerated. Crusting usually present	Yes	Sun-exposed areas; usually head and neck		Can metastasize Refer for biopsy
Basal cell	Raised, pearly edges; may be more pigmented in patients with darker skin	Yes	Sun-exposed areas; usually head and neck		Rarely metastasize Refer for biopsy
Melanoma	A asymmetry B border irregularity C color variations D diameter E evolving lesion	Yes	Men upper back, women upper back and lower legs		Can metastasize Refer for biopsy

Used with permission from Weber, J. R., Kelley, J. (2017). *Health Assessment in Nursing*. Philadelphia: Wolters Kluwer.

suggest that, for every report of abuse, 24 cases go unreported, possibly because the elder may be unable to report the abuse and health care providers do not always recognize signs and symptoms of abuse. Risk factors associated with this problem include dementia, poor physical health, functional impairment, poverty, low social support, and lack of a spouse or partner (Hall et al., 2016).

The cutaneous signs of elder physical abuse are purpura and petechiae, wounds in various stages of healing, multiple difficult-to-explain scars, defensive wounds, bilateral or parallel injuries on the extremities indicating restraint, severe IAD, and pressure injuries.

Timely and appropriate intervention is required in cases of suspected elder abuse. While the reporting rate is higher in nursing homes, most elder abuse occurs in the home and the community (Chang et al., 2013b). It is the responsibility of every nurse to:

1. Develop an awareness of elder abuse and neglect
2. Recognize the signs and symptoms of elder abuse
3. Learn how to appropriately and comfortably talk with possible victims
4. Identify resources for reporting suspected abuse and neglect

Wound care nurses are frontline staff who are frequently involved in the care of vulnerable elderly individuals. They can play an important role in identification and reporting of suspected abuse. Signs of elder abuse are sometimes subtle, and the wound care nurse needs to remember that it is not necessary to substantiate the abuse before reporting.

KEY POINT

Elder abuse is common. The wound care nurse needs to be alert to any indicators of abuse and should know that prompt reporting of any suspected abuse is a legal mandate.

DELIRIUM

Delirium, an acute decline in cognitive functioning, is a common and serious reversible disorder that affects up to 50% of hospitalized elders and costs 164 billion per year in U.S. dollars. It is an acute disorder with a relatively rapid onset and it is preventable in 30% to 40% of cases. Accumulating evidence has shown that some patients progress from delirium to permanent cognitive decline and dementia. The highest incidence rates are in intensive care, postoperative care, and palliative care units (Inouye et al., 2014). While delirium can occur in all age groups, it occurs more frequently in the elderly (Marcantonio, 2017; Robinson et al., 2009; Rudolph & Marcantonio, 2011). Development depends on a vulnerable patient being exposed to noxious insults or precipitating factors. Predisposing and precipitating factors are shown in **Table 14-3** (Inouye et al., 2014; Szokol, 2010).

Wound care nurses interact with the family and patient to assess for skin problems, determine risk for pressure injuries, and develop an individualized treatment plan. If the patient has unrecognized delirium, the plan cannot effectively address the needs of the patient, family, or caregivers. Wound care nurses must become knowledgeable regarding basic cognitive assessment and must modify their management plans based on assessment findings.

TABLE 14-3 PREDISPOSING AND PRECIPITATING FACTORS OF DELIRIUM

PREDISPOSING FACTORS	PRECIPITATING FACTORS
Dementia/cognitive impairment	Polypharmacy
History of delirium	Psychoactive medications
Functional Impairment	Sedatives or hypnotics
Sensory deficits	Inadequate pain control
Multiple comorbid illnesses	Infection
Depression	Surgery
History of TIA or stroke	Trauma
Alcohol misuse	Use of physical restraints
Advanced age (>74 y)	Increased serum urea
Low educational level	Use of a bladder catheter

Delirium has a number of different clinical presentations. Hyperactive delirium is rare but more easily recognized because its symptoms of restlessness, irritability, antagonism, or agitation are more easily identified. The majority of patients (over 70%) present with hypoactive delirium, with less obvious symptoms of lethargy, decreased alertness, and poor motivation. In 29% of cases, the clinical presentation involves a combination of hyperactive and hypoactive symptoms (Marcantonio et al., 2002). Postoperative delirium (POD) typically occurs between 1 and 3 days postoperatively and the etiology remains unclear (Bryson & Wyand, 2006). These patients often emerge from anesthesia smoothly and may be lucid in the postanesthesia care unit. After this initial lucid interval, the patient develops the classic fluctuating mental status (Chang et al., 2013b; Deiner & Silverstein, 2009). Of importance to wound care nurses, patients with delirium were three times more likely than patients who did not experience delirium to develop a wound infection during hospitalization (Redelmeier et al., 2008).

Assessment and Recognition

Staff may fail to assess cognitive status, despite the fact that delirium significantly increases the risk of complications (e.g., decreased oral intake, pressure injuries, aspiration, and pulmonary emboli) and the likelihood of discharge to a long-term care facility (Chen et al., 2011; Rudolph & Marcantonio, 2011). The most widely used instrument for detecting delirium is the Confusion Assessment Method (CAM). This tool considers four features of the patient's behavior: acute onset or fluctuating course, inattention, disorganized thinking, and altered level of consciousness (Inouye et al., 1990, 2014; Oh et al., 2017).

KEY POINT

Delirium affects up to 50% of all hospitalized elderly. At least 30% to 40% of these cases are preventable through measures such as judicious use of pain medications, measures to improve sleep, and maintenance of fluid and electrolyte balance, glycemic control, and oxygenation.

Prevention and Intervention

Prevention is the most effective strategy for minimizing the occurrence of delirium and its adverse outcomes (Fong et al., 2009; Siddiqi et al., 2007). The basic interventional options for delirium prevention and management are nonpharmacological measures and pharmacological interventions. Nonpharmacologic strategies include environmental measures to optimize sleep, maintenance of fluid and electrolyte balance, glycemic control, prevention of hypoxia, and infection prevention and reorientation when indicated. Involve family members in care and have them bring in familiar objects from home. Assure that patients have glasses, hearing aids, and dentures. Communicate to the patient their schedule of care. Pharmacological interventions include judicious use of pain medication and avoidance of psychoactive medications (e.g., benzodiazepines) (Inouye et al., 2014). The practice of prophylaxis with antipsychotics should be avoided due to increased risk of death, delirium, and complications in older patients attributed to this class of drugs (Morimoto et al., 2009; Rudolph & Marcantonio, 2011; Yang et al., 2011).

Educational programs should be implemented that increase staff awareness of effective preventive measures, early recognition, and both nonpharmacologic and pharmacologic strategies for management of delirium.

MALNUTRITION

Nutritional management is of particular importance to the wound care nurse. Malnutrition is an independent risk factor for single and multiple skin tears in hospitalized elders (Munro et al., 2018). A systematic review of the literature (Favaro-Moreira et al., 2016) found multiple risk factors associated with malnutrition in older adults: age, frailty, polypharmacy, decline in health and physical function, Parkinson disease, constipation, poor or moderate self-reported health status, cognitive decline, dementia, eating dependencies, loss of interest in life, poor appetite, dysphagia, and institutionalization. The wound care nurse is in a position to recognize many of these risk factors and make the appropriate referrals and recommendations.

Harris and Fraser (2004) identified the following as factors that delay healing and increase the risk of pressure injury development in institutionalized elderly (**Box 14-2**). Practical suggestions for long-term care would include making restrictive diets more liberal, encouraging family and friends to bring foods from home, making adjustments for favorite foods, and referrals to speech pathologist for suspected swallowing problems. See Chapter 7 for more information regarding

| BOX 14-2 | RISK FACTORS FOR MALNUTRITION, DELAYED HEALING, AND INCREASED RISK OF PRESSURE INJURIES IN ELDERLY |

- Dependency on others for help with eating
- Impaired cognition and/or communication
- Poor positioning
- Frequent acute illnesses with nausea, vomiting, and/or diarrhea
- Medications that decrease appetite or increase nutrient losses
- Polypharmacy
- Decreased thirst response, decreased ability to concentrate urine
- Psychosocial factors such as isolation and depression
- Intentional fluid restriction because of fear of incontinence or choking (dysphagia)
- Monotony of diet
- Higher nutrient density requirements along with the demands of age, illness, and disease on the body

nutritional needs for wound healing and implications for assessment and intervention.

KEY POINT

Measures to improve nutrient intake among institutionalized elderly include liberalization of diets, encouraging friends and family to bring food from home, and prompt referral to speech pathology for suspected swallowing problems.

POLYPHARMACY

There are a wide range of definitions for the term polypharmacy, with the most common being taking five or more medications (Masnoon et al., 2017). Endo et al. (2013) define polypharmacy as (1) unintentionally prescribing too many medications; (2) taking medications with duplicate mechanisms of action; or (3) inadvertently adding medications that interact with others. The truth remains that 10% of hospital admissions are related to adverse drug reactions (ADRs). According to multivariate analysis, it is not the patients' age alone that predicts adverse drug events, it is the total number of medications they take or the extent of their comorbid conditions. Polypharmacy is an important cause of morbidity and mortality. Many duplications and potential interactions occur as a result of multiple transitions among various providers and care settings. Polypharmacy increases the risk of drug-induced autoimmune cutaneous diseases (Milgrom & Huang, 2014).

ADVERSE DRUG REACTIONS IN THE ELDERLY

The prevalence of ADRs in the elderly is 11%, ADRs leading to hospitalization is 10%, and ADRs occurring during hospitalization is 11.5%. The most common categories of medications implicated in ADRs are antihypertensives,

antithrombotics, antibiotics, nonsteroidal anti-inflammatory drugs (NSAIDs), antidiabetic agents, and psycholeptics (Alhawassi et al., 2014). Skin reactions account for 7.9% of adverse events. Women have a 1.5- to 1.7-fold greater risk of developing an ADR, including adverse skin reactions, as compared to men (Gallelli et al., 2017; Rademaker, 2001).

Advanced practice providers (APPs) are frequently asked to assess and manage elderly individuals with dermatologic conditions and should consider the following physiologic principles when prescribing: (1) thinning of the skin and compromise of the barrier function means that topical agents will be absorbed more effectively; (2) changes in distribution of the adipose tissue and reduced muscle mass can also affect drug absorption; and (3) alterations in renal and hepatic function can render the elder more susceptible to drug toxicity. These aspects of pharmacokinetics are typically not emphasized in drug labeling and dosing recommendations. The APP must also be aware that the most common drug-to-drug interactions occur with nonprescription medications. It is therefore important to carefully review all medications including over-the-counter (OTC) medication and integrative therapies such as herbs, vitamins and minerals, and probiotics. They are widely marketed, readily available to consumers, and often sold as dietary supplements. The American Geriatric Society (AGS) publishes a useful tool, updated in 2019, to assist providers with making informed prescribing decisions while caring for elders, the Beers Criteria for Potentially Inappropriate Medication Use in Older Adults (AGS, 2019). This evidence-based document is designed for use with persons aged 65 and older, in all settings of care except hospice and palliative care, to improve drug selection and reduce adverse events.

KEY POINT

Consider an ADR as a potential cause of any new symptom. In this case, it is better to discontinue the problematic drug than to add another drug.

PERSISTENT PAIN

Pain management is a key intervention in a comprehensive wound care plan designed for any patient. Pain in the elderly is typically underreported and undertreated. Each interaction the wound care nurse has with an elderly patient should include a pain assessment. Three commonly used scales are the 0 to 10 Numeric Rating Scale, the Wong-Baker (1998) FACES Pain Rating Scale, and the Pain Assessment in Advanced Dementia (PAINAD) scale (Warden et al., 2003). While there are a number of analgesics that are safe for elders, careful selection is advised. Pain medications should be started at a low dose and carefully titrated upward, with frequent

BOX 14-3 ACETAMINOPHEN USE IN GERIATRIC PATIENTS

- Starting dose of 325 to 500 mg every 4 hours or 500 to 1,000 mg every 6 hours
- The maximum safe dose from all sources is <4 g/24 hours (evaluate all RX and OTC medications taken by the patient for the presence of this ingredient)
- Reduce maximum dose by 50% to 75% in persons with hepatic insufficiency or a history of alcohol abuse
- Caution with renal impairment, hypovolemia, chronic malnutrition; contraindicated with liver failure
- Severe skin reactions can occur
- Acetaminophen and warfarin can interact to create an elevated INR and subsequent hemorrhaging (Lopes et al., 2011)

reassessments for relief and adverse effects. In some instances, a combination of drugs may work synergistically to provide greater pain relief with less toxicity than a higher dose of a single agent. The AGS recommends acetaminophen as first-line therapy for pain. It is not as effective for inflammatory pain (e.g., rheumatoid arthritis) as NSAIDs. **Boxes 14-3 and 14-4** contain information to consider when recommending acetaminophen or NSAIDs (AGS, 2009, 2019; Epocrates, 2019).

Opioids may be considered for those patients with persistent pain who are at particular high risk for complications from use of NSAIDs and nonopioid pain relievers. They should be prescribed on a trial basis with a clear treatment plan that also includes functional restorative and psychosocial modalities. Though the risks of opioid

abuse are low in elderly patients without previous history of substance abuse, it is important to consider risk factors for future misuse. For example, risk factors identified by the Opioid Risk Tool (ORT) are personal or family history of substance abuse, relatively young age, mental illness, and history of preadolescent sexual abuse (Webster & Webster, 2005). If the wound care nurse identifies risk factors, the patient should be referred to a pain specialist.

Elders with persistent pain may also benefit from adjuvant drugs, either alone or co-administered with nonopioid or opioid analgesics. Examples of these are antidepressants (selective serotonin reuptake inhibitors, or serotonin–norepinephrine inhibitors) and anticonvulsants (e.g., gabapentin). As with pain medications, these must be carefully titrated, and their effects monitored. Long-term systemic corticosteroids should only be used to control pain caused by inflammatory disorders or metastatic bone pain (AGS, 2009). Monitor for hyperglycemia if using corticosteroids.

The wound care nurse should also be familiar with available topical analgesics. Lidocaine or mixtures of lidocaine and prilocaine are useful for localized neuropathic and nonneuropathic pain but should not be applied to wounds. Plain capsaicin cream has shown to have benefits treating both neuropathic and nonneuropathic pain but 30% of users stop treatment due to a burning sensation. Capsaicin creams combined with aspirin, NSAIDs, local anesthetics, or tricyclic antidepressant preparations are reported to have less burning sensation. Diclofenac sodium gel, available as a topical analgesic preparation, has shown to have minimal systemic absorption and low toxicity, when used at recommended dosages (AGS, 2009).

BOX 14-4 NONSTEROIDAL ANTI-INFLAMMATORY DRUG (NSAID) USE IN GERIATRIC PATIENTS

- Avoid or use extreme caution in patients with low creatinine clearance (kidney disease), gastropathy (peptic ulcer disease), cardiovascular (CV) disease, and congestive heart failure
- Increased risk for cardiovascular thrombotic events; may increase blood pressure
- One study of elders hospitalized with ADRs found NSAIDs implicated in 23.5% of cases
- Gastrointestinal (GI) complications increase in frequency and severity as age increases
- If GI toxicity risks are low, consider ibuprofen (200 mg t.i.d.) or naproxen (220 mg b.i.d.); if risk is moderate, add a proton pump inhibitor (PPI); for high GI & CV, risk consider Cyclooxygenase-2 (COX-2) inhibitor plus low-dose aspirin
- Risk of gastrointestinal bleeding increased when NSAIDs are combined with low-dose aspirin (often taken for cardioprotective reasons) or warfarin
- Several studies found naproxen sodium to have less cardiovascular toxicity
- Ibuprofen can inhibit aspirin's antiplatelet effect
- Diclofenac sodium may have higher cardiovascular risk compared to other traditional NSAIDs

KEY POINT

NSAIDs are the drugs most commonly associated with cutaneous reactions. Ibuprofen is a common cause of erythema multiforme and Stevens-Johnson syndrome (Patel & Marfatia, 2008).

 CONCLUSION

Skin and wound care for the elderly presents a number of challenges. The wound care nurse must assure appropriate routine care to reduce the risk of xerosis, pruritus, and skin tears. The wound nurse must be knowledgeable about common benign skin conditions and their management and should refer any patient with any evidence of skin malignancy. The wound care nurse must recognize the factors leading to delayed healing in the elderly and the importance of evidence-based wound management. The wound care nurse must be aware of geriatric syndromes such as delirium, malnutrition, elder abuse, and polypharmacy and should contribute to prevention and prompt detection of these conditions.

REFERENCES

Alhawassi, T. M., Krass, I., Bajorek, B. V., et al. (2014). A systematic review of the prevalence and risk factors for adverse drug reactions in the elderly in the acute care setting. *Clinical Interventions in Aging, 9*, 2079–2086. doi: 10.2147/CIA.S71178.

Ali, S. M., & Yosipovitch, G. (2013). Skin pH: From basic science to basic skin care. *Acta Dermato-Venereologica, 93*(3), 261–267.

American Geriatric Society (AGS). (2009). Pharmacological management of persistent pain in older persons. *Journal of the American Geriatrics Society, 57*(8), 1331–1346. doi: 10.1111/j.1532-5415.

American Geriatric Society (AGS). (2019). American Geriatrics Society 2019 updated AGS Beers Criteria for potentially inappropriate medication use in older adults. *Journal of the American Geriatrics Society, 67*(4), 674–694. doi: 10.1111/jgs.15767.

Ansari, S. A. (2014). Skin pH and skin flora. In A. O. Barel, M. Paye, & H. I. Maibach (Eds.), *Handbook of Cosmetic Science and Technology* (4th ed., pp. 163–174). Boca Raton, FL: CRC Press.

Archer, D. F. (2012). Postmenopausal skin and estrogen. *Gynecological Endocrinology, 28*(Suppl 2), 2–6. doi: 10.3109/09513590.2012.705392.

Armstrong, D. G., & Meyr, A. J. (2020). Basic principles of wound healing. In R. S. Berman, J. F. Eidt, J. L. Mills Sr (Eds.), *UpToDate*. Waltham, MA: UpToDate Inc. Accessed April 13, 2020.

Ashcroft, G. S., Greenwell-Wild, T., Horan, M. A., et al. (1999). Topical estrogen accelerates cutaneous wound healing in aged humans associated with an altered inflammatory response. *American Journal of Pathology, 155*(4), 1137–1146. doi: 10.1016/S0002-9440(10)65217-0.

Balato, A., Balato, N., Di Costanzo, L., et al. (2011). Contact sensitization in the elderly. *Clinics in Dermatology, 29*(1), 24–30.

Bains, S. N., Nash, P., & Fonacier, L. (2019). Irritant contact dermatitis. *Clinical Reviews in Allergy & Immunology, 56*(1), 99–109. https://doi.org/10.1007/s12016-018-8713-0

Berger, T. G., Shive, M., & Harper, G. M. (2013). Pruritus in the older patient: A clinical review. *JAMA, 310*(22), 2443–2450.

Bieber, T., Leung, D., Gamal, Y. E., et al., (2013). Atopic eczema. In R. Pawankar, S. T. Holgate, G. W. Canonica, et al. (Eds.), *WAO White Book on Allergy Update*. Milwaukee, WI: World Allergy Organization.

Bonte, F., Girard, D., Archambault, J., et al. (2019). Skin changes during ageing. In: J. R. Harris, & V. I. Korolchuk (Eds.), *Subcellular Biochemistry: Biochemistry and Cell Biology of Ageing: Part II Clinical Science* (pp. 249–280). Singapore: Springer Nature.

Brooks, J., Cowdell, F., Ersser, S. J., et al. (2017). Skin cleansing and emolliating for older people: A quasi-experimental pilot study. *International Journal of Older People Nursing, 12*(3). https://doi.org/10.1111/opn.12145

Brown-O'Hara, T. (2013). Geriatric syndromes and their implications for nursing. *Nursing, 43*(1), 1–3. doi: 10.1097/01.NURSE.0000423097.95416.50

Bruckenthal, P., & Barkin, R. L. (2013). Options for treating postherpetic neuralgia in the medically complicated patient. *Therapeutics and Clinical Risk Management, 9*, 329–340. doi.org/10.2147/TCRM.S47138

Bryson, G. L., & Wyand, A. (2006). Evidence-based clinical update: General anesthesia and the risk of delirium and postoperative cognitive dysfunction. *Canadian Journal of Anesthesia, 53*(7), 669–677.

Campisi, J., & d'Adda di Fagagna, F. (2007). Cellular senescence: When bad things happen to good cells. *Nature Reviews Molecular Cell Biology, 8*(9), 729–740. doi: 10.1038/nrm2233.

Centers for Disease Control and Prevention (CDC). (2013). *The State of Aging and Health in America*. Atlanta, GA: Centers for Disease Control and Prevention, US Dept of Health and Human Services.

Cesari, M., Marzetti, E., Canevelli, M., et al. (2017). Geriatric syndromes: How to treat. *Virulence, 8*(5), 577–585. https://doi.org/10.1080/21505594.2016.1219445

Chang, A. L. S., Wong, J. W., Endo, J. O., et al. (2013a). Geriatric dermatology review: Major changes in skin function in older patients and their contribution to common clinical challenges. *Journal of the American Medical Directors Association, 14*(10), 724–730. doi: 10.1016/j.jamda.2013.02.014.

Chang, A. L. S., Wong, J. W., Endo, J. O., et al. (2013b). Geriatric dermatology: Part II. Risk factors and cutaneous signs of elder mistreatment for the dermatologist. *Journal of the American Academy of Dermatology, 68*(4), 533.e1–533.e10; quiz 543–534. doi: 10.1016/j.jaad.2013.01.001.

Chen, C. C. H., Chiu, M. J., Chen, S. P., et al. (2011). Patterns of cognitive change in elderly patients during and 6 months after hospitalization: A prospective cohort study. *International Journal of Nursing Studies, 48*(3), 338–346. doi: 10.1016/j.ijnurstu.2010.03.011.

Deiner, S., & Silverstein, J. H. (2009). Postoperative delirium and cognitive dysfunction. *British Journal of Anaesthesia, 103*(Suppl 1), i41–i46. doi: 10.1093/bja/aep291.

Demling, R. H. (2005). The role of anabolic hormones for wound healing in catabolic states. *Journal of Burns and Wounds, 4*, 46–62.

Eckhart, L., Tschachler, E., & Gruber, F. (2019). Autophagic control of skin aging. *Frontiers in Cell and Developmental Biology, 7*, 143.

Endo, J. O., Wong, J. W., Norman, R. A., et al. (2013). Geriatric dermatology: Part I. Geriatric pharmacology for the dermatologist. *Journal of the American Academy of Dermatology, 68*(4), 521.e1–521.e10; quiz 531–522. doi: 10.1016/j.jaad.2012.10.063.

Epocrates - Acetaminophen. (2019). Epocrates essentials for Apple iOS (Version 5.1) [Mobile application software]. Retrieved from http://www.epocrates.com/mobile/iphone/essentials

European Pressure Ulcer Advisory Panel, National Pressure Injury Advisory Panel, and Pan Pacific Pressure Injury Alliance [EPUAP/NPIAP/PPPIA]. (2019). In E. Haesler (Ed.), *Prevention and treatment of pressure ulcers/injuries: Clinical Practice Guideline*. The International Guideline.

Farage, M. A., Miller, K. W., Berardesca, E., et al. (2009). Clinical implications of aging skin: Cutaneous disorders in the elderly. *American Journal of Clinical Dermatology, 10*(2), 73–86. doi: 10.2165/00128071-200910020-00001.

Farage, M. A., Miller, K. W., Elsner, P., et al. (2008). Intrinsic and extrinsic factors in skin ageing: A review. *International Journal of Cosmetic Science, 30*(2), 87–95. doi: 10.1111/j.1468-2494.2007.00415.x.

Fávaro-Moreira, N. C., Krausch-Hofmann, S., Matthys, C., et al. (2016). Risk factors for malnutrition in older adults: A systematic review of the literature based on longitudinal data. *Advances in Nutrition, 7*(3), 507–522. doi: 10.3945/an.115.011254.

Fong, T. G., Tulebaev, S. R., & Inouye, S. K. (2009). Delirium in elderly adults: Diagnosis, prevention and treatment. *Nature Reviews Neurology, 5*(4), 210–220.

Gallelli, L., Siniscalchi, A., Palleria, C., et al., & G&SP Working Group. (2017). Adverse drug reactions related to drug administration in hospitalized patients. *Current Drug Safety, 12*(3), 171–177. https://doi.org/10.2174/1574886312666170616090640

Gilliver, S. C., Ashworth, J. J., & Ashcroft, G. S. (2007). The hormonal regulation of cutaneous wound healing. *Clinics in Dermatology, 25*(1), 56–62. doi: 10.1016/j.clindermatol.2006.09.012.

Gosain, A., & DiPietro, L. A. (2004). Aging and wound healing. *World Journal of Surgery, 28*(3), 321–326.

Hahnel, E., Blume-Peytavi, U., Trojahn, C., et al. (2017). Associations between skin barrier characteristics, skin conditions and health of aged nursing home residents: A multi-center prevalence and correlation study. *BMC Geriatrics, 17*(263). doi: 10.1186/s12877-017-0655-5.

Hall, J. E., Karch, D. L., Crosby, A. E. (2016). *Elder abuse surveillance: Uniform definitions and recommended core data elements for use in elder abuse surveillance*, Version 1.0. Atlanta, GA: National Center for Injury Prevention and Control, Centers for Disease Control and Prevention.

Harris, C. L., & Fraser, C. (2004). Malnutrition in the institutionalized elderly: The effects on wound healing. *Ostomy/Wound Management, 50*(10), 54–63.

Heron, M. (2018). Deaths: Leading causes for 2016. *National Vital Statistics Reports, 67*(6), Hyattsville, MD: National Center for Health Statistics.

Hess, K. T. (2020). *Product Guide to Skin & Wound Care* (8th ed.). Philadelphia, PA: Wolters Kluwer.

Inouye, S., van Dyck, C., Alessi, C., et al. (1990). Clarifying confusion: The confusion assessment method. *Annals of Internal Medicine, 113*(12), 941–948.

Inouye, S. K., Studenski, S., Tinetti, M. E., et al. (2007). Geriatric syndromes: Clinical, research, and policy implications of a core geriatric concept. *Journal of the American Geriatrics Society, 55*(5), 780–791.

Inouye, S. K., Westendorp, R. G. J., & Saczynski, J. S. (2014). Delirium in elderly people. *Lancet, 383*, 911–922. doi: 10.1016/S0140-6736(13)60688-1.

Jiang, L., Zhang, E., Yang, Y., et al. (2012). Effectiveness of apoptotic factors expressed on the wounds of patients with stage III pressure ulcers. *Journal of Wound Ostomy & Continence Nursing, 39*(4), 391–396.

Kish, T. D., Chang, M. H., & Fung, H. B. (2010). Treatment of skin and soft tissue infections in the elderly: A review. *The American Journal of Geriatric Pharmacotherapy, 8*(6), 485–513.

Kopera, D. (2015). Impact of testosterone on hair and skin. *Endocrinology & Metabolic Syndrome, 4*(3), 187. doi: 10.4172/2161-1017.10000187.

Kottner, J., Lichterfeld, A., & Blume-Peytavi, U. (2013). Maintaining skin integrity in the aged: A systematic review. *British Journal of Dermatology, 169*(3), 528–542.

Lachs, M. S., & Pillemer, K. A. (2015). Elder abuse. *New England Journal of Medicine, 373*, 1947–1956. doi: 10.1056/NEJMra1404688.

Langan, S. M., Smeeth, L., Hubbard, R., et al. (2008). Bullous pemphigoid and pemphigus vulgaris—incidence and mortality in the UK: population based cohort study. *British Medical Journal, 337*, a180. doi: 10.1136/bmj.a180.

LeBlanc, K., & Baranoski, S. (2009). Prevention and management of skin tears. *Advances in Skin & Wound Care, 22*(7), 325–332.

Lichterfeld-Kottner, A., Lahmann, N., Blume-Peytavi, U., et al. (2018). Dry skin in home care: A representative prevalence study. *Journal of Tissue Viability, 27*, 226–231. doi: 10.1016/j.jtv.2018.07.001.

Lopes, R. D., Horowitz, J. D., Garcia, D. A., et al. (2011). Warfarin and acetaminophen interaction: A summary of the evidence and biological plausibility. *Blood, 118*(24), 6269–6273. doi: 10.1182/blood-2011-335612.

Mancuso, P., & Bouchard, B. (2019). The impact of aging on adipose function and adipokine synthesis. *Frontiers in Endocrinology, 10*, 137. doi: 10.3389/fendo.2019.00137.

Marcantonio, E. R. (2017). Delirium in hospitalized older adults. *The New England Journal of Medicine, 377*(15), 1456–1466. doi.org/10.1056/NEJMcp1605501

Marcantonio, E., Ta, T., Duthie, E., et al. (2002). Delirium severity and psychomotor types: Their relationship with outcomes after hip fracture repair. *Journal of American Geriatrics Society, 50*(5), 850–857.

Masnoon, N., Shakib, S., Kalisch-Ellett, L., et al. (2017). What is polypharmacy? A systematic review of definitions. *BMC Geriatrics, 17*, 230. doi: 10.1186/s12877-017-0621-2.

Mather, M., Jacobsen, L. A., & Pollard, K. M. (2015). Aging in the United States. *Population Bulletin, 70*(2).

McHugh, D., & Gil, J. (2018). Senescence and aging: Causes, consequences, and therapeutic avenues. *The Journal of Cell Biology, 217*(1), 65–77. https://doi.org/10.1083/jcb.201708092

McNichol, L. L., Ayello, E. A., Phearman, L. A., et al. (2018). Incontinence-associated dermatitis: State of the science and knowledge translation. *Advances in Skin & Wound Care, 31*(11), 502–513.

Meehan, M., & Penckofer, S. (2014). The role of vitamin D in the aging adult. *Journal of Aging and Gerontology, 2*(2), 60–71. doi: 10.12974/2309-6128.2014.02.02.1.

Milgrom, H., & Huang, H. (2014). Allergic disorders at a venerable age: A mini-review. *Gerontology, 60*(2), 99–107. doi: 10.1159/000355307.

Morimoto, Y., Yoshimura, M., Utada, K., et al. (2009). Prediction of postoperative delirium after abdominal surgery in the elderly. *Journal of Anesthesia, 23*(1), 51–56. doi: 10.1007/s00540-008-0688-1.

Munro, E. L., Hickling, D. F., Williams, D. M., et al. (2018). Malnutrition is independently associated with skin tears in hospital inpatient setting—findings of a 6-year point prevalence audit. *International Wound Journal, 15*(4), 527–533. doi: 10.1111/iwj.12893.

Oh, E. S., Fong, T. G., Hshieh, T. T., et al. (2017). Delirium in older persons: advances in diagnosis and treatment. *JAMA, 318*(12), 1161–1174. doi.org/10.1001/jama.2017.12067

Ortiz, A., & Grando, S. A. (2012) Smoking and the skin. *International Journal of Dermatology, 51*, 250–262.

Pappas, A. (2009). Epidermal surface lipids. *Dermato-Endocrinology, 1*(2), 72–76.

Patel, R. M., & Marfatia, Y. S. (2008). Clinical study of cutaneous drug eruptions in 200 patients. *Indian Journal of Dermatology, Venereology and Leprology, 74*(4), 430.

Picardo, M., Ottaviani, M., Camera, E., et al. (2009). Sebaceous gland lipids. *Dermato-Endocrinology, 1*(2), 68–71.

Pierwola, K. K., Patel, G. A., Lambert, W. C., et al. (2017). Skin disease and old age. In H. M. Fillit, K. Rockwood, & J. B. Young (Eds.), *Brocklehurst's Textbook of Geriatric Medicine and Gerontology*, (8th ed.). Philadelphia, PA: Elsevier.

Prakash, A. V., & Davis, M. D. P. (2010). Contact dermatitis in older adults. *American Journal of Clinical Dermatology, 11*(6), 373–381.

Purnamawati, S., Indrastuti, N., Danarti, R., et al. (2017). The role of moisturizers in addressing various kinds of dermatitis: A review. *Clinical Medicine & Research, 15*(3–4), 75–87. doi: 10.3121/cmr.2017.1363.

Rademaker, M. (2001). Do women have more adverse drug reactions? *American Journal of Clinical Dermatology, 2*(6), 349–351.

Ratliff, C. R., Yates, S., McNichol, L., et al. (2016). Compression for primary prevention, treatment, and prevention of recurrence of venous leg ulcers: An evidence and consensus-based algorithm for care across the continuum. *Journal of Wound, Ostomy, and Continence Nursing, 43*(4), 347.

Rawlings, A. V. (2006). Ethnic skin types: Are there differences in skin structure and function? *International Journal of Cosmetic Science, 28*(2), 79–93.

Redelmeier, D. A., Thiruchelvam, D., & Daneman, N. (2008). Delirium after elective surgery among elderly patients taking statins. *Canadian Medical Association Journal, 179*(7), 645–652. doi: 10.1503/cmaj.080443.

Reszke, R., Pelka, D., Walasek, A., et al. (2015). Skin disorders in elderly subjects. *International Journal of Dermatology, 54*, e332–e338.

Robinson, T. N., Raeburn, C. D., Tran, Z. V., et al. (2009). Postoperative delirium in the elderly: Risk factors and outcomes. *Annals of Surgery, 249*(1), 173–178. doi: 10.1097/SLA.0b013e31818e4776.

Rudolph, J. L., & Marcantonio, E. R. (2011). Review articles: Postoperative delirium: Acute change with long-term implications. *Anesthesia and Analgesia, 112*(5), 1202–1211. doi: 10.1213/ANE.0b013e3182147f6d.

Rzepecki, A. K., & Blasiak, R. (2018). Stasis dermatitis: Differentiation from other common causes of lower leg inflammation and management strategies. *Current Geriatrics Reports, 7*(4), 222–227.

Sasseville, D. (2018). Seborrheic dermatitis in adolescents and adults. In J. Fowler, & R. Corona, (Eds.), *UpToDate*. Waltham, MA: UpToDate. Retrieved November 16, 2019, from www.uptodate.com.

Saunders, C. W., Scheynius, A., & Heitman, J. (2012). Malassezia fungi are specialized to live on skin and associated with dandruff, eczema, and other skin diseases. *PLoS Pathogens, 8*(6). doi: 10.1371/journal.ppat.1002701

Schmader, K., (2016). Herpes zoster. *Clinics in Geriatric Medicine, 32*, 539–553. doi: 10.1016/j.cger.2016.02.011.

Seyfarth, F., Schliemann, S., Antonov, D., et al. (2011). Teaching interventions in contact dermatitis. *Dermatitis, 22*(1), 8–15.

Shevchenko, A., Valdes-Rodriquez, R., & Yosipovitch, G. (2018). Causes, pathophysiology, and treatment of pruritus in the mature patient. *Clinics in Dermatology, 36*, 140–151. doi:10.1016/j.clindermatol.2017.10.005.

Shi, V. Y., Tran, K., & Lio, P. A. (2012). A comparison of physiochemical properties of a selection of modern moisturizers: Hydrophilic index and pH. *Journal of Drugs in Dermatology, 11*(5), 633–636.

Shu, Y. Y., & Maibach, H. I. (2011). Estrogen and skin: Therapeutic options. *American Journal of Clinical Dermatology, 12*(5), 297–311. doi: 10.2165/11589180-000000000-00000.

Siddiqi, N., Stockdale, R., Britton, A. M., et al. (2007). Interventions for preventing delirium in hospitalized patients. *Cochrane Database of Systematic Reviews*, (2), CD005563. doi: 10.1002/14651858.CD005563.pub2.

Stojadinovic, O., Gordon, K., Lebrun, E., et al. (2012). Stress-induced hormones cortisol and epinephrine impair wound epithelialization. *Advances in Wound Care, 1*(1), 29–35.

Szokol, J. W. (2010). Postoperative cognitive dysfunction. *Conferencias Magistrales, 33*(Suppl 1), S249–S253.

Tobin, D. J. (2017). Introduction to skin aging. *Journal of Tissue Viability, 26*(1), 37–46.

Toncic, R. J., Kezic, S., Hadzavdic, S. L., et al. (2018). Skin barrier and dry skin in the mature patient. *Clinics in Dermatology, 36*, 109–115. doi: 10.1016/j.clindermatol.2017.10.0020738-081X.

Warden, V., Hurley, A. C., & Volicer, V. (2003). Development and psychometric evaluation of the Pain Assessment in Advanced Dementia (PAINAD) Scale. *Journal of the American Medical Directors Association, 4*, 9–15.

Webster, L. R., & Webster, R. (2005). Predicting aberrant behaviors in opioid-treated patients: Preliminary validation of the Opioid Risk Tool. *Pain Medicine, 6*(6), 432–442.

Wend, K., Wend, P., & Krum, S. A. (2012). Tissue-specific effects of loss of estrogen during menopause and aging. *Frontiers in Endocrinology, 3*, 19.

Wertenteil, S., Garg, A., Strunk, A., et al. (2018). Prevalence estimates for pemphigoid in the United States: A sex-adjusted and age-adjusted population analysis. *Journal of the American Academy of Dermatology, 80*(3), 655–659. doi: 10.1016/j.jaad.2018.08.030.

White-Chu, E. F., & Reddy, M. (2011). Dry skin in the elderly: Complexities of a common problem. *Clinics in Dermatology, 29*(1), 37–42. doi: 10.1016/j.clindermatol.2010.07.005.

Williamson, S., Merritt, J., & De Benedetto, A. (2019). Atopic dermatitis in the elderly: A review of clinical pathophysiological hallmarks. *British Journal of Dermatology, 182*(1), 47–54. doi: 10.1111/bjd.17896.

Wong, D. L. & Baker, C. M. (1988). Pain in children: Comparison of assessment scales. *Pediatric Nursing, 14*(1), 9–17.

Wound Ostomy Continence Nurses Society (WOCN). (2019). *Guideline for Management of Wounds in Patients with Lower-Extremity Venous Disease. WOCN Clinic Practice Guideline Series*. Mt. Laurel, NJ: Author.

Yaar, M. (2006). Clinical and histological features of intrinsic versus extrinsic skin aging. In B. A. Gilchrest, J. Krutmann (Eds.), *Skin Aging* (1st ed.), p. 198). Germany: Springer.

Yang, R., Wolfson, M., & Lewis, M. C. (2011). Unique aspects of the elderly surgical population: An anesthesiologist's perspective. *Geriatric Orthopaedic Surgery & Rehabilitation, 2*(2), 56–64. doi: 10.1177/2151458510394606.

Young, D. L., & Chakravarthy, D. (2014). A controlled laboratory comparison of 4 topical skin creams moisturizing capability on human subjects. *Journal of Wound, Ostomy, and Continence Nursing, 41*(2), 168–174. doi: 110.1097/WON.0000000000000011.

QUESTIONS

1. The wound care nurse is assessing patients in a long-term care facility for pressure injuries. What adverse age-related changes may contribute to the development of these wounds?
   A. Cell strains with longer telomeres that undergo significantly fewer doublings than younger subjects' cells
   B. Progressive increase of fibroblasts and increased proliferative capacity of the remaining fibroblasts
   C. Increased inflammatory response due to a decreased production of mast cells
   D. Loss of telomeres resulting in cellular senescence or spontaneous cellular death

2. Which age-related skin alteration may interfere with the Langerhans cells' ability to eradicate carcinogenic cells?
   A. Reduced melanocyte function
   B. Thinning of adipose layer
   C. Reduced vitamin D production
   D. Altered fibroblast function

3. What age-related alteration, critical to maintenance of normal dermal function, is a common cause of delayed wound healing in the elderly?
   A. Altered melanocyte function
   B. Thinning of adipose layer
   C. Reduced vitamin D production
   D. Altered fibroblast function

4. An elderly patient presents with documented symptoms of prodromal pain, itching, and a sharp stabbing pain, followed by a vesicular rash. What skin alteration is most likely the cause of these symptoms?
   A. Candidiasis
   B. Contact dermatitis
   C. Herpes zoster
   D. Scabies

5. An elderly patient with a partial-thickness pressure ulcer is experiencing delayed wound healing. What age-related factor may contribute to this condition?
   A. Increased keratinocyte proliferative capacity
   B. Reduced cell-to-cell communication
   C. Increased blood flow
   D. Tripling of repetition time for fibroblasts

6. Which statement accurately describes an age-related skin alteration that may delay full-thickness wound healing?
   A. There is reduced fibroblast function.
   B. An increased degranulation of platelets and release of growth factors and platelet-derived growth factor occurs.
   C. There are increased numbers of macrophages, which partially explains the diminished inflammatory response that is typically seen.
   D. Age-related stress can result in decreased production of cortisol, glucocorticoids, and epinephrine, which delays wound healing.

7. An elderly patient with a full-thickness wound is experiencing a delayed remodeling phase of wound repair. What is a usual causative factor?
   A. Failure to develop collagen tensile strength
   B. Increased perfusion to the wound
   C. Increased epithelial migration and resurfacing
   D. Increased rate of granulation tissue formation

8. The wound care nurse visiting a patient in a nursing home suspects that the patient is a victim of elder abuse. In this situation the nurse should:
   A. Investigate the nursing home staff.
   B. Substantiate the abuse before reporting to the proper authorities.
   C. Report the suspected abuse to legal authorities.
   D. Inform the elder of his or her legal right to report the abuse.

9. A patient in a long-term care facility is experiencing a disturbance of consciousness and change in cognition developing over a short period of time. Symptoms include restlessness, irritability, and agitation. What condition would the nurse suspect?
   A. Alzheimer disease
   B. Hyperactive delirium
   C. Hypoactive delirium
   D. Dementia

10. Which statement accurately describes a recommendation for pain management in the elderly?
   A. NSAIDs should be given routinely for chronic pain.
   B. Opioids cannot be safely used in older adults.
   C. Acetaminophen is the first-line treatment option.
   D. High doses of NSAIDs should be given for acute pain.

ANSWERS AND RATIONALES

1. D. Rationale: The loss of telomeres results in cellular senescence (the inability to reproduce) or in spontaneous cellular death (apoptosis). The hallmark of senescent cells is their inability to initiate DNA replication and subsequent cell division.

2. A. Rationale: The most obvious effect of melanocyte dysfunction in aging is the graying of hair. A more significant effect is interference with the Langerhans cells' ability to eradicate carcinogenic cells.

3. D. Rationale: The two factors that have the greatest negative impact on angiogenesis and collagen synthesis (granulation tissue formation) are impaired perfusion and diminished fibroblast function.

4. C. Rationale: Herpes zoster often presents with prodromal pain, itching or burning, or a sharp stabbing pain that occurs before the onset of rash.

5. B. Rationale: Partial-thickness wound healing is frequently prolonged in the elderly, due to reduced keratinocyte proliferative capacity and reduced cell-to-cell communication.

6. A. Rationale: The two factors that have the greatest negative impact on angiogenesis and collagen synthesis (granulation tissue formation) are impaired perfusion and diminished fibroblast function.

7. A. Rationale: The elderly are at risk for defective remodeling that results in failure to develop tensile strength. This may be due in part to compromised fibroblast function and also to comorbidities affecting tissue oxygenation and nutritional status.

8. C. Rationale: Signs of elder abuse are sometimes subtle, and the wound care nurse needs to remember that it is not necessary to substantiate the abuse before reporting.

9. B. Rationale: Hyperactive delirium is rare but more easily recognized because its symptoms of restlessness, irritability, antagonism, or agitation are more easily identified.

10. C. Rationale: The AGS recommends acetaminophen as first-line therapy for pain. It is not as effective for inflammatory pain (e.g., rheumatoid arthritis) as NSAIDs.

CHAPTER 15

SKIN AND WOUND CARE FOR THE BARIATRIC POPULATION

Susan Gallagher

OBJECTIVES

1. Describe common skin and wound issues associated with excess adiposity.
2. Discuss prevention and treatment of pressure injury.
3. Describe the value of preplanning for care.
4. Explore weight bias such as discrimination, prejudice, and insensitivity.

TOPIC OUTLINE

● INTRODUCTION

In 2013, the American Medical Association classified obesity as a disease. Although an imbalance between caloric intake and activiiy (energy expenditure) remains the primary etiologic factor for obesity, it is now recognized that genetic, metabolic, environmental, and other factors also play a role in the development of this disease (Gallagher, 2020).

The number of individuals with excess adiposity is increasing, and skin and wound care associated with the person of size presents specific challenges. Factors such as standard measurements and definitions, demographics, health consequences of excess adiposity, skin and wound challenges, and preplanning for care are discussed. Sensitivity as an element of care is presented.

MEASUREMENT AND DEFINITION

There are a number of ways to measure and define excess weight and atypical weight distribution. The Centers for Disease Control (CDC) refers to individuals whose weight exceeds the ranges generally considered healthy for one's height as obese and overweight. Like the CDC, the National Institutes of Health (NIH) defines the terms overweight and obesity as a body weight that is greater than what is considered normal or healthy for a certain height. The NIH suggests that overweight is generally due to extra body fat. The NIH recognizes that overweight may also be due to extra muscle, bone, or water. People who have obesity usually have excess body adiposity (NIDDK, 2019).

Body Mass Index (BMI) is a mathematical formula that assigns relative risk for mortality and morbidity (See **Table 15-1** BMI) (Nuttall, 2015). Although BMI is the most accepted and widely used measurement of obesity, there are others. For example, the Body Adiposity Index (BAI) uses hip width measurement instead of weight with a different formula for calculation (de Oliveira et al., 2019). The BAI may provide a more accurate measurement of body adiposity and may be a better indicator for adiposity-related health conditions.

Although the Bedside Mobility Assessment Tool (BMAT) is not a weight-specific assessment tool, the BMAT does help health care providers quantify mobility status using a one to four score based on mobility level. The BMAT is a validated functional mobility assessment tool and is designed to combine mobility status with other assessment criteria to develop a more relevant focused plan of care (Boynton et al., 2014).

For the purpose of developing criteria-based protocols, programs may use the following tools for measurement and definitions: actual weight, BMI, patient width at widest point, and mobility level. These four measurement criteria are not exclusive but are designed to assist wound care nurses identify patients who are at risk for the immobility-related consequences of care, one of which is pressure injury.

DEMOGRAPHICS

In 2020, the CDC reported 2017–2018 data indicating the prevalence of obesity in the United States (U.S.) was 42.4% and affected about 93.3 million adults (Hales et al., 2020). Hispanics (44.8%) and non-Hispanic blacks (49.6%) had the highest age-adjusted prevalence of obesity, followed by non-Hispanic whites (42.2%) and non-Hispanic Asians (17.5%). The rate of obesity among young adults aged 20 to 39-years-old was 40.0% and 44.8% among middle-aged adults aged 40 to 59 years. The prevalence of obesity among adults aged 60 and older was 42.8%.

Rates of obesity are increasing not only in the United States, but worldwide. According to the World Health Organization (WHO), at least 35% of adults who are over 20 years of age are overweight. In 2008, 10% of men and 14% of women worldwide were classified as obese (WHO, 2017). Researchers are recognizing that obesity is not limited to the adult population. The prevalence of obesity for those 2 to 19 years old was 18.5% and affected about 13.7 million children and adolescents. The rate of obesity was 13.9% among 2- to 5-year-old, 18.4% among 6- to 11-year-old, and 20.6% among 12- to 19-year-old. These rates very somewhat depending on region, demographic, ethnicity, family history, and other criteria. Most would agree this rate is significant and although there are many programs available to help curb the rising rate of childhood obesity, studies indicate that most children who are overweight and obese carry that weight into adulthood (Hales et al., 2017). The implication to wound care nurses is that the numbers of individuals with obesity will likely continue to increase and planning for care will become increasingly important.

TABLE 15-1 CLASSIFICATION OF OVERWEIGHT AND OBESITY BY BMI, WAIST CIRCUMFERENCE, AND ASSOCIATED DISEASE RISKS				
	BMI (kg/m²)	OBESITY CLASS	DISEASE RISK[†] RELATIVE TO NORMAL WEIGHT AND WAIST CIRCUMFERENCE	
			MEN 102 cm (40 INCHES) OR LESS WOMEN 88 cm (35 INCHES) OR LESS	MEN >102 cm (40 INCHES) WOMEN >88 cm (35 INCHES)
Underweight	<18.5		—	—
Normal	18.5–24.9		—	—
Overweight	25.0–29.9		Increased	High
Obesity	30.0–34.9	I	High	Very high
	35.0–39.9	II	Very high	Very high
Extreme Obesity	40.0[*]	III	Extremely high	Extremely high

[*]Increased waist circumference also can be a marker for increased risk, even in persons of normal weight.
[†]Disease risk for type 2 diabetes, hypertension, and CVD.
Source: National Heart, Lung, and Blood Institute. Retrieved from https://www.nhlbi.nih.gov/health/educational/lose_wt/BMI/bmi_dis
BMI calculator available at https://www.nhlbi.nih.gov/health/educational/lose_wt/BMI/bmicalc.htm

KEY POINT

Rates of obesity are increasing not only in the United States but worldwide. Most children who are overweight and obese carry the increased weight into adulthood.

HEALTH CONSEQUENCES

The disease of excess weight is associated with a number of adverse health conditions. A number of professional organizations and professionals suggest that health consequences associated with obesity be described as adiposity-based chronic disease (ABCD). The reason for this designation pertains to the impact of a hyperinflammatory state on overall health, and skin. Adiposity, especially that which is located in the abdominal region, leads to the release of cytokines, adipokines, that place the patient in this hyperinflammatory state (Bednarska-Makaruk et al., 2017; Ryu et al., 2019). This state of sustained physiologic stress contributes to a number of comorbid conditions including type 2 diabetes mellitus, hypertension, dyslipidemia, cardiovascular disease, nonalcoholic fatty liver disease, reproductive dysfunction, respiratory abnormalities, psychiatric conditions, risk for certain types of cancer, and cognitive impairment (Barone et al., 2019).

ECONOMIC IMPACT

The disease of obesity not only threatens the health and longevity of a majority of the population, it also adds an economic burden to the U.S. health care system. A recent study suggests that costs of obesity have historically been underestimated. Eight primary diseases related to metabolic dysfunction account for 75% of the health care costs in the United States. These primary obesity-related diseases include type 2 diabetes, lipid disorders, hypertension, heart disease, nonalcoholic fatty disease, some cancers, dementia, and polycystic ovarian syndrome. Of note, 30% of Americans reportedly have nonalcoholic fatty liver disease and 10% of American women have polycystic ovarian syndrome (Sasaki et al., 2014).

The obesity epidemic in the United States has cost the U.S. economy $1.72 trillion, which includes hundreds of billions of dollars in health care costs and more than a trillion dollars in lost productivity, according to a report published by the Milken Institute, a California-based economic think tank. The report, titled America's Obesity Crisis: The Health and Economic Impact of Excess Weight, draws on an analysis of data from federal health institutions, the U.S. Agency for Healthcare Research and Quality (AHRQ), and the Bureau of Labor Statistics (Graf & Waters, 2018).

The report indicates that Americans spent approximately $480.7 billion in direct health care costs in 2016 on conditions related to risk factors of obesity and overweight. Lost economic productivity was calculated at

$1.24 trillion. Those dollars reflect the monetary cost of obesity and its related diseases. The greater cost is that of life with as many as 300,000 obesity-related deaths occurring each year (Wise, 2019).

THE SKIN

The number of obese and overweight individuals accessing care in health care facilities and at home is increasing. These individuals are admitted with more comorbidities and require longer lengths of stay than do the nonbariatric patients (Temple et al., 2017). Increased weight, limited mobility, excessive moisture from increased perspiration, and reduced tissue perfusion and oxygenation all contribute to increased risk for skin injury (Shipman & Millington, 2011). The systemic effects of hormones and cytokines may also play a contributing role in skin breakdown (Guo & de Pieto, 2010). Prevention of skin breakdown and treatment of preexisting skin conditions become a primary focus in caring for the patient who has obesity.

ASSESSMENT

The first step in prevention of skin injury is a comprehensive assessment including history, comorbid conditions, risk assessment, and thorough inspection of the skin. The Braden Scale for Predicting Pressure Sore Risk® (Braden Scale) is a guide that combined with other findings including history and comorbid conditions guide the nurse in developing an assessment-based plan of care (Bergstrom, 1987).

Factors known to contribute to compromised skin integrity include excess weight, moisture issues, reduced tissue perfusion, and comorbidities. Bariatric patients are at risk for damage associated with friction and shear because of manually executed lateral transfers. They are also at risk for skin tears that occur when soft tissue (arms, legs and feet) rub against side rails or other equipment that may not be wide enough to accommodate the patient's body width. The patients may be at risk for pressure injury due to excess weight and difficulty in turning and repositioning themselves. The majority of bariatric patients are at risk for moisture-associated skin damage (MASD), friction and shear injuries, skin tears, and pressure injury. A comprehensive preventive care plan is necessary to maintain skin integrity (Gallagher et al., 2020).

KEY POINT

The majority of bariatric patients are at risk for MASD, friction and shear injuries, skin tears, and pressure injury.

Skin and risk assessment should occur daily including areas such as rehabilitation where risk assessment is generally performed less often. In critical care areas, skin and risk assessment should be performed more frequently because of the quickly changing and high-risk nature of the patient's physical condition.

MAINTAINING SKIN HEALTH

Maintaining the integrity of the skin is central to prevention of skin breakdown. The basic elements of skin care should be provided to every patient and include the following: (1) daily inspection, (2) routine cleansing, (3) moisturization, and (4) protection. Patients who are not at risk for skin breakdown and who have no mobility or moisture issues may not require daily inspection unless their at-risk status changes. Individuals with compromised circulation, moisture problems related to incontinence or diaphoresis, or issues with activity, mobility, or sensory function require frequent skin assessment and routine skin care protocols, whether at home or in a health care facility. Discharge planning for obese patients should include instructions for daily skin inspection and proper skin care. Because adequate maintenance of skin may be difficult in the presence of abdominal obesity or limited mobility, discharge planning and education should include assistive devices for self-care or have in place individual(s) who will assist with care at home.

Daily skin care should include any areas with excessive moisture loss or moisture accumulation within skin folds. Protecting the pH balance of the skin is important to skin integrity. Cleansing with a pH-balanced liquid soap or skin cleanser or disposable pH-balanced cleansing wipes is recommended. Cleansing agents should be free of perfumes and other skin irritants. The skin should be gently washed without scrubbing; drying should involve patting but not rubbing, which could irritate the skin. A hair dryer on the cool setting may also be used to dry the skin, especially in areas that are more difficult to access (Blackett et al., 2011). Disposable cleansing wipes are generally pH balanced, do not require rinsing, and dry quickly without the use of a towel or hair dryer; they are preferred by many for those reasons.

Hygienic care for the obese patient is no different than for nonbariatric patients with at-risk skin. The same principles for washing and drying apply to both groups. Care for the bariatric patient must include measures to assure adequate cleansing and drying of deep skin folds. Because the area within the skin folds remains moist due to perspiration, these areas should be examined periodically throughout the day and cleaned and dried if moist (Black et al., 2011; Gray et al., 2011). The nurse should use wicking or absorptive products to keep skin folds dry. Another reason to routinely clean the areas is to reduce bacteria that could contribute to skin breakdown. More shallow skin folds are often easier to access and clean. Deeper skin folds on the abdomen under the pannus and on the back may require assistance with lifting to enable proper cleaning. To facilitate safe elevation of the pannus, lifting devices should be used. The use of a pannus sling promotes patient comfort and dignity and helps prevent staff injury. Slings are available that can be used with either an overhead or a floor lift. If intertriginous dermatitis (ITD) or a wound is present on either surface of the pannus, dressings or medication should be applied prior to removal of the pannus sling.

KEY POINT

Skin folds represent high-risk areas for the bariatric patient. The skin must be cleansed and dried, and wicking fabrics should be routinely used to prevent maceration and friction.

In addition to appropriate cleansing, maintenance of skin integrity includes routine use of appropriate moisturizers (Beitz, 2014). Moisturizers may contain emollients or humectants or a combination of the two (Black et al., 2011). Humectants attract water to the stratum corneum from the dermis and are indicated for extremely dry rough skin. They are not appropriate for skin folds and areas of trapped moisture. Emollients smooth flaky skin cells by replacing intercellular lipids in the stratum corneum, which helps maintain integrity of the skin barrier. These products are appropriate for general use, even on fragile skin that is frequently moist (Black et al., 2011; O'Lenick, 2009). Like cleansing products, lotions and creams should be free of fragrance and other irritants. They can be applied multiple times during the day to maintain healthy skin. If profuse sweating is present, the skin should be cleansed prior to application of the lotion or cream, and the nurse should assure that the product is nonocclusive. Agents containing dimethicone or ceramides are usually a good choice.

Damage associated with friction may occur when moist or fragile skin surfaces are exposed to superficial abrasive rubbing force, such as when the sides of a skin fold rub against each other. Basic care include wicking moisture away from body folds, gentle handling during bathing and positioning, separation of skin folds with either wicking textiles or absorptive pads, and protective dressings to vulnerable sites, such as the use of silicone adhesive foam dressings to the point of contact between the soft tissue and the support surface or mattress.

Protection of skin that is exposed to excessive moisture from urine or stool consists of moisture barrier products such as zinc, dimethicone, or petrolatum-based products or liquid acrylates. Chapters 18 and 19 provide an in-depth discussion of prevention and management of MASD, specifically incontinence-associated dermatitis (IAD) and ITD. The discussion in this chapter will be limited to specific considerations for the bariatric patient.

MOISTURE-ASSOCIATED SKIN DAMAGE

Although the person who is obese may be affected by one of the many categories of MASD, those commonly experienced include IAD and ITD.

Incontinence-Associated Dermatitis

Patients at risk for IAD will require prevention measures beyond normal skin cleansing and moisturizing. Moisture-barrier ointments applied to the perineal and buttocks areas provide protection from both moisture and chemical irritants. The ointment should be applied after initial cleaning and reapplied after each toileting or incontinence episode. Caregivers should know that it is not necessary to remove barrier ointment after each toileting or incontinent episode. They should wipe away any soiled ointment and replace with additional barrier ointment. If skin is not visible under ointments, a perineal cleanser or wipe should be used to gently remove the ointments once daily to inspect the skin.

Routine protection of the perineal area should continue after discharge from a facility. Although the bariatric patient may not complain of incontinence, it may be difficult for the bariatric or obese person to properly clean self after toileting. The importance of routine cleansing and protection of the skin in the perineal area and buttocks should be discussed with the patient prior to discharge. If self-application of protective ointments is difficult for the individual, he or she may be instructed to use a three-in-one product that provides cleansing, moisturizing, and protection in a disposable wipe. An occupational therapist may help locate personal hygiene accessories that can assist the patient in cleansing and in application of ointments to the perineal and buttocks areas.

KEY POINT

Personal hygiene accessories are available that assist the patient to cleanse the perineal area and to provide protective creams and ointments.

Intertriginous Dermatitis

Excess perspiration, a more alkaline pH at the skin surface, and decreased capillary flow interfere with the skin's moisture barrier (Black et al., 2011; Gray et al., 2011). This is more apparent deep within skin folds. Areas underneath the pannus or breasts generate and trap excess moisture, which can result in ITD. If not adequately cleansed and dried, the skin will become macerated, which promotes bacterial, viral, and fungal growth. Odor may develop, which may be stressful for the patient. Maintaining skin folds that are clean and dry may be challenging. The use of soft absorbent fabric (e.g., cloth diapers) or soft absorptive pads such as abdominal pads or sanitary pads placed within the skin folds and under

the breasts may be helpful. When using abdominal pads or sanitary pads, make sure they do not create undue pressure in the skin fold. When proper precautions are in place, these products absorb the moisture and also separate the skin folds, thus protecting against frictional forces. Absorbent fabric and pads should be changed frequently to prevent moisture damage and odor. It may be necessary to find ways to stabilize the absorptive fabric or pad when the patient is out of bed.

There is a textile product (e.g., InterDry®) made specifically to absorb and wick away moisture from skin folds. The textile is a polyurethane-coated polyester material impregnated with 0.19% antimicrobial silver. The antimicrobial reduces the colonization of bacteria and yeast, such as *Staphylococcus aureus*, *Staphylococcus epidermidis*, *Pseudomonas aeruginosa*, and *Candida albicans*. One end of the fabric sheet should be placed at the base of the fold, and the other end should extend at least 2 inches beyond the fold. This provides for wicking and evaporation of moisture on a continual basis. Creams or ointments used in conjunction with this fabric may reduce efficacy of the product and are not recommended. The fabric also provides for separation of the folds and the low coefficient of friction (CoF) of the fabric surface protects against skin to skin injury. Because the fabric is a single layer and thin, it generally remains in place in the skin fold when the patient gets out of bed. It may be secured by tucking it into clothing or using a small amount of tape (Hess, 2020).

If bacterial or fungal infection develops within the folds, appropriate medicated cream should be applied sparingly. While this may address the infection, there is still a need for absorption of excess moisture. Previously discussed measures should be initiated after treatment with medication.

PRESSURE INJURY

Pressure injuries are addressed in Chapters 20 and 21. It is important for all caregivers to recognize that obese individuals are at increased risk for pressure injury in all care settings.

PRESSURE INJURY PREVENTION

Prevention is a cost-effective alternative to treatment. Use of pressure injury risk assessment tools such as the Braden Scale is extremely useful in determining risk for pressure injury development. While the total score provides an overall summary of risk, subscale scores provide specific opportunities to mitigate predicted risk.

When assessing a bariatric patient for pressure injury risk status, attention should be paid to the subscale areas of sensory perception, moisture, activity, mobility, nutrition, and friction and shear. The following discusses ways to mitigate risk associated with the Braden subscales.

Sensory perception may be impaired by medications, fatigue, medical issues, or diminished tissue perfusion and should be assessed routinely. The wound care nurse should observe skin around tubes, compression devices, and other devices that may lead to medical device–related pressure injury (MDRPI). Wrinkled sheets, excess fabric, and incontinence pads may also contribute to increased pressure and increased risk for skin breakdown. The nurse should determine if the patient can sense discomfort related to medical devices or other objects that create pressure.

When assessing exposure to moisture, the wound care nurse should carefully examine the skin between body folds, such as under the breasts, under the pannus, and in the perineal area. It is important to be gentle when examining the pannus. The wound care nurse should carefully lift the pannus and should examine both the upper and lower surfaces of the skin fold at the innermost junction. Lifting a pannus that is very heavy may require use of lifting equipment. Skin folds in the neck, upper arms, legs, ankles, inguinal and gluteal areas are often overlooked. A patient may deny incontinence but still exhibit signs of irritation and moisture damage in the perineal area, which may be due to inadequate cleansing as opposed to incontinence. Visual inspection of the perineal skin is essential; it is not sufficient to simply ask the patient about incontinence.

Accurate assessment of activity requires the nurse to do more than ask the patient about the patient's ability to walk. Patients may state that they are not restricted when they walk, have no difficulty getting around or transferring, and generally need no assistance with these activities. That may not be the situation at home. When admitted into the health care setting, the patients may be medicated, fatigued, or in pain. They are in an unfamiliar place, often in a room filled with medical equipment and little space to move around, surroundings quite different than those at home. Activity is evaluated by a rehabilitation specialist. They may ask the patient to transfer from the bed to a chair, to walk to the bathroom, or to ambulate in the room and hall, and to carefully observe the patient during performance of these activities Use of a properly sized walker or walking sling and lift can facilitate confident, safe activity.

Asking the patient to turn in bed for skin assessment provides an opportunity to assess how well the patient moves in bed and the adequacy of the current bed. Wiggermann et al. (2017) conducted a study with obese volunteers; waist circumference was the best predictor of the surface width required for the individual to turn from one side to the other. BMI was also correlated with the surface width required to turn (Wiggermann et al., 2017). Additional assessment should include the following: is the patient able to turn independently, is there sufficient room in the bed for the patient to turn unassisted or with

assistance, and is there a need for a trapeze or other mobility equipment? When evaluating mobility, assess the patient's ability to sit up in bed, move to the side of the bed, and transfer or stand. The bedside nurse should also evaluate the need for safe patient handling equipment, transfer and repositioning devices, and bariatric bed frame with support surface. A support surface with enhanced pressure redistribution, shear reduction, and microclimate features is recommended for the patient who is obese. The support surface selection should also consider the patient's body dimensions, ensuring there is adequate space for repositioning (EPUAP/NPIAP/PPPIA, 2019; McNichol et al., 2015). A decision support tool for support surface selection is available at algorithm.wocn. org and additional information on support surfaces can be found in Chapter 22.

Many individuals with obesity are also malnourished. The patient should have a complete nutritional assessment to determine if protein, carbohydrate, fluid, and other nutritional requirements for health and healing are being met (EPUAP/NPIAP/PPPIA, 2019). Monitoring intake and output for 48 hours is helpful when a nutritional consult is not immediately available. See Chapter 7 for additional information about nutrition and obesity.

Obese patients are also at risk for shear and friction injury. They tend to drag their heels and sacrum when getting out of bed, increasing risk for friction injuries. Obese patients have impaired diaphragmatic movement and may require head of bed elevation, increasing their risk for shear injury. Pressure injury prevention must include attention to prevention of shear damage, which occurs when the patient slides down in bed. The deep tissue layers move down in response to gravity, while the superficial layers remain adherent to the sheets. The intervening tissue layers undergo shear force, which causes compression of the vessels passing through the soft tissue. Shear damage commonly involves the buttocks area but has been noted occasionally over the coccyx and ischial tuberosity areas (EPUAP/NPIAP/PPPIA, 2019). For more information on shear injury, see Chapter 20.

The skin of the obese patient may be poorly vascularized, may be dry and fragile, is prone to maceration from excess sweating, and is also exposed to friction and shear, all of which contribute to increased risk for pressure injury. Immobility, poor nutrition and inadequate equipment can further add to the risk (Gallagher, 2020). Pressure results in tissue hypoperfusion due to the weight applied to the tissue in contact with the bed or chair. This results in significant cell deformation and increased likelihood of pressure injury and other pressure-related skin damage. Considerable deformations and strains may occur within the skin and deeper tissues in weight-bearing postures, such as when lying in bed or sitting in a chair (EPUAP/NPIAP/PPPIA, 2019). Atypical pressure injuries may develop in obese patients at any site where pressure, moisture, friction, and shear are present, such as in the skin folds, on the buttocks, at the neck, upper back, upper medial thigh, flanks, and posterior legs and ankles (Beitz, 2014; Gallagher, 2020). Those who are overweight to obese are at a higher risk for pressure injury compared to those individuals with a normal BMI range (EPUAP/NPIAP/PPPIA, 2019).

> **KEY POINT**
>
> Those who are overweight to obese are at a higher risk for pressure injury compared to those individuals with a normal BMI range.

Selection of the appropriate bed frame and support surface is important for the bariatric patient (**Fig. 15-1**). Many manufacturers provide standard bed frames and support surfaces to support weight up to 500 pounds to accommodate the majority of these individuals. The width of the obese person should also be considered when making bed and support surface decisions. There must be adequate space on each side of the patient for comfort, prevention of injury and to facilitate turning. Wiggermann et al. (2017) found that, when lying in the center of a standard 91-cm-wide (36 inches) hospital bed, a patient with a BMI > 35 kg/m^2 would have insufficient space to be turned in either direction without lateral repositioning. A patient with a BMI > 45 kg/m^2 would have insufficient space to be turned at all. Wound care

nurses should consider placing patients who are unable to laterally reposition themselves on a wider bed when BMI is >35 kg/m^2 and should consider placing all patients >45 kg/m^2 on a wider bed regardless of mobility. This will provide adequate space for the patient to turn unassisted in bed and for the staff to assist with safely turning the patient (Wiggermann et al., 2017).

> **KEY POINT**
>
> Wound care nurses should consider placing patients who are unable to laterally reposition themselves on a wider bed when BMI is >35 kg/m^2 and should consider placing all patients >45 kg/m^2 on a wider bed regardless of mobility.

PRESSURE INJURY TREATMENT

Pressure injury treatment is outlined in Chapter 8. For the individual who is obese and has a pressure injury, there are a few additional considerations. Pressure injury prevention interventions must be considered and each element applied to the treatment plan. Ensure the health care team understands and preplans for supplies and equipment needed for care delivery including longer gloves to ensure access to deep folds.

When filling wounds with depth, it is important to record number and type of wound fillers used to make sure all are removed and changed. Risk of infection is higher in this population, and the wound care nurse

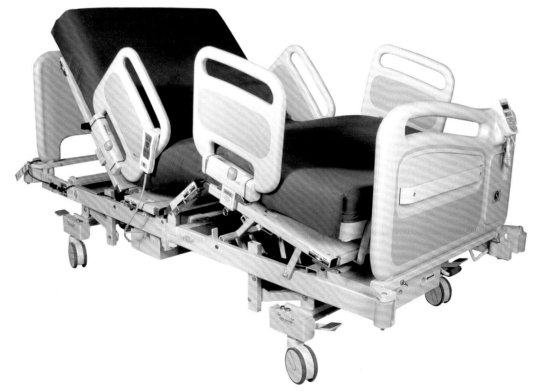

FIGURE 15-1. Bariatric Bed. Proper selection of a bed and support surface for the bariatric patient is determined by height, weight, and width of the patient as well as the need for prevention and/or treatment of skin integrity issues. (Reprinted with permission from Sizewise.)

should be alert to the signs and symptoms of infection and should observe for early signs of wound deterioration and sepsis. Patient and family education should include the need for frequent repositioning and wound care.

 WOUND CARE

Because of the chronic sustained stress associated with the hyperinflammatory state that defines ABCD, the patient is at particular risk for wound formation and delays in healing. This population has particular risk related to surgical site infections, wound dehiscence, and lower leg pathology.

SURGICAL SITE CONCERNS

A recent study suggested that hospital acquired infections kill more patients each year than breast, prostate, and lung cancers; HIV; and car accidents combined. In 2018, The Centers for Medicare and Medicaid (CMS) reported that costs associated with hospital-acquired infections have reached $28 to 45 billion annually. Excess adiposity and ABCD are associated with a higher incidence of surgical site challenges, such as surgical site infection and wound dehiscence. A factor that contributes to obesity-related surgical site issues is hypoperfusion of adipose tissue due to the higher ratio of tissue mass to capillaries within the adipose tissue. Decreased oxygen tension in adipose tissue is inadequate to meet the oxygen needs of the healing surgical incision (Pierpont et al., 2014). Additional factors that contribute to the increased rate of surgical site infections include perioperative hyperglycemia (obesity is associated with insulin resistance and hyperglycemia), prolonged operative time (operative time is an independent predictor of surgical site infection), and suboptimal doses of prophylactic antibiotics to achieve therapeutic tissue concentrations (Anaya & Dellinger, 2006). Reduced perfusion and oxygenation of the adipose tissue places the individual at risk for wound infection and wound breakdown. Adequate oxygen levels are required for normal WBC function, protection against infection, and for all aspects of wound healing, including collagen synthesis (Garwood & Mizuo, 2017). Garwood and Mizuo (2017) explain that the increased weight of the abdominal wall creates increased mechanical stress along the incision, further increasing the risk of incisional breakdown.

The wound care nurse must provide ongoing monitoring of the incision for any evidence of infection or excess mechanical stress. An abdominal binder may be used to manage local pain and to offset the effects of increased adipose tissue, which places tension on the suture line and may result in wound dehiscence (Zhang et al., 2016). It is important to ensure proper sizing of the abdominal binder. Proper sizing is important to prevent elevated intra-abdominal pressure, pulmonary compromise, MDRPI, and the risk for compartment syndrome (Barnouti, 2016).

MASSIVE LOCALIZED LYMPHEDEMA

Because of the increasing rates of morbid obesity, wound care clinics are reporting increasing frequency of a unique presentation of secondary lymphedema. Massive localized lymphedema (MLL) is described as a benign lymphoproliferative overgrowth. MLL is a form of secondary lymphedema that is caused by the obstruction of lymphatic flow. The mass is commonly found in the medial region of the upper leg but can be found elsewhere (Chopra et al., 2015). Clinically, patients often present with classic skin changes often accompanied by lymphatic weeping. The precise cause of MLL is unknown, but the most distinguishing clinical characteristic of MLL is morbid obesity.

A diagnosis of MLL is likely made based on clinical history and presentation. Standard diagnostic studies may not be advisable because of the person's morbid obesity. Diagnostic tests such as magnetic resonance imaging (MRI) may be impossible due to the patient's hip width, girth, lower leg dimensions, or weight limit of the MRI. Some clinics are equipped to perform complete decongestive physiotherapy (CDP), which is recommended (Fife, 2014). Surgical removal of the MLL collection may be possible, but surgery can be technically difficult and not always advisable due to the risk of perioperative complications, including wound dehiscence. (Hou et al., 2019). Considering the increasing number of MLL cases, the comorbidities and complexities of treating morbidly obese patients, and associated complications, wound care nurses need a heightened awareness of this condition.

There is little literature to describe the exact local skin and wound care necessary in the presence of MLL. The role of the wound care nurse is to advocate for the patient's complex emotional and physical needs. Preplanning for care, regardless of the care setting, is important to protect the patient from further skin injury and prevent staff injury in handling and moving the patient. The basic principles of skin and wound are important, especially if the patient has been admitted to the facility for an unrelated situation such as childbirth, trauma, or unanticipated surgical procedure. Frequent assessment, adequate nutrition, size-appropriate equipment, training, protection of vulnerable skin, and sensitivity are principles of care that can be provided for or monitored by the wound care nurse.

 PREPLANNING FOR CARE

In managing the skin and wound care, preplanning for equipment is an essential first step. Equipment alone is not sufficient to prevent the complications that can occur. A comprehensive, multidisciplinary patient care approach is necessary to provide safe skin and wound care in a timely, cost-effective manner. This multidisciplinary approach to preplanning should include (1) an multidisciplinary task force, (2) a criteria-based protocol, which includes preplanning equipment with policies and procedures, (3) training to include competencies, and (4) outcome management efforts.

BARIATRIC PROGRAM DEVELOPMENT TEAM

The bariatric program development team consists of champions or stakeholders who serve as influencers to promote excellence in bariatric skin and wound care. The wound care team, safe patient handling professionals, pharmacists, physical, occupational and respiratory therapists, advanced practice providers, dietitians, and others are involved in planning and delivering care.

BARIATRIC PROTOCOL

An evidence-based protocol should be in place regardless of practice setting. This protocol is preplanning based on specifically designated criteria and specifies resources such as size-appropriate equipment. The patient's weight, BMI, body width, mobility level (BMAT) and clinical condition serve as the criteria (Gallagher, 2016). Actual weight is particularly useful because breakage, failure to function properly, or patient or caregiver injury can occur if the weight limit of equipment is exceeded (Gallagher, 2016). Body width is described as the patient's body at the widest point, which could be at the hips, the shoulders, across the belly when side-lying, or ankle-to-ankle. Any clinical condition that interferes with mobility, such as pain, sedation, fear, or resistance to participating in care, places the patient at risk. Criteria-based protocols should be designed to meet the needs of the patient by ensuring access to resources, such as

specialty equipment and clinical experts, in a timely, cost-effective manner (Blackett et al., 2011; Temple et al., 2017).

Standard-sized equipment, for example, walkers, wheelchairs, commodes, lifts, slings, bedside chairs, and recliners, are inadequate for the bariatric patient (**Fig. 15-2**). These products must also accommodate the weight and width of the bariatric patient and should be considered when ordering a bariatric bed. Including elements of weight or weight distribution on the protocol is encouraged. Family and visitors may be obese as well, so furniture in the room should have extended-capacity weight limits.

There are many bed frames and mattresses available for the bariatric patient. When selecting a bariatric bed, the nurse must verify that the weight of the patient falls within the weight limits of the frame and mattress as specified by the manufacturer. The use of a low bed is frequently beneficial since it will allow the bariatric patient assistance in egress from the bed. The wound care nurse should assure that guidelines regarding bed selection are readily available to those ordering the equipment (Gallagher, 2015). Consider patient weight and weight distribution (width) in determining the need for a bariatric mattress and appropriate bed frame. When choosing between a mattress and an overlay, consider fall and entrapment risk associated with use of overlays (McNichol et al., 2015). A decision support tool for support surface selection is available at algorithm.wocn.org, and additional information on support surfaces can be found in Chapter 22.

A few points about selection of a support surface for a bariatric patient will be considered here. The requirement of a bariatric bed frame does not always necessitate

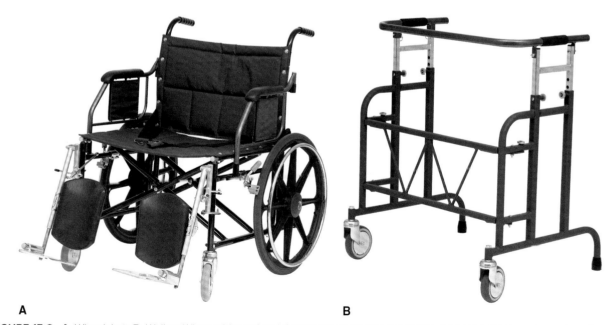

A **B**

FIGURE 15-2. A. Wheelchair. **B.** Walker. When additional mobility equipment is needed for the bariatric patient, equipment must meet the weight capacity of the intended patient and be single-patient use only. (Reprinted with permission from Sizewise.)

a specialty support surface. Foam and enhanced foam mattresses are available and can be used when mobility, exposure to moisture, sensory status, and level of consciousness are within normal limits. If the patient is at-risk in any of these areas, a therapeutic air support surface should be considered. A low air loss mattress with or without alternating pressure therapy can address moisture issues (microclimate) and provide pressure redistribution to prevent pressure injury occurrence.

If pulmonary or respiratory conditions exist, a mattress with lateral rotation can be provided for the bariatric patient. It is important to understand the specific qualities of the turning product. Although this type of surface provides pulmonary therapy and can be used to either turn or assist in turning the patient, it must be remembered that this type of support surface may not provide adequate pressure redistribution for prevention of pressure injuries. A plan must be in place for regularly scheduled repositioning of the skin and tissue. Pillows placed between the patient's legs and under the pannus or breasts will further support body weight distribution.

Hospital gowns and other clothing needs can be obtained in a variety of larger sizes and should be readily available. The use of size-appropriate slippers, identification bands, blood pressure cuffs, antiembolism stockings, sequential compression devices, and even gait belts may need to be available (VHA CEOSH, 2015). These are just a few items that not only contribute to patient comfort, safety, and dignity but are added protection from pressure injury formation or tissue deterioration.

STAFF EDUCATION

Basic care can be challenging in the presence of a complex patient. Straightforward tasks such as patient repositioning and bathing can require several staff members and various skills to accomplish these tasks safely and effectively. Education to ensure basic skills or competencies is important (Gallagher, 2013). There are several steps that facilitate learning in this situation. For example, consider a needs assessment to determine gaps in knowledge. Members of the bariatric program development team can serve as a pool of experts who develop lesson plans and education addressing identified education/training/competence needs. For example, when clinicians are seeking information on patient handling and mobility, a physical/occupational therapist, nurse expert, risk manager, and consumer member of the program development team could develop a hands-on learning tool to teach skills (Gallagher, 2016).

QUALITY AND OUTCOME MANAGEMENT

To better understand the results of the bariatric skin and wound care effort, a structured data measurement tool should be put in place. This tool should examine current and baseline data as a means of collecting relevant patient outcomes. Patient and staff satisfaction, safety, and adverse outcomes are among the measures that should be monitored. When determining outcomes, consider some of the direct and indirect outcomes influenced by preplanning. For example, properly sized sequential compression devices reduce the rate of device-related pressure injury. If the devices fit properly, they work properly. The direct impact is fewer device-related pressure injuries, and the indirect impact is fewer cases of embolic events (Gallagher, 2016; Temple et al., 2017). It makes sense to consider the direct and indirect measures that align with the facility's performance indicators (Gallagher, 2013).

⬤ PATIENT HANDLING AND MOBILITY

The effects of immobility associated with the person who is obese may be more serious and happen more quickly (Gallagher, 2015). Early, progressive, and ongoing mobility not only reduces the risk for immobility-related skin and wound issues but also promotes overall health and wellness. Mobilizing the obese patient may be time consuming. Health care workers may report a fear of personal injury, patient falls, or other patient injury. The fear of personal injury is realistic. In a study, a team found that those patients with a BMI > 30 represented 10% of the patient population. This 10% accounted for 30% of lost work days, injuries, and costs associated with the handling injuries. These common concerns are especially prevalent if mobility tasks are performed manually (Randall et al., 2009).

Many health care facilities have implemented programs to protect patients and staff from handling injuries (Gallagher, 2020). A safe patient handling and mobility program is important when caring for bariatric patients. Wound care requires staff members to turn and reposition patients, elevate the limbs, inspect the interior surfaces of the skin folds, assist from bed to chair, ambulate, toilet, and more, all of which are associated with risk of occupational injury (Gallagher, 2015). In males, the human leg weighs 16.68% of the total body weight, and in females, it is 18.43%. When one considers the weight of a patient's leg, the act of lifting the leg exceeds the recommended safe lift loads for health care workers, increasing the risk for musculoskeletal disorder (MSD) injury (Gallagher, 2015). There are a number of assistive devices to facilitate with basic care for the bariatric patient, such as pannus and limb slings (**Figs. 15-3 and 15-4**).

KEY POINT

Safe patient handling of bariatric patients requires the use of lifts and slings; even lifting the leg of a bariatric patient exceeds safe lifting limits.

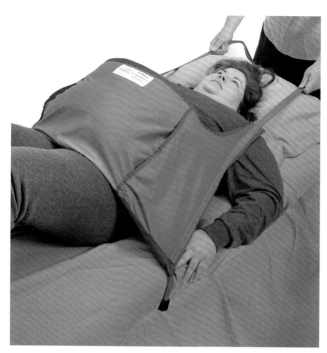

FIGURE 15-3. Pannus Sling. Use of pannus sling allows safe elevation of pannus for examination of skin without discomfort to the patient or risk of injury to health care provider. (Reprinted with permission from Alpha Modalities LLC—Sling Specialists in Safe Patient Mobility.)

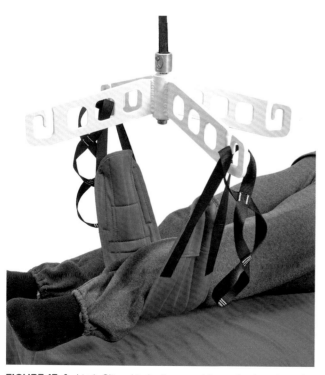

FIGURE 15-4. Limb Sling. Limb sling provides safe elevation of an arm or leg for examination or treatment; it enhances comfort for the patient and safety for the health care provider. (Reprinted with permission from Alpha Modalities LLC—Sling Specialists in Safe Patient Mobility.)

 BARIATRIC SENSITIVITY

Studies suggest that prejudice and discrimination toward the person who is obese is common in the community, in schools, in churches, and in health care settings. Insensitivities are expressed irrespective of gender, ethnicity, age, or socioeconomic status (Puhl et al., 2017, 2018, 2019).

Preconceived ideas about the causes of obesity, confirmation bias, and a belief that the obese person lacks motivation have all been identified as contributing factors to weight bias. Patients and their families are aware of the patient's size and the prejudice that many health care workers exhibit toward them (Pervez & Ramonaledi, 2017).

These insensitivities impact care. Patients often delay care as long as possible because of past experiences of prejudice and discrimination (Gallagher, 2020; Temple et al., 2017). A patient at home with lower leg cellulitis may delay access to care until the area has opened and the wound becomes infected.

Research suggests that prejudice and discrimination stem from lack of equipment, training, and adequate number of staff members to support care. Kaminsky and Gadaleta (2002) explained that those units where staff members did not have access to size-appropriate equipment and resources held the highest level of insensitivity.

Bariatric sensitivity programs are a requirement at many health care facilities and have some impact on weight bias. Use of a bariatric simulation suit has reportedly been effective in helping even the most insensitive person better understand numerous struggles associated with being a person who has obesity. One facility administrator reported, "I feel awful for some of the things I've said not meaning to cause harm." Another clinician stated, "This was life changing for me. Thank you."

Wound care nurses have the opportunity to work closely with the bariatric patient population and to provide sensitive care and treatment. They have additional opportunities to educate others in understanding of the bariatric patient. This education starts with appropriate attitude and care provided by the wound care nurse as a role model.

 CONCLUSION

The rate of overweight and obesity has increased dramatically over the past five decades. Skin and wound care is a significant concern. Few health care facilities have kept pace with this epidemic, which provides the wound care nurse an opportunity to make changes that impact the lives of many patients. Bariatric preplanning, proper equipment, multidisciplinary teamwork, and sensitivity are important aspects to provide appropriate care. Understanding the pathophysiology of obesity and its impact on skin breakdown and wound formation is important in planning for care across the continuum.

CASE STUDY

Annette is a relatively healthy 32-year-old mother who was recently on a hiking trip with her extended family. While hiking on a single-track trail, she tripped and fell 10 feet into the canyon. The airlift was delayed because of the weight limits on the rescue equipment. She has been in the Trauma ICU for 4 weeks. Today, her Braden Score is 8. She is intubated and unable to communicate. The wound care nurse has been called because she has bilateral stage 4 pressure injuries on both buttocks. Her body weight is 342 pounds.

Plan of care:

1. Reevaluate for proper bed frame and support surface. Consider ordering a bariatric bed with appropriate surface. Weight limit may be within limit for facility bed, but consider width of patient in bed and if sufficient space for patient to be turned and repositioned on the surface.

2. Examine Braden subscale scores to determine if the patient is at risk in each category rather than basing need for prevention only on total score. Braden subscale scores: Sensory Perception 1, Moisture 2, Activity 1, Mobility 1, Nutrition 2, Friction and Shear 1.

3. Assess under breasts, within abdominal folds, and the perineal area to determine presence of MASD and initiate proper treatment.

4. Assess erythema in perianal area to determine treatment (will probably need moisturizer–moisture barrier combination product)

5. Initiate enhanced skin care regimen to include addressing excess moisture and dry skin.

6. Evaluate need for additional equipment to facilitate safe handling of the patient when turning and repositioning. Order equipment with weight capacity sufficient to accommodate the weight and width of the patient.

7. Apply principles of pressure injury treatment to the buttocks pressure injury (see Chapter 8).

8. Apply principles of pressure injury prevention with attention to atypical pressure injury, such as deep tissue pressure injury (DTPI) within skin folds and MDRPI due to tubes and catheters (see Chapter 20).

REFERENCES

Anaya, D. A., & Dellinger, E. P. (2006). The obese surgical patient: a susceptible host for infection. *Surgical infections, 7*(5), 473–480.

Barnouti, H. N. (2016). The effect of different types of abdominal binders on intra-abdominal pressure. *Saudi Medical Journal, 37*(7), 815–816.

Barone, I., Giordano, C., Bonofiglio, D., et al. (2019). The weight of obesity in breast cancer progression and metastasis: Clinical and molecular perspectives. *Seminars in Cancer Biology, 19*(3), S1044–S1579.

Bednarska-Makaruk, M., Graban, A., Wiśniewska, A., et al. (2017). Association of adiponectin, leptin and resistin with inflammatory markers and obesity in dementia. *Biogerontology, 18*(4), 561–580.

Beitz, J. (2014). Providing quality skin and wound care for the bariatric patient: An overview of clinical challenges. *Ostomy/Wound Management, 60*(1), 12–21.

Bergstrom, N. (1987). The Braden Scale for predicting pressure sore risk. *Nursing Research, 36*(4), 205–210.

Black, J., Gray, M., Bliss, D., et al. (2011). MASD Part 2: Incontinence-associated dermatitis and intertriginous dermatitis. *Journal of Wound, Ostomy, and Continence Nursing, 38*(4), 359–370.

Blackett, A., Gallagher, S., Dugan, S., et al. (2011). Caring for persons with bariatric health care issues. *Journal of Wound, Ostomy, and Continence Nursing, 38*(2), 133–138.

Boynton, T., Kelly, L., & Perez, A. (2014). Implementing a mobility assessment tool for nurses. *American Nurse Today, 9*, 13–19.

Chopra, K., Tadisina, K. K., Brewer, M., et al. (2015). Massive localized lymphedema revisited: A quickly rising complication of the obesity epidemic. *Annals of Plastic Surgery, 74*(1), 126–132.

de Oliveira, C. M., Pavani, J., Krieger, J. E., et al. (2019). Body adiposity index in assessing the risk of type 2 diabetes mellitus development: The Baependi Heart Study. *Diabetology & Metabolic Syndrome, 11*(1), 76.

European Pressure Ulcer Advisory Panel, National Pressure Injury Advisory Panel, and Pan Pacific Pressure Injury Alliance [EPUAP/NPIAP/PPPIA]. (2019). In E. Haesler (Ed.), *Prevention and treatment of pressure ulcers/injuries: Clinical Practice Guideline*. The International Guideline.

Fife, C. (2014). Massive localized lymphedema, a disease unique to the morbidly obese: a case study. *Ostomy/Wound Management, 60*(1), 30–35.

Gallagher, S. M. (2013). *American Nurses Association implementation guide to safe patient handling and mobility interprofessional National standards*. Silver Spring, MD: ANA Nursing World.

Gallagher, S. M. (2015). *A practical guide to bariatric safe patient handling and mobility: Improving safety and quality for the patient of size*. Sarasota, FL: Visioning Publishers.

Gallagher, S. M. (2016). Skin care needs of the obese patient. In R. A. Bryant, & D. Nix (Eds.), *Acute and chronic wounds: Current management concepts* (5th ed.). St Louis, MO: Elsevier Inc.

Gallagher, S. M. (2020). Skin and wound care in the bariatric patient. In S. Baranowski, & E. Ayello (Eds.), *Wound care essentials* (5th ed.). Philadelphia, PA: Wolter Kluwer.

Gallagher, S. M., Alexandrowitz, M., Kumpar, D., et al. (2020). Bariatric space, technology and design: A round table. *Workplace Health & Safety, 68*(7), 313–319.

Garwood, C., & Mizuo, C. (2017). Managing lower extremity wounds in obese patients. *Podiatry Today, 30*(8), 28–35.

Graf, M., & Waters, H. (2018). *America's obesity crisis: The health and economic costs of excess weight.* Santa Monica, CA: Milken Institute.

Gray, M., Black, J. M., Baharestani, M. M., et al. (2011). Moisture-associated skin damage: Overview and pathophysiology. *Journal of Wound, Ostomy, and Continence Nursing, 38*(3), 233–241.

Guo, S., & de Pieto, L. (2010). Factors affecting wound healing. *Journal of Dental Research, 89*(3), 219–229.

Hales, C. M., Carroll, M. D., Fryar, C. D., et al. (2020). Prevalence of obesity and severe obesity among adults: United States, 2017–2018. *NCHS Data Brief*, no. 360. Hyattsville, MD: National Center for Health Statistics.

Hess, C. T. (2020). *Product guide to skin and wound care* (8th ed.). Philadelphia, PA: Wolters Kluwer.

Hou, L. G., Prabakaran, A., Rajan, R., et al. (2019). Concurrent bariatric surgery and surgical resection of massive localized lymphedema of the thigh. A case report. *Annals of Medicine and Surgery, 47*, 53–56.

Kaminsky, J., & Gadaleta, D. (2002). A study of discrimination within the medical community as viewed by obese patients. *Obesity Surgery, 12*(1), 14–18.

McNichol, L., Watts, C., Mackey, D., et al. (2015). Identifying the right surface for the right patient at the right time: generation and content validation of an algorithm for support surface selection. *Journal of Wound, Ostomy, and Continence Nursing, 42*(1), 19.

NIDDK. (2019). Adult overweight and obesity: Definitions and facts. Retrieved December 10, 2019 from https://www.niddk.nih.gov/health-information/weight-management/adult-overweight-obesity/definition-facts

Nuttall, F. Q. (2015). Body mass index: Obesity, BMI, and health: A critical review. *Nutrition Today, 50*(3), 117–128.

O'Lenick, A. (2009). Comparatively speaking: Humectants vs Emollients vs Occlusive Agents. Retrieved July 11, 2014 from http://www.cosmeticsandtoiletries.com

Pervez, H., Ramonaledi, S. (2017). Nurses' attitudes towards obese patients: A review of the literature. *Nursing Times, 113*(2), 42–45.

Pierpont, Y. N., Dinh, T. P., Salas, R. E., et al. (2014). Obesity and surgical wound healing: A current review. *ISRN Obesity, 2014*, 638936.

Puhl, R. M., Himmelstein, M. S., Gorin, A. A., et al. (2017). Missing the target: including perspectives of women with overweight and obesity to inform stigma-reduction strategies. *Obesity Science & Practice, 3*(1), 25–35.

Puhl, R. M., Himmelstein, M. S., Pearl, R. L., et al. (2019). Weight stigma among sexual minority adults: Findings from a matched sample of adults engaged in weight management. *Obesity, 27*(11), 1906–1915.

Puhl, R. M., Himmelstein, M. S., & Quinn, D. M. (2018). Internalizing weight stigma: Prevalence and sociodemographic considerations in US adults. *Obesity, 26*(1), 167–175.

Randall, S. B., Pories, W. J., Pearson, A., et al. (2009). Expanded Occupational Safety and Health Administration 300 log as metric for bariatric patient-handling staff injuries. *Surgery for Obesity and Related Diseases, 5*(4), 463–68.

Ryu, J., Loza, C. A., Xu, H., et al. (2019). Potential roles of adiponectin isoforms in human obesity with delayed wound healing. *Cells, 8*(10), 1134.

Sasaki, A., Nitta, H., Otsuka, K., et al. (2014). Bariatric surgery and non-alcoholic Fatty liver disease: Current and potential future treatments. *Frontiers in Endocrinology, 5*, 164.

Shipman, A., & Millington, G. (2011). Obesity and the skin. *British Journal of Dermatology, 165*(4), 743–750.

Temple, G., Gallagher, S., Doms, J., et al. (2017). Bariatric readiness: Clinical and economic implications. *Bariatric Times, 14*(8), 10–16.

VHA Center for Engineering & Occupational Safety and Health (CEOSH). (2015). Bariatric safe patient handling and mobility guidebook: A resource guide for care of persons of size. St. Louis, MO: CEOSH. Available at http://www.tnpatientsafety.com/pubfiles/Bariatric_Toolkit%20for%20THA.pdf

Wiggermann, N., Bunnell, S., Hildebrand, C., et al. (2017). Anthropometric data for medical equipment design: A sample of patients with high body mass. *Surgery for Obesity and Related Diseases, 13*(10), S152.

Wise, B. (2019). Obesity facts, figures and guidelines. State of West Virginia. Retrieved December 10, 2019 from https://www.wvdhhr.org/bph/oehp/obesity/credits.htm

World Health Organization (WHO). (2017). Obesity and overweight. Retrieved from www.who.int/mediacenter/fatsheets. Accessed December 10, 2019.

Zhang, H. Y., Liu, D., Tang, H., et al. (2016). The effect of different types of abdominal binders on intra-abdominal pressure. *Saudi Medical Journal, 37*(1), 66–72.

QUESTIONS

1. The wound care nurse is developing an evidence-based skin care protocol for patients with a BMI >50. Which intervention would the nurse include?

   A. Scrub the skin thoroughly to remove harmful bacteria from perspiration.
   B. Make full bathing with antibacterial soap daily requirement.
   C. Use liquid bar soap with alkaline pH and a gentle cloth to cleanse the skin.
   D. Lift all skin folds; pat dry or use a hair dryer on cool setting to assure complete drying.

2. A bariatric patient presents with a rash diagnosed as intertriginous dermatitis. In what area of the body is this condition usually found?

   A. Perineal area
   B. Under the breasts and pannus
   C. Arms and legs
   D. On the scalp

3. A wound care nurse is caring for a patient who is at risk for friction injury. Which of the following is a preventive measure for this type of skin alteration?

   A. Separating skin folds with wicking fabric
   B. Using powder under skin folds
   C. Using moisturizers in skin folds
   D. Avoiding the use of adhesive foam dressings

4. For which patient is the risk for massive localized lymphedema (MLL) greater than the general population?

   A. A patient with a body mass index (BMI) <30.
   B. A patient with a body mass index (BMI) between 30 and 40.
   C. A patient with a body mass index (BMI) >40.
   D. Body mass index is not an indicator for massive localized lymphedema.

5. The wound care nurse is choosing a bed for a bariatric patient who has orders for bed rest. What factor would the nurse consider when making the choice?
   A. The bed should be raised to accommodate turning and repositioning.
   B. A foam mattress is the product of choice for this patient.
   C. A mattress with a continuous lateral rotation feature is required.
   D. There should be extra space on each side of the patient to accommodate turning in bed.

6. Which area of the body is most prone to shear damage?
   A. Back of the head
   B. Buttocks
   C. Knees
   D. Shoulders

7. The wound care nurse applies an appropriately sized abdominal binder. What complication might this intervention prevent?
   A. Pressure injury
   B. Wound infection

C. Moisture-associated skin damage
D. Wound dehiscence

8. When choosing equipment for a bariatric patient, the major consideration is:
   A. Patient preference
   B. Patient and staff safety
   C. Cost-effectiveness
   D. Patient and staff compliance

9. What is a common reason that bariatric patients may put off needed medical attention?
   A. Lack of motivation
   B. Lack of financial means
   C. Fear of rejection, judgment, and insensitivities
   D. Lack of transportation

10. A wound care nurse is implementing a skin care program for a bariatric patient with intertriginous dermatitis. The nurse should pay particular attention to:
   A. Routine repositioning
   B. Maintaining a moist environment
   C. Reduction of calories
   D. Odor control

ANSWERS AND RATIONALES

1. **D. Rationale:** Care for the bariatric patient must include measures to assure adequate cleansing and drying of deep skin folds.

2. **B. Rationale:** Areas underneath the pannus or breasts generate and trap excess moisture, which can result in ITD.

3. **A. Rationale:** Skin folds represent high-risk areas for the bariatric patient. The skin must be cleansed and dried, and wicking fabrics should be routinely used to prevent maceration and friction.

4. **C. Rationale:** The precise cause of MLL is unknown, but the most distinguishing clinical characteristic of MLL is morbid obesity (BMI ≥ 40).

5. **D. Rationale:** Wound care nurses should consider placing patients who are unable to laterally reposition themselves on a wider bed. This will provide adequate space for the patient to turn unassisted in bed and/or for the staff to assist with safely turning the patient.

6. **B. Rationale:** Shear damage commonly involves the buttocks area but has been noted occasionally over the coccyx and ischial tuberosity areas.

7. **D. Rationale:** An abdominal binder may be used to offset the effects of increased adipose tissue that places tension on the suture line and may result in wound dehiscence.

8. **B. Rationale:** Appropriately sized equipment is important to protect the patient from further skin injury and prevent staff injury in handling and moving the patient.

9. **C. Rationale:** Patients often delay care as long as possible because of past experiences of prejudice and discrimination.

10. **D. Rationale:** Areas underneath the pannus or breasts generate and trap excess moisture, which can result in ITD. The skin becomes macerated, and odor may develop.

CHAPTER 16

SKIN AND WOUND CARE FOR THE SPINAL CORD-INJURED PATIENT

Laurie Rappl and David M. Brienza

OBJECTIVES

1. Describe factors that increase the risk for pressure injuries among SCI individuals and implications for prevention.
2. Describe factors that negatively impact healing among SCI individuals.
3. Select/recommend appropriate pressure redistribution devices for bed, chair, and heels.
4. Describe guidelines for comprehensive management of a pressure injury in an SCI individual.

TOPIC OUTLINE

INTRODUCTION

People who sustain spinal cord injuries (SCIs) develop pressure injuries (PIs) at an increased rate in the days and weeks immediately following their injury and throughout their lifetimes (Brienza & Karg, 2012; Brienza et al., 2018a; Chen et al., 2005). The effects of these wounds go beyond acute medical complications to negatively impact quality of life and physical, psychological, emotional, and financial status (Krishnan, 2014). In this chapter, we explore the incidence and prevalence of PIs in this population, SCI-specific risk factors, causes of impaired healing, recommendations for preventive care and support surface selection, treatment options, and strategies to reduce recurrence. Most prevention and treatment strategies developed for other high-risk populations also apply to the SCI population; however, there are considerations unique to the neurological deficits associated with SCI that make wheelchair seating and general repositioning critically important for people with SCIs.

> **KEY POINT**
>
> Individuals with SCIs are at high risk for PI development and for impaired healing throughout their lifespan.

DEMOGRAPHICS

Spinal Cord Injury Population

The number of people with SCIs is substantial. While statistics for incidence and prevalence of SCI have not been directly determined in the course of the past 30 years, based on extrapolations from several sources, the injury rate is presently estimated to be 54 per million of population, resulting in 17,730 new SCIs annually in the United States. The estimated number of people living with SCIs in the United States is presently estimated at 291,000. This information is an estimate based on extrapolations from several studies and is from the National Spinal Cord Injury Statistics Center (NSCISC) (www.spinalcord. uab.edu). Males presently account for 78% of SCIs. The average age at injury has risen from 28.7 years in the 1970s to 43 years currently. This trend appears to be at least partially attributable to the aging of the U.S. population. Vehicular crashes constitute the predominant cause (39.3%), particularly for teens and young adults; the incidence of SCIs caused by vehicular accidents declines in the middle-aged population and decreases rapidly with advancing age. Falls constitute the dominant cause of SCIs for those above 60 years. The incidence of SCIs attributable to violence and sports-related injuries also decreases with advancing age.

Incidence and Prevalence of Pressure Injuries

PIs are a common and costly complication of SCI (Hsieh et al., 2020). An analysis of the National Spinal Cord Injury Database (NSCID) indicates that PIs occur in 33.5% of cases (Cardenas et al., 2004; NSCISC, 2011). The second leading cause of death in individuals with SCIs is septicemia (88.6%), which is usually associated with urinary tract infections (UTIs), pneumonia, and/or presence of PIs (NSCISC, 2011). Of the estimated 249,000 to 363,000 individuals with SCIs in the United States, up to 85% will develop a PI at some point during their life (Mawson et al., 1988; National Spinal Cord Injury Statistical Center, 2018; Richardson & Meyer, 1981).

Differences in incidence and prevalence trends have been noted related to the time postinjury for people with SCIs. According to data collected from the Model System Knowledge Translation Center (MSKTC) SCI section, one third of individuals with SCIs will develop at least one PI during their initial acute or inpatient rehabilitation stay (www.msktc.org). In a prospective clinical trial, Brienza found 37.5% of participants developed a PI during inpatient acute and inpatient rehabilitation care (Brienza et al., 2018b). Chen and colleagues found the risk of developing a PI to be relatively constant during the first 10 years postinjury (prevalence rate of 11.5% to 14.3% for Stage 2 or higher PIs); however, rates tended to increase 15 years postinjury (prevalence rate of 21.0% for Stage 2 or higher PI) (Chen et al., 1999). In Italy, Pagliacci and colleagues found that 26.9% of 684 people in 32 rehabilitation centers had one or more PIs upon admission (Pagliacci et al., 2003).

> **KEY POINT**
>
> One third of SCI patients develop at least one PI during their initial acute or inpatient rehabilitation stay.

Associations between PI risk and neurological level of injury and impairment category have been reported (Brienza & Karg, 2012; Brienza et al., 2018b). Brienza found that participants with severity classification of ASIA A developed pressure injuries at higher rates than did those classified as ASIA B or C (Brienza et al., 2018b). Saladin and Krause (2009) also found an association between severity of injury and increased risk. Hitzig reported results from a self-reported incidence study where incidence rates for complete tetraplegia and paraplegia were 42.7% and 44.9%, respectively, compared to 20.4% and 20.7% for incomplete tetraplegia and paraplegia, respectively (Hitzig et al., 2008). The 2006 NSCID analysis revealed that those with complete tetraplegia were at highest risk for developing PIs (53.4%), followed by those with complete paraplegia (39%), incomplete tetraplegia (28.7%), and incomplete paraplegia (18.3%) (NSCISC, 2011).

 PRESSURE INJURY PREVENTION

The high risk of developing PIs for people with SCIs is most commonly attributed to decreased mobility and sensation and physiological changes after SCI, but literature suggests that factors such as diabetes and depression are also important (Smith et al., 2008).

RISK FACTORS

The complete list of potential factors is very long, with more than 200 individual factors mentioned in the literature (Byrne & Salzberg, 1996). Cardiac disease and renal disease have been shown to be associated with increased risk of developing PIs (Salzberg et al., 1998). Those with traumatic injury appear to be at higher risk compared to those with nontraumatic SCIs (McKinley et al., 2002). Males with SCIs have a higher risk than do females (Chen et al., 1999). A history of smoking, alcohol or drug use (Krause et al., 2001), medical comorbidities such as diabetes mellitus (Çakmak et al., 2009; Salzberg et al., 1996), impaired oxygenation or hypotension (Wilczweski et al., 2012), and infections such as pneumonia, UTIs, osteomyelitis, and other bacterial infections (Fogerty et al., 2008; Salzberg et al., 1998) have all been shown to increase risk. Dependence on mechanical ventilators (Manzano et al., 2010) and use of steroids (Wilczweski et al., 2012) are additional risk factors. As is the case for the broader populations of people at risk, moisture and/or urinary and fecal incontinence, hypo/hyperthermia, friction, and shear have been shown to increase risk, especially in acute and intensive care unit patients (Banks et al., 2012; Marin et al., 2013; Peerless et al., 1999; Reddy et al., 2006; Salzberg et al., 1996; Stover et al., 1995; Watts et al., 1998; Wilczweski et al., 2012). Compromised nutrition, low serum albumin levels, decreased mobility and sensation, and impaired cognitive function have been shown to increase risk for PI in people with SCIs (Çakmak et al., 2009; Salzberg et al., 1996).

The delivery of oxygen and other nutrients to damaged and at-risk tissue is critical to prevention of PIs and repair of damaged tissue. In SCI, the circulatory system below the level of injury is significantly and adversely affected. Significant changes include reduced blood pressure due to loss of supraspinal control of the vascular bed (Inskip et al., 2009; Teasell et al., 2000) and impaired vascular function (Thijssen et al., 2010). In addition to immobility and inactivity, individuals with SCIs are at risk for pressure damage due to impaired blood flow and oxygenation below the level of the injury.

Other physiological changes that affect PI risk relate directly to the mechanical characteristics of the soft tissues and how those mechanical characteristics affect loading and the concentrations of stress and strain in the soft tissues. These changes are particularly relevant to the potential of developing deep tissue pressure injury (DTPI). Direct damage of tissue leading to PIs occurs when tissue cells are deformed to a point in where the cell membrane diffusion characteristics are disrupted causing cell death (Gefen, 2008). Direct damage from cellular deformation occurs at a faster rate compared to

tissue damage due to ischemia (Linder-Ganz et al., 2008). Deformation damage occurs in a matter of minutes to an hour versus 2 hours plus for ischemic damage (Oomens et al., 2015). Pathoanatomical and pathophysiological changes occur in the buttocks, as tissues adapt to the chronic sitting and inactivity and to muscular denervation. These changes include bone shape adaptation (loss of cortical bone and flattening of the tips of the ischial tuberosities) as well as muscular atrophy, fat infiltration into muscles, and sometimes muscle spasms (Castro et al., 1999; de Bruin et al., 2000; Gefen, 2014; Giangregorio & McCartney, 2006; Rittweger et al., 2006). These alterations in the weight-bearing structures affect the loading and weight-bearing properties of the internal tissues. The mechanical loading properties around these anatomical interfaces have a critical effect on the risk of DTI. The biomechanical interaction is person specific and influenced by individual anatomy, tissue mechanics, and the body–support interfaces such as cushion and mattresses (Agam & Gefen, 2008; Brienza et al., 2018a; Gefen, 2008; Levy et al., 2014; Linder-Ganz & Gefen, 2009; Linder-Ganz et al., 2008; Portnoy et al., 2011).

KEY POINT

Muscle atrophy and changes in the shape of the bony prominences adversely affect normal weight bearing and tissue loading in the SCI individual.

Risk Assessment

The most commonly used and studied risk assessment scales (Braden Scale [Bergstrom et al., 1987], Norton Scale [Norton, 1996], and Waterlow Scale [Kottner et al., 2009]) have not been validated for people with SCIs and are likely not completely appropriate given the population's unique combination of risk factors. Mortenson and colleagues undertook a systematic review of risk assessment scales for use in an SCI population (Mortenson & Miller, 2007). Seven scales (Abruzzese, Braden, Gosnell, Norton, SCIPUS, SCIPUS-A, and Waterlow) were evaluated. Of the seven scales reviewed, concurrent validity was assessed for only three of the scales, the Norton Scale, Waterlow Scale, and Braden Scale. For reasons including reliability, validity, administrator burden, and respondent burden, each of these three scales was determined to have poor to adequate predictive validity for the SCI population.

Salzberg attempted to develop a risk assessment scale for people with SCIs, The Pressure Ulcer Assessment Scale for the Spinal Cord Injured (Salzberg Scale). This scale is composed of 15 risk factors: level of activity; degree of mobility; completeness of SCI; urinary incontinence; diagnosis of autonomic dysreflexia (AD); age; comorbidities such as those pertaining to cardiac, pulmonary, and renal pathophysiology; level of cognition;

diagnosis of diabetes; history of cigarette smoking; residency; and diagnosis of hypoalbuminemia and anemia (Byrne & Salzberg, 1996). This scale has not been validated and has yet to be recommended for use pending completion of further psychometric evaluation (Consortium for Spinal Cord Medicine Clinical Practice Guidelines, 2001; Krishnan et al., 2016). The Salzberg Scale was included in the evaluation undertaken by Mortenson, but despite its higher sensitivity (74.7%) and specificity (56.6%) scores, it could not be deemed the best assessment tool since it has not been validated. Mortenson recommended the use of either the Braden Scale or Waterlow Scale, despite their apparent lack of content validity for the SCI population. He based this recommendation on the similar performance and closeness to the Salzberg Scale scoring associated with these tools and on their performance on psychometric evaluation. The Spinal Cord Injury Pressure Ulcer Scale (SCIPUS) is another risk assessment scale specific to the SCI population. SCIPUS is a 15-item scale specifically designed to assess the risk of developing a PI in persons with SCI. The majority of items are scored dichotomously as either present or absent (0/1 or 0/2). Four items have three response options that have weighted scores (1/1/4 or 0/1/3). A summary score is calculated by adding the scores of individual items. Scoring ranges from 0 (best prognosis) to 25 (worst prognosis) with a high-risk cutoff score at ≥6 (Higgins et al., 2019).

Preventive Measures

Because the causes of PIs include biological, behavioral, and social factors, prevention and patient education must address all of these issues. The person with an SCI has to become aware of body systems that normally require no thought at all. The range of new things the person must learn to do and monitor can be overwhelming, especially in the acute phases of SCI. Emotional support is a critical aspect of management and must extend well beyond the acute phase. Support involves much more than verbal instruction and pointing out negative behaviors; encouragement, assistance with problem solving, and advocacy are essential strategies in helping the patient to successfully incorporate the new lifestyle and behaviors.

Prevention has to become a lifestyle, incorporating not only the interventions and behaviors discussed below but, more broadly, an awareness of the body and self-respect; a belief that personal health is important and can be achieved; adjustment of social environments; acquiring needed attendant care, equipment, and transportation; readiness for change; and self-efficacy. Many team members play a role in assisting the person with an SCI to become self-sufficient in PI prevention. Medicine, nursing, and physical and occupational therapy are givens, as well as certified durable medical equipment and seating specialists. Social workers, psychologists, and nutritionists may be required as well. Skill in the areas of

counseling, problem solving, and motivational interviewing may be helpful.

> ### KEY POINT
> Effective PI prevention requires multiple lifestyle adaptations and a 24 hours a day/7 days a week commitment that is very difficult to maintain long term; thus, multidisciplinary patient-focused care and counseling is essential.

There are a number of resources available to both clinicians and patients in the area of PI prevention. The Paralyzed Veterans of America (PVA) and the Consortium for Spinal Cord Medicine have published a very complete Clinical Practice Guideline "Pressure Ulcer Prevention and Treatment Following Spinal Cord Injury." The Consortium began an update of this extensive monograph in 2014. All monographs written or sponsored by the PVA are available free of charge from the PVA (Consortium for Spinal Cord Medicine Clinical Practice Guidelines, 2001).

The Spinal Cord Injury Rehabilitation Evidence project (www.scireproject.com) is a collaborative effort involving Canadian researchers, clinicians, scientists and consumers, health centers, and universities. The project involves review and rating of articles on a wide variety of topics related to SCI, including PI prevention and treatment. In addition, the Model Systems Knowledge Translation Center (https://msktc.org/sci/sci-resources) has an extensive list of very helpful brochures, articles, and "how to" videos designed to teach patients self-care, specifically in regard to prevention of PIs (MSKTC, 2020) **(Table 16-1)**. Many commonly recommended preventive interventions, especially those involving patient behaviors, have only poor-to-moderate quality of evidence supporting their usefulness in preventing PIs. Attempts to study behavioral and educational interventions in preventing pressure injuries have met with considerable methodological problems with recruitment, intervention consistency, and participation and have shown no efficacy in preventing pressure injuries in persons with SCI (Cogan et al., 2017). At this time, prevention must be guided by expert opinion (Guihan & Bombardier, 2012). Despite the lack of objective evidence, behavioral strategies are consistently regarded as essential to good health and positive outcomes; therefore, prevention practices should continue to be taught, reinforced, and supported.

Patient education must fit the patient's learning style and be tailored to the unique needs and constraints of that patient. Individualizing the material and the recommended interventions has been shown to improve effectiveness (Vaishampayan et al., 2011).

Activity/Mobility/Transfers

This aspect of prevention includes all types of activity, from self-repositioning in bed to quality of transfers to general mobility. People should be encouraged to move as often

TABLE 16-1 FACTSHEETS FOR SPINAL CORD INJURY EDUCATION FROM MODEL SYSTEMS KNOWLEDGE TRANSLATION CENTER (MSKTC)

Adaptive Sports and Recreation

Adjusting to Life after Spinal Cord Injury

Aging and SCI

Autonomic Dysreflexia

Bladder Management Options Following Spinal Cord Injury

Bowel Function after Spinal Cord Injury

Depression and Spinal Cord Injury

Driving after Spinal Cord Injury

Employment after Spinal Cord Injury

Exercise after Spinal Cord Injury

Maintenance Guide for Users of Manual and Power Wheelchairs

Pain after Spinal Cord Injury

Pregnancy and Women with Spinal Cord Injury

Respiratory Health and Spinal Cord Injury

Safe Transfer Technique

Sexuality and Sexual Functioning after Spinal Cord Injury

Skin Care and Pressure Sores (6-Part Series)

Spasticity and Spinal Cord Injury

Spinal Cord Injury and Gait Training

Surgical Alternatives for Bladder Management Following Spinal Cord Injury

The Wheelchair Series: What the SCI Consumer Needs to Know (3-Part Series)

Understanding Spinal Cord Injury—Part 1: The Body before and after Injury

Understanding Spinal Cord Injury—Part 2: Recovery and Rehabilitation

Urinary Tract Infection and Spinal Cord Injury

From https://msktc.org/sci/factsheets

as possible and should be provided the means to be as independent in repositioning as possible. This may entail use of an overhead trapeze or side rail bars when in bed, a firmer mattress, wheelchair modifications, and cushion choices. The more independent and mobile a person is, the more likely they are to effectively and routinely off-load bony prominences. In addition, mobility and activity improve overall health, increasing resistance to PIs.

Transfers are the first skill learned after an SCI and are a major source of tissue trauma due to inconsistencies in technique and challenging surfaces and situations. All individuals need to be taught and encouraged to do "clean" transfers (i.e., transfers that avoid sliding or bumping against objects such as wheels, skirt guards, toilet seats, or shower bench edges). Gentle landings on the intended surface are encouraged because initial contact with the seat puts very high tissue loads on the skin and at the edges of any scars, as opposed to the slow and constant rate at which fat loads (Levy et al., 2013). Sliding boards can be particularly dangerous to the skin and tissue, because sliding of the body against the hard transfer board can cause shearing. DeJong et al. (2014) studied the factors associated with risk of PI

development while in acute rehabilitation, and one of the two variables most predictive of PI development was the need for at least moderate assistance to perform a transfer on admission. Gaining as much independence as possible is a key goal in rehabilitation. If the person is unable to self-transfer, the patient needs to know how to properly educate an assistant or attendant to transfer him or her safely.

KEY POINT

Transfers are a major source of tissue trauma; individuals must be assisted and taught to do "clean" transfers.

Off-Loading Bony Prominences

Excessive weight on bony prominences is a prime cause of PIs. The person without protective sensation must pay attention to bony prominences that are sustaining pressure when in bed, in a wheelchair, on a sliding board, or in a standing frame. When in bed, the person needs to be alert to the length of time in one position and needs to know how and be able to shift their weight to alternate positions. Frequent position changes are recommended, and off-loading the posterior surface of the body is advised if at all possible; sleeping in the prone position is optimal, and a variety of side-lying positions is recommended for those who are unable to sleep in the prone position. Physical or occupational therapy may be able to assist with ideas for positioning and assistive devices such as wedges and molded pillows that can help maintain off-loaded positions. This should be considered no matter what support surface is being used; no support surface can protect the tissue as effectively as positioning off the bony prominence. The National Pressure Injury Advisory Panel (2018) has developed standards and definitions for support surfaces available on their Web site (https://npiap.org).

Weight Shifts

Weight shifts in the sitting position involve changing body posture to significantly reduce pressure over the ischial/sacral area. Most rehabilitation programs teach a complete off-loading, which involves lifting the body off the seat cushion using the armrests or wheels for leverage ("push-up"). Off-loading is meant to restore blood flow to areas that are ischemic due to closure of the capillaries, with the goal of returning the transcutaneous partial pressure of oxygen ($TcPO_2$) to unloaded levels.

The mean duration of a weight shift required to return $TcPO_2$ and full recovery of tissue perfusion to unloaded levels following upright sitting is approximately 2 minutes (Bader, 1990; Coggrave & Rose, 2003). The duration of off-weighting required to restore transcutaneous oxygen levels to normal is much longer than the time frame commonly recommended for push-ups; most clinicians and guidelines recommend 30- to 60-second push-ups every 15 to 30 minutes. In addition, push-ups are difficult to accomplish and difficult to maintain for even one full minute for most individuals, let alone at the recommended frequencies. Guihan & Bombardier (2012) found that only about 50% of people with SCI perform regular pressure relief maneuvers. Alternative means of reducing pressures such as forward leaning with the elbows or chest on the knees, side leaning with the shoulder and elbow over the wheel or further, and tilting the seat-and-back unit to >65 degrees for 1 minute have been shown to result in major reductions in ischial interface pressures and significant increases in buttock blood flow and $TcPO_2$ (Coggrave & Rose, 2003; Makhsous et al., 2007; Sonenblum & Sprigle, 2011; Sprigle & Sonenblum, 2011). The specific frequency of weight shifts required to reduce PI incidence has not been determined. Clinically, excessive pressure on any part of the body must be relieved periodically to restore normal hemodynamic and $TcPO_2$ levels. Alternative approaches to encouraging routine behaviors to prevent pressure injuries including off-loading must be explored in research and with the individual (Sprigle et al., 2019). Any relief of pressure is beneficial.

KEY POINT

Current evidence suggests that the commonly recommended "wheelchair push-ups" must be maintained for 2 minutes to effectively restore perfusion—which may not be possible. Alternative approaches to off-loading must be explored with the individual.

Substance Abuse Avoidance

Tobacco, street drugs, and excessive alcohol are known to cause tissue changes that increase susceptibility to tissue breakdown and to inhibition of wound healing. In addition, substance abuse may reflect a lifestyle that is not conducive to good health or social adaptation. Substance abuse has a negative effect on psychosocial adaptation to disability and further compromises the ability to carry out PI prevention measures. Therefore, the clinician should provide education and counseling regarding smoking cessation, drug avoidance, and moderation in alcohol use.

Skin Checks

Most rehabilitation programs recommend visual examination at least once daily to include all bony prominences, especially the sitting surfaces of the sacrum, coccyx, ischium, and posterior thighs. Any changes in skin integrity or color may be noted by a caregiver or attendant or with the use of a mirror or cell phone camera. Reddened areas that do not return to color within a minimum of 1 hour require immediate response and

intervention. Differentiate blanchable versus nonblanchable erythema using either finger pressure or transparent disk method and evaluate the extent of the erythema. It is not always possible to identify erythema on darkly pigmented skin (EPUAP/NPIAP/PPPIA, 2019).

Visual inspection alone is not enough. Most PIs begin in the subdermal tissues because these tissues are more susceptible than the skin to ischemic damage (EPUAP/NPIAP/PPPIA, 2019). Patients and caregivers often report a PI appeared suddenly with no visible warning; the damage was taking place in the deep tissues and produced no visible changes in the skin, so the problem was undetected and unaddressed. This is an example of the development of deep tissue PIs or DTPIs discussed in Chapter 20. It is important for the SCI individual (and/or caregiver) to use palpation as well as visual inspection. They need to become familiar with the normal texture of their tissue; they can then be taught to gently pinch the skin and tissues to detect any changes in integrity (much like the premise of breast self-examinations, where the woman is taught to palpate the tissues on a routine basis and to assess for any changes over time). Changes in tissue consistency may be noted as areas of firmness or softness in comparison to the surrounding tissue. The area may also feel warmer to touch as compared to the contralateral side or to the upper leg. Early identification of changes in skin and tissue color, temperature, and consistency enable implementation of an appropriate prevention and treatment plan (EPUAP/NPIAP/PPPIA, 2019).

KEY POINT

A key component of care and education is careful skin inspection at least daily with immediate response to changes in skin and tissue color, temperature, and consistency.

Hygiene

Daily bathing is not necessary, nor always feasible due to the possible need for attendant care to accomplish. The best approach to cleansing is to use pH-balanced no-rinse cleansers; baby wipes can be used for perineal cleansing. Strong alkaline soaps and cleansers should not be used on a regular basis because they strip the skin of the protective acid mantle formed by the normal skin secretions of sweat and sebum. The normal skin pH is 4 to 5.5, and this normal acidity protects against bacterial or fungal overgrowth and contributes to skin health.

Management of Bowel and Bladder Incontinence

Bowel incontinence and bladder incontinence are commonly reported in the SCI population, which supports the need for routine assessment and management (Park et al., 2017). Bladder incontinence can keep the skin in the vulnerable ischial area constantly wet, which makes it more susceptible to breakdown (Gray & Giuliano, 2018). Neurogenic bladder can be managed in a variety of ways. Fecal contamination of the skin further increases the risk of skin breakdown, due to the enzymes and bacteria in the stool. Bowel and bladder incontinence is anecdotally regarded as more debilitating than the inability to walk. Establishment of an effective bladder and bowel management program is as essential to skin health as it is to psychosocial adaptation. For additional resources see https://msktc.org/sci/factsheets/Bowel_Function and https://msktc.org/sci/factsheets/bladderhealth.

Nutrition

Proper nutrition levels and healthy eating patterns are essential for optimum health. The constant state of inflammation present in chronic SCI has been linked to reduced albumin and hematocrit levels. Salzberg et al. (1998) identified two nutritional parameters as indicators of increased risk for breakdown: albumin <3.4 or total protein < 6.4 and hematocrit <36% or hemoglobin < 12.0. These data further underscore the importance of a healthy diet and normal weight for the SCI person. An added challenge to maintenance of normal weight is the fact that many people with SCI live a relatively sedentary lifestyle; the resulting tendency to weight gain is further compounded by poor eating habits. Farkas et al. (2019) conducted a systematic review and meta-analysis to investigate nutritional status in chronic SCI and compare macronutrient and micronutrient intake to the recommended values by the US Department of Agriculture (USDA) 2015–2020 Dietary Guidelines for Americans (2015).

Individuals with SCI are at risk for multiple nutritional deficiencies. The causes are often multifactorial and result in an elevated risk of obesity and obesity-related diseases. Results from this review provide weighted averages for variables associated with the nutritional status of individuals with chronic SCI. They also demonstrate that the majority of the available literature focuses solely on the role of total energy intake. Protein intake in individuals with SCI exceeds current USDA guidelines. Regardless of age, individuals with SCI also consume a significantly greater quantity of carbohydrates than what is recommended values. Fat intake remains within the recommended daily allowance for men with chronic SCI. Females over 31 years of age may be consuming a greater quantity, which contrasts previous literature suggesting that individuals with chronic SCI consume an amount of fat that approaches or exceeds that recommended by the USDA guidelines. Fiber intake in this population has been demonstrated as low. This review demonstrates deficiencies in vitamins A, B5, B7, B9, D, and E, and the minerals potassium and calcium (Farkas et al., 2019). In addition, there is a natural increase in visceral adipose tissue after the SCI. Ongoing attention to a nutritious diet and to weight control is another factor that

must be consciously addressed by the SCI person. See Chapter 7 for additional information on nutrition.

Management of Systemic Comorbidities

As with the general population, many persons with SCI are dealing with multiple medical comorbidities including diabetes, pulmonary disease, cardiac disease, and renal failure, and any comorbidities add to the constant demands related to the SCI. The natural increase in visceral adipose tissue noted above increases the SCI individual's susceptibility to development of all of these comorbidities. Those with SCI are at 1.4- and 2-fold higher risk of mortality from diabetes and congestive heart failure, respectively, than are able-bodied persons (Edwards et al., 2008). Any coexisting condition affects overall health and can increase the risk for PI development.

With advances in general medical practices, there has been an increase in longevity with SCI and increased risk for developing chronically acquired diseases. Several risk factors for all-cause cardiovascular disease (CVD) and comorbid endocrine disorders have become more widely identified, including component disorders of central obesity, significant dyslipidemia, hypertension (depending on the extent and level of neurological injury), and insulin resistance. The clustering of these risks—described as the cardiometabolic syndrome (CMS)—is also widely reported after SCI and is thought to worsen the CVD risk prognosis. CVD is a leading cause of mortality in chronic SCI (Bigford & Nash, 2017).

KEY POINT

Effective management of all comorbid conditions is an important component of a comprehensive PI prevention strategy.

Autonomic Dysreflexia

AD is a debilitating disorder producing episodes of extreme hypertension in patients with high-level SCI. Factors leading to AD include loss of vasomotor baroreflex control to regions below injury level, changes in spinal circuitry, and peripheral changes. For example, a hyperreflexic detrusor often evolves, thermoregulation is impaired, and cardiovascular problems such as AD can also develop in patients with injuries in the high thoracic or cervical spinal segments.

Exaggerated sympathetic activity causes increased vasoconstriction below the injury, resulting in dangerous high blood pressure, which leads to headaches, bradycardia, and cold extremities. Additional symptoms occur due to compensatory baroreflex-mediated vasodilation in blood vessels above the injury level, inducing flushing and sweating (Laird et al., 2008). While the most common triggers are overdistension of the bowel or bladder, other noxious stimuli including skin lacerations, ingrown toenails, PIs, tight clothing, and certain medical procedures such as bladder catheterization and cystometry are also reported to cause AD. During an episode of AD, arterial blood pressure can reach devastating levels, with systolic values as high as 325 mm Hg, exemplifying that AD is a hypertensive crisis that requires immediate medical attention. Severe cases that do not receive rapid and appropriate treatment can have serious consequences such as hypertensive encephalopathy, stroke, cardiac arrest, seizure, and even death (Eldahan & Rabchevsky, 2018). (https://msktc.org/sci/factsheets/autonomic_dysreflexia).

KEY POINT

Skin damage can trigger AD in the individual with an SCI; this is a medical emergency.

Impaired cognitive function will affect the person's ability to carry out all of the prevention strategies required. While most individuals with SCI have normal cognition, the clinician must always be alert to indicators of cognitive impairment and, if noted, should conduct a cognitive assessment. For the SCI person who does have cognitive impairment, it is essential to provide instruction and guidance regarding prevention strategies in a way that the person can understand, internalize, and act upon.

Spasticity Management
Spasticity causes uncontrollable movements of the body and is a common complication of SCI. The movement can be as limited as a bouncing leg that rubs against part of the wheelchair or as extensive as full body extension or flexion. Spasticity can prevent maintenance of an upright posture, put the limbs at risk for injury, or be so difficult to manage that the person is not able to focus any attention on other issues, such as PI prevention (McKinley et al., 1999). The care team must work together with the person to ensure effective management of spasticity. (https://msktc.org/sci/factsheets/Spasticity)

Maintenance of Durable Medical Equipment
Prescribed equipment must be maintained in order to perform as intended. Hogaboom et al. (2018) evaluated the relation between wheelchair breakdowns, their immediate consequences, and secondary health complications after SCI. They surveyed 610 participants who were fulltime wheelchair users regarding incidence of self-reported wheelchair breakdowns within the past 6 months that did or did not result in immediate consequences (i.e., injury, being stranded, missing a medical appointment, or an inability to attend school/work). They found that participants who reported 1 or more breakdowns with immediate consequence scored worse on self-perceived health status scale, pain severity scale,

rehospitalizations, and self-reported PI development within the past 12 months. They found that wheelchair breakdowns that resulted in injury, being stranded, missing medical appointments, and/or an inability to attend work/school appear to have far-reaching impacts on health and secondary injury. Preventing wheelchair breakdowns, through either better maintenance or manufacturing, may be a means of decreasing secondary disability (Hogaboom et al., 2018).

There must be personal responsibility and accountability for the proper functioning of all durable medical equipment. A malfunctioning or worn-out seat cushion can be dangerous not just because it has lost its protective properties but also because the user believes they are protected because "I'm sitting on my cushion." The seat cushion and the wheelchair work as a unit to protect the patient and provide mobility. The importance of a properly selected and maintained wheelchair and seat cushion is reflected by the fact that 42% of all PIs occur over the ischial tuberosities and sacrum (Wannapakhe et al., 2015).

Assistive technology is the term given to durable medical equipment that helps provide accommodation to a disability, including wheelchairs, seat cushions, environmental controls, and a variety of other devices. There are a large number and variety of devices available, and effective use requires a clear understanding of the indications, contraindications, and utilization guidelines for each. There are certified specialists (assistive technology professionals [ATP]) who possess the in-depth knowledge to effectively match products and individuals. It is beneficial for any person with an SCI to be seen by an ATP in order to be evaluated and fitted for the appropriate equipment. ATPs can be found through the search feature on the Web site (www.resna.org).

Most centers that specialize in SCI have seating clinics that provide a comprehensive evaluation, including range of motion, mobility, pressure mapping, equipment trials, education in maintenance and usage, repairs, equipment prescription, options, and reimbursement. These clinics have been shown to reduce the incidence of PIs and readmission rates of persons with recurrent PIs (Kennedy et al., 2003; Stobl, 2013).

Seat cushions are a primary intervention for both prevention and treatment of sitting-related PIs. The primary mechanism of action is redistribution of *pressure* off the prominent ischial tuberosities, with the goal of reducing tissue interface pressures, preventing harmful deformation, and thereby minimizing tissue damage. Cushions can also help to reduce deformation inducing *shearing forces*, the opposing forces that cause the soft tissue layers to slide against one another when the skin is pulled in one direction and the bone and muscle pulls in the opposite direction. Shaped cushions can help to maintain an upright sitting *position* to reduce sliding that can cause shearing. The upright position improves function and movement and keeps the body structurally aligned. Some cushions address *microclimate* (heat and moisture), improving skin health and decreasing risk for skin injury.

In addition to these therapeutic considerations, there are practical issues that should be considered. For example, flatter cushions facilitate dressing because pants can be pulled up and down easily. Flatter cushions are also easier to transfer onto as they do not have higher outer edges that require a bigger lift. Cushions should be easy to keep clean as incontinence is a comorbidity for many wheelchair users. Ease of maintenance must be considered because if the cushion is not maintained, it can lose its protective properties and put the user at risk.

KEY POINT

A correctly sized wheelchair and an optimal pressure redistribution cushion are critical components of an effective PI prevention program; the individual with an SCI should be referred to a seating clinic or ATP.

Tissue deformation occurs when the soft tissues are compressed by the bony prominences internally and a hard or firm surface externally. The deformation causes internal stresses, compression of capillaries, prevention of blood and lymph flow and waste removal, and cellular damage or death. Managing this deformation is key to maintaining healthy tissue (Sonenblum et al., 2018). Two common approaches to managing body weight include envelopment and off-loading. With an enveloping design, the buttocks immerse into the wheelchair cushion and the cushion envelops the tissue to increase contact area and minimize pressure gradients. An off-loading cushion will redistribute body mass away from particular bony prominences, ideally to tissue better suited to withstand the load. One metric of cushion performance that can be used across designs of wheelchair cushions is shape compliance. Shape compliance describes the ability of a cushion to support the buttocks with minimal buttocks deformation.

The results from the study demonstrate that in every sitting condition there is some deformation present at the ischium, but that the regions of greatest deformation tend to vary. Paying attention to those regions is important. Significant loading of the sacrum and coccyx occurs, even in upright sitting (Sonenblum et al., 2018).

Standards have been developed to measure the ability of a cushion to immerse and conform to the bony prominences to protect the ischial tuberosities. While these standards are not based on clinical outcomes in regard to PI prevention, they are an objective way to compare cushions against a standard cushion and in relation to each other. These standards have been used

to group cushions into codes for Medicare coverage. The groups of codes are (1) general use, (2) skin protection, (3) positioning, (4) skin protection and positioning, (5) skin protection adjustable, (6) skin protection and positioning adjustable, and (7) custom. In comparing the criteria, each subsequent group (from 1 to 6) has increasingly difficult standards to meet and in general is increasingly complex in design. Some of the criteria include depth when loaded using a standard loading device, deflection when overloaded, and peak interface pressures at the ischial tuberosities compared to a standard reference cushion. The positioning cushions are required to have structural features such as supports around the medial and lateral thighs or a ridge in front of the ischial tuberosities to prevent forward migration (Palmetto—Medicare Pricing, Data Analysis and Coding [PDAC], 2019).

Interface pressures are used to compare devices and are sometimes used in clinical practice to evaluate seat cushion efficacy for specific patients. To measure interface pressures, a mat that contains hundreds of pressure sensors is placed between the person and the seat cushion and connected to a computer screen. This provides a visual display of interface pressures across the entire seating surface. (Pressure distribution can be displayed in numbers or colors, with either approach clearly indicating points of higher pressure.) These data can then be used to modify the equipment as needed and/or to select the best cushion for a particular patient.

Shearing may be as destructive to tissues as pressure since deformation occurs more readily as a result of shear forces (see Chapters 17 and 20). Shearing occurs when tissues move in horizontal planes or across each other and across bony prominences, in contrast to interface or direct pressures, which are exerted perpendicularly onto the soft tissue and bony prominence. As tissues are moved horizontally across each other, they exert deforming and tearing forces on each other and between each other. Shearing is thought to be the causative factor for the undermining that is typical of PIs on those with SCI. Support surfaces that move with body movement may reduce some shearing by absorbing the horizontal movement.

Shearing also occurs internally as a result of normal pressure even in the absence of external horizontal forces due to friction at the interface and resistance between tissue components. Frictional force is the resistance to motion in a parallel direction relative to the common boundary of the skin and contacting surface. The magnitude of the frictional force is dependent on the coefficient of friction between the two surfaces. Moisture is an important factor relative to shearing because the coefficient of friction between skin and most textiles increases as moisture levels increase. Cushions and cushion covers that limit the buildup of moisture will reduce the risks related to friction (Berke, 2019).

Types of Cushions

There is a large variety of commercially available cushion designs that are aimed at reducing the risk for PIs, but no objective, standard and quantitative criteria exist yet, to determine which sitting solution is adequate for protecting the tissues of individuals, particularly the subcutaneous tissues, from a PI. Cushion range from simple foam pads to air- or gel-filled bladders to powered alternating pressure seat cushions (Peko Cohen & Gefen, 2017). General descriptors for each type of cushion are as follows.

Foam

Foam is made in a chemical process that can be manipulated to produce various levels of density, stiffness, conformability, and memory. Foams are measured by the indentation load deflection (ILD), the ability of the foam to permit a disc of standard weight to indent the mattress by 25% or 65% of its standard thickness. Foams are usually layered to provide support in the lower levels and softness for immersion in the upper levels. Foams can be shaped, are lightweight, and facilitate transfers and dressing. However, the time frame for which they are effective (performance life) may be shorter, and their ability to effectively envelop (conform to) the body may be limited.

Air

There are simple air cushions made of a single chamber or more complex ones made with multiple cells that offer better immersion and envelopment (**Fig. 16-1**). Air cushions without flow restrictions provide less stability when the person is moving or leaning. They may require maintenance to prevent holes and to detect slow leaks. They can also make transfers and dressing more difficult due to instability.

Gel

No standards have been developed to help the ATP or consumer compare gels to each other or to predetermine what kind of gel is being used. Gels depend on flowability to conform to the body, a property called viscosity. Low-viscosity gels are more fluid and flow easily but may bottom out unless they are contained in a thick-walled bladder, which limits the flow but increases the interface pressure. Moderate-viscosity gels have a slower flow rate and are more conformable; they are more appropriate for use in the SCI population (**Fig. 16-2**). High-viscosity gels have no flow properties at all and have little to offer in terms of immersion and envelopment. They are not used for SCI individuals as full-time wheelchair cushions but may be used for short-term use such as in cars or on shower benches. Gel cushions can be heavy and can retain heat and moisture.

Active

Active cushions that automatically change pressures at regular intervals to redistribute pressure are available. A small study showed that one of these cushions relieved pressure enough to provide complete recovery of tissue perfusion and demonstrated slower vascular recovery among individuals with SCI as opposed to controls (Makhsous et al., 2007). Wu and Bogie (2014) demonstrated the benefits of an alternating pressure air cushion including increased skin blood flow, increased transcutaneous oxygen, and lower mean interface pressure.

KEY POINT

The field of durable medical equipment is increasingly complex; an assistive technology provider (ATP) can provide invaluable guidance in selection of the best equipment for a specific individual.

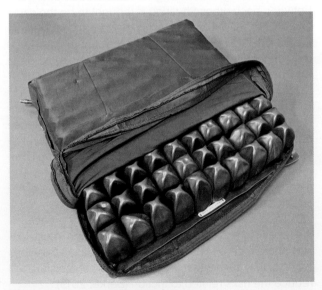

FIGURE 16-1. Segmented Air Cell Cushion.

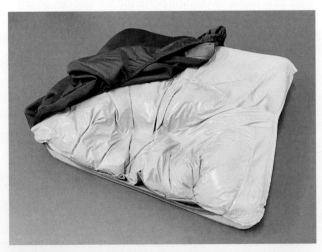

FIGURE 16-2. Moderate-Viscosity Gel Cushion (also Referred to as Viscous Fluid-Filled Cushion).

Telehealth

Telehealth may be a valuable modality for monitoring patients' skin, providing encouragement and instruction, and treating and preventing PIs. Many people live long distances from a center or clinician specializing in SCI care, and transportation difficulties or the need to remain off-weighted in bed prevent timely assessment and treatment. Consultation using cell phone cameras, tablets, Skype, and commercially available cameras and computers are helping to connect clinicians and patients (Mathewson et al., 1999). Houlihan and colleagues (2017) evaluated the impact of "My Care My Call" (MCMC), a peer-led, telephone-based health self-management intervention in adults with chronic SCI. Participants averaged 12 calls over 6 months, each lasting an average of 21.8 minutes. They found that the program had a positive impact on self-management to prevent secondary conditions in adults with SCI (Houlihan et al., 2017).

Measures to Reduce Recurrence

Jones and colleagues (2003) studied the effects of various approaches to positive reinforcement for prevention of recurrent ulcers. They found that the addition of monetary rewards for ulcer prevention or improvement led to positive results. They concluded that PI recurrence may be linked to insufficient positive consequences for prevention as well as to insufficient negative consequences (pain) for failure to adhere to prevention interventions. Individuals with SCIs remain at high risk of incurring medically serious (stage 3 or stage 4) PIs even after receiving education and training in prevention techniques (e.g., pressure redistribution practices, skin checks, incontinence management) during rehabilitation (Carlson et al., 2019).

Bates-Jensen and colleagues (2009) analyzed data from a cohort of 24 patients with SCIs and pressure ulcers to describe the characteristics associated with recurrent pressure ulcers. The patients had been part of larger prospective RCT. The 24 patients had 29 recurrent pressure ulcers. Two thirds of the patients (*n* = 16/67%) with recurrent ulcers had their pressure ulcer initially treated with flap surgery, and 10 (63%) of those patients had recurrent ulcers at the same site where surgery was performed. The median time to recurrence was 4 months. The investigators reported the majority of all recurrent pressure ulcers were located on the ischium (*n* – 17/59%) with 7 (24%) ulcers recurring at the sacrum. Of the ulcers that recurred at the same anatomic site, 11 (73%) were on the ischium (WOCN, 2016).

Di Prinzio and colleagues (2019) conducted a systematic review to identify the studies that detected risk factors for the development and recurrence of pressure injuries in patients with SCIs. Twenty-five articles met the eligibility criteria and were included for analysis. A total of 30 risk factors were identified: 4 were demographic factors, 8 were related to the injury, 5 belonged to medical comorbidities, 3 to nutritional factors, 9 were psychological, cognitive, contextual and social factors,

and 1 was related to support surface. However, 57% of the risk factors were classified as nonmodifiable. However, the authors were not able to synthesize the evidence due to the heterogeneity of the articles included in this review (Di Prinzio et al., 2019).

Community Support for Prevention

Prevention must become a lifestyle incorporating the necessary interventions and behaviors. Incorporating body awareness, self-respect, a belief in success, and self-efficacy and readiness to change are less tangible but just as important. Social support may be needed to acquire needed attendant care, equipment and transportation, and reasonable living accommodations. Community- and home-based programs support persons with SCI to make the physical, social, and psychological adjustments required for a prevention lifestyle. Examples include regular phone support, telehealth, supportive social networks, and psychological assistance. The complexity of these programs and difficulties in implementation have hampered clear measurement of outcomes. Additional information on resources is available at https:// unitedspinal.org/disability-publications.

 INCREASED RISK FOR IMPAIRED HEALING

The high recurrence rates and slow rate of healing for PIs in SCI patients have led many to question whether there are additional physiological factors in addition to lack of protective sensation, possible patient behaviors that compromise healing, and the reduced tensile strength of scar tissue. Rappl (2008) outlined physiologic factors that impact wound healing. See **Table 16-2**.

TABLE 16-2 PHYSIOLOGICAL CHANGES IN SCI LEADING TO IMPAIRED HEALING
Vascular Changes
• Abnormal vascular response
• Reduced density of adrenergic receptors
• Decreased blood flow
• Decreased blood pressure
• Decreased blood supply
• Decreased rate of reperfusion after unweighting
Reduced TcPO$_2$ levels five times lower than levels in innervated tissues
Decreased collagen and collagen precursors
• Increased collagen catabolism
• Increase in urinary excretion of glycosaminoglycans (GAGs)
• Decreased concentration of amino acids
• Decrease in levels of enzymes involved in biosynthesis
Reduced quality of collagen
• Decrease in proportion of type I to type III collagen
Impaired fibroblast activity
• Decreased fibronectin, a glycoprotein
Constant inflammatory state

Source: Rappl, L. M. (2008). Physiological changes in tissues denervated by spinal cord injury tissues and possible effects on wound healing. *International Wound Journal, 5*(3), 435–444.

VASCULAR CHANGES

SCI interrupts the spinal vasomotor pathway, specifically the input from sympathetic system that arises in the thoracic and lumbar spine. The counterbalancing parasympathetic nerves originate from the cranial nerves and the sacral area and are not affected by the SCI (Claus-Walker et al., 1977; Guttmann, 1976). This impairment in sympathetic stimulation leads to a loss of tone in the vascular bed, generalized vasodilation, and decreased vascular resistance, which results in decreased blood pressure and diminished blood flow. The loss of sympathetic innervation causes a reduction in the density of both alpha- and beta-adrenergic receptors, which explains the abnormal vascular reactions and tendency toward vasodilation. Vasodilation results in decreased blood pressure, which adversely affects tissue perfusion.

Makhsous and colleagues (2007) found that, compared to controls, persons with SCI had a significantly slower rate of reperfusion of tissues following off-loading. Bogie and colleagues (1995) found that subjects with SCIs below T6 showed a progressive loss in maintaining adequate blood flow in the sitting position, indicating that paraplegics are at higher risk than tetraplegics. These findings suggest an altered or slowed blood flow response to pressure, which can lead to tissue damage since diminished tissue perfusion limits the delivery of nutrients, enzymes, and oxygen to the tissues. A normal inflammatory response depends on vasodilation. This response is most likely impaired in the SCI individual since there is chronic vasodilation throughout the entire lower body and loss of the ability to regulate blood flow in response to metabolic demands.

AD can lead to stroke and death. Exaggerated sympathetic activity causes increased vasoconstriction below the injury, resulting in dangerous high blood pressure, which leads to headaches, bradycardia, and cold extremities. Additional symptoms occur due to compensatory baroreflex-mediated vasodilation in blood vessels above the injury level, inducing flushing and sweating (Eldahan & Rabchevsky, 2018).

DECREASED TRANSCUTANEOUS OXYGEN LEVELS

Several studies from the 1990s provide comparable findings in terms of transcutaneous oxygen levels ($TcPO_2$) in SCI patients; specifically, they found $TcPO_2$ levels to be up to five times lower below the level of injury than above (Bogie et al., 1995; Mawson et al., 1993; Patterson et al., 1993). Keratinocytes require oxygen for building epithelium, and fibroblasts need oxygen to synthesize collagen. In addition, oxygen is needed for phagocytosis and prevention of infection and to meet the metabolic demands of the tissue. The hypoxia normally found within the wound (as compared to the surrounding tissue) stimulates angiogenesis and collagen synthesis. Both of these responses may be impaired by the reduced oxygen gradient between the healthy tissue and the wound.

Lemmer and colleagues (2019) investigated differences between PI history, muscle composition, and tissue health responses under physiologically relevant loading conditions for 38 individuals with SCIs. They found that ischial region mean interface pressures are the same for individuals with or without a PI history. Tissue oxygenation is lower during sitting for persons with a PI history. Individuals with >15% gluteal intramuscular fat were highly likely ($p < 0.001$) to have a history of severe or recurrent PI. Intramuscular adipose tissue (IMAT) levels within the gluteal muscle may remain low over time or muscle tissue in the gluteal muscle region may be almost entirely replaced by IMAT. In the current study cohort, it was found that muscle composition also continues to change over time even for individuals with long-standing SCI (Lemmer et al., 2019).

DECREASED COLLAGEN, EXTRACELLULAR MATRIX, AND THEIR PRECURSORS

Collagen is broken down in denervated, insensate tissues, resulting in increased excretion of collagen catabolites and glycosaminoglycans (GAGs) in the urine of persons with SCIs (Claus-Walker et al., 1977). Those on bed rest are vulnerable, excreting three to four times more than an ambulatory adult. This is significant as collagen is the primary component of the new extracellular matrix (ECM) that must be created to fill the defect. Collagen attracts leukocytes, macrophages, monocytes, and fibroblasts for tissue building. In the ongoing breakdown and excretion of collagen in SCI patients, the tissues below the level of injury have been found deficient in some amino acids and enzymes needed to synthesize collagen (Claus-Walker et al., 1977). Without the necessary resources for production of normal collagen, the body can make only defective collagen, resulting in a weakened ECM.

Kostovski et al. (2015) compared alterations in bone mineral density (BMD) and serum biomarkers of bone turnover in 31 recent motor-incomplete to -complete SCI men, as well as described their physical activity and spasticity. The men with motor-incomplete SCI developed significant proximal femur bone loss 12 months after injury and exhibited increased bone resorption throughout the first year after the injury. Compared with complete SCI men, incomplete SCI men show attenuated bone resorption. The authors' pooled data showed increased turnover of ECM after injury and that increased exercise before and after injury correlated with reduced bone loss (Kostovski et al., 2015).

ECM in new scar tissue is composed primarily of type III collagen, which has very minimal tensile strength. Type III collagen is gradually converted to type I collagen during the maturation phase, which provides tensile strength.

SCI tissues below the level of injury have been shown to have a greater proportion of type III to type I collagen (Rodriguez & Markowski, 1995). Both the scar tissues in newly healed or closed PIs and in the uninjured tissues surrounding those scars have poor tensile strength. This may be one of the factors leading to the high frequency of recurrence of PI in this population.

KEY POINT

Both the scar tissues in newly healed or closed PIs and in the uninjured tissues surrounding those scars have poor tensile strength. This may be one of the factors leading to the high frequency of recurrence of PI in this population.

DECREASED FIBRONECTIN

SCI patients with poorly healing wounds were found to have a significantly lower concentration of fibronectin, a large glycoprotein (Vaziri et al., 1992). Fibronectin facilitates phagocytosis; promotes neovascular growth; promotes fibroblast migration, attachment, and proliferation; and supports the production of collagen. Fibronectin is also part of the scaffold for the new ECM. In addition to the decreased levels of fibronectin in SCI tissues, Cruse and colleagues (2002) found reduced adhesion or binding capacities among lymphocytes, impaired cellular interaction, and a lack of structural and functional protein in the ECM.

CONSTANT INFLAMMATORY STATE

Persons with chronic SCI show serologic evidence of a systemic inflammatory state resulting in increased C-reactive protein (CRP) levels in patients who were both symptomatic and asymptomatic (Edwards et al., 2008; Frost et al., 2005). Frost et al. (2005) found the inflammatory state to be significant in those with indwelling catheters and existing PIs. Increased CRP was also correlated with lower albumin and hemoglobin levels (Frost et al., 2005). Edwards and colleagues (2008) found that CRP in those with SCI was nearly double that of matched non-SCI subjects. He also found that the level of visceral adipose tissue was 58% higher and total adipose tissue was 26% higher in those with SCI compared to those without SCI. Adipose tissue produces and releases proinflammatory molecules that have been implicated in many health problems including diabetes and CVD (Fantuzzi, 2005). This inflammatory state negatively affects the health of the entire body.

Allison and Ditor (2015) described SCI as being characterized by a low-grade inflammatory state due to a number of factors. Damage to the autonomic nervous system may induce immune dysfunction directly, through the loss of neural innervation of lymphoid organs, or indirectly by inducing endocrine impairment. Damage to the somatic nervous system and the corresponding loss of motor and sensory function increases the likelihood of developing a number of secondary health complications and metabolic disorders, like obesity, associated with a state of inflammation. Numerous related disorders associated with a state of chronic inflammation have been found to be at a substantially higher prevalence following SCI. Together, such factors help explain the chronic inflammatory state and immune impairment typically observed following SCI (Allison & Ditor, 2015).

Edsberg and colleagues (2015) conducted a pilot study to determine whether the biochemistry of chronic pressure ulcers differs between the patients with and without SCI through measurement and comparison of the concentration of wound fluid inflammatory mediators, growth factors, cytokines, acute phase proteins, and proteases. The researchers demonstrated for the first time that the biochemical profile of the wound environment is markedly different in pressure ulcers of people with SCI ($n = 29$) compared to a group of elderly individuals without SCI ($n = 9$). They found significant differences between individuals with and without SCI in all categories of proteins known to be involved in wound healing (growth factors, MMPs, TIMPs, and inflammatory mediators) (Edsberg et al., 2015).

KEY POINT

There are many physiological changes that occur as a result of an SCI that contribute to delayed wound healing despite appropriate management: these include reduced perfusion, reduced synthesis of collagen and fibronectin, and persistent inflammation.

MANAGEMENT GUIDELINES SPECIFIC TO SCI POPULATION

Pressure injuries in persons with SCI are difficult to heal. This may be due to the multiple physiological changes that occur as a result of the SCI, the alterations in the cells and processes involved in repair, and the difficulties in keeping these wounds off-loaded. Effective management begins with the basic principles of prevention and treatment of PIs. Since healing in the SCI individual is impaired, earlier use of advanced wound therapies may be required to provide scaffolding for migrating cells and to promote granulation tissue formation.

OFF-LOADING

Reducing or eliminating pressure to the wound is a priority in PI healing. PIs often occur on the ischial tuberosities and sacrum/coccyx in those with SCI, often treated with extended periods of bed rest (Biglari et al., 2013). The sequelae of immobility must be addressed; clinicians must remember that bed rest negatively impacts every aspect of the individual's life. Patients must be motivated to adhere to this aspect of the treatment plan.

Some programs (e.g., https://www.sci-info-pages.com/top-rehabilitation-hospitals/) now allow limited sitting, up to 1 hour three times per day, with the goals of increasing compliance, decreasing emotional depression caused by isolation and inactivity, and minimizing the pulmonary complications to which those with SCI are particularly vulnerable. Their data indicate that wounds will heal with limited sitting with a pressure redistribution chair cushion, if there is a comprehensive wound care program that includes appropriate positioning in bed, bowel/bladder management, and wound management.

ELECTRICAL STIMULATION (E-STIM)

E-stim has been studied more than any other modality for healing PIs in those with SCIs. E-stim for wound healing has been studied since the 1940s, but we still lack a clear understanding of the mechanism of action. E-stim has been credited with reducing infection, increasing perfusion, and accelerating wound healing (Thakral et al., 2013; WOCN, 2016). There is evidence that e-stim increases collagen synthesis and wound tensile strength, increases the rate of wound epithelialization, and increases oxygen delivery and bactericidal activity. It is believed that e-stim imitates or enhances the natural electrical current that occurs in the body; when applied to injured tissues, e-stim increases migration of neutrophils and macrophages into the wound bed and stimulates fibroblast activity.

There are different ways to deliver e-stim including direct current (DC), alternating current (AC), high-voltage pulsed current (HVPC), and low-intensity direct current (LIDC). The parameters of the stimulation (wave form, pulse, frequency, phase duration, and voltage) also vary, as does placement of the electrodes around the wound and use of positive versus negative polarity. It has been proposed that optimal parameters for the e-stim and for electrode placement may vary depending on the phase of wound healing and wound characteristics. Frequency of application and total time of treatment per day and week also vary. Despite variations in the type and application, studies have shown benefits of e-stim to wound healing (WOCN, 2016).

One randomized clinical trial examined anodal or cathodal HVPC and the effect on cytokines and growth factors in PIs in persons with neurological deficits. They found that anodal HVPC increases the ratio of anti-inflammatory IL-10 to pro-inflammatory TNF-alpha, and that the decrease in TNF-alpha correlated positively with the decrease in PI size (Polak et al., 2019).

In a systematic review on e-stim for prevention or for treatment of wounds in SCI individuals, Liu and colleagues (2014) reviewed randomized controlled trials (RCTs), non-RCTs, prospective cohort studies, case series, case–controls, and case reports. Of the 11 studies reviewed, 6 were RCTs. All 11 studies showed enhanced PI healing. The authors concluded that the combined evidence supports use of this therapy. The types of e-stim used in the six RCTs illustrate the variety in e-stim delivery (Liu et al., 2014).

NEGATIVE PRESSURE WOUND THERAPY

While negative pressure wound therapy (NPWT) is widely used for treating PIs, there are few studies examining the effects in SCI individuals. Benefits include dressing changes every 2 to 3 days rather than daily and better management of exudate as compared to absorbent dressings. The patient will continue to require offloading of the wound since the foam or gauze within the wound can become a source of pressure, as can the tubing. Bridging technique may be used to assure that the pressure control pad and tubing are placed over non–weight-bearing surfaces.

Ho and colleagues (2010) compared wound healing in 33 wounds managed with NPWT and 53 wounds managed with standard wound care. They found no significant difference in healing rates as evidenced by reduction in wound surface area between the two groups. DeLaat and colleagues (2011) analyzed outcomes for the SCI subgroup in a prospective RCT designed to evaluate the impact of NPWT for difficult-to-treat wounds. Their results showed that the SCI group had the same outcomes as did the entire study group; wounds managed with NPWT healed twice as fast as did those managed with sodium hypochlorite gauze dressings.

Dwivedi and colleagues (2017) conducted an RTC to assess the level of matrix metalloproteinase-8 (MMP-8) and wound-healing outcome measures (length, width, and depth, exudate amount, and tissue type) in PIs of spinal cord–injured patients treated with NPWT using a novel negative pressure device versus PI treated with wet to moist gauze (conventional wound care). Forty-four SCI patients with stage 3 and 4 sacral PI participated in the study. Significantly lower levels of MMP-8 were observed in the NPWT group at week 6 and week 9. There were no significant changes in the length and width of PIs between the groups until week 3. Significant reduction in length and width were observed in PIs of patients in the NPWT group at week 6 ($p = 0.04$) and week 9 ($p = 0.001$). Similarly, significant reduction in the depth of PIs was observed in the NPWT group at week 9 ($p < 0.05$). At the end of week 9, levels of MMP-8 showed a positive correlation with reduction in the length, width, and depth of PIs in the NPWT group (Dwivedi et al., 2017). See Chapter 12 for additional information on NPWT.

ULTRAVIOLET C

Ultraviolet light is easy to apply, and ultraviolet C (UVC) has been shown to be effective against multidrug-resistant microorganisms including MRSA and VRE

(Conner-Kerr et al., 1998; Dai et al., 2012). Nussbaum and colleagues (2013) conducted a double blind RCT (N = 43) to compare the effects of UVC with placebo-UVC on pressure ulcer healing in individuals with SCI (n = 58 stage 2 to 4). Ulcers and periwound skin were irradiated 3 times per week using UVC or placebo. Overall UVC- and placebo-treated ulcers had similar decreases in size from weeks 1 to 6. Data are insufficient about the benefit of light therapy for healing PIs (WOCN, 2016).

PLATELET-RICH PLASMA AND PRP GEL

Platelet-rich plasma (PRP) is also known as platelet-enriched plasma, platelet rich concentrate, autogenous platelet gel, or platelet releasate. PRP is autologous blood that has a high platelet concentration and a high concentration of growth factors. To create the PRP, blood is drawn from the patient and centrifuged to separate the red and white blood cells. This creates plasma that has high concentration of platelets. Additional centrifugation is conducted to further concentrate the platelets. Growth factors are then activated from the platelets using a number of different chemical processes that promote physical lysis through disruption of the cell membrane. The resulting plasma gel is then applied to the wound (EPUAP/NPIAP/PPPIA, 2019).

Two studies have evaluated PRP in management of SCI wounds, though each study used a different formulation. Scevola et al. (2010) conducted a prospective randomized trial involving 13 patients with 16 stage 3 or 4 PIs comparing the use of a high-concentration cryopreserved PRP against standard protocol, which included iodoform packing, sodium/alginate foam dressing, or NPWT. In this study, the PRP group had a statistically significant faster time to granulation (p = 0.025), indicating that the PRP promoted faster healing as compared to the non-PRP group. At the end of the study, no statistically significant difference was found in volume reduction between the two groups (p = 0.76), and all wounds showed significant volume reduction compared to the start of the study (p < 0.001). The second study involved the use of a low concentration, nonfrozen PRP in a case series of 20 wounds on 20 patients; wound volume, area, undermining, and tunneling were measured over time. In this study, wound volume (baseline 53.4 cm³) was reduced by 56% in 3.4 weeks with four treatments; all figures are averages (Rappl, 2011). Ramos-Torrecillas and colleagues (2015) evaluated the effectiveness of PRP and hyaluronic acid applied separately and together for the treatment of 100 patients with 124 PIs. Both groups had about 30% complete healing in the 36-day study period. Per 2019 International Guideline, consider pulsed electrical stimulation to facilitate wound healing in recalcitrant PIs or consider applying PRP gel to promote healing in PIs (EPUAP/NPIAP/PPPIA, 2019). See Chapter 12 for additional information on advanced therapies.

Tools commonly used to monitor PI healing, such as the Pressure Ulcer Scale for Healing (PUSH) Tool and the Bates-Jensen Wound Assessment Tool (BWAT) have not been widely studied in the SCI population. See Chapter 4 for additional information on these tools. The Spinal Cord Impairment Pressure Ulcer Monitoring Tool (SCI-PUMT) has been developed and validated and is recommended for use in SCI wounds (Thomason et al., 2014, 2016). This tool was tested for validity and reliability on a convenience sample of 66 veterans (Thomason et al., 2014, 2016). The investigators defined pressure ulcer healing as the reduction in volume of the pressure ulcer and complete healing as resurfacing of the wound. Volume was an estimate obtained by calculating the surface area (multiplied length by width by depth). Content and construct validity identified a set of seven variables for inclusion in the SCI-PUMT: wound surface area, depth, edges, tunneling, undermining, exudate type, and amount of necrotic tissue. These variables are divided into two subscales including geometric factors and substance factors. Subscale scores are added to calculate the total SCI-PUMT score with a range from 2 (healed) to 26 (most severe). In the clinical setting, interrater reliability of the SCI-PUMT was 0.79 and intrarater reliability ranged from 0.81 to 0.99 (Thomason et al., 2014, 2016). When scores of the SCI-PUMT were compared to the PUSH and BWAT scores, SCI-PUMT explained more variance in pressure ulcer volume (59%) than the PUSH (57%) or BWAT (24%) tools. The investigators concluded that the SCI-PUMT was a reliable, valid, and sensitive measure of pressure ulcer healing in patients with SCIs (WOCN, 2016).

SKIN OR TISSUE FLAP SURGERY

Operative procedures for pressure injury repair include direct closure (rarely indicated or used), skin grafts, and local and sensate flaps (Biering-Sørensen et al., 2004). Types of flaps used to cover PIs are classified according to the type of vascular supply and type of tissue in the flap. Generally, fasciocutaneous or myocutaneous flaps are used for reconstruction of full-thickness pressure injuries (EPUAP/NPIAP/PPPIA, 2019). Fasciocutaneous flaps include epidermis, dermis, subcutaneous tissue, and fascia; and can provide padding and superficial coverage. Myocutaneous flaps involve skin, subcutaneous tissue, fascia, and muscle; and provide optimal coverage for bony prominences (Black & Black, 2016). Myocutaneous flaps include arterial and venous blood supply. Myocutaneous flaps are the treatment of choice in full-thickness pressure injury because they provide good protection and blood supply to the area (Black & Black, 2016; Biering-Sørensen et al., 2004). High rates of pressure injury recurrence and postoperative complications have been reported after surgery for pressure injuries. Suture line dehiscence is the most common complication after surgery (EPUAP/NPIAP/PPPIA, 2019).

Kenneweg et al. (2015) retrospectively reviewed the medical records of 49 patients with 102 pressure ulcers who were surgically treated to identify perioperative risk factors that might predict improved outcomes and reduced complications with flap reconstructive surgeries. Ninety percent of the patients had SCIs and were male; mean age was 45 years. There were 59 primary ulcers and 43 recurrent ulcers; 54 were reconstructed with myocutaneous and/or fasciocutaneous flaps and five were closed by primary closure. There was an overall wound dehiscence rate of 37.6%. The most common location for flap breakdown was the ischium with recurrence rates of 89.29%. The analysis indicated that pressure ulcer closure was positively correlated with lower BMI, smaller surface area, fewer debridements, hemoglobin, hematocrit, and prealbumin. Closure was negatively correlated with creatinine, total protein, CRP, platelet count, wound dehiscence, infection, and delayed healing. In the final model to predict wound closure after flap reconstruction, creatinine, hematocrit, hemoglobin, and prealbumin levels successfully predicted closure outcome in 83.6% of cases. The investigators concluded that these tests could be valuable in determining a patient's healing potential and risk for postoperative complications and useful in patient counseling and selection prior to reconstructive surgery (WOCN, 2016).

Venous congestion has been associated with incision line dehiscence and flap failure. Monitoring for increasing warmth and edema as well as discoloration is recommended. NPWT is commonly used post flap surgery to minimize edema and promote perfusion. Effective off-loading of the flap is also important. Patients must be positioned off of the surgical site for up to 6 weeks and may be placed on support surfaces to minimize the risk of developing other PIs.

Support surfaces with an air fluidized feature were considered standard of care during the immediate postoperative period for many years but presented challenges. There is limited evidence on their relative effectiveness compared to other support surfaces. In a small pilot study (N = 37), Finnegan and colleagues (2008) compared healing following pressure injury flap surgery between an air fluidized bed and an alternating pressure air mattress. In short-term follow-up, 98% of the patients on air fluidized therapy had an intact surgical incision while 87% of those on alternating pressure air mattress had an intact incision. Patients and health care professionals rated both surfaces as comfortable, but air fluidized therapy was 52% more expensive. For additional information on support surfaces, see Chapter 22.

The patient undergoing myocutaneous flap surgery requires meticulous postoperative care including consistent pressure and shear reduction, nutritional support, and monitoring for indicators of flap ischemia or congestion. Acute post-op care includes assistance in bed mobility and positioning, bowel and bladder management, range of motion, and resistive exercise. Sitting usually begins 3 to 6 weeks after surgery. Patients are instructed in safe transfer techniques and limiting hip flexion until advised by the surgeon. Evaluate the patient's seating and sleeping surfaces at home to optimize pressure redistribution. To prevent flap failure, discuss with the patient the importance of off-loading and transfer techniques.

● CONCLUSION

People who sustain SCIs develop PIs at an increased rate immediately following their injury and throughout their lifetime. These wounds negatively impact physical, psychological, emotional, and financial status. Physiological changes occur due to the SCI alter the tissues below the level of injury. The wound care nurse contributes to the comprehensive plan of care by providing emotional and social support as well as evidence-based wound care.

REFERENCES

Agam, L., & Gefen, A. (2008). Toward real-time detection of deep tissue injury risk in wheelchair users using Hertz contact theory. *Journal of Rehabilitation Research and Development, 45*(4), 537–550.

Allison, D., & Ditor, D. (2015). Immune dysfunction and chronic inflammation following spinal cord injury. *Spinal Cord, 53*, 14–18. doi: 10.1038/sc.2014.184.

Bader, D. L. (1990). The recovery characteristics of soft tissues following repeated loading. *Journal of Rehabilitation Research and Development, 27*(2), 141–150.

Banks, M. D., Graves, N., Bauer, J. D., et al. (2012). Cost effectiveness of nutrition support in the prevention of pressure ulcer in hospitals. *European Journal of Clinical Nutrition, 67*, 42–46.

Bates-Jensen, B. M., Guihan, M., Garber, S. L., et al. (2009). Characteristics of recurrent pressure ulcers in veterans with spinal cord injury. *Journal of Spinal Cord Medicine, 32*(1), 34–42.

Bergstrom, N., Braden, B. J., Laguzza, A., et al. (1987). The Braden Scale for predicting pressure sore risk. *Nursing Research, 36*(4), 205–210.

Berke, C. T. (2019). Friction injury versus deep tissue injury: Level of tissue involvement: A comparison of 2 cases. *Journal of Wound Ostomy Continence Nursing, 46*(6), 539–542. doi: 10.1097/WON.0000000000000596.

Biering-Sørensen, F., Hansen, R. B., & Biering-Sørensen, J. (2004). Mobility aids and transport possibilities 10–45 years after spinal cord injury. *Spinal Cord, 42*(12), 699–706.

Bigford, G., & Nash, M. S. (2017). Nutritional health considerations for persons with spinal cord injury. *Topics in Spinal Cord Injury Rehabilitation, 23*(3), 188–206. doi: 10.1310/sci2303-188.

Biglari, B., Büchler, A., Reitzel, T., et al. (2013). A retrospective study on flap complications after pressure ulcer surgery in spinal cord-injured patients. *Spinal Cord, 52*(1), 80–83.

Black, J. M., & Black, J. S. (2016). Reconstructive surgery. In R. A. Bryant, & D. P. Nix (Eds.), *Acute and chronic wounds: Current management concepts* (5th ed.). St. Louis, MO: Elsevier, Inc.

Bogie, K., Nuseibeh, I., & Bader, D. (1995). Early progressive changes in tissue viability in the seated spinal cord injured subject. *Spinal Cord, 33*(3), 141–147.

Brienza, D., & Karg, P. (2012). Pressure ulcers in people with spinal cord injury. In B. Pieper with the National Pressure Ulcer Advisory Panel (NPUAP). (Ed.), *Pressure ulcers: Prevalence, incidence, and implications for the future.* Washington, DC: NPUAP.

Brienza, D., Krishnan, S., Karg, P., et al. (2018a). Predictors of pressure ulcer incidence following traumatic spinal cord injury: A secondary analysis of a prospective longitudinal study. *Spinal Cord, 56*(1), 28–34. doi: 10.1038/sc.2017.96.

Brienza, D., Vallely, J., Karg, P., et al. (2018b). An MRI investigation of the effects of user anatomy and wheelchair cushion type on tissue deformation. *Journal of Tissue Viability, 27*(1), 42–53. doi: 10.1016/j.jtv.2017.04.

Byrne, D., & Salzberg, C. (1996). Major risk factors for pressure ulcers in the spinal cord disabled: A literature review. *Spinal Cord, 34*(5), 255–263.

Çakmak, S. K., Gül, Ü., Özer, S., et al. (2009). Risk factors for pressure ulcers. *Advances in Skin & Wound Care, 22*(9), 412–415.

Cardenas, D. D., Hoffman, J. M., Kirshblum, S., et al. (2004). Etiology and incidence of rehospitalization after traumatic spinal cord injury: A multicenter analysis. *Archives of Physical Medication and Rehabilitation, 85*(11), 1757–1763.

Carlson, M., Vigen, C. L., Rubayi, S., et al. (2019). Lifestyle intervention for adults with spinal cord injury: Results of the USC–RLANRC pressure ulcer prevention study. *The Journal of Spinal Cord Medicine, 42*(1), 2–19. doi: 10.1080/10790268.2017.1313931.

Castro, M. J., Apple, D. F. Jr, Staron, R. S., et al. (1999). Influence of complete spinal cord injury on skeletal muscle within 6 months of injury. *Journal of Applied Physics, 86*, 350–358.

Chen, D., Apple, D. F. Jr, Hudson, L. M., et al. (1999). Medical complications during acute rehabilitation following spinal cord injury—current experience of the Model Systems. *Archives of Physical Medicine and Rehabilitation, 80*(11), 1397–1401.

Chen, Y., Devivo, M. J., & Jackson, A. B. (2005). Pressure ulcer prevalence in people with spinal cord injury: Age-period-duration effects. *Archives of Physical Medicine and Rehabilitation, 86*(6), 1208–1213.

Claus-Walker, J., Singh, J., Leach, C. S., et al. (1977). The urinary excretion of collagen degradation products by quadriplegic patients and during weightlessness. *The Journal of Bone and Joint Surgery, 59*(2), 209–212.

Cogan, A. M., Blanchard, J., Garber, S. L., et al. (2017). Systematic review of behavioral and educational interventions to prevent pressure ulcers in adults with spinal cord injury. *Clinical Rehabilitation, 31*(7), 871–880.

Coggrave, M., & Rose, L. (2003). A specialist seating assessment clinic: Changing pressure relief practice. *Spinal Cord, 41*(12), 692–695.

Conner-Kerr, T. A., Sullivan, P. K., Gaillard, J., et al. (1998). The effects of ultraviolet radiation on antibiotic-resistant bacteria in vitro. *Ostomy and Wound Management, 44*(10), 50–56.

Consortium for Spinal Cord Medicine Clinical Practice Guidelines. (2001). Pressure ulcer prevention and treatment following spinal cord injury: A clinical practice guideline for health-care professionals. *The Journal of Spinal Cord Medicine, 24*, S40.

Cruse, J. M., Wang, H., Lewis, R. E., et al. (2002). Cellular and molecular alterations in spinal cord injury patients with pressure ulcers: A preliminary report. *Experimental and Molecular Pathology, 72*(2), 124–131.

Dai, T., Vrahas, M. S., Murray, C. K., et al. (2012). Ultraviolet C irradiation: An alternative antimicrobial approach to localized infections? *Expert Review of Anti-Infective Therapy, 10*(2), 185–195.

de Bruin, E. D., Herzog, R., Rozendal, R. H., et al. (2000). Estimation of geometric properties of cortical bone in spinal cord injury. *Archives of Physical Medicine and Rehabilitation, 81*(1), 150–156.

de Laat, E. H., van den Boogaard, M. H., Spauwen, P. H., et al. (2011). Faster wound healing with topical negative pressure therapy in difficult-to-heal wounds: A prospective randomized controlled trial. *Annals of Plastic Surgery, 67*(6), 626–631.

De Jong, G., Hsieh, C. H. J., Brown, P., et al. (2014). Factors associated with pressure ulcer development in spinal cord injury rehabilitation. *American Journal of Physical Medicine and Rehabilitation, 93*(11), 971–986.

Di Prinzio, M. F., Argento, F. J., Barbalaco, L., et al. (2019). Factores de riesgo para la aparición y/o recurrencia de úlceras por pre-

siónensujetos con lesiónmedular: Revisiónsistemática [Risk factors for the development and recurrence of pressure ulcers in patients with spinal cord injury: A systematic review]. *Revista de la Facultad de CienciasMédicas de Córdoba, 76*(4), 242–256. doi: 10.31053/1853.0605.v76.n4.24906.

Dwivedi, M. K., Bhagat, A. K., Srivastava, R. N., et al. (2017). Expression of MMP-8 in pressure injuries in spinal cord injury patients managed by negative pressure wound therapy or conventional wound care. *Journal of Wound, Ostomy and Continence Nursing, 44*(4), 343–349. doi: 10.1097/WON.0000000000000333.

Edsberg, L. E., Wyffels, J. T., Ogrin, R., et al. (2015). A pilot study evaluating protein abundance in pressure ulcer fluid from people with and without spinal cord injury. *The Journal of Spinal Cord Medicine, 38*(4), 456–467. doi: 10.1179/2045772314Y.0000000212.

Edwards, L. A., Bugaresti, J. M., & Buchholz, A. C. (2008). Visceral adipose tissue and the ratio of visceral to subcutaneous adipose tissue are greater in adults with than in those without spinal cord injury, despite matching waist circumferences. *The American Journal of Clinical Nutrition, 87*(3), 600–607.

Eldahan, K. C., & Rabchevsky, A. G. (2018). Autonomic dysreflexia after spinal cord injury: Systemic pathophysiology and methods of management. *Autonomic Neuroscience, 209*, 59–70. doi: 10.1016/j.autneu.2017.05.002.

European Pressure Ulcer Advisory Panel, National Pressure Injury Advisory Panel and Pan Pacific Pressure Injury Alliance (EPUAP/NPIAP/PPPIA). (2019). Prevention and treatment of pressure ulcers/injuries: Clinical Practice guideline. In E. Haesler (Ed.), *The International Guideline*.

Fantuzzi, G. (2005). Adipose tissue, adipokines, and inflammation. *Journal of Allergy and Clinical Immunology, 115*(5), 911–919.

Farkas, G. J., Pitot, M. A., Berg, A. S., et al. (2019). Nutritional status in chronic spinal cord injury: A systematic review and meta-analysis. *Spinal Cord, 57*(1), 3–17. doi: 10.1038/s41393-018-0218-4.

Finnegan, M. J., Gazzerro, L., Finnegan, J. O., et al. (2008). Comparing the effectiveness of a specialized alternating air pressure mattress replacement system and an air-fluidized integrated bed in the management of post-operative flap patients: A randomized controlled pilot study. *Journal of Tissue Viability, 17*(1), 2.

Fogerty, M. D., Abumrad, N. N., Nanney, L., et al. (2008). Risk factors for pressure ulcers in acute care hospitals. *Wound Repair and Regeneration, 16*(1), 11–18.

Frost, F., Roach, M. J., Kushner, I., et al. (2005). Inflammatory C-reactive protein and cytokine levels in asymptomatic people with chronic spinal cord injury. *Archives of Physical Medicine and Rehabilitation, 86*(2), 312–317.

Gefen, A. (2008). The compression intensity index: A practical anatomical estimate of the biomechanical risk for a deep tissue injury. *Technology and Health Care, 16*(2), 141–149.

Gefen, A. (2014). Tissue changes in patients following spinal cord injury and implications for wheelchair cushions and tissue loading: A literature review. *Ostomy and Wound Management, 60*(2), 34–45.

Giangregorio, L., & McCartney, N. (2006). Bone loss and muscle atrophy in spinal cord injury: Epidemiology, fracture prediction, and rehabilitation strategies. *The Journal of Spinal Cord Medicine, 29*, 489–500.

Gray, M., & Giuliano, K. K. (2018). Incontinence-associated dermatitis, characteristics and relationship to pressure injury: A multisite epidemiologic analysis. *Journal of Wound Ostomy and Continence Nursing, 45*(1), 63–67. doi: 10.1097/WON.0000000000000390.

Guihan, M., & Bombardier, C. H. (2012). Potentially modifiable risk factors among veterans with spinal cord injury hospitalized for severe pressure ulcers: A descriptive study. *Journal of Spinal Cord Medicine, 35*(4), 240–250.

Guttmann, L. (1976). *Spinal cord injuries: Comprehensive management and research* (Vol. 6). Oxford, England: Blackwell Scientific Publications.

Higgins, J., Laramée, M. T., Harrison, K. R., et al. (2019). The spinal cord injury pressure ulcer scale (SCIPUS): An assessment of validity using Rasch analysis. *Spinal Cord, 57*(10), 874–880. doi: 10.1038/s41393-019-0287-z.

Hitzig, S. L., Tonack, M., Campbell, K. A., et al. (2008). Secondary health complications in an aging Canadian spinal cord injury sample. *American Journal of Physical Medicine and Rehabilitation, 87*(7), 545–555. doi: 10.1097/PHM.0b013e31817c16d610.1097/PHM.0b013e31817c16d6.

Ho, C. H., Powell, H. L., Collins, J. F., et al. (2010). Poor nutrition is a relative contraindication to negative pressure wound therapy for pressure ulcers: Preliminary observations in patients with spinal cord injury. *Advances in Skin and Wound Care, 23*(11), 508–516.

Hogaboom, N. S., Worobey, L. A., Houlihan, B. V., et al. (2018). Wheelchair breakdowns are associated with pain, pressure injuries, rehospitalization, and self-perceived health in full-time wheelchair users with spinal cord injury. *Archives in Physical Medicine Rehabilitation, 99*(10), 1949–1956. doi: 10.1016/j.apmr.2018.04.002.

Houlihan, B. V., Brody, M., Everhart-Skeels, S., et al. (2017). Randomized trial of a peer-led, telephone-based empowerment intervention for persons with chronic spinal cord injury improves health self-management. *Archives of Physical Medicine & Rehabilitation, 98*(6), 1067–1076. doi: 10.1016/j.apmr.2017.02.005.

Hsieh, J., Benton, B., Titus, L., et al. (2020). Skin integrity and pressure injuries following spinal cord injury. In J. J. Eng, R. W. Teasell, W. C. Miller, et al. (Eds.), *Spinal cord injury rehabilitation evidence.* Version 7.0. 1–123. Retrieved March 2, 2020 from https://scireproject.com/evidence/rehabilitation-evidence/skin-integrity-pressure-injuries/

Inskip, J. A., Ramer, L. M., Ramer, M. S., et al. (2009). Autonomic assessment of animals with spinal cord injury: Tools, techniques and translation. *Spinal Cord, 47*, 2–35.

Jones, M. L., Mathewson, C. S., Adkins, V. K., et al. (2003). Use of behavioral contingencies to promote prevention of recurrent pressure ulcers. *Archives of Physical Medicine & Rehabilitation, 84*(6), 796–802.

Kennedy, P., Berry, C., Coggrave, M., et al. (2003). The effect of a specialist seating assessment clinic on the skin management of individuals with spinal cord injury. *Journal of Tissue Viability, 13*(3), 122–125.

Kenneweg, K. A., Welch, M. C., & Welch, P. J. (2015). A 9-year retrospective evaluation of 102 pressure ulcer reconstructions. *Journal of Wound Care, 24*(Suppl 4a), S12–S21.

Kostovski, E., Hjeltnes, N., Eriksen, E. F., et al. (2015). Differences in bone mineral density, markers of bone turnover and extracellular matrix and daily life muscular activity among patients with recent motor-incomplete versus motor-complete spinal cord injury. *Calcified Tissue International, 96*(2), 145–154. doi: 10.1007/s00223-014-9947-3.

Kottner, J., Dassen, T., & Tannen, A. (2009). Inter- and intrarater reliability of the Waterlow pressure sore risk scale: A systematic review. *International Journal of Nursing Studies, 46*(3), 369–379. doi: 10.1016/j.ijnurstu.2008.09.01010.1016/j.ijnurstu.2008.09.010.

Krause, J. S., Vines, C. L., Farley, T. L., et al. (2001). An exploratory study of pressure ulcers after spinal cord injury: Relationship to protective behaviors and risk factors. *Archives of Physical Medicine and Rehabilitation, 82*(1), 107–113.

Krishnan, S. (2014). Factors associated with occurrence and early detection of pressure ulcers following traumatic spinal cord injury. Doctoral Dissertation, University of Pittsburgh.

Krishnan, S., Brick, R. S., Karg, P. E., et al. (2016). Predictive validity of the Spinal Cord Injury Pressure Ulcer Scale (SCIPUS) in acute care and inpatient rehabilitation in individuals with traumatic spinal cord injury. *NeuroRehabilitation, 38*(4), 401–409. doi: 10.3233/NRE-161331.

Laird, A. S., Finch, A. M., Waite, P. M., et al. (2008). Peripheral changes above and below injury level lead to prolonged vascular responses following high spinal cord injury. *American Journal of Physiology-Heart and Circulatory Physiology, 294*(2), H785–H792. doi: 10.1152/ajpheart.01002.2007.

Lemmer, D. P., Alvarado, N., Henzel, K., et al. (2019). What lies beneath: Why some pressure injuries may be unpreventable for individuals with spinal cord injury. *Archives of Physical Medicine and Rehabilitation, 100*(6), 1042–1049. doi: 10.1016/j.apmr.2018.11.006.

Levy, A., Kopplin, K., & Gefen, A. (2013). Simulation of skin and subcutaneous tissue loading in the buttocks while regaining weight bearing after a pushup in wheelchair users. *Journal of Mechanical Behavior of Biomedical Materials, 28*, 436–447.

Levy, A., Kopplin, K., & Gefen, A. (2014). An air-cell-based cushion for pressure ulcer protection remarkably reduces tissue stresses in the seated buttocks with respect to foams: Finite element studies. *Journal of Tissue Viability, 23*(1), 13–23.

Linder-Ganz, E., & Gefen, A. (2009). Stress analyses coupled with damage laws to determine biomechanical risk factors for deep tissue injury during sitting. *Journal of Biomechanical Engineering, 131*(1), 011003.

Linder-Ganz, E., Shabshin, N., Itzchak, Y., et al. (2008). Strains and stresses in sub-dermal tissues of the buttocks are greater in paraplegics than in healthy during sitting. *Journal of Biomechanics, 41*, 567–580.

Liu, L. Q., Moody, J., Traynor, M., et al. (2014). A systematic review of electrical stimulation for pressure ulcer prevention and treatment in people with spinal cord injuries. *Journal of Spinal Cord Medicine, 37*(6), 703–718.

Makhsous, M., Priebe, M., Bankard, J., et al. (2007). Measuring tissue perfusion during pressure relief maneuvers: Insights into preventing pressure ulcers. *Journal of Spinal Cord Medicine, 30*(5), 497–507.

Manzano, F., Navarro, M. J., Roldán, D., et al., & Granada UPP Group. (2010). Pressure ulcer incidence and risk factors in ventilated intensive care patients. *Journal of Critical Care, 25*(3), 469–476.

Marin, J., Nixon, J., & Gorecki, C. (2013). A systematic review of risk factors for the development and recurrence of pressure ulcers in people with spinal cord injuries. *Spinal Cord, 51*(7), 522–527.

Mathewson, C., Adkins, V. K., Lenyoun, M. A., et al. (1999). Using telemedicine in the treatment of pressure ulcers. *Ostomy and Wound Management, 45*(11), 58–62.

Mawson, A. R., Biundo, J. J., Neville, P., et al. (1988). Risk factors for early occurring pressure ulcers following spinal cord injury. *American Journal of Physical Medicine and Rehabilitation, 67*(3), 123–127.

Mawson, A., Siddiqui, F., & Biundo, J. (1993). Enhancing host resistance to pressure ulcers: A new approach to prevention. *Preventive Medicine, 22*(3), 433–450.

McKinley, W. O., Jackson, A. B., Cardenas, D. D., et al. (1999). Long-term medical complications after traumatic spinal cord injury: A regional model systems analysis. *Archives of Physical Medicine and Rehabilitation, 80*(11), 1402–1410.

McKinley, W., Tewksbury, M., & Godbout, C. (2002). Comparison of medical complications following nontraumatic and traumatic spinal cord injury. *Journal of Spinal Cord Medicine, 25*(2), 88.

Model Systems Knowledge Translation Center. (2020). Retrieved January 30, 2020, from https://msktc.org/sci/sci-resources.

Mortenson, W., & Miller, W. (2007). A review of scales for assessing the risk of developing a pressure ulcer in individuals with SCI. *Spinal Cord, 46*(3), 168–175.

National Pressure Injury Advisory Panel. (2018). National Pressure Injury Advisory Panel Support Surface Standards Initiative (S3I)—Terms and Definitions Related to Support Surfaces. Retrieved February 15, 2020, from https://npiap.com/general/custom.asp?page=S3I.

National Spinal Cord Injury Statistical Center. (2018). *Facts and figures at a glance*. Birmingham, AL: University of Alabama at Birmingham. Retrieved March 2, 2020, from https://www.nscisc.uab.edu/Public/Facts%20and%20Figures%20-%202018.pdf

Norton, D. (1996). Calculating the risk: Reflections on the Norton scale. *Advances in Skin & Wound Care, 9*(6), 38–43.

NSCISC. (2011). *Annual report for the model spinal cord injury care systems*. Birmingham, AL: NSCISC.

Nussbaum, E. L., Flett, H., Hitzig, S. L., et al. (2013). Ultraviolet C irradiation in the management of pressure ulcers in people with spinal cord injury: A randomized placebo-controlled trial. *Archives of Physical Medicine & Rehabilitation, 94*(4), 650–659.

Oomens, C. W., Bader, D. L., Loerakker, S., et al. (2015). Pressure induced deep tissue injury explained. *Annals of biomedical Engineering, 43*(2), 297–305.

Pagliacci, M. C., Celani, M. G., Zampolini, M., et al. (2003). An Italian survey of traumatic spinal cord injury. The Gruppo Italiano studio epidemiologicoMielolesioni study. *Archives of Physical Medicine and Rehabilitation, 84*(9), 1266–1275.

Palmetto—Medicare Pricing, Data Analysis and Coding (PDAC). (2019). Application and Checklist for PDAC HCPCS Coding Verification Request: Wheelchair Cushions. Retrieved March 2, 2020, from https://www.dmepdac.com/palmetto/PDAC.nsf/DID/B723EU24.

Park, S. E., Elliott, S., Noonan, V. K., et al. (2017). Impact of bladder, bowel and sexual dysfunction on health status of people with thoracolumbar spinal cord injuries living in the community. *Journal of Spinal Cord Medicine, 40*(5), 548–559. doi: 10.1080/10790268.2016.1213554.

Patterson, R. P., Cranmer, H. H., Fisher, S. V., et al. (1993). The impaired response of spinal cord injured individuals to repeated surface pressure loads. *Archives of Physical Medicine and Rehabilitation, 74*(9), 947–953.

Peerless, J. R., Davies, A., Klein, D., et al. (1999). Skin complications in the intensive care unit. *Clinics in Chest Medicine, 20*(2), 453–467.

Peko Cohen, L., & Gefen, A. (2017). Deep tissue loads in the seated buttocks on an off-loading wheelchair cushion versus air-cell-based and foam cushions: Finite element studies. *International Wound Journal, 14*(6), 1327–1334. doi: 10.1111/iwj.12807.

Polak, A., Kloth, L. C., Paczula, M., et al. (2019). Pressure injuries treated with anodal and cathodal high-voltage electrical stimulation: The effect on blood serum concentration of cytokines and growth factors in patients with neurological injuries. A randomized clinical study. *Wound Management & Prevention, 65*(11), 19–32.

Portnoy, S., Vuillerme, N., Payan, Y., et al. (2011). Clinically oriented real-time monitoring of the individual's risk for deep tissue injury. *Medical and Biological Engineering and Computing, 49*(4), 473–483.

Ramos-Torrecillas, J., García-Martínez, O., De Luna-Bertos, E., et al. (2015). Effectiveness of platelet-rich plasma and hyaluronic acid for the treatment and care of pressure ulcers. *Biological Research for Nursing, 17*(2), 152–158.

Rappl, L. M. (2008). Physiological changes in tissues denervated by spinal cord injury tissues and possible effects on wound healing. *International Wound Journal, 5*(3), 435–444.

Rappl, L. M. (2011). Effect of platelet rich plasma gel in a physiologically relevant platelet concentration on wounds in persons with spinal cord injury. *International Wound Journal, 8*(2), 187–195.

Reddy, M., Gill, S. S., & Rochon, P. A. (2006). Preventing pressure ulcers: A systematic review. *Journal of the American Medical Association, 296*(8), 974–984.

Richardson, R. R., & Meyer, P. R. (1981). Prevalence and incidence of pressure sores in acute spinal cord injuries. *Spinal Cord, 19*(4), 235–247.

Rittweger, J., Gerrits, K. H., Altenburg, T. M., et al. (2006). Bone adaptation to altered loading after spinal cord injury: A study of bone and muscle strength. *Journal of Musculoskeletal and Neuronal Interactions, 6*, 269–276.

Rodriguez, G., & Markowski, J. (1995). Changes in skin morphology and its relationship to pressure ulcer incidence in spinal cord injury [ACRM abstract]. *Archives of Physical Medicine and Rehabilitation, 76*(6), 593.

Saladin, L. K., & Krause, J. S. (2009). Pressure ulcer prevalence and barriers to treatment after spinal cord injury: Comparisons of four groups based on race-ethnicity. *NeuroRehabilitation, 24*(1), 57–66. doi: 10.3233/NRE-2009-0454.

Salzberg, C. A., Byrne, D. W., Cayten, C. G., et al. (1996). A new pressure ulcer risk assessment scale for individuals with spinal cord injury. *American Journal of Physical Medicine and Rehabilitation, 75*(2), 96–104.

Salzberg, C. A., Byrne, D. W., Cayten, C. G., et al. (1998). Predicting and preventing pressure ulcers in adults with paralysis. *Advances in Skin and Wound Care, 11*(5), 237–246.

Scevola, S., Nicoletti, G., Brenta, F., et al. (2010). Allogenic platelet gel in the treatment of pressure sores: A pilot study. *International Wound Journal, 7*(3), 184–190.

Smith, B. M., Guihan, M., LaVela, S. L., et al. (2008). Factors predicting pressure ulcers in veterans with spinal cord injuries. *American Journal of Physical Medicine and Rehabilitation, 87*(9), 750–757. doi: 10.1097/PHM.0b013e3181837a50.

Sonenblum, S. E., Ma, J., Sprigle, S. H., et al. (2018). Measuring the impact of cushion design on buttocks tissue deformation: An MRI approach. *Journal of Tissue Viability, 27*(3), 162–172. doi: 10.1016/j.jtv.2018.04.001.

Sonenblum, S. E., & Sprigle, S. H. (2011). The impact of tilting on blood flow and localized tissue loading. *Journal of Tissue Viability, 20*(1), 3–13.

Sprigle, S. H., & Sonenblum, S. E. (2011). Assessing evidence supporting redistribution of pressure for pressure ulcer prevention: A review. *Journal of Rehabilitation Research & Development, 48*(3), 203–213.

Sprigle, S. H., Sonenblum, S. E., & Feng, C. (2019). Pressure redistributing in-seat movement activities by persons with spinal cord injury over multiple epochs. *PLoS One, 14*(2), e0210978. doi: 10.1371/journal.pone.0210978.

Strobl, W. M. (2013). Seating. *Journal of Children's Orthopaedics, 7*(5), 395–399.

Stover, S. L., DeLisa, J. A., & Whiteneck, G. G. (1995). *Spinal cord injury: Clinical outcomes from the model systems*. Gaithersburg, MD: Aspen Publishers.

Teasell, R. W., Arnold, J. M. O., Krassioukov, A., et al. (2000). Cardiovascular consequences of loss of supraspinal control of the sympathetic nervous system after spinal cord injury. *Archives of Physical Medicine and Rehabilitation, 81*(4), 506–516.

Thakral, G., LaFontaine, J., Najafi, B., et al. (2013). Electrical stimulation to accelerate wound healing. *Diabetic Foot & Ankle, 4*(1), 22081.

Thijssen, D. H. J., Maiorana, A. J., O'Driscoll, G., et al. (2010). Impact of inactivity and exercise on the vasculature in humans. *European Journal of Applied Physiology, 108*, 845–875.

Thomason, S. S., Luther, S. L., Powell-Cope, G. M., et al. (2014). Validity and reliability of a pressure ulcer monitoring tool for persons with spinal cord impairment. *Journal of Spinal Cord Medicine, 37*(3), 317–327.

Thomason, S. S., Powell-Cope, G., Peterson, M. J., et al. (2016). A multisite quality improvement project to standardize the assessment of pressure ulcer healing in veterans with spinal cord injuries/disorders. *Advances in Skin &Wound Care, 29*(6), 269–276.

U.S. Department of Health and Human Services and U.S. Department of Agriculture. (2015). *2015–2020 Dietary Guidelines for Americans*. (8th Ed.). Washington, DC: USDA. Available at http://health.gov/dietaryguidelines/2015/guidelines/

Vaishampayan, A., Clark, F., Carlson, M., et al. (2011). Preventing pressure ulcers in people with spinal cord injury: Targeting risky life circumstances through community-based interventions. *Advances in Skin & Wound Care, 24*(6), 275–84.

Vaziri, N. D., Eltorai, I., Gonzales, E., et al. (1992). Pressure ulcer, fibronectin, and related proteins in spinal cord injured patients. *Archives of Physical Medicine and Rehabilitation, 73*(9), 803–806.

Wannapakhe, J., Arrayawichanon, P., Saengsuwan, J., et al. (2015). Medical complications and falls in patients with spinal cord injury during the immediate phase after completing a rehabilitation program. *Journal of Spinal Cord Medicine, 38*(1), 84–90. doi: 10.1179/2045772313Y.0000000173.

Watts, D., Abrahams, E., MacMillan, C., et al. (1998). Insult after injury: Pressure ulcers in trauma patients. *Orthopaedic Nursing, 17*(4), 84–91.

Wilczweski, P., Grimm, D., Gianakis, A., et al. (2012). Risk factors associated with pressure ulcer development in critically ill traumatic spinal cord injury patients. *Journal of Trauma Nursing, 19*(1), 5–10. doi: 10.1097/JTN.0b013e31823a4528.

Wound Ostomy & Continence Nurses Society (WOCN). (2016). *Guideline for prevention and treatment of pressure ulcer (Injuries)*. Mt. Laurel, NJ: Author.

Wu, G. A., & Bogie, K. M. (2014). Effects of conventional and alternating cushion weight-shifting in persons with spinal cord injury. *Journal of Rehabilitation Research and Development, 51*(8), 1265–1276. doi: 10.1682/JRRD.2014.01.0009.

QUESTIONS

1. The wound care nurse is teaching a patient with a spinal cord injury (SCI) how to accomplish a clean transfer. What intervention is recommended for this procedure?
   A. Using a sliding board
   B. Using extra attendants for the transfer if needed
   C. Learning how to off-load bony prominences
   D. Choosing a softer mattress and chair pad

2. The wound care nurse is teaching pressure injury prevention to a patient with a spinal cord injury (SCI). What teaching point reflects a recommended intervention for patients with SCI to restore normal blood flow and oxygen levels?
   A. Sleep in the prone position if possible.
   B. Off-loading by leaning backward with the elbows on a flat surface.
   C. Tilt the seat-and-back unit to <65 degrees for 1 minute.
   D. Perform wheelchair push-ups for 60 seconds every 30 minutes.

3. The wound care nurse recommends skin checks for a paraplegic being transferred to a rehabilitation facility. What sign would indicate that a pressure injury is developing?
   A. Blanchable erythema that is present 15 minutes following off-loading.
   B. Warmth persisting 30 minutes following off-loading.
   C. An area of the skin feels cool to the touch compared to the rest of the skin.
   D. A reddened area does not return to normal color when off-loading 1 hour.

4. What assessment technique must the SCI individual (or caregiver) use to ensure a pressure injury is not developing unnoticed in the subdermal tissues?
   A. Observation
   B. Palpation
   C. Auscultation
   D. Percussion

5. The wound care nurse is teaching hygienic measures to protect the skin to a patient with a recently diagnosed spinal cord injury (SCI). What statement reflects a recommended guideline for this population?
   A. Bathe daily to remove perspiration.
   B. Use pH-balanced no-rinse cleansers on the skin.
   C. Do not use baby wipes on the perineal area.
   D. Remove bowel or bladder incontinence with alcohol wipes.

6. For what two comorbidities does the risk of mortality increase for the person with a spinal cord injury (SCI) by 1.4- and 2-fold, respectively?
   A. Diabetes mellitus and congestive heart failure
   B. Diabetes mellitus and renal failure
   C. Pulmonary disease and bladder cancer
   D. Renal failure and hypertension

7. The wound care nurse is aware that 47% of all pressure injuries occur over the ischial tuberosities and sacrum. What intervention would the nurse institute based on this statistic?
   A. Have the patient lie in a side-lying position to sleep.
   B. Tell the patient to stay out of the wheelchair as much as possible.
   C. Maintain the wheelchair and seat cushion in proper working order.
   D. Pad the bony prominences with foam overlays.

8. The wound care nurse is inspecting the wheelchair of a patient who just returned from a seating clinic. What is a recommended guideline for choosing a wheelchair seat?
   A. Shaped cushions are always contraindicated.
   B. A slightly reclined position should be maintained to improve function and prevent shearing forces.
   C. Thicker cushions should be used to facilitate dressing and transfers to other surfaces.
   D. The cushion should envelop the skeleton, spreading interface pressure across the whole seating surface.

9. The wound care nurse is investigating why modalities and treatments used in the management of wounds are less effective with spinal cord–injured patients. What is one reason that has surfaced?
   A. There is an increase in sympathetic innervation causing enhanced perfusion of the skin and soft tissues.
   B. TcPO$_2$ levels may be up to five times lower below the level of injury than above, decreasing oxygen to the wound.
   C. Collagen is not excreted as quickly through the urine of a person with SCI causing a buildup in the wound bed.

   D. SCI patients have a significantly higher concentration of fibronectin, which counteracts the function of collagen.

10. The wound care nurse is preparing a patient who has a spinal cord injury for tissue flap surgery to heal a pressure injury. What intervention is a recommended guideline for postsurgical care?
   A. Monitoring the site for ischemic changes
   B. Off-loading the site every 2 hours for 6 weeks
   C. Placing the patients on an alternating pressure overlay
   D. Initiating sitting 1 week after surgery

ANSWERS AND RATIONALES

1. B. Rationale: If the person is unable to self-transfer, the patient needs to know how to properly educate an assistant or attendant to transfer him or her safely.

2. A. Rationale: Frequent position changes are recommended, and off-loading the posterior surface of the body is advised if at all possible; sleeping in the prone position is optimal, and a variety of side-lying positions is recommended for those who are unable to sleep in the prone position.

3. D. Rationale: Reddened areas that do not return to color within a minimum of 1 hour require immediate response and intervention. Differentiate blanchable versus nonblanchable erythema using either finger pressure or transparent disk method and evaluate the extent of the erythema.

4. B. Rationale: It is important for the SCI individual (and/or caregiver) to use palpation as well as visual inspection.

5. B. Rationale: The best approach to cleansing is to use pH-balanced no-rinse cleansers; baby wipes can be used for perineal cleansing.

6. A. Rationale: Those with SCIs are at 1.4- and 2-fold higher risk of mortality from diabetes and congestive heart failure, respectively, than are able-bodied persons.

7. C. Rationale: The importance of a properly selected and maintained wheelchair and seat cushion is reflected by the fact that 47% of all PIs occur over the ischial tuberosities and sacrum.

8. D. Rationale: The cushion should effectively envelop (conform to) the bony prominences, redistributing interface pressure across the whole seating surface.

9. B. Rationale: Studies have shown TcPO$_2$ levels to be up to five times lower below the level of injury than above.

10. A. Rationale: The patient undergoing myocutaneous flap surgery requires meticulous postoperative care including consistent pressure and shear reduction, nutritional support, and monitoring for indicators of flap ischemia or congestion.

CHAPTER 17

GENERAL CONCEPTS RELATED TO SKIN AND SOFT TISSUE INJURY CAUSED BY MECHANICAL (EXTERNAL) FACTORS

Joyce Pittman

OBJECTIVES

1. Define the following terms: friction, shear, and pressure.

2. Explain the pathology and clinical presentation of each of the following:

   a. Moisture-associated skin damage

   b. Friction injuries

   c. Shear injuries

   d. Pressure injuries

3. Explain the concept of partial thickness versus full-thickness tissue damage.

4. Explain the importance of accurate classification of pressure and nonpressure injuries.

5. Identify the parameters most critical to accurate differential assessment of trunk wounds.

6. Utilize patient history, wound location, and wound characteristics to determine probable wound etiology.

7. Discuss current challenges in accurate wound classification.

TOPIC OUTLINE

● INTRODUCTION

The first portion of the Wound Management core curriculum focused on general concepts related to skin and soft tissue anatomy, physiology of wound healing, guidelines for wound assessment, and principles of wound management, to include both systemic factors and topical therapy. In addition, chapters devoted to wound healing and wound management for specific patient populations were included. In this portion of the core curriculum, we will delve deeper and focus on specific types of wounds and their management. We will discuss wounds caused by mechanical (external) factors, vascular and metabolic disease, infectious processes, dermatologic conditions, oncologic conditions, and trauma.

Mechanical (external) factors contributing to skin and soft tissue breakdown include, but are not limited to, friction, shear, pressure, and moisture. Trauma and other etiologies are addressed later in this section. Management of mechanical external factors is essential for prevention of skin damage, which is a key nursing responsibility in all care settings. This chapter will provide an overview of these mechanical external factors and the differences in skin damage that occurs specific to the anatomical layer of the skin. Partial thickness injury affects epidermal and dermal layers versus full thickness affecting deeper dermal or subcutaneous tissue. This is sometimes referred to the "top down" or "bottom up" pathway of soft tissue damage. Guidelines for differential assessment are provided, and current gaps in our knowledge and research base are addressed.

OVERVIEW OF MECHANICAL FACTORS CAUSING SKIN AND SOFT TISSUE DAMAGE

Moisture-associated skin damage, including incontinence-associated dermatitis, intertriginous dermatitis, friction lesions, skin tears, and shear/pressure injuries, are all examples of skin and soft tissue damage caused by external factors. Effective management of these factors can significantly reduce the incidence of skin and soft tissue damage. Most wounds caused by external factors are considered avoidable or preventable. Thus, the wound care nurse must educate health care professionals regarding the adverse effects of moisture, friction, shear, and pressure on tissue viability. Specific strategies must be emphasized to mitigate the effects of these external factors.

MOISTURE-ASSOCIATED SKIN DAMAGE

Normally hydrated skin is resistant to injury caused by external factors. However, overhydrated skin is associated with reduced tensile strength and increased vulnerability to damage caused by friction, shear, pressure, or exposure to pathogens, irritants, and enzymes (Gray et al., 2012). Various studies report histopathologic findings revealing inflammation of the upper dermis, dermal and epidermal disruption, and partial thickness erosion (Gray et al., 2012). These findings support that moisture-associated skin damage is a result of partial thickness damage to the skin caused by chemical and physical irritation at the stratum corneum layer (Beeckman et al., 2016).

Recent consensus sessions and documents have introduced the concept of "moisture plus" in the etiology of skin and soft tissue breakdown (Gray et al., 2011, 2012). Overhydration (maceration) results in increased permeability of the cell wall. This renders the epithelium more vulnerable to invasion by pathogens, irritants, or enzymatic agents. In addition, overhydration increases the friction coefficient between the skin and the underlying linen or absorptive pads. This translates into increased "drag"

(frictional forces and shear forces) when the patient is repositioned. Finally, multiple studies confirm the link between overhydration and pressure injury development, probably because macerated tissues are less able to provide normal pressure distribution (Doughty et al., 2012; Gray et al., 2011, 2012; Mahoney et al., 2013). As a result of increased understanding of the effect of moisture on skin health, a new focus on "skin microclimate control" has emerged (Kottner et al., 2018; Oomens et al., 2015); this will be addressed in more depth in the chapter on support surfaces (Chapter 22).

> **KEY POINT**
>
> Overhydrated skin is more vulnerable to invasion by pathogens, irritants, or enzymatic agents, is at greater risk for friction and shear damage, and is also at greater risk for pressure injury development.

The four most common types of moisture-associated skin damage are incontinence-associated dermatitis; intertriginous dermatitis; peristomal moisture-associated skin damage; and periwound moisture-associated skin damage (Gray et al., 2011). Each of these will be addressed in detail in Chapter 18 along with implications for management.

FRICTION

Friction (frictional force) is defined as the "resistance to motion in a parallel direction relative to the common boundary of two surfaces" (EPUAP/NPIAP/PPPIA, 2019). Specifically, when related to pressure injuries, friction is defined as "the contact force parallel to the skin surface due to internal bodyweight loads or forces exerted by a medical device" (EPUAP/NPIAP/PPPIA, 2019). For example, a situation when friction occurs is when skin is dragged across a coarse surface, such as bed linens. This type of skin damage should not be confused with or classified as a pressure injury. In the 2019 International Pressure Injury Prevention and Treatment Guideline, friction is described as "continuous or repetitive movement, rubbing or sliding of a material ... and can result in redness, inflammation or a lesion referred to as a friction blister. These blisters are not considered to be pressure injuries" (EPUAP/NPIAP/PPPIA, 2019).

SHEAR

There are two components to shear, shear stress and shear strain. Shear stress is defined as the "the force per unit area exerted parallel to the perpendicular plane of interest." Shear strain is defined as the distortion or deformation of tissue as a result of shear stress (EPUAP/NPIAP/PPPIA, 2019). In contrast, when normal forces (body weight) and shear forces are generated between the body and the support surface, the loaded

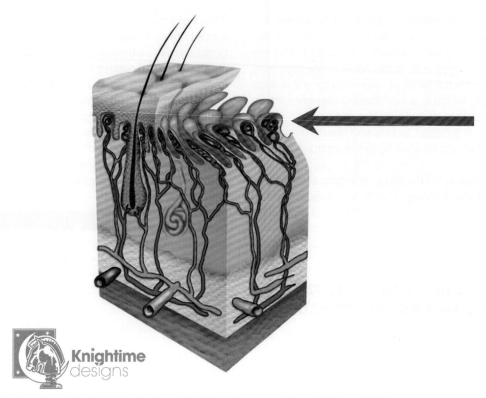

FIGURE 17-1. Shear is a Force Parallel to the Surface of the Skin. (Courtesy of Laura Edsberg, PhD.)

soft tissues distort and deform due to the mechanical load and strain. This distortion and deformation leads to impairment of the cell cytoskeleton or plasma membrane and impaired transport processes. Perfusion reduction, impaired lymphatic function, and altered transport in the interstitial spaces occur, resulting in cell death and inflammation. Continued damage is evident with increased permeability of the vasculature, which results in inflammatory edema, and increased interstitial pressures, which further increase the mechanical loads on the cells and tissues (EPUAP/NPIAP/PPPIA, 2019).

The specific cell and tissue damage caused by mechanical loads and strain is complex and depends on the individual anatomical structure and morphology, tissue properties, and magnitude and distribution of the mechanical forces applied (EPUAP/NPIAP/PPPIA, 2019) (**Figs. 17-1 and 17-2**).

Shear strain can cause either superficial damage, as occurs with skin tears, or deeper damage, as occurs with pressure injuries (Bryant, 2016). Skin tears most commonly involve shearing of the epidermal layer from the dermal layer, as a result of patient handling or adhesive removal; this type of superficial shear force usually creates a partial-thickness wound. Occasionally, the dermal layer is sheared from the underlying subcutaneous tissue, creating a shallow full-thickness wound. The pathology, prevention, and management of skin tears are discussed further in Chapter 18.

KEY POINT

Superficial shear can cause skin tears (due to shearing of epidermal layer from dermal layer). Deep shear is a causative or contributing factor to pressure injury development.

Deep shear strain occurs when the subcutaneous tissue shears against the dermal layer, creating distortion of the blood vessels (see **Figs. 17-1 and 17-2**). This type of shear occurs when the patient slides down in the bed or chair or when the patient is pulled up in bed without the use of safe patient handling equipment or low-friction coefficient linens (Bryant, 2016; Pieper, 2016). Deep tissue pressure injuries may occur in these instances and are due to the effects of shear force, anatomical and tissue properties, and magnitude and distribution of the mechanical load/strain.

PRESSURE

Pressure is defined as the "force per unit area exerted perpendicular to the plane of interest" (EPUAP/NPIAP/PPPIA, 2019). Sustained pressure (mechanical load) applied to soft tissues causes tissue deformation and ischemia and eventual tissue necrosis. The sustained tissue deformations may impair lymphatic function and obstruct interstitial fluid flow, which increases the risk of cell and tissue death (**Fig. 17-3**). When pressure is relieved and blood flow is restored, there is the risk of reperfusion injury, which can further compromise the

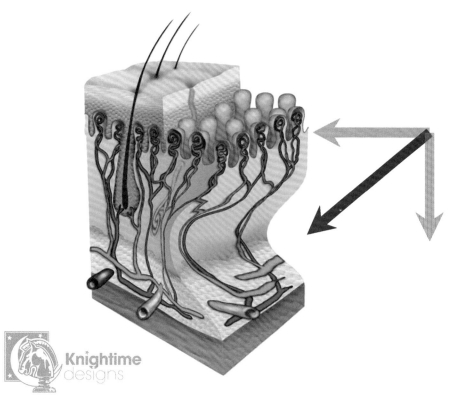

FIGURE 17-2. Tissue Distortion as a Result of Shear Force. The total force is the combination of both pressure and shear forces applied to the tissue. Depending on the magnitude of the components (pressure and shear), this force can significantly impact deep tissues. (Courtesy of Laura Edsberg, PhD.)

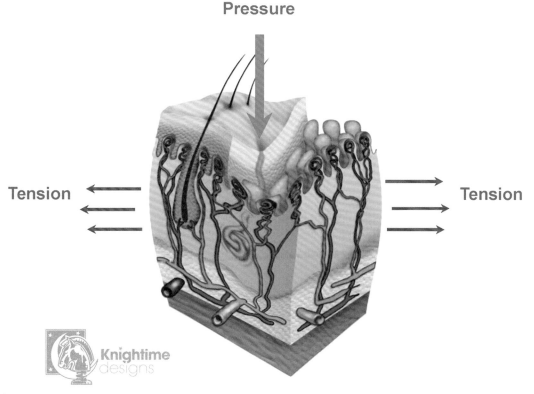

FIGURE 17-3. Pressure and Tension: Vertical Compression of Tissues Leading to Ischemia. Pressure (in pressure injuries) is typically defined as force perpendicular to the skin. When pressure is applied to the tissue, it is compressed and also experiences tension. (Courtesy of Laura Edsberg, PhD.)

already damaged tissues through the release of harmful oxygen free radicals and proinflammatory cytokines (EPUAP/NPIAP/PPPIA, 2019). Thus, pressure injuries typically present as ischemic wounds with significant tissue loss (see Chapter 20 for an in-depth explanation of pressure injury pathology and presentation).

> **KEY POINT**
>
> Sustained pressure causes tissue deformation, inflammation, and ischemia; thus, pressure injuries typically present as ischemic wounds with significant tissue loss.

DIFFERENTIATION OF SKIN INJURY

For many years, there was no attempt to differentiate between wounds caused by moisture and/or friction versus those caused by pressure and/or shear; any wound located in the trunk area was typically labeled a "pressure injury" (Bouten et al., 2003; Ceelen et al., 2008; Oomens et al., 2015).

IMPORTANCE OF ACCURATE CLASSIFICATION

Over the past decade, there has been increasing recognition that most pressure injuries are avoidable. As a result, third-party payers no longer provide reimbursement for facility-acquired pressure injuries, and the incidence of facility-acquired pressure injuries is a reportable quality-of-care indicator. Benchmarking of quality indicators is now standard, and such benchmarking data are available to the public. This means that facilities/organizations need to accurately assess and document any pressure injuries present on admission and to accurately differentiate between pressure injuries and other types of skin damage. Failure to accurately classify wounds based on etiology compromises the accuracy of benchmarking data and can potentially increase a facility's risk for fiscal penalties related to perceived poor quality of care. It is therefore critical for the wound care nurses to accurately classify wounds and to educate and assist their staff to classify wounds correctly (Mahoney et al., 2013). However, this is sometimes difficult to achieve since etiology is often unknown, and since some wounds are of mixed or unclear etiology.

ORIGINATION OF INJURY

One approach to assist the wound care nurse to differentiate pressure injuries from non–pressure-related wounds (those caused by moisture and/or friction) is the source of the injury. This approach reflects the primary location and source of skin damage. The damage from moisture and friction occurs at the upper most layers of the skin. This usually begins as a result of chronic or repeated exposure of the skin to a chemical irritant (urine or feces) or friction (Beeckman et al., 2016). In contrast,

damage occurring at the deeper tissue layers as a result of mechanical load and strain causes deformation, inflammation, and ischemia to the tissues (EPUAP/NPIAP/PPPIA, 2019). Current evidence indicates that most pressure injuries develop because the muscle layer is much more vulnerable to ischemia than the epidermis, dermis, and subcutaneous tissue. Thus, reduced perfusion will have the greatest effects at the muscle layer. Cell death actually begins within minutes of high mechanical loads causing intense tissue deformation. Tissue damage varies due to individual anatomical variation, tissue tolerance, and confounding factors (EPUAP/NPIAP/PPPIA, 2019). In contrast, nonpressure wounds develop because overhydration and friction primarily affect the exposed surface of the skin (Sibbald et al., 2011). Thus, most pressure/shear wounds are full-thickness wounds that exhibit evidence of ischemic damage, while most nonpressure wounds present as superficial wounds with evidence of abrasive force (and possibly maceration) but no evidence of tissue ischemia. In teaching clinicians to distinguish between pressure wounds and nonpressure wounds, it is sometimes instructive to have them ask: Is there evidence of ischemic damage or significant tissue loss? or Does this wound appear to have been caused by superficial mechanical damage that removed the skin one layer at a time?

> **KEY POINT**
>
> Pressure wounds develop because the muscle layer is more vulnerable to ischemia than the skin layers and subcutaneous tissue; in contrast, wounds caused by moisture and/or friction present as superficial wounds with evidence of abrasive force (and possibly maceration) but no evidence of ischemia.

GUIDELINES FOR DIFFERENTIAL ASSESSMENT

As noted, accurate classification of wounds according to etiology is critical in today's health care environment, and this is frequently very challenging for the wound care nurse. There are new technologies to enhance visual physical assessment and improve accurate prediction of skin damage. Thermography and subepidermal moisture measurement are two such technologies that are becoming more available to the clinician (EPUAP/NPIAP/PPPIA, 2019). The wound care nurse is therefore challenged to determine probable etiology based on comprehensive wound assessment, patient history, and understanding of the mechanisms of injury involved in each type of wound.

The assessment parameters to differential assessment of wounds include (1) location; (2) wound depth (partial vs. full thickness) and characteristics (indicators of pressure vs. indicators of maceration and/or friction); and (3) patient history (**Table 17-1**). The mechanism of injury

TABLE 17-1 DIFFERENTIAL ASSESSMENT FRICTION WOUNDS, MASD, AND PRESSURE INJURIES

WOUND TYPE	LOCATION	DEPTH	CHARACTERISTICS	PATIENT HISTORY
Friction	Body surfaces exposed to repetitive rubbing	Usually partial thickness (superficial)	Wound bed usually pink/red with no evidence of necrosis Edges may be well defined or irregular	Restlessness Frequent sliding in bed or chair Patient may be malnourished, diaphoretic, or on steroids
Moisture-associated skin damage	IAD: perineal area, inner and posterior thighs, buttocks ITD: between skin folds, particularly in a patient who is diaphoretic and/or obese	Usually partial thickness (superficial)	IAD: edges frequently indistinct; associated fungal rash common Both: Wound bed usually pink/red with no evidence necrosis ITD: linear breaks in skin at base of fold *or* superficial "kissing lesions"	IAD: prolonged or recurrent exposure to urine and/or stool ITD: trapped moisture beneath skin folds often due to diaphoresis or obesity
Pressure/shear injury	Over bony prominences Under medical devices Atypical: over nonbony prominences exposed to prolonged pressure (e.g., in a patient who was "found down")	Usually full thickness (Stage 3, Stage 4, unstageable, or deep tissue pressure injury)	Well-defined lesions with distinct borders Tunneling and undermining common, especially when shear involved Tissue necrosis usually evident (i.e., purple discoloration, blood-filled blister, slough or eschar, significant tissue loss)	Prolonged immobility Exposure to shear (sliding) force Use of medical device in area of damage May have periods of hypotension and/or vasopressor administration

for pressure injuries is deformation of soft tissue caused by mechanical load or strain, which leads to inflammation, ischemia, and ultimate tissue necrosis (EPUAP/NPIAP/PPPIA, 2019). Thus, pressure injuries are most likely to occur over bony prominences or under medical devices (where soft tissue deformation occurs more readily). In terms of wound characteristics, pressure injuries are often full-thickness (because damage usually begins at the muscle–bone interface), they typically demonstrate evidence of necrosis (significant tissue loss, purple discoloration, or blood-filled blisters), and they usually are well-defined lesions with distinct borders. Patient history reveals prolonged immobility, exposure to shear force, or use of a medical device associated with wound development (Pieper, 2016). Occasionally, pressure injuries occur over nonbony prominences in patients who have been immobile for a prolonged period of time or who have experienced a combination of unrelieved pressure and hypotension; however, the clinician will observe indicators of pressure damage such as well-defined areas of purplish discoloration. In contrast, friction injuries are typically located over nonbony prominences exposed to repetitive "rubbing" force as the patient moves around in the bed or chair. The wounds are usually superficial with no evidence of ischemic damage; the edges may be well defined or irregular (**Figs. 17-4 to 17-6**). Patient history reveals that the patient is restless or that the patient frequently slides down in the bed or chair and may reveal that the patient is malnourished, on steroids, or diaphoretic; however, the patient does not experience prolonged immobility (Mahoney et al., 2013). Moisture-associated skin damage occurs either between skin folds (in a patient with diaphoresis) or in the perineal area, inner thighs, and buttocks (in a patient with incontinence). The lesions are typically superficial (partial thickness), and the edges are frequently indistinct and irregular. The surrounding skin is macerated, and the patient history includes either diaphoresis or incontinence (Mahoney et al., 2013) (see **Figs. 17-1 and 17-3**).

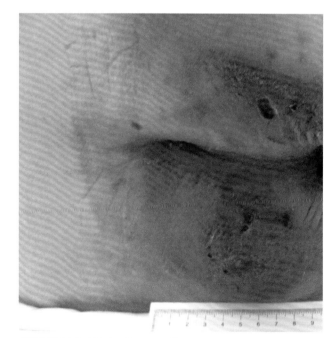

FIGURE 17-4. Friction Damage Characterized by Hyperkeratosis, Ridging, Lichenification, Scaling, Blanching Erythema, Shallow Full-Thickness Wounds, and Tissue Deformation. (Courtesy of Chris Berke.)

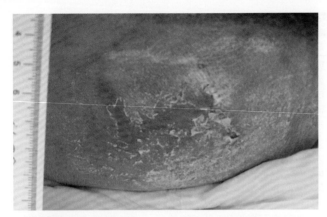

FIGURE 17-5. Mild Friction Damage Characterized by Hyperkeratosis, Scaling, Blanching Erythema. (Courtesy of Chris Berke.)

KEY POINT

Differential assessment of wounds includes (1) location; (2) wound depth (partial vs. full thickness); (3) characteristics (indicators of pressure vs. indicators of maceration and/or friction); and (4) patient history.

In some cases, wounds are of mixed etiology; in this case, that is, superficial skin loss with evidence of underlying pressure-related soft tissue damage. Patient history will reveal exposure to more than one mechanical stressor, for example, pressure and moisture.

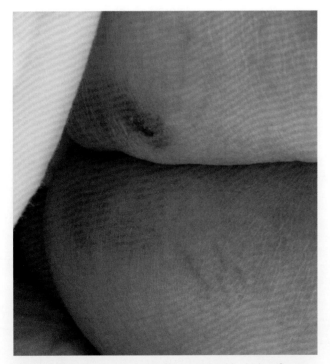

FIGURE 17-6. Friction Damage Characterized by Lichenification, Ulcer Formation, and Scaling. (Courtesy of Chris Berke.)

 CURRENT GAPS

There are gaps in the science related to the accurate determination of wound etiology. One gap is the incomplete understanding of the specific mechanisms of damage leading to both superficial and deep injury. There is increasing evidence that pressure injuries are caused by deformation of tissues that leads to inflammation and ischemia, and ultimately tissue necrosis (EPUAP/NPIAP/PPPIA, 2019). This cellular damage begins within minutes of the pressure event and often at the interface between soft tissue and bone. There is growing evidence to support the impact of skin microclimate (humidity and temperature) on the development of both superficial and deep breakdown. However, more evidence is needed to determine the specific interplay between skin moisture and friction and between skin moisture and pressure/shear injury. Evidence demonstrates that thermography, subepidermal moisture measurement, and ultrasound can augment visual physical assessment and determine the presence of tissue damage and provide early and accurate determination of superficial versus deep damage. These devices are not yet widely used in all health care settings. Currently, clinicians must base wound classification on the parameters discussed in this chapter (location, depth, characteristics, and patient history).

KEY POINT

There is a growing body of evidence to support the impact of skin microclimate on both superficial and deep breakdown.

 CONCLUSION

External factors (moisture, friction, shear, and pressure) are common causative and contributing factors to skin damage. Accurate identification of the specific etiologic factors helps ensure accurate wound classification, management, benchmarking, and reimbursement. However, accurate classification is not always easy, because many patients are at risk for multiple types of wounds, and accurate diagnostic tools are not widely available for determining depth of injury. Wound care nurses are reminded to consider the following questions when assessing a particular wound: does this wound appear to involve pressure damage or does it appear to be caused by external forces (moisture and/or friction) that remove the skin one layer at a time? The factors most critical to accurate differential assessment of wound etiology include location, depth, characteristics, and patient history.

REFERENCES

Beeckman, D., Van Damme, N., Schoonhoven, L., et al. (2016). Interventions for preventing and treating incontinence-associated dermatitis in adults. *Cochrane Database of Systematic Reviews*, (11), CD011627. doi: 10.1002/14651858.CD011627.pub2.

Bouten, C. V., Oomens, C. W., Baaijens, F. P., et al. (2003). The etiology of pressure ulcers: Skin deep or muscle bound? *Archives of Physical Medicine and Rehabilitation, 84*(4), 616–619.

Bryant, R. (2016). Types of skin damage and differential diagnosis. In R. Bryant & D. Nix (Eds.), *Acute and chronic wounds: Current management concepts* (5th ed.). St. Louis, MO: Elsevier Mosby.

Ceelen, K. K., Oomens, C. W., & Baaijens, F. P. (2008). Microstructural analysis of deformation-induced hypoxic damage in skeletal muscle. *Biomechanics and Modeling in Mechanobiology, 7*(4), 277–284.

Doughty, D., Junkin, J., Kurz, P., et al. (2012). Incontinence associated dermatitis: Consensus statements, evidence-based guidelines for prevention and treatment, and current challenges. *Journal of Wound, Ostomy, and Continence Nursing, 39*(3), 303–315.

European Pressure Ulcer Advisory Panel, National Pressure Injury Advisory Panel, and Pan Pacific Pressure Injury Alliance [EPUAP/NPIAP/PPPIA]. (2019). In E. Haesler (Ed.), *Prevention and treatment of pressure ulcers/injuries: Clinical Practice Guideline*. The International Guideline.

Gray, M., Beeckman, D., Bliss, D. Z., et al. (2012). Incontinence associated dermatitis: A comprehensive review and update. *Journal of Wound, Ostomy, and Continence Nursing, 39*(1), 61–74.

Gray, M., Black, J., Baharestani, M., et al. (2011). Moisture associated skin damage: Overview and pathophysiology. *Journal of Wound, Ostomy, and Continence Nursing, 38*(4), 359–370.

Kottner, J., Black, J., Call, E., et al. (2018). Microclimate: A critical review in the context of pressure ulcer prevention. *Clinical Biomechanics, 59*, 62–70.

Mahoney, M., Rozenboom, B., & Doughty, D. (2013). Challenges in classification of gluteal cleft and buttock wounds: Consensus session reports. *Journal of Wound, Ostomy, and Continence Nursing, 40*(3), 239–245.

Oomens, C. W., Bader, D. L., Loerakker, S., et al. (2015). Pressure induced deep tissue injury explained. *Annals of Biomedical Engineering, 43*(2), 297–305.

Pieper, B. (2016). Pressure ulcers: Impact, etiology, and classification. In R. Bryant & D. Nix (Eds.), *Acute and chronic wounds: Current management concepts* (5th ed.). St. Louis, MO: Elsevier Mosby.

Sibbald, G., Krasner, D., & Woo K. (2011). Pressure ulcer staging revisited: Superficial skin changes and deep pressure ulcer framework. *Advances in Skin and Wound Care, 24*(12), 571–580.

QUESTIONS

1. The wound care nurse is assessing a patient whose wounds were caused by external factors. Which of the following is an example of this type of injury?
   A. A pressure injury
   B. A venous leg ulcer
   C. Eczema
   D. A malignant wound

2. What is the best descriptor of tissue damage caused by shear strain?
   A. Superficial skin loss caused by separation of epidermal and dermal layers
   B. Tissue compression caused by sustained pressure
   C. Edema caused by impaired lymphatic function resulting from unrelieved pressure
   D. Subcutaneous tissue damaged by distortion of the blood vessels

3. Which type of wounds develop at the muscle–bone interface?
   A. Friction wounds
   B. Pressure injuries
   C. Wounds associated with incontinence
   D. Wounds caused by intertriginous dermatitis

4. What is the initial effect of sustained pressure on a body part?
   A. Tissue necrosis
   B. Tissue loss
   C. Tissue deformation
   D. Tissue remodeling

5. What is the driving force for the collection of data regarding facility-acquired pressure injuries?
   A. Patient satisfaction
   B. Quality indicators
   C. Infection control
   D. Minimizing staff workload

6. Which statement accurately describes an assumption wound care nurses can use when differentiating pressure wounds from nonpressure wounds?
   A. Current evidence indicates that most pressure wounds develop at the muscle–bone interface.
   B. Most pressure/shear wounds are partial-thickness wounds that exhibit evidence of ischemic damage.
   C. Most nonpressure wounds present as superficial wounds with evidence of friction and tissue ischemia.
   D. Diagnostic tools and imaging technology are readily available for use by clinicians in all care settings.

7. Which assessment parameter is of greatest value to differential assessment of wounds?
   A. Indicators of pressure versus indicators of maceration or friction
   B. Wound size
   C. Type of eschar involved
   D. Indicators of infected versus noninfected wounds

8. Which condition might the wound care nurse observe as an indicator of pressure injury?
   A. Maceration of surrounding tissue
   B. Excessive granulation tissue
   C. Edema
   D. Purple discoloration

9. A wound care nurse documents a wound as being of mixed etiology. What is the nurse describing?
   A. Patient history reveals exposure to only one mechanical stressor.
   B. The wound is limited to the superficial skin and tissue layers.
   C. Features of both superficial and deeper injury are manifested.
   D. Patient positioning affected the development of the wound.

10. What skin condition is associated with increased risk for pressure injuries?
   A. Dry skin
   B. Macerated skin
   C. Hyperkeratotic skin
   D. Skin manifesting a rash

ANSWERS AND RATIONALES

1. A. Rationale: Mechanical (external) factors contributing to skin and soft tissue breakdown include friction, shear, pressure, and moisture.

2. D. Rationale: Shear strain disrupts blood vessels from deeper structures and causes deep tissue damage, as occurs with pressure injuries.

3. B. Rationale: Shear strain disrupts blood vessels from deeper structures and causes deep tissue damage, as occurs with pressure injuries.

4. C. Rationale: Pressure injuries are most likely to occur over bony prominences or under medical devices where soft tissue deformation occurs more readily.

5. B. Rationale: Benchmarking of facility acquired pressure injury rates reflects quality of care and identifies opportunities to improve care.

6. A. Rationale: Pressure injuries are often full-thickness because damage usually begins at the muscle–bone interface.

7. A. Rationale: One approach to assist the clinician to differentiate pressure injuries from nonpressure related wounds (those caused by moisture and/or friction) is the source of the injury. The damage from moisture and friction occurs at the upper most layers of the skin.

8. D. Rationale: Pressure injuries typically demonstrate evidence of ischemia.

9. C. Rationale: Superficial skin loss with evidence of underlying pressure-related soft tissue damage.

10. B. Rationale: Maceration decreases the resistance of the skin to external pressure sources.

CHAPTER 18

PREVENTION AND MANAGEMENT OF MOISTURE-ASSOCIATED SKIN DAMAGE (MASD), MEDICAL ADHESIVE–RELATED SKIN INJURY (MARSI), AND SKIN TEARS

Debra Thayer, Barbara J. Rozenboom, and Kimberly LeBlanc

OBJECTIVES

1. Explain the pathology and clinical presentation of each of the following:

   a. Incontinence-associated dermatitis (IAD) (Refer to Chapter 19)

   b. Intertriginous dermatitis (ITD)

   c. Peristomal moisture-associated skin damage (PMASD)

   d. Periwound moisture-associated skin damage (PWMASD)

   e. Medical adhesive–related skin injury (MARSI)

   f. Skin tears (Type 1, Type 2, Type 3)

2. Describe strategies for prevention and management of each of the following:

   a. Incontinence-associated dermatitis (IAD) (Refer to Chapter 19)

   b. Intertriginous dermatitis (ITD)

   c. Peristomal moisture-associated skin damage (PMASD)

   d. Periwound moisture-associated skin damage (PWMASD)

   e. Medical adhesive–related skin injury (MARSI)

   f. Skin tears (Type 1, Type 2, Type 3)

TOPIC OUTLINE

INTRODUCTION

In this chapter, we will explore three common types of skin injuries: moisture-associated skin damage (MASD), medical adhesive–related skin injury (MARSI), and skin tears.

MOISTURE-ASSOCIATED SKIN DAMAGE

In 2010 a panel of nine clinicians and researchers met to discuss the etiologic factors resulting in chronic inflammation and erosion of the skin. The panel recognized that there were known etiologic factors resulting in skin damage, for example, pressure and shear that resulted in ischemia and ulceration, and peripheral vascular disease resulting in lower extremity ulcers. The panel's purpose was to increase attention to moisture as an etiologic factor in skin damage (Gray et al., 2011).

MASD is the term given to a group of dermatological conditions in which the integrity of the skin is compromised by prolonged exposure to moisture (Browning et al., 2018). MASD is characterized by inflammation and erosion of the skin caused by prolonged exposure to various sources of moisture, including urine or stool, perspiration, wound exudate, and mucus or saliva (Gray et al., 2011). The four most common forms of MASD have been identified as: incontinence-associated dermatitis (IAD), intertriginous dermatitis (ITD), peristomal moisture-associated skin damage (PMASD), and periwound moisture-associated skin damage (PWMASD). Wound care nurses are frequently consulted to identify and mitigate the source of moisture and recommend interventions to treat the skin damage, prevent further skin damage, and promote healing (Haesler, 2018).

A variety of terms have been used to describe MASD including irritant dermatitis, diaper rash, perineal dermatitis, moisture lesions, skin erosion, and perineal maceration. The skin changes associated with prolonged exposure to moisture have been traditionally linked to incontinence, but it is now realized that prolonged exposure to moisture from any source can cause skin damage (Voegeli, 2012; Woo et al., 2017).

Healthy skin serves to prevent the entry of harmful pathogens and also prevents excess fluid loss from the body. Excessive moisture from any source can cause overhydration, particularly of the outermost stratum corneum, which can precipitate inflammation and facilitate the passage of irritants into the skin, leading to dermatitis. Patients with MASD experience intense, persistent symptoms such as pain, burning, and pruritus, especially where skin breakdown involves partial-thickness erosions and denudement. Emerging evidence highlights the association between MASD and other skin conditions such as dermatitis, cutaneous fungal and bacterial infection, and pressure injuries (Woo et al., 2017). Skin damage is attributable to overhydration complicated by one of the following: chemical irritants within the moisture source; mechanical factors such as friction; and/or invasion of pathogenic microorganisms. For example, when the skin is exposed to liquid stool, the enzymes and irritants in the stool may cause inflammation and skin damage. Similarly, persistent urinary and/or fecal incontinence may create an environment favorable to overgrowth of yeast, and candidiasis is commonly seen in patients with IAD. The combination of overhydrated skin and minor friction can cause skin loss (Berke, 2015; Gray et al., 2011; Mahoney & Rozenboom, 2019) (**Fig. 18-1**).

KEY POINT

Moisture alone causes maceration. Intense inflammation and skin loss are usually due to a combination of maceration and some other source of injury (chemical irritant, friction, or pathogenic invasion).

When friction is added to moist skin, the skin is more vulnerable to the erosive forces of friction. Macerated skin has less tolerance to the friction forces (Black et al., 2011). The overhydrated stratum corneum allows

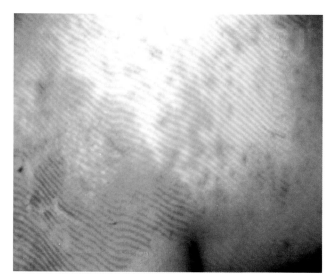

FIGURE 18-1. Candidiasis.

common pathogens such as *Candida* and *Staphylococcus* to enter, potentially leading to a secondary infection (Voegeli, 2012).

Other factors that affect the protective barrier of the skin include age, obesity, and the environment. As people age, the skin becomes thinner and dryer, and the barrier function is compromised due to increased adipose tissue. Obese persons store heat longer than do lean individuals resulting in less efficient heat loss when challenged by a warm, humid environment or physical activity (Gray et al., 2011). Obese individuals produce more sweat, and this exposes the skin to increased moisture, especially in skin folds.

Microclimate is defined as the temperature and humidity in a specified location. It manifests as an interaction between skin temperature and moisture at the skin surface. Environmentally, the relative humidity affects transepidermal water loss (TEWL) (Gray et al., 2011). When humidity is reduced, TEWL is increased and the stratum corneum becomes drier. If the humidity is increased, the rate of TEWL decreases and the stratum corneum becomes overhydrated, impairing its mechanical integrity and its ability to act as an effective barrier (Falloon et al., 2018).

The National Pressure Injury Advisory Panel (NPIAP) defines friction as the resistance to motion in a parallel direction relative to the common boundary of two surfaces (NPIAP, 2020). Skin injury by friction initially appears as erythema and progresses to an abrasion. Friction primarily affects superficial layers and thus does not result in tissue necrosis, while shearing forces mainly affect deeper tissue layers (Berke, 2015; Bryant, 2016). Friction occurs when caregivers use vigorous rubbing during cleansing of the perineal area or when the skin rubs against incontinence garments or bed or chair surfaces. Caregivers should be instructed to use gentle cleansing techniques and soft cloths (McNichol, 2018). Turn sheets

and lift devices should be used to reduce friction during repositioning or transfer. Prevention and treatment of MASD may encompass a variety of options including specialized equipment or surfaces, incontinence products, customized linen and fabrics, dressings, and skin cleansing agents, in addition to topical application of barriers and moisturizers to protect or strengthen the skin (Woo et al., 2017).

PREVALENCE AND INCIDENCE

A quality improvement project by Werth and Justice (2019) looking at the prevalence of multiple forms of MASD in an acute care setting revealed the prevalence of MASD was 4.34% (62 out of 1,427 patients). Twenty-two (1.54%) were found to have IAD, thirty-eight (2.66%) had ITD, and two (0.14%) had PMASD (Lachenbruch et al., 2016; Werth & Justice, 2019). Arnold-Long & Johnson (2019) measured the prevalence of IAD and ITD upon admission to hospital and the incidence of hospital-acquired IAD and ITD in acutely ill adults from January 1, 2014, to December 31, 2016. The mean prevalence of IAD present on admission was 16%. The mean incidence of hospital-acquired IAD during the data collection period was 23%. Patients classified as normal weight from their body mass index and patients 60 years and older had the highest incidence of hospital-acquired IAD. The mean prevalence of ITD for patients admitted to the hospital was 40%. The mean incidence of hospital-acquired ITD was 33%. The incidence of ITD was higher in patients classified as obese based on body mass index in patients 60 years and older. The most common location was the gluteal cleft (Arnold-Long & Johnson, 2019). Globally, the incidence of IAD is between 3.4% and 50% and the prevalence of IAD is estimated to be between 5.7% and 27%, with the highest prevalence in acute care settings. While certain patient populations may be more vulnerable to IAD, wide variations in the prevalence of IAD may be explained by the lack of internationally agreed diagnostic criteria (Beeckman, 2017).

Beeckman et al. (2018) developed the Ghent Global IAD Categorization Tool (GLOBIAD) and evaluated its psychometric properties. The GLOBIAD consists of two categories based on the presence of persistent redness (category 1) and skin loss (category 2), both of which are subdivided based on the presence of clinical signs of infection. More research is needed to evaluate the reliability of GLOBIAD and to find out whether better classification skills would improve IAD prevention and treatment (Beeckman et al., 2018).

Gray and Giuliano (2018) measured the prevalence of IAD among incontinent persons in the acute care setting, characteristics of IAD in this group, and associations among IAD, urinary, fecal, and dual incontinence, immobility, and pressure injury in the sacral area. The overall prevalence rate of IAD was 21.3% (1,140/5,342); the prevalence of IAD among patients with incontinence was

45.7% (1,140/2,492). Slightly more than half of the IAD was categorized as mild (596/1,140, 52.3%), 27.9% (318/1,140) was categorized as moderate, and 9.2% (105/1,140) was deemed severe. In addition, 14.8% (169/1,140) of patients with IAD also had a fungal rash. The prevalence of pressure injury in the sacral area among individuals with incontinence was 17.1% (427/2,492), and the prevalence of full-thickness pressure injury in this population was 3.8% (95/2,492). The authors concluded that their research supported clinically relevant association between IAD and pressure injury of the sacral area and even after controlling for immobility, IAD may be an independent risk factor for pressure injury occurrence.

INCONTINENCE-ASSOCIATED DERMATITIS

IAD is the most common form of MASD. A 2005 consensus statement defined IAD as inflammation of the skin that occurs when urine or stool comes in contact with perianal or perigenital skin (Gray et al., 2007). Gray and colleagues subsequently updated the definition to an irritant dermatitis that develops from chronic exposure to urine or liquid stool (Gray et al., 2011). Skin exposed to urine and stool, especially liquid stool, is at risk for IAD. The term dermatitis denotes inflammation and erythema with or without erosion or denudation; IAD specifically identifies the source of the irritant (urine or fecal incontinence) and acknowledges that the area of the skin affected commonly extends beyond the perineum (Beeckman et al., 2016; Gray et al., 2012) (**Fig. 18-2**).

Refer to Chapter 19 for a comprehensive review of IAD.

INTERTRIGINOUS DERMATITIS

ITD, also referred to as intertrigo, is an inflammatory skin condition that affects opposing skin surfaces. This condition can develop in any area of the body where two skin surfaces are in contact (Arnold-Long et al., 2018).

Pathology

Intertrigo is a common skin condition in all care settings including care homes and home care. Obese and diabetic patients and patients needing help with hygiene and getting dressed are at particular high risk. Adequate skin care strategies might be helpful to prevent this skin problem (Kottner et al., 2020; Mitchell & Hill, 2020). Intertrigo is thought to be caused by a combination of two factors: overhydration of the skin due to trapped moisture and friction between the opposing skin folds (i.e., skin rubbing against skin). The overhydrated stratum corneum drags rather than glides over opposing skin surfaces, which leads to increased friction and the risk of skin damage. Intertrigo can coexist with IAD (Arnold-Long & Johnson, 2019; Gray, 2004). ITD can also present as a linear skin tear at the base of the skin fold. The tear may occur when the overhydrated skin is stretched during routine assessment and skin care requiring separation of the skin folds. Contributing factors to ITD include reduced perfusion (common in adipose tissue), diabetes, and concomitant administration of steroids and antibiotics. Obese individuals are at high risk for ITD due to increased perspiration and the physical challenges to performing skin care (Voegeli, 2013). Obese individuals may have deep folds with constant skin to skin contact. These folds may be difficult to separate for effective cleansing and drying (Gabriel et al., 2019).

Clinical Presentation

ITD is commonly seen in the axillae, intergluteal cleft, inguinal region, inframammary region, and abdominal folds. Obese individuals often develop ITD under an abdominal or pubic pannus (Voegeli, 2012). ITD can also occur in the neck folds of infants, where moisture from drooling is trapped in the deep creases of the neck (Janniger et al., 2005; Tüzün et al., 2015).

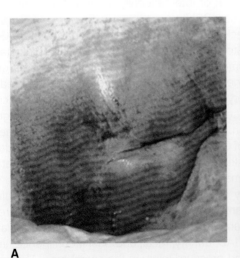
A

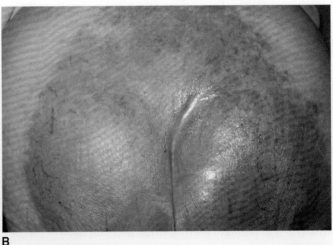
B

FIGURE 18-2.   A, B. Incontinence-Associated Dermatitis (IAD). Note diffuse erythema, patchy areas of denudation, and coexisting candidiasis. (Courtesy of KDS Consulting.)

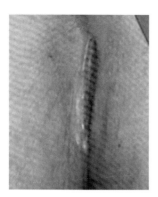

FIGURE 18-3. Intertriginous Dermatitis (ITD): Linear Lesions Located at Base of Skin Fold in Area of Maceration.

The earliest indicator of ITD is mild erythema. If left untreated, the condition may progress to severe inflammation with mirrored areas of skin erosion or linear fissure formation (**Fig. 18-3**). ITD lesions are typically partial thickness, though there are anecdotal reports of progression to full-thickness lesions when treatment is delayed or ineffective. The patient may report pain, itching, burning, and odor. Macerated skin can become inflamed and denuded, which produces a breeding ground for many microorganisms. These organisms thrive in the moist, warm environment created by trapped moisture and skin loss (Voegeli, 2012). The most common fungal organisms in ITD are *Candida* (Takahashi et al., 2020). Interdigital ITD is commonly complicated by the presence of dermatophytes. If ITD is not well managed, the bacteria present on damaged skin increases the risk for soft tissue infections such as cellulitis and/or panniculitis. Complications of ITD include secondary infections including *Pseudomonas*, *Staphylococcus*, *Streptococcus*, and antibiotic-resistant infections (Black et al., 2011; Gabriel et al., 2019; Tammel et al., 2019; Voegeli, 2012, 2013). If secondary infection is suspected, it is appropriate to perform a culture and sensitivity. Skin lesions with atypical clinical presentations or lesions that are not responsive to treatment should be referred to dermatology for diagnosis (Arnold-Long & Johnson, 2019; Janniger et al., 2005). (See Chapter 11 for more information about infection.)

KEY POINT

ITD is caused by trapped perspiration in a skin fold causing maceration, and friction or slight mechanical stretch that may cause superficial breakdown or a linear fissure (i.e., erosion) at the base of the fold.

Prevention

There is limited evidence to support any specific preventive measures (Janniger et al., 2005; Mistiaen & van Halm-Walters, 2010). There is currently no formal risk assessment tool available. Because of recent increases in obesity rates, intertrigo has been assigned a specific code within the International Classification of Diseases (ICD). Prevention of ITD should be focused on measures to keep skin folds clean and dry and measures to reduce friction. Skin folds should be cleansed gently with a soft cloth and a pH-balanced spray cleanser or pre-moistened no-rinse cloth. The skin fold should be patted dry or dried with a handheld dryer on a cool setting. The patient should be encouraged to wear lightweight and loose-fitting clothing in order to wick moisture away from the skin and should be taught to avoid the use of plain gauze pads, paper towels, or coffee filters between the skin folds, since these can actually trap the moisture and increase the risk for maceration of the skin. In the patient care setting, effective strategies include positioning to enhance air flow to the area and placement of wicking textile or absorptive padding between the skin folds (Black et al., 2011; Kalra et al., 2014).

Treatment

Treatment of ITD begins with a thorough and complete examination of all skin folds. Conventional treatment, much like preventive measures, should focus on minimizing moisture and friction. Topical treatments such as powders and barrier creams have little or no proven benefits (Janniger et al., 2005).

A moisture wicking fabric with antimicrobial silver (Interdry®) can be used in skin folds to wick away moisture. The fabric is placed between the folds of skin and should extend from the base of the fold to at least 2 inches beyond the fold to allow for wicking and evaporation. The antimicrobial agent is intended to reduce the risk of cutaneous infections including candidiasis. The silver within the textile provides antimicrobial action for up to 5 days. Placement of the low coefficient of friction (CoF) textile provides separation of the body folds and reduces the risk of friction damage. In the past, multiple interventions have been used unsuccessfully, including feminine hygiene products, washcloths, deodorant, powders, and abdominal pads. These products do not wick moisture away from the skin fold. When using the wicking textile, the use of powders and creams should be avoided (Kalra et al., 2014). Treatment should continue until the ITD has resolved. Continued use of the wicking textile may prevent reoccurrence (Gray et al., 2007).

ITD complicated by fungal infection may also be managed with topical antifungals. Nystatin is effective only for candidal intertrigo. Clotrimazole, ketoconazole, oxiconazole (Oxistat®), or econazole may be used for both *Candida* and dermatophyte infections. Topical treatments are applied twice daily until the rash resolves. Fluconazole (Diflucan®) 100 to 200 mg daily for 7 days, is used for resistant fungal infections, although patients who are obese may require an increased dosage. Oral azoles may potentiate the effects of hypoglycemic agents, leading to low blood glucose levels, and patients with diabetes should be instructed to monitor their blood glucose levels with concomitant use of these medications (Kalra et al., 2014).

PERIWOUND MOISTURE-ASSOCIATED SKIN DAMAGE

The literature defines periwound skin as the area within 4 cm of a wound edge, which is at the greatest risk for skin damage caused by exposure to wound exudate. Cases of more extensive PWMASD have been noted when there is caustic drainage from a wound or fistula (Colwell et al., 2017). Periwound skin is vulnerable to MASD when drainage volume exceeds the fluid-handling capacity of a dressing (Mitchell & Hill, 2020; Woo et al., 2017).

Pathology

The etiology and pathophysiology of PWMASD are not well understood but are likely due to a combination of overhydration (maceration), inflammation, and friction. The production of exudate is normal during the inflammatory phase of wound healing due to osmotic and hydrostatic forces that cause fluid to leak from the blood vessels. The exposed stratum corneum responds by absorbing the exudate (Gray et al., 2011). As a result, the underlying epidermal layers become overhydrated and macerated; this renders the periwound skin more vulnerable to friction damage and to penetration by pathogens and irritants. Macerated skin is more prone to MARSI that is, epidermal stripping with removal of adhesive dressings (McNichol et al., 2013). The resultant loss of the epidermal layer causes denudement, which further increases exposure of the periwound tissue to moisture (Colwell et al., 2011).

Current evidence indicates a greater risk of PWMASD with chronic wounds as opposed to acute wounds due to differences in chronic wound exudate. All wound exudate contains cellular debris and enzymes, which are potentially damaging to the skin. The enzymes in acute wounds tend to be inactive, and there are lower levels of cellular debris. In contrast, the exudate produced by chronic wounds contains higher levels of active proteolytic enzymes such as matrix metalloproteinases (MMPs) and proinflammatory cytokines. Chronic wounds are more likely to become infected, which further increases the volume of enzymatic exudate (Colwell et al., 2011; Cutting & White, 2002).

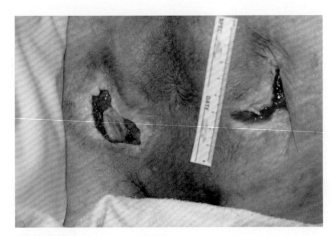

FIGURE 18-4. Periwound MASD.

Clinical Presentation

Clinical indicators of PWMASD include erythema, maceration, and skin loss. Macerated skin typically appears wet, hyperhydrated, and wrinkled. It is important to realize that the initial presentation may be different in patients with darker skin tones. Erythema may be masked, and maceration may present as gray-white, wrinkled skin (Voegeli, 2013) (**Fig. 18-4**).

Prevention

The goal in the prevention of PWMASD is to maintain a moist wound bed while keeping the periwound skin dry (Colwell et al., 2011). Strategies to prevent PWMASD include (1) confining the filler dressing to the wound bed, (2) the selection of dressings that provide effective exudate control, (3) appropriate frequency of dressing change to prevent overhydration and leakage of exudate onto the periwound skin, and (4) protection of the periwound skin with moisture barrier products. Staff and caregivers should be educated to change saturated or leaking dressings rather than reinforcing them. Wet dressings will trap moisture against intact skin and lead to the development of PWMASD (Gray & Weir, 2007). (See Chapters 8 and 9 for additional information about protection of periwound skin and dressing selection.)

Management

Dressings designed to absorb moisture such as alginates, hydrofibers, foams, hydrocolloids, and antimicrobial dressings should be considered for treatment options. While it would be ideal for dressings to pull fluid up into the dressing (vertical wicking) and minimize the risk of fluid exposure to the periwound skin, be aware that dressings may differ in their capacity to wick and absorb fluid (Okan et al., 2007). Negative pressure wound therapy (NPWT) can be effective in removing edema and wound exudate, reducing the risk of periwound moisture. Clinical experience demonstrates that inappropriately sized or applied NPWT can paradoxically promote PWMASD. Applying hydrocolloid products or transparent films may be used to protect the periwound skin from exposure to exudate. Pouching systems should be considered for wounds with >200 mL of exudate/day (Colwell et al., 2011). Many of these systems have detachable windows that provide access to the wound for assessment and care while containing the drainage and providing protection of the periwound skin (Hess, 2020). Extra caution is needed with patients who are incontinent to avoid soiled or saturated dressings from coming in contact with the skin (Woo et al., 2017).

Gray and Weir reviewed evidence on the prevention and management of PWMASD and found a reduced risk of maceration with application of a liquid acrylate skin protectant or a petrolatum- or zinc-based skin protectant (Gray & Weir, 2007). Moisture barrier ointments may be effective in preventing exposure of periwound skin to exudate but may interfere with the adherence of the dressing. They may be more appropriate for wounds managed with nonadhesive dressings. Liquid acrylate skin protectant may be used for wounds requiring periwound protection. A study by Cameron and associates compared a zinc-based product and a no-sting barrier film for prevention of periwound maceration and irritation associated with venous leg ulcers (VLUs). Both products proved effective. The no-sting barrier films were found to be easier to apply and were transparent. The zinc-based product was messy to apply and difficult to remove, which increases nursing time for wound care (Cameron et al., 2005).

O'Connor and Murphy (2014) estimated the clinical and cost-effectiveness of using a skin protectant (Cavilon No Sting Barrier Film [NSBF] or Cavilon Durable Barrier Cream [DBC]; 3M) compared with not using a skin protectant in the management of VLUs. There was a significantly greater reduction in wound size among patients in the NSBF group. The authors concluded that use of NSBF leads to significantly greater wound size reduction than that observed in the other groups and it may facilitate the healing of larger wounds without increasing costs (O'Connor & Murphy, 2014).

PERISTOMAL MOISTURE-ASSOCIATED SKIN DAMAGE

PMASD is inflammation and erosion of the skin related to moisture that begins at the stoma/skin junction and can extend to include all skin under the pouching system (Colwell et al., 2011; Gray et al., 2013).

Pathology

PMASD can occur when there is prolonged or recurrent exposure of the peristomal skin to the effluent from any type of stoma including urine and fecal ostomies, tracheostomies, and gastrostomies. The most common cause of peristomal skin damage is prolonged exposure to stool or urine. Peristomal skin damage can also be caused by prolonged exposure to perspiration, outside water sources (bathing, swimming), or wound drainage.

Several studies have been done on the prevalence and incidence of peristomal skin damage. A descriptive study performed in 2014 involved 796 wound, ostomy and continence nurses in the United States and Canada who are currently caring for patients with ostomies. Study results reported that participants estimated approximately 77.7% of their patients developed peristomal skin issues. The most commonly identified problem was irritant contact dermatitis (PMASD). Contributing factors include inappropriate sizing of pouching system and lack of follow-up after hospital discharge (Colwell et al., 2017). One study reported that the majority of peristomal complications occur within the first 2 weeks following discharge (Persson et al., 2010). Patient education is often limited in the postoperative phase as a result of short acute care stays and limited options for ostomy education once the patient is discharged home (Colwell et al., 2011, 2016).

When the skin barrier of the ostomy appliance is dislodged or leaks, it allows effluent from the stoma to have contact with the skin around the stoma. The greatest risk occurs when the skin is exposed to highly enzymatic liquid stool, such as the effluent from an ileostomy. Enzymes from the small intestine cause erosion of the skin when the effluent is in contact for even a short period of time, and bacteria in the stool may lead to a secondary infection (Colwell et al., 2011). Fecal stomas with liquid output, such as ileostomies, are associated with a higher degree of skin breakdown complications (Ratliff, 2010). Thicker or formed stool contains less moisture and fewer enzymes and is less likely to lead to skin damage. Urine does not contain enzymes and so is less damaging to the skin than liquid stool; however, prolonged exposure of the peristomal skin to urine can cause maceration, compromise of the epidermal barrier, and other complications.

There are factors other than the effluent that can contribute to PMASD. For example, perspiration can become trapped under the skin barrier and interfere with an effective seal. The skin under the barrier can become macerated, with increased TEWL (Gray et al., 2013; Omura et al., 2010). Prolonged exposure to outside water sources may also contribute to the development of PMASD. Pouching systems may require more frequent changes when the water-resistant adhesive on the ostomy appliance becomes impaired. Frequent appliance changes may cause mechanical stripping of the epidermal layer of skin. Inflammatory skin ulcerations that develop around the stoma and cause drainage may lead to impaired peristomal skin integrity due to exposure to wound exudate. The skin becomes overhydrated, which interferes with maintenance of an effective seal between the skin barrier and the skin (Colwell et al., 2011; Gray et al., 2013).

Clinical Presentation

Assessment should begin with determining the source of the moisture. Assessment of PMASD should include the integrity of the skin, the location of the affected area, and the distribution of the skin damage. PMASD is usually manifested by areas of maceration and erythema. Superficial skin loss is common. The ostomy pouching system should be assessed after removal to help determine the cause and location of the leakage. The patient's technique for pouch removal and application should also be assessed.

Prevention

Prevention of PMASD begins with a thorough clinical assessment and product selection by a wound and ostomy care nurse. Patients should be educated on proper peristomal skin care and application of the skin barrier. The goal in preventing peristomal skin complications is to establish an appropriate pouching system that provides a reasonable wear time and maintains a seal that protects the peristomal skin.

Treatment

Treatment of PMASD should focus on identifying and eliminating the cause of the moisture. The pouching system should be modified to eliminate exposure of the skin to urine or stool (or other sources of moisture). PMASD should be treated with topical products that will promote adherence of the barrier seal. Skin protectants containing cyanoacrylates have the ability to adhere to moist damaged skin surfaces and to protect and facilitate pouch adherence. Alcohol-free barrier films may be used in conjunction with stoma powder as part of a crusting technique to provide protection for the peristomal skin. Ostomy pouching systems may require more frequent changes until the skin damage has healed. For additional information on PMASD, see the clinical tool at **psag.wocn.org.**

Treatment may also include dietary modifications or pharmacologic interventions to thicken the stool output, wound care for the peristomal ulcerations, and treatment of secondary infections (Colwell et al., 2011). Prevention and management of PMASD are discussed further in the Ostomy Core Curriculum textbook.

CASE STUDIES

CASE STUDY FOR MASD

Ms. Green is a 25-year-old female who is being seen at the outpatient wound center for treatment of an open abdominal surgical wound post cesarean section. Assessment reveals the skin distal to the incision is moist and white and has a wrinkled appearance. The patient reports that with a newborn she is not always able to change her wound packing twice a day as ordered. The packing and cover dressing is noted to be saturated with serosanguinous fluid.

Any of the following treatment options would be appropriate for Ms. Green's wound:

- An absorbent wound filler such as an alginate or hydrofiber may be considered. An absorbent cover dressing such as a silicone foam could extend wear time and provide gentle removal.
- Negative-pressure wound therapy (NPWT) may be effective in removing edema and wound exudate, reducing the risk of PMASD.
- Periwound protection can also be accomplished with application of a liquid alcohol-free skin protectant or a petrolatum- or zinc-based skin protectant. Ointments may be effective in preventing exposure of periwound skin to exudate but can interfere with the adherence of the dressing. They are more appropriate for wounds managed with non-adhesive dressings.

⬤ MEDICAL ADHESIVE–RELATED SKIN INJURY

MARSI is defined as an occurrence in which erythema and/or other manifestation of cutaneous abnormality (including, but not limited to, vesicle, bulla, erosion, or tear) persists 30 minutes or more after removal of the adhesive (McNichol et al., 2013).

There are five types of MARSI:

- Mechanical
  - skin tears
  - epidermal stripping
  - tension blisters
- Maceration
- Folliculitis
- Irritant contact dermatitis
- Allergic contact dermatitis

Figures 18-5 to 18-12 demonstrate the clinical presentations of MARSI.

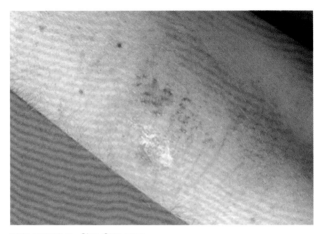

FIGURE 18-5. Skin Stripping.

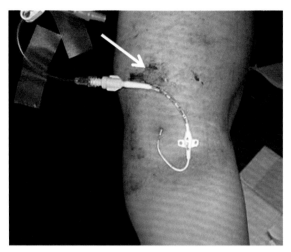

FIGURE 18-6. Skin Tear Adjacent to PICC Line.

---

9. USING BOTH HANDS, REMOVE SKIN BARRIER AT A LOW ANGLE PARALLEL TO THE SKIN, SLOWLY WHILE SUPPORTING THE SKIN AT THE SKIN-BARRIER INTERFACE.

Teaching Points
- Two hands are used to remove an ostomy skin barrier
- One hand removes the ostomy skin barrier by pulling downwards and parallel to the skin, the other hand is continuously repositioned to support the peristomal skin at the ostomy skin-barrier interface
- This minimizes potential skin stripping, trauma, and discomfort

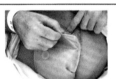

Figure 10. Pouch removal technique to minimize injury.

10. CONSIDER REMOVAL OF THE POUCHING SYSTEM MORE FREQUENTLY OR USE A DIFFERENT POUCHING SYSTEM WHEN ABDOMINAL DISTENTION OCCURS OR IS EXPECTED (EG, FOLLOWING LAPAROSCOPIC OR ROBOTIC ASSISTED SURGERY).

Teaching Points
- Abdominal distention may occur following colorectal surgery; this may be more prominent following laparoscopic or robotic assisted cases
- There may be rapid change to abdominal contours following laparoscopic or robotic assisted surgery that can contribute to PMARSI
- More frequent pouching system changes allow assessment of the peristomal skin and reduce the risk of PMARSI as abdominal distention resolves

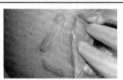

Figure 11. Blisters—in an area where previous barrier had a taped edge.

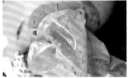

Figure 12. Ruptured blisters.

Discussion
Peristomal medical adhesive–related skin injury can occur in association with abdominal distention occurring after laparoscopic or robotic assisted surgery, and some panelists speculated about possible causes. The panelists discussed the possible role of skin barrier types and the timing of first postoperative pouch changes. The panelists discussed the implications for frequency of barrier removal and the selection of the pouching system *(1-piece, 2-piece, with or without adhesive border)*. This consensus statement begins with "consider" rather than being directive, given the variability in opinions about the topic.

11. LIMIT OR AVOID THE USE OF ADDITIONAL TACKIFIERS (ADHESIVE ENHANCERS) UNDER OSTOMY PRODUCTS.

Teaching Points
- Using additional tackifiers requires extra teaching to ensure they are used appropriately

Discussion
Some panel members required clarification on the definition of tackifiers and how they are used to increase adhesion. Other global members stated they never use tackifiers. Following these clarifications, the statement was agreed upon in the initial vote.

12. AVOID USE OF ADDITIONAL ADHESIVE PRODUCTS NOT DESIGNED FOR USE ON THE PERISTOMAL SKIN (EG, NONMEDICAL TAPES).

Teaching Points
- Discourage patients from using nonmedical adhesives such as duct tape
- If required, there are purpose-designed, skin-friendly adhesives that are available to secure the edges of the ostomy skin barrier

Discussion
Minimal dialogue was required to reach consensus on this statement on the initial vote. All nonmedical tapes and adhesives should be avoided.

Abbreviation: PMARSI, peristomal medical adhesive–related skin injury.

FIGURE 18-7. Tension Blister. (From LeBlanc, K., et al. (2019) Peristomal MASD. *Journal of Wound Ostomy and Continence Nursing*, *46*(2), 125–136.)

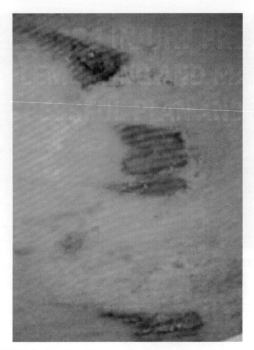

FIGURE 18-8. Tension Blister at Periphery of Dressing.

PREVALENCE AND INCIDENCE

Early data on skin damage attributed to adhesives comes from orthopedic populations with reported incidence between 13% and 35% (Cosker et al., 2005; Jester et al., 2000; Koval et al., 2003; McNichol et al., 2013; Polatsch et al., 2004; Sellæg et al., 2012).

Despite the universal and frequent use of adhesive dressings and tapes in clinical settings, only one study has evaluated prevalence and incidence of adhesive injury in a general patient population. Farris et al. (2015) reported daily prevalence of MARSI on two inpatient units in an academic medical center in the United States. Mean prevalence was 13.0% (range 3.4% to 25%). By age, median prevalence was highest for those 65 to 74 years

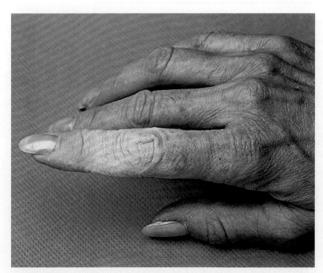

FIGURE 18-9. Maceration.

at 21.2% (range 0% to 60%). Erythema was the most commonly observed alteration. Prevalence of mechanical injuries ranged between 0.6% (skin tears) and 1.2% (stripping and tension blisters). The authors also reported skin damage by product category with the highest being surgical closures (type of product not specified), followed by electrodes and surgical dressings.

A study conducted in an ICU setting in Taiwan found a MARSI prevalence of 31% with 86% of injuries associated with tube securement. Use of elastic tape for endotracheal tube securement was identified as the most common cause, and the cheek and jaw were the most common locations (Hsu, 2015).

Wang (2019) reported MARSI in a pediatric intensive care population in China. Mean prevalence was 37.15% with stripping and skin tears the most common type of injury. The face was the most common location, resulting most often from securement of endotracheal tubes. Independent risk factors were age <2 years, presence of infection and edema, surgery and female gender. Earlier pediatric studies done by Noonan et al. (2006) and McLane et al. (2004) showed a prevalence rate for epidermal stripping of 8% and 17% respectively.

Ratliff (2017) observed a MARSI frequency of 5.8% in an outpatient vascular clinic population. For 6 of the 7 patients experiencing skin damage, removal of paper tape was identified as the causal factor. Damage for one patient was associated with use of surgical closure strips in combination with tincture of benzoin.

In a study of 155 long-term care residents 65 years and older, Konya and colleagues (2010) reported a cumulative incidence rate of 15.5%. Maene (2013) reported on a European survey, in which an incidence of 7.1% was reported, with skin stripping being the most common type of injury.

For patients with type 1 diabetes, ostomies and specific infusion therapy needs, the wear of adhesive products is a lifelong or long-term requirement. Adhesive-related skin problems associated with the wear of continuous glucose monitors (CGM) and continuous subcutaneous insulin infusions (CSII) have been described as occurring in 34% to 90% of patients (Berg, 2018a, 2018b; Ross et al., 2016; Schober & Rami, 2009). In these papers, skin damage is described as erythema, eczema, blisters, wounds and scarring.

In ostomy populations, irritant dermatitis (PMASD) is the most common skin injury, but peristomal MARSI (PMARSI) is also a concern. In the survey done by Colwell et al. (2017) ostomy specialists identified excessive use of tape as a key contributing cause and >50% of patients using a tape bordered product. LeBlanc et al. (2019) defined PMARSI as erythema, epidermal stripping or skin tears, erosion, bulla, or vesicle observed after removal of an adhesive ostomy pouching system. Unlike the MARSI definition, no time frame for observation was included.

---

13. CONTINUE PREVENTION INTERVENTIONS WHILE MANAGING PMARSI.

Teaching Points
- When PMARSI has been identified, appropriate treatment actions should be started
- Reeducate the patient on PMARSI prevention strategies

Discussion
The panelists agreed on the ongoing importance of prevention strategies when dealing with PMARSI. They clarified the wording to achieve consensus on this statement.

---

14. IDENTIFY AND MANAGE PERISTOMAL SKIN INFECTIONS/CONDITIONS (EG, FOLLICULITIS, CANDIDIASIS).

Teaching Points
- Folliculitis can occur in those who require shaving of the peristomal skin in order to maintain the pouch seal or when trauma from pouch removal results in hairs being pulled out
- Bacterial infection causes erythema and red pustules
- Appropriate hair removal, cleansing, and hair clipping techniques can decrease folliculitis
- Peristomal folliculitis may require antibacterial skin cleansing or treatment with an appropriate antibiotic powder
- Peristomal skin provides a warm, dark, and often moist environment for *Candida* to proliferate
- Over-the-counter antifungal creams may interfere with pouch adhesion
- An antifungal powder can be rubbed into the skin and sealed with barrier film spray
- Occasionally, a prescription may be required if the infection is severe or unresponsive to over-the-counter medications

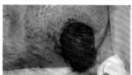 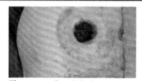

Figure 13. Folliculitis.   Figure 14. Candidiasis.

Discussion
The initial statement reviewed by the panel did not include examples, and the group felt it could be strengthened. They acknowledged that the goal was to provide information to help readers identify when an issue was present so that the reader could appropriately make referrals to a WOC nurse. Similarly, the panelists agreed to use the term "peristomal" skin infections/conditions rather than "secondary" skin infections/conditions.

---

15. MANAGEMENT OF PERISTOMAL SKIN DAMAGE FROM ADHESIVES MAY INCLUDE:

A. Application of stoma powder, additional stoma seal/ring/nonalcohol paste, or wound dressings to absorb excess moisture
B. Selection of skin barrier with more absorptive properties
C. Application of liquid barrier film *(eg, protective barrier film, cyanoacrylate)*
D. Avoidance of products *(eg, creams, ointments)* that interfere with ostomy barrier adherence
E. Use of antimicrobial cleansing for skin with folliculitis
F. Change product if known allergy to skin barrier
G. Consider topical steroid for hypersensitivity responses *(eg, allergy, secondary inflammation)*
H. Consider use of a nonadhesive product

Discussion
The panelists took considerable time to extensively debate the points for inclusion in this statement. Some items were removed and others expanded, reworked, and reordered. There was deliberation on whether all peristomal skin damage could be resolved by the measures included in the statement. Some panel members requested clarification that the focus of this statement was only for the treatment of PMARSI and not for PMASD. Consensus was achieved on the second vote.

---

16. PROVIDE PATIENT EDUCATION TAILORED TO INDIVIDUAL LEARNING NEEDS.

Teaching Points
- Assess patient learning styles and individualize their education and training

---

17. CONSULT A WOC NURSE IF CONDITION DOES NOT IMPROVE WITH TREATMENT WITHIN 3-7 DAYS.

Teaching Points
- Nurses should be advised to refer PMARSI to a stoma care nurse if there is not satisfactory improvement following the implementation of treatment
- Patients should contact a WOC nurse if PMARSI does not improve

Discussion
The panelists discussed the importance of reassessment for patients with PMARSI, and the timing of follow-up. There are differences in global expectations regarding time frame for referral, with some panelists believing referral should be immediate while others suggest escalation only if the condition does not improve and referral within 7 days is warranted.
The group came to agreement that a 3- to 7-day referral time meets global expectations.

FIGURE 18-10. Folliculitis. (From LeBlanc, K., et al. (2019). Peristomal MASD. *Journal of Wound Ostomy and Continence Nursing,* *46*(2):125–136.)

KEY POINT

The definition for peristomal medical adhesive–related skin injury (PMARSI) does not include the 30-minute time parameter and specifies that skin alternation is apparent after removal of an adhesive ostomy pouching system.

MARSI is common in vascular access populations. Zhao and colleagues (2018) measured MARSI prevalence in 697 oncology patients with peripherally inserted central catheters (PICCs). Total prevalence was 19.7% (137/697). Irritant contact dermatitis was the most frequently observed injury occurring in 76% (*n* = 103 of 137).

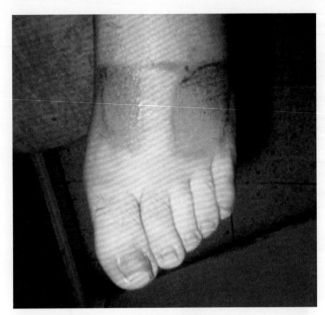

FIGURE 18-11. Irritant Contact Dermatitis.

TABLE 18-1 INTRINSIC AND EXTRINSIC FACTORS INCREASING RISK OF MARSI

INTRINSIC RISK FACTORS

- Age: the very young and the very old are at increased risk; extremes of age impact not only how individuals heal but also their susceptibility to developing a wound
- Skin changes: dermal and subcutaneous tissue loss, epidermal thinning, reduced levels of skin lipids/skin moisture content, reduced elasticity and tensile strength of skin
- Dehydration, poor nutrition, cognitive impairment, altered mobility, and decreased sensation
- Neonates: decreased epidermal-to-dermal cohesion, deficient stratum corneum, impaired thermoregulation

EXTRINSIC RISK FACTORS

- Increased risk of mechanical trauma during ADLs
- Use of soap (reduces the skin's natural lubrication)
- Dry skin more susceptible to friction and shearing
- Inability to reposition independently
- Sharp corners/edges that are not padded to protect

Mechanical injury represented 26% (35/137) followed by MASD (presumably maceration) in 7% (9/137). Age over 50, history of MARSI, and type of transparent film used emerged as independent and significant risk factors. Twenty-three percent of 92 adult oncology outpatients reported MARSI occurring during their treatment period. While the study did not specifically address vascular access–related injury, chemotherapy infusion was the most common reason for patient visits (Yates et al., 2017).

RISK FACTORS

Numerous intrinsic and extrinsic risk factors have been identified (McNichol et al., 2013), but a risk assessment tool has yet to be developed and additional work is needed to identify relevant population-specific determinants of risk (**Table 18-1**, Risk Factors for Skin Tears).

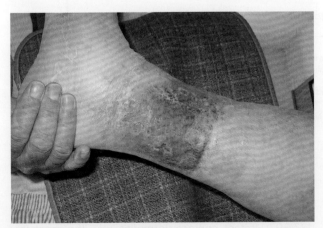

FIGURE 18-12. Allergic Contact Dermatitis (Patient with Sensitivity to Hydrocolloid Adhesive).

Age has been considered a significant risk factor, with the very young and very old being at greatest risk. The elderly are at risk due to changes in the dermal–epidermal junction that compromise the attachment of the epidermis to the dermis including flattening of the rete ridge and reduction in number of rete pegs. Reduced cohesion between skin layers significantly increases the risk of adhesive-related injury particularly from mechanical forces (Farage et al., 2009). Recent research using skin models suggests that age-related changes including the extent of *skin wrinkling* are risk factors for the development of superficial skin lesions (Sopher & Gefen, 2011). In preterm infants and especially those <27 weeks, maturation of skin structures has not yet occurred; as a result, the barrier function of the stratum corneum is absent or diminished, and there is very poor cohesion of the skin layers. In addition, the skin is much thinner in these infants (AWHONN, 2018; Visscher, 2015). These factors place these infants at increased risk for MARSI. (Please refer to Chapters 13 and 14 for additional details on age-related skin characteristics.)

Patients in intervention-intense settings such as critical care, perioperative care, or the emergency department are exposed to numerous adhesive products that may require repeated application and removal over the course of therapy. Individuals with central venous catheters, especially devices at jugular and femoral sites, may require frequent dressing changes increasing their risk for MARSI (Timsit et al., 2013). Patients with dermatologic diseases that disrupt epidermal barrier function are also at increased risk for adhesive injury. Patients who have degenerative, atrophic skin changes from long-term corticosteroid administration have fragile skin and are also at high risk for MARSI (Hadfield et al., 2019).

Oncology patients receiving cytotoxic therapy represent another high-risk group. Similar to patients with dermatologic conditions, those receiving targeted therapies also experience severe acneiform skin reactions increasing their risk for adhesive injury. These therapies are designed to block epidermal growth factor receptors causing severe skin reactions. Radiation therapy is also associated with high incidence of adverse skin changes (radiodermatitis). Early changes are due to inflammation and loss of epidermal cells, and late changes are due to chronic ischemia and fibrosis (Seité et al., 2017). As a result, these patients are likely more vulnerable to MARSI when adhesive products are needed. (Please refer to Chapter 31 for additional information on effects of cancer treatments.)

TYPES OF INJURY

Five types of MARSI have been identified (Bryant, 2016; McNichol et al., 2013). The wound care nurse needs to understand mechanisms of injury and the key assessment findings for each type of MARSI to develop and provide appropriate preventive care and treatment.

Mechanical Trauma

All adhesive products used in clinical practice can be expected to detach layers of cells to some degree (Alikahn & Maibach, 2009; Cutting, 2008; Dykes et al., 2001; Zhai et al., 2007). In some cases, this can result in significant disruption of the epidermis. TEWL is a sensitive indicator of stratum corneum integrity and barrier function, with TEWL levels rising as the skin's barrier function diminishes. TEWL can be measured with specialized instruments and has been used in tape studies to show that TEWL increases in direct proportion to the extent of stratum corneum damage (Grove et al., 2013, 2019; Hoffman & Maibach, 1976; Shah et al., 2005).

The term skin stripping is used to describe delamination of epidermal layers (McNichol et al., 2013). Any degree of stripping triggers cell division in the stratum germinativum (basal layer of the epidermis) in an effort to repair the disrupted barrier. No obvious injury will be seen with removal of just a few cell layers if the patient can initiate a healing response and if the recovery time (i.e., time between adhesive removal episodes) is sufficient for cell regeneration. A moist glistening surface is observed when sufficient layers are removed to expose the lower portion of the epidermis (Lund & Tucker, 2003) (**Fig. 18-8**).

Time to healing has not been reported for stripping sustained in clinical situations. Data from healthy volunteers have demonstrated return of barrier function (as evidenced by normal TEWL) within 6 to 12 days after stripping injury (Hoffman & Maibach, 1976.)

Within the MARSI framework, complete detachment of the epidermis from the dermis is described as a skin tear (McNichol et al., 2013). Complete epidermal loss creates a partial-thickness wound. The underlying moist dermis is visible, and significant discomfort can be expected as nerve endings are exposed (**Fig. 18-9**).

Several factors are implicated in the development of skin stripping and adhesive-related skin tears. Skin-related factors include overall health of the skin and the cohesive competence between the epidermal layers or between the epidermis and dermis (the degree to which the cell layers are attached).

Adhesive-related factors include type of adhesive, amount of tack to skin or aggressiveness of the adhesive, and the peel force, angle, and speed of adhesive product removal (Dykes, 2007; Jackson, 1988; Klode et al., 2010; Lund & Tucker, 2003; Tokumura et al., 2005; Waring et al., 2011). The use of aggressive adhesives can strip the epidermis, especially when the epidermis is immature or fragile and poorly anchored. Occlusive adhesives cause excessive hydration and increase the risk of cell disruption (Tokumura et al., 1999). Data comparing different manufacturers' adhesive products within a category have not been reported. Indiscriminate use of adhesion promoters (referred to as tackifiers) is believed to increase risk of stripping (INS, 2016; McNichol et al., 2013). Adhesive removal can disrupt epidermal cohesion and can create stripping injuries. It is important to use the correct technique for adhesive removal.

Tension Blisters

The term tension blisters describes another variation of mechanical injury (McNichol et al., 2013) (**Fig. 18-10**). When a shearing force is applied to skin and the skin to adhesive attachment is greater than that of skin layer to skin layer, the epidermis lifts from the dermis (Polatsch et al., 2004). Development of edema and the accompanying distortion of skin are key factors contributing to tension underlying the adhesive. Tension blisters have been shown to form when adhesive dressings or tapes are stretched or strapped during application (**Fig. 18-11**). When the tape is released following application under tension, the adhesive backing resumes its normal configuration. The resulting tension, that is shearing force, pulls the epidermis away from the dermis, causing a blister to form. The blisters are typically unroofed when the adhesive is removed, resulting in a partial-thickness wound that is painful. Tension blisters have primarily been reported in the orthopedic population (Cosker et al., 2005; Jester et al., 2000; Koval et al., 2003; Polatsch et al., 2004; Sellæg et al., 2012) but have also been associated with intravenous securement dressings and ostomy pouching systems (LeBlanc et al., 2019; Thayer, 2012). Key properties of adhesives contributing to tension blisters include lack of conformability and elasticity, and lack of breathability (Sivamani et al., 2003).

Distortion of the skin caused by edema, distention, or movement of the skin under an adhesive can increase the risk of skin injury. Highly mobile areas such as the neck, torso, joints, and upper extremities are at greater risk for injury. At these sites, skin moves along with underlying structures and could cause adhesive movement along the skin surface. Micro-trauma is described as adhesive dressing–mediated small magnitude cell and skin extracellular matrix damage (Rogers et al., 2013). This may manifest as erythema without blister formation at the periphery of adhesive dressings and tapes. This may result from frictional forces generated by skin movement under nonconformable adhesives (Tokumura et al., 2005). Frictional forces are increased when skin is moist or wet with an accompanying increase in the likelihood of skin injury (Sivamani et al., 2003). In a patient with significant diaphoresis, moisture and friction likely combine to contribute to skin injury. These factors underscore the need for proper skin preparation and application techniques for adhesives.

Maceration

Maceration is another type of MARSI (McNichol et al., 2013). The mechanism of damage involves overhydration of the skin under tape and has already been described in the section on MASD. Excessive hydration causes the epidermal cells (corneocytes) to swell with loss of the normal tight intercellular junctions (Zhai & Maibach, 2001). Overhydration reduces tensile strength and increases the risk of skin disruption with adhesive removal. Overhydration presents clinically as wrinkling of the skin surface and a change in skin color (to white or gray or a tone lighter than the surrounding skin) (**Fig. 18-7**).

Maceration is promoted by the use of occlusive or minimally breathable adhesive products or by adhesive products being left in place for extended periods of time. It is also influenced by the skin's microclimate. Increases in skin surface moisture can contribute to maceration, even when breathable adhesive products are used.

Folliculitis

Folliculitis is a dermatologic condition also included in the MARSI framework (McNichol et al., 2013). It is characterized by inflammation of hair follicles but is not exclusively associated with adhesive use. Causes include physical or chemical irritation or infection. Staphylococcal species are the most common offending organisms for infectious folliculitis (Dinulos, 2020). Assessment findings include erythema that is localized to the follicles (**Fig. 18-12**).

Pustules are noted in the presence of infection. The distinct localized lesions of folliculitis should be differentiated from candidiasis, a yeast-like fungus that manifests as an area of diffuse erythema with pinpoint maculopustular or maculopapular lesions at the periphery of the affected area. PMARSI with folliculitis may occur in those who require shaving of the peristomal skin in order to maintain the pouch seal or when trauma from pouch removal results in hairs being pulled out (LeBlanc et al., 2019).

Irritant Contact Dermatitis

The term irritant contact dermatitis describes cutaneous inflammation that is triggered by exposure to an irritant. The response is nonallergic and comprises a group of complex reactions that are not completely understood. Reaction threshold and severity are influenced by the offending irritant and vary from person to person (Bains et al., 2019). Reactions to products commonly used in clinical settings generally develop over hours to days. Erythema and edema are initial assessment findings (**Fig. 18-5**).

Vesicles may be present in addition to erythema and edema. Repeated exposure may result in a cumulative irritant contact dermatitis, which may persist for an extended period even if the offending substance has been discontinued (Widmer et al., 1994). The time required for resolution of adhesive-induced dermatitis in clinical settings has not been documented. Data from healthy volunteers have demonstrated return of normal barrier function, as evidenced by normal TEWL, within 6 to 12 days after injury (Hoffman & Maibach, 1976).

Adverse cutaneous reactions to skin care products (SCP) are becoming increasingly common and may be indicative of defective permeability barrier function. Liu et al. (2020) studied the differences in TEWL between skin patch positive versus negative to SCP in women. Out of 65 subjects, 24 (37%) displayed positive reactions to one or more SCP. The occurrence of positive reactions to patch tests did not correlate with either TEWL rates or hydration levels. The authors concluded that though many normal females display adverse reactions to SCP, the problem cannot be attributed to differences in the qualities of their epidermal permeability barriers. The reactions more likely reflect the potential adverse events of the SCP themselves (Liu et al., 2020).

Allergic Contact Dermatitis

Allergic contact dermatitis is a well-defined immune-mediated inflammatory response. The initial phase, sensitization, occurs when tiny protein molecules called haptens or nonprotein molecules penetrate the stratum corneum. The Langerhans cells normally present in the epidermis for immune surveillance bind to the invading allergen (the antigen) and then transport the bound antigen to the lymph nodes for presentation to T lymphocytes. If the T cell possesses a receptor that is complementary for the antigen, the T cell becomes sensitized to that antigen. The sensitized T cells then proliferate, returning to the skin and circulating through the bloodstream. As a result, areas of skin distant to the site of exposure can become populated with sensitized T cells. During the elicitation phase, sensitized T lymphocytes accumulate at the site of exposure. When repeat exposure to the offending substance occurs, proinflammatory mediators (cytokines and lymphokines) are produced by both antigen-specific and nonspecific T cells.

Some cytokines (e.g., tumor necrosis factor-beta [TNF-β]) exert significant, destructive effects on cells including epidermal lysis. Other inflammation-promoting chemicals such as histamine are released by mast cells and basophils during allergic contact dermatitis (Rietschel & Fowler, 2008).

Allergy has been described as consisting of two distinct phases with elicitation occurring as a result of previous exposure. It is recognized that these phases can occur simultaneously in some patients upon initial exposure to the antigen. Allergy does require antigen-specific susceptibility. Sensitization is more easily induced in individuals whose barrier integrity of the skin is already compromised. The presence of irritant contact dermatitis may increase risk for an allergic response in a susceptible individual (Lima et al., 2019).

In both irritant and allergic contact dermatitis, there is erythema of variable severity, which manifests as shades of pink to red. Primary lesions such as macules, papules, and vesicles are often present in the form of a diffuse rash (**Fig. 18-6**). Wheals may also be noted. It is important to recognize that distinguishing allergic contact dermatitis from irritant contact dermatitis on clinical assessment alone is difficult (Bains et al., 2019; Belsito, 2000; Marzulli & Maibach, 2008). Patch testing can provide definitive confirmation of allergy.

Shelanski et al. (1996) observed that every topically applied product has the potential to cause an adverse reaction in some individual. The diversity of individual immune response and skin sensitivity provides a meaningful perspective for wound care nurses who routinely apply a wide variety of topical products including adhesives to the skin. Other potential etiologies of dermatitis should be considered if similar lesions are noted beyond or distant from the adhesive footprint. A referral to dermatology may be indicated in these situations.

In many clinical situations, assessment of the skin is conducted rapidly after adhesive removal. It is common for bedside nurses to presume an allergic reaction when erythema is observed. This erroneous conclusion has resulted in many patients reporting they are allergic to adhesives. Transient erythema (also known as transient hyperemia) is commonly observed in light-skinned individuals when adhesives are removed. This represents a short-term inflammatory response triggered by corneocyte disruption and typically resolves within several minutes (Pinkus, 1952). The 30-minute time factor within the MARSI definition has provided clarity in differentiating this transient color change from actual injury (McNichol et al., 2013).

Data on incidence of contact dermatitis related to adhesive product use are limited. Anecdotally, wound care nurses report allergic contact dermatitis to be much less common than irritant contact dermatitis. In a study of ostomy patients, allergic contact dermatitis occurred in only 0.7% (Lyon et al., 2000). Within the extensive literature on occupational dermatitis, 90% to 95% of occupational skin damage is estimated to be irritant versus allergic (NIOSH, 2013). Based on available data and expert opinion, an adverse skin response that persists for >30 minutes is more likely to be the result of a contact irritation or mechanical damage than true allergy.

KEY POINT

Common types of MARSI include mechanical trauma (skin stripping, tension blisters, and skin tears), macerations, folliculitis, irritant contact dermatitis, and allergic contact dermatitis.

Prevention of MARSI

Five key interventions form the essential clinical approach to MARSI prevention (see **Box 18-1**).

Assessment

A thorough assessment should be conducted to (1) identify risk factors associated with MARSI development (see **Table 18-1**) and (2) inspect the skin. Two areas of risk warrant special attention. A focused patient history should be obtained to identify known or potential allergies and sensitivities (McNichol et al., 2013). Patch testing may be beneficial for patients: (1) undergoing chemotherapy or a surgical procedure requiring extended aftercare; (2) with complex skin problems; or (3) with a history of multiple allergies. Patch testing allows the wound care nurse to evaluate the commonly used adhesive products for patient tolerance and reactivity.

Assessment should also be focused on identifying patients at risk for mechanical injury (McNichol et al., 2013). In addition to the elderly and very young, patients of any age with significant edema (e.g., anasarca) or distention are at high risk for stripping or tension blister formation.

Selection of Correct Adhesive Product Based on Clinical Requirements and Patient Characteristics

Adhesives will adhere most effectively to a clean, dry, flat, immobile surface. Skin presents a challenging surface due to its unique characteristics. The epidermal surface is contaminated by the presence of dead corneocytes and surface oil. The skin's microclimate—a combination of skin surface temperature and moisture—varies with body temperature and environmental humid-

BOX 18-1   PREVENTION OF MARSI

1. Assess the patient.
2. Select the correct adhesive product based on clinical requirements and patient characteristics.
3. Prepare the skin.
4. Apply the adhesive product correctly.
5. Remove the adhesive product correctly.

ity and can produce moist or dry skin. Skin has contours and is mobile creating an uneven surface for adhesion. Elasticity allows accommodation of mobile surfaces (e.g., over joints) but presents a major challenge to adhesives. Adhesive products are better tolerated and less likely to fail in areas that are static.

Medical adhesive technology must accommodate these characteristics in order to provide effective clinical products. Understanding the fundamentals of this technology enables the wound care nurse to optimize product selection for securement and avoidance of skin injury.

How Adhesives Work

The majority of adhesive products consist of at least two components: the adhesive coating that attaches to the skin and the material or backing to which the adhesive is applied (**Fig. 18-13**). The combination of these components determines the characteristics of the product. Some tapes may incorporate additional layers, for example, a release coating that allows easier release or unwinding from a roll.

KEY POINT

One key intervention for MARSI prevention is selection of the best adhesive product based on clinical requirements and patient characteristics. In selecting adhesive products, the wound care nurse must consider both the adhesive coating and the adhesive backing.

While there is evidence of adhesive use in ancient times, the first modern tapes for medical care incorporated natural rubber and appeared in the late 1800s. World War II created a shortage of rubber and spurred development of synthetic polymers. Modern medical adhesives were introduced in the 1960s. These newer acrylates offered

good tack, material stability, and greater adaptability than did rubber adhesives (Lucast, 2000). Currently, the majority of medical products incorporate acrylate or silicone polymers, with natural rubber still used for some tapes. Other categories of adhesives include hydrocolloids (ostomy skin barriers and hydrocolloid dressings), hydrogels (incorporated into some electrodes), and zinc oxide–containing formulations (used in tapes).

Acrylate adhesives are considered pressure-sensitive adhesives. Pressure-sensitive adhesives behave like liquids and flow into the skin's irregular contours due to viscoelastic properties. When using pressure-sensitive adhesive products, the wound care nurse should apply with gentle warming hand pressure to promote adhesion of the adhesive product to the skin (Yates et al., 2017). Pressure-sensitive adhesives should ideally demonstrate a strong holding force, remaining attached for the desired time period, while also allowing atraumatic removal with no adhesive residue on the skin (Lund & Tucker, 2003).

KEY POINT

Acrylate adhesives (found on most tape products) are pressure-sensitive adhesives. They should be applied with gentle warming hand pressure, with the adhesive bond increasing over time. They may not be a good choice for situations in which only short-term adhesion is needed.

The adhesion of acrylate pressure-sensitive adhesives builds over time. This illustrates the importance of understanding adhesive product characteristics and matching those features to the desired clinical wear time. The risk of skin trauma is increased when adhesives are removed during peak adhesion. They may not be a good choice for clinical situations in which only short-term adhesion is needed.

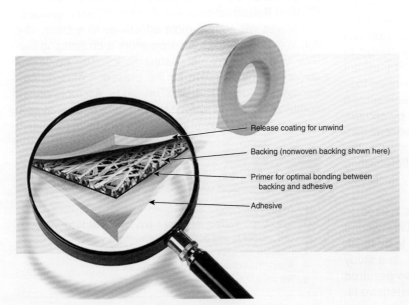

Release coating for unwind

Backing (nonwoven backing shown here)

Primer for optimal bonding between backing and adhesive

Adhesive

FIGURE 18-13. Common Component Layers of Medical Tape. (Used with permission, 3M.)

Adhesives characterized as aggressive typically have thick adhesive coatings. While they may utilize acrylates, natural or synthetic rubber–based agents may be used. Common backings used for adhesive tapes and dressings include paper and paper blends, plastic, paper/plastic blends, fabric (cotton or woven polyesters), foam, and polyurethane film.

The breathability of an adhesive product may greatly impact the skin's normal TEWL. Occlusive products create a barrier on the skin surface and may cause overhydration. Overhydration causes the cells to swell, with an accompanying decrease in the cohesive strength between cells. As a result, removal of the adhesive product is more likely to create a stripping injury (Tokumura et al., 1999). The combination of the adhesive and backing will determine breathability, gentleness, potential for sensitization, strength, conformability, ability to stretch, ability to be torn, wear time, and optimal clinical uses.

The introduction of an acrylate adhesive coating onto a porous paper backing in the 1960s has been described as the single most important technical innovation in decreasing tape dermatitis (Hoffman & Maibach, 1976). In addition to being breathable, this tape was the first minimally sensitizing and residue-free tape available for clinical use.

Matching Adhesive Product to Clinical Situation (Table 18-2)

Clinical considerations that influence adhesive product selection include clinical purpose, type of device to be secured (especially with consideration of weight and rigidity), location on the body, duration of securement, and skin condition (Lund & Tucker, 2003; McNichol et al., 2013). Patient or intrinsic factors include epidermal integrity, amount of skin surface oil (sebum), dryness, or moisture, typically perspiration (Matsumura, 2014). Product properties such as tack, gentleness, breathability, stretch, conformability, and ability to tear should also be considered.

While maintenance of skin integrity is an important consideration, it must be balanced against the need for reliable securement of critical devices such as endotracheal tubes and vascular access devices. Dislodgment or detachment of life-sustaining or supporting devices due to adhesive failure is unacceptable. In these situations, securement is the priority, and products with higher adhesion are indicated. Traditional cloth tapes coated with zinc oxide–containing adhesives or synthetic rubber or woven polyester (silk) coated with acrylate adhesives are still in use. Because of the challenges associated with use of these adhesive products, commercial securement devices with minimal adhesive for endotracheal tubes have been adopted by many facilities in the United States. When adhesive securement is desired or the only option available, critical tubes and devices should be anchored using a strong but conformable and breathable adhesive product.

TABLE 18-2 GUIDELINES FOR TAPE SELECTION

CLINICAL NEED	ADHESION LEVEL	BACKING/ ADHESIVE	EXAMPLES
Securing critical or heavy devices and tubes (dry or moist skin)	High to very high	Polyester ("silk")/acrylate; cloth/acrylate; cloth/latex rubber	"Silk" tape; cloth adhesive tape; "athletic tape"
Securing dressings; reinforcing dressings	Moderate	Cloth–paper combo/ acrylate; cloth/ acrylate; variable backings/ silicone	Soft cloth tape; paper tape; paper–plastic blend tape
Securement of medium-light size/weight tubes/devices	Moderate	Cloth–paper combo/ acrylate; cloth/ acrylate; variable backings/ silicone	Soft cloth tape; paper tape; paper–plastic blend tape
Noncritical securement on sensitive, compromised or at-risk skin; situations where removal anticipated to be traumatic (e.g., pediatric population, cognitive impairment)	Lower	Variable backings/ silicone	Silicone tape
Securement where movement/ edema/ distention is anticipated	Moderate	Cloth/acrylate	Soft cloth tape
Noncritical securement where skin is moist/damp	Moderate	Paper/acrylate; paper–plastic blend/acrylate	Paper tape

With higher adhesion correlated with increased risk of skin injury and pain (Bryant, 2016; Dykes et al., 2001), alternative adhesive coatings have been developed. Silicone adhesives provide an effective solution for securement on fragile skin or where frequent adhesive product changes are required. In contrast to acrylate adhesives, silicone adhesives attach to skin with lower surface tension, and adhesion does not build over time. Silicone adhesives detach fewer cells during removal (Cutting, 2006; Grove et al., 2013). Silicone adhesive tapes are best suited for securement of dressings and lightweight tubing. They do not provide sufficient adhesion for securing critical or heavy devices.

Medical tapes that are intended for a range of dressing securement or splinting needs are referred to as multipurpose and typically feature a gentle acrylate adhesive on a backing such as polyester (silk) or soft cloth fabric. Some silicone tapes may also be suitable for multipurpose use.

KEY POINT

Silicone adhesive products are gentle adhesives in which the adhesion does not build over time; they are appropriate for application of dressings and securement of light tubing to fragile skin. Suitability of silicone adhesive products for securement of critical devices should be based on manufacturer's data.

Achieving adhesion over contoured areas or within folds requires soft, conformable backings with adequate tack to skin. A backing that stretches is necessary over areas of the body that move or where edema or distention is anticipated. Even if a stretchable adhesive product has been appropriately selected and applied, the product should be removed and replaced if underlying tension is noted. Silicone adhesives are the exception to this rule as they allow repositioning (**Fig. 18-13**).

Adhesives perform optimally on dry surfaces. Some pressure sensitive adhesives are formulated to adhere to moist surfaces but will not adhere optimally when skin is wet. This property reinforces the need to create as dry a surface as possible prior to adhesive application.

Skin Preparation

Skin preparation is essential for successful adhesive product use. Attention to skin preparation can prevent adhesive failures that create patient discomfort, increase workload, and waste supplies.

Hair adversely impacts adhesion as well as increases discomfort during removal. Hair follicles are a reservoir for microbes. The effect of shaving has not been studied in the ostomy or chronic wound population. In a surgical population, shaving has been shown to increase infection risk (Tanner et al., 2006) and is associated with folliculitis (Dinulos, 2020). Recommendations include removal of excessive or coarse hair with scissors or surgical clippers and avoidance of shaving. For the infusion therapy population where sterile technique is required, Infusion Nurses Society (INS) guidelines recommend hair removal using sterile scissors or a clipper with disposable head (INS, 2016).

Next, skin should be cleansed and dried. The optimal product for skin preparation has not been identified,

but principles of cleansing directed at maintaining normal skin pH and minimizing barrier disruption should be followed (Schmid & Kortig, 1995). Gentle, no-rinse pH-balanced cleansers or pH-balanced soaps are desirable based on their ability to remove dead skin cells, excessive oil, and adhesive or dressing residue. Cleansing formulations containing barrier or moisturizing ingredients (e.g., dimethicone) can potentially interfere with adhesion. Most bar soaps are alkaline and should be avoided. After cleansing, the skin should be gently dried (Lichterfeld et al., 2015).

The wound care nurse may be consulted on MARSI prevention in patients receiving infusion therapy. In this population, considerations for skin preparation are different from those of ostomy or wound care patients. Antiseptic preparations, typically chlorhexidine gluconate (CHG) in alcohol must be allowed to completely dry prior to application of an adhesive securement dressing or device. The risk of irritant contact dermatitis or MASD is believed to increase when a wet solution is trapped under an adhesive product.

Adhesive removal may strip cell layers of the stratum corneum. Wound care nurses have used liquid skin protectants to minimize this effect and to prevent stripping injuries associated with adhesive use. The effectiveness of this practice is supported by several small studies and by expert opinion (Bryant, 2016; Campbell et al., 2000; Korber et al., 2007; McNichol et al., 2013; Sanders et al., 2007).

KEY POINT

Skin preparation is an important element in MARSI prevention and includes the following: removal of hair, gentle cleansing with no-rinse cleanser, thorough drying, and protection with liquid skin protectant that is allowed to dry prior to tape application.

Liquid skin protectants consist of either a copolymer or terpolymer dissolved in a liquid solvent. When applied to the skin, the solvent evaporates, and the polymer dries on the skin as a transparent coating that provides a protective interface between the epidermis and the adhesive. When the adhesive product is removed, the film is lifted from the skin rather than skin cells. They are useful to help prevent stripping injuries and may contribute to prevention of tension blisters. It is unknown if they provide any benefit in preventing irritant contact dermatitis.

Formulations of liquid skin protectants differ, and this should be considered when selecting a product. Traditional formulations, while inexpensive, utilize alcohol as a solvent. Alcohol is a potent irritant that is unsuitable for use on compromised skin. Alcohol can also elicit a sting or pain response on intact skin in some individuals (Rietschel & Fowler, 2008). Most liquid skin protectant formulations currently utilize alcohol-free, nonstinging solvents that can be applied to damaged or sensitive skin.

Polymers in liquid skin protectants also differ. The polymer should create a waterproof, transparent coating that allows TEWL. Once on the skin, many barrier films tend to be brittle and fail over time by forming microcracks. This compromises barrier function and results in failure of the coating. The incorporation of an additional polymer called a plasticizer is advantageous in that it softens the film, which allows it to flex with skin movement. This characteristic helps to maintain an intact coating over the desired area of protection.

Based on McNichol et al. (2013), the INS Standards of Practice (INS, 2016) call for routine use of liquid skin protectants around central venous access devices. The polymer in the liquid skin protectant should also be compatible with CHG antiseptic preps when used for infusion therapy site protection.

The liquid skin protectant should be applied to any skin that will contact the adhesive product. As with antiseptics, liquid skin protectant should be allowed to dry completely prior to adhesive application. Most liquid skin protectants are removed when the adhesive product is lifted from the skin and require reapplication prior to placement of a new adhesive tape, dressing, or device.

The wound care nurse may be asked about skin protection under other types of medical devices. The appropriateness of liquid skin protectants under electrodes and grounding pads should be verified with the device manufacturer prior to application, because the presence of a liquid skin protectant may increase skin impedance and reduce effectiveness of the device.

Preventive use of liquid skin protectants may be an underutilized tool for PMARSI prevention. Application under tape collars or supplemental tape can allay concerns about potential interference with barrier adhesion. Adhesion promoters such as compound tincture of benzoin or gum mastic are commonly referred to as tackifiers. It is important to distinguish these products from liquid skin protectants as their chemistry and indications differ. Adhesion promoters enhance or promote adhesion between the skin and adhesive product. Use should be based on specific patient need, and routine or indiscriminate use of these compounds should be avoided to prevent MARSI (INS, 2016; McNichol et al., 2013; Yates et al., 2017). This is especially important in patients with fragile skin. Sensitization to both compounds has been reported in the literature (Rietschel & Fowler, 2008). In a 2015 consensus conference, the WOCN Society endorsed the following statement regarding use of tackifiers:

- Limit or avoid the use of additional tackifiers (adhesive enhancers) under ostomy products.

Correct Application of Adhesive Product

Adhesive products should be applied without tension or stretch of the adhesive product to avoid deformation of the underlying skin and to prevent tension blisters or irritation at the product's periphery. Selection of an appropriately sized adhesive product reduces the inclination to stretch a dressing to fit the desired coverage area. Stretching an adhesive does not improve or increase tack. Most adhesives used in clinical practice are pressure sensitive. Gentle warming hand pressure upon application activates the viscoelastic polymers so that they act like a liquid and flow into the sulci cutis (i.e., contours) of the epidermis. This assures optimal surface area contact.

Even with proper application, edema or distention of the underlying tissue can develop, resulting in deformation or compression of the skin. Acrylate adhesive products must be replaced when this occurs, whereas most silicone adhesive products can be repositioned.

Removal of Adhesive Product

Inappropriate removal technique is believed to be a common contributor to MARSI.

Technique for removal is important for maintenance of skin integrity, with attention directed to the peel angle, support of the peel line, and speed of removal.

Peel force is associated with skin injury and is governed by the angle at which the adhesive is removed from the skin (Lund & Tucker, 2003). Removal at a 90-degree angle (i.e., perpendicular) to the skin surface generates significantly greater forces than narrow-angle or horizontal removal where the adhesive remains close to the skin surface (Breternitz et al., 2007; Jackson, 1988). The peel line describes the point where the adhesive separates from the skin (**Fig. 18-14**).

In a 2015 consensus conference the WOCN Society endorsed the following statement regarding removal of adhesive products:

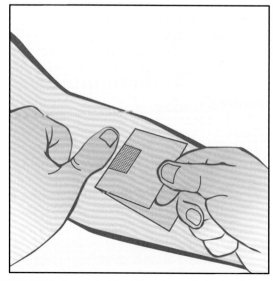

FIGURE 18-14. Support of Peel Line during Adhesive Removal.

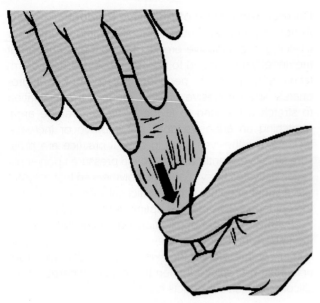

FIGURE 18-15. "Stretch and Release" Technique for Tape Removal.

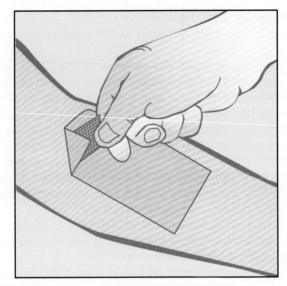

FIGURE 18-16. "Tape Tab" Technique for Tape Removal.

- Using two hands, remove adhesives at a low angle, parallel to skin, slowly while supporting the skin at the skin–tape interface (Yates et al., 2017)

Most adhesive products can be safely removed in this manner, but the approach requires patience. Wound care nurses should teach this technique and emphasize its importance to all caregivers.

An alternative stretch and release or stretch and relax technique may be used to remove nonbordered transparent film dressings. The edge of the film is gently pulled, allowing the film to lift from the skin (**Fig. 18-15**).

Placement of a small piece of tape at the edge or corner of the adhesive product can facilitate removal. A portion of this tape tab is gently pressed onto the underlying adhesive product. The free edge of the tab serves as a handle to help lift the adhesive product and begin removal, thus avoiding the need to scratch or pick at the skin (**Fig. 18-16**).

Use of adhesive removers should be considered, especially when removing aggressive adhesives or adhesive residue from skin (McNichol et al., 2013). Ethanol, isobutene, naphtha, mineral spirits, and silicone are common ingredients in adhesive removal products. Other removers contain a chemical called D-limonene, which is a citrus-derived oil. While this agent is naturally occurring, it can remove skin lipids, disrupt the skin barrier, and serve as an irritant (Tornier et al., 2008). No studies have been conducted to show the benefit of one formulation over another. Because formulations may contain both water-soluble and water-insoluble ingredients (e.g., isobutene), wound care nurses should review specific product instructions to determine if the adhesive remover should

be removed from skin prior to application of a new adhesive product. Products containing an ingredient called hexamethyldisiloxane (HMDS) will remove silicone. Isobutene can be removed with mineral oil. Prior to adhesive reapplication, the skin should be washed with a surfactant-containing cleanser or gentle soap to remove any residual oil.

In a 2015 consensus conference the WOCN Society endorsed the following statement regarding use of adhesive removers:

- Follow manufacturer's recommendations for removal of adhesive-based catheter securement devices (e.g., alcohol or commercially available releasers) (Yates et al., 2017).

CREATING A MARSI-FREE ENVIRONMENT

Adhesive Alternatives

Alternatives to adhesives should be considered for dressing securement when skin is fragile or silicone adhesives are not available. Options for nonadhesive dressing securement are listed in **Table 18-3**.

Both open weave wrap gauze and elastic bandages (e.g., ACE wraps) are commonly used as adhesive alternatives but are not ideal choices as both have the potential for slippage.

Adhesive alternatives are an excellent approach for securing products to very fragile skin (e.g., wrap gauze, elastic net dressings, and commercial securement devices).

Nonadhesive stabilizing devices are available for a variety of tubes and devices including dressings and indwelling urinary catheters. There are also specifically designed feeding tubes with stabilizing bumpers or discs that avoid the need for adhesive securement.

TABLE 18-3 ADHESIVE ALTERNATIVES FOR DRESSING SECUREMENT

DEVICE DESCRIPTION	EXAMPLES ONLY (NOT ALL INCLUSIVE)
Tubular elastic net dressing	Curad Tubular Elastic Retention Netting, Curad Hold Tite Tubular Stretch Bandage (Medline Industries Inc.); Medi-Pak Performance Tubular Elastic Net Dressing Retainer (McKesson Corp.); Surgilast Tubular Elastic Dressing Retainer (DermaSciences, Inc.); Stretch Net tubular elastic bandage (DeRoyal Industries Inc.); Spandage (MEDI-TECH International Corporation)
Elastic tubular bandage	Tubigrip Multi-Purpose Tubular Bandage, Tubifast 2-Way Stretch Elasticated Tubular Bandage (Molnlycke Health Care); Medigrip Elasticated Tubular Bandage (Medline Industries Inc.)
Self-adherent elastic bandages	3M Coban Self-Adherent Wrap (3M Health Care); CoFlex Self-Adherent Wrap (Milliken Healthcare Inc.); Medi-Rip Self-Adherent Compression Bandage, Co-Lastic LF, Co-Wrap (Hartmann USA)
Conforming bandages (gauze)	Kling Conforming Bandage (Johnson & Johnson); Curity Stretch Bandage (Covidien); Conform Stretch Bandages (Covidien); Duflex Synthetic Conforming Bandage (Derma Sciences Inc.)
Abdominal dressing holders	Medfix Montgomery Straps (Medline Industries Inc.); Montgomery Straps Adhesive Retention Dressing (DeRoyal Industries Inc.)

Routine use of these products should be encouraged as they typically provide both better securement for these devices and protection against MARSI.

In a 2015 consensus conference the WOCN Society endorsed the following statement regarding use of nonadhesive stabilizing devices:

- Consider nonadhesive tube securement devices for indwelling urinary catheters (Yates et al., 2017).

Clinical Leadership for Improved Outcomes

Adding MARSI surveillance to internal safety reporting systems or to pressure injury prevalence and incidence surveys may quantify the scope of the problem and target prevention efforts where needed. Education on adhesive injury and preventive strategies may be built into orientation and ongoing training (McNichol et al., 2013). All disciplines that apply or remove adhesive products should be educated on securement protocols and prevention techniques.

Infection control should also be considered. Convenience practices that can contribute to cross-contamination should be identified. These include keeping tape rolls on stethoscopes or in pockets and tearing off tape strips and attaching them to the bed rail or overbed table for ease of use.

Acute care facilities commonly stock a wide variety of adhesive products and an array of medical tapes. Often the characteristics and indicated uses of these adhesive products are not well understood. They may be inappropriately used, increasing the risk for MARSI (McNichol et al., 2013). Adhesive products should be aligned to protocols, and available where clinically needed. Unit-based skin champions may play a key role in choosing adhesive products needed in their clinical population. Procedures should be developed to guide adhesive product use.

The wound care nurse should work with key clinical stakeholders (nurse managers, clinical specialists, skin team members) as well as relevant procurement decision makers to assure that tapes and other adhesive products are systematically identified and evaluated for performance characteristics and matched to the clinical needs of the organization. Product decisions based solely on cost without clinical input can result in not only wasted resources but adverse patient outcomes. A process of standardization can be beneficial in reducing the number of adhesive products and clarifying appropriate use of each. In addition to clinical benefits, this deliberate collaborative approach can result in reduced waste, improved inventory control, and reduced supply costs.

Beyond typical populations of concern, the wound care nurse can provide valuable consultation to those serving other clinical populations such as those with type 1 diabetes (wearing continuous monitoring or infusion devices) and patients receiving vascular access. Collaborating with these care providers to share information and expertise on MARSI prevention and management has the potential to improve clinical outcomes and resource utilization (Messer, 2018).

MANAGEMENT OF MARSI

Adhesive-related skin injury should be managed according to the type of damage. When irritant contact dermatitis develops, the etiology must be determined, and treatment is based on assessment. In situations where more than one product was used on the skin (e.g., an antiseptic, a liquid skin protectant and an adhesive product), products should be removed and reintroduced systematically. For allergic contact dermatitis confirmed by patch testing or when allergic contact dermatitis is strongly suspected, the offending topical product should be discontinued. Allergic contact dermatitis may be treated with a limited course of low- to mid-potency topical corticosteroids (McNichol et al., 2013). If ongoing adhesive product use is required, the steroid should be provided in a vanishing base or liquid formulation. A dermatology referral should be considered for failure to respond to this first-line therapy.

Partial-thickness injuries associated with skin stripping and tension blisters should be managed using principles of topical wound therapy (Bryant, 2016; McNichol et al., 2013). See Chapter 9 for additional information about topical wound therapies.

Maceration can be improved by discontinuing adhesive product use and allowing the affected skin to dry. In the event that adhesive securement cannot be discontinued, a more breathable adhesive product should be used.

Antibiotics (topical and oral) are used to treat folliculitis complicated by infection (Dinulos, 2020; McNichol et al., 2013). Other nursing considerations include (1) modification of hair removal technique (eliminate shaving, or modify shaving technique to leave hair longer) (Dinulos, 2020); (2) skin preparation to assure a clean surface; and (3) selection of a more breathable adhesive product.

The wound care nurse may be consulted for MARSI at vascular access sites. The need for antiseptic site preparation, site visibility, and strict aseptic technique presents requirements and challenges not ordinarily present in wound and skin care. Best practice guidelines for management of skin damage at central venous access device sites have been developed by the World Congress of Vascular Access (WoCoVA) (Broadhurst et al., 2017).

SKIN TEARS

Skin tears were first defined by Payne and Martin (1990) as traumatic wounds occurring principally on the upper limbs as a result of friction alone or shearing and friction forces, which separate the epidermis from the dermis (partial-thickness wounds) or which separate both the epidermis and the dermis from underlying structures (full-thickness wounds). Skin tears are reported to be common, especially on fragile exposed skin such as that encountered among older adults, disabled populations and neonates. Skin tears can be found on all areas of the body. Skin tears have a prevalence of up to 41% in acute and long-term care settings (LeBlanc et al., 2014; Woo & LeBlanc, 2018).

BACKGROUND

In 1990, Payne and Martin established a classification system for skin tears (Payne & Martin, 1993). They published a descriptive clinical nursing research study on the epidemiology and management of skin tears in older adults. The Payne-Martin Classification System for Skin Tears describes three categories and two subcategories of injury. The Payne-Martin classification is based on the level or amount of tissue loss from the skin tear, that is, without tissue loss, with partial-thickness skin loss, and with full-thickness skin loss. In the partial-thickness category, an estimate of the percentage of tissue loss was required (Ratliff & Fletcher, 2007).

Problems associated with interrater reliability testing of the Payne and Martin classification system and its poor utility in Australia led to a study that resulted in the Skin Tear Audit Research (STAR) Classification System (Carville et al., 2007). This system comprises three categories and two subcategories of skin tears like the Payne Martin but omits the percentage estimation of tissue loss and adds an assessment of flap tissue color.

Both the Payne-Martin and STAR classification systems have been used for categorization of skin tears. In 2011, the International Skin Tear Advisory Panel (ISTAP) skin tear classification was developed and has since been validated. Like its predecessors, it identifies three categories of skin injury but deleted the subcategories. It is important to know which classification tool is being used in your facility, so documentation is consistent (LeBlanc & Baranoski, 2011; LeBlanc et al., 2014; Zulkowski, 2017).

DEFINITION AND OVERVIEW

A skin tear is a tear or laceration of the skin caused by shear or friction or by minor blunt force trauma. Skin tears result in a separation of the epidermis from the dermis or of the epidermis and dermis from the underlying connective tissue, with creation of a flap or pedicle of skin. The skin flap may or may not be viable. Skin tears can produce either a partial- or a full-thickness injury. Van Tiggelen et al. (2019) defined a skin tear skin flap as a portion of the skin (epidermis/dermis) that is unintentionally separated from its original place due to shear, friction, and/or blunt force (Van Tiggelen et al., 2019). Skin tears are often jagged or irregular and usually occur in high-risk areas, such as the extremities. These wounds may be dry with little or no drainage or may produce moderate amounts of drainage, depending on the location and extent of injury (LeBlanc et al., 2018; McNichol et al., 2013).

ISTAP CLASSIFICATION SYSTEM

ISTAP defines skin tears as traumatic wounds caused by mechanical forces, including removal of adhesives. Severity may vary by depth (not extending through the subcutaneous layer). The scheme involves three categories of skin tears:

Type 1
No skin loss—linear or flap tear that can be repositioned to cover the wound bed

Type 2
Partial flap loss—partial flap loss that cannot be repositioned to cover the wound bed

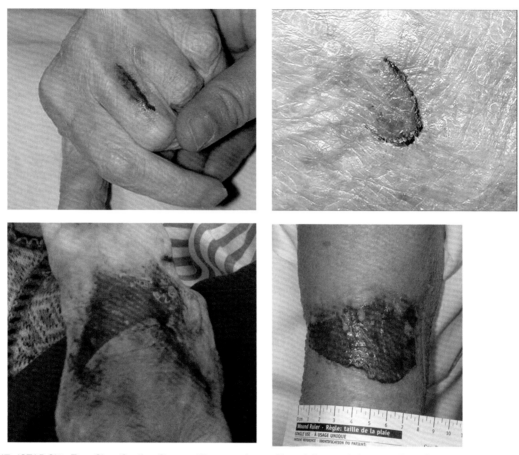

FIGURE 18-17. ISTAP Skin Tear Classification System. Top two photos: Type 1; Bottom left photo: Type 2; Bottom right photo: Type 3.

Type 3

Total flap loss—total flap loss exposing the entire wound bed (**Fig. 18-17**).

ETIOLOGY AND RISK FACTORS

Serra et al. (2018) conducted a scoping review of articles from January 1990 to June 2017 using the keywords of skin tears and risk factors, which resulted in 17 articles that were included in the qualitative synthesis. They found the risk factors included age-related skin changes, dehydration, malnutrition, sensory changes, mobility impairment, pharmacological therapies, and mechanical factors related to skin care practices.

Age

Preterm and newborn infants are susceptible to skin tears. Neonates have underdeveloped skin, and their decreased epidermal-to-dermal cohesion, deficient stratum corneum, impaired thermoregulation, body surface/weight ratio that is nearly five times greater than an adult, and immature immune system place them at an increased risk for skin tears (Serra et al., 2018).

In the elderly, the skin has less collagen, elastin, and fatty tissue with decreased skin elasticity and reduced subcutaneous tissue that causes wrinkles and folds to appear. Skin also has decreased sebaceous gland and sweat gland activity that causes the skin to dry out (xerosis), becoming more fragile. Arteriosclerotic changes in the small and large vessels cause thinning of vessel walls and a reduction in the blood supply to the extremities, and to the skin microcirculation. The vascular capillaries become more fragile, which can lead to vascular lesions, such as ecchymosis (bruising) and senile purpura. These changes make the skin less able to withstand normal wear and tear.

Dehydration and Nutrition

Infants and children are more susceptible to dehydration than young adults because of their smaller body weights and higher turnover of water and electrolytes. The elderly and those with illnesses are at a higher risk. The hydration status may influence the protective function of the skin, which depends on hygroscopic proteins, osmotically active elements, and the integrity of the lipid–water barrier.

The elderly are at an increased risk of developing malnutrition due to medical, psychological, physiological, social, and economic difficulties (Serra et al., 2018). Patients with wounds often experience nutrition deficiency. Energy, carbohydrate, protein, fat, vitamin, and

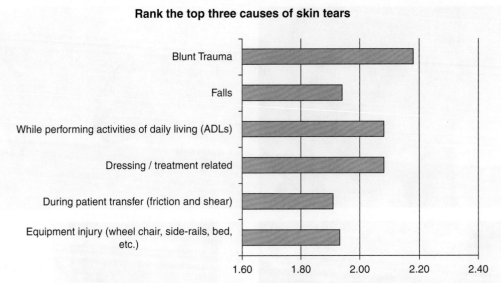

FIGURE 18-18. Top Causes of Skin Tears.

mineral metabolism can all affect skin integrity and the healing process (Dorner et al., 2009). For additional information on hydration and nutrition, see Chapter 7.

Sensory Changes and Mobility Impairment

Sensory and cognitive deficits including communication difficulties, impaired decision making, cognitive impairments, decreased tactile sensation, hearing impairment, and visual deficits appear to be related to the onset of skin tears. History of falls, impaired mobility, and inability to perform activities of daily living (ADLs) increase risk. For example, individuals who require assistance for bathing, dressing, toileting, and transferring are at increased risk for skin tears (Baranoski & Ayello, 2014; Thayer et al., 2016).

Skin tears are frequently linked to blunt trauma from accidentally bumping into objects (Bank & Nix, 2006; LeBlanc et al., 2008). In the 2011 survey conducted by LeBlanc and colleagues, the most common causes of skin tears included blunt trauma, falls, patient transfers, equipment injury, and medical adhesives (LeBlanc & Baranoski, 2011).

Pharmacological Therapies

Chronic use of corticosteroids, for their potential side effects in collagen synthesis inhibition, as well as the use of anticoagulant agents, for their potential side effects in determining ecchymosis and senile purpura, appear to be related to the onset of skin tears. Chemotherapeutic agents are a particular risk factor because they interfere with epidermal regeneration and collagen synthesis (Reddy, 2008).

Polypharmacy lacks a standard definition but includes the use of multiple medications (five or more) that might predispose patients to drug interactions and reactions. It is common among older adults (Nguyen et al., 2020). Polypharmacy has also been found to be an independent risk factor for falls. Individuals receiving five or more medications, or any medication associated with cognitive impairment, reduced mobility, hypotension, dizziness, or drowsiness increases risk of falls and resultant skin tears. Alcohol consumption may be an additional risk factor (Wong et al., 2016).

Mechanical Factors Related to Skin Care Practices

Shear and friction forces associated with transfer activities of patients and those associated with wound dressings and medical adhesives used may be responsible for the onset of skin tears. The most common cause of skin tears in the elderly population is from traumatic injury due to wheelchair injuries, bumping into objects, transfers, and falls (LeBlanc & Baranoski, 2011). In the neonatal and pediatric population, skin tears are a common skin injury, along with medical device–related skin injury (MDRPI) and pressure injury on the occiput (Baharestani, 2007; Irving et al., 2006). A key component to the prevention of skin tears in these populations is to recognize fragile, thin, vulnerable skin and to modify care accordingly (Carville et al., 2007; LeBlanc et al., 2018; Payne & Martin, 1993). **Figure 18-18** ranks the top causes of skin tears (**Table 18-4**) (see **Box 18-2**).

RISK ASSESSMENT

Validated risk assessment tools are available to predict pressure injury and are well utilized, but the same is not true for skin tears. Several tools have been proposed in the literature, but none have been validated and none are in common use. The ISTAP Skin Tear Risk Assessment pathway (**Fig. 18-19**) was developed to identify patients who are at risk. This tool focuses on three main categories of identified risk factors (General Health, Mobility, and Skin) (LeBlanc et al., 2013).

TABLE 18-4 STRATEGIES FOR PREVENTION OF SKIN TEARS

- Determine and remove potential causes for trauma. Ensure a safe environment with adequate lighting.
- Remove objects that can be a source of blunt trauma; declutter area; remove scatter rugs and excessive furniture.
- Hydrate skin with moisturizer at least twice a day, especially after bathing, with the skin still damp, not wet.
- Utilize soapless, no-rinse, and pH-balanced skin cleansers; tepid water; and gentle technique for bathing.
- Use appropriate lifting, turning aids, slide sheet, when moving patients; never drag the patient across bed.
- Encourage the patient to wear long sleeves, long trousers or knee high socks; provide shin guards for those who experience repeat skin tears; provide gloves for those in wheelchairs to protect the hands.
- Pad edges of furniture and equipment.
- Finger and toe nails should be kept cut short and filed to remove rough edges to prevent self-inflicted skin tears. (Good idea for health care workers to keep nail short as well)
- Avoid adhesive products on frail skin. If dressings or tapes are required, use paper tapes or soft nonadherent dressings to avoid skin stripping or tearing the skin with the removal of adhesives.
- Label dressings showing removal pulling away from the skin flap.
- Educate staff on the importance of "gentle care."

BOX 18-2   RISK FACTORS FOR SKIN TEARS

- Very young and very old (>75 years of age)
- Gender (female)
- Race (Caucasian)
- Immobility (chair or bed bound)
- Inadequate nutritional intake
- Long-term corticosteroid use
- History of previous skin tears
- Altered sensory status
- Cognitive impairment
- Stiffness and spasticity
- Neuropathy
- Having blood drawn
- Polypharmacy
- Presence of ecchymosis
- Dependence for activities of daily living
- Using assistive devices
- Applying and removing stockings
- Removing tape
- Vascular problems
- Cardiac problems
- Pulmonary problems
- Visual impairment
- Transfers and falls
- Prosthetic devices
- LE skin tears
- Continence/incontinence
- Skin cleansers
- Improper use of skin sealants

PREVENTION

Skin tears can be effectively prevented if individuals at risk are appropriately identified and if a comprehensive prevention program is implemented. Ratliff and Fletcher (2007) found that identification of at-risk individuals and implementation of prevention measures reduced the incidence of skin tears. Bank and Nix (2006) also demonstrated the ability of a prevention program to reduce the incidence of skin tears.

Patients and caregivers should keep their fingernails short to prevent mechanical trauma, should use no-rinse, pH-balanced cleansers for bathing, should use gentle technique and caution in assisting the patient to dress, and should moisturize the skin with creams rather than lotions (Shevchenko et al., 2018; Stephen-Haynes et al., 2011). Carville et al. (2014) found that twice-daily application of a moisturizer to the extremities of residents in a long-term care facility in Australia reduced the incidence of skin tears almost 50%.

Caregivers should be educated on gentle handling of elderly patients with frail skin. Any firm movement or pulling can create a skin tear. Patients and families

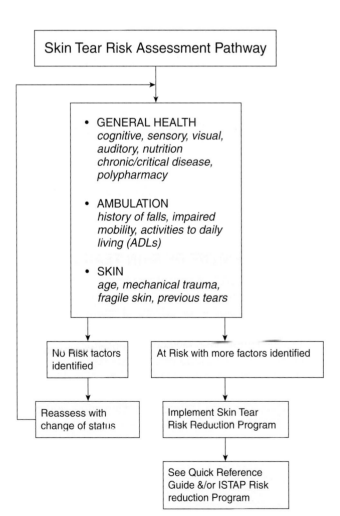

FIGURE 18-19. Skin Tear Risk Assessment Pathway.

should understand the importance of proper positioning, turning, lifting, and transferring. Lift sheets or underpads (if designed for that purpose) should be used to move patients up in bed, and padding should be added to hard objects, including side rails, wheelchair arm and leg supports, and other equipment. Protective arm sleeves or wraps and trousers/pants or shin guards should be routinely used to protect the extremities (Baranoski & Ayello, 2014; Benbow, 2009; LeBlanc & Baranoski, 2009). A best practice document is available at https://www.woundsinternational.com/resources/details/istap-best-practice-recommendations-prevention-and-management-skin-tears-aged-skin.

KEY POINT

Strategies for preventing mobility-related skin tears include padding corners and edges in the patient environment, use of shin guards and gloves for wheelchair-bound patients, and eliminating environmental clutter to prevent falls.

Implementation of a best practice fall prevention program has proven to be successful in reducing falls (and skin tears) in elderly long-term care patients. Successful implementation requires adequate planning, resources, organization, and administrative support (Hawk & Shannon, 2018).

KEY POINT

Measures for prevention of skin tears related to handling during daily care include protective arm sleeves, short nails for patient and caregivers, routine use of moisturizers, gentle approach when assisting with bathing and mobility, and appropriate medical adhesive removal technique.

MANAGEMENT OF SKIN TEARS

The same principles of topical therapy used to manage other wounds should be employed when treating skin tears. See Chapter 9 for additional information about dressing selection.

The first step in developing a treatment plan for skin tears is to assess the wound. Key assessment factors include presence and viability of the skin flap (pedicle), type of skin tear according to ISTAP Classification System, amount of exudate, signs of infection, and periwound condition.

Recommendations will vary according to the type of skin tear, but include the following:

- Control bleeding.
- Cleanse the wound.
- Realign skin flap (pedicle) if viable; gently ease flap back into place using a dampened cotton tip applicator or gloved finger; if flap is difficult to align, consider moistening the flap with saline and soft gauze to rehydrate; if necrotic or dried, the flap may need debridement.
- Classify, measure, and document the skin tear.
- Select a dressing that absorbs exudate, maintains moist surface, and provides atraumatic removal. Mark dressing with an arrow indicating the direction of the tear.
- Consider administration of tetanus immunoglobulin if source of skin tear is unknown, especially if full thickness or contaminated.
- At each dressing change, gently lift and remove the dressing in the direction of the tear.
- Monitor and observe for any changes, signs or symptoms of infection, and poor healing.

Based on available evidence, the recommended dressing options for skin tears include nonadherent dressings such as nonadhesive foam secured with wrap or roll gauze, nonadherent contact layers secured with wrap or roll gauze, impregnated mesh, silicone mesh, hydrogel, alginate, hydrofiber, and clear acrylic dressings and those dressings with gentle adhesive properties. Dressings with aggressive adhesives and limited absorptive capacity may be problematic and should be avoided, for example, hydrocolloids, and transparent film dressings (LeBlanc et al., 2018).

KEY POINT

Consider drawing an arrow on the dressing to show best direction for removal to protect the flap from disruption.

CONCLUSION

MASD, MARSI, and skin tears constitute three types of skin injury commonly encountered in clinical practice. The wound care nurse is responsible for providing expert care for skin injury and for creating a culture where risk is recognized, and best practice interventions are focused on prevention.

CASE STUDY

CASE STUDY FOR SKIN TEAR MANAGEMENT

Mr. P was a 75-year-old with a history of cardiac, pulmonary, and renal comorbidities. His skin was easily damaged due to the nature of his illnesses and longstanding use of Coumadin.

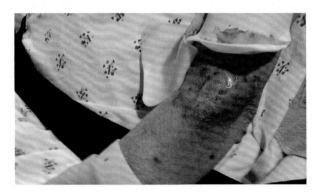

Day 1.

The skin tear seen on his left arm is from the staff pulling him onto a stretcher to go to x-ray. As Mr. P was pulled to the stretcher, his skin was torn in the area where the health care worker was holding his arm. Wound care nurse was consulted.

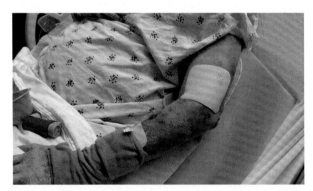

Nonadherent dressing.

The skin tear was cleansed with saline and the wound was assessed by the wound care nurse as being a type 3 skin tear. No flap or pedicle was present. A nonadherent foam dressing was applied and ordered to be changed every 3 to 4 days.

On Day 2, the wound care nurse stopped by and found the dressings saturated and in need of being changed. She changed the dressings while educating the nurse taking care of Mr. P. It was also decided to use a protective sleeve to reduce the risk of further injury to the area and to secure the dressing. The wound care nurse followed up 1 week later and found the skin tear much improved and healing.

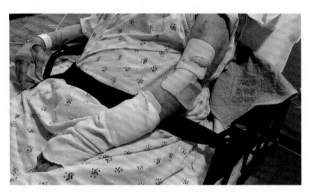

Day 2

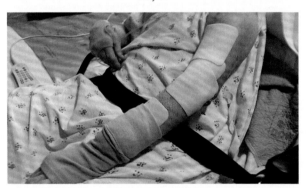

Protective sleeve

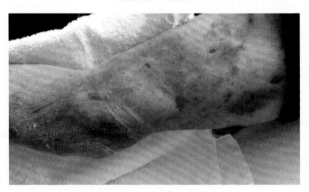

One week later

REFERENCES

Alikahn, A., & Maibach, H. I. (2009). Biology of the stratum corneum: Tape stripping and protein quantification. In M. A. Firage, H. I. Maibach, & K. W. Miller (Eds.), *Textbook of aging skin* (pp. 401–408). New York, NY: Springer-Verlag.

Arnold-Long, M., Emmons, K., & Chovan, J. D. (2018). Incontinence-associated dermatitis and intertriginous dermatitis as nurse-sensitive quality indicators: A Delphi study. *Journal of Wound, Ostomy and Continence Nursing, 45*(3), 221–226. https://doi.org/10.1097/WON.0000000000000427

Arnold-Long, M., & Johnson, E. (2019). Epidemiology of incontinence-associated dermatitis and intertriginous dermatitis (intertrigo) in an acute care facility. *Journal of Wound, Ostomy and Continence Nursing, 46*(3), 201–206.

Association of Women's Health, Obstetric and Neonatal Nurses (AWHONN). (2018). *Neonatal Skin Care: Evidence-Based Clinical Practice Guideline.* (4th ed.). Washington, DC: AWHONN.

Baharestani, M. (2007). An overview of neonatal and pediatric wound care knowledge and considerations. *Ostomy & Wound Management, 53*(6), 34–55.

Bains, S. N., Nash, P., & Fonacier, L. (2019). Irritant contact dermatitis. *Clinical Reviews in Allergy & Immunology, 56*(1), 99–109. https://doi.org/10.1007/s12016-018-8713-0

Bank, D., & Nix, D. (2006). Preventing skin tears in a nursing and rehabilitation center: An interdisciplinary effort. *Ostomy Wound Management, 52*(9), 38–46.

Baranoski, S., & Ayello, E. A. A. (2014). Skin an essential organ. In S. Baranoski, & E. A. A. Ayello (Eds.), *Wound Care Essentials: Practice Principles* (pp. 60–85). Philadelphia, PA: Lippincott Williams & Wilkins.

Beeckman, D. (2017). A decade of research on Incontinence-Associated Dermatitis (IAD): Evidence, knowledge gaps and next steps. *Journal of Tissue Viability, 26*(1), 47–56. https://doi.org/10.1016/j.jtv.2016.02.004

Beeckman, D., Van Damme, N., Schoonhoven, L., et al. (2016). Interventions for preventing and treating incontinence-associated dermatitis in adults. *Cochrane Database of Systematic Reviews, 11*(11), CD011627. doi: 10.1002/14651858.CD011627.pub2.

Beeckman, D., Van den Bussche, K., Alves, P., et al. (2018). Towards an international language for incontinence-associated dermatitis (IAD): Design and evaluation of psychometric properties of the Ghent Global IAD Categorization Tool (GLOBIAD) in 30 countries. *The British Journal of Dermatology, 178*(6), 1331–1340. https://doi.org/10.1111/bjd.16327

Belsito, D. V. (2000). The diagnostic evaluation, treatment and prevention of allergic contact dermatitis in the new millennium. *Journal of Allergy and Clinical Immunology, 105*(3), 409–420.

Benbow, M. (2009). Skin tears. *Journal of Community Nursing, 23*(1), 14–18.

Berg, A. K., Norgaard, K., Thyssen, J. P., et al. (2018a). Skin problems associated with insulin pumps and sensors in adults with type 1 diabetes: A cross-sectional study. *Diabetes Technology & Therapeutics, 20*(7), 475–482. doi.org/10.1089/dia.2018.0088

Berg, A. K., Simonsen, A. B., & Svensson, J. (2018b). Perception and possible causes of skin problems to insulin pump and glucose sensor: Results from pediatric focus groups. *Diabetes Technology & Therapeutics, 20*(8), 566–570. doi.org/10.1089/dia.2018.0089

Berke, C. T. (2015). Pathology and clinical presentation of friction injuries: Case series and literature review. *Journal of Wound Ostomy & Continence Nursing, 42*(1), 47–61.

Black, J. M., Gray, M., Bliss, D. Z., et al. (2011). MASD Part 2: Incontinence-associated dermatitis and intertriginous dermatitis. *Journal of Wound, Ostomy, and Continence Nursing, 38*(4), 359–370.

Breternitz, M. Flach, M. Präßler, J., et al. (2007). Acute barrier disruption by adhesive tapes is influenced by pressure, time and anatomical location: Integrity and cohesion assessed by sequential tape stripping: A randomized controlled study. *British Journal of Dermatology, 156*, 231–240.

Broadhurst, D., Moureau, N., Ullman, A. J., & World Congress of Vascular Access (WoCoVA) Skin Impairment Management Advisory Panel. (2017). Management of central venous access device-associated skin impairment: An evidence-based algorithm. *Journal of Wound, Ostomy and Continence Nursing, 44*(3), 211–220. https://doi.org/10.1097/WON.0000000000000322

Browning, P., Beeckman, D., White, R. et al. (2018). Report of the proceedings of a UK skin safety advisory group. *British Journal of Nursing, 27*(20), S34–S40. https://doi.org/10.12968/bjon.2018.27.Sup20.S34

Bryant, R. A. (2016). Types of skin damage and differential diagnosis. In R. A. Bryant & D. P. Nix (Eds.), *Acute and Chronic Wounds: Current Management Concepts* (5th ed.). St Louis, MO: Elsevier Inc.

Cameron, J., Hoffman, D., Wilson, J., et al. (2005). Comparison of two peri-wound skin protectants in venous leg ulcers: A randomized controlled trial. *Journal of Wound Care, 14*, 233–236.

Campbell, K., Woodbury, M. G., Whittle, H., et al. (2000). A clinical evaluation of 3M Cavilon No Sting Barrier Film. *Ostomy & Wound Management, 46*(1), 24–30.

Carville, K., Lewin, G., Newall, N., et al. (2007). STAR: A consensus for skin tear classification. *Primary Intention, 15*(1), 8–28.

Carville, K., Osseiran-Moisson, R., Newall, N., et al. (2014). The effectiveness of a twice-daily skin moisturizing regimen for reducing the incidence of skin tears. *International Wound Journal, 11*(4), 446–453.

Colwell, J. C., Kupsick, P. T., & McNichol, L. L. (2016). Outcome criteria for discharging the patient with a new ostomy from home health care. *Journal of Wound, Ostomy and Continence Nursing, 43*(3), 269–273.

Colwell, J. C., McNichol, L., & Boarini, J. (2017). North America wound, ostomy, and continence and enterostomal therapy nurses current ostomy care practice related to peristomal skin issues. *Journal of Wound, Ostomy, and Continence Nursing, 44*(3), 257.

Colwell, J. C., Ratliff, C. R., Goldberg, M., et al. (2011). MASD Part 3: Peristomal moisture–associated dermatitis and periwound moisture–associated dermatitis: A consensus. *Journal of Wound Ostomy & Continence Nursing, 38*(5), 541–553.

Cosker, T., Elsayed, S., Gupta, S., et al. (2005). Choice of dressing has a major impact on blistering and healing outcomes in orthopedic patients. *Journal of Wound Care, 14*(1), 27–29.

Cutting, K. F. (2006). Silicone and skin adhesives. *Journal of Community Nursing, 20*(11), 36–37.

Cutting, K. F. (2008). Impact of adhesive surgical tape and wound dressing on the skin with reference to skin stripping. *Journal of Wound Care, 17*(4), 157–162.

Cutting, K., & White, R. (2002). Avoidance and management of periwound maceration of the skin. *Journal of Professional Nursing, 18*(33), 35–36.

Dinulos, J. G. H. (2020). *Habif's clinical dermatology* (7th ed.). St. Louis, MO: Elsevier.

Dorner, B. D., Posthauer, M. E., & Thomas, D. (2009). Role of nutrition in pressure ulcer healing clinical practice guideline. In National Pressure Ulcer Advisory Panel and European Pressure Ulcer Advisory Panel. *Prevention and treatment of pressure ulcers: Clinical practice guideline.* Washington, DC: National Pressure Ulcer Advisory Panel.

Dykes, P. (2007). The effect of adhesive dressing edges on cutaneous irritancy and skin barrier function. *Journal of Wound Care, 16*(3), 97–100.

Dykes, P. J., Heggie, R., & Hill, S. A. (2001). Effects of adhesive dressings on the stratum corneum of the skin. *Journal of Wound Care, 10*(2), 7–9.

Falloon, S. S., Abbas, S., Stridfeldt, C., et al. (2018). The impact of microclimate on skin health with absorbent incontinence product use: An integrative review. *Journal of Wound Ostomy & Continence Nursing, 45*(4), 341–348.

Farage, M. A., Miller, K. W., Berardesca, E., et al. (2009). Clinical implications of aging skin: Cutaneous disorders in the elderly. *American Journal of Clinical Dermatology, 10*(2), 73–86. doi: 10.2165/00128071-200910020-00001.

Farris, M. K., Petty, M., Hamilton, J., et al. (2015). Medical adhesive-related skin injury prevalence among adult acute care patients: A single-center observational study. *Journal of Wound Ostomy & Continence Nursing, 42*(6), 589–598.

Gabriel, S., Hahnel, E., Blume-Peytavi, U., et al. (2019). Prevalence and associated factors of intertrigo in aged nursing home residents: A multicenter cross-sectional prevalence study. *BMC Geriatrics, 19*(1), 105.

Gray, M. (2004). Preventing and managing perineal dermatitis: A shared goal for wound and continence care. *Journal of Wound Ostomy & Continence Nursing, 31*(suppl 1), S2–S9.

Gray, M., Beeckman, D., Bliss, D. Z., et al. (2012). Incontinence-associated dermatitis: A comprehensive review and update. *Journal of Wound Ostomy & Continence Nursing, 39*(1), 61–74.

Gray, M., Black, J. M., Baharestani, M. M., et al. (2011). Moisture-associated skin damage: Overview and pathophysiology. *Journal of Wound Ostomy & Continence Nursing, 38*(3), 233–241.

Gray, M., Bliss, D. Z., Doughty, D. B., et al. (2007). Incontinence-associated dermatitis: A consensus. *Journal of Wound Ostomy & Continence Nursing, 34*(1), 45–54.

Gray, M., Colwell, J. C., Doughty, D., et al. (2013). Peristomal moisture–associated skin damage in adults with fecal ostomies: A comprehensive review and consensus. *Journal of Wound Ostomy & Continence Nursing, 40*(4), 389–399.

Gray, M., & Giuliano, K. K. (2018). Incontinence-associated dermatitis, characteristics and relationship to pressure injury: A multisite epidemiologic analysis. *Journal of Wound, Ostomy, and Continence Nursing, 45*(1), 63–67.

Gray, M., & Weir, D. (2007). Prevention and treatment of moisture-associated skin damage (maceration) in the periwound skin. *Journal of Wound Ostomy & Continence Nursing, 34*, 153–157.

Grove, G., Houser, T., Sibbald, G., et al. (2019). Measuring epidermal effects of ostomy skin barriers. *Skin Research and Technology, 25*(2), 179–186.

Grove, G. L., Zerweck, C. R., Houser, T. P., et al. (2013). A randomized and controlled comparison of gentleness of 2 medical adhesive tapes in healthy human subjects. *Journal Wound Ostomy & Continence Nursing, 40*(1), 51–59.

Hadfield, G., De Freitas, A., & Bradbury, S. (2019). Clinical evaluation of a silicone adhesive remover for prevention of MARSI at dressing change. *Journal of Community Nursing, 33*(3), 36–41.

Haesler, E. (2018). Moisture associated skin damage: Classification and assessment. *Wound Practice & Research: Journal of the Australian Wound Management Association, 26*(2), 113.

Hawk, J., & Shannon, M. (2018). Prevalence of skin tears in elderly patients: A retrospective chart review of incidence reports in 6 long-term care facilities. *Ostomy & Wound Management, 64*(4), 30–36.

Hess, C. T. (2020). *Product guide to skin and wound care* (8th ed.). Philadelphia, PA: Wolters Kluwer.

Hoffman, H., & Maibach, H. (1976). Transepidermal water loss in adhesive tape induced dermatitis. *Contact Dermatitis, 2*, 171–177.

Hsu, S. (2015). Decrease medical adhesive related skin injuries (MARSI) in ICU setting. *Journal Wound Ostomy & Continence Nursing, 42*(3S), S46.

Infusion Nurses Society (INS). (2016). Infusion therapy standards of practice. *Journal of Infusion Nursing, 39*(1S), S1–S159.

Irving, V., Bethell, E., & Burtin, F. (2006). Neonatal wound care: Minimizing trauma and pain. *Wounds UK, 2*(1), 33–41.

Jackson, A. P. (1988). The peeling of pressure-sensitive adhesives at different angles. *Journal of Materials Science Letters, 7*, 1368–1370.

Janniger, C., Schwartz, R., Szepietowski, J., et al. (2005). Intertrigo and common secondary skin infections. *American Family Physician, 72*(5), 833–838.

Jester, R., Russell, L., Fell, S., et al. (2000). A one hospital study of the effect of wound dressings and other related factors on skin blistering following total hip and knee arthroplasty. *Journal of Orthopaedic Nursing, 4*, 71–77.

Kalra, M. G., Higgins, K. E., & Kinney, B. S. (2014). Intertrigo and secondary skin infections. *American Family Physician, 89*(7), 569–573.

Klode, J., Schöttler, L., Stoffels, I., et al. (2010). Investigation of adhesion of modern wound dressings: A comparative analysis of 56 different wound dressings. *Journal of European Academy of Dermatology and Venereology, 25*, 933–939.

Konya, C., Sanada, H., Sugama, J., et al. (2010). Skin injuries caused by medical adhesive tape in older people and associated factors. *Journal of Clinical Nursing, 19*, 1236–1242.

Korber, A., Holze, K., Grabbe, S., et al. (2007). Protection of wound edges with 3M cavilon no sting barrier film during vacuum-assisted closure therapy: Results of a clinical investigation in patients with chronic leg ulcers. *Zeitshrift for Wundheilung, 12*(1), 6–11.

Kottner, J., Everink, I., van Haastregt, J., et al. (2020). Prevalence of intertrigo and associated factors: A secondary data analysis of four annual multicentre prevalence studies in the Netherlands. *International Journal of Nursing Studies, 104*, 103437. https://doi.org/10.1016/j.ijnurstu.2019.103437

Koval, K. J., Egol, K. A., Polatsch, D. B., et al. (2003). Tape blisters following hip surgery: A prospective, randomized study of two types of tape. *Journal of Bone and Joint Surgery (American), 85-A*(10), 1884–1887.

Lachenbruch, C., Ribble, D., Emmons, K., et al. (2016). Pressure ulcer risk in the incontinent patient. *Journal of Wound, Ostomy and Continence Nursing, 43*(3), 235–241.

LeBlanc, K., Whitely, I., McNichol L., et al. (2019). Peristomal medical adhesive-related skin injury. *Journal Wound Ostomy & Continence Nursing, 46*(2), 125–136.

LeBlanc, K., Campbell, K. E., Wood, E., et al. (2018). Best practice recommendations for prevention and management of skin tears in aged skin: An overview. *Journal of Wound Ostomy & Continence Nursing, 45*(6), 540–542.

LeBlanc, K., & Baranoski, S. (2009). Prevention and management of skin tears. *Advances in Skin & Wound Care, 22*(7), 325–334.

LeBlanc, K., & Baranoski, S. (2011). Skin tears: State of the science: Consensus statements for the prevention, prediction, assessment, and treatment of skin tears. *Advances in Skin & Wound Care, 24*(9S), 2–15.

LeBlanc, K., Baranoski, S., Christensen, D., et al. (2013). International skin tear advisory panel: A tool kit to aid in the prevention, assessment, and treatment of skin tears using a simplified classification system. *Advances in Skin & Wound Care, 26*(10), 459–476.

LeBlanc, K., Baranoski, S., Holloway, S., et al. (2014). A descriptive cross-sectional study to explore current practices in the assessment, prevention, and treatment of skin tears. *International Wound Journal, 11*(4), 424–430.

LeBlanc, K., Christensen, D., Orstead, H., et al. (2008). Best practice recommendations for the prevention and treatment of skin tears. *Wound Care Canada, 6*(8), 14–32.

Lichterfeld, A., Hauss, A., Surber, C., et al. (2015). Evidence-based skin care. *Journal of Wound, Ostomy and Continence Nursing, 42*(5), 501–524.

Lima, A. L., Timmermann, V., Illing, T., et al. (2019). Contact dermatitis in the elderly: Predisposing factors, diagnosis, and management. *Drugs & Aging, 36*(5), 411–417. https://doi.org/10.1007/s40266-019-00641-4

Liu, D., Wen, S., Huang, L. N., et al. (2020). Comparison of transepidermal water loss rates in subjects with skin patch test positive vs negative to skin care products. *Journal of Cosmetic Dermatology, 19*(8), 2021–2024.

Lucast, D. (October 2000). Skin tight: Adhesive considerations for developing stick-to-skin products. *Adhesives Age*, 36–39.

Lund, C. H., & Tucker, J. A. (2003). Adhesion and newborn skin. In S. Hoath, & H. I. Maibach (Eds.), *Neonatal skin: Structure and function* (pp. 299–324). New York, NY: Marcel Dekker, Inc.

Lyon, C. C., Smith, A. J., Griffiths, C. E. M., et al. (2000). The spectrum of skin disorders in abdominal stoma patients. *British Journal of Dermatology, 143*, 1248–1260.

Maene, B. (2013). Hidden cost of medical tape-induced injuries. *Wounds UK, 9*, 46–50.

Mahoney, M. F., & Rozenboom, B. J. (2019). Definition and characteristics of chronic tissue injury: A unique form of skin damage. *Journal of Wound Ostomy & Continence Nursing, 46*(3), 187–191.

Marzulli, F. N., & Maibach, H. I. (2008). Allergic contact dermatitis. In H. Zhai, K.-P Wilhelm, & H. I. Maibach (Eds.), *Marzulli and Maibach's dermatotoxicology* (pp. 155–157). Boca Raton, FL: CRC Press.

Matsumura, H., Imai, R., Ahmatjan, N., et al. (2014). Removal of adhesive wound dressing and its effects on the stratum corneum of the skin: Comparison of eight different adhesive wound dressings. *International Wound Journal, 11*(1), 50–54. doi: 10.1111/j.1742-481X.2012.01061.x.

McLane, K., Bookout, K., McCord, S., et al. (2004). The 2003 national pediatric pressure ulcer and skin breakdown prevalence survey: Multisite study. *Journal of Wound Ostomy & Continence Nursing, 31*(4), 168–178.

McNichol, L. L., Ayello, E. A., Phearman, L. A., et al. (2018). Incontinence-associated dermatitis: State of the science and knowledge translation. *Advances in Skin and Wound Care, 31*(11), 502–513.

McNichol, L., Lund, C., Rosen, T., et al. (2013). Medical adhesives and patient safety: State of the science: Consensus statements for the assessment, prevention, and treatment of adhesive-related skin injuries. *Journal Wound Ostomy & Continence Nursing, 40*(4), 365–380.

Messer, L. H., Berget, C., Beatson, C., et al. (2018). Preserving skin integrity with chronic device use in diabetes. *Diabetes Technology & Therapeutics, 20*(S2), S2–S54.

Mistiaen, P., & van Halm-Walters, M. (2010). Prevention and treatment of intertrigo in large skin folds of adults: A systematic review. *BMC Nursing, 9*(1), 12.

Mitchell, A., & Hill, B. (2020). Moisture-associated skin damage: An overview of its diagnosis and management. *British Journal of Community Nursing, 25*(3), S12–S18. https://doi.org/10.12968/bjcn.2020.25.Sup3.S12

National Institute for Occupational Safety and Health (NIOSH). (2013). Skin exposure and effects. Retrieved December 1, 2019 from http://www.cdc.gov/niosh/topics/skin/

National Pressure Injury Advisory Panel (NPIAP). (2020). National Pressure Injury Advisory Panel Support Surface Standards Initiative (S3I) https://cdn.ymaws.com/npiap.com/resource/resmgr/website_version_terms_and_de.pdf

Nguyen, T., Wong, E., & Ciummo, G. (2020). Polypharmacy in older adults: Practical applications alongside a patient case. *JNP–The Journal for Nurse Practitioners, 16*(3), 205–209. https://doi.org/10.1016/j.nurpra.2019.11.017

Noonan, C., Quigley, S. & Curley, M. A. Q. (2006). Skin integrity in hospitalized infants and children a prevalence survey. *Journal of Pediatric Nursing, 21*(6), 445–453.

O'Connor, S., & Murphy, S. (2014). Chronic venous leg ulcers: Is topical zinc the answer? A review of the literature. *Advances in Skin & Wound Care, 27*(1), 35–44.

Okan, D., Woo, K., Ayello, E. A., et al. (2007). The role of moisture balance in wound healing. *Advances in Skin & Wound Care, 20*(1), 39–53.

Omura, Y., Yamabe, M., & Anazawa, S. (2010). Peristomal skin disorders in patients with intestinal and urinary ostomies: Influence of adhesive forces of various hydrocolloid wafer skin barriers. *Journal of Wound Ostomy & Continence Nursing, 37,* 289–298.

Payne, R. L., & Martin, M. C. (1990). The epidemiology and management of skin tears in older adults. *Ostomy & Wound Management, 26*(1), 26–37.

Payne, R. L., & Martin, M. C. (1993). Defining and classifying skin tears: Need for a common language. *Ostomy Wound Management, 39*(5), 16–26.

Persson, E., Berndtsson, I., Carlsson, E., et al. (2010). Stoma-related complications and stoma size a two year follow up. *Colorectal Diseases, 12,* 971–976.

Pinkus, H. (1952). Examination of the epidermis by the strip method. II. Biometric data on regeneration of the human epidermis. *Journal of Investigative Dermatology, 19,* 431–446.

Polatsch, D. B., Baskies, M. A., Hommen, J. P., et al. (2004). Tape blisters that develop after hip fracture surgery: A retrospective series and a review of the literature. *American Journal of Orthopedics (Belle Mead, N.J.), 33*(9), 452–456.

Ratliff, C. (2010). Early peristomal skin complications reported by WOC nurses. *Journal Wound Ostomy & Continence Nursing, 37*(5), 505–510.

Ratliff, C. R. (2017). Descriptive study of the frequency of medical adhesive–related skin injuries in a vascular clinic. *Journal of Vascular Nursing, 35*(2), 86–89.

Ratliff, C. R., & Fletcher, K. R. (2007). Skin tears: A review of the evidence to support prevention and treatment. *Ostomy Wound Management, 53*(3), 32–42.

Reddy, M. (2008). Skin and wound care: Important considerations in the older adult. *Advances Skin Wound Care, 21*(9), 424–436.

Rietschel, R., & Fowler, J. F. (2008). *Fisher's contact dermatitis.* Hamilton, ON: B.C. Decker.

Rogers, A. A., Rippon, M., & Davis, P. (2013). Does "micro-trauma" of tissue play a role in adhesive dressing-initiated damage? *Wounds UK. 9*(4), 128–134.

Ross, P., Gray, A. R., Milburn, J., et al. (2016). Insulin pump-associated adverse events are common, but not associated with glycemic control, socio-economic status, or pump/infusion set type. *Acta Diabetologica, 53*(6), 991–998.

Sanders, C., Young, A., McAndrews, H. F., et al. (2007). A prospective randomized trial on the effect of a soluble adhesive on the ease of dressing removal following hypospadias repair. *Journal of Pediatric Urology, 3*(3), 209–213.

Schmid, M. H., & Kortig, H. C. (1995). The concept of the acid mantle of the skin: Its relevance for the choice of skin cleansers. *Dermatology, 191,* 276–280.

Schober, E., & Rami, B. (2009). Dermatological side effects and complications of continuous subcutaneous insulin infusion in preschool-age and school-age children. *Pediatric Diabetes, 10*(3), 198–201.

Seité, S., Bensadoun, R. J., & Mazer, J. M. (2017). Prevention and treatment of acute and chronic radiodermatitis. *Breast Cancer: Targets and Therapy, 9,* 551.

Sellæg, M. S., Romild, U., & Kuhry, E. (2012). Prevention of tape blisters after hip replacement surgery: A randomized clinical trial. *International Journal of Orthopaedic and Trauma Nursing, 16*(1), 39–46.

Serra, R., Ielapi, N., Barbetta, A., et al. (2018). Skin tears and risk factors assessment: A systematic review on evidence-based medicine. *International Wound Journal, 15*(1), 38–42. https://doi.org/10.1111/iwj.12815

Shah, J. H., Zhai, H., & Maibach, H. I. (2005). Comparative evaporimetry in man. *Skin Research and Technology, 11,* 205–208.

Shelanski, M. V., Phillips, S. B., & Potts, C. E. (1996). Evaluation of cutaneous reactivity to recently marketed dermatologic products. *International Journal of Dermatology, 35*(2), 137–140.

Shevchenko, A., Valdes-Rodriquez, R., & Yosipovitch, G. (2018). Causes, pathophysiology, and treatment of pruritus in the mature patient. *Clinics in Dermatology, 36,* 140–151. doi: 10.1016/j.clindermatol.2017.10.005.

Sivamani, R. K., Goodman, J., Gitis, N. V., et al. (2003). Friction coefficient of skin in real-time. *Skin Research and Technology, 9*(3), 235–239.

Sopher, R., & Gefen, A. (2011). Effects of skin wrinkles, age and wetness on mechanical loads in the stratum corneum as related to skin lesions. *Medical and Biological Engineering and Computing, 49*(1), 97–105.

Stephen-Haynes, J., Callaghan, R., Bethell, E., et al. (2011). The assessment and management of skin tears in care homes. *British Journal of Nursing, 20*(11), S12–S22.

Takahashi, H., Oyama, N., Amamoto, M., et al. (2020). Prospective trial for the clinical efficacy of anogenital skin care with miconazole nitrate-containing soap for diaper candidiasis. *The Journal of Dermatology, 47*(4), 385.

Tammel, K., Benike, D., & Sievers, B. (2019). A novel approach to treating moderate to severe incontinence-associated dermatitis and intertiginous dermatitis: A case series. *Journal of Wound Ostomy & Continence Nursing, 46*(5), 446–452.

Tanner J., Woodings, D., & Moncaster, K. (2006). Perioperative hair removal to reduce surgical site infection. *Cochrane Database Systematic Reviews*, (3), CD004122.

Thayer, D. (2012). Skin damage associated with intravenous therapy: Common problems and strategies for prevention. *Journal of Infusion Nursing, 36*(6), 390–401.

Thayer, D. M., Rozenboom, B., & Baranoski, S. (2016). "Top Down" injuries: Prevention and management of moisture-associated skin damage (MASD), medical adhesive-related skin injury (MARSI), and Skin Tears. In D. B. Doughty, & L. L. McNichol (Eds.), *WOCN Core Curriculum Wound Management*. Philadelphia, PA: Wolters Kluwer.

Timsit, J. F. et al. (2013). Jugular versus femoral short-term catheterization and risk of infection in intensive care unit patients. Causal analysis of two randomized trials. *American Journal of Respiratory and Critical Care Medicine, 188*(10), 1232–1239.

Tokumura, F., Ohyama, K., Fujisawa, H., et al. (1999). Time-dependent changes in dermal peeling force of adhesive tapes. *Skin Research and technology, 5*(1), 33–36.

Tokumura, F., Umekage, K., Sado, M., et al. (2005). Skin irritation due to repetitive application of adhesive tape: The influence of adhesive strength and seasonal variability. *Skin Research and Technology, 11*(2), 102–106.

Tornier, C., Rosdy, M., & Maibach, H. I. (2008). *In vitro* skin irritation testing on SkinEthic™-Reconstituted Human Epidermis: Reproducibility for fifty chemicals tested with two protocols. In H. Zhai, K.-P. Wilhelm, & H. I. Maibach (Eds.), *Marzulli and Maibach's dermatotoxicology* (pp. 927–944). Boca Raton, FL: CRC Press.

Tüzün, Y., Wolf, R., Engin, B., et al., (2015). Bacterial infections of the folds (intertiginous areas). *Clinics in Dermatology, 33*(4), 420–428. https://doi.org/10.1016/j.clindermatol.2015.04.003

Van Tiggelen, H., LeBlanc, K., Campbell, K., et al. (2019). Standardizing the classification of skin tears: Validity and reliability testing of the International Skin Tear Advisory Panel Classification System in 44 countries. *British Journal of Dermatology, 183*(1), 146–154. doi: 10.1111/bjd.18604. Retrieved April 5, 2020 from https://onlinelibrary.wiley.com/doi/epdf/10.1111/bjd.18604

Visscher, M. O., Adam, R., Brink, S., et al. (2015). Newborn infant skin: physiology, development, and care. *Clinics in Dermatology, 33*(3), 271–280.

Voegeli, D. (2012). Moisture-associated skin damage: Aetiology, prevention and treatment. *British Journal of Nursing, 21*(9), 517–521.

Voegeli, D. (2013). Moisture-associated skin damage: An overview for community nurses. *British Journal of Community Nursing, 18*(1), 6, 8, 10–12.

Wang, D., Xu, H., Chen, S., et al. (2019). Medical adhesive-related skin injuries and associated risk factors in a pediatric intensive care unit. *Advances in Skin Wound Care, 32*(4),176–182. doi: 10.1097/01.ASW.0000553601.05196.fb

Waring, M., Bielfeldt, S., Matzold, K., et al. (2011). An evaluation of the skin stripping of wound dressing adhesives. *Journal of Wound Care, 20*(9), 412–422.

Werth, S. L., & Justice, R. (2019). Prevalence of moisture-associated skin damage in an acute care setting: Outcomes from a quality improvement project. *Journal of Wound Ostomy & Continence Nursing, 46*(1), 51–54.

Widmer, J., Elsner, P., & Burg, G. (1994). Skin irritant reactivity following experimental cumulative irritant contact dermatitis. *Contact Dermatitis, 199*(30), 33–39.

Wong, H., Heuberger, R., Logomarsino, J., et al. (2016). Associations between alcohol use, polypharmacy and falls in older adults. *Nursing Older People, 28*(1), 30–36.

Woo, K. Y., Beeckman, D., & Chakravarthy, D. (2017). Management of moisture-associated skin damage: A scoping review. *Advances in Skin & Wound Care, 30*(11), 494–501. https://doi.org/10.1097/01.ASW.0000525627.54569.da

Woo, K., & LeBlanc, K. (2018). Prevalence of skin tears among frail older adults living in Canadian long-term care facilities. *International Journal of Palliative Nursing, 24*(6), 288–294.

Yates, S., McNichol, L., Heinecke, S. B., et al. (2017). Embracing the concept, defining the practice, and changing the outcome. *Journal of Wound, Ostomy and Continence Nursing, 44*(1), 13–17.

Zhai, H., & Maibach, H. I. (2001). Skin occlusion and irritant and allergic contact dermatitis: An overview. *Contact Dermatitis, 44*, 201–206.

Zhai, H., Dika, E., Goldovsky, M., et al. (2007). Tape-stripping method in man: Comparison of evaporimetric methods. *Skin Research and Technology, 13*, 207–210.

Zhao H, He Y, Wie, Q, et al. (2018). Medical adhesive-related skin injury prevalence at the peripherally inserted central catheter insertion site: A cross-sectional, multiple center study. *Journal Wound Ostomy and Continence Nursing, 45*(1):22–25.

Zulkowski, K. (2017). Understanding moisture-associated skin damage, medical adhesive-related skin injuries, and skin tears. *Advances in Skin & Wound Care, 30*(8), 372–381.

QUESTIONS

1. A home care patient is found to have a linear skin tear at the base of her abdominal skin fold. Which of the following are risk factors in developing this type of skin injury?
A. Obesity
B. Diabetes
C. Perspiration
D. All of the above

2. Strategies to prevent PWMASD include
A. The selection of dressings that provide effective exudate control
B. Reinforcing saturated dressings instead of changing
C. Using a tackifier in place of a liquid skin protectant around the periwound skin
D. Applying a pouching system for wounds with <100 mL of exudate

3. Which product would be an appropriate choice to treat PMASD?
A. Zinc-based protective barrier
B. Skin protectant with cyanoacrylate
C. Antibiotic ointment
D. Stoma paste

4. The wound care nurse documents a type 2 skin tear. What are the characteristics of this type of skin tear?
A. No skin loss; flap tear that can be repositioned to cover the wound bed
B. Partial flap loss that cannot be repositioned to cover the wound bed
C. Partial flap loss that can be repositioned to cover the wound bed
D. Total flap loss exposing entire wound bed

5. Which anatomical skin change related to aging predisposes the elderly to skin tears?
A. Thickening of the epidermis
B. Increased production of skin lipids
C. Loss of subcutaneous tissue
D. Increased "anchoring" of the epidermis to the dermis

6. The wound care nurse is managing an elderly patient who has a skin tear. Which of the following is a recommended guideline?
A. Do not remove the skin flap even if it is necrotic.
B. Cleanse the wound with hydrogen peroxide.
C. Administer antibiotics prophylactically.
D. Select a dressing that absorbs exudate.

7. What type of dressing is recommended for type 2 and type 3 skin tears?
A. Nonadhesive foam dressings secured with wrap gauze.
B. Hydrocolloid dressings.
C. Transparent film dressings.
D. Dressings should not be used for skin tears.

8. Which of the following patients is most susceptible to an epidermal stripping injury?
A. A 62-year-old female
B. A 42-year-old male
C. A 6-year-old female
D. An 82-year-old male

9. During application, which of the following facilitates adhesion of most medical adhesive products?
A. Heat
B. Light
C. Pressure
D. Tension

10. A liquid skin protectant may be applied under an adhesive product to
A. Increase initial tack of the adhesive product
B. Increase wear time of the adhesive product
C. Form a protective interface between the skin and the adhesive product
D. Reduce the likelihood of an allergic contact dermatitis

ANSWERS AND RATIONALES

1. D. Rationale: Contributing factors to ITD include the following: reduced perfusion (common in adipose tissue), diabetes, and concomitant administration of steroids and broad-spectrum antibiotics. Obese individuals are at high risk due to increased perspiration and the challenges of personal hygiene resulting from restricted dexterity and limited ability to reach the necessary areas to cleanse.

2. A. Rationale: Prevention and management of periwound MASD include selection of dressings (and dressing change frequency) to effectively manage wound exudate.

3. B. Rationale: Skin protectants containing cyanoacrylates have the ability to attach to and protect wet, damaged skin surfaces and allow pouch adherence.

4. B. Rationale: Description of a type 2 skin tear per the ISTAP Classification System is partial flap loss that cannot be repositioned to cover the wound.

5. C. Rationale: Subcutaneous tissue provides protection against shear force. Loss of subcutaneous tissue increases skin vulnerability to minor trauma, especially over the face, dorsum of the hands, and shins.

6. D. Rationale: Skin tears are optimally managed with a dressing that will manage exudate and promote a healing environment.

7. A. Rationale: The recommended dressing options for skin tears include nonadherent dressings such as nonadhesive foam secured with wrap or roll gauze, nonadherent contact layers secured with wrap or roll gauze, impregnated mesh, silicone mesh, hydrogel, alginate, hydrofiber, and clear acrylic dressings and those dressings with gentle adhesive properties.

8. D. Rationale: Age has been considered a significant risk factor, with the very young and very old being at greatest risk. The elderly are at risk due to changes in the dermal–epidermal junction that compromise the attachment of the epidermis to the dermis including flattening of the rete ridge and reduction in number of rete pegs.

9. C. Rationale: The majority of medical adhesive products are coated with pressure sensitive adhesives. The application of gentle warming hand pressure enhances adhesion to the skin.

10. C. Rationale: When applied to the skin, the liquid skin protectant dries on the skin as a transparent coating that provides a protective interface between the epidermis and the adhesive.

CHAPTER 19

INCONTINENCE-ASSOCIATED DERMATITIS

Debra Thayer and Denise Nix

OBJECTIVES

1. Explain the pathology and clinical presentation of incontinence-associated dermatitis (IAD).

2. Describe strategies for prevention and management of incontinence-associated dermatitis (IAD).

TOPIC OUTLINE

DEFINITION

Incontinence-associated dermatitis (IAD) is a type of top-down injury and the most common form of moisture–associated skin damage (MASD). IAD is characterized by erythema and edema of the surface of the skin, sometimes accompanied by serous exudate, erosion, or secondary cutaneous infection (Beeckman et al., 2016; Gray et al., 2012). See **Figure 19-1**.

The term dermatitis denotes inflammation and erythema with or without erosion or denudation. The term IAD specifically identifies the source of the irritant (urine or fecal incontinence) and acknowledges that the area of the skin affected commonly extends beyond the perineum (Bryant, 2012). Further, the term is not limited to an anatomical location (e.g., perineum) or persons using body worn absorbent products (BWAP) such as diapers, or briefs (Gray et al., 2007).

KEY POINT

Incontinence-associated dermatitis (IAD) is characterized by erythema and edema of the surface of the skin, sometimes accompanied by serous exudate, erosion, or secondary cutaneous infection. It involves only the superficial layers of the skin thereby reflecting a "top-down" injury.

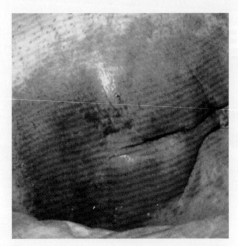

FIGURE 19-1. Incontinence-Associated Dermatitis (IAD). Note diffuse erythema, patchy areas of denudation, and coexisting candidiasis. (Courtesy of KDS Consulting.)

 SIGNIFICANCE

IAD can result in pain, discomfort, infection, pressure injuries, depression, loss of independence, disruption in activities and/or sleep, reduced quality of life, and undue burden of care (Beeckman et al., 2015; Campbell et al., 2016; Demarre et al., 2015; Minassian et al., 2013). The prevalence and clinical relevance of IAD has been measured in a variety of health care settings.

In a large sample of 5,342 adults in *acute care* facilities in 36 states in the United States, 46.6% of patients were incontinent of urine, stool, or both. In that sample, the prevalence of IAD was 45.7% with 14.8% of the patients with IAD also presented with secondary fungal infections (Gray & Giuliano, 2018). In *long-term care*, researchers combined data from two electronic databases, the MDS, and practitioners' orders, and reported a 5.5% incidence of IAD in a group of 10,713 nursing home residents newly diagnosed with incontinence (Bliss et al., 2017). A large study ($N=3,406$) of residents in German nursing homes reported a 5.2%-point prevalence for individuals with incontinence (Boronat-Garrido et al., 2016). A *long-term acute care* setting in the United States reported a 22.8%-point prevalence of IAD and a 7.6% incidence based on direct observation of 171 patients (Long et al., 2012). In a study of 189 *community-dwelling* individuals with fecal or fecal and urinary incontinence (dual), more than half (52.5%) reported recurring episodes of IAD (Rohwer et al., 2013).

IAD was identified as an independent risk factor for pressure injuries ($p = 0.001$) in a secondary analysis of a randomized clinical trial with 610 patients with incontinence (Demarre et al., 2015). A meta-analysis of 58 studies showed a statistically significant association between incontinence and pressure injuries and a statistically significant ($p < 0.05$) relationship between IAD and full-thickness pressure injuries (Beeckman et al., 2014). Data from a study of 176,689 patients cared for in predominately acute care facilities over 2 years showed a 53%

prevalence of incontinence. The likelihood of developing pressure injuries among incontinent patients was higher (6.3%) compared to patients without incontinence (4.1%). Of the subjects with facility-acquired pressure injuries, 6% had incontinence, while 1.6% did not (Lachenbruch et al., 2016). Similarly, in the large sample of acute care patients ($N = 2,492$) mentioned earlier, Gray and Giuliano (2018) reported that the patients with IAD were also more likely to experience a facility-acquired sacral area pressure injury (32.3%) compared to only 6.3% of patients without IAD ($p < 0.001$). Further, the subjects with IAD were more likely to develop a facility-acquired full-thickness sacral pressure injury (6.4%) compared to 1.5% of patients without IAD ($p < 0.001$). Not surprisingly, occurrence of pressure injuries has been positively related to the severity of IAD (Park & Kim, 2014).

> **KEY POINT**
>
> IAD is quite a prevalent condition especially in acute care facilities; it is an *independent risk factor* for pressure injury development.

 PATHOLOGY

Overhydration of the stratum corneum (SC) compromises the brick-and-mortar configuration of the epidermal layer and permits penetration by irritants found in urine and stool, which results in inflammation and impaired tensile strength. As urea in urine breaks down, highly alkaline ammonia is produced and changes pH from acid to alkaline compromising the protective acidic mantle of the skin. Gray and Giuliano (2018) demonstrated that individuals exposed to urine and stool or liquid stool are at higher risk for IAD, than those exposed to formed stool ($p < 0.001$). The pH properties of formed stool are more neutral and have fewer active enzymes than liquid stool.

> **KEY POINT**
>
> Overhydration of the stratum corneum compromises the brick-and-mortar configuration of the epidermal layer and permits penetration by irritants found in urine and stool; urine urea changes into ammonia causing elevated skin pH creating a conducive environment for microbial growth.

Friction is the resistance to motion in a parallel direction relative to the common boundary of two surfaces. Skin injury by friction initially appears as erythema and progresses to an abrasion. Friction primarily affects superficial layers and thus does not result in tissue necrosis (Bryant, 2012). Incontinence care involves the use of friction for skin cleansing. Forces of friction, shear or drag, against an underlying surface (bed, chair, linen, containment garments) facilitate deformation of tissue layers and injures the skin allowing pathogens such as *Candida* and *Staphylococcus* to invade and cause secondary infections (Voegeli, 2012).

KEY POINT

Skin injury by friction initially appears as erythema and progresses to an abrasion. Friction primarily affects superficial layers and thus does not result in tissue necrosis. Forces of friction include incontinence care, shear, or drag against an underlying surface facilitating tissue layer deformation that leads to skin injury.

RISK FACTORS

Risk factors for developing IAD include incontinence, frequent episodes of incontinence, poor skin condition, compromised mobility, diminished cognitive awareness, inability to perform personal hygiene, pain, raised body temperature, select medications, poor nutritional status, and critical illness (Beeckman et al., 2015). Dual fecal and urinary incontinence, loose stools, and diarrhea increase the likelihood of IAD. Although increased age is associated with higher prevalence of incontinence, age does not appear to be an independent risk factor for IAD (Kottner et al., 2014). Raised body temperature causes the body to sweat and store heat longer impairing moisture evaporation or transepidermal water loss (TEWL). Environmental humidity also impairs TEWL. When environmental humidity decreases, TEWL is likely to increase (Gray et al., 2011). As previously described, exposure to urine and stool or liquid stool are at greater risk for IAD due to the more neutral pH properties and fewer active enzymes in formed stool (see **Fig. 19-2**).

KEY POINT

Dual urinary and fecal incontinence, loose stools, and diarrhea increase the likelihood of IAD.

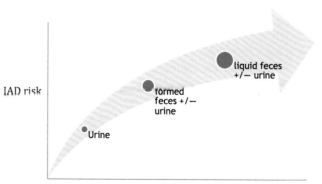

FIGURE 19-2. IAD Risk. (From Beeckman, D., et al. (2015). Proceedings of the Global IAD Expert Panel. Incontinence-associated dermatitis: Moving prevention forward. *Wounds International*. Reproduced with kind permission of Wounds International, London, UK.)

RISK

Pressure injury risk assessment tools are not designed to predict the risk for IAD. Risk assessment tools for IAD have been developed and tested for validity and reliability (Li et al., 2019; Nix, 2002; Shiu et al., 2013). IAD risk assessment tools, however, are not widely used in clinical practice. Much like pressure injury risk assessment tools, IAD risk assessment tools do not capture all known risk factors.

CLINICAL PRESENTATION AND SKIN ASSESSMENT

IAD appears initially as erythema ranging from pink to red. Darker skin tones may present with paler, yellow, or dark discoloration (Bliss et al., 2014). Affected skin can look patchy with nondistinct edges. IAD can be located at any anatomical location exposed to urine and/or stool. Vesicles, papules, or pustules may be present, or the epidermis may be eroded exposing moist, weeping dermis (see **Fig. 19-3**). IAD-affected skin maybe warm or firm on palpation due to the underlying inflammation. Whether the IAD presents as intact erythema or severely eroded skin, patients often complain of burning, itching, tingling, or pain. A red rash with pinpoint satellite lesions (papules or pustules) indicative of a candidiasis (a secondary infection) is not uncommon (Beeckman et al., 2015). Bacterial infections secondary to IAD are not commonly reported in peer review literature.

KEY POINT

IAD presents as intact erythema or severely eroded skin, patients often complain of burning, itching, tingling, or pain. A red rash with pinpoint satellite lesions (papules or pustules) indicative of a candidiasis (a secondary infection).

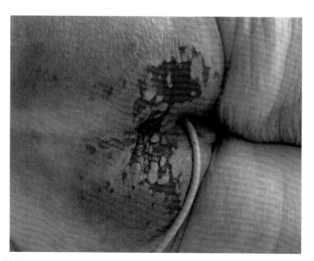

FIGURE 19-3. Severe IAD-Note Areas of Denudement Surrounded by Erythema. (From Beeckman, D., et al. (2015). Proceedings of the Global IAD Expert Panel. Incontinence-associated dermatitis: Moving prevention forward. *Wounds International*. Reproduced with kind permission of Wounds International, London, UK.)

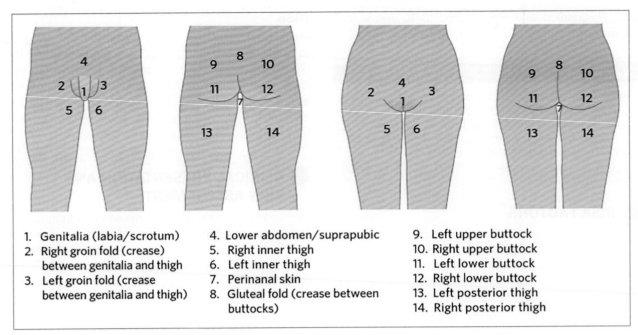

1. Genitalia (labia/scrotum)
2. Right groin fold (crease) between genitalia and thigh
3. Left groin fold (crease between genitalia and thigh)
4. Lower abdomen/suprapubic
5. Right inner thigh
6. Left inner thigh
7. Perinanal skin
8. Gluteal fold (crease between buttocks)
9. Left upper buttock
10. Right upper buttock
11. Left lower buttock
12. Right lower buttock
13. Left posterior thigh
14. Right posterior thigh

FIGURE 19-4. Anatomic Locations Susceptible to IAD. (From Beeckman, D., et al. (2015). Proceedings of the Global IAD Expert Panel. Incontinence-associated dermatitis: Moving prevention forward. *Wounds International*. Reproduced with kind permission of Wounds International, London, UK.)

All patients with urinary and/or fecal incontinence should have their skin assessed regularly to check for signs of IAD. This should be done at least once daily but may be indicated more often based on contributing factors such as frequent or loose stools. In a critical care population, Coyer et al. (2017) observed that IAD developed rapidly and resulted in moderate to severe skin damage. IAD can develop in any anatomical location exposed to urine and feces such as anus, vulva, scrotum, labia, groin folds, lower abdomen, thighs, gluteal folds, gluteal cleft, buttocks, and the sacrococcygeal region (see **Fig. 19-4**).

Decision-making for managing IAD is dependent on visual skin assessment and determination of the severity of skin damage. Tools have been developed to guide visual assessment of IAD and have various degrees of validity and reliability testing (Beeckman et al., 2015, 2018; Borchert et al., 2010). However, they are not yet routinely used in clinical practice.

DIFFERENTIAL DIAGNOSIS

IAD, moisture lesions, stage 2 pressure injuries, and friction injury are superficial "top-down" wounds. Full-thickness wounds from pressure and shear are considered "bottom up" (Sibbald et al., 2011). These types of wounds can occur alone or in combination on or near the perineal, perianal, sacral, and buttocks region making differential assessment a challenge. Careful attention must be paid to exact anatomical location, pain descriptions, patterns, distribution of lesions, and risk factors not only for IAD and pressure but also other skin conditions

that may occur near the perineal, perianal, sacral, and buttocks region (see **Table 19-1**).

PREVENTION AND MANAGEMENT OF INCONTINENCE-ASSOCIATED DERMATITIS

All patients who are incontinent are at risk for developing skin damage. Because of the adverse clinical outcomes associated with IAD (pressure injury development, secondary infection, and pain), the continence nurse specialist needs to create and implement a robust prevention strategy. This includes establishing guidance for care, creating a product formulary, and educating of bedside caregivers to recognize risk, assess skin condition, and consistently implement relevant interventions.

A guideline for IAD prevention and treatment has not been developed, but a set of best practice principles has been established (Beeckman et al., 2015). Key interventions include risk assessment, continence management, skin assessment, and skin care.

As discussed previously, risk for IAD is primarily driven by the type of incontinence with patients who have fecal and dual incontinence at higher risk than those incontinent of urine alone. In their study, Park and Kim (2014) reported that all patients with fecal incontinence had some evidence of IAD. More recently, intensive prevention efforts for catheter-associated urinary tract infection (CAUTI), especially in the acute care setting, have led to reduced usage of indwelling catheters. As a result, dual incontinence is more common and places patients at higher risk of skin damage.

TABLE 19-1 DIFFERENTIAL DIAGNOSIS OF PERINEAL/PERIANAL SKIN CONDITIONS

	IAD	CANDIDIASIS	HERPES ZOSTER	PRESSURE
Location	Perineum Buttocks Inner thighs Groin Lower abdominal skin folds	Perineum Buttocks Inner thighs Groin Lower abdominal skin folds	Perianal Buttocks Genitals	Near bony prominences Coccyx, sacrum, ischium Under device/tube
Confirmed Risk Factors	Urinary and/or fecal incontinence	Moisture Antibiotics Immunosuppression	Immunosuppression Elderly Stress	Limited mobility or activity Dependent on others for repositioning, transferring, etc.
Blisters	Yes	No	Initially vesicles then pustules	Sometimes (Stage II)
Distribution Pattern	Confluent or patchy Irregular edges with erythema Shallow denudement, and/or maceration Fleshy part of buttocks	Confluent or patchy rash Small round pustules, plaques, and/or satellite lesions	Grouped unilateral distribution of rash or ulcerations along dermatome Pustules erode into ulcerations Clusters or isolated individual shallow lesions or blisters	Isolated individual lesions on or near bony prominence or pressure-causing device Damage ranges from intact discoloration to partial- or full-thickness wounds
Color	Pink/red	Pink/red	Initial: Pink/red Ulcer may have yellow slough Later: Crust Severe cases: Necrosis	Pink, red, yellow, tan, gray, brown, black
Discomfort	Pain may be mild to severe	Itching, burning	Tingling sometimes noted initially Often very painful	Pain may be absent to severe
Diagnostic Tests	None	Potassium hydroxide preparation scraping (KOH)	DNA polymerase chain reaction assay and direct immunofluorescent stain of skin scraping for VZV antigen Tzanck preparation Tissue culture	None

With permission: Bryant, R. A. (2012). Types of skin damage and differential diagnosis. In R. A. Bryant & D. P. Nix (Eds.), *Acute and chronic wounds: Current management concepts* (5th ed.). St Louis, MO: Mosby Elsevier.

KEY POINT

People who suffer dual incontinence (urine and stool) are at higher risk for IAD, especially with liquid stool.

KEY POINT

The most effective way to prevent IAD is to eliminate or reduce incontinent episodes. This removes the primary factors (moisture, irritants, and friction) that contribute to skin injury.

The most effective way to prevent IAD is to eliminate or reduce incontinent episodes. This removes the primary factors (moisture, irritants, friction) that contribute to skin injury. In any setting, the continence nurse should be able to perform a basic continence evaluation and implement a plan of care to address reversible problems such as urinary retention, urinary tract infection, and fecal impaction. Additionally, identification of problematic medications that are continence-disruptive can be accomplished through collaboration with a pharmacist; alternatives can be identified and suggested to the primary care provider. For patients in acute care who are nonambulant but able to toilet, toileting schedules and equipment (e.g., commodes) should be built into the plan of care in order to formalize incontinence as a health care problem and continence as a goal.

In post-acute settings, more comprehensive continence management programs can be undertaken. Behavioral programs including bowel and/or bladder training programs should be considered for patients with the potential for bladder or bowel rehabilitation. Attention to mobility improvement and dietary modifications can also be implemented. Refer to Chapter 6 for more information on bladder and bowel health measures and conservative continence management.

During continence restoration or whenever continence is intractable, containment or diversion should be used to protect skin from stool or urine. Use of body worn absorbent products (BWAPs) remains the most common approach to containment (Gray et al., 2018). Briefs, pull-ons and pads comprise the most common designs with products typically composed of four layers. The "coverstock" is the layer contacting skin, an "acquisition" layer facilitates fluid movement, the absorbent core sequesters fluid, and an outer barrier layer prevents egress of fluid from the product into the environment. Modern absorbent cores contain superabsorbent polymers (SAPs), molecules that are designed to absorb many times their weight and retain fluid away from the skin. Increasingly, products are designed with a breathable outer barrier to improve moisture and heat transfer.

Concern over the effect of occlusive absorbent products on skin began with observations regarding the effect of infant diapers (Berg, 1988). While absorbent products do not cause IAD, product composition and construction can contribute to altered microclimate and skin damage (Falloon et al., 2018). Adult products with poorly absorbent core material such as fluff or pulp do not sequester liquid, resulting in skin contact with moisture. Occlusive outer layers have been shown to trap moisture and increase heat at the product–skin interface. The practice of leaving briefs unfastened and the skin "open to air" evolved from concerns that briefs trapped moisture. Many clinicians believe that this is beneficial for skin health, but no evidence exists to support this assumption. This practice is of questionable value when BWAPs containing materials that support normal microclimate are used. Additionally, a brief that is not positioned on the patient as designed nor fastened can move and bunch potentially creating a source of friction or pressure.

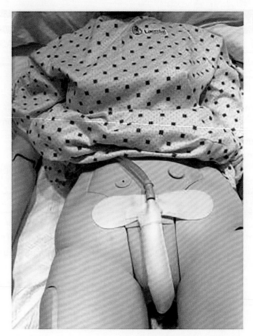

FIGURE 19-5. Female External Collection Device. (From Beeson, T., & Davis, C. (2018). Urinary management with an external female collection device. *Journal of Wound Ostomy and Continence Nursing, 45*(2), 187–189.)

> **KEY POINT**
>
> Absorbent products do not cause IAD, product composition and construction can contribute to altered microclimate and skin damage.

Layering of pads and linens under the patient has been identified not only as a risk factor for pressure injuries but also for IAD (Kayser et al., 2019). As with occlusive body worn products, normal microclimate is compromised by heat and excessive hydration. Increasing from 1 to 6 layers has been shown to double the risk of pressure injury development (Schwartz et al., 2018).

> **KEY POINT**
>
> Layering of pads and linens under the patient has been identified not only as a risk factor for pressure injuries but also for IAD.

With the reduction in indwelling catheter use, use of female external urinary containment devices has grown. See **Figure 19-5**. Intended for bed and chair-bound individuals, these devices are positioned over the urethral meatus and labia and connected to suction. Urine moves across the absorbent interface and is absorbed into material within the device. Two devices have been commercialized, one with a latex outer covering, the other covered in silicone. Early published experience (Beeson & Davis, 2018) suggests benefits not only for skin but also in minimizing the sleep disruptive effects of incontinence. As with any device with rigid components, patients are at risk for medical device–related pressure injury.

Based on available published evidence and expert opinion, external collection devices (ECDs) can be safely used for urine diversion in males (Gray et al., 2016). ECDs include latex and nonlatex sheath devices (i.e., "condom" catheters). Sheath devices should be available in a range of sizes, and staff should be trained in principles and techniques of application and removal in order to prevent medical adhesive–related skin injury (MARSI). Other ECD options include a retracted penile pouch and a glans-adherent device.

Options for stool diversion and containment remain limited with BWAPs engineered to primarily manage urine (i.e., fluid). Fecal management systems are used for diversion of liquid stool in non- or minimally ambulant patients. A silicone catheter with a soft inflatable cuff is retained in the rectum and connected to bedside drainage. These devices offer the advantage of stool diversion and containment providing benefits for both skin health and infection control. Benoit and Watts (2007) reported a 30.5% reduction in prevalence and incidence of pressure injuries when a fecal management system was used as part of a comprehensive pressure ulcer prevention program. Echols et al. (2007) reported fewer UTIs and skin and soft tissue infections in a burn population. Because leakage can occur around the catheter, skin protection is an essential intervention (see Fig. 22-3, Chapter 22).

A fecal pouch applied to the perianal area can provide an alternative to an indwelling fecal management device (see Fig. 22-2, Chapter 22). While a noninvasive approach, application can be difficult due to anatomic contours and available space between the vagina/scrotum and the anus. The pouch can also be easily disrupted with patient movement or repositioning. Devices are most successful when connected to bedside drainage. As with female urinary devices, attention to prevention of device-related pressure injury is required.

SKIN CARE

Recent data have identified a relationship between IAD and pressure injury (Barakat-Johnson et al., 2018; Demarre et al., 2015; Gray & Giuliano, 2018). Considering this, it is important to think of skin care not merely as a tool for IAD prevention, but rather as an essential and complementary component of a successful PI prevention bundle.

First described by Lyder et al. (1992), a "structured skin care regimen" is still considered a best practice approach to prevention *and* treatment of IAD (Beeckman et al., 2009; Park & Kim, 2014). This term describes a standardized approach to care and product selection based on skin condition. A protocol or algorithm guides care while simplifying decision-making for bedside staff and helping to ensure compliance with best practice (Beeckman et al., 2015). Cleansing and protection comprise the two key interventions within a structured skin care regimen (Beeckman et al., 2015). Product choice for these interventions is primarily based on clinician preference and increasingly, contractual agreements. Unlike other medical products or even a consumer product like sunscreen, there are no accepted standards or criteria by which to evaluate and compare efficacy of cleansers, moisturizers, or protective products. From a regulatory perspective, most skin care products used for IAD prevention and treatment fall into one of three FDA categories: (1) over-the-counter ("OTC") products (many moisture barriers, antifungals, and some multifunctional products); (2) cosmetics (moisturizers, some moisture barriers, and cleansers), or (3) medical devices (barrier films and skin protectants). Rules for labeling and claims differ for each category. For both OTC drugs and cosmetics, efficacy is primarily based on composition. Only OTC drugs are required to identify an "active" ingredient.

> **KEY POINT**
>
> Think of "structured skin care regimen" not merely as a tool for IAD prevention and treatment, but rather as an essential and complementary component of a successful pressure injury prevention bundle.

Two recent reviews have evaluated the quality of evidence for incontinence-related skin care. A total of 18 papers were included in final analyses with 5 studies included in both reviews. Prather et al. (2017) reported on 10 studies, noting significant deficiencies including weak methodologies, wide variation in "comparators [and] outcomes," ambiguous or incomplete data, and a range of measurement tools. A 2016 Cochrane review by Beekman and colleagues set out to "assess and compare the effectiveness of various products and procedures to prevent and treat IAD in adults." Authors reported that the majority of trials suffered from small sample size and lack of blinding. Based on these limitations, pooling of data and meta-analysis was not possible in either review, and the Cochrane review concluded that "there is little evidence of very low to moderate quality, on the effectiveness of interventions for preventing and treating IAD in adults" (Beeckman et al., 2016, p. 34).

Best practice guidance for cleansing advocates use of no rinse, "pH balanced" liquid cleansers. Similar in principle to cosmetic facial cleansers, cleansers for incontinence are water-based solutions that contain ingredients ("surfactants") to reduce surface tension and allow cleansing with a minimum of friction. "Gentleness" has consistently been identified as an important criterion for cleanser selection, and the term, while somewhat vague, is generally interpreted to mean lack of potential to induce irritation. While the category of surfactant (anionic, cationic, nonionic) has been often cited as an important decision criterion, product safety should be assessed based on the *overall formulation*.

> **KEY POINT**
>
> Cleansing the skin following an incontinence episode is the *first* step in a structured skin care program. Cleansers for incontinence should be pH balanced, contain surfactants to reduce surface tension, and friction with incontinence skin cleansing practices.

While the benefit of these products for incontinence cleansing is widely accepted, this is largely based on formulation science and expert opinion. A small crossover trial (Byers et al., 1995) evaluated 10 nursing home patients comparing a no-rinse liquid cleanser to (1) liquid soap, (2) liquid cleanser plus skin protectant, (3) soap and water plus skin protectant, and (4) soap and water. No skin breakdown was observed in any group, but in the cleanser group, positive effects were noted for the parameters of pH and TEWL. In their systematic review, Prather et al. evaluated two studies that compared foam cleansers to soap and water (Cooper & Gray, 2001; Park & Kim, 2014) They concluded that the foam cleanser appeared to be "slightly more effective than soap in water in preventing IAD or skin breakdown that may lead to pressure ulcers."

Cleansers are typically classified as cosmetics. Suitability for use on damaged skin should not be assumed and should be evaluated using manufacturer's data.

Cleansers are delivered as sprays, as foams, or in premoistened wipes. For liquids and foams, use with soft, nonlinting cloths is recommended. In settings where concentrated formulations are used, it is critical that staff understand and follow instructions for dilution. From an ease of use perspective, cleansers and multifunctional products are convenient and reduce nursing time required as opposed to basins and cloths (Beeckman et al., 2015; Lewis-Byers et al., 2002; Warshaw et al., 2002).

In settings where cleansers are not available, a liquid soap formulated for sensitive skin can be an option. No published trials have compared sensitive-skin formulation soaps (liquid or bar) to liquid cleansers. Plain water can be an acceptable alternative for cleansing (Beeckman et al., 2015). When skin is denuded and pain is present, water gently delivered by syringe may be better tolerated than a spray cleanser or wipes. Use of standard bath bar soaps is discouraged as they are considered to be pH disruptive, drying, and irritating based on their formulation.

Evidence to support routine use of antiseptics for incontinence cleansing has not been published. The continence nurse should carefully evaluate cleansers promoted as antimicrobial or antibacterial. This labeling may be referencing ingredients (e.g., benzalkonium hydrochloride, benzethonium hydrochloride) that are incorporated to preserve the formulation and that do not provide an antimicrobial therapeutic benefit.

KEY POINT

Plain water can be an acceptable alternative for cleansing especially if the skin is denuded, and water gently delivered by syringe may be better tolerated than a spray cleanser or wipes. Use of standard bath bar soaps is discouraged as they are pH disruptive, drying, and irritating based on their formulation.

Bedside staff should understand that patients experiencing incontinence are at risk for *preventable* skin injury and intervene accordingly. Recent evidence has shown that exposure to synthetic urine rapidly creates adverse changes to barrier function, even with the presence of a

wicking absorbent pad (Phipps et al., 2019). When stool and especially liquid stool is present, removal of irritants is even more critical, reinforcing the importance of prompt cleansing.

KEY POINT

Bedside staff should understand that patients experiencing incontinence are at risk for *preventable* skin injury and need to intervene with prompt cleansing. Research reports that exposure to synthetic urine rapidly creates adverse changes to barrier function, even with the presence of a wicking absorbent pad and more so with liquid stool.

Protection of skin is the *second* critical step in a structured skin care regimen. For a product to provide protection, *minimally* it must repel moisture (i.e., be waterproof) and remain in place over the affected area. Protection from liquid stool, or dual stool and urine, require a substantive barrier that is capable of protecting skin from an irritant (i.e., fecal enzymes) in addition to moisture remaining in place over the affected area.

The terms skin protectant, moisture barrier, and skin barrier are used interchangeably to describe these products. Recently, the term "leave-on" (as opposed to products that are rinsed off) has been applied to moisture barriers (Kottner & Surber, 2016).

KEY POINT

Protection of the skin with a "leave-on" moisture barrier is the *second* critical step in a structured skin care regimen. Several terms are used to describe skin barrier products: moisture barrier, skin barrier, and skin protectant, but "moisture barrier" is the preferred term.

Several characteristics are desirable for a protective product (see **Table 19-2**). Beyond barrier capability, the ability to allow evaporation from the skin surface, often referred to as breathability, is critical for normal SC function. Skin is constantly transpiring moisture vapor, and occlusive materials have been shown to trap moisture within hours of application. This results in an impaired epidermal barrier and reduced skin breaking strength. Additionally, frictional forces are increased when skin is wet (Gerhardt et al., 2008; Schaefer et al., 2002; Zhai & Maibach, 2002). Increased friction can not only result in superficial injury but also contributes to shear strain.

Polymer-based liquids, creams, ointments, and pastes are the most common forms of barrier products. Because standard measures of barrier performance have not been established, comparisons of different forms are difficult at best (Beeckman, 2017). In this chapter, the term *moisture barrier* will be used as a generic descriptor to describe protective products.

TABLE 19-2 DESIRABLE MOISTURE BARRIER PRODUCT CHARACTERISTICS

DESIRABLE MOISTURE BARRIER PRODUCT CHARACTERISTICS	RATIONALE
Provides durable protection	Minimally should be waterproof, should be capable of protection from fecal enzymes if used for protection from liquid stool
Breathable	To allow normal moisture-vapor transmission from skin
Close to skin pH	Note—pH value not relevant to chemistry of most polymeric films
Low irritant potential	Previously referred to as "hypoallergenic," dye-free, fragrance-free
Nonstinging and/or comfortable during wear	Promotes patient comfort
Transparent	Allows skin inspection
Does not require removal or easily removed	Minimizes friction required for cleansing, promotes patient comfort ease of use
Does not contribute to skin damage (e.g., does not increase friction)	Minimizing friction at skin surface will reduce risk of tissue deformation associated with shear strain
Does not interfere with absorption of incontinence products	Enables function of BWAPs or external female devices

Modified from general characteristics of the ideal product for prevention and treatment of IAD (Beeckman et al., 2015).

KEY POINT

The term "skin protectant" may be used as a generic descriptor or may refer to a specific FDA category of over-the-counter (OTC) drugs. Only OTC skin protectants designate an "active" ingredient, and a document called a "monograph" recognizes 21 ingredients that may be identified as an "active." Specific guidance for labeling and claims based on the ingredient(s) used are provided for manufacturers. Creams, ointments, and pastes not labeled as OTC drug skin protectants are typically cosmetics; cosmetics are not considered to have active ingredients.

Liquid barriers include barrier films and skin protectants. Modern barrier films contain polymers (large molecules composed of monomers) dissolved in a nonstinging, alcohol-free solvent delivered via an applicator or spray. The solvent acts as a carrier to deliver the polymer and then evaporates, leaving a thin, transparent waterproof coating on the skin. Products are similar in appearance but vary in protective ability. Film products

that are described by the manufacturer as "easy to remove" with soap and water are not waterproof and will fail to form a durable barrier.

KEY POINT

While the term "skin sealant" is often used to describe barrier films, it more accurately describes early formulations containing copolymers and alcohol primarily used for ostomy care.

Barrier films do not readily attach to wet surfaces. When using the product to protect a damaged surface that is also wet, many Wound Ostomy Continence (WOC) nurses employ a technique called "crusting." Ostomy powder is dusted onto the damaged surface to create a dry platform. Excess powder is removed, and the barrier film is then sprayed or blotted onto the powder and allowed to dry creating a protective barrier. The process is then repeated two or more times depending on preference. Anecdotally, the technique is reported to be effective but can be labor-intensive and difficult for bedside staff to replicate. Data evaluating the efficacy of crusting versus other forms of moisture barriers have not been reported.

Film-forming liquid skin protectants differ from barrier films. Two products are commercially available: a cyanoacrylate monomer and a polymer–cyanoacrylate complex. Long available as tissue sealants, cyanoacrylates impart the ability to attach to wet, surfaces. As such, they offer an option for protection of severely damaged skin where weeping is present. A nonrandomized prospective study (Brennan et al., 2017) evaluated the polymer–cyanoacrylate formulation in 16 patients with IAD. Skin condition improved in 13 of 16 patients. Pain reduction was noted in those patients able to self-report. In a randomized, prospective trial of 21 healthy volunteers (Mathisen et al., 2018), the polymer–cyanoacrylate product showed superior durability to repeated washing as compared to two commercially available barrier films and the cyanoacrylate monomer product.

KEY POINT

Film-forming liquid skin protectants differ from traditional barrier films. Two products are commercially available: a cyanoacrylate monomer and a polymer–cyanoacrylate complex that adhere well to weeping skin and resist washing off.

Traditional moisture barrier formulations used for skin protection include nonmedicated creams, ointments, and pastes. The term cream describes an emulsion of water in oil, or oil in water. Creams may be a vehicle for moisturizers, barriers, or combination products. Barrier function is achieved by adding common ingredients such as zinc oxide, petrolatum, and dimethicone alone or in combination. Formulations may vary from thin liquids to extremely thick semisolids. Some liquid creams are formulated to be breathable. Creams can also be made to vanish into the epidermis as opposed to remaining on the skin surface; this provides the benefit of visualization of the underlying surface. Because creams contain water, they require preservatives to prevent microbial growth during their shelf-life.

KEY POINT

The term cream describes an emulsion of water in oil, or oil in water; may be a vehicle for moisturizers, barriers (zinc oxide, petrolatum, and dimethicone), or combination products. Dimethicone is a cream moisture barrier that is breathable.

Ointments are moderately thick, semisolids formed from a "base," often petrolatum. As such, they typically have an oilier feel than creams. Ointments are *always* occlusive. Formulations for incontinence skin protection are intended to sit on the skin and do not vanish. Ointments do not contain water, and some products are formulated without preservatives.

KEY POINT

Ointments are moderately thick, semisolids formed from a "base," often petrolatum and are *always* occlusive, altering TEWL of the skin.

Pastes emerged from the early practice of clinicians compounded mixtures of zinc oxide and ostomy powder in an effort to create a material that would attach to and protect moist, denuded skin. Today, "bedside compounding" is discouraged; not only it is outside the scope of nursing practice, but it yields a product of unknown safety and stability. Pastes are now commercially manufactured semisolids (typically an ointment) to which an absorbent (e.g., carboxymethylcellulose) has been added. The absorbent can impart a gritty texture to the finished product, making it uncomfortable for application to damaged skin. Pastes are intended to be applied in a thick layer in order to provide a physical barrier to irritants. The degree to which the coating remains intact during wear varies by formulation. Some products can dry and crack yet remain firmly adherent to the underlying surface. This creates an ineffective barrier, yet one that is difficult to remove.

Difficulty in removing moisture barriers can negatively impact the burden of care for bedside staff particularly when caring for patients with acute fecal incontinence with diarrhea (AFID). In the FIRST study (Bayon-Garcia et al., 2012), 60% of clinicians estimated that management of a single episode of AFID required between 10 and 20 minutes. Heidegger et al. (2016) reported the average time needed for management of an AFID episode was 17 minutes, 33 seconds and involved an average of 1.4 nurses and 0.8 aides. In both studies, the majority of time was required by the cleansing and removal of thick barriers.

To mitigate the challenges associated with removal of semisolid barriers, clinicians resort to "work-around" practices such as applying products in a thin layer (i.e., less than the recommended amount) and/or attempting to wipe only stool from the surface in order to avoid damage to the underlying injured skin. Neither practice has been studied for effectiveness or infection control implications.

KEY POINT

Pastes are intended to be applied to damaged skin in a thick layer to provide a physical barrier to irritants; they adhere to the skin and are difficult and time consuming to remove. Inappropriate use of pastes can further skin damage.

Clinical efficacy of barrier products should not be assumed based on labeling or ingredients. Viscosity (i.e., thickness) and visibility do not correlate to protective ability. Unfortunately, no well-designed comparative study has demonstrated the superiority of any barrier cream, ointment, or paste. In the absence of published evidence, the continence nurse should request manufacturer's data demonstrating barrier capability. At a minimum, testing in healthy volunteers should show that the material is waterproof and resistant to removal with soap and water. Protection from diarrhea requires a substantive barrier that can hold up to fecal enzymes as well as wetness. Products that are intended for protection (i.e., "treatment") of denuded skin should be non- or minimally cytotoxic.

KEY POINT

No well-designed comparative study has demonstrated the superiority of any barrier cream, ointment, or paste. The continence care nurse should request manufacturer's data demonstrating barrier capability.

Additional important considerations when selecting a moisture barrier include impact on BWAPs and effect on friction. Ointments, pastes, and nonvanishing barrier creams sit on the surface of the skin and can transfer off, interfering with the coverstock of the absorbent product. Impaired wicking and functionality of absorbent products has been shown with use of these types of moisture barriers (Zehrer et al., 2005) although in three other studies which acknowledged some product transfer to the coverstock but no major effect on absorption (Bolton et al., 2004; Dykes & Bradbury, 2016; Fleming et al., 2014). All four studies were performed in a nonclinical setting and deemed to be of low quality, and thus, more research is needed to verify if ointments reduce product absorption in a clinical setting (Gray et al., 2018). At this time, vanishing barrier creams and polymer-based barriers attach to the skin and appear to not transfer to other surfaces, maintaining functionality of BWAP.

Many incontinent patients are also at risk for pressure injury. Emerging data from a laboratory model suggests that some ointments and pastes have the potential to increase friction (Asmus et al., 2018). With friction being an important contributor to shear strain and tissue deformation, use of a barrier that does not increase friction is desirable.

While moisturization has long been advocated as an essential second step in incontinence skin care, the relative contribution of moisturizers to IAD prevention has not been studied. As with barriers, guidance regarding moisturizers in the incontinence care literature can be confusing with the terms moisturizer and emollient used interchangeably. Moisturizers are typically formulated as lotions and creams, both of which contain water. Based on their ingredients, they function by (1) retaining available moisture in the epidermis-through incorporation of humectants such as glycerin or urea or (2) softening and improving the appearance and feel of the epidermis through inclusion of ingredients called emollients. Occlusive skin conditioners comprise another category of ingredients sometimes used for moisturization; they retard evaporative loss by laying down a greasy film on the skin.

KEY POINT

Ingredients can be confusing: Urea is a humectant, whereas diazolidinyl urea is a preservative. Humectants should be avoided in incontinence skin care products since they draw moisture into the skin that is already compromised from moisture (urine).

By design, moisturizers are intended to work on the epidermis. *Excessive wetness* is known to be a key contributing factor for IAD development and places IAD within the MASD framework. When the epidermis is excessively hydrated or absent (i.e., denuded), moisturizers provide *no benefit* and have the potential to add *undesirable* hydration. While SC lipid replenishment

(also referred to as "restoration") has been advocated (Beeckman et al., 2015) and may be beneficial to aid barrier repair, not all moisturizers and specifically emollients are capable of this. Lipid replenishment requires a formulation that incorporates relevant SC lipids (e.g., ceramides) and is capable of epidermal permeation. This should be supported by manufacturer's data, minimally with data from healthy volunteers.

KEY POINT

Not all moisturizers are able to provide lipid replenishment (restoration). Restoration requires a formulation that incorporates relevant SC lipids (e.g., ceramides) and is capable of epidermal permeation. *Principles of a structured skin care therefore include cleansing, protecting, and restoring as needed to promote perigenital skin health.*

Multifunction products (also referred to as "3-in-1" products) gained attention in the 1990s. These products are intended to cleanse, moisturize, and protect the skin in a single step, replacing the early and confusing practice of using three separate products. Initially delivered in the form of spray-on lotions, premoistened wipes are now the most common delivery format. Dimethicone is commonly used to provide barrier function; other ingredients will include one or more surfactants and skin conditioning ingredients. Driver (2007) reported that IAD developed in 19% of a group that received a 3-in-1 wipe as compared to 50% of subjects treated with a no rinse cleanser and a zinc oxide ointment with menthol. Beeckman et al. (2011) observed superior skin outcomes when a "3-in-1" wipe was compared to soap and water for incontinence care. No barrier was used for the soap and water group. After 120 days, there was a 27.1% incidence of IAD in the soap and water group compared to an 8.1% incidence in the intervention group. Another study (Brunner et al., 2012) compared a 3-in-1 wipe to a no-rinse cleanser and barrier film. In this study, the wipe group did not demonstrate superior outcomes with 27.3% of subjects developing IAD as compared to 22.6% in the cleanser/barrier film group. Additionally, patients in the cleanser/barrier film group took longer to develop IAD (213.3 vs. 91.1 hours). As with other skin care products, effectiveness should not be judged based on ingredients alone. Because the product is delivered by wiping across the skin, data on barrier retention is needed to evaluate effectiveness.

KEY POINT

Products that cleanse and protect are often combined to provide an effective but simplified structured skin care program.

TREATMENT OF IAD AND SECONDARY INFECTIONS

As with prevention, care should be focused on prompt removal of irritants and protection of the affected area to promote healing. Use of nonirritating and noncytotoxic products is important when skin is damaged even if the epidermis is intact. Unlike treatment for other forms of irritant contact dermatitis, use of topical corticosteroids for management of IAD is rare. Reasons for this may include clinician's lack of familiarity with potency of various steroids and/or lack of prescriptive authority. Pain from IAD has not been studied, but clinician experience validates that it is a significant concern. Application of topical barriers may mitigate discomfort, but analgesics should be considered when skin injury is severe.

Guidance for management of concomitant fungal infections is based on expert opinion and information extrapolated from the skin and nail care literature. Topical antifungal medications are common first-line treatments for candidiasis. They are available as a prescription formulation (nystatin) or OTC preparations. Miconazole is a broad-spectrum antifungal and the most common active ingredient incorporated into OTC medications. Systemic antifungals are preferred by some providers.

Some general guidance for application of topical antifungals can be considered: an antifungal powder may be helpful in reducing moisture if the affected area is wet. The powder should be applied or "dusted" on in a thin coating to cover the entire affected area. Creams and lotions contain water and can add undesirable moisture when skin is wet or macerated. When the affected area is dry, a cream or ointment can be used. Ointments may provide some barrier function, but additional protection should be considered especially where ongoing exposure to liquid stool is likely. The common practice of "sealing in" antifungal powders under a barrier film or semisolid moisture barrier ointment or paste is a long-standing practice based on expert opinion as opposed to manufacturer's recommendation. It is important to understand that this may constitute "off-label" use of both products. The ideal duration of treatment for IAD-related fungal infections has not been established. In women, vaginal infection may accompany cutaneous infection and should be evaluated. If initial treatment was based on clinical assessment and the patient is not improving, an appropriate skin specimen should be obtained for culture. Referral to a provider skilled in dermatology may be indicated. While bacterial infections have been anecdotally described as associated with IAD, incidence is not known, and best practice guidance has not been established.

INFECTION CONTROL CONSIDERATIONS

Collaboration with infection prevention colleagues is essential to identify how goals for skin integrity can align to or be balanced with infection control requirements. With the emphasis on CAUTI prevention, use of antiseptic agents for "catheter care" is becoming more common and the compatibility of antiseptics and skin care products must be considered. In settings where chlorhexidine gluconate (CHG) bathing is routine and includes application of CHG in the perineal/buttocks region, the compatibility of "leave-on" protective products with CHG should be determined. Additionally, all antiseptics are cytotoxic to some degree; use on damaged skin can potentially interfere with repair.

Environmental contamination is another consideration. Most products used for skin care are multiuse. During incontinence care and especially when diarrhea is present, there is potential for micro- and macro-contamination of tubes or bottles with fecal material. This can raise the risk of spreading pathogens to other surfaces in the patient room and beyond. Consideration of product packaging that minimizes the risk of cross contamination is desirable and especially in settings where pathogens like *Clostridium difficile* have been problematic.

PROFESSIONAL PRACTICE CONSIDERATIONS

In many organizations, the WOC nurse is responsible for outcomes related to skin integrity. With this in mind, it is important to monitor incidence of IAD. Frequent consults for severe IAD (GLOBIAD Category 2/2A, Beeckman et al., 2018) should trigger a review of incontinence skin care practice and products.

A number of quality improvement projects have demonstrated improvement in IAD outcomes. Gates et al. (2019) implemented a skin care algorithm in a surgical intensive care unit. Seventy-nine (79) and 132 patients were included in the pre- and postassessment, respectively. They reported a 24% decrease in IAD over a 4-month period. Prather and Hines (2016) implemented nursing education and product standardization. Improvements included a 40% increase of staff ability to differentiate IAD from PI and a 41% increase in correct application of skin protectants. When the project was initiated, 100% of staff were using multiple products. Following implementation, 70% of staff were using the standard protocol. Skin outcomes were not reported. Hall and Clark (2015) implemented an online education program on IAD and hospital acquired pressure injuries (HAPIs) along with a one-step product for skin care. Pre intervention, 29.4% of incontinent patients ($N = 5$) developed IAD with all developing a HAPI. Post intervention, no patients developed either IAD or a PI ($p = 0.017$).

Additional important information on process elements was provided by Nix and Ermer-Seltun (2004). They asked staff nurses to identify factors contributing to the development of IAD. Participants responded that absence of, or incomplete protocols, inadequate product knowledge and lack of convenient access to products were felt to be precursors to IAD. These data support the creation of facility-relevant protocols or algorithms for IAD prevention and treatment. The continence nurse should consider type and patterns of incontinence in order to create population-appropriate interventions. Processes and products should be clearly identified and understood by all levels of staff providing care.

Additionally, the continence nurse must create and maintain a formulary of products to support care delivery. This requires knowledge of products used for IAD care. In many organizations, this also involves collaborative work with business buyers including health value analysts. In the absence of published evidence on efficacy, product decisions can be based on a well-designed product evaluation. Performance criteria should be specific and measurable and consistent with indications for use. If bedside staff participate, they should have clinical assessment expertise and be trained on product use.

The Institute for Healthcare Improvement (2011) has identified that *bedside accessible* skin care supplies are key to prevention efforts for pressure injuries. Within the four principles of health care ethics (Beauchamp & Childress, 2001), the concept of beneficence states that "health care providers must do all they can to benefit the patient in each situation." When applied to IAD prevention and treatment, this thinking calls for products to be available to staff whenever patient need arises. **Box 19-1** calls the continence care nurse to evaluate current "State of Affairs" in their care setting if they have the protocols, product formulary, accessible products, and knowledgeable staff to implement and optimize an IAD prevention program.

Beyond skin care, the acquisition of basic continence care knowledge and skills can be a valuable addition to the consultative services that the continence nurse provides. In addition to improved patient outcomes and satisfaction, the continence nurse may be able to show improved resource utilization and potential cost savings.

⬤ CONCLUSION

IAD is an avoidable and preventable health care–associated skin injury that impacts quality of care often leading to pain, infection, pressure injuries, and patient dissatisfaction. Health care organizations need to acknowledge that all

---

BOX 19-1   IAD PREVENTION CHECK LIST

- Does my facility have a written protocol for IAD prevention?
- Does the staff know what it says and what is required of them?
- Does the staff understand how to use the products specified in the protocol?
- Can bedside staff access products 24 hours per day, 7 days per week?

---

patients with incontinence are at risk for IAD and know the incidence of IAD in their organizations. Caregivers require education and infrastructure support that facilitates understanding of etiology, risk, and differential diagnosis for IAD. Structured protocols are critical to decreasing IAD in health care. Protocols must address reversible causes of incontinence, skin cleansing, application of a moisture barrier, and if indicated, treatment of secondary infection. As with most clinical challenges, patient and family education and engagement must be included with any care plan to prevent and manage IAD.

REFERENCES

Asmus, R., Bodkhe, R., Ekholm, B., et al. (November 2018; March 2019). The effect of a high endurance polymeric skin protectant on friction and shear stress. Poster presentation at 2018 Symposium on Advanced Wound Care Las Vegas NV and 2019 National Pressure Ulcer Advisory Panel Annual Conference St Louis MO.

Barakat-Johnson, M., Barnett, C., Lai, M., et al. (2018). Incontinence, incontinence-associated dermatitis, and pressure injuries in a health district in Australia: A mixed-methods study. *Journal of Wound, Ostomy, and Continence Nursing, 45*(4), 349–355.

Bayon-Garcia, C., Binks, R. M., DeLuca, E., et al. (2012). Prevalence, management and financial challenges associated with acute fecal incontinence in the ICU and critical care settings: The FIRST™ cross-sectional descriptive survey. *Intensive and Critical Care Nursing, 28*, 242–250.

Beauchamp, T. L., & Childress, J. F. (2001). *Principles of biomedical ethics* (5th ed.). New York, NY: Oxford University Press.

Beeckman, D. (2017). A decade of research on Incontinence-associated Dermatitis (IAD): Evidence, knowledge gaps and next steps. *Journal of Tissue Viability, 26*, 47–56.

Beeckman, D., Campbell, J., Campbell, K., et al. (2015). Incontinence-associated dermatitis: Moving prevention forward. Proceedings of the Global IAD Expert Panel. *Wounds International*, Retrieved October 21, 2019, from https://www.academia.edu/12441496/Proceedings_of_the_Global_IAD_Expert_Panel._Incontinence_associated_dermatitis_Moving_prevention_forward

Beeckman, D., Schoonhoven, L., Verhaeghe, S., et al. (2009). Prevention and treatment of incontinence-associated dermatitis: Literature review. *Journal of Advanced Nursing, 65*(6), 1141–1154.

Beeckman, D., Van Damme, N., Schoonhoven, L., et al. (2016). Interventions for preventing and treating incontinence associated dermatitis in adults. *Cochrane Database of Systematic Reviews, 10*, 11, CD011627.

Beeckman, D., Van den Bussche, K., Alves, P., et al. (2018). Towards an international language for incontinence-associated dermatitis (IAD): Design and evaluation of psychometric properties of the Ghent Global IAD Categorization Tool (GLOBIAD) in 30 countries. *British Journal of Dermatology, 178*(6), 1331–1340.

Beeckman, D., Van Lancker, A., Van Hecke, A., et al. (2014). A systematic review and meta-analysis of incontinence-associated dermatitis, incontinence, and moisture as risk factors for pressure ulcer development. *Research in Nursing and Health, 37*(3), 204–218.

Beeckman, D., Woodward, S., Rajpaul, K., et al. (2011). Clinical challenges of preventing incontinence-associated dermatitis. *British Journal of Nursing, 20*(13), 784–786, 788, 790.

Beeson, T., & Davis, C. (2018). Urinary management with an external female collection device. *Journal of Wound, Ostomy, and Continence Nursing, 45*(2), 187–189.

Benoit, R. A., Jr, & Watts, C. (2007). The effect of a pressure ulcer prevention program and the bowel management system in reducing pressure ulcer prevalence in an ICU setting. *Journal of Wound, Ostomy, and Continence Nursing, 34*(2), 163–175.

Berg, R. W. (1988). Etiology and pathophysiology of diaper dermatitis. *Advances in Dermatology, 3*, 75–98.

Bliss, D. Z., Hurlow, J., Defalu, J., et al. (2014). Refinement of an instrument for assessing incontinent-associated dermatitis and its severity for use with darker-toned skin. *Journal of Wound, Ostomy, and Continence Nursing, 41*(4), 365–370.

Bliss, D. Z., Mathiason, M. A., Gurvich, O., et al. (2017). Incidence and predictors of incontinence associated skin damage in nursing home residents with new onset incontinence. *Journal of Wound, Ostomy, and Continence Nursing, 44*(2), 165–171.

Bolton, C., Flynn, R., Harvey, E., et al. (2004). Assessment of pad clogging. *Journal of Community Nursing, 18*(6), 18–20.

Borchert, K., Bliss, D. Z., Savik, K., et al. (2010). The incontinence-associated dermatitis and its severity instrument: Development and validation. *Journal of Wound Ostomy & Continence Nursing, 37*(5), 527–535.

Boronat-Garrido, X., Kottner, J., Schmitz, G., et al. (2016). Incontinence-associated dermatitis in nursing homes: Prevalence, severity, and risk factors in residents with urinary and/or fecal incontinence. *Journal of Wound, Ostomy, and Continence Nursing, 43*(6), 630–635.

Brennan, M. R., Milne, C. T., Agrell-Kann, M., et al. (2017). Clinical evaluation of a skin protectant for the management of incontinence-associated dermatitis: An open-label, nonrandomized, prospective study. *Journal of Wound Ostomy & Continence Nursing, 44*(2), 172–180.

Brunner, M., Droegemueller, C., Rivers, S., et al. (2012). Prevention of incontinence-related skin breakdown for acute and critical care patients: Comparison of two products. *Urologic Nursing, 32*(4), 214–219.

Bryant, R. A. (2012). Types of skin damage and differential diagnosis. In R. A. Bryant & D. P. Nix (Eds.), *Acute and chronic wounds: Current management concepts* (pp. 83–107). St Louis, MO: Mosby Elsevier.

Byers, P. H., Ryan, P. A., Regan, M. B., et al. (1995). Effects of incontinence care cleansing regimens on skin integrity. *Journal of Wound Ostomy & Continence Nursing, 22*(4), 188–192.

Campbell, J. L., Coyer, F. M., & Osborne, S. R. (2016). Incontinence-associated dermatitis: A cross-sectional prevalence study in the Australian acute care hospital setting. *International Wound Journal, 13*(3), 403–411.

Cooper, P., & Gray, D. (2001). Comparison of two skin care regimes for incontinence. *British Journal of Nursing, 10*(6), S7–S20.

Coyer, F., Gardner, A., & Doubrovsky, A. (2017). An interventional skin care protocol (InSPIRE) to reduce incontinence-associated dermatitis in critically ill patients in the intensive care unit. *Intensive and Critical Care Nursing, 40*, 1–10.

Demarre, L., Verhaeghe, S., Van Hecke, A., et al. (2015). Factors predicting the development of pressure ulcers in an at-risk population who receive standardized preventive care: Secondary analyses of a multicenter randomized controlled trial. *Journal of Advanced Nursing, 71*(2), 391–403.

Driver, D. S. (2007). Perineal dermatitis in critical care patients. *Critical Care Nurse, 27*, 42–46.

Dykes, P., & Bradbury, S. (2016). Incontinence pad absorption and skin barrier creams: A non-patients study. *British Journal of Nursing, 25*(22), 1244–1248.

Echols, J., Friedman, B. C., Mullins, R. F., et al. (2007). Clinical utility and economic impact of introducing a bowel management system. *Journal of Wound Ostomy & Continence Nursing, 34*(6), 664–670.

Falloon, S. S., Abbas, S., Stridfeldt, C., et al. (2018). The impact of microclimate on skin health with absorbent incontinence product use: An integrative review. *Journal of Wound Ostomy & Continence Nursing*, *45*(4), 341–348. doi: 10.1097/WON.0000000000000449.

Fleming, L., Zala, K., & Ousey, K. (2014). Investigating the absorbency of LBF barrier cream. *Wounds UK, 10*(2), 24–30.

Gates, B. P., Vess, J., Long, M. A., et al. (2019). Decreasing incontinence-associated dermatitis in the surgical intensive care unit. *Journal of Wound, Ostomy, and Continence Nursing, 46*(4), 327–331.

Gerhardt, L. C., Strassle, V., Lenz, A., et al. (2008). Influence of epidermal hydration on the friction of human skin against textiles. *Journal of the Royal Society Interface, 5*, 12.

Gray, M., Beeckman, D., Bliss, D. Z., et al. (2012). Incontinence associated dermatitis: A comprehensive review and update. *Journal of Wound, Ostomy, and Continence Nursing, 39*(1), 61–74.

Gray, M., Black, J., Baharestani, M., et al. (2011). Moisture-associated skin damage: Overview and pathophysiology. *Journal of Wound, Ostomy, and Continence Nursing, 38*(3), 233–241.

Gray, M., Bliss, D., Doughty, D., et al. (2007). Incontinence-associated dermatitis: A consensus. *Journal of Wound, Ostomy, and Continence Nursing, 34*(1), 45–54.

Gray, M., & Giuliano, K. K. (2018). Incontinence-associated dermatitis, characteristics and relationship to pressure injury: A multisite epidemiologic analysis. *Journal of Wound, Ostomy, and Continence Nursing, 45*(1), 63–67.

Gray, M., Kent, D., Ermer-Seltun, J., et al. (2018). Assessment, selection, use, and evaluation of body-worn absorbent products for adults with incontinence: A WOCN® Society Consensus Conference. *Journal of Wound, Ostomy, and Continence Nursing*, *45*(3), 243–264.

Gray, M., Skinner, C., & Kaler, W. (2016). External collection devices as an alternative to the indwelling urinary catheter: Evidence-based review and Expert Clinical Panel Deliberations. *Journal of Wound, Ostomy, and Continence Nursing, 43*(3), 301–307.

Hall, K., & Clark, R. A. (2015). Prospective, descriptive, quality improvement study to decrease incontinence-associated dermatitis and hospital-acquired pressure ulcers. *Ostomy Wound management, 61*(7), 26–30.

Heidegger, P., Graf, S., Perneger, T., et al. (2016). The burden of diarrhea in the intensive care unit (ICU-BD). A survey and observational study of the caregivers opinions and workload. *International Journal of Nursing Studies, 59*, 163–168.

How-to guide: Prevent pressure ulcers. (2011). Cambridge, MA: Institute for Healthcare Improvement. Retrieved November 14, 2019, from www.ihi.org.

Kayser, S. A., Phipps, L., VanGilder, C. A., et al. (2019). Examining prevalence and risk factors of incontinence-associated dermatitis using the international pressure ulcer prevalence survey. *Journal of Wound, Ostomy, and Continence Nursing, 46*(4), 285–290.

Kottner, J., Blume-Peytavi, U., Lohrmann, C., et al. (2014). Associations between individual characteristics and incontinence-associated dermatitis: A secondary data analysis of a multi-center prevalence study. *International Journal of Nursing Studies, 51*, 1372–1380.

Kottner, J., & Surber, C. (2016). Skin care in nursing; a critical discussion of nursing practice and research. *International Journal of Nursing Studies, 61*, 20–28.

Lachenbruch, C., Ribble, D., Emmons, K., et al. (2016). Pressure ulcer risk in the incontinent patient: Analysis of incontinence and hospital-acquired pressure ulcers from the International Pressure Ulcer Prevalence™ Survey. *Journal of Wound, Ostomy, and Continence Nursing, 43*(3), 235–241.

Lewis-Byers, K., Thayer, D., & Kahl, A. M. (2002). An evaluation of two incontinence skin care protocols in a long-term care setting. *Ostomy Wound Management, 48*(12), 44–51.

Li, Y., Lee, H., Lo, Y., et al. (2019). Perineal assessment tool (pat-c): Validation of a Chinese language version and identification of a clinically validated cut point using roc curve analysis. *Journal of Wound, Ostomy, and Continence Nursing, 46*, 150–153.

Long, M. A., Reed, L. A., Dunning, K., et al. (2012). Incontinence-associated dermatitis in a long-term acute care facility. *Journal of Wound, Ostomy, and Continence Nursing, 39*(3), 318–327.

Lyder, C. H., Clemes-Lowrance, C., Davis, A., et al. (1992). Structured skin care regimen to prevent perineal dermatitis in the elderly. *Journal of ET Nursing: Official Publication, International Association for Enterostomal Therapy, 19*, 12–16.

Mathisen, M., Grove, G., Houser, T., et al. (2018). Durability of an advanced skin protectant compared with other commercially available products in healthy human volunteers. *Wounds, 30*(9), 269–274.

Minassian, V., Devore, E., Hagan, K., et al. (2013). Severity of urinary incontinence and effect on quality of life in women, by incontinence type. *Obstetrics and Gynecology, 121*(5), 1083–1090.

Nix, D. H. (2002). Validity and reliability of the perineal assessment tool. *Ostomy Wound Management, 48*(2), 43–49.

Nix, D., & Ermer-Seltun, J. (2004). A review of perineal skin care protocols and skin barrier product use. *Ostomy/Wound Management, 50*(12), 59–67.

Park, K. H., & Kim, K. S. (2014). Effect of a structured skin care regimen on patients with fecal incontinence: Comparison cohort study. *Journal of Wound, Ostomy, and Continence Nursing, 41*(2), 161–167.

Phipps, L., Gray, M., & Call, E. (2019). Time of onset to changes in skin condition during exposure to synthetic urine: A prospective study. *Journal of Wound, Ostomy, and Continence Nursing, 46*(4), 315–320.

Prather, P., & Hines, S. (2016). Best practice nursing care for ICU patients with incontinence-associated dermatitis and skin complications resulting from faecal incontinence and diarrhea. *International Journal of Evidence-Based Healthcare, 14*(1), 15–23.

Prather, P., Hines, S., Kynoch, K., et al. (2017). Effectiveness of topical skin products in the treatment and prevention of incontinence-associated dermatitis: A systematic review. *JBI Database of Systematic Reviews and Implementation Reports, 15*(5), 1473–1496.

Rohwer, K., Bliss, D. Z., & Savik, K. (2013). Incontinence-associated dermatitis in community-dwelling individuals with fecal incontinence. *Journal of Wound, Ostomy, and Continence Nursing, 40*(2), 181–184.

Schaefer, P., Berwick-Sonntag, C., Capri, M. G., et al. (2002). Physiological changes in skin barrier function in relation to occlusion level, exposure time and climactic conditions. *Skin Pharmacology and Applied Skin Physiology, 15*, 7–19.

Schwartz, D., Magen, Y. K., Levy, A., et al. (2018). Effects of humidity on skin friction against medical textiles as related to prevention of pressure injuries. *International Wound Journal, 15*(6), 1–9.

Shiu, S. R., Hsu, M. Y., Chang, S. C., et al. (2013). Prevalence and predicting factors of incontinence-associated dermatitis among intensive care patients. *Journal of Nursing & Healthcare Research, 9*(3), 210.

Sibbald, G., Krasner, D., & Woo, K. (2011). Pressure ulcer staging revisited: Superficial skin changes and deep pressure ulcer framework. *Advances in Skin & Wound Care, 24*(12), 571–580.

Voegeli, D. (2012). Moisture-associated skin damage: Etiology, prevention and treatment. *British Journal of Nursing, 21*(9), 517–521.

Warshaw, E., Nix, D., Kula, J., et al. (2002). Clinical and cost effectiveness of a cleanser protectant lotion for treatment of perineal skin breakdown in low-risk patients with incontinence. *Ostomy Wound Management, 48*(6), 44–51.

Zehrer, C., Grove, G., Newman, D., et al. (2005). Assessment of diaper-clogging potential of petrolatum moisture barriers. *Ostomy Wound Management, 51*(12), 54–58. http://www.o-wm.com/content/assessment diaper-clogging-potential-petrolatum-moisture-barriers

Zhai, H., & Maibach, H. (2002). Occlusion versus skin barrier function. *Skin Research and Technology, 8*, 1–6.

CASE STUDY

Mr. Jones is an 80-year-old male who was admitted to home health care services following a recent hospitalization for pneumonia. Mr. Jones lives at home with his wife who is his primary caregiver. Mr. Jones' medical history includes Parkinson disease and hypertension. He has occasional fecal incontinence with episodes of loose stool. He wears a pull-on BWAP. In addition to his prehospitalization medication regimen, he was prescribed an oral antibiotic for 7 days.

Mr. Jones had been ambulatory in his home prior to this illness but now requires assistance to stand and transfer from his bed to the chair or commode. He sits in a recliner chair when up. His appetite is poor, but he has adequate fluid intake. He drinks one can of liquid nutritional supplement daily. He has had a 5-pound weight loss since his recent illness. Mrs. Jones provides daily hygiene and incontinence care. Personal care is often difficult for her to provide due to his weakness and limited mobility.

The home health nurse visits Mr. Jones twice a week. Upon assessment, the nurse observed that the scrotum was erythemic. The skin was moist and shiny, and Mr. Jones reported that this area was sore.

It was noted that the buttocks and intergluteal area were also reddened and moist, with scattered superficial lesions present. The home health care nurse requested a consultation from the Wound Ostomy Continence (WOC) nurse to determine the etiology of the skin breakdown and develop a plan to manage incontinence and skin care.

CASE STUDY QUESTIONS

1. What are the key factors contributing to skin breakdown?

   The key factors contributing to Mr. Jones skin breakdown include the following:

   - The skin is exposed to moisture and irritants from liquid stool. Stool may contain enzymes as well as other irritants that are damaging to the skin. Alteration in normal skin pH (change from acidic to alkaline) is also common. The presence of microbes can trigger a secondary infection.
   - Decreased mobility makes toileting difficult and incontinence care a challenge for his caregiver.

- Friction from aggressive cleansing, moist or soiled incontinence garments, and transferring from a sitting to standing position contributes to skin breakdown. Moist skin is more prone to damage.

2. What are the clinical characteristics that will help the WOC nurse determine that this is IAD versus a pressure injury?

   The characteristics most critical to differential assessment include location, depth and distribution of the damage, and patient history. Mr. Jones' breakdown involved areas exposed to urine and stool, the lesions were superficial and scattered, and his history includes multiple episodes of fecal incontinence; all of these findings are consistent with IAD. Pressure injuries are generally distinct open lesions that are located over and localized to a bony prominence.

3. What interventions must be included in the WOC nurse's management plan?

   - Gentle cleansing with pH-balanced no-rinse cleanser
   - Protect skin with:
     - A polymer–cyanoacrylate skin protectant or
     - Pectin powder followed with an alcohol-free barrier film ("crusting") or

- A moisture barrier ointment or
- A moisture barrier paste

   A pH-balanced no-rinse cleanser and disposable soft cloth would be appropriate. Application of a polymer–cyanoacrylate skin protectant provides a durable barrier that is easy to clean and does not require removal, easing the caregiver burden. "Crusting" is an alternative but may be difficult for home health staff to replicate. A moisture barrier ointment or paste may also be used but will require family to remove and reapply periodically.

   Additional measures would include the following:

- Establish cause of diarrhea: perform basic continence assessment including gentle rectal examination to rule out impaction.
- Review findings with primary care provider.
- Use of a polymer-based absorptive product that wicks liquid away from the skin.
- Bedside commode to facilitate toileting; scheduled toileting if indicated.
- Consider physical therapy consult to provide strengthening exercises.
- Nutritional assessment and modifications as indicated.

QUESTIONS

1. Which of the following statement is true?
   A. IAD and MASD are used interchangeably.
   B. IAD is nonblachable erythema.
   C. IAD is incontinence-associated inflammation and erythema with or without erosion or denudation.
   D. IAD will become infected without antibiotics.

2. Pathophysiology of IAD includes
   A. Overhydration of the stratum corneum
   B. Penetration by environmental irritants
   C. pH changes from alkaline to acid
   D. Presence of friction

3. What role does friction play in the development of IAD?
   A. Friction is associated with pressure injuries, not IAD.
   B. IAD causes friction.
   C. Incontinence skin cleansing causes friction.
   D. All moisture barrier skin protectants cause friction.

4. How does IAD present differently depending on skin tone?
   A. IAD appears initially as erythema in lighter skin, while darker skin tones may present with paler, yellow, or dark discoloration.
   B. IAD appears patchy on lighter skin while darker skin tones present with distinct edges.
   C. IAD presents as partial thickness skin breakdown with lighter skin, while darker skin tones can have full-thickness IAD.
   D. None of the above.

5. On a patient with IAD, a red rash with pinpoint satellite lesions (papules or pustules) in the perineal region is most likely indicative of:
   A. *Staphylococcus aureus*
   B. Herpes zoster
   C. Candidiasis
   D. Tinea pedis

6. The WOC nurse is preparing a teaching plan for prevention and treatment of incontinence-associated dermatitis (IAD) in long-term care facilities. What teaching point should the nurse include?
   A. Cleanse the skin vigorously twice per day using a soft cloth and antibacterial soap.
   B. Apply a moisturizer to any skin that is red.
   C. Always leave briefs open to air.
   D. Use a moisture barrier to protect skin from urine and stool.

7. A WOC nurse is preparing a treatment plan for a patient with IAD and denuded skin. Which intervention is not recommended for this patient?
   A. Using an ointment containing glycerin and petrolatum on denuded skin
   B. Leaving the area open to air
   C. Using a moisture barrier paste
   D. Using a polymer–cyanoacrylate skin protectant

8. Desirable characteristics for a moisture barrier include
   A. Durable, breathable, and transparent
   B. Transparent, antifungal, and antibacterial
   C. pH balanced, breathable, and vanishing
   D. Noncytotoxic, pH balanced, and visible

9. For IAD prevention, multifunction ("3-in-1") products are used to
   A. Cleanse, disinfect, and protect
   B. Cleanse, protect, and restore if needed
   C. Cleanse, moisturize, and treat
   D. Cleanse, protect, and soothe

10. When designing a program for IAD prevention and treatment, the continence care nurse should incorporate which of the following elements:
   A. Staff autonomy in determining skin care protocol for each patient
   B. Formulary with at least three cleansers and three moisture barriers
   C. Structured skin care regimen (protocol) and bedside accessible supplies
   D. Engagement of medical staff for guidance

ANSWERS AND RATIONALES

1. C. Rationale: IAD is a type of top-down injury and the most common form of moisture-associated skin damage (MASD). IAD is characterized by erythema and edema of the surface of the skin, sometimes accompanied by serous exudate, erosion, or secondary cutaneous infection.

2. A. Rationale: Overhydration of the stratum corneum compromises the brick-and-mortar configuration of the epidermal layer and permits penetration by irritants found in urine and stool, which results in inflammation and impaired tensile strength. As urea in urine breaks down, highly alkaline ammonia is produced, and changes pH from acid to alkaline and compromised the protective acidic mantle of the skin.

3. C. Rationale: Incontinence care involves the use of friction for skin cleansing. Forces of friction and shear against an underlying surface (bed, chair, linen, containment garments) wounds the skin and allows pathogens such as *Candida* and *Staphylococcus* to enter, invade and cause secondary infections.

4. A. Rationale: IAD appears initially as erythema ranging from pink to red. Darker skin tones may present with paler, yellow or dark discoloration. All skin effected by IAD can look patchy with nondistinct edges. Current evidence suggests that IAD is limited to partial thickness skin breakdown.

5. C. Rationale: A red rash with pinpoint satellite lesions (papules or pustules) is indicative of a candidiasis (a secondary infection) and is not uncommon. Bacterial infections secondary to IAD are not commonly reported in peer review literature. Herpes Zoster is an important differential diagnosis for IAD but presents without satellite lesions and are generally grouped unilaterally along dermatomes.

6. D. Rationale: Cleansing skin vigorously is never appropriate. When skin is red, IAD is already present and a moisture barrier versus moisturizer is indicated. The practice of leaving briefs open to air may provide some benefit but would not be a recommendation for all residents. All incontinent patients are at risk for IAD so use of a moisture barrier to protect skin is always advisable.

7. B. Rationale: Once IAD has been observed and especially if denudement is present, the objective of care is to protect the skin from further exposure to stool and/or urine and create an environment that promotes healing. This is accomplished with application of a moisture barrier. Leaving the area open to air will not provide skin protection.

8. A. Rationale: Important characteristics for a moisture barrier include durability (to assure protection over time), breathability (to allow moisture vapor transmission from the skin), and transparency (allows for skin assessment). The presence of an antifungal or antibacterial is not necessary unless an infection is present. While visible barriers are desired by some clinicians, visible barriers can interfere with skin assessment.

9. B. Rationale: Multifunction products contain ingredients "to cleanse" and "to protect" by utilization of a moister barrier skin protectant, and some products contain ceramides to help replace lipids lost to the skin thus "restoring" barrier function. They do not contain antifungals or antibacterials. Because of formulation characteristics, they are best used for prevention of IAD. When used in patients at *high risk* for IAD (i.e., frequent or continuous liquid stool), skin should be observed often as a more protective barrier may be required.

10. C. Rationale: A structured skin care regimen and bedside accessible supplies are considered essential to effective IAD prevention efforts. Improved outcomes have been demonstrated when staff follows an established protocol for skin care, individualizing a care plan can then occur as needed. Stocking multiple products within a single category can prove confusing to staff and can add unnecessary cost. While support of the medical staff is always desirable, the wound care nurse can provide valuable guidance on IAD prevention and treatment to physician colleagues.

CHAPTER 20

PRESSURE AND SHEAR INJURIES

Laura Edsberg

OBJECTIVES

1. Explain the role of each of the following in pressure injury development:
   a. Prolonged or intense pressure
   b. Shear force
   c. Compromised tissue tolerance
2. Discuss current theories of pressure injury pathogenesis, to include each of the following:
3. Vessel compression and tissue ischemia
   a. Lymphatic vessel compression and edema

b. Reperfusion injury
   c. Direct damage to cytoskeleton of muscle cell
4. Correctly stage a pressure injury using the currently accepted staging system.
5. Identify limitations of the current classification system and implications for practice.
6. Describe the etiology and pathology of DTPI lesions, and address implications for documentation and management.

TOPIC OUTLINE

INTRODUCTION

Pressure-induced injuries impose a significant burden not only on the patient but on the entire health care system. Reducing their frequency is an important component of current goals for patient safety, as evidenced by the Institute for Healthcare Improvement (IHI) 5 Million Lives Campaign and the decision by the U.S. Centers for Medicare and Medicaid Services (CMS) to not reimburse hospitals for the treatment of hospital-acquired pressure-related injuries (Berlowitz, 2020a, 2020b). Estimates approach 11.6 billion U.S. dollars annually for pressure injury care in the United States (Russo et al., 2006; WOCN, 2016).

Pressure-induced skin and soft tissue injuries are among the most common conditions encountered in acutely hospitalized patients or those requiring long-term residential care. The incidence varies widely by clinical setting (Bauer et al., 2016; Russo et al., 2006; Stevenson et al., 2013). An estimated 2.5 million pressure-induced injuries are treated each year in acute care facilities in the United States alone (Bauer et al., 2016; Stevenson et al., 2013).

Methods of studying and reporting pressure injury incidence and prevalence include direct patient examination, use of databases, and surveys. These studies tend to be small and often involve only a single facility, making it difficult to generalize results. Shorter hospital length of stays may also mean that many pressure-induced injuries are missed. Caution is required when interpreting the reported incidence and prevalence rates since the methodology and duration of follow-up varies between studies. Studies have also differed on whether they included Stage 1 injuries. Stage 1 pressure injuries are frequently encountered, but many epidemiological studies have elected not to include them since they are difficult to detect. The most accurate estimates are derived from studies where the wound care nurses have directly examined the patients.

Increased morbidity and mortality are associated with the presence of pressure injuries (Bauer et al., 2016). Pressure injuries (Pls) are common in vulnerable populations including people with spinal cord injuries, neonates and children, critically ill individuals, and individuals in aged care and rehabilitation settings (Coyer et al., 2017; Habiballah & Tubaishat, 2016; Houghton & Campbell, 2013; Stevenson et al., 2013). Pls cause extensive pain, impede recovery, prolong hospitalization, and substantially increase the risk of sepsis and overall patient mortality (Sullivan & Schoelles, 2013).

The superficial skin is noted to be less susceptible to pressure-induced damage than deeper tissues, and the external appearance may underestimate the extent of damage (Kosiak, 1961). Lesions are typically related to immobility (i.e., bed-bound or chair-bound individuals) but can also result from poorly fitting casts or other medical equipment or devices.

The clinical staging that guides treatment of pressure-induced skin and soft tissue injuries is reviewed here.

> **KEY POINT**
>
> Pls are a very costly and preventable complication associated with extensive pain, prolonged hospitalization, and significant increased risk for sepsis and death.

CLASSIFICATION AND TERMINOLOGY

Pressure injuries were considered a pressure or occlusion/ischemic injury, but ongoing research has sought to describe other factors involved in the development of pressure injuries. The National Pressure Injury Advisory Panel (NPIAP) Pressure Injury staging definitions included the role of other factors including shear and moisture in the definition of pressure injuries. A pressure injury is localized damage to the skin and underlying soft tissue usually over a bony prominence or related to a medical or other device. The injury can present as intact skin or an open ulcer and may be painful. The injury occurs as a result of intense and/or prolonged pressure or pressure in combination with shear. The tolerance of soft tissue for pressure and shear may also be affected by microclimate, nutrition, perfusion, comorbidities, and condition of the soft tissue (NPIAP, 2016).

Superficial lesions (e.g., skin maceration, moisture-associated dermatitis, abrasions) are primarily the result of moisture and friction and should not be considered pressure-induced injuries. Exposure to moisture in the form of perspiration, feces, or urine with resulting skin maceration may predispose to superficial ulceration.

● ETIOLOGY AND RISK FACTORS

Understanding of the etiology of pressure injuries has evolved from a tissue tolerance injury caused by pressure to include intrinsic and extrinsic factors contributing to the development of PI (EPUAP/NPIAP/PPPIA, 2019). The tissue's response to loading results in either tissue tolerance or tissue damage. Deformation is a normal occurrence in tissue, but if deformation exceeds the tissue's tolerance or ability to respond to the external forces, then damage may occur (Bergstrom et al., 1988; Braden & Bergstrom, 1987). The type of loading (compressive and shear) and the magnitude and duration and tissue tolerance will determine if there will be an injury, how long before injury is apparent, and the severity of injury. Tissue tolerance is unique to each individual and is composed of a number of variables including internal anatomy (shape of bony prominences), mechanical properties of the tissue, tissue's response to external forces, thermal properties, and the perfusion of the tissue (EPUAP/NPIAP/PPPIA, 2019) (**Fig. 20-1**).

Tissues vary in their susceptibility to pressure-induced injury, with muscle being the most susceptible, followed by subcutaneous fat and then dermis. Deep tissue damage can occur with little or no evidence of superficial tissue injury. Stage 3 and 4 PIs may begin as an injury to the deeper layers of tissue that may progress to the skin surface. Pressure injury development is not a linear process. There is little evidence to suggest that Stage 3 and 4 PIs develop as a gradual progression from Stage 1 through Stage 4. The practice of changing the stage as healing occurs, known as reverse or back staging, is not recommended (Berlowitz, 2020a, 2020b). Pressure over a bony prominence tends to result in a cone-shaped distribution with the most affected tissues located deep, adjacent to the bone–muscle interface. The extent of injury to deep tissues is often much greater than perceived from the visible ulcer on the skin surface. The skin changes are just the tip of the iceberg.

KEY POINT

The time frame and pressure intensity required to produce irreversible damage varies from person to person depending on their clinical condition. No specific level of pressure intensity has been identified beyond which tissue damage is inevitable.

Risk factors can be divided into those that impact the magnitude and duration of pressure and those that affect individual susceptibility and tolerance. Over 100 risk factors for the development of pressure injuries have been identified in the literature. **Box 20-1** highlights additional risk factors. The most important risk factors, immobility, reduced perfusion, and sensory loss are discussed below.

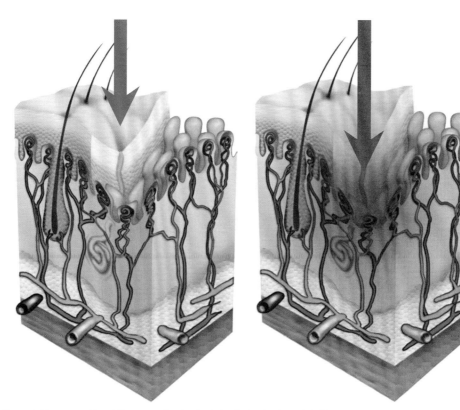

FIGURE 20-1. Tissue Tolerance—Equal Pressure Applied to Two Individuals with Differing Tissue Tolerance.

BOX 20-1 COMMON RISK FACTORS FOR PRESSURE INJURY DEVELOPMENT

- General medical conditions, such as diabetes, stroke, multiple sclerosis, cognitive impairment, cardiopulmonary disease, cancer, hemodynamic instability, peripheral vascular disease, malnutrition, and dehydration
- Smoking
- History of a previous pressure ulcer (since scar tissue is weaker than the skin it replaced and will break down more rapidly than intact skin)
- Increased facility length of stay
- Prolonged surgical procedures (i.e., >3 hours)
- Significant weight loss
- Prolonged time on a stretcher, such as in the emergency room
- Medications, such as sedatives and analgesics
- Refusal of care, such as when a patient refuses to be turned or moved despite education
- Edema
- Obesity
- An ICU stay, due to the high acuity of illness, presence of multiple comorbid conditions, and
  - Mechanical ventilation
  - Vasopressors and hemodynamic instability
  - Multiple surgeries
  - Increased length of stay
  - Inability to report discomfort

Immobility is the most important risk factor that contributes to development of PI. Immobility may be permanent or temporary. Any individual with significant immobility is at risk, specifically those who are wheelchair bound or bedbound and those for whom turning and repositioning requires significant effort, such as those who are morbidly obese. The prevalence of Stage 3, Stage 4, and unstageable PI is greater among those who are completely immobile (Lahmann & Kottner, 2011).

Sensory loss is caused by neurologic diseases such as dementia, delirium, spinal cord injury, and peripheral neuropathy. It is an important risk factor for the development of PI. When a patient has sensory perception limitations, often they have limitations in mobility and activity. Patients may not perceive pain or discomfort from prolonged pressure. Mobility may be affected by spasticity and contractures from neurologic diseases (WOCN, 2016).

Another risk factor for PI development is decreased perfusion. In the setting of poor perfusion, pressure applied to the skin for <2 hours may be sufficient to cause severe tissue damage. When organs such as the kidneys and the gastrointestinal tract are not adequately perfused, blood flow to the skin will also be decreased, increasing the risk for the development of PI. Factors that contribute to reduced perfusion include volume depletion, hypotension, vasomotor failure, and vasoconstriction secondary to shock, heart failure, or medications, and underlying peripheral artery disease (Berlowitz, 2020a, 2020b).

While moisture alone may not be a direct causative factor, overhydrated skin is much more vulnerable to friction and shear damage and is also less able to distribute weight normally. Moisture contributes to PI development by decreasing tissue tolerance (Braden & Bergstrom, 1987) and by increasing susceptibility to friction, pressure, and shear (EPUAP/NPIAP/PPIAP, 2019). Moisture decreases stratum corneum stiffness and mechanical strength and increases the coefficient of friction so that skin is more adherent to its contact surface. This results in greater deformation and shear forces being transmitted to the subcutaneous tissues with increased likelihood of deep tissue injury. Urinary incontinence is frequently cited as a predisposing factor to PI development, with some studies suggesting that incontinent patients have up to a fivefold higher risk. Lachenbruch et al. (2016) reported that the presence of incontinence was strongly associated with Stage 3, Stage 4, DTPI, and unstageable rather than Stage 1 or Stage 2 PI (Lachenbruch et al., 2016). Gray and Giuliano (2018) found that incontinence-associated dermatitis (IAD) was an independent risk factor for PI, after accounting for immobility as a confounding risk factor (Gray & Giuliano, 2018). A national survey of nursing home discharges found that 94% of incontinent patients with PI were bed- or chair-bound (Berlowitz, 2020a, 2020b; Gray & Giuliano, 2018; Lachenbruch et al., 2016).

Microclimate is the temperature and moisture that exists on the tissue surface interface. The microclimate can be modified using support surface selection with features that control moisture or temperature, as well as the support surface cover selection. Vapor permeable surface covers draw moisture and heat away from the skin interface. Adding pads or products between the patient and the surface of the bed may impact the properties of the support surface by blocking or impeding the features that mitigate negative microclimates. Synthetic silk-like fabrics have been shown to reduce shear and friction, as well as decrease the development of PI (EPUAP/NPIAP/PPPIA, 2019; Smith et al., 2013; Twersky et al., 2012). These fabrics are moisture wicking and evaporating, which facilitates water loss from the fabric.

Certain populations have multiple risk factors that predispose them to PI development. These include individuals who are critically ill, have spinal cord injury, reside in long-term care (LTC) and rehabilitation settings, receiving palliative care, have diabetes, and who have undergone >3 hours of surgery. Standard care with these populations should include prompt implementation of preventive measures (EPUAP/NPIAP/PPPIA, 2019).

KEY POINT

The purpose of risk assessment is to provide early detection of the at-risk individual, followed by prompt implementation of preventive measures.

RISK ASSESSMENT TOOLS

Risk assessment tools have been developed to assist the nurse to identify individuals at risk for PI development.

Braden Scale

The most widely used risk assessment tool is the Braden Scale for Predicting Pressure Sore Risk® (Bergstrom et al., 1988). The theoretical framework for the Braden Scale is based on a physiological model depicting factors that contribute to the development of PI. It includes factors affecting intensity and duration of pressure (decreased mobility, decreased activity, and decreased sensory perception) and other extrinsic factors (increased moisture, increased friction, and increased shear forces), as well as intrinsic factors (e.g., nutrition) that affect tissue tolerance (Reddy et al., 2006). A total Braden Scale score ranges from 6 to 23. Lower scores on the Braden Scale indicate greater risk for PI development; very high risk = 9 or below; high risk = 10 to 12; moderate risk = 13 to 14; mild risk = 15 to 18; and not at risk = 19 or more. Braden suggests that if a person has other risk factors, for example, advanced age, fever, or hemodynamic instability, the score should be advanced to the next highest level of risk. Observational studies suggest that this is not routinely done by nurses. Studies suggest that nurses frequently underestimate the level of PI risk (Ayello & Braden, 2002; Bergstrom, 1987; Braden & Bergstrom, 1987; Stotts & Gunningberg, 2007). See Chapter 21 for additional information on Braden Scale and other risk assessment tools.

KEY POINT

Braden recommends that for persons with major risk factors not addressed by the Braden Scale (e.g., advanced age, fever, or hemodynamic instability), the score should be advanced to the next highest level of risk.

PATHOGENESIS

The development of a PI is a complex process that requires the application of external forces to the skin. To understand the role of the forces in the deformation of the tissue, it is important to understand the types of forces, specifically pressure, shear, and friction.

PRESSURE

Pressure is a compressive force defined as perpendicular to the surface of the skin (**Fig. 20-2**).

Friction describes surfaces sliding with respect to each other. It is a contact force parallel to the skin surface. Static friction is the force resisting movement between two bodies when they are not moving. It keeps the body from sliding out of bed when the head of bed is raised. Dynamic friction is the force resisting movement between two bodies when they are moving, such as a person sliding down in bed.

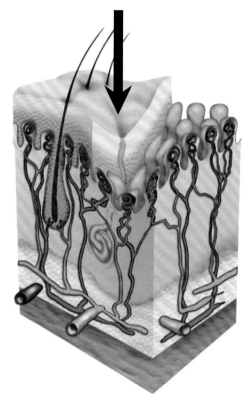

FIGURE 20-2. Illustration of Tissue Deformation under Pressure.

SHEAR

Shear is the force parallel to the surface of the tissue. As friction increases, shear may increase. Studies have shown that in the presence of shear, less pressure is required to cause a pressure injury (Goldstein & Sanders, 1998). Shearing forces occur when patients are placed on an inclined surface (**Fig. 20-3**). Deeper tissues, including muscle and subcutaneous fat, are pulled downward by gravity, while the superficial epidermis and dermis remain fixed through contact with the external surface. The result is stretching, angulation, and trauma to local blood vessels and lymphatics along with additional tissue deformation. Shear forces have an additive effect such that in the presence of pressure, more severe tissue damage will occur (Berlowitz, 2020a, 2020b).

Sustained compression of the tissue may cause development of deep tissue damage, without the visible changes at the skin surface. This sustained compression form is considered especially detrimental because the subcutaneous, fascia, and muscle layers can suffer substantial necrosis, with only minor signs of tissue breakdown at the skin surface. Deformation of deep tissues resulting from pressure and shear may directly cause cell death as a result of loss of cytoskeletal integrity. Deformation-induced cell death combines with tissue hypoxia, edema, and reperfusion injury to result in additional injury (Berlowitz, 2020a, 2020b). Pressure and shear

Shearing forces and pressure ulcers

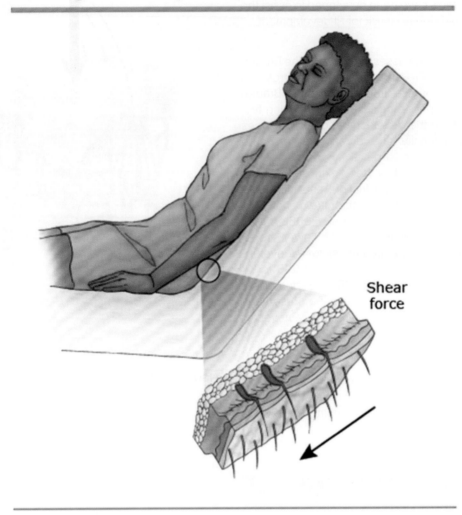

Shear force

FIGURE 20-3. Shear. (Used with permission from Taylor CR, Lillis C, LeMone P, et al. (2008). *Fundamentals of nursing: The art and science of nursing care* (6th ed.). Philadelphia, PA: Lippincott Williams & Wilkins. Copyright © 2008 Lippincott Williams & Wilkins.)

forces act together, and the resulting force is the combination of the pressure and shear (**Fig. 20-4**).

PRESSURE INTENSITY AND DURATION

Research on PI has focused on determining the minimal degree of loading that will consistently lead to tissue damage. These studies all show an inverse relationship between the magnitude and duration of loading, indicating that higher loads (pressure levels) require less time to cause deep tissue breakdown. No specific level of pressure intensity has been identified as the cut point beyond which ischemic damage is inevitable. Pressure-related damage may occur within a short period of time, and the specific time frame and pressure intensity required to produce irreversible damage likely varies from person to person depending on their clinical condition. The data indicate that PI prevention must include strategies

to reduce both the magnitude of loading (intensity of pressure) and the duration of loading, specifically pressure redistribution surfaces and routine repositioning. These two strategies are the primary components of all recommended PI prevention protocols.

 PATHOLOGY OF PRESSURE/SHEAR DAMAGE

The literature on PI etiology and pathology identifies four major factors hypothesized to cause this type of tissue damage:

1. Occlusion of blood vessels resulting in tissue ischemia (Edsberg et al., 2000)
2. Occlusion of lymph vessels resulting in impaired removal of waste products and increased risk of edema (Krouskop, 1983)

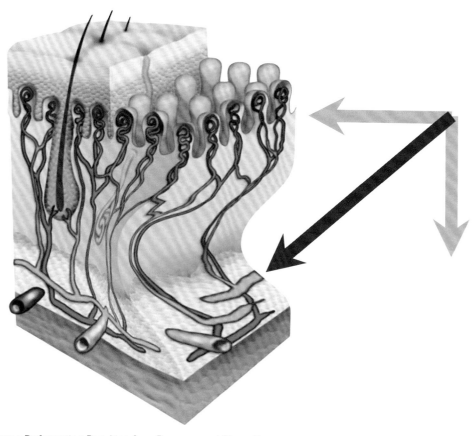

FIGURE 20-4. Tissue Deformation Resulting from Pressure and Shear Forces.

3. Ischemia/reperfusion damage resulting from an accumulation of oxygen free radicals during the ischemic period (Peirce et al., 2000)
4. Direct deformation damage of the cytoskeleton of muscle cells in situations involving high-pressure loads (Loerakker et al., 2011)

VESSEL COMPRESSION RESULTING IN TISSUE ISCHEMIA

Even at relatively low pressures, there can be some reduction in perfusion related to vessel compression. Smaller or damaged blood vessels may be totally occluded. As the tissue load (pressure) increases, the degree of interference to perfusion becomes greater and can lead to significant reduction in blood flow to the tissues. At very high tissue loads, even larger vessels can be completely occluded. The reduced blood flow causes tissue ischemia with the delivery of oxygen and nutrients to the cells compromised. The removal of metabolic waste products from the cells is also impaired. This does not cause immediate damage to the tissues, because the cells can and will shift from aerobic to anaerobic metabolism. Anaerobic metabolism is less effective and generates more waste products (lactate).

Anaerobic metabolism can meet the energy needs of the cells for a period of time. Metabolic waste products accumulate in the intercellular space and reduce the pH levels, which will eventually damage the cells. In animal experiments, cell damage becomes evident after a period of 2 to 3 hours.

LYMPH VESSEL OCCLUSION AND EDEMA FORMATION

Lymphatic vessels play an important role in removal of waste products from the interstitial space and control of the amount of free water in the interstitial space. The exact point at which pressure and shear forces begin to occlude the blood vessels and lymphatics is unknown. Failure of the lymphatic system results in increased accumulation of cellular waste and accumulation of fluid in the interstitial space (edema).

REPERFUSION INJURY

Rapid reperfusion after a period of ischemia can add to the damage caused by the ischemic episode. The period of reduced blood flow can result in formation of small clots that obstruct small vessels once blood flow is reestablished. Ischemia results in the accumulation of

Sites associated with pressure-induced injury

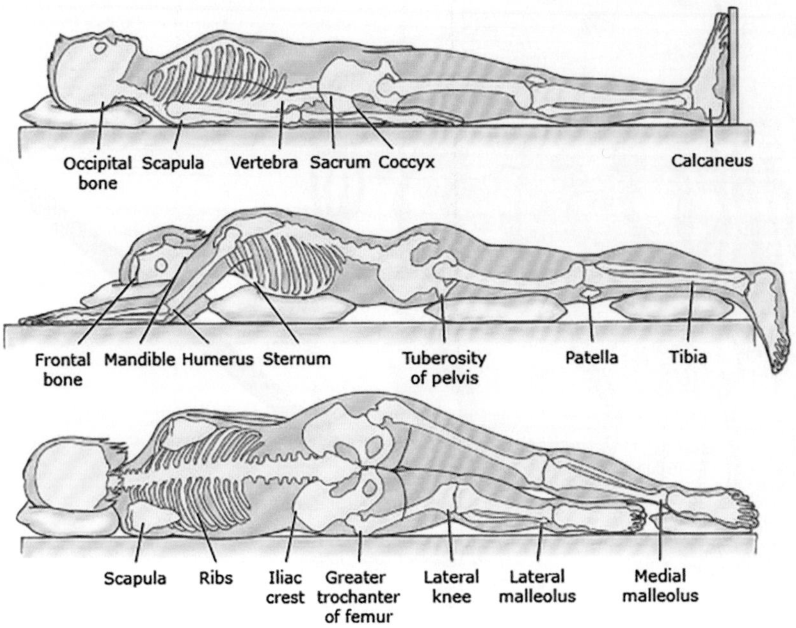

Common sites for development of pressure-induced skin and soft tissue injury.

FIGURE 20-5. Common Sites of Development of PI. (Used with permission from Taylor CR, Lillis C, LeMone P, et al. (2008). *Fundamentals of nursing: The art and science of nursing care* (6th ed.). Philadelphia, PA: Lippincott Williams & Wilkins. Copyright © 2008 Lippincott Williams & Wilkins.)

oxygen free radicals. When oxygen becomes available, a chemical reaction damages cells and tissue. A slower rate of reperfusion may reduce these negative effects. The exact role that reperfusion injury plays in PI development remains unknown (Peirce et al., 2000).

> **KEY POINT**
>
> The pathology of PI development is thought to involve the following four factors: vascular compression with reduced perfusion and tissue ischemia, lymph vessel compression and edema, reperfusion injury, and direct damage to the cytoskeleton of the muscle cell.

DIRECT DAMAGE TO CYTOSKELETON OF MUSCLE CELL

Muscle deformation may cause direct damage to the cytoskeleton of the cell. Studies using cultured cells and tissue engineered muscle indicate that even moderate levels of deformation can compromise the cytoskeleton of the muscle cell. Extensive studies in which deformation was combined with different degrees of ischemia indicate that deformation damage occurs faster than ischemic damage. The causes of the deformation damage are not clear but may include cell membrane damage,

rupture of the cytoskeleton, or activation of a biochemical pathway triggered by the deformation (Loerakker et al., 2013). Animal studies confirm the phenomenon of deformation damage and have shown that the amount of damage is correlated to the degree of deformation. In vivo studies found that damage only occurred at high levels of strain and deformation. The level of strain associated with muscle cell damage is most likely to occur near the bony prominence of a person sitting or lying on a hard surface (**Fig. 20-5**). This level of strain and deformation can also be caused by folds in the clothing or sheets or from hard objects in pockets (Loerakker et al., 2011). Clinically, it is hard to completely protect the soft tissue from the ischemic effects of tissue loading. It is important to change the areas exposed to mechanical loading regularly by repositioning the patient. It is often possible to minimize deformation damage through the use of proper support surfaces.

> **KEY POINT**
>
> PI prevention must include strategies to reduce both the magnitude of loading, intensity of pressure, and the duration of loading, specifically pressure redistribution surfaces and routine repositioning. These two strategies are the primary components of all recommended PI prevention protocols.

Healthy Skin – Lightly Pigmented

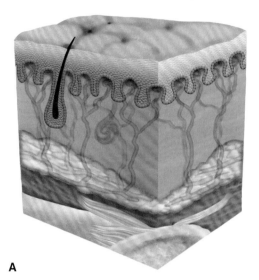

Healthy Skin – Darkly Pigmented

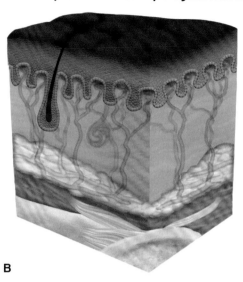

A

B

FIGURE 20-6. A, B. Healthy Lightly Pigmented and Darkly Pigmented Skin (Diagram). (Used with permission of the National Pressure Injury Advisory Panel, 2020. Copyright © NPIAP.)

 STAGING OF PRESSURE INJURIES

Pressure injuries are classified and described through the use of staging systems. The most commonly used staging system is from the NPIAP (Berlowitz, 2020a, 2020b). The NPIAP Pressure Injury Staging System was revised in 2016 to incorporate the current scientific and clinical understanding of the etiology of pressure injuries, as well as to clarify the anatomical features present or absent in each stage of injury. The term ulcer does not accurately describe the physical presentation of a Stage 1 pressure injury or a deep tissue pressure injury (DTPI), which present as intact skin. An injury can be present without an ulcer, but an ulcer cannot be present without an injury. Histopathological studies have shown that small changes in pressure-related injuries start in the tissue prior to the changes being visible on physical examination of the epidermis (Arao et al., 1998; Edsberg, 2007; Witkowski & Parish, 1982). Diagrams of normal skin are provided for comparison before describing the NPIAP staging system (**Fig. 20-6A and B**).

KEY POINT

Only PIs should be staged with the NPIAP Pressure Injury Staging System.

 STAGE 1 PRESSURE INJURY

DEFINITION

Intact skin with a localized area of nonblanchable erythema, which may appear differently in darkly pigmented skin. Presence of blanchable erythema or changes in sensation, temperature, or firmness may precede visual changes. Color changes do not include purple or maroon discoloration; these may indicate DTPI (NPIAP, 2016) (**Fig. 20-7A–C**).

Although the term heralding sign is no longer part of this revised definition, Stage 1 pressure injuries are often the first visible change in the skin and their presence signals a concern regarding the tissue's tolerance for the conditions it is undergoing. Scar tissue and DTPI should not be classified as a Stage 1 PI. The blanche response of skin can be assessed by pressing the skin with a finger to close the capillary bed and releasing the pressure. The skin should immediately return to the native skin color when the pressure is released. This can also be done using a clear disc pressed on the skin (**Figs. 20-8A and B and 20-9**).

 STAGE 2 PRESSURE INJURY: PARTIAL-THICKNESS SKIN LOSS WITH EXPOSED DERMIS

DEFINITION

Partial thickness loss of skin with exposed dermis. The wound bed is viable, pink or red, moist, and may also present as an intact or ruptured serum-filled blister. Adipose (fat) is not visible, and deeper tissues are not visible. Granulation tissue, slough, and eschar are not present. These injuries commonly result from adverse microclimate and shear in the skin over the pelvis and shear in the heel (NPIAP, 2016) (**Fig. 20-10A–C**).

Since the appearance of a Stage 2 PI can closely resemble moisture-associated skin damage (MASD),

Stage 1 Pressure Injury – Lightly Pigmented

Stage 1 Pressure Injury – Darkly Pigmented

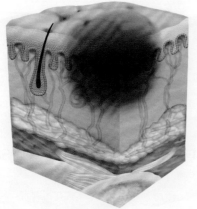

A

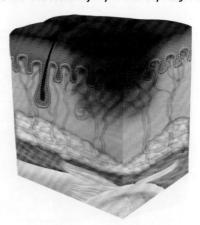

B

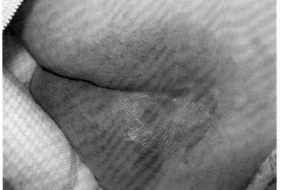

C

FIGURE 20-7. A–C. Stage 1 PI Lightly Pigmented and Darkly Pigmented Diagram and Photo. (Used with permission of the National Pressure Injury Advisory Panel, 2020. Copyright © NPIAP.)

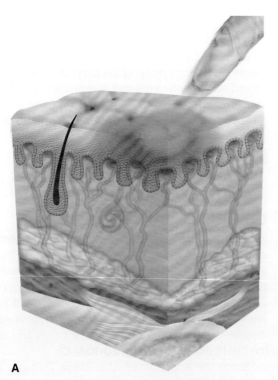

A

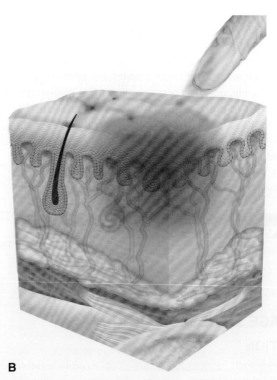

B

FIGURE 20-8. A. Blanchable Erythema. **B.** Nonblanchable Erythema. (Used with permission of the National Pressure Injury Advisory Panel, 2020. Copyright © NPIAP.)

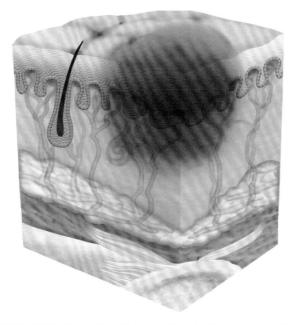

FIGURE 20-9. Stage 1 PI with Edema. (Used with permission of the National Pressure Injury Advisory Panel, 2020. Copyright © NPIAP.)

the presence or history of pressure and shear should be confirmed so that MASD may be ruled out as an etiology. Stage 2 PI should not be used to describe MASD including IAD, intertriginous dermatitis (ITD), medical adhesive related skin injury (MARSI), or traumatic wounds (skin tears, burns, and abrasions) (Edsberg et al., 2016).

⬤ STAGE 3 PRESSURE INJURY: FULL-THICKNESS SKIN LOSS

DEFINITION

Full-thickness skin loss, in which adipose (fat) is visible in the ulcer and granulation tissue, and epibole (rolled wound edges) are often present. Slough and/or eschar may be visible. The depth of tissue damage varies by anatomical location; areas of significant adiposity can develop deep wounds. Undermining and tunneling may occur. Fascia, muscle, tendon, ligament, cartilage, or bone are not exposed. If slough

Stage 2 Pressure Injury

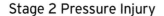

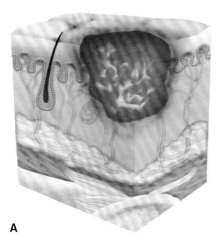

A

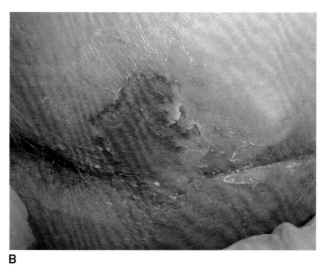

B

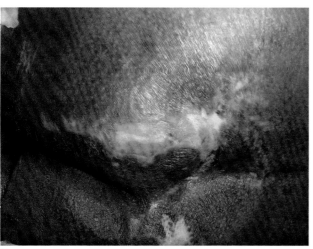

C

FIGURE 20-10. A–C. Stage 2 PI Diagram and Two Photos. (Used with permission of the National Pressure Injury Advisory Panel, 2020. Copyright © NPIAP.)

Stage 3 Pressure Injury

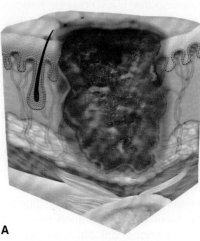
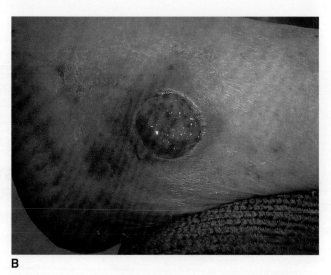

A   **B**

FIGURE 20-11. A, B. Stage 3 PI Diagram and 1 Photo. (Used with permission of the National Pressure Injury Advisory Panel, 2020. Copyright © NPIAP.)

or eschar obscures the extent of tissue loss, this is an unstageable PI (NPIAP, 2016) (**Figs. 20-11A and B and 20-12**).

It is important to note that depth of injury is not an actual depth measurement, but instead a way of describing the extent of deepest layer of tissue visible or palpable. Anatomical location and differences between individuals can lead to differences in measurable depths of injury, and areas of significant adiposity can develop deep wounds. Undermining and tunneling may occur.

Fascia, muscle, tendon, ligament, cartilage, or bone are not exposed in Stage 3 injuries. If slough or eschar obscures the extent of tissue loss, this is a unstageable PI, not a Stage 3 injury.

Stage 3 Pressure Injury with Epibole

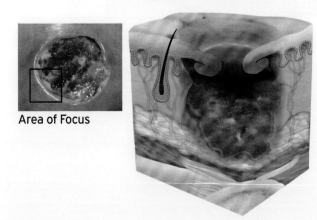

Area of Focus

FIGURE 20-12. Stage 3 PI with Epibole. (Used with permission of the National Pressure Injury Advisory Panel, 2020. Copyright © NPIAP.)

🔴 STAGE 4 PRESSURE INJURY: FULL-THICKNESS SKIN AND TISSUE LOSS

Full-thickness skin and tissue loss with exposed or directly palpable fascia, muscle, tendon, ligament, cartilage, or bone in the ulcer. Slough and/or eschar may be visible. Epibole (rolled edges), undermining, and/or tunneling often occur. Depth varies by anatomical location. If slough or eschar obscures the extent of tissue loss, this is an unstageable PI (NPIAP, 2016) (**Fig. 20-13A and B**).

🔴 UNSTAGEABLE FULL-THICKNESS PRESSURE INJURY: OBSCURED FULL-THICKNESS SKIN AND TISSUE LOSS

Full-thickness skin and tissue loss in which the extent of tissue damage within the ulcer cannot be confirmed because it is obscured by slough or eschar. If slough or eschar is removed, a Stage 3 or Stage 4 PI will be revealed. Stable eschar, that is, dry, adherent, intact without erythema or fluctuance, on ischemic limb or heels should not be softened or removed (NPIAP, 2016) (**Figs. 20-14 and 20-15**).

A PI is staged as unstageable due to the wound care nurse's inability to visualize the wound base because it is obscured by slough and/or eschar and not the clinician's inability to determine the injury stage. Stable eschar in poorly perfused areas should not be removed as it results in an open wound that may expose the limb to infection and disrupt the ability to heal. Stable eschar should be treated similarly to dry gangrene; it should not be moistened or softened. Pressure redistribution is the most important intervention with stable eschar. As eschar loosens from the wound bed, the edges should

Stage 4 Pressure Injury

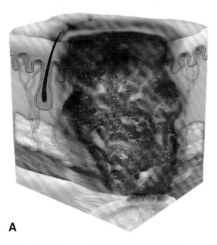

A

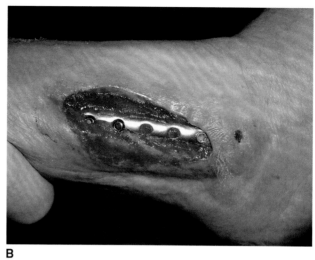

B

FIGURE 20-13.   A, B. Stage 4 PI Diagram and 1 Photo. (Used with permission of the National Pressure Injury Advisory Panel, 2020. Copyright © NPIAP.)

be trimmed to avoid inadvertent removal (Edsberg et al., 2016).

KEY POINT

Stable eschar in poorly perfused areas should not be removed as it results in an open wound that may expose the limb to infection and disrupt the ability to heal. Stable eschar should be treated similarly to dry gangrene; it should not be moistened or softened.

⬤ DEEP TISSUE PRESSURE INJURY

DEEP TISSUE PRESSURE INJURY: PERSISTENT NONBLANCHABLE DEEP RED, MAROON, OR PURPLE DISCOLORATION

Intact or nonintact skin with localized area of persistent nonblanchable deep red, maroon, purple discoloration,

or epidermal separation revealing a dark wound bed or blood-filled blister. Pain and temperature change often precede skin color changes. Discoloration may appear differently in darkly pigmented skin. This injury results from intense and/or prolonged pressure and shear forces at the bone–muscle interface. The wound may evolve rapidly to reveal the actual extent of tissue injury or may resolve without tissue loss. If necrotic tissue, subcutaneous tissue, granulation tissue, fascia, muscle, or other underlying structures are visible, this indicates a full-thickness PI (unstageable, Stage 3, or Stage 4). Do not use DTPI to describe vascular, traumatic, neuropathic, or dermatologic conditions (NPIAP, 2016) (**Fig. 20-16A–C**).

It must be confirmed that the purple skin present with DTPI which may appear as ecchymosis or bruising is due to pressure or shear and not related to a medication or trauma. DTPI can rapidly deteriorate. Timing and setting of the pressure and shear that lead to injury should be

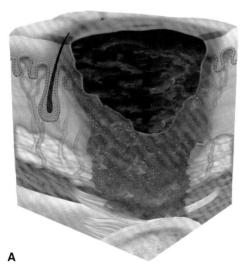

A

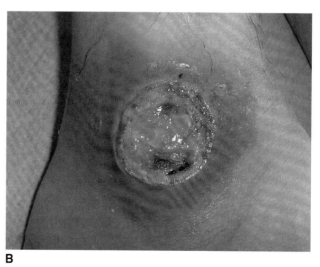

B

FIGURE 20-14.   A, B. Unstageable PI with Photo. (Used with permission of the National Pressure Injury Advisory Panel, 2020. Copyright © NPIAP.)

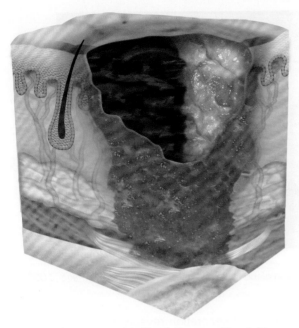

evaluated. Following identification of a DTPI, evolution of the injury should be documented since these injuries often slough the epidermis to reveal deeper tissue damage. If the injury becomes full thickness, the Stage of the resultant injury (Unstageable, Stage 3, or Stage 4) should be documented (Edsberg et al., 2016).

The phases of DTPI evolution have been described as purple intact tissue, purple discoloration with a thin blister covering a dark wound bed, a blood blister, or necrotic tissue. When the DTPI has necrotic tissue obscuring the wound bed, it is classified as unstageable. The wound care nurse should document the origin of the injury as DTPI for root cause analysis and continuous quality improvement purposes (Black et al., 2016). A study by Sullivan and Schoelles (2013) examined risk factors, presentation, and outcomes in 77 patients with documented DTPI. Average length of follow-up was 6 days (range 1 day to 14 weeks). At the final assessment, 85 DTPIs (66.4%) completely resolved or were progressing toward resolution, 31 remained unchanged and were still documented as purple-maroon discoloration or a blood-filled blister, and 12 (9.3%) had deteriorated

FIGURE 20-15. Unstageable PI with Focus on Slough Diagram. (Used with permission of the National Pressure Injury Advisory Panel, 2020. Copyright © NPIAP.)

Deep Tissue Pressure Injury

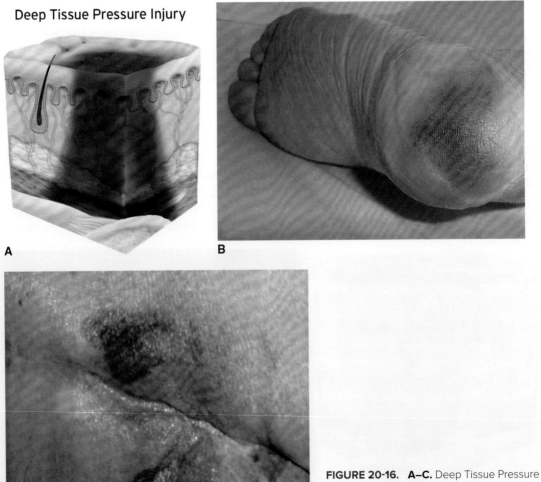

FIGURE 20-16. A–C. Deep Tissue Pressure Injury Diagram with Two Photos. (Used with permission of the National Pressure Injury Advisory Panel, 2020. Copyright © NPIAP.)

to full-thickness tissue loss (Sullivan & Schoelles, 2013). These observations offer insights into the evolution of DTPIs, since the majority of these lesions had resolved or were improving (Sullivan & Schoelles, 2013).

Pressure injuries should be staged according to their deepest depth. An understanding of anatomy is important when evaluating the type of tissue present in the wound, since the NPIAP staging system is based on the extent of tissue damage. To perform an accurate visual assessment, PI staging should take place only after the wound bed has been cleansed. If the wound is not of uniform depth, the portion that extends deeper requires classification of the injury at a higher stage. Stage 3 PIs can be shallow in areas without subcutaneous tissue, which include the bridge of the nose, ear, occiput, and the malleolus. The gluteal region can develop very deep ulcers that remain Stage 3. The depth of a Stage 4 PIs also varies by anatomic location. As with Stage 3 PIs, the bridge of the nose, ear, occiput, and malleolus do not have subcutaneous tissue, and Stage 4 PIs in these locations can be shallow. The extent of Stage 3 and 4 PIs is often underestimated due to undermining and fistula formation. A relatively small superficial skin defect may mask extensive deep tissue necrosis. Stage 4 PIs that extend into supporting structures, including fascia, tendon, or joint capsule, may be associated with osteomyelitis. DTPI and Stage 1 PIs may be difficult to detect in individuals with darker skin tones. The area may be painful, firm or spongy, boggy, warm, or cool compared with the surrounding tissue (Berlowitz, 2020a, 2020b).

 MEDICAL DEVICE–RELATED PRESSURE INJURIES

The NPIAP defines MDRPIs as PIs that result from the use of devices designed and applied for diagnostic or therapeutic purposes, noting that on the skin such PIs tend to take on the pattern or shape of the device and should be staged using the NPIAP staging system. Alternate terminology for the phenomenon includes omitting the word medical, becoming device-related pressure injury (DRPI) (EPUAP/NPIAP/PPPIA, 2019). It includes PIs from common devices such as cutlery, pens, and phones that have inadvertently applied pressure to the skin. The preferred term remains MDRPI. It is suggested that the actual item be included in the record to allow for root and common cause analysis (Edsberg et al., 2016).

Medical devices may be in place for extended periods of time resulting in sustained mechanical loads. The device can also alter the microclimate beneath it. Risk for MDRPI may increase as a result of impaired sensation, moisture under the device, poor perfusion, altered tissue tolerance, poor nutritional status, and edema. Other factors that contribute to the formation of MDRPI include poor positioning and ill-fitting devices. If the device must

remain, strategies to reduce risk of injury should be utilized (EPUAP/NPIAP/PPPIA, 2019). Thin dressings applied between the device and the skin redistributes the pressure beneath medical devices (Huang et al., 2009; Kuo et al., 2013; Weng, 2008). Children and neonates are at significant risk of MDRPI. Adjusting or modifying the device may be necessary to prevent PI (EPUAP/NPIAP/PPPIA, 2019). Additional information on pediatric pressure injury is available in Chapter 13.

KEY POINT

Risk for MDRPI may increase as a result of impaired sensation, moisture under the device, poor perfusion, altered tissue tolerance, poor nutritional status, and edema. Other factors that contribute to the formation of MDRPI include poor positioning and ill-fitting devices.

 MUCOSAL MEMBRANE PRESSURE INJURY

Mucosal membrane (MM) pressure injuries are found on mucous membranes with a history of a medical device in use at the location of the injury. Due to the anatomy of the tissue, these injuries cannot be staged (NPIAP, 2016). The histologic characteristics of mucosal tissue do not allow wound care nurses to distinguish partial from full-thickness tissue loss (Delmore & Ayello, 2017; Edsberg et al., 2016) (**Figs. 20-17 and 20-18**).

Nonblanchable erythema cannot be seen in mucous membranes and superficial tissue loss of the nonkeratinized epithelium cannot be distinguished from deeper, full thickness injuries by the naked eye (Edsberg et al., 2016). Examination of the lips, tongue, and mouth during oral care is important since injured MM often appears inflamed and may be tender and edematous (Edsberg et al., 2016). The soft coagulum that may remain loosely attached after forming is not slough. Mucous membranes line the tongue, oral mucosa, GI tract, nasal passages, urinary tract, tracheal lining, and vaginal tract. They are especially vulnerable to pressure from medical devices such as oxygen tubing, endotracheal tubes, bite blocks, orogastric and nasogastric tubes, urinary catheters, and fecal containment devices. Medical devices should be positioned to reduce pressure on mucous membranes. Using stabilizing systems to secure indwelling urinary catheters or nasogastric tubes without pressure can protect the tissues (Edsberg et al., 2016). The healing of wounds on MMs typically does not result in a scar since the scar tissue is remodeled.

Development of a classification system for MM pressure injuries has been undertaken with testing of reliability performed in an intensive care setting (ICU). The

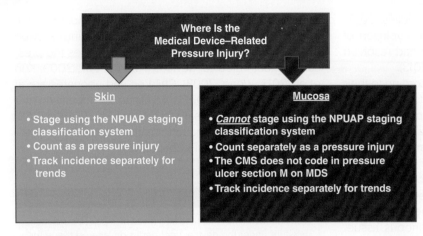

Where Is the Medical Device–Related Pressure Injury?

Skin

- Stage using the NPUAP staging classification system
- Count as a pressure injury
- Track incidence separately for trends

Mucosa

- *Cannot* stage using the NPUAP staging classification system
- Count separately as a pressure injury
- The CMS does not code in pressure ulcer section M on MDS
- Track incidence separately for trends

FIGURE 20-17. Staging and Classification Differences between Skin and Mucosal Pressure Injuries. CMS, Centers for Medicare and Medicaid Services; MDS, Minimum Data Set; NPUAP, National Pressure Ulcer Advisory Panel. (Used with permission from © 2016 EA Ayello and BA Delmore.)

Reaper Oral Mucosa Pressure Injury Scale (ROMPIS), which describes three stages of MM pressure injury, showed moderate interrater reliability. This classification system is undergoing further validation (Reaper et al., 2015, 2017).

Staging is based on visual and palpable clinical observation of the area. This has limits for diagnosing an injury before it is visible on the surface of the skin. Localized heat, edema, and changes in tissue consistency in relation to surrounding tissue (e.g., induration or hardness) have been identified as warning signs for PI development. Early identification of changes in skin and tissue color, temperature, and consistency enables implementation of an appropriate prevention and treatment plan. Accurate assessment is also important on admission, transfer within the facility as well as at discharge. Adjuncts to skin assessment are emerging including ultrasound, photoplethysmogram (PPG), laser Doppler flowmetry (LDF), and measures of transcutaneous oxygen and other biophysical variables. Their use in clinical practice is increasingly popular as devices become more accessible.

Mucous Membrane

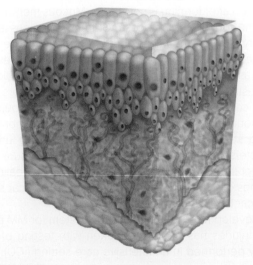

FIGURE 20-18. Mucous Membrane Diagram.

Objective measures of skin temperature using infrared imaging have become more accessible to health professionals. These techniques can be used as an adjunct to clinical examination skills to assess skin temperature (Koerner et al., 2019). Bates-Jensen et al. (2008, 2009) introduced the concept of subepidermal moisture (SEM) as a tissue parameter. SEM is a measure of soft tissue edema below the skin surface. Hydration of subepidermal tissues is normal. Inflammatory processes associated with tissue damage lead to increases in SEM in soft tissues. Change in SEM is a marker for inflammation and tissue damage.

In a study by Raizman et al. (2018), subepidermal (SEM) scores were taken in two groups of patients, but only used to determine interventions and care planning in the second group. The SEM Scanner made the nonvisible damage detectable by providing a numerical readout, alerting clinicians to implement stronger prevention measures. This change in practice resulted in a decrease in HAPIs by 93% between the two evaluation periods. Clinicians were able to target interventions, lower incidence, affect earlier recovery, save considerable pain, and lower costs of care (Raizman et al., 2018).

PRESSURE INJURIES PRESENT ON ADMISSION

On July 31, 2008, in the inpatient prospective payment system (IPPS) fiscal year 2009 Final Rule, CMS included 10 categories of conditions that were selected for the hospital-acquired conditions (HAC) payment provision. Stages 3 and 4 were included in this list. This payment system led to CMS ceasing payment for these complications considered reasonably preventable (e.g., catheter-associated urinary tract infections (CAUTIs), central line–associated blood stream infections [CLABSIs], surgical site infections [SSIs], Stage 3 and 4 PIs). Present on admission (POA) is defined as follows:

- Present at the time of the order for inpatient admission occurs. PI that develop during an outpatient encounter, including the emergency department, observation, or outpatient surgery is considered POA.

- PI diagnosis documented by provider. A provider is a physician or any qualified health care practitioner who is legally accountable for establishing the patient's diagnosis.
- Determination of whether the PI was POA is based on the provider's best clinical judgment anytime during the hospital stay.
- Inconsistent, missing, or conflicting documentation issues are resolved by the physician.
- PI is POA when the patient is discharged with a facility-acquired pressure injury and later readmitted with a different diagnosis.

The POA rule establishes a baseline for the patient so that subsequent pressure-related abnormalities in the skin can be identified and captured as hospital acquired (CMS, 2019). The wound care nurse should provide education for the skills needed for those conducting skin assessments. Consideration should be given for the use of diagnostic technology to augment visual and palpatory evaluation.

 ## AVOIDABLE VERSUS UNAVOIDABLE PRESSURE INJURIES

The same payment system change that led to CMS ceasing payment for these complications considered reasonably preventable led to conversation regarding the ability to prevent all pressure injuries. While many studies support the use of prevention strategies to decrease pressure injuries, no strategies have been shown to eliminate all pressure injuries.

In 2004, the CMS wrote regulatory language addressing PI prevention in LTC; stating that the facility must assure that an individual who enters the facility without PI does not develop PI unless the individual's clinical condition demonstrates that they were unavoidable. This statement did not apply to hospitalized or home care patients. In 2007, CMS classified full-thickness PI (Stage 3 and Stage 4) as never events in acute care, meaning these injuries should not occur and can be prevented.

In 2009, the WOCN Society issued a position statement refuting the position by Centers for Medicare & Medicaid Services (CMS) that all hospital-acquired PIs are avoidable (Schmitt et al., 2017; WOCN, 2009). In 2010, the NPIAP provided broader support of the avoidable versus unavoidable nomenclature, which could be applied to all clinical practice settings instead of just LTC settings.

An avoidable pressure injury may develop when the provider did not do one or more of the following:

- Evaluate the individual's clinical condition and pressure injury risk factors

- Define and implement interventions consistent with individual needs, individual goals, and recognized standards of practice
- Monitor and evaluate the impact of the interventions
- Revise the interventions as appropriate.

An unavoidable pressure injury may develop even though the provider did the following:

- Evaluated the individual's clinical condition and pressure injury risk factors
- Defined and implemented interventions consistent with individual needs, goals, and recognized standards of practice
- Monitored and evaluated the impact of the interventions
- Revised the approaches as appropriate.

The NPIAP further evaluated the issue of unavoidable PIs considering the complexities of nonmodifiable intrinsic and extrinsic risk factors (Black et al., 2011). Some of the nonmodifiable risk factors included cardiopulmonary status, hemodynamic stability, the impact of head-of-bed elevation, septic shock, anasarca, burns, immobility, medical devices, spinal cord injury, terminal illness, and nutrition (Edsberg et al., 2014). Consensus was achieved that unavoidable PIs do occur.

END-OF-LIFE SKIN INJURIES

With advanced illness and at end of life, significant changes in bodily systems occur, each of which has an impact on skin integrity. Many health care providers believe that PIs which occur at the end of life are often not preventable due to multiple risk factors, comorbid conditions, and the frail condition of the patient. Physiologic changes that occur with the dying process, over days to weeks, may affect the skin and soft tissues and manifest as observable changes in the skin's color, turgor, or integrity, or as subjective symptoms such as localized pain. These changes may be unavoidable and may occur even with the application of appropriate interventions that meet or exceed the standard of care (EPUAP/NPIAP/PPPIA, 2019; Schmitt et al., 2017). Several authors have proposed nomenclature to describe this phenomenon. Examples have been documented over 100 years ago (decubitus ominous) (Charcot, 1877) with more recent contributions including the Kennedy Terminal Ulcer (KTU), Trombley-Brennan Terminal Tissue Injury (TB-TTI), and Skin changes at life's end (SCALE) (Ayello et al., 2019; Kennedy, 1989; Trombley et al., 2012). Some but not all PIs in individuals receiving end of life or palliative care will heal (EPUAP/NPIAP/PPPIA, 2019; Tippett, 2005).

PI prevention and care should not be abandoned. Documentation of care should support that all measures are taken to prevent and treat PIs to support that the PI is unavoidable.

CLINICAL CHALLENGES IN PI STAGING

IDENTIFYING DTPI AND STAGE 1 PIs IN DARKLY PIGMENTED SKIN

The detection of DTPI and Stage 1 PIs in patients with darkly pigmented skin is especially challenging. Wound care nurses should increase their awareness of the disparity that exists in skin assessments between patients with light and darkly pigmented skin (Lyder, 2009). Tips for staging darkly pigmented skin include the following:

- Moisten the skin.
- Inspect for changes in pigmentation.
- Palpate for edema.
- Ask about pain in the area.
- Use indirect light to examine skin (Black, 2018).

It should be noted that when PIs in patients with darkly pigmented skin heal, the pigmentation may be absent, lighter, or darker than the surrounding skin. Newer technologies may augment visual and palpatory assessments and should be considered.

SKIN CHANGES WITH REPEATED FRICTION INJURY

Differentiating wounds that have friction as a primary or contributing cause from those caused by pressure and shear is sometimes difficult and continues to be a challenge for wound care nurses. Friction can cause minor to substantial skin impairment, but friction alone is not a direct cause of a PI. It is a risk factor that may contribute to or exacerbate PI development.

In distinguishing wound types that have friction as a factor, other factors that contribute to PI should be considered including moisture. If the cause is solely a frictional force, which leads to visible skin impairment, it would not be categorized as a PI. Superficial friction wounds can occur in the same location as PI due to the surface effects combined with the deeper effects of shear and pressure. In these circumstances, interventions should reduce both pressure and friction (Brienza et al., 2015). Chronic friction skin injuries are characterized by blanchable erythema or violaceous (i.e., purple) skin discoloration, lichenification related to repeated scratching or rubbing, hypertrophy of wound edges, skin scaling, and shallow skin ulcerations or skin tags (Berke, 2015; Berke, 2019; Mahoney et al., 2011; Mahoney & Rozenboom, 2019). They do not typically regress or resolve. This presentation may be confused with both Stage 1 PI and DTPI.

PRESSURE INJURIES OVER LOCATION OF PREVIOUSLY HEALED PRESSURE INJURIES

Loss of skin integrity over areas of previously healed full-thickness PIs may be difficult to classify. The NPIAP recommends that these injuries be classified as reopened, recurrent, or new depending on the length of time since the previous pressure injury closed and the maturation of the scar tissue (EPUAP/NPIAP/PPPIA, 2019).

 CONCLUSION

Pressure injuries are a life-threatening problem among vulnerable individuals, including those who are bedbound, or chair bound and those who are critically ill. The pathology of PI development is thought to include vessel occlusion and ischemia, lymphatic vessel compression and edema, reperfusion injury, and possibly direct damage to the cytoskeleton of the muscle cell. The major etiologic factors for PI development are prolonged or high-intensity pressure and shear force, and individuals with multiple comorbid conditions adversely affecting tissue tolerance are at greater risk. Pressure injury severity ranges from preulcerative conditions (such as Stage 1 lesions) to full-thickness tissue loss (Stage 3 and 4 PIs). Pressure injuries of particular interest include DTPI, which are rapidly developing lesions typically associated with very high-intensity or prolonged pressure, perioperative pressure injuries, and medical device–related pressure injuries. Pressure injury prevention requires prompt identification of the at-risk individual followed by prompt initiation of an evidence-based prevention protocol.

REFERENCES

Agam, L., & Gefen, A. (2008). Toward real-time detection of deep tissue injury risk in wheelchair users using Hertz contact theory. *Journal of Rehabilitation Research & Development, 45*(4), 537–550.

Arao, H., Obata, M., Shimada, T., & Hagisawa, S. (1998). Morphological characteristics of the dermal papillae in the development of pressure sores. *Journal of Tissue Viability, 8*(3), 17–23.

Ayello, E. A., & Braden, B. (2002). How and why to do pressure injury risk assessment. *Advances in Skin & Wound Care, 15*(3), 125–131.

Ayello, E. A., Levine, J. M., Langemo, D., et al. (2019). Reexamining the literature on terminal ulcers, SCALE, skin failure, and unavoidable pressure injuries. *Advances in Skin & Wound Care, 32*(3), 109–121.

Bates-Jensen, B. M., McCreath, H. E., & Pongquan, V. (2009). Sub-epidermal moisture is associated with early pressure ulcer damage in nursing home residents with dark skin tones: Pilot findings. *Journal of Wound, Ostomy, and Continence Nursing, 36*(3), 277.

Bates-Jensen, B. M., McCreath, H. E., Pongquan, V., et al. (2008). Sub-epidermal moisture differentiates erythema and stage I pressure ulcers in nursing home residents. *Wound Repair and Regeneration, 16*(2), 189–197.

Bauer, K., Rock, K., Nazzal, M., et al. (2016). Pressure ulcers in the United States' inpatient population from 2008 to 2012: Results of a Retrospective Nationwide Study. *Ostomy Wound Management, 62*(11), 30–38.

Bergstrom, N. (1987). The Braden Scale for predicting pressure sore risk. *Nursing Research, 36*(4), 205–210.

Bergstrom, N., Braden, B., Norvell, K., et al. (1988). Diminished tissue tolerance: Influence on pressure sore development in the institutionalized elderly. *Applied Nursing Research, 1*(2), 96.

Berke, C. T. (2015). Pathology and clinical presentation of friction injuries: Case series and literature review. *Journal of Wound Ostomy & Continence Nursing, 42*(1), 47–61.

Berke, C. T. (2019). Friction injury versus deep tissue injury: Level of tissue involvement: A comparison of 2 cases. *Journal of Wound Ostomy & Continence Nursing, 46*(6), 539–542.

Berlowitz, D. (2020a). Clinical staging and management of pressure-induced skin and soft tissue injury. In K. E. Schmader, R. S. Berman, & A. Cochran (Eds.), *UpToDate*. Waltham, MA: UpToDate Inc. Retrieved from https://www-uptodate-com.proxy.lib.duke.edu. Accessed on April 25, 2020.

Berlowitz, D. (2020b). Epidemiology, pathogenesis, and risk assessment of pressure-induced skin and soft tissue injury. In K. E. Schmader, R. S. Berman, & A. Cochran (Eds.), *UpToDate*. Waltham, MA: UpToDate Inc. Retrieved from https://www-uptodate-com.proxy.lib.duke.edu. Accessed on April 25, 2020.

Black, J. (2018). Using thermography to assess pressure injuries in patients with dark skin. *Nursing, 48*(9), 60–61.

Black, J. M., Brindle, C. T., & Honaker, J. S. (2016). Differential diagnosis of suspected deep tissue injury. *International Wound Journal, 13*(4), 531–539.

Black, J. M., Edsberg, L. E., Baharestani, M. M., et al. (2011). Pressure ulcers: Avoidable or unavoidable? Results of the national pressure ulcer advisory panel consensus conference. *Ostomy Wound Management, 57*(2), 24.

Braden, B., & Bergstrom, N. (1987). A conceptual schema for the study of the etiology of pressure sores. *Rehabilitation Nursing, 12*(1), 8–16.

Brienza, D., Antokal, S., Herbe, L., et al. (2015). Friction-induced skin injuries—are they pressure ulcers? An updated NPUAP white paper. *Journal of Wound Ostomy & Continence Nursing, 42*(1), 62–64.

Centers for Medicare and Medicaid Services (CMS). (2019). Hospital acquired conditions (POA Indicator) CMS. Last updated March 10, 2019. Retrieved from https://www.cms.gov/Medicare/Medicare-Fee-for-Service-Payment/HospitalAcqCond. Accessed April 25, 2020.

Charcot, J. M. (1877). *Lectures on the Diseases of the Nervous System*. London: The New Sydenham Society.

Coyer, F., Miles, S., Gosley, S., et al. (2017). Pressure injury prevalence in intensive care versus non-intensive care patients: A state-wide comparison. *Australian Critical Care, 30*(5), 244–250.

Delmore, B. A., & Ayello, E. A. (2017). Pressure injuries caused by medical devices and other objects: A clinical update. *American Journal of Nursing, 117*(12), 36–45.

Edsberg, L. E. (2007). Pressure ulcer tissue histology: An appraisal of current knowledge. *Ostomy Wound Management, 53*(10), 40–49.

Edsberg, L. E., Black, J. M., Goldberg, M., et al. (2016). Revised National Pressure Ulcer Advisory Panel pressure injury staging system: Revised pressure injury staging system. *Journal of Wound, Ostomy, and Continence Nursing, 43*(6), 585.

Edsberg, L. E., Cutway, R., Anain, S., et al. (2000). Microstructural and mechanical characterization of human tissue at and adjacent to pressure ulcers. *Journal of Rehabilitation Research and Development, 37*(4), 463–472.

Edsberg, L. E., Langemo, D., Baharestani, M. M., et al. (2014). Unavoidable pressure injury: State of the science and consensus outcomes. *Journal of Wound Ostomy & Continence Nursing, 41*(4), 313–334.

European Pressure Ulcer Advisory Panel, National Pressure Injury Advisory Panel, and Pan Pacific Pressure Injury Alliance [EPUAP/NPIAP/PPPIA]. (2019). In E. Haesler (Ed.), *Prevention and treatment of pressure ulcers/injuries: Clinical Practice Guideline*. The International Guideline.

Goldstein, B., & Sanders, J. (1998). Skin response to repetitive mechanical stress: A new experimental model in pig. *Archives of Physical Medicine and Rehabilitation, 79*(3), 265–272.

Gray, M., & Giuliano, K. K. (2018). Incontinence-associated dermatitis, characteristics and relationship to pressure injury: A multisite epidemiologic analysis. *Journal of Wound, Ostomy, and Continence Nursing, 45*(1), 63.

Habiballah, L., & Tubaishat, A. (2016). The prevalence of pressure ulcers in the paediatric population. *Journal of Tissue Viability, 25*(2), 127–134. doi: 10.1016/j.jtv.2016.02.001.

Houghton, P. E., Campbell, K. E., CPG Panel. (2013). Canadian best practice guidelines for the prevention and management of pressure ulcers in people with spinal cord injury. A resource handbook for clinicians. Retrieved April 24, 2020, from https://onf.org/wp-content/uploads/2019/04/Pressure_Ulcers_Best_Practice_Guideline_Final_web4.pdf

Huang, T. T., Tseng, C. E., Lee, T. M., et al. (2009). Preventing pressure sores of the nasal ala after nasotracheal tube intubation: From animal model to clinical application. *Journal of Oral and Maxillofacial Surgery, 67*(3), 543–551.

Kennedy, K. L. (1989). The prevalence of pressure ulcers in an intermediate care facility. *Advances in Skin & Wound Care, 2*(2), 44–47.

Koerner, S., Adams, D., Harper, S. L., et al. (2019). Use of thermal imaging to identify deep-tissue pressure injury on admission reduces clinical and financial burdens of hospital-acquired pressure injuries. *Advances in Skin & Wound Care, 32*(7), 312–320.

Kosiak, M. (1961). Etiology of decubitus ulcers. *Archives of Physical Medicine and Rehabilitation, 42*, 19–29.

Krouskop, T. A. (1983). A synthesis of the factors that contribute to pressure sore formation. *Medical Hypotheses, 11*(2), 255–267.

Kuo, C. Y., Wootten, C. T., Tylor, D. A., et al. (2013). Prevention of pressure ulcers after pediatric tracheotomy using a Mepilex Ag® dressing. *Laryngoscope, 123*(12), 3201–3205.

Lachenbruch, C., Ribble, D., Emmons, K., et al. (2016). Pressure ulcer risk in the incontinent patient. *Journal of Wound, Ostomy, and Continence Nursing, 43*(3), 235–241.

Lahmann, N. A., & Kottner, J. (2011). Relation between pressure, friction and pressure ulcer categories: A secondary data analysis of hospital patients using CHAID methods. *International Journal of Nursing Studies, 48*(12), 1487–1494.

Loerakker, S., Manders, E., Strijkers, G. J., et al. (2011). The effects of deformation, ischemia, and reperfusion on the development of muscle damage during prolonged loading. *Journal of Applied Physiology, 111*(4), 1168–1177.

Loerakker, S., Solis, L. R., Bader, D. L., et al. (2013). How does muscle stiffness affect the internal deformations within the soft tissue layers of the buttocks under constant loading? *Computer Methods in Biomechanics and Biomedical Engineering, 16*(5), 520–529.

Lyder, C. (2009). Closing the skin assessment disparity gap between patients with light and darkly pigmented skin. *Journal of Wound Ostomy & Continence Nursing, 36*(3), 285.

Mahoney, M. F., & Rozenboom, B. J. (2019). Definition and characteristics of chronic tissue injury: A unique form of skin damage. *Journal of Wound Ostomy & Continence Nursing, 46*(3), 187–191.

Mahoney, M., Rozenboom, B., Doughty, D., et al. (2011). Issues related to accurate classification of buttocks wounds. *Journal of Wound Ostomy & Continence Nursing, 38*(6), 635–642.

National Pressure Injury Advisory Panel (NPIAP). (2016). NPIAP Pressure Injury Stages. Retrieved from https://cdn.ymaws.com/npiap.com/resource/resmgr/online_store/npiap_pressure_injury_stages.pdf

Peirce, S. M., Skalak, T. C., & Rodeheaver, G. T. (2000). Ischemia-reperfusion injury in chronic pressure ulcer formation: A skin model in the rat. *Wound Repair and Regeneration, 8*(1), 68–76.

Raizman, R., MacNeil, M., Rappl, L. (2018). Utility of a sensor-based technology to assist in the prevention of pressure ulcers: A clinical comparison. *International Wound Journal, 15*(6), 1033–1044. doi: 10.1111/iwj.12974.

Reaper, S., Green, C., Gupta, S., et al. (2015). Development and validation of a scale for the assessment of pressure injuries in the mouth and oral mucosa: The Reaper Oral Mucosa Pressure Injury Scale (ROMPIS). *Australian Critical Care, 28*(1), 42.

Reaper, S., Green, C., Gupta, S., et al. (2017). Inter-rater reliability of the Reaper Oral Mucosa Pressure Injury Scale (ROMPIS): A novel scale for the assessment of the severity of pressure injuries to the mouth and oral mucosa. *Australian Critical Care, 30*(3), 167–171.

Reddy, M., Gill, S. S., & Rochon, P. A. (2006). Preventing pressure ulcers: A systematic review. *JAMA, 296*(8), 974–984.

Russo, C. A., Steiner, C., & Spector, W. (2006). Hospitalizations related to pressure ulcers among adults 18 years and older, 2006: Statistical brief# 64. In *Healthcare cost and utilization project (HCUP) statistical briefs.*

Schmitt, S., Andries, M. K., Ashmore, P. M., et al. (2017). Avoidable versus unavoidable pressure ulcers/injuries: WOCN society position paper. *Journal of Wound, Ostomy, and Continence Nursing, 44*(5), 458–468.

Smith, A., McNichol, L. L., Amos, M. A., et al. (2013). A retrospective, nonrandomized, before and-after study of the effect of linens constructed of synthetic silk-like fabric on pressure ulcer incidence. *Ostomy Wound Management, 59*(4), 28–30.

Stevenson, R., Collinson, M., Henderson, V., et al. (2013). The prevalence of pressure ulcers in community settings: An observational study. *International Journal of Nursing Studies, 50*(11), 1550–1557.

Stotts, N. A., & Gunningberg, L. (2007). Predicting pressure ulcer risk. *American Journal of Nursing, 107*(11), 40–48.

Sullivan, N., & Schoelles, K. M. (2013). Preventing in-facility pressure ulcers as a patient safety strategy: A systematic review. *Annals of Internal Medicine, 158*(5), 410–416.

Tippett, A. W. (2005). Wounds at the end of life. *Wounds, 17*(4), 91–98.

Trombley, K., Brennan, M. R., Thomas, L., et al. (2012). Prelude to death or practice failure? Trombley-Brennan terminal tissue injuries. *American Journal of Hospice and Palliative Medicine®, 29*(7), 541–545.

Twersky, J., Montgomery, T., Sloane, R., et al. (2012). A randomized, controlled study to assess the effect of silk-like textiles and high-absorbency adult incontinence briefs on pressure ulcer prevention. *Ostomy Wound Management, 58*(12), 18.

Weng, M. H. (2008). The effect of protective treatment in reducing pressure ulcers for non-invasive ventilation patients. *Intensive and Critical Care Nursing, 24*(5), 295–299.

Witkowski, J. A., & Parish, L. C. (1982). Histopathology of the decubitus ulcer. *Journal of the American Academy of Dermatology, 6*(6), 1014–1021.

Wound Ostomy and Continence Nurses Society (WOCN). (2009). Position statement on avoidable versus unavoidable pressure ulcers. *Journal of Wound Ostomy & Continence Nursing, 36*, 378–381.

Wound Ostomy and Continence Nurses Society (WOCN). (2016). *Guideline for management of pressure ulcers. WOCN clinical practice guidelines series # 2.* Mt. Laurel, NJ: Author.

CASE STUDY

Mr. M. is a 68-year-old male with type 2 diabetes was admitted to the hospital following a fall at home. He fell off a 6-feet ladder onto the ground. He could move all extremities, but he is a large man and was unable to stand following the accident. He stayed on his back on the ground for approximately 6 hours until his grandson came to his home to check on him. Mr. M. was transported by EMS to the ED of the local hospital where his blood glucose was regulated and radiographic studies were performed overnight. He was diagnosed with a left femur fracture. He was held in the ED on a stretcher and was transported to the larger hospital the following morning for surgery. The admitting nurse on the orthopedic unit noted a 6 × 8 cm purple-red discoloration at the apex of the gluteal cleft, or coccyx. It presented as symmetrical in appearance and did not blanch. The staff nurse who noted the abnormality in the skin indicated in the electronic medical record that it was an area of ecchymosis from trauma sustained during the fall. Mr. M. went for surgery (an open reduction and internal fixation, or ORIF) within an hour after being admitted. The sur-

gery lasted just under 3 hours. Mr. M. recovered for about an hour in the post anesthesia care unit and returned to the orthopedic unit. Within 72 hours following admission, the area surrounding Mr. M's coccyx was indurated and the top layer of skin was peeling away from the discolored area. The tissue revealed beneath was dark purple with a black center. A wound care nurse was consulted for suggestions for topical care. It was determined that Mr. M. required a bariatric bed with a low air loss feature for turning. A silicone foam dressing was placed over the affected area with instructions for the nursing staff to peel it back twice daily to inspect the ulcer and document their findings. The dressing was to be changed twice weekly and PRN for loosening of dressing edges or strike-through of drainage. Mr. M. complained of pain in this area. The dark center of the area evolved into a dry eschar. On post-op day 5, wound care was changed to an enzymatic debriding agent topped with a saline-dampened gauze dressing and covered with dry dressing. Mr. M. was discharged to home with a home health nurse and physical therapy. On day 9, Mr. M.'s home health nurse called the orthopedic surgeon to report that the DTPI ulcer had opened as a Stage 4 PI. The measurements were 6 × 8 × 2.5 cm. The surgeon referred Mr. M. to the outpatient wound care center where he underwent serial debridements, pulsatile lavage sessions, and continued topical wound care using moisture retentive dressings. Home health care was continued for 12 weeks. The Stage 4 PI closed. His home health nurse recommended Mr. M. to limit the time he spends in his recliner chair and use a pressure redistribution chair cushion. He subsequently returned to work.

DISCUSSION POINTS

1. No documentation exists for the turning and repositioning of Mr. M. in the ED, although we have to assume he was moved for the radiographic procedures. There is no notation of an alteration in his integumentary system. We know that the focus of his stay there was to regulate his blood glucose level and to determine the extent of his LE injury. Might a comprehensive skin assessment have revealed a tissue abnormality at that point of care?

2. Mr. M. was transported via EMS twice following his fall, once from his home to the ED and a second time to the community hospital for his surgery.

3. Upon admission to the orthopedic unit at the community hospital, the red-purple area of discoloration that did not blanch is not documented as an area of DTPI nor was it documented as a PI that was present on admission (POA). Do you think this is a common error? Do you think that having two members of the nursing staff perform skin assessment on admission might have resulted in different documentation?

4. Patients who undergo operative procedures lasting >3 hours have an increased incidence of pressure injury. Do you think that this particular operative procedure contributed to the tissue injury and subsequent PI sustained by Mr. M?

5. What role would having a sleep surface of the appropriate size play in the adequate turning and repositioning of this patient off of an area that is known to be compromised?

6. Areas of DTPI typically evolve and occasionally resolve. There is no specific time frame for evolution, but some suggest that it is between 3 and 10 days, even with appropriate interventions. Does Mr. M.'s presentation and evolution occur during this time frame?

7. Mr. M. is considering litigation pertaining to his "bedsore" after talking to neighbors, parishioners, and some of his care providers. Was this PI avoidable? Do you think that there is enough information provided to substantiate a claim that any care providers were negligent?

QUESTIONS

1. What is the greatest risk factor for the development of pressure injuries?
   A. Diabetes mellitus that is long-standing (>10 years)
   B. Immobility
   C. Exposure to excessive moisture
   D. African American ethnicity

2. Which of the following is NOT considered an etiologic factor for pressure injury?
   A. Shear force
   B. Prolonged pressure
   C. Friction
   D. Medical device–related injury

3. Which statement accurately describes one of the four major factors hypothesized to cause pressure and shear damage?

   A. Excessive perfusion of blood vessels resulting in tissue ischemia
   B. Increased risk of dehydration due to occlusion of lymph vessels
   C. Edema resulting from accumulation of oxygen free radicals
   D. Direct deformation damage of muscle cells during high-pressure loads

4. Which area of the body is the most difficult to protect using pressure redistribution surfaces?
   A. Sacrum
   B. Heel
   C. Ischial spine
   D. Skull

5. The wound care nurse is responsible for staging pressure injuries for hospitalized patients. Which statement accurately describes a guideline for staging?
   A. DTPI lesions should always be considered as Stage I pressure injuries.
   B. DTPI presents as a partial-thickness wound that heals predictably.
   C. Visual inspection alone is prone to error in pressure injury staging.
   D. Tissue damage should be inspected at the initial point of injury for staging.

6. The wound care nurse is assessing the development of a potential DTPI on a patient in the critical care unit. How do these pressure injuries present initially?
   A. Deep purple or maroon bruised area
   B. Open full-thickness wound
   C. Open wound covered with black eschar
   D. Reddened patch of skin

7. Which statement describes the primary focus of management of DTPI lesions?
   A. Surgical debridement
   B. Topical therapy
   C. Use of appropriate dressings
   D. Reducing pressure and shear forces

8. Which surgical patient would the wound care nurse consider high risk for the development of pressure injuries?
   A. A patient whose surgery lasted >2 hours
   B. A patient having a cesarean birth
   C. A patient with a BMI < 18
   D. A patient with a BMI > 30

9. The wound care nurse is planning care for a patient with a tracheostomy tube. What intervention would the nurse institute to prevent a medical device-related pressure injury?
   A. Avoid using tape to secure the device.
   B. Pad the device with a foam dressing.
   C. Remove or reposition the device every day.
   D. Use antiseptic cleansers on the skin surrounding the device.

10. Which patient would the wound care nurse classify as high risk for developing an unavoidable pressure injury while hospitalized?
   A. A patient who is at end of life and has severely impaired perfusion
   B. A patient with long-standing diabetes mellitus and peripheral neuropathy
   C. A patient with a spinal injury
   D. A patient with a cardiac condition

ANSWERS AND RATIONALES

1. B. Rationale: Immobility is the most important risk factor that contributes to development of pressure injury. Immobility may be permanent or transient.

2. C. Rationale: Superficial lesions (e.g., skin maceration, moisture-associated dermatitis, abrasions) are primarily the result of moisture and friction and should not be considered pressure-induced injuries.

3. D. Rationale: Deformation of deep tissues resulting from pressure and shear may directly cause cell death as a result of loss of cytoskeletal integrity. Deformation-induced cell death combines with tissue hypoxia, edema, and reperfusion injury to result in additional injury.

4. B. Rationale: The data indicate that PI prevention must include strategies to reduce both the magnitude of loading (intensity of pressure) and

the duration of loading, specifically pressure redistribution surfaces and routine repositioning. The anatomy of the heel with bony prominences having little subcutaneous tissue makes it difficult to offload.

5. C. Rationale: Staging is based on visual and palpable clinical observation of the area. This has limits for diagnosing an injury before it is visible on the surface of the skin.

6. A. Rationale: DTPI is intact or nonintact skin with localized area of persistent nonblanchable deep red, maroon, purple discoloration or epidermal separation revealing a dark wound bed or blood-filled blister.

7. D. Rationale: The most important initial intervention when DTPI is detected is to redistribute shear and pressure forces from the area.

8. C. Rationale: The patient who is underweight is considered to be high risk for PI development. Obese patients over BMI of 40 are also at risk.

9. B. Rationale: Thin dressings applied between the device and the skin redistribute the pressure beneath medical devices.

10. A. Rationale: Unavoidable PIs may occur, hemodynamic stability, head-of-bed elevation, septic shock, anasarca, burns, medical devices, and terminal illness.

CHAPTER 21

PRESSURE INJURY PREVENTION: IMPLEMENTING AND MAINTAINING A SUCCESSFUL PLAN AND PROGRAM

Kathleen Borchert

OBJECTIVES

1. Utilize evidence-based risk assessment tool to accurately identify patients at risk for pressure injury development.
2. Describe technique and frequency of comprehensive skin assessments.
3. Identify strategies to prevent medical device–related pressure injuries.

4. Provide best-practice strategies implemented for pressure injury prevention.
5. Design a process to monitor incidence of facility-acquired pressure injuries.

TOPIC OUTLINE

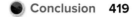

INTRODUCTION

The body of knowledge advancing our understanding of pressure injury (PI) prevention has grown significantly but knowledge alone does not prevent pressure injuries. Every facility and health care organization should have a comprehensive pressure injury prevention program (PIPP). Programmatically, it should include a best practice bundle along with the infrastructure to support it. The wound care nurse is often the coordinator of these efforts and provides leadership and clinical expertise in the content of the program. The PIPP will not be successful without the full support of administration at all levels. All care providers and administrators should believe that pressure injuries represent a negative outcome and that all health care providers play an integral role in their prevention.

Pressure injury prevention is the best defense against pressure injuries. The goal is a well-developed, evidence-based prevention plan that can be tailored to the individual's specific needs, effectively implemented, and revised according to the patient's response to care (AHRQ, 2014).

A pressure injury prevention plan focused on the patient should be based on knowledge and assessment data related to (1) clinical condition (current health state and comorbidities), (2) current skin condition, (3) overall pressure injury risk status and specific risk factors, and (4) resource availability (people and environmental) (AHRQ, 2014). Knowledge pertaining to the patient's clinical presentation, skin condition, and specific risk factors provides information needed to determine what should be done to prevent the development of pressure injuries. Knowledge pertaining to the available resources helps to determine what can be done. What will be done depends largely upon the knowledge base, motivation, commitment, and involvement of the entire health care team (i.e., patient, family, provider, nurse, therapists [e.g., respiratory, physical, occupational, or speech], pharmacist, dietitian, and nursing assistants). The goals of this chapter are to provide current information regarding pressure injury prevention with strategies for ensuring that preventive care is routinely incorporated into patient care.

MAINTENANCE OF SKIN HEALTH

Skin care including bathing, moisturizing, and incontinence management are basic elements of nursing care with the aim to maintain or restore healthy skin. Routine skin assessment is needed to identify issues with skin integrity promptly. The wound nurse should review and offer guidance on the general skin care products available for use. Protocols that describe general care of patients related to bathing and incontinence care should promote efforts to maintain the protective function of the skin. Common skin issues like dry skin and moisture-associated dermatitis (MASD) should be addressed (Brennan-Cook & Turner, 2019; Rahn et al., 2016). (See Chapter 2 for more information about the skin.)

ROUTINE SKIN CARE

Maintaining healthy skin and early detection of skin injury are nursing responsibilities. Regular cleansing assists in keeping the skin healthy but can be damaging if harsh, alkaline soaps are used. Often warm water is all that is needed to cleanse the skin adequately (Maklebust & Sieggreen, 2001). Moisturizing agents applied immediately after bathing, while the skin is still damp but not wet, will help to keep the skin supple. With respect to cleansing equipment, the washbasin has historically been standard equipment used by nurses. Research has shown that washbasins are a source of bacteria and may be linked to the transmission of hospital-acquired infections (HAIs) (Johnson et al., 2009; Marchaim et al., 2012; Sturgeon et al., 2019). Using prepackaged, premoistened, rinse-free, disposable cleansing cloths as an alternative to conventional bath basins and washcloths is recommended. These cleansing wipes help maintain skin health and reduce the risk of infection associated with use of bath basins. There is evidence to support that daily bathing with cleansing wipes that contain chlorhexidine gluconate (CHG), especially in the intensive care units, reduces the spread of infections (Reynolds et al., 2019). CHG can cause mild skin rash, allergic reaction, and skin dryness. The use on mucous membranes is not recommended (Wang & Layon, 2017).

SKIN ASSESSMENT

Head-to-toe skin inspection for integrity and color should be performed by staff regularly with the frequency specified by care setting (e.g., on admission, every shift on medical/surgical units, and every 4 hours in ICU). A comprehensive skin assessment includes a methodical head-to-toe, front and back inspection of bony prominences and examination under and around medical devices. Assessment is not a visual skin inspection alone. It also includes palpation of the tissue to check for temperature, edema, and tissue consistency. These assessments assist in determining if the patient has tissue damage. Assessment of the skin should also include identification of factors that may decrease the resilience of the skin, such as age-related thinning of the skin, malnutrition and dehydration, exposure to moisture, excessive dryness, and the individual's overall health status (Dealy, 2009; WOCN, 2016). The EPUAP/NPUAP/PPPIA (2019) recommends the following to the timing of a skin assessment: (1) as soon as possible upon admission/transfer (2) at the same time as pressure injury risk assessment, (3) periodically as indicated by the individual's degree of pressure injury risk and (4) prior to discharge from the facility.

Consideration should be given to using a subepidermal moisture/edema measurement device as an adjunct to routine clinical skin assessment, when assessing darkly pigmented skin for pressure injury as early signs of visual color changes are not as apparent for this population. Use of subepidermal moisture and/or a color chart should be considered as adjunctive assessment strategies (EPUAP/NPIAP/PPPIA, 2019; Ross & Gefen, 2019).

For patients at risk for pressure injuries, the skin assessment should focus attention to the skin over bony prominences (e.g., sacrum and coccyx, ischial tuberosities, greater trochanters, and heels) and the skin in contact with medical devices (EPUAP/NPIAP/PPPIA, 2019; WOCN, 2016). The health care provider should be alert to foreign objects in the bed when repositioning (e.g., needle covers, rolls of tape, ink pens and covers, disposable instruments). Stockings, heel protectors, and anything covering the skin including prophylactic dressings should be removed to allow for comprehensive skin assessment.

KEY POINT

Anything covering the skin must be removed to allow for a comprehensive skin assessment including stockings, heel protectors, and prophylactic dressings.

Inspection of the lateral and medial malleoli should be conducted during heel assessments. A body diagram may be used to accurately document the location of any abnormal findings such as abrasions and other skin lesions. It is important to use anatomical nomenclature to describe location including the bony prominences under areas of pressure injury (e.g., trochanter instead of hip, medial malleolus instead of inner ankle, ischial tuberosity or sacrum instead of buttock).

 # PRESSURE INJURY RISK ASSESSMENT

Risk assessment for pressure injury includes identification of subjective, objective, and psychosocial factors to determine the risk and care needs of the patient. It aims to identify individuals with characteristics that increase their probability of developing a PI. There is no agreed-upon best approach to assessing risk. The assessment of risk seems intuitive but the variability in training and experience of health care providers make intuition unreliable for predicting risk as evidence in several studies (García-Fernández et al., 2014).

GENERAL PRINCIPLES

Risk assessment should be performed on admission, following any change in the patient's condition and on transfer to a different level of care, and at regular intervals (EPUAP/NPIAP/PPPIA, 2019). The frequency of reassessment of risk is every 24 hours for acute care patients. More frequent reassessments may be needed based upon the patient's clinical presentation or institutional policy. Determinations about risk and sources of risk should be based upon data obtained from completion of a valid and reliable PI risk assessment tool. Additional data obtained from a comprehensive clinical assessment including a skin assessment informs decisions about risk status including perfusion, skin temperature, and the presence of medical devices (Bryant & Nix, 2016). A structured risk assessment is important in identifying the patient at risk for PI development but does not replace clinical judgment.

KEY POINT

Risk assessment should be performed on admission, following any change in the patient's condition and on transfer to a different level of care, and at regular intervals as specified by facility policy.

RISK ASSESSMENT TOOLS

In the United States, health care providers use pressure injury risk assessment tools that have been proven valid and reliable, such as the Braden Scale for Predicting Pressure Sore Risk© (Braden Scale) for adult patients (Braden & Bergstrom, 1987), Braden QD for pediatric patients (Curley et al., 2003), and Neonatal Skin Risk Assessment Scale (NSRAS) for patients born at 26 to 40 weeks of gestation (Huffines & Lodgson, 1997). Pressure injury risk assessment tools are usually composed of subscales that are scored and added to yield a total score. Variations in the total score are used to determine the level of risk from low to high. The total risk assessment score does not provide information concerning specific risk factors and should not be used as the basis for development of an appropriately individualized prevention program (EPUAP/NPIAP/PPPIA, 2019). Subscale scores should be used to identify the specific factors contributing to risk for the individual, and the prevention program should be designed to address those risk factors as well as any other factors determined as contributing to overall risk (EPUAP/NPIAP/PPPIA, 2019).

KEY POINT

Prevention protocols should not be based only on the total risk assessment score. Subscale scores should be used to identify specific risk factors for the individual patient.

Risk assessment tools were developed in an attempt to incorporate multiple factors into a simple assessment tool that would accurately identify patients at greatest risk, permitting appropriate allocation of prevention equipment and interventions. At least 40 PI risk assessment scales have been developed by researchers and clinicians from the United States and Europe (Nixon et al., 2005). The relationship between PI risk assessment scores and PI incidence is not firmly established. Risk assessment scales are recommended for use in prevention guidelines because they provide a systematic means of assessing sources of risk (EPUAP/NPIAP/PPPIA, 2019).

Pancorbo-Hildago and colleagues (2006) conducted a systematic review of risk assessment scales for PI prevention with specific attention to their effectiveness in clinical practice, the degree to which they had been validated, and their effectiveness as indicators of risk for developing a PI (Pancorbo-Hildago et al., 2006). In this review, there was no evidence that use of risk assessment scales decreased PI incidence. There was evidence that use of a risk assessment tool enhances identification of at-risk individuals, which provides guidance in use of preventive resources. Three PI risk assessment scales used for adult patients have been determined to have validity and reliability: the Braden Scale (Bergstrom et al., 1987a), the Norton Pressure Sore Risk-Assessment Scale Scoring System (Norton, 1989), and the Waterlow Score Card (Waterlow, 1985). The Braden Scale offers the best balance between sensitivity (57.1%) and specificity (67.5%) and the best PI risk prediction (Defloor & Grypdonck, 2005; Pancorbo-Hidalgo et al., 2006). Sensitivity and specificity are two terms utilized in statistical testing to indicate validity. In statistical testing, sensitivity refers to how accurately the tool predicts pressure injury risk, whereas specificity refers to how well the tool identifies those who are not at risk for pressure injury. Ideally the tool would generate 100% sensitivity and 100% specificity, indicating that use of the tool is exceptional at predicting who is at risk and accurately identifies individuals not at risk. Bolton (2007) conducted an integrated review of the literature to determine the most reliable and valid scale for assessing pressure injury risk in the clinical set-

ting. The Braden Scale was found to be a valid instrument for determining pressure injury risk in a variety of health care settings when the assessment was conducted by a registered nurse (RN) (Bolton, 2007; Halfens et al., 2000). All three risk assessment scales (Braden Scale, Norton Score, and Waterloo Scale) were developed more than 30 years ago, without benefit of insights from recent studies. The older risk assessment tools do not include assessment of certain key factors contained in the more recently developed tools, including tissue perfusion/oxygenation, general skin status, and medical device–related risk (WOCN, 2016).

The Braden Scale

The Braden Scale for Predicting Pressure Sore Risk© was introduced into the literature in 1987 by Braden and Bergstrom (Braden & Bergstrom, 1987; Bergstrom et al., 1987a, 1987b) and was based on a conceptual model of the etiologic factors contributing to pressure injury development. Their schema (**Fig. 21-1**) included two main etiologic factors: pressure against the tissue and the tissue's ability to tolerate pressure. Together, these two etiologic factors were theorized to determine a person's likelihood for developing a pressure injury. Individual risk factors either increased the likelihood of prolonged pressure or reflected reduced tissue tolerance to pressure.

The Braden Scale (**Fig. 21-2**) directs health care providers to assess and score six specific risk factors that contribute to pressure injury risk: sensory perception level, skin exposure to moisture, activity level, mobility ability, nutritional intake, and exposure to friction and shear. Each of these risk factor subscales are scored between 1 and 4, except the friction/shear subscale, which is rated from 1 to 3. Each rating is accompanied by a brief description of the criteria for assigning the rating. When the six subscales are added, the total Braden Scale score ranges from 6 to 23.

Braden Scale scores reflect five levels of pressure injury risk: no risk (19 to 23), mild risk (15 to 18), moderate risk (13 to 14), high risk (10 to 12), and very high risk ($\leq$9) (Bergstrom & Braden, 2002; Braden & Maklebust, 2005). The Braden Scale score is an inverse measurement of risk; lower Braden Scale score indicates higher risk for developing a pressure injury. A cutoff score of 18 or below is considered predictive of pressure injury in all care settings and all ethnic groups (Bergstrom & Braden, 2002; Braden & Bergstrom, 1994; Braden & Maklebust, 2005; Lyder et al., 1999). Detailed information and training materials are available at https://bradenscale.com/.

Since its 1987 inception, the Braden Scale has undergone extensive reliability and validity testing. Validity refers to the ability of an instrument to accurately reflect or represent that which it is intended to measure (Polit & Beck, 2011). The ability of the Braden Scale to accurately predict pressure injury has been studied extensively across settings including intensive care, acute care, multisite, acute tertiary care, Veterans Administration

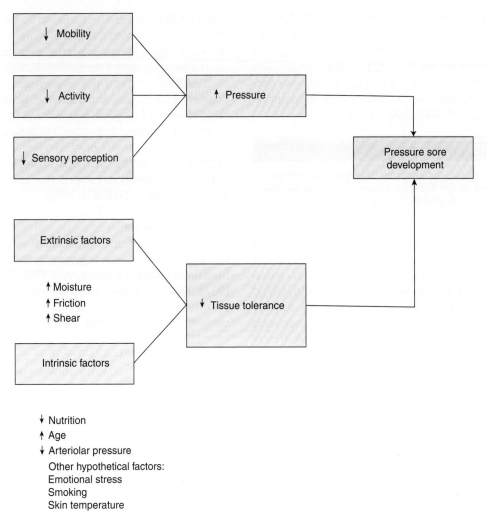

FIGURE 21-1. Braden Scale Schema. (Reprinted from Braden, B. (1987). A conceptual schema for the study of the etiology of pressure sores. *Rehabilitation Nursing, 12*(1), 9, with permission of the Association of Rehabilitation Nurses. Copyright © 1987 by the Association of Rehabilitation Nurses.)

Medical Center (VAMC), skilled rehabilitation, home care, and nursing home settings (Bergstrom et al., 1987a, 1987b, 1995, 1998; Berquist & Frantz, 2001; Braden & Bergstrom, 1987; 1994). It has also been tested among diverse ethnic groups, including black and white subjects, ethnic minorities, black and Latino/Hispanic elders, and Asian patients, including those in rehabilitation hospitals and acute care hospitals in China (Bergstrom & Braden, 2002; Kwong et al., 2005; Lyder, 1996; Lyder et al., 1999; Pang & Wong, 1998).

When compared to other risk assessment tools, the Braden Scale has demonstrated high ratings for reliability related to total score, ranging from 0.72 to 0.95. Reliability refers to the capacity of a measuring device to produce consistent measures when performed by different reviewers (Polit & Beck, 2011). Support for reliability of the Braden Scale as a screening tool in clinical practice is based on five studies, the majority in nursing home settings (EPUAP/NPIAP/PPPIA, 2019).

Common Errors in Use of Braden Scale

Support for the reliability of the Braden Scale when used by RNs in acute care settings is sparse. Magnan and Maklebust (2008) conducted a quasi-experimental study of staff RNs' use of the Braden Scale in three different hospital systems in Michigan. The results showed the gravity of the number and type of measurement errors on pressure injury risk assessments made by nurses using the Braden Scale in clinical practice. Results of the study suggest that training in proper use of the Braden Scale is needed and that correct use of the scale should be evaluated periodically.

Clinical nurse specialists, wound care nurses, and other wound team members report staff nurses make errors and misapplications of the Braden Scale in daily clinical practice (Kalisch et al., 2009). Staff must be reminded to avoid shortcuts such as (1) copying the score obtained by a previous caregiver, (2) using the same score every day, (3) choosing a subscale score without comparing the

BRADEN SCALE FOR PREDICTING PRESSURE SORE RISK

Patient's Name _____ Evaluator's Name _____ Date of Assessment

SENSORY PERCEPTION Ability to respond meaningfully to pressure-related discomfort	1. Completely Limited Unresponsive (does not moan, flinch, or grasp) to painful stimuli, due to diminished level of consciousness or sedation, OR limited ability to feel pain over most of body.	2. Very Limited Responds only to painful stimuli. Cannot communicate discomfort except by moaning or restlessness, OR has a sensory impairment which limits the ability to feel pain or discomfort over ½ of body.	3. Slightly Limited Responds to verbal commands but cannot always communicate discomfort or the need to be turned, OR has some sensory impairment which limits ability to feel pain or discomfort in one or two extremities.	4. No Impairment Responds to verbal commands. Has no sensory deficit which would limit ability to feel or voice pain or discomfort.				
MOISTURE Degree to which skin is exposed to moisture	1. Constantly Moist Skin is kept moist almost constantly by perspiration, urine, etc. Dampness is detected every time patient is moved or turned.	2. Very Moist Skin is often but not always moist. Linen must be changed at least once a shift.	3. Occasionally Moist Skin is occasionally moist, requiring an extra linen change approximately once a day.	4. Rarely Moist Skin is usually dry; linen only requires changing at routine intervals.				
ACTIVITY Degree of physical activity	1. Bedfast Confined to bed.	2. Chairfast Ability to walk severely limited or non-existent. Cannot bear own weight and/or must be assisted into chair or wheelchair.	3. Walks Occasionally Walks occasionally during day, but for very short distances, with or without assistance. Spends majority of each shift in bed or chair.	4. Walks Frequently Walks outside room at least twice a day and inside room at least once every 2 hours during waking hours.				
MOBILITY Ability to change and control body position	1. Completely Immobile Does not make even slight changes in body or extremity position without assistance.	2. Very Limited Makes occasional slight changes in body or extremity position but unable to make frequent or significant changes independently.	3. Slightly Limited Makes frequent though slight changes in body or extremity position independently.	4. No Limitations Makes major and frequent changes in position without changes.				
NUTRITION Usual food intake pattern	1. Very Poor Never eats a complete meal. Rarely eats more than 1/3 of any food offered. Eats two servings or less of protein (meat or dairy products) per day. Takes fluids poorly. Does not take a liquid dietary supplement, OR is NPO and/or maintained on clear liquids or IV for more than 5 days.	2. Probably Inadequate Rarely eats a complete meal and generally eats only about ½ of any food offered. Protein intake includes only three servings of meat or dairy products per day. Occasionally will take a dietary supplement OR receives less than optimum amount of liquid diet or tube feeding.	3. Adequate Eats over half of most meals. Eats a total of four servings of protein (meat, dairy products) each day. Occasionally will refuse a meal, but will usually take a supplement when offered, OR is on a tube feeding or TPN regimen, which probably meets most of nutritional needs.	4. Excellent Eats most of every meal. Never refuses a meal. Usually eats a total of four or more servings of meat and dairy products. Occasionally eats between meals. Does not require supplementation.				
FRICTION & SHEAR	1. Problem Requires moderate to maximum assistance in moving. Complete lifting without sliding against sheets is impossible. Frequently slides down in bed or chair, requiring frequent repositioning with maximum assistance. Spasticity, contractures, or agitation leads to almost constant friction.	2. Potential Problem Moves feebly or requires minimum assistance. During a move, skin probably slides to some extent against sheets, chair, restraints, or other devices. Maintains relatively good position in chair or bed most of the time but occasionally slides down.	3. No Apparent Problem Moves in bed and in chair independently and has sufficient muscle strength to lift up completely during move. Maintains good position in bed or chair.					
				Total Score				

FIGURE 21-2. Braden Scale. (Copyright © Barbara Braden and Nancy Bergstrom, 1988. All rights reserved.)

clinical data to the defined subscale criteria, (4) choosing a numerical rating from the subscale without reading the criteria, (5) interpreting the criteria definition differently than intended (e.g., linen meaning full linen change, and not considering the incontinent underpad as linen and overscoring the moisture subscale score), and (6) choosing poor nutrition with 1 day of NPO status.

KEY POINT

Common errors in risk assessment include copying results obtained by a previous caregiver, underestimation of risk, and choosing a subscale score without comparing clinical data to the defined criteria.

Measures to Improve Accuracy in Risk Assessment

Strategies that may be used to improve accuracy in risk assessment include ongoing education for nurses using interactive teaching strategies and emphasizing that when in doubt, choose the lower score to assure

that at-risk patients are identified and protected. Posting the detailed descriptors in the subscales or having them available electronically in the electronic health record provides nurses with a reference when selecting the risk level. It is also helpful to conduct periodic spot audits of Braden Scale score accuracy by comparing Braden subscale scores with those of an expert validator. Some wound care nurses incorporate Braden Scale risk assessment and prevention planning into annual skills days by creating a patient scenario and having nurses complete a risk assessment and select prevention measures for the scenario patient. Data obtained from audits and skills fairs can be used to enhance ongoing staff education related to pressure injury prevention.

KEY POINT

One strategy for improving accuracy in risk assessment is to emphasize that when in doubt, choose the lower score to assure that at-risk patients are identified and protected. Another is to teach risk assessment using interactive strategies.

Pediatric Risk Assessment

Specialized risk assessment tools have been developed that focus on a population or care setting.

Braden Q

The Braden Scale provided the conceptual basis for the Braden Q Scale, developed by Quigley and Curley (1996) to predict immobility-related pediatric pressure injury risk. The primary difference between the Braden Scale and the Braden Q Scale concerns the addition of the tissue perfusion and oxygenation subscale to the Braden Q Scale. The Braden Q Scale has two distinct limitations. First, the instrument did not address device-related pressure injuries. Second, initial validation testing excluded several pediatric cohorts, such as neonates younger than three weeks of age, children over age eight, and patients diagnosed with congenital heart disease (Quigley & Curley, 1996).

Braden QD

The Braden Q has continued to evolve while pediatric nurses made significant progress in preventing pressure-related injuries in vulnerable infants and children. Immobility-related pressure injuries have decreased significantly, and most hospital-acquired pressure injuries are currently associated with the use of medical devices creating pressure against the patient's skin or mucous membranes (Curley et al, 2018; Murray et al., 2013). Neonates are at higher risk than other populations, due to their undeveloped skin and lack of adipose tissue, both of which result in pressure injuries quickly evolving to full thickness. See Chapter 13 for additional information on neonatal and pediatric populations.

Identification of the need for medical device–related risk assessment resulted in the Braden Q risk assessment tool being modified. The revised tool, the Braden QD, provides pediatric nurses with a single instrument by which to assess both immobility-related and medical device–related pressure injury risk (Curley, 2018). The Braden QD eliminated the activity subscale and scoring for the remaining six subscales was simplified to a score of 0 to 2 (higher score indicating higher risk) (**Fig. 21-3**). A section on medical devices was added (up to eight devices are recorded) and repositionability of devices is scored. The Braden QD was validated in a multicenter prospective cohort study of 625 patients, ages preterm to 21 years, who were on bed rest for at least 24 hours with a medical device in place. At a cutoff score of 13, the Braden QD Scale was found to have a sensitivity of 86% and a specificity of 59%.

Neonatal Skin Risk Assessment Scale

In response to the limitations of the Braden Q Scale, the Neonatal Skin Risk Assessment Scale (NSRAS) was developed by Huffines and Logsdon (1997) specifically for the neonatal population. As with the Braden Q Scale, the NSRAS is based on the Braden Scale. The NSRAS is composed of six subscales: general physical condition, mental status, mobility, activity, nutrition, and moisture. Each subscale is scored from 1 to 4 points for a total of 6 through 24, with a higher score indicative of higher risk. It differs from the Braden and Braden Q scoring. The sensitivity and reliability of the NSRAS was piloted on 32 neonates. It was found to be reliable for the subscales of general physical condition, activity, and nutrition. Evidence for predictive validity was noted, with sensitivity at 83% and specificity at 81%. The NSRAS is a useful tool for predicting risk of developing skin breakdown among neonates (WOCN, 2016).

Risk Assessment in Specialized Populations

Examples of population-based tools include spinal cord injury (Spinal Cord Injury Pressure Ulcer Scale [SCI-PUS]), palliative care (Performance Palliation Scale [PPS]) (EPUAP/NPIAP/PPPIA, 2019; WOCN, 2016). Care setting-specific tools include perioperative risk assessment tools aimed to identify risks particular to the care setting itself. Both the Munro Pressure Ulcer Risk Assessment Scale for Perioperative Patients and Scott Triggers are used in the perioperative period (Munro, 2010; Park et al., 2019).

⬤ MANAGEMENT OF RISK FACTORS

LIMITATIONS IN MOBILITY

Immobility has been identified as the primary contributing factor to the development of pressure injury. It is a common issue with patients in all care settings. Patients may be sedated rendering them immobile, or may have a medical device preventing movement, or they may have a medical condition such as a stroke that makes movement difficult. Any of these cases would result in a low score in the mobility subscale of the Braden Scale.

Magnitude and Duration of Pressure

Research has established the damaging effects of pressure as being related to both the magnitude of the pressure and the duration of the pressure. This was demonstrated as early as 1959 in Kosiak's work with animals showing that pressure injuries occurred when tissues were exposed to high-pressure loads for short periods of time and when exposed to low-pressure loads for longer periods (Kosiak, 1959). Reswick and Rogers (1976) studied time–pressure relationships in human subjects with a spinal cord injury and found the same time–pressure relationship in humans that Kosiak observed in dogs. The Reswick-Rogers curve is shown in **Figure 21-4**. Evidence also indicates that intense pressure to a small surface area results in greater damage than the same pressure load applied to a larger surface area (Reswick & Rogers, 1976).

Insights into time–pressure relationships have established that off-loading pressure and limiting the time tissues are exposed to pressure are important components of pressure injury prevention. Individuals with normal

Braden QD Scale

Intensity and Duration of Pressure				Score
Mobility The ability to independently change & control body position	**0. No Limitation** Makes major and frequent changes in body or extremity position independently.	**1. Limited** Makes slight and infrequent changes in body or extremity position OR <u>unable</u> to reposition self independently (includes infants too young to roll over).	**2. Completely Immobile** Does not make even slight changes in body or extremity position independently.	
Sensory Perception The ability to respond meaningfully, in a <u>developmentally</u> appropriate way, to pressure-related discomfort	**0. No Impairment** Responsive **and** has no sensory deficits which limit ability to feel or communicate discomfort.	**1. Limited** Cannot always communicate pressure-related discomfort OR has some sensory deficits that limit ability to feel pressure-related discomfort.	**2. Completely Limited** Unresponsive due to diminished level of consciousness or sedation OR sensory deficits limit ability to feel pressure-related discomfort over most of body surface.	
Tolerance of the Skin and Supporting Structure				
Friction & Shear *Friction:* occurs when skin moves against support surfaces *Shear:* occurs when skin & adjacent bony surface slide across one another	**0. No Problem** Has sufficient strength to completely lift self up during a move. Maintains good body position in bed/chair at all times. Able to completely lift patient during a position change.	**1. Potential Problem** Requires **some** assistance in moving. Occasionally slides down in bed/chair, requiring repositioning. During repositioning, skin often slides against surface.	**2. Problem** Requires **full** assistance in moving. Frequently slides down and requires repositioning. Complete lifting without skin sliding against surface is impossible OR spasticity, contractures, itching or agitation leads to almost constant friction.	
Nutrition *Usual* diet for age – assess pattern over the most recent 3 consecutive days	**0. Adequate** Diet for age providing **adequate** calories & protein to support metabolism and growth.	**1. Limited** Diet for age providing **inadequate** calories OR **inadequate** protein to support metabolism and growth OR receiving supplemental nutrition any part of the day.	**2. Poor** Diet for age providing **inadequate** calories **and** protein to support metabolism and growth.	
Tissue Perfusion & Oxygenation	**0. Adequate** Normotensive for age, & oxygen saturation ≥ 95%, & normal hemoglobin, & capillary refill ≤ 2 seconds.	**1. Potential Problem** Normotensive for age **with** oxygen saturation <95%, OR hemoglobin <10 g/dl, OR capillary refill > 2 seconds.	**2. Compromised** Hypotensive for age OR hemodynamically unstable with position changes.	
Medical Devices				
Number of Medical Devices	Score 1 point for each medical device* up to 8 (Score 8 points maximum) *Any diagnostic or therapeutic device that is currently attached to or traverses the patient's skin or mucous membrane.*			
Repositionability/ Skin Protection	**0. No Medical Devices**	**1. Potential Problem** All medical devices can be repositioned OR the skin under each device is protected.	**2. Problem** Any one or more medical device(s) can**not** be repositioned OR the skin under each device is not protected.	
			Total (≥ 13 considered at risk)	

© Curley MAQ; Adapted with permission from B. Braden and N. Bergstrom, Braden Scale for Predicting Pressure Sore Risk, (1987)

FIGURE 21-3. Braden QD Scale. (© Curley MAQ: Adapted with permission from B. Braden and N. Bergstrom, Braden Scale for Predicting Pressure Sore Risk, 1987.)

sensation and no limitations in mobility will independently off-load pressures as often as needed to prevent tissue damage. For example, after sitting in one position for a time, the unimpaired person will sense discomfort in the buttocks and independently change position even a minor shift to off-load or redistribute pressure. This off-loading or redistribution occurs during sleep in unimpaired individuals. Those with limited mobility may sense

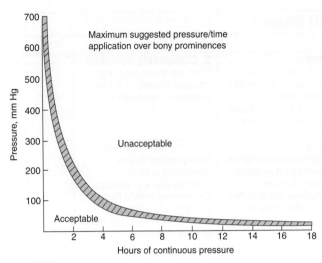

FIGURE 21-4. Reswick-Rogers Curve.

discomfort but will need assistance because they may not have the ability to off-load pressure independently. Those with limited sensation may not notice the discomfort and will not move independently.

KEY POINT

Reducing the intensity of pressure through use of off-loading support surfaces and reducing the duration of pressure through repositioning are important strategies in pressure injury prevention.

Limitations in Mobility, Activity, and Sensory Perception

Interventions to address the mobility and activity subscale categories are very similar. When a patient has sensory perception limitations, he or she also often has limitations in mobility and activity. Limited and impaired mobility increases the potential for exposure of tissues to prolonged and intense pressure (WOCN, 2016). The prevalence of more severe injuries (stage 3, stage 4, and unstageable) is greater among those who are completely immobile (Lahmann & Kottner, 2011).

Preventive Measures for Limited Mobility, Activity, and Sensory Perception

Individuals on bed rest are at higher risk for pressure injury. Implementation of an early mobilization program that increases activity and mobility results in positive patient outcomes. It is important to use appropriate mobilization techniques to avoid increased shear forces (EPUAP/NPIAP/PPPIA, 2019). PI prevention for persons with limited mobility, activity, and sensory perception must focus on proactively limiting the magnitude of pressure (load) over bony prominences and limiting the duration (length of time) the tissue is exposed to pressure.

Routine Repositioning and Early Mobility

Repositioning (e.g., turning) patients is a well-recognized and long-standing nursing intervention and is a consistent element of evidence-based PI prevention guidelines in the United States, Europe, and Australia (EPUAP/NPIAP/PPPIA, 2019). Repositioning is commonly understood as manually moving the patient into another position to alleviate pressure on one part of the body and redistribute pressure to another body part. The ideal schedule for repositioning should be individualized to the patient, considering other risk factors and the surface on which he or she is resting. Many organizations support a range of repositioning every 2 to 4 hours.

The bony prominence of the neonate and pediatric patient at highest risk for PI is the occiput, due to its comparatively large bony surface and weight. Off-loading the head is an important component of a PI prevention plan for the immobile infant and child. Refer to Chapter 13 for additional information regarding pediatric PI risk.

The sacrum is the bony prominence of an adult at highest risk for PI. Pressure to the sacral area is present while supine in bed, reclining in a chair or on a stretcher. Consideration should be given to the repositioning schedule your facility follows. Using the clock method (left, supine, right, supine, etc. every 2 hours) results in the bedridden patient being supine 12 hours a day, right 6 hours a day, and left 6 hours a day. It is reasonable to explore implementing a repositioning schedule, especially in the ICU, of left to right positioning, avoiding supine position except during meals. Meta-analysis by Gillespie et al. (2014) noted evidence supporting the use of repositioning to prevent pressure injuries is low. This does not mean that repositioning is ineffective or unnecessary (Gillespie et al., 2014). A PI prevention program that does not include a repositioning schedule would be deemed deficient based on current best practice prevention guidelines (EPUAP/NPIAP/PPPIA, 2019).

Pressure intensity and the amount of time body tissues are exposed to pressure work together to cause PIs. The twofold aim of repositioning should be to (1) reduce or relieve pressure at the interface between bony prominences and the support surface or medical device and skin and (2) limit the amount of time the tissues are exposed to pressure. Early best practice guidelines commonly recommended repositioning at least every 2 hours for bedridden patients and hourly for chair-bound/wheelchair patients (McInnes et al., 2015). Advances in technology have led to improved support surfaces that redistribute body weight more evenly (Hermans et al., 2014; Moore et al., 2014). Researchers are attempting to determine whether the frequency of repositioning of bedridden patients might be extended from every 2 hours to every 3 or 4 hours (without adverse effect), depending upon the type of support surface being used.

In a multisite randomized clinical trial (RCT) involving nursing home patients ($N = 942$) in the United States and Canada, Bergstrom and colleagues (2013) compared the effects of repositioning at 2-, 3-, and 4-hour intervals on the incidence of PIs. In this study (the TURN study), all nursing homes were using high-density foam mattresses, and patients were admitted to the study if their age was 65 years or older and at moderate (Braden score = 13 or 14) or high (Braden score = 10 to 12) risk for developing PIs. Findings showed an overall low incidence (2% of participants) of superficial PIs, stage 1 or stage 2, and no statistically significant difference in the incidence of PIs observed by risk category or turning schedule. When nursing home patients are placed on high-density foam mattresses, turning at 3- and 4-hour intervals seems to be as effective in preventing pressure injuries as turning every 2 hours. The study protocol called for consistent and careful documentation every time the patient was repositioned. This documentation included position, checks for incontinence, skin condition, and skin care provided. The authors speculated that the level of documentation required may have acted as an effective reminder for the caregivers, adding a dimension of safety and contributing to the low incidence of pressure injuries observed (Bergstrom et al., 2013). In a similar study involving nursing home patients ($N = 235$) placed on a viscoelastic foam (7 cm) mattress, patients in the experimental group were repositioned at varying intervals (2 hours lateral, then 4 hours supine, and then 2 hours lateral), whereas patients in the control group were repositioned at equal intervals (4 hours lateral, then 4 hours supine, and then 4 hours lateral) (Vanderwee et al., 2007). Patients in both the experimental and control group developed pressure injuries, but between the two groups, there was no statistically significant difference in the incidence, severity, or time to development of pressure injuries (Vanderwee et al., 2007; WOCN, 2016).

In another well-designed study of nursing home patients, Defloor and colleagues (2004) reported a low incidence (3%) of stage 2 and higher PIs among patients placed on viscoelastic foam mattresses and turned every 4 hours, as compared to incidence ranging from 14.3% to 24.1% among patients on a standard nursing home mattress who were turned every 2, 3, and 6 hours.

The results of these studies question the value of more frequent turning (e.g., every 2 hours) and suggest that repositioning at 4-hour intervals is an effective preventative intervention when nursing home patients are placed on a pressure redistribution foam mattress. Findings may be generalizable for patients in other care settings. Published research is currently lacking to support changing every 2 hour routine repositioning schedules for the hospitalized patient (WOCN, 2016).

While research may help to define general parameters for turning and repositioning intervals, all preventive care must be tailored to the specific needs of individuals and their unique responses to the care provided. Blanchable, reactive hyperemia is an expected response when tissue is exposed to pressure loads that compromise arteriolar flow to the tissues (Maklebust & Sieggreen, 1996). This normal reactive hyperemia should resolve within 20 to 30 minutes of off-loading pressure with no residual effects. Evidence of nonblanchable erythema that persists following off-loading is a stage 1 pressure injury (Maklebust & Sieggreen, 1996) and an indication that the intervals between repositioning need to be shortened. One method to confirm the area of erythema is nonblanchable is to press one finger to the area of erythema for 3 seconds and release. Upon release of the pressure, healthy skin should immediately return to native skin color. Reminder strategies should be implemented for repositioning to promote adherence (EPUAP/NPIAP/PPIAP, 2019). Turning clocks placed in the patient's room at the head of the bed are helpful reminders for repositioning (Magnan & Maklebust, 2009; Maklebust & Sieggreen, 1996) and may be of benefit whenever a patient's repositioning interval varies from the agency's routine repositioning intervals. Another repositioning reminder is continuous bedside pressure mapping. This commercially available device provides a visual cue to guide repositioning and monitors patient movement. (Gunningberg, et al., 2017; Hultin et al., 2017).

Maintaining head of bed elevation as low as possible, at or below 30 degrees, minimizes soft tissue deformity (EPUAP/NPIAP/PPPIA, 2019). Slumped positions increase pressure and shear on the coccyx and sacrum and should be avoided. Elevating the head of the bed may be medically necessary to facilitate breathing and prevent aspiration and ventilator-associated pneumonia (Krapfl et al., 2017). Positioning patients to prevent sliding down in bed is essential to shear prevention. Flexing the knees and positioning pillows under the arms may help to prevent, or at least reduce, sliding (EPUAP/NPIAP/PPPIAP, 2019).

Repositioning for Hemodynamically Unstable Patients

Repositioning of critically ill and hemodynamically unstable patients is another area of concern. Critical care nurses have reported unstable vital signs and low levels of respiratory and energy reserves as reasons for not repositioning patients (Winkleman & Peereboom, 2010). Decisions made about repositioning critically ill patients often are based on the nurse's perception of what might happen rather than on a test of the patient's tolerance to repositioning (Brindle et al., 2013). Experts recommend that most critically ill patients, even those receiving vasoactive medications, undergo repositioning trials to evaluate their tolerance to repositioning (Brindle et al., 2013; Dammeyer et al., 2013; Vollman, 2012). The mobility restriction may also be related to concern of dislodging a medical device, for example extracorporeal membrane oxygenation (ECMO) cannula in the neck more than hemodynamic instability.

Repositioning hemodynamically unstable patients does frequently result in changes in BP and heart rate. Research has shown that these changes are usually transient, and most patients return to baseline within 5 minutes of completing the turn (Winslow et al., 1995). Experts suggest that critically ill patients be monitored for time to recovery to baseline hemodynamic parameters. Timely recovery is a better indicator of tolerance to repositioning than the immediate changes seen. The patient's ability to tolerate a position change should not be assessed until 5 to 10 minutes after repositioning (Vollman, 2012).

Repositioning is important for hemodynamically unstable patients, and slow small shifts may be tolerated even when major repositioning is not tolerated. Recovery to baseline within 10 minutes should be used as the measure of tolerance to repositioning.

KEY POINT

Current evidence suggests that repositioning is important for hemodynamically unstable patients and that slow small shifts may be tolerated when major repositioning is not tolerated. Recovery to baseline within 10 minutes should be used as the measure of tolerance to repositioning.

Repositioning even hemodynamically unstable patients should be attempted shortly after admission to the ICU. Vollman (2012) has noted that orthostatic tolerance to repositioning deteriorates quickly with immobility and failure to reposition. The longer the patient is left immobile in a supine position, the more apt he or she is to develop what has been referred to as gravitational disequilibrium. Gravitational disequilibrium inhibits the patient's ability to adapt to position changes. This situation can be aggravated by turning the patient too rapidly. Turning the critically ill patient slowly and in small increments gives the body time to adjust to the position change.

Critically ill patients appear to tolerate the right lateral tilt position better than the left lateral position (Vollman, 2012). While the reasons for this difference are not clear, experts recommend beginning with a supine to right lateral tilt and incorporating the left lateral position as repositioning tolerance improves (Bush et al., 2015; Powers, 2016; Vollman, 2012). Using positioning wedges may help to achieve small incremental lateral position changes of 15 degrees before moving the patient to the 30-degree lateral position. Repositioning from the 30-degree lateral position to the supine position may require a similar incremental approach.

There is no consensus regarding contraindications to repositioning the critically ill patient. It has been suggested that the presence of life-threatening arrhythmias, active fluid resuscitation to maintain systemic blood pressure, and active hemorrhage may render the patient too unstable to tolerate turning. Unstable spinal fractures and fractures of the pelvis are also considered contraindications to turning (Brindle et al., 2013; Bush et al., 2015; Krapfl et al., 2017). For patients who fail repositioning trials due to hemodynamic instability, the use of a lateral rotation bed should be considered. This surface should not be considered an alternative to repositioning because the trunk is minimally affected by a lateral rotation bed. Repositioning should be implemented as soon as possible.

There are occasions when critically ill patients must be placed in a prone position for an extended period, up to 20 hours with acute respiratory distress syndrome (ARDS). Indications for prone positioning include poor oxygenation, mobilization of secretions, and pressure relief (Gattinoni et al., 2001; Vollman, 2004). These patients should be assessed for evidence of facial injuries as well as injuries in other areas of the body (e.g., breast region, knees, toes, penis, clavicles, anterior iliac crests, symphysis pubis) that are usually considered low risk or no risk for PI development (EPUAP/NPIAP/PPPIA, 2019). Special attention is required under and around medical devices on the anterior body surface. Small, incremental lateral position changes using positioning wedges can be implemented for the prone patient. Use of a fluidized positioner under the chest can help to raise the head off the mattress, resulting in less pressure on tube/skin interface from feeding and respiratory tubing. Best practice for head positioning when an intubated patient is prone in the ICU involves a minor repositioning of the head hourly and turning the head side to side every 2 hours (Powers et al., 2016). NPIAP (2020) developed a best practice document for preventing pressure injury when using the prone position. It is available at https://cdn.ymaws.com/npiap.com/resource/resmgr/online_store/posters/npiap_pip_tips_-_proning_202.pdf (NPIAP, 2020).

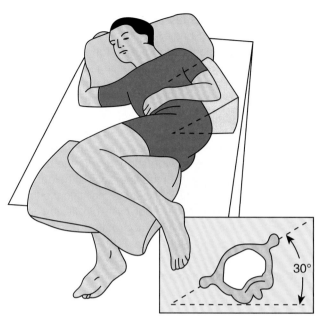

FIGURE 21-5. 30-Degree Tilt For Side-Lying Position.

Side-Lying Tilt

To avoid pressure on the trochanters, patients at risk for pressure injuries should not be placed in a 90-degree lateral position (EPUAP/NPIAP/PPPIA, 2019; WOCN, 2016). Instead, the 30-degree lateral tilt position is recommended for lateral positioning (**Fig. 21-5**). When using the 30-degree lateral tilt position, it is prudent to ensure the correct position has been achieved by observing the angle of the hips in relation to the long axis of the bed. Pillows or wedges can be used to help maintain the desired position. Whenever patients are positioned laterally, separating opposing bony prominences such as the knees and ankles with a pillow is recommended. Any positioning device behind the individual should not be positioned directly over the coccyx/sacrum.

KEY POINT

A 30-degree lateral tilt is recommended for the side-lying position. This position protects both the trochanter and the sacrococcygeal area.

Repositioning Individuals in the Operating Room

The increased risk of pressure injuries in individuals undergoing surgery suggests that additional diligence in positioning this population is indicated. It is usually not possible to reduce the length of surgery or reposition the patient in the operating room once surgery has started. Positioning the individual to distribute pressure over a larger surface area and protecting bony prominences are key strategies in preventing operating room–acquired pressure injuries (Goudas & Bruni, 2019).

A pressure injury prevention plan in the OR includes (1) positioning the individual preoperatively and postoperatively in a position different than the operative position (e.g., side-lying if supine on the OR), (2) avoiding positioning an individual on a medical device, (3) when possible, repositioning during surgery. This need not be full body movement, (4) using pressure redistribution surfaces and padding to assist in positioning (e.g., facial and chest pads when positioned prone), (5) consideration of the use of prophylactic dressings to bony prominences, and (6) off-loading heel from OR table that does not provide pressure to the Achilles tendon (Engels et al., 2016; EPUAP/NPIAP/PPPIA, 2019; Riemenschneider, 2018; Wang et al., 2018).

Support Surfaces in Bed

Support surfaces play an important role in both the prevention and the treatment of pressure injuries (Thompson et al., 2009; WOCN, 2016). The National Pressure Injury Advisory Panel (NPIAP) defines support surface as a specialized device for pressure redistribution designed for management of tissue loads, microclimate, and/or other therapeutic functions (i.e., any mattresses, integrated bed system, mattress replacement, overlay or seat cushion, or seat cushion overlay) (NPIAP, 2019).

When used appropriately, support surfaces help prevent pressure injuries by cushioning vulnerable parts of the body, redistributing body weight, and managing microclimate. They should be used in conjunction with other preventive measures including repositioning, moisture management, nutritional support, and protection from friction and shear (McNichol et al., 2015; Thompson et al., 2008; WOCN, 2016). The use of a support surface alone will not prevent pressure injury. As a part of PI prevention best practice bundle, the wound care nurse should understand the different support surfaces available in the institution and the process to obtain alternate surfaces as needed. Chapter 22 provides in-depth information regarding off-loading support surfaces for the chair and bed.

Support Surfaces in the Chair

Seating surfaces and cushions constitute a special class of support surfaces. They are primarily static and made of foam, gel, air, or some combination. Seating surfaces play an important role in preventing sitting-induced pressure injuries especially for individuals who are wheelchair bound. When selecting a seating support surface, consideration should be given to the (1) individual's body size and habitus, (2) effects of posture and deformity on pressure distribution, and (3) patient's mobility and lifestyle needs (EPUAP/NPIAP/PPPIA, 2019).

A seating surface for long-term use by wheelchair-bound individuals (e.g., those with spinal cord injury) must address patient comfort, pressure relief, microclimate, heat accumulation and loss, and the patient's postural stability (Brienza & Geyer, 2000). It is best if the seating surface and the wheelchair are ordered at the same time, and selection should be done by a seating specialist who can use real-time pressure mapping to guide decision making about seat cushion selection (Bain & Ferguson-Pell, 2002). See Chapter 16 for further discussion regarding options and considerations for selection of wheelchair cushions for spinal cord–injured individuals.

Patients in long term care (LTC) are particularly vulnerable to pressure injuries when in a seated position because they often spend long hours seated or confined to a wheelchair. The risk increases considerably if mobility is impaired and they are unable to reposition themselves independently (Shaw & Taylor, 1991). Characteristics of the patient, the wheelchair, and the support surface work together to influence the development of PI in seated position.

Obese individuals are not always more vulnerable to sitting-induced PIs. Obese individuals typically have more fat and muscle padding, which provides a larger seating surface over which the weight of the upper body can be distributed. In comparison, emaciated individuals

with flaccid gluteal tissues are at greater risk for PIs in the seated position (Sprigle, 2000). The combination of decreased padding and poor muscle tone contributes to poor weight distribution over the seating surface. Tissues over the ischial tuberosities are at greater risk for PI. Positioning the individual to distribute weight evenly across the seating surface is important for preventing PIs. Even when a pressure-redistribution cushion is used, care should be taken to ensure that (1) the depth of the chair seat (back to front) is sufficient to provide support from the buttocks to the back of the knees, (2) the floor-to-seat height (from floor-to-seating surface) is sufficient to maintain the thighs in a position parallel to the floor (with hip flexion at 90 degrees), and (3) the pelvis is not rotated posteriorly or obliquely (Maklebust & Sieggreen, 2001) (**Fig. 21-6**).

Protecting the Heels from PI

The heel is one of the two most common anatomical sites for PI. Older individuals, patients in critical care, children, and neonates are at particularly high risk for heel

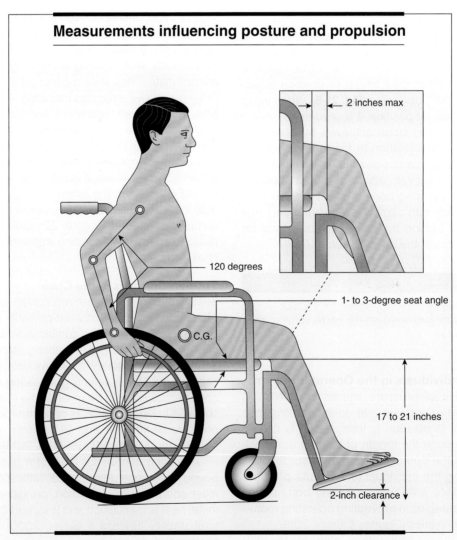

Measurements influencing posture and propulsion

2 inches max

120 degrees

1- to 3-degree seat angle

C.G.

17 to 21 inches

2-inch clearance

FIGURE 21-6. Proper Position for Wheelchair Seating.

PI. The prevalence of heel PI among individuals in acute care has been reported to be between 21% and 46% (Tubaishat et al., 2018). The reduction of pressure and shear at the heel is an important consideration in clinical practice. Because the heel is covered with a small volume of subcutaneous tissue, mechanical loads are transmitted directly to the bone. Heels have a small surface area and a heavy bony structure resulting in high compressive force. Redistributing the load off the heel is challenging. Particular attention should be paid to assessment of the heel for PI especially in individuals who are medically complex (EPUAP/NPIAP/PPPIA, 2019).

Heel protection should be a high priority for all at-risk patients. Heels should be elevated using a specifically designed heel suspension device or a pillow or foam cushion. The heels should be off-loaded completely in such a way as to distribute the weight of the leg along the calf without placing pressure on the Achilles tendon and the popliteal vein. This is often referred to as floating. Determining whether to implement placement of pillows under the calf or using an off-loading boot depends on whether the patient has lateral foot rotation and whether the position can be maintained. Prolonged lateral foot rotation in bed can result in pudendal nerve damage. Use of an off-loading boot should be considered if the patient has a prolonged bed rest restriction. Staff should ensure that the device effectively elevates the heel off the bed each time the patient is repositioned (EPUAP/NPIAP/PPPIA, 2019; WOCN, 2016).

Prophylactic dressings are dressings that are applied to intact skin over a pressure point with the aim of preventing a PI. Use of prophylactic dressings should be an adjunct to rather than a replacement for heel elevation. Different types of prophylactic dressings are available, including those designed specifically for application to the heel. Dressings should be selected based on their ability to manage microclimate, ease of application and removal, access required to assess the skin, and correct size (EPUAP/NPIAP/PPPIA, 2019; WOCN, 2016).

KEY POINT

Heels are the second most common site for PI development. Heel protection must be a high priority.

Foam Positioning Wedges

Pressure reduction occurred in the sacral region with the pillow and wedge systems. This reduction resulted in increased pressures in the posterolateral regions of the buttocks and thighs.

Positioning devices are often used to facilitate repositioning in critical care. In many facilities, pillows are positioned behind the patient to maintain the lateral recumbent position. Pillows come in various sizes, shapes, and densities, with various moisture-proof coverings. They tend to flatten when used over time. Powers

(2016) examined 60 participants and demonstrated that a 20-degree turn was achieved when pillows were used, but this angle declined to an average of 15 degrees when reassessed after 1 hour. This study did not measure interface pressures, and it is unknown if effective sacral off-loading occurred with only a 15- to 20-degree tilt. Thirty-degree wedges were also evaluated for repositioning. Results showed that a 30-degree turn was consistently achieved and maintained for 1 hour when a wedge was employed.

Peterson and colleagues (2010) reported that sacral and buttock interface pressures were increased in area and degree with the use of a wedge. This finding supports the importance of proper wedge placement. Bush and colleagues (2015) reported that use of foam wedges was the most effective in reducing pressures on the sacral area; however, higher pressures were identified on the buttock and thigh with wedge use.

MINIMIZE EXPOSURE TO FRICTION AND SHEAR

An early definition of PI included both friction and shear as contributing to PI. It was later determined that friction injuries to the superficial layers of the skin were not PIs (Brienza et al., 2015). The NPIAP modified the definition of PI and removed friction from the definition of PI. In the 2019 International Guideline, friction is defined as continuous or repetitive movement, rubbing or sliding of a material … and can result in redness, inflammation or a lesion referred to as a friction blister. These blisters are not considered to be PIs (EPUAP/NPIAP/PPPIA, 2019).

There are two components to shear: shear stress and shear strain. Shear stress is defined as the force per unit area exerted parallel to the perpendicular plane of interest. Shear strain is defined as the distortion or deformation of tissue as a result of shear stress (EPUAP/NPIAP/PPPIA, 2019). In contrast, when normal forces (body weight) and shear forces are generated between the body and the support surface, the loaded soft tissues distort and deform due to the mechanical load and strain. Strain can cause either superficial damage, as occurs with skin tears, or deeper damage, as occurs with pressure injuries. Shear strain occurs when the subcutaneous tissue shears against the dermal layer, creating distortion of the blood vessels. This type of shear occurs when the patient slides down in the bed or chair or when the patient is pulled up in bed without the use of safe patient handling equipment or low-friction coefficient linens. (See Chapters 17 and 20 for additional information).

Friction

Friction occurs when skin rubs against an external surface. Many patient care situations may cause friction. For example, friction occurs when a patent is pulled or dragged up in bed rather than lifted. Friction may also occur when an orthotic device rubs against the skin (Antokal et al., 2012). Potential for a friction injury exists during the placement and removal of bedpans, especially if care is not taken to ensure that the surface of the bedpan is not dragged across the skin. Agitated patients, and those who are resistant to care, may be unduly exposed to friction as a result of repetitive and resistive movement. Abrasive fabrics used in washcloths and vigorous rubbing during cleansing care are additional sources of friction.

Some body locations and body types are more vulnerable to the mechanical forces of friction. Berke (2015) summarized results of skin injuries in 45 patients that were primarily related to friction. The injuries occurred over the fleshy parts of the buttocks and posterior proximal thighs secondary to prolonged semirecumbent positioning (sliding, slumping, or slouching) in a bed or reclining chair. They often occurred in conjunction with impaired mobility that resulted in dragging of the buttocks or posterior thigh skin over a seat surface during transfers. The resulting lesions were usually lichenified with skin ridging or skin surface deformation. Shallow, full-thickness ulcerations were frequently observed, but they were limited to the dermis and none progressed to deeper ulceration. None of these areas of damage occurred over palpable bony prominences. Moisture was a factor for most of the patients and likely contributed to the skin damage (Berke, 2015).

The heels and elbows are particularly vulnerable to friction (Hanson et al., 2010). It is problematic for patients who use their elbows and heels to reposition themselves in bed. Wearing long sleeves on the arms and socks on the feet can help to minimize the frictional forces on these areas, as can protective dressings such as a transparent film dressings or thin silicone foam dressing. Obesity may increase the risk of friction damage. Research suggests that low scores on the friction and shear subscale of the Braden Scale are more highly associated with PI development among obese patients (BMI $\geq$ 30) than among patients with a BMI < 30 (Swanson et al., 2011). This does not mean that friction is not a problem for thin patients. Laboratory research suggests that among very thin patients with protruding bony prominences, the magnitude of the mechanical forces of friction can be quite severe and damaging, especially over protruding bony prominences (Ohura, 2013).

KEY POINT

There is evidence to support the use of silicone foam dressings as one component of a comprehensive prevention program.

Shear

Shear is defined as the force per unit area exerted parallel to the plane of interest (EPUAP/NPIAP/PPPIA, 2019; Maklebust, 1987). Shear is further defined as a mechanical force that acts on an area of the skin in a direction parallel to the body's surface. Shear is affected by the amount of pressure exerted, the coefficient of friction (CoF) between the materials contacting each other, and the extent to which the body contacts the support surface (Bergstrom et al., 1995). In the body, tissue consists of several layers or planes including the skin, adipose tissue, fascia, muscle, periosteum, tendon, and bone. Shearing forces cause one layer of tissue to move in relation to one or more of the other layers (Ohura, 2013), distorting the tissues involved (Nakagami et al., 2006). For example, when a patient is sitting in a less than fully upright position, the skin and surface tissues adhere to the surface of the bed while the skeleton and attached muscle slides downward inside the skin. It is the adipose tissue and perfusing blood vessels that are most often involved in this type of shear damage. Shear injuries may also occur when the patient is repositioned by being dragged up toward the head of the bed instead of being lifted completely off the bed surface. Using slide boards to transfer from bed to chair can cause shearing injuries in the deep body tissue, especially if the patient sticks to the sliding surface. Patients are advised not to use a slide board against their bare skin. If the patient is not wearing pants, a sheet or blanket or pillowcase can be used to cover the slide board before use to mitigate the tendency of the skin to adhere to the sliding surface (Maklebust, 1987). A shear injury will not be immediately visible at the skin surface because the damage occurs in deeper tissue planes. Individuals are at risk for shear damage when they slide down in bed or when they use sliding boards against the bare skin for transfers.

It is difficult to separate friction and shear for clinical research purposes. The Braden Scale (Braden & Bergstrom, 1987), used widely to assess the risk for pressure injury, combines the assessment of friction and shear into one subscale. A number of studies have demonstrated a significant relationship between low scores on the friction and shear subscale and pressure injury development. Management of friction and shear is an important component of a PIPP (Lahmann & Kottner, 2011; Lahmann et al., 2010, 2011).

Prevention Strategies

Strategies used to minimize the adverse effects of friction should be directed at lowering the CoF. One important strategy is to keep the skin dry. Wet skin is known to have a much higher CoF (Gerhardt et al., 2008; Zhong et al., 2006). An effective moisture management program can help minimize the friction problem. Use of protective dressings such as transparent film dressings, silicone foam dressings, and sheet hydrogel dressings may be of benefit. There is evidence to support the use of silicone foam dressings as one component of a comprehensive prevention program (Brindle & Wegelin, 2012; Kalowes et al., 2016; Santamaria et al., 2015).

Low-Friction Textiles

Silk-like low CoF textiles, such as bed linens and patient gowns, have received increased recognition as a significant contributor to skin health. Traditional bed linens can compromise the skin by increasing the friction coefficient and abrasive force and trapping heat and moisture against the skin, adversely affecting the skin's microclimate (Coladonato et al., 2012; Smith et al., 2013; Zhong et al., 2006, 2008). Tissue tolerance to friction and shear is reduced when moisture accumulates at the skin surface, common among febrile and diaphoretic patients (Pan & Sun, 2011; Zhong et al., 2006). Textiles that wick moisture away from the skin, and linens that reduce CoF forces can both contribute to pressure injury prevention and overall skin health.

Clinical research demonstrating the effectiveness of these special textiles in pressure injury prevention is growing. In a study involving 46 male nursing home residents, Twersky and colleagues (2012) reported significantly fewer pressure injuries among residents bedded on silk-like fabric sheets constructed from nylon and polyester yarns and using high-absorbency briefs compared to residents bedded on conventional cotton–polyester sheets (approximately 50% cotton and 50% polyester) and usual care adult incontinence brief. The number of new non–stage 1 injuries was significantly lower in the intervention group. Smith et al. (2013) used a retrospective research design to examine pressure injury incidence in an acute care setting before and after introducing hospital-wide use of synthetic silk–like fabric bed linens and patient gowns. The researchers reported the number of patients with hospital-acquired pressure injuries in the group using the silk-like fabric textiles was statistically significantly less for all pressure injuries than the number of patients with pressure injuries in the group using traditional cotton-blend linens. Results of these studies provide an early indication that using low CoF textiles for bedding and gowns may help prevent PIs. While further research is needed, especially among special needs groups (e.g., neonates, infants, paraplegic patients, obese patients), current evidence-based guidelines list use of therapeutic linens as an adjunct to PIPP (EPUAP/NPIAP/PPPIA, 2019).

Lifting and Positioning

Strategies used to minimize the adverse effects of shearing forces should be directed at minimizing the contralateral movement between tissue planes. Proper lifting, positioning, and repositioning techniques are the best defense against injury from shearing forces. The use of lift sheets, lateral assist devices, low CoF bed linen, and having sufficient help (i.e., manpower or electronic lift assistance) to actually lift not drag patients when moving them to the head of the bed is important (Nelson et al., 2003). When positioning in a semi-Fowler position, elevating the head of the bed to 30 degrees or less will minimize the risk for shearing that comes from sliding down in bed. Measures to reduce the CoF between the skin and the bed or chair surface will also reduce shear force. Strategies to keep the skin cool and dry, use of therapeutic linens, support surfaces with low-friction low-shear covers, and use of multilayered silicone foam protective dressings can help to reduce both superficial friction damage and shear damage.

MOISTURE

Moisture alone will not cause PI (Gray et al., 2011). Overhydrated skin is much more vulnerable to friction and shear damage and is also less able to distribute weight normally. Moisture contributes to pressure injury development by decreasing tissue tolerance (Braden & Bergstrom, 1987) and by increasing susceptibility to friction, pressure, and shear (EPUAP/NPIAP/PPIAP, 2019). A comprehensive PIPP should include measures to protect the skin from excessive exposure to moisture from urinary and fecal incontinence, wound exudate, perspiration, oropharyngeal secretions, and ostomy output (Gray et al., 2011).

Exposure to moisture from urine and stool can alter the skin pH, which compromises tissue tolerance (Gray et al., 2011). Tissue tolerance may be further compromised by exposure to fecal contents including fecal enzymes and intestinal flora (Beeckman et al., 2011; Gray et al., 2011). Strategies for moisture management should include strategies for managing urine, stool, perspiration, and wound exudate. Moisture barrier products include liquid skin protectant applied using spray, wipe, and applicator and moisture barrier ointments (e.g., dimethicone, petrolatum, zinc oxide). Aggressively rubbing skin that is at risk for pressure injury should be avoided (EPUAP/NPIAP/PPPIA, 2019).

See Chapters 18 and 19 for an in-depth discussion of prevention and management of MASD and IAD. Other strategies for protecting the skin against stool and urine include diverting devices such as urinary catheters and fecal containment devices. The risk of catheter-associated urinary tract infections makes the use of internal urinary catheters a less desirable strategy for moisture management. Alternatives such as frequent toileting, skin protection with barrier creams, and incontinence briefs or absorbent underpads that wick moisture away from the skin are preferred. For male patients, external containment devices including condom-type sheath catheters or pouches may be an effective way of diverting urine away from the skin, but care must be taken to apply and remove them properly. For female patients, an external collection device can be effective for containment but may restrict mobility. External fecal incontinence collectors (e.g., pouches) may be used to limit perianal skin exposure to stool. These devices may be challenging to apply and may require two caregivers to place the device properly (Scardillo & Aronovitch, 1999). Bowel management systems (BMS) may be used for containment and diversion of stool that is of liquid or semiliquid consistency. BMS use requires patient to have adequate sphincter tone. Irritation and erosion of the rectal mucosa with subsequent bleeding is a safety risk whenever any device is inserted into the rectum. Evidence indicates that intra-anal bowel management system provides a viable option for fecal incontinence management and these devices reduce incontinence-associated dermatitis and/or pressure injuries (Beeson et al., 2017). (See Chapter 19.)

Minimizing skin contact with effluent is a component of any moisture management program. The longer the skin is exposed to incontinence moisture and the contaminants in the effluent, the greater the risk of skin damage. Skin care for the individual who requires use of absorptive products must include frequent checks of briefs and absorbent underpads if the individual is unable to self-report an incontinent episode. Absorptive products should be left open under the patient to avoid an occlusive environment that results from closure of the brief around the patient. It is difficult to make recommendations regarding the timing and frequency of checks for incontinence. Clinical judgment must be used in making decisions, and this information should be communicated in handoff reports. The time from moisture exposure to skin damage cannot be predicted accurately but may be short, especially if the pH of the moisture is alkaline and proteolytic enzymes are present and active. Absorptive products should be composed of super absorbent polymers that wick moisture away from the skin, and a check and change program should be used in conjunction with the use of moisture barrier products (Gray et al., 2018). The importance of prompt cleaning after incontinence cannot be overstated. Patients who are both incontinent and immobile are at great risk for tissue damage and in need of conscientious nursing care.

Use of soap and water to cleanse the skin may be damaging to the skin. Soaps often have an alkaline pH that is not compatible with the normal acid mantle of the skin (Lambers et al., 2006). Alkaline products can dry the skin and alter the surface pH, making it more vulnerable to skin damage. Cleansers that are pH adjusted and no-rinse or soft disposable cloths are recommended for perineal cleansing. Impregnated cleansing wipes that also contain moisturizers and moisture barriers simplify the incontinence care regimen. Implementing an all-in-one product (i.e., cleanser, moisturizer, and barrier ointment) ensures barrier ointment application with each incontinence clean-up episode.

NUTRITION

Both inadequate nutritional intake and undernutrition are linked to the development of pressure injuries, pressure injury severity, and prolonged healing (EPUAP/NPIAP/PPPIA, 2019). Consensus supports nutritional management as an important aspect of a comprehensive care plan for pressure injury prevention and treatment (Carter & Lecko, 2018; Pinchofsky-Devin & Kaminski, 1986; Thomas, 2007). Nutrition should be addressed with every patient with a pressure injury because adequate calories, protein, fluids, vitamins, and minerals are required for healing. These nutrients are also required for health and tissue maintenance.

> **KEY POINT**
>
> Consensus supports nutritional management as an important aspect of a comprehensive care plan for pressure injury prevention and treatment.

While evidence regarding the specific impact of nutritional status on pressure injury risk is limited, consensus supports nutritional assessment and nutritional intervention as an important component of pressure injury prevention. To make sure that nutrition is not overlooked during hospitalization, a registered dietitian nutritionist (RDN) should be a member of the pressure injury prevention team. Nursing staff should be taught the meaning of each Braden scale rating criterion, and a house-wide Braden subscale trigger should be established for a nutrition consult (e.g., a nutrition subscale score <3 initiates a nutrition consult). For a more in-depth review of nutrition and nutritional needs of individuals with protein energy malnutrition (PEM), please see Chapter 7.

MEDICAL DEVICES

Medical device–related pressure injuries (MDRPIs) result from the use of medical devices designed and applied for diagnostic or therapeutic purposes. Nonmedical devices (e.g., bed clutter, furniture, and equipment) can also result in a pressure injury when they usually inadvertently remain in contact with skin and tissues (EPUAP/NPIAP/PPPIA, 2019). Common sources of MDRPI include respiratory devices (tracheostomy, CPAP mask), orthopedic devices (cervical collar, immobilizer, splint), repositioning devices (heel boots, transfer sling), tubing (urinary catheter, fecal management device, chest tube, nasogastric tube), and miscellaneous devices (restraints, bedpan). Schindler et al. (2011) analyzed risk factors for pressure injuries in intensive care units and trauma centers. The patients at highest risk for pressure injury were those on mechanical ventilation, BiPAP or CPAP, and ECMO.

In a survey of almost 100,000 individuals from 115 facilities in the United States and Canada, most MDRPIs were superficial (58% were Stage 1 or 2), 15% were deep-tissue PIs, and 22% were full-thickness PIs (Stage 3 or 4 or unstageable). The most common anatomic locations for MDRPIs were the ears (29%) and the feet (12%). The most common devices associated with MDRPIs were nasal oxygen tubes, 26%; other, 19%; cast/splints, 12%; and continuous positive airway pressure/bilevel positive airway pressure masks, 9%. Fifty-one percent of the MDRPIs occurred on the face or head (Kayser et al., 2018).

Key principles related to MDRPI prevention include (1) discontinuation of the device when no longer medically necessary, (2) appropriately sizing the device for the individual (i.e., condom catheter sheath), (3) application of the device according to manufacturer's instruction, (4) appropriate stabilization (i.e., without tension to tubes), (5) rotating or repositioning the device, when able, (6) replacement of a firm device (i.e., rigid field cervical collar) with a padded option, as soon as medically feasible, (7) use of a prophylactic dressing under a medical device to reduce risk of pressure injury, and (8) alternating between two devices that have different device/skin interfaces if appropriate and safe (i.e., oxygen delivery mask vs. nasal prongs) (EPUAP/NPIAP/PPPIA, 2019).

Critically ill patients and neonates are particularly vulnerable to MDRPIs. Wound care nurses need to be aware of the medical devices used in their institution, the correct application of these devices, expected points of contact with skin, areas of skin that need additional protection from pressure (e.g., edematous or fragile tissue under a medical device), and ways of cushioning the devices to redistribute pressure (Black et al., 2010).

KEY POINT

Medical device–related pressure injuries (MDRPIs) are common. Prevention includes proper fit, padding, retaping/repositioning when possible, and daily inspection.

 ## PATIENT AND FAMILY EDUCATION

Formal programs for patient and family education in PI prevention are important to reduce the incidence of PI in any care setting. Certain populations such as spinal cord injury (SCI) or stroke patients require intensive education as they will remain at high risk throughout their life. The education should help the patient and family understand the importance of repositioning and why it should not be delayed (AHRQ, 2014). Information provided should include risk factors, skin inspection, repositioning schedule, nutrition, and equipment needed such as support surface for bed and chair. A variety of teaching methods should be available to accommodate a variety of learning styles and literacy levels (Bryant & Nix, 2016). For more comprehensive information about patient education, see Chapter 6.

 ## PRESSURE INJURY PREVENTION PLAN

The assertion has been made that the best defense against pressure injuries is a well-developed, evidence-based prevention plan that is tailored to the individual's specific needs, conscientiously implemented, and revised as needed based on the patient's response. A pressure injury prevention plan should be based on knowledge and assessment data related to the following: clinical condition (current health state and comorbidities), current skin condition, overall pressure injury risk status and specific risk factors, and resource availability (human and environmental). **Table 21-1** provides an example of an individualized plan of care, based on the principles discussed this far.

PROGRAM MANAGEMENT

Creating a PIPP is a complex process that involves many areas of the organization. It takes a coordinated effort by many people with specialized knowledge and skill. An effective program requires the organization to develop an integrated program at the institutional level, across departments (e.g., transportation, radiology, OR, ED, PACU, etc.) and among multiple disciplines as well as at the unit level. The Agency for Health Care Research and Quality (AHRQ) published a toolkit in 2014 to guide hospitals in the development of PIPPs. This comprehensive toolkit is available online at: https://www.ahrq.gov/patient-safety/settings/hospital/resource/pressureulcer/tool/index.html (Berlowitz et al., 2014).

KEY POINT

The AHRQ published a toolkit to guide hospitals in the development of PIPP. Many of the principles and components addressed in the AHRQ toolkit can be adapted for use in other settings.

Wound care nurses are well positioned to establish or modify a PIPP. Jankowski and Nadzam (2011) con-

TABLE 21-1 EXAMPLE OF INDIVIDUALIZED PRESSURE INJURY PREVENTION PLAN

RISK FACTORS	DATA	INTERVENTION	SUPPORTIVE RATIONALE FROM EPUAP/NPIAP/PPPIA GUIDELINES (2019) AND THE LITERATURE
Limitations in mobility/activity	**PI Risk assessment data**: Braden mobility score = 1 Braden activity score 1 **Clinical presentation data**: BMI = 45; poor tolerance of lateral positioning, heart rate increase from 120 up to >200 with repositioning **Skin condition data**: Blanchable erythema right heel	Place the patient on a bariatric bed with alternating pressure low air loss mattress. Start progressive bed mobility by alternating between supine position and right lateral 15-degree tilt (monitor tolerance by assessing vital signs 10 minutes after lateral positioning). Reposition slowly to optimize adaptation to position change. Use a foam wedge (with special textile covering) to help maintain position. Reposition every 2 hours; post a turning clock at the head of the bed and adjust frequency of repositioning based upon tolerance. Apply protective boots to both feet. Remove protective boots daily for heel inspection.	Select a support surface that meets the individual's needs. Consider the individual's need for pressure redistribution based on the following factors: level of immobility and inactivity, need for microclimate control and shear reduction, size and weight of the patient (EPUAP/NPIAP/PPPIA, 2019, p. 156) Use an active support surface (overlay or mattress) for individuals at higher risk of pressure injury development when frequent manual reposition is not possible (EPUAP/NPIAP/PPPIA, 2019, p. 29). Consider the need for additional features such as ability to control moisture and temperature when selecting a support surface (EPUAP/NPIAP/PPPIA, 2019, p. 158). Consider selecting a support surface with enhanced pressure redistribution, shear reduction, and microclimate control for bariatric individuals (EPUAP/NPIAP/PPPIA, 2019, p. 158). Consider use of a high-specification reactive single layer foam mattress or overlay in preference to foam mattress without high-specification qualities for individuals at risk of developing a pressure injury (EPUAP/NPIAP/PPPIA, 2019, p. 160). Consider using a reactive air mattress or overlay for individuals at risk for developing pressure injuries (EPUAP/NPIAP/PPPIA, 2019, p. 163). Ensure the bed surface area is sufficiently wide to allow turning of the individual (EPUAP/NPIAP/PPPIA, 2019, p. 157). Use heel suspension devices or a pillow/foam cushion to ensure that the heels are free from the surface of the bed. Off-load the heel in such a way as to distribute the weight of the leg along the calf without placing pressure on the Achilles tendon and popliteal vein (EPUAP/NPIAP/PPPIA, 2019, p. 147). Remove the heel suspension device periodically to assess skin integrity (EPUAP/NPIAP/PPPIA, 2019, p. 146).
Skin exposure to moisture	**PI risk assessment data**: Braden moisture score = 1 **Clinical presentation**: Sweating profusely, frequent liquid diarrhea stools contaminated with *Clostridium difficile* **Skin condition data**: Perianal skin and skin on the buttocks intact but fire-engine red with blanchable erythema Skin under the breast and pannus intact, moist, and red	Change sheets as needed to minimize moisture contact with the skin. Insert FDA-approved internal bowel management system to divert stool away from the skin. Apply moisture barrier cream to the buttocks and perianal area t.i.d. and p.r.n. Use prepackaged, pH-adjusted wipes for cleaning as needed. Place wicking textile or surgical pads under the breasts and pannus to interrupt skin-to-skin contact and wick moisture away.	Develop and implement an individualized continence management program (EPUAP/NPIAP/PPPIA, 2019, p. 86). Protect the skin from exposure to excessive moisture with a barrier product in order to reduce the risk of pressure damage. Differentiate intertriginous dermatitis from category I/stage 1 and 2 pressure injuries (EPUAP/NPIAP/PPPIA, 2019, p. 88).

TABLE 21-1 EXAMPLE OF INDIVIDUALIZED PRESSURE INJURY PREVENTION PLAN (Continued)

RISK FACTORS	DATA	INTERVENTION	SUPPORTIVE RATIONALE FROM EPUAP/NPIAP/PPPIA GUIDELINES (2019) AND THE LITERATURE
Skin exposure to friction and shear	**PI risk assessment data**: Braden friction/shear score = 1 **Clinical presentation data**: BMI = 45; requires maximum assistance for positioning (3 to 4 care givers) **Skin condition data**: Elbows red and chafed	Use special textile sheets only. Use a lift sheet (special textile) to lift patient up toward the head of the bed. Use a lift team of 3 to 4 nursing personnel to move patient up in bed. Contact materials management regarding bariatric lift system. Apply transparent protective dressing to both elbows.	Avoid subjecting the skin to pressure and shear forces (p. 17). Consider using textiles with low friction coefficient rather than cotton or cotton-blend fabrics to reduce shear and friction (EPUAP/NPIAP/PPPIA, 2019, p. 88). Consider applying a polyurethane foam dressing to bony prominences for the prevention of pressure injuries in anatomical areas frequently subjected to friction and shear. When selecting a prophylactic dressing consider ability of the dressing to manage microclimate, ease of application and removal, ability to regularly assess the skin, anatomical location where the dressing will be applied, etc. (EPUAP/NPIAP/PPPIA, 2019, p. 89).
Nutrition	**PI risk assessment data**: Braden nutrition score = 1 **Clinical presentation data**: NPO since admission 4 days ago, increased metabolic demands from fever and agitation, fresh surgical wound	**Consult dietitian for nutritional screening.**	Screen nutrition status for each individual at risk of or with a pressure injury with each significant change of clinical condition (EPUAP/NPIAP/PPPIA, 2019, p. 95)

ducted a study involving four hospitals and identified commonly occurring gaps: (1) use of an abbreviated version of the Braden Scale scoring form that provides only the risk factor but does not include the rating criteria for the levels of risk, (2) failure to include Braden Scale risk score information during RN handoff reports, (3) lack of communication between RNs and nursing assistants, (4) pressure injury prevention equipment not readily available, and (5) physicians unaware of PIPP. Wound care nurses are well equipped to address each of these issues.

PIPPs should be evidence based. A variety of pressure injury prevention guidelines are available (e.g., EPUAP/NPIAP/PPPIA, WOCN). When prevention guidelines are implemented, the prevalence of pressure injuries decreases (Lahmann et al., 2010). Wound care nurses should use current guidelines when developing or updating a PIPP. They should determine which agency-wide prevention measures must be implemented immediately and which measures can be implemented later. These determinations should be based upon an evaluation of the organization's readiness for change, existing threats to patient safety, and the availability of human and environmental resources. It may not be feasible to initiate a complete prevention program all at once. Careful planning and feedback

will provide guidance in terms of program success and readiness for the next phase of implementation. Important indicators include the amount of resistance to the program, the amount of acceptance for the program, and the trend in the incidence of hospital-acquired pressure injuries.

MONITORING PRESSURE INJURY PREVALENCE AND INCIDENCE

An important component of a PIPP is to ensure the facility has a process for reporting a facility-acquired pressure injury (i.e., through the institution's safety reporting structure). An effective monitoring (i.e., surveillance) process is needed to provide periodic assessment of PI prevalence and incidence across the entire facility to ensure the self-reporting process is effective. The wound care nurse should monitor the degree to which best practices for PI prevention are being used throughout the facility. To understand the severity of a PI problem and the degree to which preventive care is being incorporated, information should be collected and analyzed by nursing as well as those responsible for quality care and performance improvement. This information includes the number and percentage of patients with pressure injuries and whether these injuries occurred before or after admission to the facility. Determining the number and percentage of patients with pressure injuries provides information about the frequency of pressure injury per unit. Determining the number and percentage of injuries that developed following admission provides important information regarding the effectiveness of the current PIPP. This information contributes to a pressure injury best practice program for the health care facility. The data need to be collected periodically (usually quarterly but may be monthly) to determine whether the PIPP is working or needs some improvement.

ROOT CAUSE ANALYSIS

Many facilities find it helpful to track facility-acquired PIs on an ongoing basis and to analyze the preventive care provided to identify improvements needed. The facility may require root cause analysis (RCA) on any facility-acquired PI. RCA is an important study method to help determine the exact cause of a serious problem (**Box 21-1** provides a sample form). It requires a team who were involved in the patient's care to review the case and ensure an appropriate pressure injury prevention plan of care was implemented. Documentation is reviewed and staff interviews are conducted to identify the underlying reason the pressure injury developed. Sample questions include the following: Was there a gap in appropriate risk assessment? Was a comprehensive skin assessment completed according to facility policy? Was the plan of care related to pressure injury prevention appropriate? The goal is not to place blame but to determine if any steps in the care process can be changed in order to avoid having the same problem recur. As changes in the process are made, they must be made clear to all who use the process. The NPIAP (2020) developed a tool kit for RCA, available online, that may prove helpful to establish or improve the current system. It may be purchased at https://npiap.com/page/RCAToolkit.

KEY POINT

Monitoring facility-acquired pressure injury incidence periodically and on an ongoing basis validates the effectiveness of the facility prevention plan.

CALCULATION OF PREVALENCE AND INCIDENCE RATES

Accurate interpretation and utilization of data regarding pressure injury rates requires a basic understanding of how these rates are determined and factors affecting accuracy. Both incidence and prevalence rates are measures of disease frequency. They each provide a perspective on the scope of the pressure injury problem in a given setting and at a given time. Prevalence is the proportion of all persons who have a pressure injury in a specific setting at a specific point in time (point prevalence), or period of time (period prevalence). Incidence

---

BOX 21-1 SAMPLE ROOT CAUSE ANALYSIS FORM

Root Cause Analysis
Unit:_____
Pressure Injury Site:_____
Date Injury First Identified:_____
Injury Stage When First Identified:_____
Risk Assessment Done on Admission? Yes (score)_____ No_____
Risk Assessment Done At Least Daily Following Admission? Yes, Consistently_____ Sometimes_____ No_____
Risk Assessment Scores Consistent with Pt Status as Documented in Record?
Yes_____ No (explain)_____
If patient found to be at risk:
Prevention Protocol Initiated Immediately? Yes_____ No_____ Not Clear_____

Trunk Wound:
Pt on appropriate support surface? Yes_____ No_____
Date patient placed on current surface: _____
- Repositioned q2 to 3h and documented? Yes_____ No_____ Partial_____
- Comprehensive Skin Assessment documented at least daily? Yes_____ No_____ Partial_____
- Nutritional consult? Yes_____ No_____ Not indicated (no evidence nutritional compromise) _____

Pressure Injury under Medical Device:
- Type of medical device:_____
- Duration of use prior to pressure injury development:_____
- Protective measures utilized? Yes_____ No_____ Yes, but inconsistently or only after breakdown noted:_____

Heel Pressure Injury:
- Heel elevation consistently maintained? Yes _____ No_____ Partial_____
- Support stockings/SCDs removed at least BID & skin status documented? Yes_____ No_____ N/A_____

Contributing Factors:
Hemodynamic instability (describe severity, duration, and time frame in relation to pressure injury development): _____
_____
Patient/family nonadherence to prevention program despite education (specify areas of program in which pt not in compliance, education provided, frequency and duration of noncompliance, time frame in relation to pressure injury development):
_____
Has pt been off unit for >4 consecutive hours within past 3 days?
Yes (specify)_____ No_____
Other: _____
_____

Conclusion:
_____ All appropriate preventive measures implemented; pressure injury not avoidable
_____ Gaps in preventive measures
Specify: _____
_____ Pressure injury most likely began when pt off unit
Recommendations:
_____

is the proportion of persons who develop a new pressure injury during a specific period of time (cumulative incidence), or who develop a new injury relative to the number of injury-free days (incidence density). While prevalence and incidence rates are a standard tool for use in epidemiology research and quality improvement, they do have limitations. Prevalence of pressure injuries provides information about the number of persons with the problem but does not tell the clinician whether or not the injuries developed following admission. To address some of these limitations, efforts to describe pressure injury rates are increasingly using a hybrid approach that incorporates elements of both prevalence and incidence studies in order to calculate what is known as the facility-acquired incidence rate (e.g., Hospital-Acquired Pressure Injury [HAPI] rate) (Berlowitz, 2012).

Formulas used to calculate prevalence and incidence rates are shown in **Table 21-2** (EPUAP/NPIAP/PPPIA, 2019). Berlowitz (2012) provided detailed information about the interpretation of prevalence, incidence, and facility-acquired rates. The most important data for the wound care nurse developing and monitoring a PIPP are the incidence or facility-acquired rates.

Some facilities have implemented a process that involves doing a brief RCA for any new injury that is pressure related. The staff immediately reports any lesion thought to be pressure related to the wound care team. A member of the wound care team then assesses the patient to determine whether the lesion is pressure related. If the lesion is determined to be pressure related, the patient's plan of care is reviewed to determine whether there were any areas in which preventive care could be improved. For example, if brief RCA reveals the heel injury was associated with failure to provide consistent heel off-loading, a targeted improvement may be initiated. In contrast, if it reveals that all preventive care is being consistently implemented and the injury occurred in a critically ill patient, no corrective action is needed. The key point of analysis is to evaluate whether the facility prevention plan was followed. If it was, and patients are developing pressure injuries, then it is time to reevaluate the facility PIPP.

KEY POINT

Root cause analysis involves assessment of the care provided to a patient with facility-acquired pressure injury to identify any gaps in care, with the intent of improving care processes.

STRATEGIES TO PROMOTE ACCURACY IN PREVALENCE AND INCIDENCE DATA COLLECTION

For the data provided by prevalence and incidence studies to be of value, the studies must be done correctly and consistently. For hospitals who participate in the National Data Base for Nursing Quality Indicators (NDNQI), directions for conducting a facility-wide pressure injury audit can be accessed (Press Ganey NDNQI). Training modules are available on the Web site. The wound care nurse must continually reinforce key points and take measures to ensure accuracy. Strategies to promote accuracy of prevalence and incidence data obtained during quarterly studies include the following: (1) ongoing education to all survey team members regarding wound classification and pressure injury staging, (2) wound team member availability during surveys to assist with classification or staging of challenging wounds, and (3) spot audits conducted by wound team members to verify the accuracy of wound classification and wound staging.

KEY POINT

Strategies to improve accuracy in prevalence and incidence studies include education of all survey team members, wound care nurse, and spot audits.

TABLE 21-2 FORMULAS USED TO CALCULATE PREVALENCE AND INCIDENCE

FORMULA NAME	CALCULATION
Pressure Injury Point Prevalence	$\dfrac{\text{Number of persons with a pressure ulcer} \times 100}{\text{Number of persons in population at a particular point in time}}$
Pressure Injury Period Prevalence	$\dfrac{\text{Number of persons with a pressure ulcer} \times 100}{\text{Number of persons in population at a particular time period}}$
Pressure Injury Cumulative Incidence	$\dfrac{\text{Number of persons developing new pressure ulcer} \times 100}{\text{Total number of persons in population at beginning of time period}}$
Pressure Injury Incidence Density	$\dfrac{\text{Number of persons developing new pressure ulcer} \times 100}{\text{Total patient days free of ulcers}}$
Facility Acquired Rate	$\dfrac{[(\text{No. of persons with a pressure ulcer}) - (\text{No. of people with same ulcer on admission})] \times 100}{(\text{No. of person in a population at a particular point}) - (\text{No. of people with same ulcer on admission})}$

European Pressure Ulcer Advisory Panel, National Pressure Injury Advisory Panel, and Pan Pacific Pressure Injury Alliance [EPUAP/NPIAP/PPPIA]. (2019). In E. Haesler (Ed.), *Prevention and treatment of pressure ulcers/injuries: Clinical Practice Guideline.* The International Guideline.

BENCHMARKING

The data obtained from facility-wide surveys should be compared to data from similar facilities as one indicator of the effectiveness of the prevention program. These benchmarking data are also used by independent quality monitoring programs as one indicator of the quality of nursing care.

PROGRAM MANAGEMENT AT THE ORGANIZATIONAL LEVEL

At the organizational level, the prevention program should include a planning and oversight committee that is strongly committed to developing and implementing an effective prevention program. The focus at this level should be on having the right level of expertise and authority involved and ensuring that the planning and oversight committee has the support of upper-level management (AHRQ, 2014). The members of the planning and oversight committee should have authority for (1) resource allocation, (2) an appropriate level of program monitoring and evaluation, (3) implementation of continuous quality improvement initiatives, (4) establishment of policies and procedures as well as standards of care and standards of practice, and (5) completion of an RCA when an HAPI is identified.

PROGRAM MANAGEMENT AT THE DEPARTMENTAL AND INTERDEPARTMENTAL LEVEL

Departmental and interdepartmental programs are needed to ensure that preventive care is not compromised while off the unit in another department (e.g., ED, OR, PACU, radiology). Each department should have its own set of policies related to pressure injury prevention. For example, emergency department polices may include statements related to (1) identification of patients who require pressure injury risk assessment at time of admission to the ED, (2) time frame a patient at high risk for pressure injury is kept on a stretcher, (3) frequency of repositioning for immobile and critically ill patients on a stretcher, and (4) documentation of skin condition at time of admission to the ED. Documentation of skin status on admission is especially important for patients admitted from nursing homes, and patients who were found down, that is, patients who fell and were on the floor for an unknown length of time. Each department should have ready access to supplies and equipment (i.e., available on the unit) needed for pressure injury prevention in their setting. For example, this may include repositioning wedges, redistribution cushion for the chair, off-loading heel boots, and silicone foam preventative dressings.

KEY POINT

An effective agency-wide program for pressure injury prevention must include all departments and all levels of personnel.

Interdepartmental collaboration and education about best practices related to pressure injury prevention are important if an agency-wide culture of prevention is to be established. For example, prevention is supported by an agency-wide standard that includes communication regarding pressure injury risk and prevention at each handoff, such as from nursing to transportation to interventional radiology. All transport stretchers should be equipped with pressure redistribution mattresses. Patient transporters need to be taught to float heels for at-risk patients. Personnel who work in radiology need to be educated regarding the potential for ischemic damage related to prolonged placement in one position on the radiology table. Radiology staff should be taught to reposition patients when possible and to assist the patient to make small shifts in body weight when a full-body rotation is not feasible. If there is a delay in transport, the patient should be repositioned. Colored wristbands may be used to readily identify at-risk patients who are in transit from one area of the hospital to another. The wristband would serve as a visual cue that the patient is at risk and in need of repositioning.

PROGRAM MANAGEMENT AT THE UNIT LEVEL

Unit-level prevention programs are needed to ensure that quality care delivered on a day-to-day basis is evidence based. Pressure injury prevention rounds are one approach for exchanging information about patients and for team building. Contact among team members should be a deliberate effort to clarify and talk about the shared goals of PI prevention and their individual responsibilities related to goal attainment.

The division of labor and responsibilities of team members may vary across institutions. It is important that team member responsibilities are communicated and understood. During pressure injury prevention rounds, team members should be able to provide information about activities that fall within their scope of responsibility and provide additional information about barriers and facilitators that impact their ability to achieve goal-specific tasks. Including patient care assistants and nursing assistants in patient care rounds is important. These providers are well positioned to provide preventative care and to observe, document, and report conditions that increase the risk for pressure injury.

Effective pressure injury prevention teams meet together on a regular basis to review the effectiveness of the prevention program on their unit. Each unit should have assigned team members who rotate on and off the team so that each nursing staff member has a chance to serve on the committee. Each member of the pressure injury prevention team should have assigned duties for the unit. Team members may include the wound care nurse, the unit manager, staff nurses (one from each shift), nursing assistants, and a representative from performance improvement and risk management. Information discussed at meetings should be shared with all unit staff.

Nurses and nursing assistants sometimes have difficulty communicating. Kalisch et al. (2009; 2011) found that the nursing activities most often missed are assisting patients to ambulate and providing mouth care, tasks that are commonly delegated to nursing assistants. All team members should work together to respond to patients' care needs, and nurses and nursing assistants recognize that each team member has an important role in pressure injury prevention. For example, nursing assistants play a critical role in both prevention and early detection of skin breakdown. They are the front-line care providers and the team members who provide direct patient care and can monitor skin for early changes.

⬤ CONCLUSION

The goal for this chapter was to provide current information regarding pressure injury prevention and strategies for ensuring that preventive care is routinely incorporated. The best defense against pressure injuries is a well-developed, evidence-based prevention plan that is tailored to the individual's specific needs. Detailed information about risk factors and specific strategies used to minimize risk was provided. An example of a pressure injury presentation plan of care was presented. A brief discussion of the concepts of incidence and prevalence is to help the reader distinguish between these concepts and recognize that facility-acquired incidence is the best indicator of the effectiveness of a PIPP. Effective program management cannot just be a unit initiative but needs to start with organizational support and guidance and extend across all departments and disciplines. Wound care nurses are well positioned to take the lead in pressure injury prevention programs.

REFERENCES

Agency for Healthcare Research and Quality (AHRQ). (2014). *Preventing pressure ulcers in hospitals: A toolkit for improving quality of care*. Content last reviewed October 2014. Rockville, MD: AHRQ. Retrieved February 2, 2020, from https://www.ahrq.gov/patient-safety/settings/hospital/resource/pressureulcer/tool/index.html

Antokal, S., Brienza, D., Bryan, N., et al. (2012). Friction induced skin injuries: Are they pressure ulcers? A National Pressure Ulcer Advisory Panel White Paper. Retrieved September 15, 2014, from http://www.npuap.org/wp-content/uploads/2012/01/NPUAP-Friction-White-Paper.pdf

Bain, D. S., & Ferguson-Pell, M. (2002). Remote monitoring of sitting behavior of people with spinal cord injury. *Journal of Rehabilitation Research and Development, 39*(4), 513–520.

Beeckman, D., Woodward, S., & Gray, M. (2011). Incontinence-associated dermatitis: Step-by-step prevention and treatment. *British Journal of Community Nursing, 16*(8), 382–389.

Beeson, T., Eifrid, B., Pike, C. A., et al. (2017). Do intra-anal bowel management devices reduce incontinence-associated dermatitis and/or pressure injuries? *Journal of Wound, Ostomy, and Continence Nursing, 44*(6), 583–588.

Bergquist, S., & Frantz, R. (2001). Braden scale: Validity in community-based older adults receiving home health care. *Applied Nursing Research, 14*(1), 36–43.

Bergstrom, N., & Braden, B. J. (2002). Predictive validity of the Braden scale among Black and White subjects. *Nursing Research, 51*(6), 398–403.

Bergstrom, N., Braden, B., Boynton, P., et al. (1995). Using a research-based assessment scale in clinical practice. *Nursing Clinics of North America, 30*(3), 539–551.

Bergstrom, N., Braden, B., Kemp, M., et al. (1998). Predicting pressure ulcer risk. A multi-site study of the predictive validity of the Braden scale. *Nursing Research, 47*(5), 261–269.

Bergstrom, N., Horn, S. D., Rapp, M. P., et al. (2013). Turning for Ulcer ReductioN: A multisite randomized clinical trial in nursing homes. *Journal of the American Geriatrics Society, 61*(10), 1705–1713.

Bergstrom, N., Braden, B. J., Laguzza, A., et al. (1987a). The Braden scale for predicting pressure sore risk. *Nursing Research, 36,* 205–210.

Bergstrom, N., Demuth, P. J., & Braden, B. J. (1987b). A clinical trial of the Braden scale for predicting pressure sore risk. *Nursing Clinics of North America, 22*(2), 417–428.

Berke, C. T. (2015). Pathology and clinical presentation of friction injuries: case series and literature review. *Journal of Wound, Ostomy, and Continence Nursing, 42*(1), 47–61.

Berlowitz, D. (2012). Prevalence, incidence and facility-acquired rates. In B. Pieper (Ed.), *Pressure Ulcers: Prevalence, Incidence, and Implications for the Future* (pp. 19–24). Washington, DC: National Pressure Ulcer Advisory Panel.

Berlowitz, D. (2014). Incidence and prevalence of pressure ulcers. In Thomas, D. R., & Compton, G. (Eds.), *Pressure Ulcers in the Aging Population* (pp. 19–26). Totowa, NJ: Humana Press.

Black, J. M., Cuddigan, J. E., Walko, M. A., et al. (2010). Medical device related pressure ulcers in hospitalized patients. *International Wound Journal, 7*(5), 358–365.

Bolton, L. (2007). Which pressure ulcer risk assessment scales are valid for use in the clinical setting? *Journal of Wound, Ostomy, and Continence Nursing, 34*(4), 368–381.

Braden, B., & Bergstrom, N. (1987). A conceptual schema for the study of the etiology of pressure sores. *Rehabilitation Nursing, 12*(1), 8–12.

Braden, B., & Bergstrom, N. (1994). Predictive validity of the Braden scale for pressure sore risk in a nursing home population. *Research in Nursing and Health, 17*(6), 459–470.

Braden, B., & Maklebust, J. (2005). Preventing pressure ulcers with the Braden scale: An update on this easy-to-use tool that assesses a patient's risk. *American Journal of Nursing, 105*(6), 70–72.

Brennan-Cook, J., & Turner, R. L. (2019). Promoting skin care for older adults. *Home Healthcare Now, 37*(1), 10–16.

Brienza, D. M., & Geyer, M. J. (2000). Understanding support surface technologies. *Advances in Skin & Wound Care, 13*(5), 237.

Brienza, D., Antokal, S., Herbe, L., et al. (2015). Friction-induced skin injuries—are they pressure ulcers? An updated NPUAP white paper. *Journal of Wound, Ostomy, and Continence Nursing, 42*(1), 62–64.

Brindle, C. T., & Wegelin, J. A. (2012). Prophylactic dressing application to reduce pressure ulcer formation in cardiac surgery patients. *Journal of Wound, Ostomy, and Continence Nursing, 39*(2), 133–142.

Brindle, C. T., Malhotra, R., O'Rourke, S., et al. (2013). Turning and repositioning the critically ill patient with hemodynamic instability: A literature review and consensus recommendations. *Journal of Wound, Ostomy, and Continence Nursing, 40*(3), 254–267.

Bryant, R. A., & Nix, D. P. (2016). Developing and maintaining a pressure ulcer prevention program. In R. A. Bryant & D.P. Nix (Eds.). *Acute & Chronic Wounds: Current Management Concepts* (5th ed.). St. Louis, MO: Elsevier Inc.

Bush, T. R., Leitkam, S., Aurino, M., et al. (2015). A comparison of pressure mapping between two pressure-reducing methods for the sacral region. *Journal of Wound, Ostomy, and Continence Nursing, 42*(4), 338–345.

Carter, R., & Lecko, C. (2018). Supporting evidence-based practice in nutrition and hydration. *Wounds UK, 14*(3), 18–21.

Coladonato, J., Smith, A., Watson, N., et al. (2012). Prospective, nonrandomized controlled trials to compare the effect of a silk-like fabric to standard hospital linens on the rate of hospital-acquired pressure ulcers. *Ostomy/Wound Management*, *58*(10), 14.

Curley, M. A. Q. (2018). Braden QD Scale for assessment of immobility and device-related pressure ulcer risk in your pediatric population. Retrieved February 2, 2020 from http://www.marthaaqcurley.com/braden-qd.html

Curley, M. A., Hasbani, N. R., Quigley, S. M., et al. (2018). Predicting pressure injury risk in pediatric patients: the Braden QD Scale. *The Journal of Pediatrics, 192*, 189–195.

Curley, M. A., Razmus, I. S., Roberts, K. E., et al. (2003). Predicting pressure ulcer risk in pediatric patients: the Braden Q Scale. *Nursing Research, 52*(1), 22–33.

Dammeyer, J., Dickinson, S., Packard, D., et al. (2013). Building a protocol to guide mobility in the ICU. *Critical Care Nursing Quarterly*, *36*(1), 37–49.

Dealy, C. (2009). Skin care and pressure ulcers. *Advances in Skin & Wound Care, 22*(9), 421.

Defloor, T., & Grypdonck, M. F. H. (2005). Pressure ulcers: Validation of two risk assessment scales. *Journal of Clinical Nursing, 14*, 373–382.

DeFloor, T., De Bacquer, D., & Grypdonck, M. H. F. (2004). The effect of various combinations of turning and pressure reducing devices on the incidence of pressure ulcers. *International Journal of Nursing Studies, 42*(1), 37–46.

Engels, D., Austin, M., McNichol, L., et al. (2016). Pressure ulcers: factors contributing to their development in the OR. *AORN Journal, 103*(3), 271–281.

European Pressure Ulcer Advisory Panel, National Pressure Injury Advisory Panel, and Pan Pacific Pressure Injury Alliance [EPUAP/NPIAP/PPPIA]. (2019). In E. Haesler (Ed.), *Prevention and treatment of pressure ulcers/injuries: Clinical Practice Guideline*. The International Guideline.

García-Fernández, F. P., Pancorbo-Hidalgo, P. L., & Agreda, J. J. S. (2014). Predictive capacity of risk assessment scales and clinical judgment for pressure ulcers: a meta-analysis. *Journal of Wound, Ostomy, and Continence Nursing, 41*(1), 24–34.

Gattinoni, L., Tognoni, G., Pesenti, A., et al. (2001). Effect of prone positioning on the survival of patients with acute respiratory failure. *New England Journal of Medicine, 345*(8), 568–573.

Gerhardt, L. C., Strässle, V., Lenz, A., et al. (2008). Influence of epidermal hydration on the friction of human skin against textiles. *Journal of the Royal Society Interface, 5*(28), 1317–1328.

Gillespie, B. M., Chaboyer, W. P., McInnes, E., et al. (2014). Repositioning for pressure ulcer prevention in adults. *Cochrane Database of Systematic Reviews*, (4), CD009958.

Goudas, L., & Bruni, S. (2019). Pressure injury risk assessment and prevention strategies in operating room patients-findings from a study tour of novel practices in American hospitals. *Journal of Perioperative Nursing, 32*(1), 33.

Gray, M., Black, J. M., Baharestani, M. M., et al. (2011). Moisture-associated skin damage: overview and pathophysiology. *Journal of Wound, Ostomy, and Continence Nursing*, *38*(3), 233–241.

Gray, M., Kent, D., Ermer-Seltun, J., et al. (2018). Assessment, selection, use, and evaluation of body-worn absorbent products for adults with incontinence. *Journal of Wound, Ostomy, and Continence Nursing*, *45*(3), 243–264.

Gunningberg, L., Sedin, I. M., Andersson, S., et al. (2017). Pressure mapping to prevent pressure ulcers in a hospital setting: A pragmatic randomised controlled trial. *International Journal of Nursing Studies, 72*, 53–59.

Halfens, R. J. G., Van Achterberg, T., & Bal, R. H. (2000). Validity and reliability of the Braden scale and the influence of risk factors: A multicentre prospective study. *International Journal of Nursing Studies*, *37*(19), 313–319.

Hanson, D., Langemo, D. K., Anderson, J., et al. (2010). Friction and shear considerations in pressure ulcer development. *Advances in Skin & Wound Care*, *23*(1), 21–24.

Hermans, M. H. E., Weyl, C., & Roger, S. I. (2014). Performance parameters of support surfaces: Setting measuring and presentation standards. *Wounds, 26*(1), 28–36.

Huffines, B., & Logsdon, M. C. (1997). The neonatal skin risk assessment scale for predicting skin breakdown in neonates. *Issues in Comprehensive Pediatric Nursing, 20*(2), 103–114.

Hultin, L., Olsson, E., Carli, C., et al. (2017). Pressure mapping in elderly care. *Journal of Wound, Ostomy, and Continence Nursing, 44*(2), 142–147.

Jankowski, I. M., & Nadzam, D. M. (2011). Identifying gaps, barriers, and solutions in implementing pressure ulcer prevention programs. *The Joint Commission Journal on Quality and Patient Safety*, *37*(6), 253–264.

Johnson, D., Lineweaver, L., & Maze, L. (2009). Patients' bath basins as potential sources of infection. A multicenter sampling study. *American Journal of Critical Care*, *118*(1), 31–38.

Kalisch, B. J.,. Landstrom, G., & Williams, R. A. (2009). Missed nursing care: Errors of omission. *Nursing Outlook*, *57*(1), 3–9.

Kalisch, B. J., Tschannen, D., & Friese, C. R. (2011). Hospital variation in missed nursing care. *American Journal of Medical Quality*, *28*(4), 291–292.

Kalowes, P., Messina, V., & Li, M. (2016). Five-layered soft silicone foam dressing to prevent pressure ulcers in the intensive care unit. *American Journal of Critical Care*, *25*(6), e108–e119.

Kayser, S. A., VanGilder, C. A., Ayello, E. A., et al. (2018). Prevalence and analysis of medical device-related pressure injuries: Results from the international pressure ulcer prevalence survey. *Advances in Skin & Wound Care, 31*(6), 276.

Kosiak, M. (1959). Etiology and pathology of ischemic ulcers. *Archives of Physical Medicine and Rehabilitation, 40*, 62–69.

Krapfl, L. A., Langin, J., Pike, C. A., et al. (2017). Does incremental positioning (weight shifts) reduce pressure injuries in critical care patients? *Journal of Wound, Ostomy, and Continence Nursing, 44*(4), 319–323.

Kwong, E., Pang, S., Wong, T., et al. (2005). Predicting pressure ulcer risk with the modified Braden, Braden, and Norton scales in acute care hospitals in mainland China. *Applied Nursing Research*, *18*(2), 122–128.

Lahmann, N. A., & Kottner, J. (2011). Relation between pressure, friction and pressure ulcer categories: A secondary data analysis of hospital patients using CHAID methods. *International Journal of Nursing Studies*, *48*(12), 1487–1494.

Lahmann, N. A., Halfens, R. J. G., & Dassen, T. (2010). The impact of prevention structures and processes on pressure ulcer prevalence in nursing homes and acute-care hospitals. *Journal of Evaluation in Clinical Practice*, *16*(1), 50–56.

Lahmann, N. A., Tannen, A., Dassen, T., et al. (2011). Friction and shear highly associated with pressure ulcers of residents in long-term care—Classification tree analysis (CHAID) of Braden items. *Journal of Evaluation in Clinical Practice*, *17*, 168–173.

Lambers, H., Piessens, S., Bloem, A., et al. (2006). Natural skin surface pH is on average below 5, which is beneficial for its resident flora. *International Journal of Cosmetic Science*, *28*(5), 359–370.

Lyder, C. H. (1996). Examining the inclusion of ethnic minorities in pressure ulcer prediction studies. *Journal of Wound, Ostomy, and Continence Nursing*, *23*(5), 257–260.

Lyder, C. H., Yu, C., Emerling, J., et al. (1999). The Braden Scale for pressure ulcer risk: Evaluating the predictive validity in Blacks and Hispanic elderly patients. *Applied Nursing Research*, *12*(2), 60–68.

Magnan, M. A., & Maklebust, J. (2008). The effect of web-based Braden Scale training on the reliability and precision of Braden scale pressure ulcer risk assessments. *Journal of Wound, Ostomy, and Continence Nursing*, *35*(2), 199–208.

Magnan, M. A., & Maklebust, J. (2009). The nursing process and pressure ulcer prevention: Making the connection. *Advances in Skin & Wound Care, 22*(2), 83–92.

Maklebust J. (1987). Pressure ulcers: Etiology and prevention, *Nursing Clinics of North America, 22*(2), 359–377.

Maklebust, J., & Sieggreen, M. Y. (1996). *Pressure Ulcers: Guidelines for Prevention and Nursing Management* (2nd ed.). Springhouse, PA: Springhouse Corporation.

Maklebust, J., & Sieggreen, M. (2001). *Pressure Ulcers: Guidelines for Prevention and Management* (3rd ed.). Springhouse, PA: Springhouse Corporation.

Marchaim, D., Taylor, A. R., Hayakawa, K., et al. (2012). Hospital bath basins are frequently contaminated with multi-drug resistant human pathogens. *American Journal of Infection Control, 40*(6), 562–564.

McInnes, E., Jammali-Blasi, A., Bell-Syer, S. E., et al. (2015). Support surfaces for pressure ulcer prevention. *Cochrane Database of Systematic Reviews,* (9), CD001735.

McNichol, L., Watts, C., Mackey, D., et al. (2015). Identifying the right surface for the right patient at the right time: generation and content validation of an algorithm for support surface selection. *Journal of Wound, Ostomy, and Continence Nursing, 42*(1), 19–37.

Moore, Z., Haynes, J. S., & Callaghan, R. (2014). Prevention and management of pressure ulcers: Support surfaces. *British Journal of Nursing, 33*(6), S636.

Munro, C. A. (2010). The development of a pressure ulcer risk-assessment scale for perioperative patients. *AORN Journal, 92*(3), 272–287.

Murray, J. S., Noonan, C., Quigley, S., et al. (2013). Medical device-related hospital-acquired pressure ulcers in children: An integrative review. *Journal of Pediatric Nursing, 28*(6), 585–595.

Nakagami, G., Sanada, H., Konya, C., et al. (2006). Comparison of two pressure ulcer preventive dressings for reducing shear force on the heel. *Journal of Wound, Ostomy, and Continence Nursing, 33*(3), 267–272.

National Pressure Injury Advisory Panel. (2019). Terms and Definitions to Support Surfaces. Retrieved January 31, 2020, from https://cdn.ymaws.com/npiap.com/resource/resmgr/terms_and_defs_nov_21_2019_u.pdf

National Pressure Injury Advisory Panel. (2020). Pressure Injury Prevention: Tips for Prone Positioning. Retrieved 4/25/2020 from https://cdn.ymaws.com/npiap.com/resource/resmgr/online_store/posters/npiap_pip_tips_-_proning_202.pdf

Nelson, A., Owen, B., Lloyd, J. D., et al. (2003). Safe patient handling and movement: Preventing back injury among nurses requires careful selection of the safest equipment and techniques. *American Journal of Nursing, 103*(3), 32–43.

Nixon, J., Thorpe, H., Barrow, H., et al. (2005). Reliability of pressure ulcer classification and diagnosis. *Journal of Advanced Nursing,* 50, 613–623. doi: 10.1111/j.1365-2648.2005.03439.x.

Norton, D. (1989). Calculating the risk: Reflections on the Norton Scale. *Decubitus, 2*(3), 24–31.

Ohura, T. (2013). External force and its clinical influence-The relationships between fundamental biomechanics and clinical findings. *World Council of Enterostomal Therapists Journal, 33*(2), 14–20.

Pan, N., & Sun, G. (2011). *Functional Textiles for Improved Performance, Protection and Health.* Cambridge, UK: Woodhead Publishing Ltd.

Pancorbo-Hidalgo, P. L., Garcia-Fernandez, F. P., Lopez-Medina, I. M., et al. (2006). Risk assessment scales for pressure ulcer prevention: A systematic review. *Journal of Advanced Nursing, 54*(1), 94–110.

Pang, S. M., & Wong, T. K. (1998). Predicting pressure sore risk with the Norton, Braden, and Waterlow Scales in a Hong Kong Rehabilitation Hospital. *Nursing Research, 47*(3), 147–153.

Park, S. K., Park, H. A., & Hwang, H. (2019). Development and comparison of predictive models for pressure injuries in surgical patients: A retrospective case-control study. *Journal of Wound, Ostomy, and Continence Nursing, 46*(4), 291–297.

Peterson, M. J., Schwab, W., Van Oostrom, J. H., et al. (2010). Effects of turning on skin-bed interface pressures in healthy adults. *Journal of Advanced Nursing, 66*(7), 1556–1564.

Pinchofsky-Devin, G. D., & Kaminski, M. V. (1986). Correlation of pressure sores and nutritional status. *Journal of the American Geriatrics Society,* 34, 435–440.

Polit, D. R., & Beck, C. T. (2011). *Nursing research: Principles and methods* (9th ed.). Philadelphia, PA: Lippincott Williams & Wilkins.

Powers, J. (2016). Two methods for turning and positioning and the effect on pressure ulcer development: a comparison cohort study. *Journal of Wound, Ostomy, and Continence Nursing, 43*(1), 46–50.

Powers, J., Dickenson, S., Vollman, K. (2016). Prone positioning procedure. In D. L. Wiegand (Ed.), *AACN Procedure Manual for High Acuity, Progressive and Critical Care* (7th ed.). St. Louis, MO: Elsevier Health Sciences.

Quigley, S. M., & Curley, M. A. (1996). Skin integrity in the pediatric population: preventing and managing pressure ulcers. *Journal for Specialists in Pediatric Nursing, 1*(1), 7–18.

Rahn, Y., Lahmann, N., Blume-Peytavi, U., et al. (2016). Assessment of topical skin care practices in long-term institutional nursing care from a health service perspective. *Journal of Gerontological Nursing, 42*(6), 18–24.

Reswick, J., & Rogers, J. (1976). Experiences at Rancho Los Amigos Hospital with devices and techniques to prevent pressure sores. In R. M. Kenedi, J. M. Cowden, & J. T. Scales (Eds.), *Bedsore Biomechanics* (pp. 301–310). Baltimore, MD: University Park Press.

Reynolds, S. S., Sova, C., McNalty, B., et al. (2019). Implementation strategies to improve evidence-based bathing practices in a neuro ICU. *Journal of Nursing Care Quality, 34*(2), 133–138.

Riemenschneider, K. J. (2018). Prevention of pressure injuries in the operating room. *Journal of Wound, Ostomy, and Continence Nursing, 45*(2), 141–145.

Ross, G., & Gefen, A. (2019). Assessment of sub-epidermal moisture by direct measurement of tissue biocapacitance. *Medical Engineering & Physics,* 73, 92–99.

Santamaria, N., Gerdtz, M., Sage, S., et al. (2015). A randomised controlled trial of the effectiveness of soft silicone multi-layered foam dressings in the prevention of sacral and heel pressure ulcers in trauma and critically ill patients: the border trial. *International Wound Journal, 12*(3), 302–308.

Scardillo, J., & Aronovitch, S. A. (1999). Successfully managing incontinence-related irritant dermatitis over the lifespan. *Ostomy/Wound Management,* 45, 36–44.

Schindler, C. A., Mikhailov, T. A., Kuhn, E. M., et al. (2011). Protecting fragile skin: nursing interventions to decrease development of pressure ulcers in pediatric intensive care. *American Journal of Critical Care, 20*(1), 26–35.

Shaw, G., & Taylor, S. J. (1991). A survey of wheelchair seating problems of the institutionalized elderly. *Assistive Technology, 3*(1), 5–10.

Smith, A., McNichol, L. L., Amos, M. A., et al. (2013). A retrospective, nonrandomized, before-and-after study of the effect of linens constructed of synthetic silk-like fabric on pressure ulcer incidence. *Ostomy/Wound Management, 59*(4), 28–34.

Sprigle, S. (2000). Effects of forces and the selection of support surfaces. *Topics in Geriatric Rehabilitation, 16*(2), 47–62.

Sturgeon, L. P., Garrett-Wright, D., Lartey, G., et al. (2019). A descriptive study of bathing practices in acute care facilities in the United States. *American Journal of Infection Control, 47*(1), 23–26.

Swanson, M. S., Rose, M. A., Baker, G., et al. (2011). Braden subscales and their relationship to the prevalence of pressure ulcers in hospitalized obese patients. *Bariatric Nursing and Surgical Patient Care, 6*(1), 21–23.

Thomas, D. R. (2007). Loss of skeletal muscle mass in aging: Examining the relationship of starvation, sarcopenia and cachexia. *Clinical Nutrition, 26*(4), 389–399.

Thompson, P., Anderson, J., Langemo, D., et al. (2008). Support surfaces: Definitions and utilization for patient care. *Advances in Skin & Wound Care, 21*(6), 264–266.

Thompson, P., Anderson, J., Langemo, D., et al. (2009). Support surfaces: Reducing pressure ulcer risk. *Nursing Management, 40*(11), 49–51.

Tubaishat, A., Papanikolaou, P., Anthony, D., et al. (2018). Pressure ulcers prevalence in the acute care setting: A systematic review, 2000-2015. *Clinical Nursing Research, 27*(6), 643–659.

Twersky, J., Montgomery, T., Sloane, R., et al. (2012). A randomized, controlled study to assess the effect of silk-like textiles and high-absorbency adult incontinence briefs on pressure ulcer prevention. *Ostomy/Wound Management, 58*(12), 18–24.

Vanderwee, K., Grypdonck, M. H. F., De Bacquer, D., et al. (2007). Effectiveness of turning with unequal time intervals on the incidence of pressure ulcer lesions. *Journal of Advanced Nursing, 57*(1), 59–68.

Vollman, K. M. (2004). Prone positioning for the patient who has acute respiratory distress syndrome: The art and science. *Critical Care Nursing Clinics of North America, 16*(3), 319–336.

Vollman, K. M. (2012). Hemodynamic instability: Is it really a barrier to turning critically ill patients? *Critical Care Nursing Quarterly, 32*(1), 70–75.

Wang, E. W., & Layon, A. J. (2017). Chlorhexidine gluconate use to prevent hospital acquired infections—A useful tool, not a panacea. *Annals of Translational Medicine, 5*(1), 14.

Wang, L., Walker, R., & Gillespie, B. M., (2018). Pressure injury prevention for surgery: Results from a prospective, observational study in a tertiary hospital. *Journal of Perioperative Nursing 31*(3), 25–28.

Waterlow, J. (1985). A pressure sore risk assessment card. *Nursing Times, 81*, 49–55.

Winkleman, C., & Peereboom, K. (2010). Staff perceived barriers and facilitators. *Critical Care Nurse, 30*(2), S13–S16.

Winslow, E. H., Lane, L. D., & Woods, R. J. (1995). Dangling, a review of relevant physiology: Research and practice. *Heart and Lung, 24*(4), 263–272.

Wound Ostomy and Continence Nurses Society (WOCN). (2016). *Guideline for Management of Pressure Ulcer/Injury. WOCN clinical practice guidelines series # 2*. Mt. Laurel, NJ: Author.

Zhong, W., Ahmad, A., Xing, M. M., et al. (2008). Impact of textiles on formation and prevention of skin lesions and bedsores. *Cutaneous and Ocular Toxicology, 27*(1), 21–28.

Zhong, W., Xing, M. M. Q., Pan, N., et al. (2006). Textiles and human skin, microclimate, cutaneous reactions: An overview. *Cutaneous and Ocular Toxicology, 25*(1), 23–39.

QUESTIONS

1. The wound care nurse in a long-term care facility is calculating the cumulative incidence of pressure injuries among the current residents. What does this ratio represent?

A. The number of persons at risk who develop new pressure injuries during a specific period of time

B. The number of persons at risk who develop new injuries relative to the number of injury-free days

C. The proportion of all persons who have a pressure injury in a specific setting at a specific point in time

D. The proportion of all persons who have a pressure injury in a specific setting over specific period of time

2. All of the following will minimize the risk of a patient developing a medical device-related pressure injury EXCEPT

A. Stabilize tubes without tension

B. Avoid moving medical devices during comprehensive skin assessment, as this creates friction against the skin

C. Remove medical devices as soon as medically no longer indicated

D. Consider use of a prophylactic dressing under a medical device

3. The wound care nurse is benchmarking the data on pressure injury incidence obtained in a critical care unit. What is the goal of this process?

A. To determine the severity of the pressure injuries discovered

B. To obtain reimbursement from third-party payers and reduce litigation risk

C. To determine pressure injury treatment protocols

D. To determine effectiveness of the prevention program by comparing outcomes to those of other (similar) agencies/settings

4. The bedside staff nurse uses a risk assessment tool to determine which patients in an acute care setting are at risk for pressure injuries. What is the primary purpose of these tools?

A. To use as a basis to design an agency-wide pressure injury prevention program

B. To obtain information as to specific risk factors throughout the agency

C. To identify other factors contributing to overall risk

D. To identify patients at risk and their particular risk factors

5. The wound care nurse assessing a patient for pressure injuries scores the patient as an 11 on the Braden Scale. What risk level does this number represent?

A. Mild risk

B. Moderate risk

C. High risk

D. Very high risk

6. What measures can a nurse take to improve accuracy in risk assessment?
   A. When in doubt, score high on the Braden Scale.
   B. Refrain from using data obtained from audits and skills fairs.
   C. Review the NDNQI module as a learning strategy.
   D. Assign a Braden Scale total score of 19 to save time with patient care.

7. A wound care nurse off-loading a patient every 2 hours notes that normal reactive hyperemia does not resolve within 30 minutes of off-loading. What is the significance of this finding?
   A. A stage 1 pressure injury is developing.
   B. This is a normal finding unrelated to pressure injury development.
   C. The nurse should discontinue off-loading and concentrate on the surface.
   D. The patient has developed a stage 2 pressure injury.

8. The bedside staff nurse is repositioning the patient in a critical care unit. Which statement accurately describes a therapeutic effect of this intervention?
   A. Critically ill patients seem to tolerate the right lateral position better than the left lateral position.
   B. Wedges should be used to achieve small incremental lateral position changes of 30 degrees before moving the patient to the 45-degree lateral position.

   C. The presence of life-threatening arrhythmias or active hemorrhage in a patient requires more frequent positioning.
   D. The use of a lateral rotation bed should be considered as an alternative to repositioning.

9. The wound care nurse uses effective strategies to protect patients from pressure injury development. What is one recommended technique?
   A. Always use a commercial foot elevation boot rather than a bed pillow to suspend the heel off the bed and prevent pressure injuries.
   B. Use a sliding board against bare skin when transferring a patient from bed to stretcher or bed to chair.
   C. Protect the sacrococcygeal area against friction damage by applying a silicone adhesive foam dressing.
   D. Take measures to keep the skin warm and moist to reduce the risk for friction and shear injury.

10. Which of the following describes an effective strategy for minimizing the adverse effects of shearing forces?
   A. Maintain the head of the bed elevation at 45 degrees unless medically contraindicated
   B. Use foam redistribution surfaces whenever possible.
   C. Use two to three layers of underpads to keep the perineal skin dry and to prevent contamination of the support surface
   D. Elevate the head of the bed to 30 degrees or less when positioning in a semi-Fowler position.

ANSWERS AND RATIONALES

1. A. Rationale: Incidence is the proportion of persons who develop a new pressure injury during a specific period of time (cumulative incidence).

2. B. Rationale: Key principles related to MDRPI prevention include discontinuation of the device when no longer medically necessary; appropriate stabilization (i.e., without tension to tubes); rotating or repositioning the device, when able; and use of a prophylactic dressing under a medical device to reduce risk of pressure injury.

3. D. Rationale: The data obtained from prevalence and incidence surveys should be compared to data from similar facilities as one

indicator of the effectiveness of the prevention program.

4. D. Rationale: Risk assessment for pressure injury includes identification of subjective, objective, and psychosocial factors to determine the risk and care needs of the patient. It aims to identify individuals with characteristics that increase their probability of developing a PI.

5. C. Rationale: Braden Scale scores reflect five levels of pressure injury risk: no risk (19 to 23), mild risk (15 to 18), moderate risk (13 to 14), high risk (10 to 12), and very high risk ($\leq$9).

6. C. Rationale: To improve accuracy of risk assessment, it is suggested that training in proper use of the Braden Scale is needed. NDNQI offers training modules for participating institutions on their Web site.

7. A. Rationale: Normal reactive hyperemia should resolve within 20 to 30 minutes of off-loading pressure with no residual effects. Evidence of nonblanchable erythema that persists following off-loading is a stage 1 pressure injury.

8. A. Rationale: Critically ill patients appear to tolerate the right lateral tilt position better than the left lateral position.

9. C. Rationale: Strategies to keep the skin cool and dry, use of therapeutic linens, support surfaces with low-friction low-shear covers, and use of multilayered silicone foam protective dressings can help to reduce both superficial friction damage and shear damage, resulting in PI.

10. D. Rationale: When positioning in a semi-Fowler position, elevating the head of the bed to 30 degrees or less will minimize the risk for shearing that comes from sliding down in bed.

CHAPTER 22

THERAPEUTIC SURFACES FOR BED AND CHAIR

Dianne Mackey and Carolyn Watts

OBJECTIVES

1. Explain the role of each of the following in pressure injury development: prolonged or intense pressure, shear force, moisture, and tissue tolerance.

2. Explain how therapeutic bed and chair surfaces contribute to prevention and management of pressure injury.

3. Select and recommend appropriate pressure redistribution devices for bed and chair.

4. Design a decision-making algorithm for appropriate use of off-loading devices and therapeutic support surfaces.

TOPIC OUTLINE

INTRODUCTION

As discussed in the chapter on pressure injury pathology and presentation (Chapter 20), key etiologic factors for pressure injuries include prolonged or high-intensity pressure, friction and shear, and warm moist skin. Each of these factors may be partially controlled by an appropriate surface for the bed and chair. Appropriate selection and use of these surfaces are the focus of this chapter. A support surface is a specialized device for pressure redistribution designed for management of tissue loads, microclimate, and/or other therapeutic functions (e.g., any mattresses, integrated bed system, mattress replacement, overlay, or seat cushion, or seat cushion overlay) (NPIAP, 2020; WOCN, 2016). Knowledge of the components of a support surface along with the product's performance is key in selecting a product that reduces pressure, shear, friction, and moisture between the patient's skin and the support surface. Support surfaces are available in a variety of sizes and shapes and include mattresses, mattress overlays, operating room (OR) surfaces, examination and procedure table surfaces, and pads for emergency and transport stretchers. For the purposes of this chapter, the term support surface refers to both horizontal surfaces (overlay, mattress, or integrated bed system) and seat cushions, unless otherwise stated.

Wound care nurses are expected to make recommendations based on current research. There is evidence that pressure redistribution devices reduce the incidence of pressure injuries by up to 60% (McInnes et al., 2018). Research related to support surface utilization is very limited, and at present, there is no evidence that one particular brand of support surface is better than another (Iglesias et al., 2006; NPIAP, 2020; WOCN, 2016). Wound care nurses must base product selection on a clear understanding of the therapeutic features of various products as compared to the patient's needs. This chapter addresses (1) risk factors and support surfaces; (2) components, categories, and features of support surfaces; (3) selection and evaluation of a support surface based on an individual patient's needs; and (4) the development and evaluation of a facility- or agency-wide support surface decision tree or algorithm. General guidelines for care of the patient requiring a support surface are provided in **Box 22-1**.

KEY POINT

Studies indicate that pressure redistribution devices may reduce the incidence of pressure injuries by up to 60%. Wound care nurses must base product selection on a clear understanding of the therapeutic features of various products as compared to the patient's needs.

BOX 22-1 GENERAL RECOMMENDATIONS FOR SUPPORT SURFACES

- Support surfaces are not a stand-alone intervention for the prevention and treatment of pressure ulcers but are to be used in conjunction with proper nutritional support, moisture management, pressure redistribution when in bed and chair, turning and repositioning, risk identification, and patient and caregiver education.
- Support surfaces do not eliminate the need for turning and repositioning.
- Consider concurrent use of a pressure redistribution seating surface or cushion of an appropriate type along with use of any support surface.
- When choosing a support surface, consider contraindications for use of specific support surfaces as specified by the manufacturer.
- In order to achieve the full benefits of a support surface, the support surface must be functioning properly and used correctly according to the manufacturer's instructions.
- When choosing a support surface, consider current patient characteristics and risk factors, including weight and weight distribution; fall and entrapment risk; risk for developing new pressure ulcers; number, severity, and location of existing pressure ulcers; as well as previous support surface usage and patient preference.
- The person who exceeds the weight limit or whose body dimensions exceed his or her current support surface should be moved to an appropriate bariatric support surface.
- For persons who are candidates for progressive mobility, consider a support surface that facilitates getting out of bed.
- Persons who meet facility protocol for a low bed frame and who have a pressure ulcer, or are at risk for developing a pressure ulcer, should also receive an appropriate support surface.
- Persons who have medical contraindications for turning should be considered for an appropriate support surface and repositioning with frequent small shifts.
- For persons experiencing intractable pain, consider providing an appropriate alternative to the current support surface.
- Persons with a new myocutaneous flap on the posterior or lateral trunk or pelvis should be provided with an appropriate support surface per facility protocol.
- Minimize the number and type of layers between the patient and the support surface.
- Support surfaces must be compatible with the care setting while meeting the individual needs of the patient.
- Consider fall/entrapment risk when choosing between a mattress and an overlay.
- A support surface that dissipates moisture (low air loss) may be indicated when moisture/incontinence cannot be managed by other means.
- At present, guidelines for prevention of heel ulcers require elevation of the heel off the bed; support surfaces cannot provide sufficient envelopment to protect the soft tissue of the heel (even very-high-level support surfaces).

Source: McNichol, L., Watts, C., Mackey, D., et al. (2015). Identifying the right surface for the right patient at the right time: Generation and content validation of an algorithm for support surface selection. *Journal of Wound, Ostomy, and Continence Nursing, 42*(1), 19–37.

RISK FACTORS ADDRESSED BY SUPPORT SURFACES

Prevention of pressure injuries is accomplished primarily by management of tissue loads and shear forces. Support surfaces are an integral component of a pressure injury prevention and treatment program because they may enhance perfusion of at-risk or injured soft tissue. Support surfaces are only one component of a comprehensive pressure injury prevention and treatment program; they should not be considered a stand-alone intervention. Pressure is not the only contributing factor to tissue breakdown and not the only factor to be addressed by a therapeutic support surface. Other causative factors include shear, friction, moisture, and heat. In most situations, pressure redistribution is the most important feature of a support surface. Research has shown that the damaging effects of pressure are related to both its magnitude and duration. Tissues can withstand higher loads for shorter periods of time and lower loads for longer periods of time (Brienza & Geyer, 2005). A surface that redistributes pressure across the entire contact surface effectively reduces the magnitude of the pressure and extends the time that the patient can safely remain in one position.

KEY POINT

Support surfaces are only one element of a comprehensive pressure injury prevention program; they should not be considered a stand-alone intervention.

The wound care nurse must remember that the risk of skin and soft tissue breakdown is affected not only by the extrinsic factors already addressed (pressure, shear, friction, moisture, and heat) but also by intrinsic risk factors such as advanced age, low blood pressure, smoking, elevated body temperature, poor protein intake, anemia, generalized edema, and hemodynamic instability. This underscores the fact that a support surface is only one element of a comprehensive management plan and does not replace attention to perfusion, nutritional support, and management of comorbidities.

TISSUE LOADING AND INTERFACE PRESSURE

Tissue interface pressure is defined as the force per unit area that acts perpendicularly between the patient's skin and the support surface (McInnes et al., 2018; NPIAP, 2020). The intensity (magnitude) and duration of pressure exerted against the skin and soft tissue is a critical factor in the risk for skin breakdown. Therapeutic support surfaces work primarily by reducing the intensity of interface pressure. Interface pressure measurements have been used for years to compare various products in terms of their pressure redistribution ability. This non-invasive test involves placement of a mat equipped with a single pressure sensor or multiple pressure sensors

between the patient's skin and the underlying support surface. The tissue interface pressure measurement provides an approximation of the pressure exerted over a specific bony prominence and the surrounding area (Le et al., 1984; Miller et al., 2013; Reger et al., 1988). In the past, research efforts have focused on establishment of a critical cutoff for interface pressure (i.e., the pressure reading beyond which pressure injuries are likely to develop). However, it has not been possible to establish a specific reading that represents the physiologic limit for the majority of patients. The value of tissue interface pressure measurements is primarily in comparison of one product to another (assuming the availability of valid interface pressure measurements for the various devices).

KEY POINT

In most situations, pressure redistribution is the most important feature of the support surface; effective pressure redistribution reduces the intensity of the pressure and extends the time the patient can safely remain in one position.

Physical Concepts

The physical concepts of life expectancy and fatigue are performance-related terms used to guide discussions and evaluations on the performance of various support surfaces. The term life expectancy refers to the period of time during which a product is expected to effectively fulfill its purpose. Life expectancy may be impacted by fatigue. Fatigue is the reduced capacity of a surface or its components to perform as specified. This change may be the result of intended or unintended use and/or prolonged exposure to chemical, thermal, or physical forces (NPIAP, 2020). Life expectancy and fatigue will impact the ability of the support surface to redistribute pressure, control friction and shear, and manage the microclimate (temperature and humidity). Staff who have the opportunity to observe support surfaces during linen or room changes should be alert to indicators that the surface is no longer performing as expected: reduced height or thickness; discoloration; altered integrity of the mattress cover, seams, zipper, zipper cover flap, or backing; degradation of internal components; or presence of odor. If any of these are observed, the surface should be referred to engineering/maintenance for evaluation, whether or not it has exceeded its stated product life span.

KEY POINT

All staff should be alert to evidence of product fatigue (e.g., reduced height or thickness, discoloration, odor, visible damage) and should have the product evaluated by engineering/maintenance, even if it is still under warranty and has not exceeded its stated life span.

Pressure Redistribution
(Immersion and Envelopment)

Support surfaces are designed to prevent pressure injuries and promote pressure injury healing through effective pressure redistribution and reduction in pressure intensity and magnitude. By conforming to the contours of the body, support surfaces redistribute pressure over a larger surface area rather than having pressure concentrated in a more circumscribed location (e.g., directly over the bony prominence), which reduces interface pressure. The therapeutic function of pressure redistribution is accomplished through immersion and envelopment.

Immersion

The term immersion refers to the penetration (sinking) into a support surface, measured by depth; as the body sinks into the surface, the pressure is spread out over the entire contact area rather than being concentrated directly over the bony prominence (NPIAP, 2020). Immersion is dependent on factors such as the stiffness and thickness of the support surface and the flexibility of the cover.

Envelopment

The term envelopment refers to the ability of a support surface to conform, so to fit or mold around irregularities in the body (e.g., clothing, bedding, bony prominences) without causing a substantial increase in pressure. By creating a very close match between the support surface and the body surface, envelopment maximizes pressure redistribution (NPIAP, 2020).

KEY POINT

Most support surfaces provide pressure redistribution through immersion and envelopment (i.e., allowing the patient to sink into the product and evenly conforming to his or her bodily contours).

Bottoming Out

In contrast to the therapeutic functions of immersion and envelopment, bottoming out is the term used to denote the state of support surface deformation beyond critical immersion whereby effective pressure redistribution is lost (NPIAP, 2020). If the surface provides inadequate support for the patient's weight, the body may sink so deeply into the surface that the patient's bony prominences are actually resting against the underlying bed frame. Whitney et al. (2006) defined bottoming out as <1 inch of material between the support surface and the skin surface. Factors that contribute to bottoming out include (1) patient weight that exceeds support surface's weight limits, according to the manufacturer; (2) disproportion between weight and size, such as with bilateral lower extremity amputations; (3) persistent head-of-bed elevation exceeding 30 degrees; and (4) inadequate support surface settings, such as over or under inflation.

An essential clinical caveat in effective use of all support surfaces is to limit the layers (sheets, briefs, and underpads) between the patient and the support surface.

Hand checks at the bedside have historically been used to assess bottoming out of static air mattress overlays. The clinician would insert a hand, palm up, beneath the support surface in the area underlying the patient's bony prominence. This practice is no longer recommended because hand checks are subjective, and they create the potential for infection risks for both the patient and the caregiver or clinician. Results vary with the elevation of the head of the bed and patient positioning and the method has not been validated as effective. This gap in the evidence indicates that additional research is needed to provide a bedside method to determine when a support surface has bottomed out (NPIAP, 2015).

KEY POINT

Bottoming out means the overlay or mattress is providing insufficient support, and the patient's bony prominences are resting on the underlying bed frame; this mandates a change in support surface.

FRICTION AND SHEAR REDUCTION

Friction and shear are physical forces that increase the risk of pressure injury formation. Shear stress refers to the force per unit area exerted parallel to the perpendicular plane of interest. It is deformation that occurs when the tissue is exposed to lateral strain (NPIAP, 2020); specifically, the patient is at risk for shear damage when exposed to the dual forces of friction and gravity. Friction is defined as the resistance to motion in a parallel direction relative to the common boundary of two surfaces. This occurs when the patient slides down in bed; typically, frictional forces hold the skin stationary while gravitational forces cause the deep tissue layers (muscle and bone) to slide down. This causes shear and deformation of the subcutaneous tissue and blood vessels, which is a major contributor to ischemic injury. Support surfaces with low friction covers (e.g., Gore-Tex type covers) reduce frictional forces and reduce tissue deformation when the patient slides down in bed (McNichol et al., 2020). Head of bed should be kept low to reduce sliding, but this is very difficult to accomplish in situations requiring head-of-bed elevation. A support surface cannot provide total protection against shear and does not eliminate the need for additional interventions to minimize friction and shear.

MICROCLIMATE (TEMPERATURE AND MOISTURE) CONTROL

Microclimate control is the temperature and humidity in a specified location. For purposes of support surfaces, microclimate refers to temperature and humidity at the support surface/body interface (NPIAP, 2020). Some support surfaces offer a therapeutic function addressing microclimate; this feature may be of particular benefit to patients who are diaphoretic. Excessively moist skin is a well-known risk factor for pressure injury development, as is abnormally warm skin. Control of temperature at the interface surface (patient–bed) helps to maintain normal skin temperature, which inhibits sweating and reduces skin moisture (McNichol et al., 2020; Nix & Mackey, 2016). An ideal support surface would be designed to help maintain normal skin hydration and temperature (Brienza & Geyer, 2005). This may be accomplished through porous covers that reduce moisture by promoting air transfer between the skin and surface, with resultant dissipation of moisture and body heat. Another approach is to provide constant airflow against the skin by pumping air through microperforations in the support surface cover.

KEY POINT

Microclimate control can be provided through airflow against the skin or by increasing the transfer of air between the skin and the support surface.

COMPONENTS OF A SUPPORT SURFACE

The most important component of a support surface is the medium used to provide pressure redistribution. Mediums include air, fluid, or solid and can be used alone or in combination. The ability to encapsulate the medium is another component of the support surface and is called a cell or bladder (NPIAP, 2020). Cells can be configured in a longitudinal or latitudinal pattern and can be individual or interconnected.

FOAM

Foam is available in chair cushions, overlays, mattresses for beds, and pads for transport gurneys, stretchers, and OR and procedure tables. Most foam overlays and cushions are indicated for single-patient use, whereas mattresses are intended for multiple-patient use. All foam products are designed for a specific weight limit and life span. Foam can be the sole medium or may be included in hybrid products that include gel, air, or other fluid materials that enhance envelopment in key areas. Benefits associated with foam support surfaces include their relatively low cost, light weight, and minimal maintenance. Disadvantages include a limited life span due to fatigue caused by flexion and compression over time. There is also a high risk for moisture penetration with potential for infection. Additional disadvantages include the cost of disposal and negative environmental impact.

Foam can be closed cell or open cell. Closed-cell foam is a nonpermeable formulation with a barrier between the cells that prevents gases or liquids from passing through the foam (NPIAP, 2020); closed-cell foam products have the potential to increase skin temperature by preventing dissipation of body heat (Nicholson et al., 1999). Open-cell foam is a permeable structure with interconnection between the cells, the majority of which are open. The interconnectedness of the cellular matrix typically results in permeability to gases and liquids. It is a higher-specification foam that has been shown to be more effective in preventing pressure injuries than closed-cell foam. Examples of higher-specification foams are elastic and viscoelastic. There is no evidence that one type of high-specification foam is better than another (NPIAP, 2020).

Elastic Foam

Elastic foam is a chemically complex polymeric product having a broad range of load bearing capability and resiliency for comfort and cushioning typically characterized by an interconnected and open cell structure; the elastic nature of this foam causes it to resist deformation and return to its original shape after the stress (external force) that made it deform is removed. It is a high-specification foam made of a porous polymer material that conforms in proportion to the applied weight; air enters and exits the open-cell foam rapidly due to its greater density (NPIAP, 2020). The surface continues to conform until the resistance to compression exceeds the weight being applied. The combination of density and hardness determines compressibility and conformability, which determines the ability of the support surface to mechanically redistribute loading force. Density refers to the weight of the foam and is reported as either pounds per cubic foot or kilograms per cubic meter. Greater density provides more durability.

Indentation force deflection (IFD), known previously as indentation load deflection (ILD), is a measure of firmness or resistance to compression. In the United States, IFD is reported as the force in pounds required to compress a specific area of foam by 25%. Surfaces can be made with a combination of foams strategically placed to optimize pressure redistribution in targeted locations (Polyurethane Foam Association [PFA], 2010). For example, a mattress or cushion may be constructed with a lower-density and more compressible foam located close to the surface to enhance conformability and a higher-density and less compressible foam located more deeply in the mattress to prevent compression or bottoming out. See **Figure 22-1** for an example of a foam pressure redistribution device.

A foam overlay is a single-use form of support surface placed on the top of a mattress. If used for pressure redistribution, an overlay should have a base height of at least 3 inches measured from the base (or bottom)

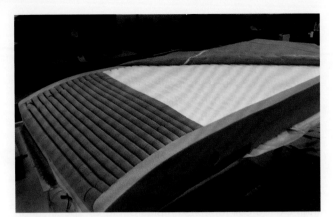

FIGURE 22-1. Foam Pressure Redistribution Surface.

to the lower level of convolution, sufficient density to ensure durability (1.3 to 1.6 pounds/feet³), and an IFD of 30 (Whittemore, 1998).

Viscoelastic (Memory) Foam

A viscoelastic foam is a type of porous polymer material which conforms in proportion to the applied weight. The material exhibits dampened elastic properties when load is applied. It is another high-specification open-cell foam made of a porous polymer material that conforms in proportion to the applied weight. Air enters and exits the foam cells slowly, which means the material responds more slowly than elastic foam. Viscoelastic foams are a subset of urethane polymer foams that exhibit a slow recovery (memory) property; these products generally have high density and low IFD, meaning they provide both conformability and support. Because of its fluid nature and low resistance, viscoelastic foam is rapidly displaced and conforms readily to the shape of any object placed on the surface. Viscoelastic foam is available in many grades and qualities; each has properties that affect pressure redistribution and microclimate performance in unique ways. Some viscoelastic foams are engineered to change hardness within a specific temperature range. These materials tend to get softer as the material warms to body temperature, resulting in conformability similar to that provided by a gel. Viscoelastic support surfaces are often used in the OR (Association of periOperative Registered Nurses [AORN], 2017) and have been shown to effectively decrease the incidence of pressure injuries in high-risk elderly patients with fractures of the neck and femur (Cullum et al., 2001). In one study of 838 patients at risk for pressure injuries, patients turned every 4 hours on a viscoelastic foam surface had lower incidence of pressure injury development than patients on a standard mattress who were turned every 2 hours. Park and Park found a significantly lower incidence of pressure injury with use of a viscoelastic foam surface (Defloor et al., 2005; Park & Park, 2017). (See **Fig. 22-2** for an example of viscoelastic foam.)

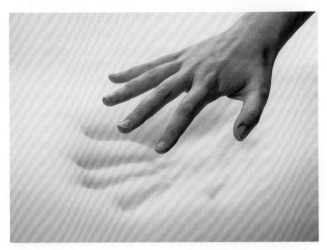

FIGURE 22-2. Viscoelastic Foam Surface. (Courtesy Tempur-Pedic.)

GEL

Gel is a semisolid system consisting of a network of solid aggregates, colloidal dispersions, or polymers which may exhibit elastic properties. Gels can range from hard to soft (NPIAP, 2020). Some gel products are called viscoelastic gel because they respond similarly to viscoelastic foam. Gel support surfaces are intended for multiple-patient use. Because of the consistency of the medium, gels have been found to be especially effective in preventing shear. Other advantages include ease of cleaning and that it is nonpowered and requires no electricity. Disadvantages of gel support surfaces are that they tend to be heavy and are difficult to repair. In addition, the nonporous nature of the gel and lack of airflow can result in increased skin moisture; although the gel is cool upon initial contact, skin temperature may rise after hours of constant contact. Gel must be carefully monitored for migration, and the material must be manually moved back to the areas under bony prominences if this has occurred (Brienza & Geyer, 2005).

FLUIDS (VISCOUS FLUID, WATER, AIR)

Fluids are considered substances whose molecules flow freely past one another. Fluids have no fixed shape, so they take on the shape of the load with less resistance than a gel or solid, providing a high degree of immersion. Fluid mediums include viscous fluid, water, and air. Moisture control characteristics are dependent on the ability of the medium to conduct heat and the composition of the product's cover.

Viscous Fluid

Viscous fluid is fluid having a molecular structure which produces sufficient internal friction to resist motion. It is composed of materials such as silicon elastomer, silicon, or polyvinyl (Brienza & Geyer, 2005). At first glance, viscous fluid can be mistaken for gel. Although many of the advantages and disadvantages are similar to those of gels, viscous fluid is free flowing and has a similar pressure redistribution response as air or water. Compared to air and water, viscous fluid is thicker, with a relatively higher resistance to flow (NPIAP, 2020).

Water

Water is a moderate-density fluid with moderate resistance to flow (NPIAP, 2020). Studies have demonstrated that water-filled support surfaces provide lower interface pressure than a standard mattress (Cullum et al., 2001). One small study (120 participants) found there was no clear difference in ulcer healing between water-filled support surfaces and foam replacement mattresses (McInnes et al., 2018). Although popular for use in the home, water mattresses are undesirable in the hospital or long-term care setting due to multiple management concerns including the need for a heater to control temperature; potential for leakage; difficulty associated with repositioning, transfers, performance of cardiopulmonary resuscitation (CPR), and the time and labor required to drain and move the bed.

Air

Air is a low-density fluid with minimal resistance to flow (NPIAP, 2020) and is frequently used medium for support surfaces. Air may be the sole redistribution medium, or it may be combined with other mediums (EPUAP/NPIAP/PPPIA, 2019). Support surfaces that incorporate air are available as chair cushions, overlays, mattresses, and bed systems. Most air support surfaces are easy to clean and can be reused. Air products have the potential to leak if damaged and require either periodic reinflation (nonpowered device) or a pump to maintain continuous inflation (powered device). Air mattresses and overlays have the advantage of being lightweight and easy to clean.

CATEGORIES AND FEATURES

Categories of pressure redistribution support surfaces include overlays, mattresses, and integrated bed systems. Pressure redistribution products may be purchased in the form of a mattress, mattress overlay, chair cushion, transport pad, procedure pad, emergency room pad, or perioperative surface. All of these surfaces may be powered or nonpowered, active or reactive. A feature is a therapeutic (functional) component of a support surface that can be used alone or in combination with other features and includes low air loss, air fluidization, lateral rotation, and alternating pressure (AP). Pressure redistribution surfaces can be either single- or multizoned surfaces; a zone is a segment with a single pressure redistribution capability. A multizoned surface has different segments with different pressure redistribution capabilities (NPIAP, 2020).

OVERLAYS

The mattress overlay is a support surface that is placed on the top of an existing mattress (NPIAP, 2020). Gel, water, and some air-filled overlays are intended for multiple-patient use and have the advantage of requiring much less storage space than mattresses and bed systems. Other overlays, such as foam and some air products, are for single-patient use and present environmental concerns relative to disposal of the product. Overlays are thinner than mattress replacements, so there is the risk for bottoming out, especially if the patient is heavy. Because they are applied over an existing mattress, mattress overlays increase the height of the sleep surface and may complicate patient transfers, alter the fit of linens, or increase the risk for patient entrapment and falls (U.S. Food and Drug Administration [U.S. FDA], 2006).

KEY POINT

Overlays should be used with caution, as they increase the risk for entrapment and falls and may permit the patient to bottom out.

MATTRESSES

A mattress is a full body support surface designed to be placed directly on the existing bed frame (NPIAP, 2020). It is composed of any medium or combination of mediums. Mattresses reduce some of the high-profile–related disadvantages experienced with overlays and generally present less risk for bottoming out. When therapeutic support surfaces were first introduced, the available options were essentially limited to rental beds (integrated support surfaces) or overlays that were rented or purchased. As the market evolved, manufacturers began to produce nonpowered mattresses that incorporated the features of pressure redistribution along with the usual features of hospital mattresses (e.g., durability, multiple-patient use following cleaning, etc.). These surfaces were initially known as replacement mattresses because agencies began to replace their standard mattresses with the therapeutic mattresses; for most agencies, this change resulted in improved skin and wound outcomes as well as reduced expenditures related to rental surfaces (Gray et al., 2001; McInnes et al., 2018). In addition, replacement mattresses eliminated wait time for delivery of bed systems and the need for staff to transfer the patient once they were identified as being at risk for pressure injury development. Most companies make mattresses that redistribute pressure, and therapeutic surfaces have become the standard of care for acute care facilities. Mattresses may provide a variety of therapeutic functions in addition to pressure redistribution, depending on the support medium and cover; selected products also provide shear and friction reduction and management of the microclimate between the patient's skin and the support surface.

INTEGRATED BED SYSTEMS

An integrated bed system is a bed frame and support surface combined into a single unit. It may be either a rented or purchased unit, but its components do not function separately (NPIAP, 2020). An integrated bed system is used in place of an existing bed. When recommending an integrated bed system, the wound care nurse must evaluate the features of both the frame and the support surface. Frames come in different heights, widths, and lengths and support a specified amount of weight. Some frames have the ability to adjust or fold for storage or for transport through narrow doors and elevators. Most frames are electric, but alternatives are available. When selecting a frame, the population to be served and the setting in which it will be used should be considered. For example, frames with bed exit alarms may be needed for patients who are confused and at risk for falls. Frames with bed scales may be needed for inpatient units and are often a standard feature.

PROCEDURE, TRANSPORT, EMERGENCY ROOM, AND OR MATTRESSES

Patients who require a support surface in bed would benefit from a support surface during transport on stretchers, while in the emergency department (ED) awaiting admission, and during special procedures (e.g., endoscopy, cardiac evaluation/procedures, or surgical procedures). Patients may be at greater risk while on these surfaces, due to the limited space for moving and repositioning in addition to their potential need for sedation or anesthesia. Pads are defined as a cushion-like mass of soft material used for comfort, protection, or positioning (NPIAP, 2020). Many ED or transport stretchers, and procedure or OR tables are now fitted with pads that provide pressure redistribution.

Prevention of perioperative pressure injuries has been identified as apriority for health care institutions across the country. International guidelines recommend that individuals at risk for perioperative pressure injury be placed on mattresses that provide higher-level pressure redistribution than standard OR mattresses (AORN, 2017; EPUAP/NPIAP/PPPIA, 2019). A standard OR mattress is defined as a 2-inch foam surface covered with a vinyl or nylon fabric (AORN, 2017). There are a number of uncontrolled variables in the surgical environment that may alter a patient's risk during the procedure, for example, reaction to anesthesia, unexpected prolongation of the surgical procedure, unanticipated hypotensive episodes, and temperature in the OR (Engels et al., 2016; Riemenschneider, 2018; Walton-Geer, 2009).

> **KEY POINT**
>
> Patients who need pressure redistribution when in bed also need pressure redistribution during transport and procedures. It is important to assure appropriate mattresses for ED or transport stretchers, and procedure or operating room (OR) tables.

A number of support surface options are now available for the OR, including air, viscoelastic polymer foam, and gel-based mattresses. The best OR surface to prevent the development of pressure injury due to surgical positioning is unknown (de Oliveira et al., 2017). McInnes et al. (2018) concluded that pressure redistribution overlays reduced the incidence of postoperative pressure injuries, but this finding may not be generalizable to all pressure-redistributing overlays. A study by Schultz et al. (1999) found that some overlays were associated with adverse postoperative skin changes. Selection of an OR support surface requires that the product provide effective pressure redistribution and be in compliance with the facility's surgical positioning procedures, safety protocols, and transfer equipment.

Pads and blankets (such as warming and cooling blankets) placed between the patient and the OR mattress will interfere with the pressure redistribution properties of the mattress. AORN (2017) specifically recommends use of a higher-grade pressure redistribution mattress when a cooling blanket is placed between the patient and the OR mattress.

CHAIR CUSHIONS

Individuals who remain seated for prolonged periods of time are predisposed to pressure injury, particularly in the ischial area. Wounds that develop from sitting are located on the ischial tuberosities during upright sitting and on the sacrum when slouching, sliding, or reclining. Pressure redistribution chair cushions should be used with seated individuals who are at risk for pressure injuries and have reduced mobility (EPUAP/NPIAP/PPPIA, 2019). General guidelines for chair cushion selection include matching the chair cushion to the individual patient, with attention to body size and configuration, postural effects, mobility, and lifestyle needs. An important aspect in product selection is to assure that the cushion and cover provide heat dissipation and air exchange at the skin–cushion interface (EPUAP/NPIAP/PPPIA, 2019). Selecting a cushion of appropriate size and depth is important. In the seated position, the weight of the body is supported by a relatively small surface area, which increases the risk for bottoming out. Cushions are available in both regular and bariatric size, and the appropriate size should be chosen based on the patient's weight and body configuration. Individuals who are wheelchair dependent should be evaluated by

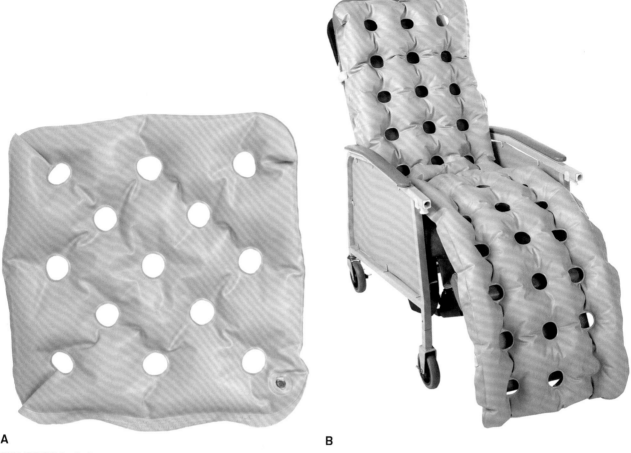

A

B

FIGURE 22-3. A. Reactive air seat cushion. **B.** A full reactive air chair cushion. (Courtesy EHOB, Inc.)

a seating specialist (if available) to assure the optimal selection of chair cushion (**Fig. 22-3**).

Chair cushions are available in a variety of support mediums, including foam, air, and gel. Some cushions also provide AP therapy. This therapy must be used with caution, that is, construction and operation of the cushion must be evaluated, and the benefits of off-loading must be weighed against the risk for instability and shear (EPUAP/NPIAP/PPPIA, 2019). The data regarding effectiveness of AP cushions are limited; their use has been studied in young spinal cord–injured patients (Makhsous et al., 2009) and in older hospitalized patients. There were mixed outcomes, leading Saha et al. (2013) to state that the strength of evidence is insufficient to draw generalizable conclusions.

Once implemented, chair cushions must be inspected regularly for wear and tear. Improper inflation, over-compression, or displaced gel can compromise pressure redistribution and lead to bottoming out. Appropriate training and maintenance must occur on a regular basis to ensure that the device is functioning properly and effectively meets the patient's needs.

Patients with existing ischial or sacral pressure injuries should avoid sitting for long periods of time until the

injury has completely healed. Individuals with existing pressure injuries should be referred to a seating specialist for evaluation if sitting is unavoidable.

Pressure redistribution chair cushions are recommended for all at-risk patients. They are available in a variety of sizes and support mediums. Ring cushions (doughnut devices) should not be used for pressure injury prevention or management (EPUAP/NPIAP/PPPIA, 2019; WOCN, 2016).

> **KEY POINT**
>
> Ring cushion (doughnut) devices increase venous congestion and edema and should not be used for pressure injury prevention and management.

ACTIVE (ALTERNATING PRESSURE)

An active support surface is a powered mattress or overlay that changes its load distribution properties with or without an applied load (NPIAP, 2020). High-risk patients should be placed on an active mattress or overlay when frequent repositioning is not possible (EPUAP/NPIAP/PPPIA, 2019).

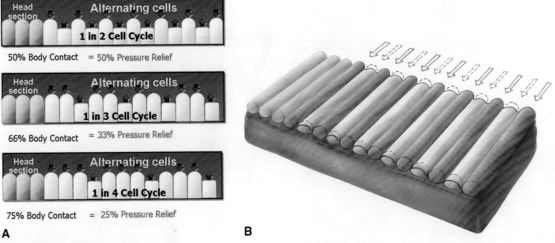

FIGURE 22-4. Alternating Pressure Device. **A.** Diagram depicting options for alternating pressure devices (2 vs. 3 vs. 4 cell models). **B.** Example of 2-cell model. (Courtesy Joerns, Inc.)

Alternating pressure is a feature found in both overlays and mattresses. These products are composed of air cells that can be cyclically inflated and deflated to provide pressure redistribution, and they periodically change the areas of the body under pressure by inflating and deflating the cells of alternating zones. They vary according to frequency, duration, amplitude, and rate of change parameters (Nixon et al., 2006; NPIAP, 2020). The individual cell that composes the alternating pressure mattress and/or overlay must be 10 cm or greater in depth to effectively redistribute pressure (EPUAP/NPIAP/PPPIA, 2019). Pulsating pressure is similar to alternating pressure but provides shorter duration inflation and higher-frequency cycling; there is less direct evidence supporting use of these products (NPIAP, 2020). Alternating pressure and pulsating pressure can be found in combination with foam and products with low air loss feature (**Fig. 22-4**).

KEY POINT

The use of an active support surface (mattress or overlay) is recommended for patients at increased risk for pressure injury where frequent manual repositioning is not possible.

REACTIVE

A reactive support surface moves or changes its load distribution properties only in response to an applied load, such as the patient's body (NPIAP, 2020). Reactive support surfaces may be either powered or nonpowered. The advantages of nonpowered surfaces are the lack of dependency on electricity or battery and the absence of noise associated with a motor. Examples of reactive support surfaces include mattresses and overlays filled with foam, air, or a combination of foam and air. Reactive surfaces are available as chair cushions, overlays, mattresses, and pads for ED or transport stretchers,

OR and procedure tables. Nonpowered air-filled support surfaces range from products that encapsulate air into a single bladder or cell to therapeutic products containing hundreds of cells. All reactive support surfaces are appropriate for pressure injury prevention in the patient who is frequently repositioned and may be appropriate for patients with existing pressure injuries. Reactive support surfaces are appropriate for use in long-term care facilities, hospitals, and home settings.

KEY POINT

Active surfaces are powered devices that change their load-bearing properties even if no weight is applied (alternating pressure devices); reactive surfaces may be powered or nonpowered devices and change their load-bearing properties only in response to applied weight (such as the patient's body).

LOW AIR LOSS

Low air loss is a feature that provides airflow to assist in managing the heat and humidity (microclimate) of the skin (NPIAP, 2020). Low air loss surfaces are composed of a series of connected pillows. A pump provides slow continuous airflow allowing for even distribution into the porous mattress and continuous airflow across the skin. The amount of pressure in each pillow can be calibrated according to height and weight distribution to meet the patient needs. As the patient sinks into the mattress, weight is evenly distributed for pressure redistribution. There may be an additional component at the base of the product, such as foam or air pillows, to prevent bottoming out. Low air loss may be used alone or in combination with alternating pressure, lateral rotation, and air-fluidized technology and may be incorporated into overlays, mattresses, bed systems, and chair cushions.

The construction of a low air loss surface that addresses the microclimate of the skin can be achieved in two ways, with airflow under the cover or with an air-permeable cover. Most familiar to clinicians is the air-permeable cover, which allows for the slow, evenly distributed release of air through the cover and directly to the skin. Low air loss surfaces with airflow under the cover addresses skin microclimate by receiving heat, gas, and water molecules through a moisture vapor-permeable cover (conducted downward from the skin), into the air stream inside the mattress, which eventually exits along the sides or ends of the mattress.

The smooth covers for low air loss surfaces are generally made of nylon or polytetrafluoroethylene fabric and have a low coefficient of friction (CoF). The covers are waterproof, impermeable to bacteria, and easy to clean. To obtain the full benefits of low air loss, layers of linen including underpads should be minimized. Underpads with a high level of moisture vapor permeability should be used rather than pads with plastic backing (McNichol et al., 2015).

Low air loss support surfaces have been reported as an effective treatment surface and may improve healing rates of pressure injuries (Saha et al., 2013). Because of the two aforementioned constructions (air-permeable cover vs. airflow under the cover), low air loss helps to reduce moisture and may help to prevent skin damage such as incontinence-associated dermatitis or maceration (McInnes et al., 2018; WOCN Society, 2016). There is some potential for wound desiccation, which may be prevented by using a hydrating rather than absorptive dressing (if necessary).

Low air loss surfaces come with safety features, such as controls that instantly inflate the cushions, facilitating patient positioning. Position sensors may adjust support for seated patients (Fowler Boost). This feature prevents bottoming out by adding more air under the buttocks when the patient's head is elevated. Controls that instantly flatten the air cushions are activated prior to administration of CPR allowing effective chest compressions.

Low air loss is contraindicated for patients with an unstable spine due to the lack of stability compared to a firmer mattress. Similarly, some patients lose their ability to effectively self-position on a low air loss surface, in part due to envelopment. Low air loss surfaces may increase the risk of bed entrapment in the bed rails, especially if the device is not properly adjusted. Clinicians and involved staff should follow the manufacturer's instructions for use. See **Figure 22-5** for example of bed with LAL feature.

AIR FLUIDIZED

The feature of air fluidization provides pressure redistribution by forcing air through a granular medium (e.g., silicone-coated beads) producing a fluid state (NPIAP,

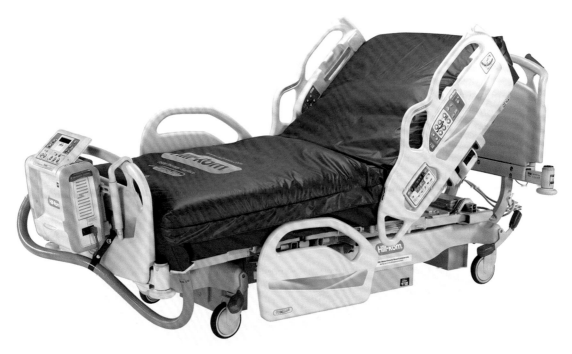

FIGURE 22-5. Surface with Low Air Loss Feature. (Courtesy Hillrom.)

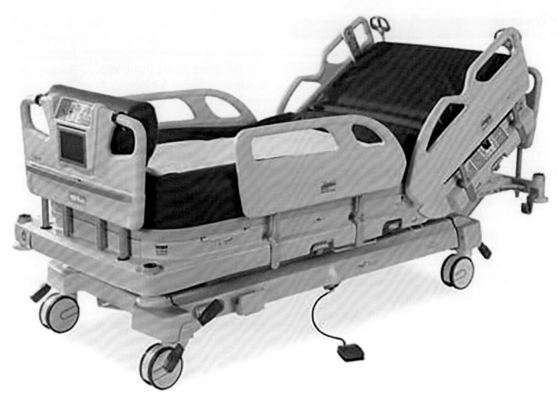

FIGURE 22-6. Bed with Air-fluidized Feature in Lower Section (Low Air Loss in Upper Section). (Courtesy Hillrom.)

2020). When air is pumped through the beads, the beads behave like a liquid. The person floats on the surface, with one third of the body above the surface and the rest of the body immersed in the warm, dry, fluidized beads. Body fluids flow freely through the sheet and cover, but contamination is prevented through continuous pressurization. When the air-fluidized bed is turned off, it quickly becomes firm enough for repositioning or CPR. Air fluidization is only available in integrated bed systems.

Air-fluidized beds are most commonly used for patients with burns, myocutaneous skin flaps, and multiple stage 3 or 4 pressure injuries. In the institutional environment, these products are not ideally suited to facility ownership because of the complexity and the high costs of maintenance (Ochs et al., 2005). An air-fluidized bed system is one of the most expensive support surfaces. Air-fluidized products have a warming feature for the pressurized air, which can be comforting or harmful depending on the overall condition of the patient. Hydration issues may be more pronounced than those experienced with low air loss surfaces. Because air-fluidized beds are heavy, they may not be safe for use in older homes. Traditional air-fluidized beds are not recommended for the patient with pulmonary disease or an unstable spine. Air-fluidized therapy in the lower half of the bed has been combined with low air loss in the upper portion of the surface to create an adjustable bed for the patient who needs to be more upright. This bed is similar in size to a hospital bed, the head of the bed is adjust-

able, and the bed weighs less than a total air-fluidized system. See **Figure 22-6** for example of air-fluidized bed.

CONTINUOUS LATERAL ROTATION THERAPY

Continuous lateral rotation therapy (CLRT) is a feature used for the prevention and treatment of selected cardiopulmonary conditions. CLRT involves rotation of the patient in a regular pattern around a longitudinal (i.e., head-to-foot) axis; rotation is limited to 40 degrees or less to each side over a prescribed length of time ranging from minutes to hours (NPIAP, 2020). Kinetic therapy is defined as the side-to-side rotation of 40 degrees or more to each side. These surfaces are primarily used to facilitate pulmonary hygiene in the patient with acute respiratory conditions, and it is difficult to draw conclusions regarding their effectiveness in pressure injury prevention.

Continuous lateral rotation therapy has been incorporated into some low air loss and air/foam mattresses, overlays, and integrated bed systems. CLRT does not eliminate the need for routine manual repositioning. Nursing care providers need to incorporate measures to protect the patient against shear, including aligning and securing the patient with bolster pads provided by the manufacturer, and frequent skin inspection for any indications of shear damage. If the staff discovers a new shear injury, the patient should be positioned off the involved area and placed on an alternative support surface if clinically feasible. If the patient remains in respiratory distress, the pulmonary benefits of CLRT should

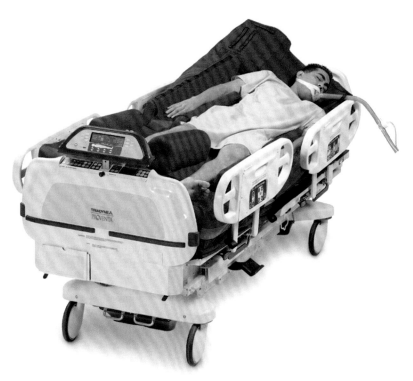

FIGURE 22-7. Continuous Lateral Rotation Therapy. (TriaDyne images courtesy of ArjoHuntleigh Inc.)

be carefully balanced against the potential for additional skin damage, with the decision based on the patient's overall condition and need for therapy (EPUAP/NPIAP/PPPIA, 2019). See **Figure 22-7** for example of continuous lateral rotation therapy.

KEY POINT

Continuous lateral rotation therapy devices are designed for pulmonary care and do not replace manual repositioning for pressure injury prevention.

 MATCHING THE PRODUCT TO THE PATIENT

Wound care nurses and other health care providers should maintain up-to-date knowledge regarding pressure redistribution along with the other therapeutic features provided by support surfaces. The wound care nurse must be familiar with the performance characteristics of support surfaces to match individual patient needs to the appropriate support surface. The wound care nurse should use a web-based clinical decision support tool such as the WOCN Evidence- and Consensus-Based Support Surface Algorithm (http://algorithm.wocn.org) to match patients to the appropriate support surfaces.

INDIVIDUAL PATIENT NEEDS

Individuals with pressure injuries or those at risk for pressure injuries should be placed on a support surface rather than on a standard hospital mattress (EPUAP/NPIAP/PPPIA, 2019; WOCN, 2016). Support surfaces should be selected based on assessment of the patient and their needs and not on the patient's wound (EPUAP/NPIAP/PPPIA, 2019). Criteria include need for microclimate control, activity and positioning limitations, risk for falls and entrapment, body habitus including height and weight, and patient comfort or discomfort on the support surface.

CLINICAL CONSIDERATIONS

All patients with existing pressure injuries should be placed on a surface that provides pressure redistribution (e.g., high-density foam, low air loss, alternating pressure, viscous fluid, or air-fluidized surface). A support surface that dissipates moisture (low air loss) may be indicated for the diaphoretic patient or the patient with large amounts of wound drainage or incontinence not contained by dressings and absorptive products (McNichol et al., 2015). Patients who require head-of-bed elevation may benefit from a surface that provides low CoF.

ACTIVITY AND POSITIONING

Patients who have been identified as being at a moderate-high level of risk for pressure injuries are typically placed on an every 2-hour turning and repositioning schedule. While this is the standard of care in most care settings, the results from a multisite RCT conducted in a long-term care setting concluded that patients lying on a high-density foam mattress may benefit from a more individualized turning schedule, for example, every 2, 3, or 4 hours. Additional benefits, including improved quality of life, increased sleep, fewer staff injuries, and more time for activities of daily living, may be seen with a less strict turning and repositioning schedule (Bergstrom et al., 2014). If frequent repositioning is not possible, an active support surface is recommended (EPUAP/NPIAP/PPPIA, 2019). When prolonged head-of-bed elevation is required, there is increased risk for bottoming out, and the wound care nurse should consider changing from an overlay to a mattress. The patient who self-repositions, gets in and out of the bed, or is attempting to increase mobility and independence should be placed on a surface that facilitates rather than impairs activity and mobility.

> **KEY POINT**
>
> Active support surfaces (alternating pressure devices) are recommended for individuals who cannot be routinely and effectively repositioned.

RISK FOR FALLS OR ENTRAPMENT

A surface that increases the patient's overall height in bed (overall distance from the underlying bed frame) or creates more distance between the mattress and side rails increases the risk for entrapment and falls. A pressure redistribution surface that also minimizes height and gaps should be selected for patients at risk for falls (U.S. FDA, 2006). Some facilities are adding fall risk assessment scores to support surface selection criteria to ensure that it is considered in the selection process. If the patient becomes at risk for falls or entrapment on a selected support surface, additional monitoring will be necessary or an alternative support surface should be selected (Nix & Mackey, 2016). Some facilities utilize bed frames that go down close to the floor (low beds). Combining a low bed with a pressure redistribution mattress addresses both safety concerns and the need for pressure injury prevention.

SIZE AND WEIGHT

Bed frame and mattress specifications for weight capacity must be considered. Low air loss products designed for adults do not provide options to accommodate the height and weight of small children (WOCN, 2016). Children and infants can sink into and between cushions, leading to risk for entrapment and falls (McLane et al., 2004).

The bariatric patient presents challenges in terms of skin integrity, including increased risk for pressure injury and for moisture-associated skin damage (MASD), specifically intertriginous dermatitis (ITD). Admission assessment and support surface selection should include the potential need for a bariatric frame and support surface. A trapeze may be used to reduce shear over the sacrum during repositioning. Bariatric support surfaces are available in foam, air, gel, and water with or without microclimate and moisture control features. Adult hospital bed frames have weight limits between 350 and 500 pounds. The width of bed frames may prevent effective repositioning of bariatric patients. In addition to weight,

the wound care nurse should consider the patient's body habitus and width when selecting a bed frame and surface. For example, shorter patients and those with truncal obesity may fall within the weight restrictions of the bed, but their width may prevent safe repositioning to prevent prolonged contact between the skin and the side rails. Bariatric patients should be educated regarding the importance of repositioning and should be encouraged to make small position changes at regular intervals and to keep the head of the bed below 30 degrees. See Chapter 15 for additional information about care of the bariatric patient.

REEVALUATING SUPPORT SURFACES

Support surfaces should be routinely reevaluated. Discontinuing or changing a support surface may be warranted when there are changes in a patient's overall condition or change in care setting. For example, the patient who was hemodynamically unstable but is improving may require a different support surface to facilitate independence with activity and mobility, including turning and repositioning. Another example is the patient who develops delirium and is at increased risk for falls. In this case, the patient may need a low bed and a pressure redistribution mattress (Nix & Mackey, 2016).

CARE SETTING–SPECIFIC FORMULARY

The development and implementation of a care setting-specific formulary describing the support surfaces available can minimize staff confusion, manage costs, and improve access to appropriate products. Considerations for particular care settings include issues of reimbursement, rental versus purchase options, product maintenance, safety features, and facility responsibilities. Once these considerations are analyzed, a formulary can be created with a range of products intended to meet the needs of the patient population. Innovative and creative decision-making tools are essential in educating staff regarding guidelines for support surface selection (McNichol et al., 2020). See **Figure 22-8** for sample algorithm for support surface selection, available to all at https://algorithm.wocn.org.

SUPPORT SURFACE INITIATIVE (S3I)

NPIAP's Support Surface Standards Initiative (S3I) has focused efforts on the definitions, objective testing, and comparable reporting of therapeutic features such as immersion, envelopment, and microclimate management. In 2017, the International Standards Organization (ISO) endorsed, approved, and published the S3I standardized test methods for immersion, envelopment, and heat and moisture dissipation. These standards help consumers in product comparisons. They also serve as a guide for manufacturers in new product development (Thurman et al., 2017).

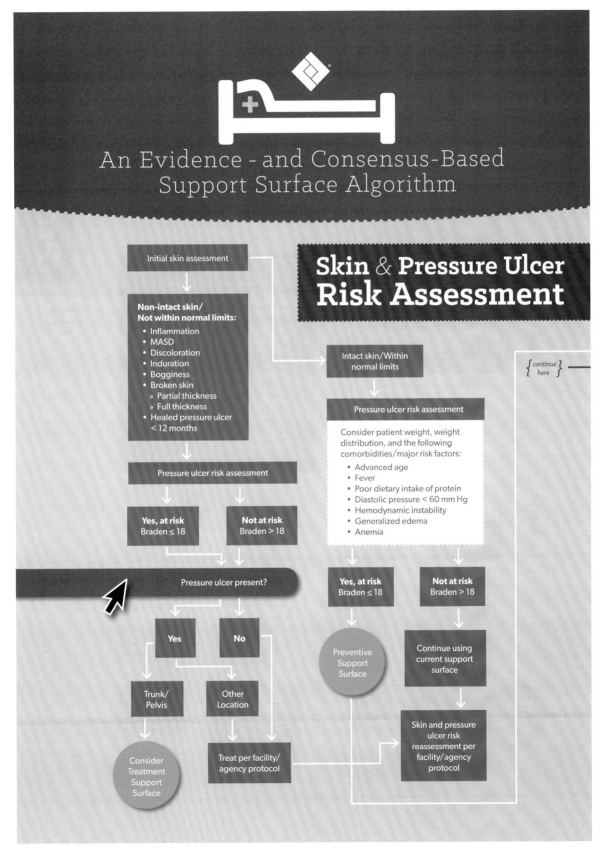

FIGURE 22-8. Algorithm for Support Surface Selection. (Copyright WOCN.)

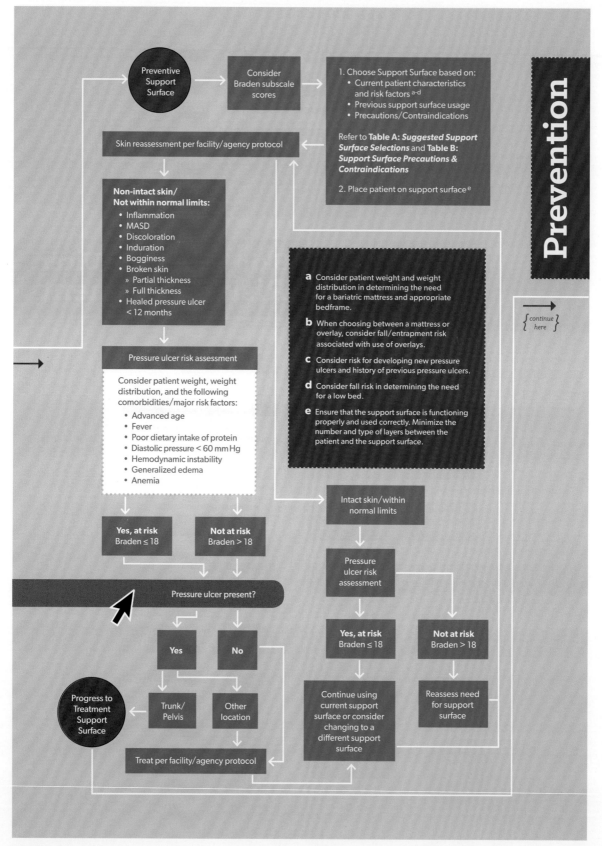

FIGURE 22-8 (*Continued*)

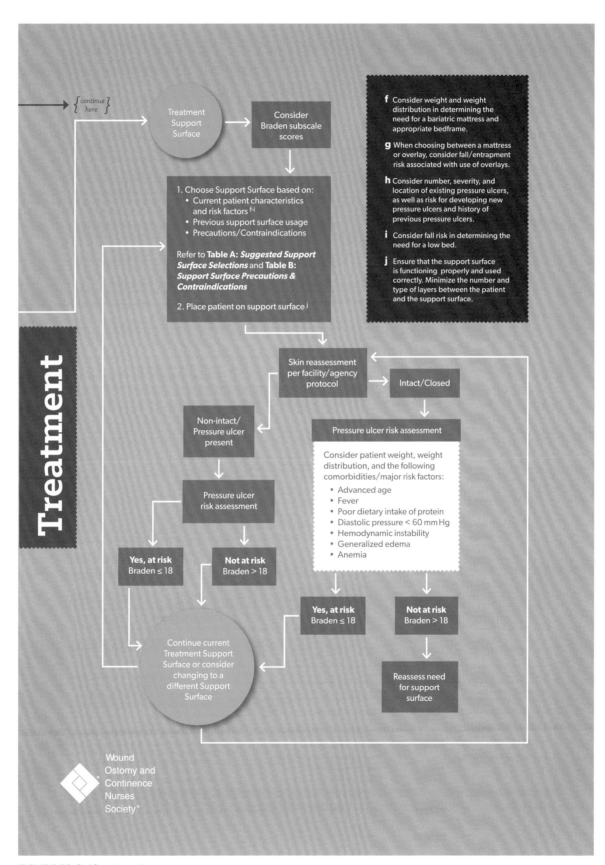

FIGURE 22-8 (*Continued*)

TABLE A:

Suggested Support Surface Overlay or Mattress Selections for Pressure Ulcer Prevention & Treatment Based on Braden Mobility & Moisture Subscores

[a] Braden B, Bergstrom N. http://bradenscale. com/images/bradenscale.pdf. Copyright 1988. Accessed August 8, 2014.

[b] In this table, Reactive/CLP refers to all types of Support Surfaces in this category with the exception of AMG sheep skin overlays, which are noted separately.

[c] AMG sheepskin is available for purchase through online suppliers.

Note: Persons with multiple Stage II, or large (of sufficient size to compromise a turning surface) or multiple Stage III or Stage IV pressure ulcers on the trunk or pelvis involving more than one available turning surface should be placed on a support surface with a low air loss or an air fluidized feature.

BRADEN MOISTURE SUBSCALE SCORES	BRADEN MOBILITY SUBSCALE SCORES[a]	
	4 or 3 No limitation or slightly limited	**2 or 1** Very limited or completely immobile
4 or 3 Rarely or occasionally moist	• Reactive/CLP[b] (air, foam, gel, fiber, or viscous fluid, or combinations) • AMG sheepskin overlay (Prevention only) [c]	• Reactive/CLP • Active with AP feature
2 Very moist	• Reactive/CLP • Reactive/CLP with LAL feature	• Reactive/CLP with LAL feature
1 Constantly moist	• Reactive/CLP • Reactive/CLP with LAL feature	• Reactive/CLP with LAL feature • Reactive/CLP with AF feature (Treatment only)

AF = air fluidized; AMG = Australian Medical grade; AP = alternating pressure; CLP = constant low pressure; LAL = low air loss.

[a] Refer to manufacturer specifications, including product lifespan. Staff who have ongoing exposure to support surfaces during bedding or room changes should practice a continual awareness and opportunity-based observation of support surface lifespan indicators, including reduced height or thickness; discoloration; altered integrity of cover, seams, zipper/ zipper cover flap, or backing; degradation of internal components, or presence of odor. If any of these are observed, it is recommended that the surface be referred to engineering/ maintenance for testing or evaluation for continued use, irrespective of stated product lifespan.

[b] High risk for moisture penetration with potential for infection.

TABLE B:
Select Support Surface Precautions & Contraindications[a]

SUPPORT SURFACE	PRECAUTIONS	CONTRAINDICATIONS
High-specification foam	• Braden moisture subscale score of 2 or 1[b]	• Weight limitations for surface–may require another product in this category with higher weight limit
Reactive/CLP	• NA	• Unstable cervical, thoracic or lumbar spine • Cervical or skeletal traction • Weight limitations for surface–may require another product in this category with higher weight limit
Active with AP feature	• NA	
Reactive/CLP with LAL feature	• Combative/restless/agitated state	
Reactive/CLP with AF feature	• Combative/restless/agitated state • Need for aggressive pulmonary toilet • Need for frequent head elevation • Need for mobilization • Claustrophobia	• Unstable cervical, thoracic or lumbar spine • Cervical or skeletal traction • Weight limitations for surface–may require another product in this category with higher weight limit • Trendelenburg positioning

AF = air fluidized; AP = alternating pressure; CLP = constant low pressure; LAL = low air loss.

FIGURE 22-8 (*Continued*)

CONCLUSION

Support surfaces are one element of a comprehensive pressure injury prevention program. They do not eliminate the need for routine repositioning. The primary therapeutic feature for all support surfaces is pressure redistribution. Selected surfaces also provide shear reduction and microclimate control. Effective use of support surfaces requires an understanding of the various features and products available, coupled with a comprehensive patient assessment. Use of a support surface algorithm guides decision-making.

REFERENCES

Association of periOperative Registered Nurses (AORN). (2017). Guideline summary: Positioning the patient. *AORN Journal, 106*(3), e1–e72. Retrieved from https://aornjournal-onlinelibrary-wiley-com.proxy.lib.duke.edu/doi/epdf/10.1016/j.aorn.2017.07.006. Accessed on March 14, 2020.

Bergstrom, N., Horn, S. D., Rapp, M., et al. (2014). Preventing pressure ulcers: a multisite randomized controlled trial in nursing homes. *Ontario Health Technology Assessment Series, 14*(11), 1031.

Brienza, D. M., & Geyer, M. J. (2005). Using support surfaces to manage tissue integrity. *Advances in Skin & Wound Care, 18*(3), 151–157.

Cullum, N., Nelson, E. A., Flemming, K., et al. (2001). Systematic reviews of wound care management: (5) beds; (6) compression; (7) laser therapy, therapeutic ultrasound, electrotherapy and electromagnetic therapy, *Health Technology Assessment, 5*(9), 1–221.

de Oliveira, K. F., Nascimento, K. G., Nicolussi, A. C., et al. (2017). Support surfaces in the prevention of pressure ulcers in surgical patients: An integrative review. *International Journal of Nursing Practice, 23*(4), e12553. doi.org/10.1111/ijn.12553.

Defloor, T., De Bacquer, D., & Grypdonck, M. H. (2005). The effect of various combinations of turning and pressure reducing devices on the incidence of pressure ulcers. *International Journal of Nursing Studies, 42*(1), 37–46.

Engels, D., Austin, M., McNichol, L., et al. (2016). Pressure ulcers: factors contributing to their development in the OR. *AORN Journal, 103*(3), 271–281. doi: 10.1016/j.aorn.2016.01.008.

European Pressure Ulcer Advisory Panel, National Pressure Injury Advisory Panel, and Pan Pacific Pressure Injury Alliance [EPUAP/NPIAP/PPPIA]. (2019). In E. Haesler (Ed.), *Prevention and treatment of pressure ulcers/injuries: Clinical Practice Guideline*. The International Guideline.

Gray, D., Cooper, P. J., & Stringfellow, S. (2001). Evaluating pressure-reducing foam mattresses and electric bed frames. *British Journal of Nursing, 10*(Suppl 22), s23.

Iglesias, C., Nixon, J., Cranny, G., et al. (2006). Pressure relieving support surfaces (PRESSURE) trial: Cost effectiveness analysis. *British Medical Journal, 332*(7555), 1416.

Le, K. M., Madsen, B. L., Barth, P. W., et al. (1984). An in-depth look at pressure sores using monolithic silicon pressure sensors. *Plastic and Reconstructive Surgery, 74*(6), 745.

Makhsous, M., Lin, F., Knaus, E., et al. (2009). Promote pressure ulcer healing in individuals with spinal cord injury using an individualized cyclic pressure-relief protocol. *Advances in Skin & Wound Care, 22*(11), 514–521.

McInnes, E., Jammali-Blasi, A., Bell-Syer, S. E., et al. (2018). Support surfaces for pressure injury prevention. *Cochrane Database of Systematic Reviews*, (94), CD009490. doi.org/10.1002/14651858. CD009490.pub2.

McLane, K. M., Bookout, K., McCord, S., et al. (2004). The 2003 national pediatric pressure ulcer and skin breakdown prevalence survey: A multisite study. *Journal of Wound, Ostomy, and Continence Nursing, 31*(4), 168–178.

McNichol, L., Mackey, D., Watts, C., et al. (2020). Choosing a support surface for pressure injury prevention and treatment. *Nursing, 50*(2), 41–44. doi.org/10.1097/01.NURSE.0000651620.87023.d5.

McNichol, L., Watts, C., Mackey, D., et al. (2015). Identifying the right surface for the right patient at the right time: generation and content validation of an algorithm for support surface selection. *Journal of Wound, Ostomy, and Continence Nursing, 42*(1), 19–37.

Miller, S., Parker, M., Blasiole, N., et al. (2013). A prospective, in vivo evaluation of two pressure-redistribution surfaces in healthy volunteers using pressure mapping as a quality control instrument. *Ostomy/Wound Management, 59*(2), 44–48.

National Pressure Injury Advisory Panel (NPIAP). (2015). Hand check method: Is it an effective method to monitor for bottoming out? A National Pressure Ulcer Advisory Position Statement. Retrieved on March 2, 2020 from https://cdn.ymaws.com/npuap.site-ym.com/resource/resmgr/position_statements/hand-check-position-statemen.pdf

National Pressure Injury Advisory Panel (NPIAP). (2020). Support surface standards initiative (S3I): Terms and definitions related to support surfaces. Retrieved on March 1, 2020, from https://cdn.ymaws.com/npiap.com/resource/resmgr/website_version_terms_and_de.pdf

Nicholson, G. P., Scales, J. T., Clark, R. P., et al. (1999). A method for determining the heat transfer and water vapour permeability of patient support systems. *Medical Engineering & Physics, 21*(10), 701.

Nix, D., & Mackey, D. (2016). Support surfaces. In R. Bryant & D. Nix (Eds.), *Acute and chronic wounds; Current management concepts* (5th ed., pp. 162–176). St. Louis, MO: Elsevier.

Nixon, J., Cranny, G., Iglesias, C., et al. (2006). Randomised, controlled trial of alternating pressure mattresses compared with alternating pressure overlays for the prevention of pressure ulcers: PRESSURE (pressure relieving support surfaces) trial. *British Medical Journal, 332*(7555), 1413.

Ochs, R. F., Horn, S. D., van Rijswijk, L., et al. (2005). Comparison of air-fluidized therapy with other support surfaces used to treat pressure ulcers in nursing home residents. *Ostomy/Wound Management, 51*(2), 38.

Park, K. H., & Park, J. (2017). The efficacy of a viscoelastic foam overlay on prevention of pressure injury in acutely ill patients. *Journal of Wound, Ostomy, and Continence Nursing, 44*(5), 440–444. doi: 10.1097/WON.0000000000000359.

Polyurethane Foam Association (PFA). (2010). Joint industry foam standards and guidelines. Indentation force deflection (IFD) standards and guidelines. Retrieved October 5, 2010, from http://www.pfa.org/jifsg/jifsgs4.html

Reger, S. I., McGovern, T. F., Chung, K.-C., et al. (1988). Correlation of transducer systems for monitoring tissue interface pressures. *Journal of Clinical Engineering, 13*(5), 365–370.

Riemenschneider, K. J. (2018). Prevention of pressure injuries in the operating room: A quality improvement project. *Journal of Wound, Ostomy, and Continence Nursing, 45*(2), 141–145. doi: 10.1097/WON.0000000000000410.

Saha, S., Smith, M. B., Totten, A., et al. (2013). *Pressure ulcer treatment strategies: Comparative effectiveness. Comparative Effectiveness Review No. 90. (Prepared by the Oregon Evidence-based Practice Center under Contract No. 290-2007-10057-I.) AHRQ Publication No. 13-EHC003-EF*. Rockville, MD: Agency for Healthcare Research and Quality.

Schultz, A. A., Bien, M., Dumond, K., et al. (1999). Etiology and incidence of pressure ulcers in surgical patients. *AORN Journal, 70*(3), 434–449.

Thurman, K., Jordan, R., & Call, E. (2017). Support Surface Standards Initiative: Standards published. *Journal of Wound, Ostomy, and Continence Nursing, 44*(3), S24–S25.

U.S. Food and Drug Administration (U.S. FDA), Center for Devices and Radiological Health. (2006). Guidance Document. Hospital Bed System Dimensional and Assessment Guidance to Reduce Entrapment. Content current as of 08/23/2018. Retrieved from https://www.fda.gov/regulatory-information/search-fda-guidance-documents/

hospital-bed-system-dimensional-and-assessment-guidance-re-duce-entrapment. Accessed March 3, 2020.

Walton-Geer, P. (2009). Prevention of pressure ulcers in the surgical patient. *AORN Journal, 89*(3), 538–552.

Whitney, J., Phillips, L., Aslam, R., et al. (2006). Guidelines for the treatment of pressure ulcers. *Wound Repair and Regeneration, 14*(6), 663–679.

Whittemore, R. (1998). Pressure-reduction support surfaces: A review of the literature. *Journal of Wound, Ostomy, and Continence Nursing, 25*, 6.

Wound Ostomy and Continence Nurses Society (WOCN). (2016). *Guideline for management of pressure injuries/ulcers, WOCN Clinical Practice Guideline Series #2*. Mt. Laurel, NJ: Author.

QUESTIONS

1. The wound care nurse is recommending a support surface for a patient at risk for pressure injury. Which of the following is true?
A. Support surfaces should be used as a stand-alone intervention for the prevention and treatment of pressure injuries.
B. Correctly using support surfaces eliminates the need for turning and repositioning.
C. Layers of linen and underpads between the patient and the support surface should be minimized.
D. Active support surfaces with an AP feature are not more effective in preventing pressure injuries than standard hospital mattresses.

2. For which patient would the wound care nurse recommend placement on a reactive support surface with a LAL or AF feature?
A. A patient with multiple stage 2 pressure injuries
B. A patient with Braden Mobility score of 2
C. A patient at risk for pressure injuries with a mobility subscale score of 1
D. A patient who exceeds the weight limit of the current support surface

3. A patient is on a continuous lateral rotation therapy (CLRT) support surface. Which of the following describes this therapy?
A. CLRT involves rotation of the patient around a latitudinal (i.e., side-to-side) axis.
B. CLRT is primarily used to prevent and treat pressure injuries.
C. CLRT rotation is limited to 90 degrees or more over a prescribed length of time.
D. CLRT is primarily used to prevent and treat cardiopulmonary conditions.

4. Which general practice point for using support surfaces follows recommended guidelines for prevention and management of patients with pressure injuries?

A. Choose a support surface based on availability within the facility and cost of product.
B. Make sure that the patient can assume a variety of positions on the surface without bottoming out.
C. Use an overlay over a mattress if the patient has a considerable risk for fall or entrapment.
D. Choose a regular mattress over a support surface when patient incontinence cannot be managed by other means.

5. In most cases what is the most important therapeutic feature of a support surface to prevent or treat pressure injuries?
A. Pressure redistribution
B. Cooling effect
C. Moisture barrier
D. Friction reduction

6. A wound care nurse recommends a support surface for a patient who is at risk for pressure injuries. The nurse explains to the patient that the mechanism works by
A. Increasing tissue load
B. Reducing fatigue
C. Decreasing interface pressure
D. Increasing air pressure

7. The wound care nurse is assessing the "envelopment" feature of a support surface being used for a patient who has a sacral pressure injury. What factor would the nurse check?
A. Depth to which the body is allowed to penetrate the surface
B. Reduced performance capacity due to use
C. Ability of the support surface to conform evenly to irregularities
D. Degree to which the surface reduces pressure

8. A wound care nurse is investigating the use of a foam overlay for a patient with chronic wounds. Which statement correctly describes a characteristic of a type of foam product?
   A. *Closed-cell* foam is a higher-specification foam that has been shown to be more effective in reeventing pressure injuries than open-cell foam.
   B. *A viscoelastic* foam allows air to enter and exit the foam cells slowly, which means the material responds more quickly than elastic foam.
   C. Gel support surfaces are intended for single-patient use and have been found to be effective in preventing shear.
   D. Indentation force deflection (IFD), known previously as indentation load deflection (ILD), is a measure of firmness or resistance to compression.

9. The wound care nurse recommends an active (alternating pressure) surface for a patient with an ischial pressure injuries. What is the advantage of this type of surface?
   A. It does not need power to operate it.
   B. It is effective for high-risk patients when frequent positioning is not available.
   C. It does not make noise when it is operating.
   D. It facilitates pulmonary hygiene in the patient with acute respiratory condition.

10. The wound care nurse is deciding on a support surface for a patient who requires head-of-bed elevation for tube feedings. What additional benefit might influence the choice?
   A. Provision of shear reduction
   B. Dissipation of moisture
   C. Facilitation of activity
   D. Minimization of the height of the bed and gaps

ANSWERS AND RATIONALES

1. C. Rationale: To obtain the full benefits of low air loss, layers of linen including underpads should be minimized. Underpads with a high level of moisture vapor permeability should be used rather than pads with plastic backing.

2. A. Rationale: All reactive support surfaces are appropriate for pressure injury prevention in the patient who is frequently repositioned and may be appropriate for patients with existing pressure injuries.

3. D. Rationale: Continuous lateral rotation therapy (CLRT) is a feature used for the prevention and treatment of selected cardiopulmonary conditions.

4. B. Rationale: Bottoming out means the overlay or mattress is providing insufficient support and the patient's bony prominences are resting on the underlying bed frame; this mandates a change in support surface.

5. A. Rationale: In most situations, pressure redistribution is the most important feature of a support surface.

6. C. Rationale: Therapeutic support surfaces work primarily by reducing the intensity of interface pressure. Interface pressure measurements have been used for years to compare various products in terms of their pressure redistribution ability.

7. C. Rationale: The term envelopment refers to the ability of a support surface to conform, so to fit or mold around irregularities in the body (e.g., clothing, bedding, bony prominences) without causing a substantial increase in pressure.

8. D. Rationale: Indentation force deflection (IFD), known previously as indentation load deflection (ILD), is a measure of firmness or resistance to compression.

9. B. Rationale: An active support surface is a powered mattress or overlay that changes its load distribution properties with or without an applied load (NPIAP, 2020). High-risk patients should be placed on an active mattresses or overlay when frequent repositioning is not possible.

10. A. Rationale: Head of bed should be kept low to reduce sliding, but this is very difficult to accomplish in situations requiring head-of-bed elevation. A support surface cannot provide total protection against shear and does not eliminate the need for additional interventions to minimize friction and shear.

CHAPTER 23

DIFFERENTIAL ASSESSMENT OF LOWER EXTREMITY WOUNDS

Laurie L. McNichol, Catherine R. Ratliff, and Stephanie S. Yates

OBJECTIVES

1. Describe critical parameters to be included in assessment of the individual with a lower extremity wound.

2. Use assessment data to determine causative and contributing factors for a lower extremity wound and to develop evidence-based individualized management plans.

3. Compare and contrast arterial, venous, neuropathic, and wounds of mixed etiology in terms of risk factors,

pathology, clinical presentation, and management guidelines.

4. Identify indications that a lower extremity wound is "atypical" and requires additional interprofessional collaboration and intervention.

5. Describe indications for referral to vascular, orthopedics, podiatry, dermatology, and prosthetics and orthotics.

TOPIC OUTLINE

INTRODUCTION

Previous chapters in this text have addressed general principles related to wound healing, wound assessment, and wound management, and the following chapters in this section will describe the pathology, clinical

presentation, and management of lower extremity wounds, including venous ulcers, arterial ulcers, and neuropathic ulcers. Chapter 27 will address the pathology and management of common "atypical" lower extremity wounds.

Lower extremity wounds are very common, especially in the older adult population, due to the increasing prevalence of the underlying disease processes associated with development of these ulcers. Venous ulcers are the most common type of lower extremity wound; approximately 70% of leg ulcers are caused by venous disease and 20% are caused by arterial insufficiency or mixed arteriovenous disease (Agale, 2013; Alavi et al., 2016; Nelson & Adderly, 2016). Approximately 85% of foot ulcers are caused by peripheral neuropathy, often complicated by arterial disease (Singer et al., 2017); however, the incidence of arterial and neuropathic ulcers is rising, due in part to the increasing prevalence of poorly controlled diabetes. Current estimates suggest that >9% of the U.S. population is affected by diabetes (CDC, 2017), and these numbers are expected to rise with the continued increase in the number and percent of adults and children who are obese or morbidly obese.

Lower extremity wounds present a major burden to the health care system; they are costly to treat, they are frequently refractory to standard wound care, and there is a high risk for recurrence. Downstream societal impact includes loss of productivity and out of pocket costs of dressings and supplies (Rice et al., 2014; WOCN, 2019a). Even with the best care currently available, 25% to 50% of leg ulcers and more than 30% of foot ulcers are not fully healed after 6 months of treatment (Singer et al., 2017). Thus, comprehensive and evidence-based management is essential, as are ongoing patient education and routine follow-up to minimize the risk of recurrence.

KEY POINT

Lower extremity wounds are costly to treat, frequently refractory and at high risk for recurrence; thus, comprehensive and evidence-based management is essential, as are ongoing patient education and routine follow-up.

 ## DIFFERENTIAL ASSESSMENT OF LOWER EXTREMITY WOUNDS

The critical "first step" in effective management of any wound is accurate determination of the etiologic factors followed by interventions to correct those factors. This step is of particular importance in management of lower extremity ulcers, because interventions that are essential to effective management of a venous ulcer (leg elevation and compression therapy) are typically *contraindicated* with an arterial ulcer and of no benefit in management of a neuropathic ulcer. Thus, accurate differential assessment is an essential skill for the wound care nurse.

ASSESSMENT OF MEDICAL HISTORY AND RISK FACTORS

Accurate differential assessment begins with the patient interview (history) and physical examination. In conducting the patient interview, the nurse must ask specific questions related to known risk factors for venous insufficiency, arterial insufficiency, and neuropathy. For example, DVT, obesity, a sedentary lifestyle, and impaired calf muscle pump are known risk factors for venous insufficiency, while coronary artery disease, hyperlipidemia, hypertension, diabetes, and tobacco use are the primary risk factors for arterial insufficiency and, in the United States, longstanding diabetes and metabolic disorders are the most common risk factors for neuropathy. The nurse should be aware that many individuals, especially elder adults, will have risk factors for all types of lower extremity wounds; thus, the history is insufficient, in and of itself, to determine the etiology of the wound. (Refer to Appendix 1, WOCN Venous, Arterial, and Neuropathic Lower-Extremity Wounds: Clinical Resource Guide (2019b).)

ASSESSMENT OF COMORBID CONDITIONS

Certain health conditions confound and complicate the treatment of lower extremity ulcers. Patients with venous ulcers may also have coexisting heart failure, lymphedema, orthopedic procedures, and hypercoagulable states. Arterial ulcers may be associated with cardiovascular disease, cerebrovascular disease, and spinal cord injury. Patients with neuropathic ulcers also often have lower extremity arterial disease and renal disease. Adjustment to treatment plan may be needed to accommodate these conditions. (Refer to Appendix 1.)

ULCER HISTORY

Additional elements of the patient history of particular benefit to differential assessment are medications, which provide additional clues regarding the individual's comorbid conditions and risk factors, and ulcer history, to include onset, triggering factors, and previous treatment and response. The patient with a venous ulcer may report that the ulcer began with a small cut or insect bite, while the patient with an arterial ulcer may report spontaneous necrosis of the toes or a traumatic injury that failed to heal and developed into a steadily worsening ulcer. The patient with a neuropathic ulcer may be unaware as to when and how the ulcer began due to loss of normal sensation. ("I just noticed I had drainage on my sock and started looking and found it.") Response to previous treatment also provides important clues (WOCN, 2012, 2014, 2019a).

PAIN HISTORY

One of the assessment parameters most critical to differential assessment is the pain history; the nurse should carefully query the patient as to the location, severity, and characteristics of any wound-related pain, and about exacerbating and relieving factors. Classic descriptors of pain for each type of ulcer are as follows:

- *Venous ulcers*: pain is typically described as aching, heavy, and dull and typically involves the entire leg. Severity is variable. Pain is usually worsened by dependency and edema and relieved by elevation. Many patients report minimal discomfort in the morning (after their legs have been elevated all night) and that pain steadily worsens throughout the day (WOCN, 2019a).
- *Arterial ulcers*: pain is typically described as intense, cramping, and throbbing and typically involves the lower leg and foot. Severity is variable and typically progressive; early in the disease process, pain occurs with significant activity and is relieved by rest (intermittent claudication), while advanced disease causes pain when the legs are placed in a horizontal and neutral position (such as for sleeping) and eventually persists even when the legs are dependent. Pain is worsened by activity and elevation and at least partially relieved by rest and dependent position. Patients may report having to sleep in a recliner or dangling the leg over the edge of the bed to relieve the pain (WOCN, 2014).
- *Neuropathic ulcers*: pain is typically described as pins and needles, stinging, burning, and electric shock and is sometimes worse at night, when the individual is trying to sleep. Severity is variable. Pain may be reduced by walking, which helps to mask the abnormal signals generated by the damaged nerves. Many individuals require pharmaceutical pain management (WOCN, 2012).

KEY POINT

Data obtained from patient history of particular importance to differential assessment include medications (which provide clues as to significant comorbidities), ulcer onset and history (to include treatment to date and response), and pain history (particularly the exacerbating and relieving factors).

PHYSICAL EXAMINATION

Physical examination of the lower extremities should include in-depth assessment of circulatory status, sensorimotor function, and ulcer status.

Circulatory Status

The nurse must assess for indicators of normal versus compromised arterial perfusion and normal versus compromised venous return. Both limbs should be assessed, with comparison of the affected to the unaffected limb. Parameters to be included in vascular assessment include status of skin, hair, and nails; skin color at rest and changes with elevation and dependency; skin temperature; capillary refill time; lower limb pulses, with particular attention to the dorsalis pedis and posterior tibialis pulses; ankle brachial index (ABI) measurement; observation for varicose veins and/or prominent ankle veins; and assessment of edema, to include distribution, type (pitting vs. nonpitting), and severity (WOCN, 2014, 2019a).

Indicators of arterial compromise include trophic changes in the skin, hair, and nails, such as thin shiny skin, diminished or absent hair growth, and thin ridged nails (which may not be visible in the patient with coexisting fungal infection of the nails); elevational pallor or ashen tone to the skin; dependent rubor; coolness of the distal limb and foot; prolonged capillary refill time (>3 seconds); diminished or absent pedal pulses; and ABI <0.9 or >1.3 (severe arterial disease, also known as critical limb ischemia [CLI], is typically manifested by ABI < 0.5). The patient who keeps his or her legs down in response to ischemic pain frequently also has some degree of dependent edema (WOCN, 2014).

Indicators of venous insufficiency include hemosiderin staining of the lower leg, pitting edema extending from the ankle to the knee, presence of varicosities and prominent ankle veins, fibrotic changes in the skin and soft tissue (lipodermatosclerosis), and venous dermatitis (erythema, pruritis, and dermatitis changes involving the gaiter area of the leg, just above the malleoli, and below the calf muscle) (WOCN, 2019a).

Indicators of lymphedema include edema (either pitting or nonpitting) extending from the toes to the groin, cobblestone texture to the skin, and, with advanced disease, papillomatous lesions.

Sensorimotor Status

The nurse must also screen for changes in sensorimotor status indicative of neuropathy. This includes assessment of sensory function using a 10-g Semmes-Weinstein monofilament; assessment of vibratory sense at the base of the great toe or medial aspect of the first metatarsophalangeal joint; assessment of proprioceptive (position) sense; observation of gait and footwear, to include appropriateness of the shoe in relation to the size and contours of the foot and abnormal wear patterns; assessment for foot deformities and callus formation; and assessment of skin hydration. Assessment of plantar surface skin temperature is also very helpful; skin temperature should be measured at multiple sites using a dermal infrared thermometer, and any site at which the temperature is >4.0°F higher than the surrounding skin must be further assessed for inflammatory changes and possible impending ulceration (WOCN, 2012).

Indicators of neuropathy include loss of protective sensation (LOPS), as evidenced by failure to sense the 10-g monofilament at one or more sites; loss of vibratory sense, which frequently precedes LOPS; loss of position sense; abnormal gait and wear patterns in footwear; foot deformities, such as hammertoes, claw toes, or Charcot deformity; very dry skin with fissure formation (or very wet skin); and areas of elevated temperature (WOCN, 2012).

After completing the history and physical assessment, the nurse should be able to determine whether the patient has arterial, venous, and/or neuropathic disease. However, many individuals have risk factors and physical manifestations of more than one pathologic process (e.g., mixed arteriovenous disease, mixed neuropathic arterial disease, or mixed venous and neuropathic disease), and it is possible that one person could present with all three disease processes (arterial, venous, and neuropathic).

Wound Assessment

Conduct a comprehensive assessment of wound status, to include location, shape, dimensions and depth, presence and extent of any tunneling or undermining, type of tissue in the wound bed, status of wound edges, status of surrounding tissue, exudate (volume, color, consistency, and odor), and any signs and symptoms of infection. Key parameters in the differential assessment are **location, wound bed appearance, exudate, and surrounding skin**. Venous ulcers are typically located superior to the medial malleolus but can be anywhere on the lower leg, are shallow and irregular in appearance, and have moderate to heavy exudate; the wound bed is usually dark red and may have a layer of yellow adherent or loose slough and/or biofilm due to high bacterial loads. Undermining or tunneling is uncommon in venous ulcers. In contrast, arterial wounds are usually located distally (toes, forefoot, and heels) because those areas are most distal to the heart; arterial wounds may also present as nonhealing traumatic injuries (because there is insufficient perfusion to support healing). Most commonly, arterial wounds have a punched out appearance, with a pale or necrotic wound bed and scant exudate. Neuropathic wounds are most commonly located on the plantar surface of the foot. Other common locations include metatarsal head of the great toe, dorsal or distal aspects of toes, interdigital areas, and interphalangeal areas of the foot. These wounds are red and have moderate to heavy exudate unless there is coexisting ischemia (WOCN, 2012, 2014, 2019a).

KEY POINT

Wound location is a major indicator as to etiology: venous ulcers are almost always located between the ankle and the knee (most commonly around the medial malleoli); arterial wounds are usually located distally (toes and forefoot) or in areas of traumatic injury that failed to heal; and neuropathic ulcers are located over the foot in areas in contact with the shoe (most commonly the plantar surface).

Surrounding Skin and Nails

Appearance of the surrounding skin can assist with the differential assessment. Common findings in venous disease include edema, hemosiderin staining, dermatitis, and lipodermatosclerosis. In arterial wounds, common findings include hair loss over the lower extremity, shiny taut skin, and dependent rubor (redness). In neuropathic wounds, the surrounding skin may demonstrate anhidrosis with fissuring or callus formation. Other conditions may include maceration and tinea pedis (fungal overgrowth), and xerosis. Toenails in patients with venous disease appear normal, while those in patients with both arterial and neuropathic disease may be dystrophic. A common finding in patients with neuropathic disease is onychomycosis.

DIFFERENTIAL ASSESSMENT AND MANAGEMENT

Determination of primary etiology is based on **predominant pain pattern, ulcer location, ulcer appearance**, and **exudate** and supported by a review of the vascular and sensorimotor assessment data. See **Table 23-1** for the classic presentation of arterial, venous, and neuropathic wounds. Some patients will clearly present with a wound resulting from a single etiology. Once the differential assessment and classification have been completed, the wound nurse will develop an individualized management plan, determined by ulcer classification, for example, leg elevation and compression therapy for venous ulcers, measures to improve perfusion for arterial ulcers, and offloading for neuropathic ulcers. Specifics for the management of each distinct type of wound will be covered in subsequent chapters.

CLINICAL PRESENTATION AND MANAGEMENT OF PATIENTS WITH WOUNDS OF MIXED ETIOLOGY

Many wounds however will demonstrate signs and symptoms indicating additional coexisting pathology. These wounds are referred to as having mixed etiology. The management plan will still be based on the primary etiology with modifications based on the coexisting conditions. Common types of mixed etiology requiring modifications include the following: arterial ulcer in patient with mixed arterial–venous disease and edema, venous ulcer in patient with mixed arterial–venous disease and ABI < 0.8, and neuropathic ulcer complicated by arterial insufficiency. Examples of assessment and management of mixed etiology wounds are included below.

Example 1: Venous Wound with Poor Arterial Perfusion

The patient presents with complaints of a nonhealing wound located just above the inner ankle that she thinks began with a small nick and has enlarged considerably over the past 8 weeks, despite daily application of

TABLE 23-1 DIFFERENTIAL ASSESSMENT ARTERIAL, VENOUS, AND NEUROPATHIC ULCERS

	PAIN PATTERN	LOCATION	APPEARANCE	ASSOCIATED FINDINGS
Arterial	• Cramping, throbbing • Worsened by activity and elevation • Relieved by rest and dependency	• Distal foot • Nonhealing traumatic injury	• Punched out • Pale or necrotic wound bed • Minimal exudate	• Diminished pulses, abnormal ABI, trophic changes • Infection common (S/S of infection may be muted)
Venous	• Dull, aching, "heavy" • Worsened by dependency • Relieved by elevation	• Ankle to knee	• Shallow with irregular edges • Wound bed dark red; may have yellow film • Highly exudative	• Edema and hemosiderin staining common • Venous dermatitis or periwound maceration common
Neuropathic	• "Pins and needles," burning, "electric shock" • Partially relieved by walking	• Plantar surface of foot • Area of foot in contact with shoe	• Red unless there is coexisting ischemia • Exudative	• LOPS and foot deformities common • Callus common (may be macerated)

From Doughty, D. B., & McNichol, L. L. (2016). Differential assessment of lower extremity wounds. In D. B. Doughty & L. L. McNichol (Eds.), *WOCN core curriculum wound management* (p. 512). Philadelphia, PA: Wolters Kluwer.

antibiotic ointment. On assessment, the ulcer bed is 70% dark red and 30% yellow; there is a moderately large volume of exudate and dark brown/gray discoloration over the lower extremity consistent with hemosiderin staining, along with 2+ edema. The patient describes two types of pain: a dull aching pain that is worse at the end of the day when the edema is worse and improves with leg elevation, and occasional cramping pain in the calf and lower leg that occurs only when she walks significant distances and is relieved by sitting down for 5 to 10 minutes. A review of the vascular and sensorimotor data reveals normal sensorimotor function, 1+ pulses on the involved leg, 2+ edema on the involved leg, and an ABI of 0.7. This patient has mixed arterial–venous disease, but the ulcer is due to venous insufficiency, as indicated by ulcer location, primary pain pattern, and ulcer appearance. Thus, management will be based on the primary etiology and involves dressings to manage exudate, leg elevation, and therapeutic-level compression therapy; however, therapeutic-level compression is contraindicated in a patient whose ABI is <0.8. If the ABI is >0.5 and <0.8, as in the patient example provided above, modified compression therapy (light compression) should be initiated with 23 to 30 mm Hg compression at the ankle (Ratliff et al., 2016). If this is poorly tolerated, the nurse should consider dynamic compression therapy (WOCN, 2014, 2019a). If the patient described above showed signs of neuropathy in addition to venous and arterial disease, compression should be used with extreme caution as patient may be unable to detect sensory changes with increasing ischemia.

Example 2: Arterial Wound with Coexisting Neuropathy

The patient presents with complaints of severe cramping pain that is worsened by activity and partially relieved by rest and dependency. Assessment reveals a nonhealing wound on the anterior lower leg that began with a small cut and progressively worsened. Assessment further reveals a wound bed that is 50% necrotic and 50% very pale pink, with minimal exudate. After assessing diminished pedal pulses, the wound nurse should establish a preliminary assessment of an arterial wound and review the vascular assessment to assure consistency with the preliminary assessment. Additional expected findings include trophic changes, diminished pulses, and abnormal ABI/TBI. The nurse also finds that the patient exhibited LOPS at 8/10 sites tested, along with loss of vibratory sense and loss of position sense. This would establish an additional nursing diagnosis of neuropathic changes but would not change the determination regarding primary wound etiology. In this situation, the patient would be determined to have an arterial (ischemic) ulcer with coexisting neuropathy (WOCN, 2012, 2014). Management would include measures to increase arterial blood flow, such as revascularization, medical management, and smoking cessation. Topical therapy would be determined by the characteristics of the ulcer and the potential for healing; for example, a very poorly perfused wound covered with dry eschar and no signs of infection would be left open to air or covered with dry gauze, while an open wound in a patient with an ABI of 0.65 would be managed according to moist wound healing principles, with particular attention to prevention of infection. To address neuropathy, education should be provided about maintaining healthy feet, preventing injury and monitoring foot skin condition (WOCN, 2012, 2014).

Example 3: Arterial Ulcer Complicated by Venous Insufficiency and Edema

The patient presents with complaints of severe cramping pain, worsened by activity and partially relieved by rest and dependency, and assessment reveals a nonhealing wound over the lateral malleolus that began with a scratch and failed to heal. Assessment reveals a wound bed that is very pale pink, with moderate exudate. The wound nurse should have high suspicion of arterial (ischemic) wound and should then review the vascular assessment to assure consistency with the preliminary assessment. Expected finding would include trophic changes, cool temperature, diminished pulses, and abnormal ABI. Further examination reveals brown/gray discoloration above the ankle and 2+ edema indicating coexisting venous disease. Initial management strategies would include measures to improve perfusion and topical therapy would be determined by the characteristics of the ulcer and the potential for healing as noted in Example 2 above. Management of edema would also be determined by the degree of arterial insufficiency; in the patient with very advanced disease in which there is no potential for healing, any form of elevation or compression would be contraindicated and edema management would not be appropriate. In contrast, if the wound is open and perfusion is borderline (e.g., ABI 0.7), edema management *would* be indicated, since edema is a known impediment to tissue oxygenation and wound healing. In this case, very simple and conservative measures to reduce edema (leg elevation or removable compression garments) should be undertaken along with monitoring for any worsening of ischemic pain; dynamic compression therapy is also sometimes beneficial for the patient with mixed disease (WOCN, 2014, 2019a).

Example 4: Neuropathic Ulcer Complicated by Poor Arterial Perfusion

The patient presents with an open wound on the plantar surface of the right foot that he found when removing his shoe. He denies pain from the wound but notes leg pain develops when he walks a long distance and pain is relieved by rest. Assessment of the wound demonstrates 2 × 1.5 × 0.5 cm with pale pink base, moderate serous drainage. Periwound skin has thick callus. LOPS noted with monofilament examination. Thin brittle nails and absence of hair is noted. ABI measurement of >1.3 indicates noncompressible vessels. Toe brachial index (TBI) is 0.25 indicating poor arterial perfusion. Management is dictated by the degree of arterial insufficiency and the characteristics of the ulcer (open vs. closed and infected vs. noninfected). If there is advanced arterial insufficiency with ABI < 0.5 and very limited potential for healing, and the wound is closed and uninfected, the wound should be left open to air or covered with dry gauze and monitored for signs of infection until perfusion is improved to a point to support healing. Offloading should be maintained to prevent worsening of the existing ulcer or development of new ulcers. If there is borderline perfusion and/or the wound is open, the principles of moist wound healing should be followed, along with consistent offloading and medical and behavioral strategies to maximize perfusion (WOCN, 2012, 2014).

REFERRALS

Referrals are frequently required for individuals with lower extremity ulcers and should be initiated in the following situations: (1) when comprehensive assessment reveals that the patient history and ulcer characteristics are inconsistent with ulcers caused by venous, arterial, neuropathic, or mixed disease; (2) when the assessment reveals mixed arterial–venous disease, but the severity of the arterial disease and potential for healing is unclear; (3) when clinical signs of infection or osteomyelitis (probe to bone) are present; (4) when additional expertise is required for optimal management, for example, total contact casting for neuropathic plantar surface ulcer or customized footwear for diabetic patient with foot deformities, or lack of response to initial treatment; and/or (5) when management of the patient's comorbid conditions is required to promote healing.

In situations where wound etiology is unclear, a dermatology referral is frequently indicated, as dermatologists specialize in difficult cutaneous wounds and they are usually the ones best prepared to provide differential diagnosis and management of atypical wounds. A vascular consult is most appropriate for situations involving mixed arterial–venous disease or mixed neuro-ischemic disease.

 ## CONCLUSION

Lower extremity wounds are common, and effective management is critical to wound healing and prevention of recurrence. The first step in optimal wound management is accurate identification of the causative and contributing factors. This can be a challenge since many patients present with wounds of mixed etiology. Thus, a comprehensive assessment and accurate synthesis of the assessment data are critical to positive outcomes and must be based on vascular assessment parameters, sensorimotor parameters, pain pattern, and the location and characteristics of the ulcer. Treatment is then based on primary etiology, with modifications as indicated based on contributing factors and comorbidities. Whenever the wound etiology is unclear, or for wounds that are refractory to initial management, appropriate referrals are mandatory.

CASE STUDIES

A 67-year-old black woman is referred to the wound clinic for a nonhealing ulcer of the left leg, which has been present for 6 months after bumping her leg on the car door. She works part-time as a teaching assistant at the local day care center. She reports that her left leg is always swollen especially at the end of the day.

Relevant medical history: Diabetes mellitus Type 2 for 20 years (last HbA$_{1C}$ 7.2); hypertension; hyperlipidemia; history of "blood clot in the left leg" following a cholecystectomy 2 years ago. She denies a history of heart problems or stroke. Medications include aspirin 81 mg daily, atorvastatin 40 mg daily, glipizide 10 mg daily, and losartan 100 mg daily. Social history: lives alone, independent in activities of daily living, cognitively intact, and no history of tobacco or alcohol abuse.

Vascular assessment: no elevational pallor or dependent rubor; pedal pulses palpable bilaterally; ABI on right 0.84; ABI on left 0.76; 2+ edema left leg with hemosiderin staining; capillary refill 3 seconds bilaterally.

Sensorimotor assessment: unable to feel the 5.07 monofilament on either foot; hammertoes second to fourth toes bilaterally; marked callus noted at first metatarsal heads bilaterally; dry feet.

Pain assessment: minimal in morning; worse at end of day; described as "aching"; relieved by elevation and ibuprofen; also reports occasional "burning" pain in legs at night.

Ulcer assessment: location medial malleolus left leg; 8.5 × 6.6 × 0.25 cm; ulcer bed 80% red and 20% yellow slough large amounts serous exudate; periwound skin very macerated.

ASSESSMENT AND PLAN

- "+" risk factors for arterial, venous, and neuropathic
- Ulcer location/characteristics, volume of exudate, and pain pattern consistent with venous
- "Standard" management venous ulcer: compression + elevation
- Review of vascular assessment data to rule out contraindications to compression: ABI < 0.8 but >0.5 so needs reduced compression (23 to 30 mm Hg)
- Topical therapy: needs protection for periwound skin (e.g., petrolatum, liquid skin barrier, etc.) and absorptive dressing (e.g., alginate, hydrofiber, and/or foam with or without antimicrobial) + modified compression
- Review of sensorimotor assessment: needs aggressive "foot care" education, correctly fitted footwear, good glucose control, careful daily inspection of feet to prevent neuropathic ulcers

REFERENCES

Agale, S. V. (2013). Chronic leg ulcers: Epidemiology, aetiopathogenesis, and management. *Ulcers, 2013.* Retrieved from https://www.hindawi.com/journals/ulcers/2013/413604/. Accessed October 12, 2019.

Alavi, A., Sibbald, R. G., Phillips, T. J., et al. (2016). What's new: Management of venous leg ulcers: Approach to venous leg ulcers. *Journal of American Academy of Dermatology, 74*(4), 627–640.

Centers for Disease Control and Prevention (CDC). (2017). *National diabetes statistics report.* Atlanta, GA: Centers for Disease Control and Prevention, US Department of Health and Human Services. Retrieved from https://www.cdc.gov/diabetes/data/statistics/statistics-report.html. Accessed October 12, 2019.

Doughty, D. B., & McNichol, L. L. (2016). Differential assessment of lower extremity wounds. In D. B. Doughty & L. L. McNichol (Eds.), *WOCN core curriculum wound management* (p. 512). Philadelphia, PA: Wolters Kluwer.

Nelson, E. A., & Adderly, U. (2016). Venous leg ulcers. *BMJ Clinical Evidence, 2016,* 1902. Retrieved from https://www.ncbi.nlm.nih.gov/pmc/articles/PMC4714578/. Accessed October 12, 2019.

Ratliff, C. R., Yates, S., McNichol, L., et al. (2016). Compression for primary prevention, treatment, and prevention of recurrence of venous leg ulcers. *Journal of Wound Ostomy & Continence Nursing, 43*(4), 347–364. doi: 10.1097/WON.0000000000000242.

Rice, J. B., Desai, U., Cummings, A. K. G., et al. (2014). Burden of diabetic foot ulcers for Medicare and private insurers. *Diabetes Care, 37*(3), 651–658.

Singer, A. J., Tassiopoulos, A., & Kirsner, R. S. (2017). Evaluation and management of lower-extremity ulcers. *New England Journal of Medicine, 377,* 1559–1567. doi: 10.1056/NEJMra1615243.

Wound Ostomy Continence Nurses Society. (2012). *Guideline for management of wounds in patients with lower extremity neuropathic disease.* Mt. Laurel, NJ: WOCN Society.

Wound Ostomy Continence Nurses Society. (2014). *Guideline for management of wounds in patients with lower extremity arterial disease.* Mt. Laurel, NJ: WOCN Society.

Wound Ostomy Continence Nurses Society. (2019a). *Guideline for management of wounds in patients with lower extremity venous disease.* Mt. Laurel, NJ: WOCN Society.

Wound, Ostomy and Continence Nurses Society. (2019b). *Venous, arterial, and neuropathic lower-extremity wounds: Clinical resource guide.* Mt. Laurel, NJ: Author.

QUESTIONS

1. The wound care nurse assesses a patient for known risk factors for venous insufficiency. These factors include
   A. Coronary artery disease
   B. Hyperlipidemia
   C. Obesity
   D. Diabetes

2. A patient with a leg ulcer describes his pain as a "cramping sensation" that gets worse in bed. What type of ulcer would the nurse suspect?
   A. Neuropathic
   B. Arterial
   C. Venous
   D. Peripheral

3. Upon assessment of a patient with leg ulcers, the wound care nurse documents venous insufficiency. What is a sign of this condition?
   A. Thin, shiny skin
   B. Elevational pallor
   C. Prolonged capillary refill time
   D. Hemosiderin stain

4. The wound care nurse is assessing vibratory sense at the base of a patient's great toe using a tuning fork. This test is used to assess for
   A. Lymphedema
   B. Neuropathy
   C. Venous deficiency
   D. Arterial deficiency

5. The wound care nurse is assessing a wound on the anterior foot of a patient. The wound presents with a "punched-out appearance with a necrotic wound bed and limited exudate." What type of wound would the nurse most likely document?
   A. Neuropathic
   B. Arterial
   C. Venous
   D. Peripheral

6. What is the most common location of neuropathic ulcers?
   A. Around the medial malleoli
   B. Tips of toes
   C. Plantar surfaces
   D. Pretibial area

7. The wound care nurse is assessing a wound on a patient's ankle that has the appearance of a venous ulcer. Which characteristic would likely be present?
   A. Pale wound bed
   B. Shallow wound with irregular edges
   C. Minimal exudate
   D. Necrotic wound bed

8. What pain pattern would most likely be assessed in a patient with an arterial wound?
   A. Dull, aching, heavy
   B. Pins and needles
   C. Cramping, throbbing
   D. Burning, electric shock

9. In which type of ulcer would callus (possibly macerated) be a common associated finding?
   A. Neuropathic
   B. Arterial
   C. Venous
   D. Peripheral

10. A patient presents with an ischemic ulcer complicated by venous insufficiency and pitting edema. The wound is covered with dry eschar, and there are no signs of infection. What would be an initial management strategy for this patient?
   A. Moist wound healing
   B. Vascular consult
   C. Therapeutic-level compression therapy
   D. Prophylactic antibiotics

ANSWERS AND RATIONALES

1. C. Rationale: Risk factors for venous insufficiency include those that increase resistance to venous return such as obesity, multiple pregnancies, or pregnancies close together.

2. B. Rationale: Rest pain in LEAD occurs in the absence of activity, most typically at night when the patient is supine or in bed.

3. D. Rationale: Common physical signs of LEVD include skin changes such as hemosiderosis or hemosiderin staining.

4. B. Rationale: Vibratory testing is a reliable and validated indicator of sensory perception.

5. B. Rationale: Classic assessment findings for wounds caused by LEAD include location on distal foot and toes, necrosis at the wound base due to ischemia, and rolled or punched out wound edges.

6. C. Rationale: Wounds caused by LEND are most commonly found on the plantar surfaces of the foot due to mechanical trauma and the loss of protective sensation (LOPS).

7. B. Rationale: Venous ulcers often have high levels of exudate and minimum necrosis with red, ruddy wound base.

8. C. Rationale: Wounds caused by LEAD are ischemic in nature and associated pain is characterized by cramping and throbbing.

9. A. Rationale: Callus formation occurs as a protective mechanism of the skin with repeated injury. In patients with LEND and loss of protective sensation, callus formation is a common finding.

10. B. Rationale: In planning care for a patient with a mixed etiology lower extremity wound, arterial blood flow should be addressed first via a vascular consult.

CHAPTER 24

LOWER EXTREMITY VENOUS DISEASE, VENOUS LEG ULCERS, AND LYMPHEDEMA

Teresa J. Kelechi, Glenda Brunette, and Joanna J. Burgess

OBJECTIVES

1. Identify risk factors, pathology, clinical presentation, and management of lower extremity venous disease and venous leg ulcers.

2. Describe essential parameters to be included in assessment of the individual with a lower extremity ulcer.

3. Use assessment data to determine causative and contributing factors for a lower extremity ulcer and to develop evidence-based, patient-centered management plans.

4. Identify indications, contraindications, options, and guidelines for implementation of compression therapy.

5. Describe correct techniques for application of compression devices including stockings, wraps, and intermittent compression therapy.

6. Describe clinical characteristics and management options for venous dermatitis.

7. Describe indications for referral to specialists such as certified wound care nurses, physical and occupational therapists, orthotists, vascular surgeons, dermatologists, lymphedema specialists, and compression specialists.

8. Describe the etiology and pathology of lymphedema, to include differentiation between primary and secondary lymphedema.

9. Describe the various stages of lymphedema, to include clinical characteristics and implications for management.

10. Identify the most efficacious therapies for management of lymphedema and lipedema.

TOPIC OUTLINE

● INTRODUCTION

This chapter addresses the prevalence and incidence, pathology, diagnosis, clinical presentation, and management of lower extremity venous disease (LEVD) and venous leg ulcers (VLUs). The chapter introduces current evidence-based recommendations for secondary prevention of ulcer recurrence and management of mixed arterial–venous disease. The prevalence, pathology, presentation, and management of lymphedema and lipedema are also addressed.

● PREVALENCE AND INCIDENCE OF LOWER EXTREMITY VENOUS DISEASE AND VENOUS LEG ULCERS

LEVD, also known as venous insufficiency, chronic venous insufficiency, and chronic venous disorders, covers a broad spectrum of morphologic and/or functional abnormalities of the venous system (Couch et al., 2017). Severity ranges from mild conditions such as edema, uncomplicated telangiectasias, or spider veins to more complex conditions such as skin changes (lipodermatosclerosis, venous eczema, hemosiderin staining, atrophy blanche) and VLUs. A common finding in LEVD, varicose veins, are present in approximately 25% of the general population of U.S. adults with increasing prevalence associated with aging (Gloviczki et al., 2011). Varicose veins are more common in females affecting 22 million, whereas half as many, or 11 million, males between the ages of 40 and 80 are affected (Hamdan, 2012). An estimated 7 million individuals worldwide have LEVD with 2 million progressing to ulceration (Alavi et al., 2016). VLUs, also known as venous stasis ulcers, and venous insufficiency ulcers, affect approximately 1% of the U.S. population with reports of two million new venous ulcers each year (Alavi et al., 2016; WOCN, 2019). VLUs account for 80% to 90% of all leg ulcers (Nelson & Adderly, 2016) and cost the U.S. health care system an estimated $14 billion per year (Rice et al., 2014). Recurrence rates of 57% to 97% reflect the chronicity of this condition and the failure of treatments to effectively manage the underlying problem (Finlayson et al., 2015). The negative impact on quality of life (QOL) is substantial and includes absence from work due to pain, frequent clinic visits, and treatment requirements (Vuylsteke et al., 2015). Findings from several studies conducted in numerous countries around the world demonstrate that even in the earlier or "mild" stages of the disease, the symptoms associated with LEVD significantly reduce physical, psychological, and social functioning, all components of QOL (Branisteanu et al., 2019). Assessment of QOL is a critical component of overall care of patients with both LEVD and VLUs.

KEY POINT

LEVD is a progressive disorder of the venous system that ranges from mild symptoms of edema to severe abnormalities of the venous system resulting in VLUs that negatively affect quality of life in physical, psychological, and social functioning.

 PATHOLOGY OF VENOUS INSUFFICIENCY AND VENOUS ULCERATION

NORMAL FUNCTION

Proper functioning of the venous system is dependent on the patency of the veins, condition of the one-way valves, and the muscle pumps in the foot and calf (Eberhardt & Raffetto, 2014). With normal venous function, blood is drained from the superficial vessels of the skin and subcutaneous fat by three major vascular pathways: the superficial veins (low-pressure system), the deep veins (high-pressure system), and the perforating veins (veins that transfer blood between the superficial and deep systems) (**Fig. 24-1**). The superficial veins are located above the deep muscular fascia and include the great saphenous and small saphenous veins. The deep veins lie within the muscle compartments (intramuscular) or between the muscles (intermuscular). The latter are more critical in the development of LEVD because they are exposed to high subfascial pressures during calf muscle contraction. The intermuscular veins parallel the lower extremity arteries and include the anterior tibial, posterior tibial, peroneal, popliteal, and femoral veins. Perforator veins, also known as communicating veins, connect the two systems, passing through the deep fascia at the mid-thigh, knee, and ankle. There are more than 90 perforating veins in each leg; the perforators are equipped with unidirectional bicuspid valves that open

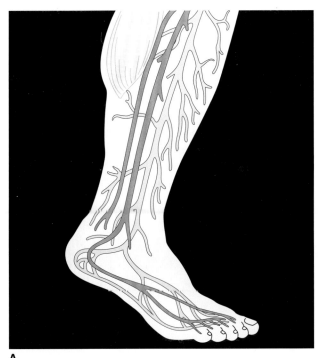

A

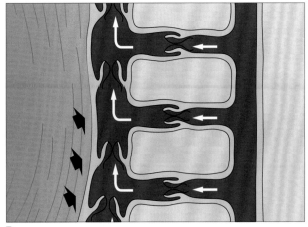

B

FIGURE 24-1. Normal Venous System. **A.** Anatomy of venous system: superficial, perforator, and deep veins. **B.** One-way valves in perforator and deep veins for prevention of venous reflux.

to permit blood flow out of the legs toward the heart and then close to prevent the return of blood toward the feet (Johnson et al., 2016). This series of valves is essential to normal venous function and unidirectional blood flow, particularly when the individual is in the upright position. The calf muscle pump and the valves normally work in concert to promote the return of blood, against gravity, to the heart (Eberhardt & Raffetto, 2014). When the calf muscle is relaxed, the valves open, allowing blood to fill the deep veins; filling increases the pressure in the deep venous system. Contraction of the calf muscle then empties the veins and reduces venous pressure.

KEY POINT

Normal function of the venous valves is essential to unidirectional blood flow and effective venous return; the one-way valves and calf muscle pump work together to promote the return of blood, against gravity, back to the heart.

PATHOLOGY OF LEVD

Pathology develops when there are abnormalities in any part of the system that result in impaired venous return and persistent high pressures within the deep venous system (venous hypertension) caused by obstruction such as venous thromboembolism (VTE), also known as deep vein thrombosis (DVT) that reduces venous return and results in valvular dysfunction (**Fig. 24-2**). Venous hypertension is the etiologic factor common to LEVD (Franks et al., 2016). Venous hypertension occurs when the venous system does not empty causing capillary bed congestion or engorgement, and leakage (extravasation) of fluid and molecules into the surrounding tissues. This impaired venous return, known as "reflux," eventually results in pathologic changes in the superficial venous system and the microvascular system (capillary bed) (Nicolaides et al., 2014). As a consequence of these high venous pressures within the superficial system, damage to the skin results in hyperpigmentation, dermatitis, tissue fibrosis, and ulcers.

PATHOLOGY OF VENOUS ULCERATION

While the pathology of LEVD is clear, the specific pathologic mechanisms resulting in venous ulceration and impaired healing are not well understood. Theories include damage to the endothelial lining of the vessels, platelet aggregation, activation of white blood cells, abnormal levels of inflammatory cytokines such as matrix metalloproteases (MMPs), inflammation, and fibrotic changes in the soft tissues, due in part to the extravasation of cells and plasma proteins into the tissue (Chi & Raffetto, 2015; McDaniel et al., 2017; Pocock et al., 2014). In addition, functional and structural mechanisms such as comorbid conditions including obesity and genetic factors have been posited to play a role in the development of VLUs.

ASSESSMENT AND DIAGNOSIS

LEVD is diagnosed based on patient history and clinical findings.

HISTORY

A thorough history should include causative and contributing factors to valvular or calf muscle pump dysfunction, prior leg ulceration, previous treatments, barriers to healing and/or treatment, prior venous procedures, as well as family history of arterial or venous disease (O'Donnell et al., 2014). In addition, it is important to differentiate from other etiologies that may require different management (Johnson et al., 2016; Pieper & Templin, 2015; Ratliff et al., 2016; WOCN, 2019). Concomitant arterial insufficiency is present in an estimated 10% to 18% of those with LEVD (Matic et al., 2016). An ABI of 0.9 or lower signals clinically significant arterial compromise (Bonham et al., 2016).

Conditions Leading to Valvular Dysfunction

Assess for factors contributing to valvular compromise including

- Conditions that increase resistance to venous return, such as obesity or multiple pregnancies
- Conditions that directly damage the valves, such as VTE/DVT or phlebitis, and conditions associated with

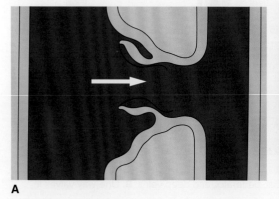

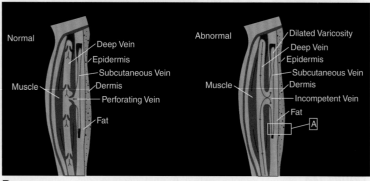

A   **B**

FIGURE 24-2. A, B. Valvular Dysfunction/Venous Reflux.

undiagnosed VTE/DVT (i.e., pulmonary embolism [PE], leg trauma, leg surgery, head injury, or other trauma)

- Thrombophilic conditions such as protein S deficiency, protein C deficiency, or factor V Leiden mutations
- Inflammatory autoimmune diseases such as systemic lupus erythematosus (SLE) and antiphospholipid syndrome, which may result in microthrombi from venous inflammation

Conditions Resulting in Calf Muscle Pump Dysfunction

Assess for factors contributing to compromised calf muscle pump function including

- Advanced age, which may lead to stiffening of the calf muscle tendon and reduced range of motion in the ankle
- Alteration in gait resulting in loss of the normal heel strike—toe-off mechanics (e.g., a "shuffling" gait). Sedentary lifestyle or reduced mobility: occupations requiring long periods of sitting or standing, mobility-limiting obesity, paralysis, arthritis, or prior surgery to the knee, ankle, or foot resulting in fixation of the joint (Franks et al., 2016; Kim et al., 2015; O'Donnell et al., 2014).

Impediments to Healing

The patient should be assessed for barriers to healing such as comorbid conditions such as arterial disease, heart failure, uncontrolled diabetes, heart failure and inflammatory diseases, location and duration of the VLU, elevated inflammatory biomarkers, inflammatory disease, tobacco or alcohol use, inadequate nutrition, social isolation, psychological distress, medications, inadequate wound treatment, activity restrictions, and impaired mobility (Finlayson et al., 2017; Parker et al., 2016; Scotton et al., 2014; Serra et al., 2013; Yim et al., 2014; WOCN, 2019).

History of Healed and/or Current Ulceration

The patient should be assessed for current and prior lower extremity ulcers to include location, description, duration, treatment including surgical intervention or biopsies, and

patient's tolerance of treatment. Individuals with prior VLUs should be carefully assessed to ensure understanding of the underlying pathology and the need for good skin care, leg elevation, and lifelong compression to control edema and avoid ulcer recurrence (Bobridge et al., 2011; Protz et al., 2016). The patient should also be asked about the use of compression garments and obstacles to obtaining, doffing, or donning them.

Triggers for Ulceration

Seventy-four percent of VLUs begin with a specific trigger. Therefore, the history should include queries related to known triggering events such as cellulitis, penetrating injury/trauma, contact dermatitis, rapid onset of leg edema, burns, dry skin with itching/scratching, and insect bites (Kelechi et al., 2015).

SYMPTOMS

The initial presentation/clinical symptomatology related to LEVD varies widely; common symptoms include aching of the legs, pain, swelling, dry skin, feelings of tightness or heaviness, skin irritation, and itching (Kelechi et al., 2018). Pain is typically reported as worsening with prolonged dependency and improving with elevation. Pain may be severe enough to limit ambulation. Sleep is often affected, and patients report other symptoms such as fatigue and depression (Edwards et al., 2014).

PHYSICAL EXAMINATION

Physical assessment includes a thorough examination of the lower extremities, to include skin integrity, perfusion status, edema, and any ulcerations. Common physical signs appear most commonly in the gaiter region around the lower aspect of the leg between the calf muscle and malleoli but can appear anywhere on the lower leg. These signs include dilated veins (telangiectasias, reticular veins, varicose veins) also known as ankle flaring (a cluster of reticular and spider veins along the ankle), edema, skin changes (hemosiderosis—brown staining, atrophie blanche—smooth white plaques, and/or venous eczema/dermatitis—red flakiness, lipodermatosclerosis—hardening), and/or ulceration (see **Table 24-1** for common

TABLE 24-1 COMMON PHYSICAL FINDINGS IN LOWER EXTREMITY VENOUS DISEASE

Telangiectasias	Small (<1 mm diameter) linear blood vessels visible under the skin, usually red or purple; commonly referred to as "spider veins"
Reticular veins	Slightly larger (1–3 mm diameter) veins that are visible under the skin, usually blue and slightly bulging in venous disease
Varicose veins	Superficial veins that are large, thickened, twisting, dilated, and often painful
Hemosiderosis	Reddish brown/black pigmentation, usually in the ankle area, resulting from extravasated red blood cells; as the cells break down, iron from the hemoglobin is released into the tissue causing the staining
Atrophie blanche	Smooth localized areas of ivory white atrophic skin with or without tiny dilated capillaries that appear as red dots throughout the area, often confused with scar tissue
Lipodermatosclerosis	Skin changes in the lower leg with induration, fibrosis, and hyperpigmentation resulting in "inverted champagne bottle" or "inverted bowling pin" appearance

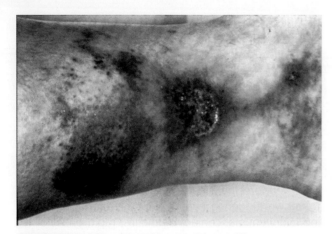

FIGURE 24-3. Hemosiderosis around Venous Ulcer.

physical findings and descriptions; see **Figure 24-3** for hemosiderosis). The presence of edema is a particularly significant finding and requires differential assessment to rule out causes other than LEVD (**Table 24-2**). The edema is often long-standing and typically worsens when the leg is in a dependent position for prolonged periods of time; edema that is venous in origin is normally reduced by elevation of the leg above the level of the heart. Venous dermatitis is another common finding and should be distinguished from cellulitis, a skin and soft tissue infection that presents as a well-demarcated red and/or highly

pigmented area of skin accompanied by systemic signs of infection including elevated temperature and white blood cells (Morton & Phillips, 2013). Scars from previous ulcers should be noted.

Perfusion status must be thoroughly assessed for any individual with a lower extremity wound; this includes assessment of pedal pulses, which are commonly palpable in patients with LEVD, and validation of perfusion status with measurement of the ankle–brachial index (ABI) (Bonham et al., 2016). ABI measurement is critical not only to rule out significant arterial disease but also to determine the level of compression therapy that can be safely used for treatment of the LEVD and or mixed arterial–venous disease (see Chapter 25 for directions on ABI testing and interpretation). Common physical findings in the patient with a VLU include edema, hemosiderosis, palpable pulses, warm feet, and possibly venous dermatitis. Signs of ischemic skin changes include thin, shiny, fragile skin, little to no hair growth, dystrophic toenails, elevational pallor and dependent rubor, cool to touch skin, and atrophy of skin, subcutaneous tissue, and muscle (Bonham et al., 2016). Findings should be documented in the medical record. Peripheral sensory neuropathy is often present in patients with LEVD; thus, physical assessment should include monofilament testing (see Chapter 26 for directions on monofilament testing and interpretation).

TABLE 24-2 DIFFERENCES BETWEEN VENOUS EDEMA, LYMPHEDEMA, AND LIPEDEMA

	SKIN AND PIGMENT ALTERATIONS	EDEMA CHARACTERISTICS	PART INVOLVED	TREATMENT
Lower Extremity Venous Disease				
Elevated venous pressures related to venous valve incompetence and/or obstruction	Skin thickens, becomes fibrotic and woody. Dark pigmentation common. Ulceration common	Insidious onset; heaviness and pain in the legs at the end of the day; increasing soft, pitting swelling; when chronic becomes hard and irregular with venous eczema common	Lower legs and feet	Skin care; compression therapy; possibly manual drainage (note limited evidence on the benefits of manual drainage for edema associated with LEVD)
Lymphedema				
Damage and/or blockage of lymph flow, which causes accumulation of high-protein edema	Skin thickened, becomes firm and fibrotic; lymphangitis and cellulitis common. Ulceration not common	May be congenital; may be sudden onset; otherwise may be gradual increase in edema over months or years; pitting if recent onset; indurated and hard if long-standing	Any extremity or body part; may be one part, one entire side, or one, two, or all extremities	Weight control; skin care; manual lymphatic drainage; exercise; compression (bandages, garments, devices)
Lipedema				
Increase in fat deposition of lower extremities ("painful fat syndrome")	Accumulation of loosely textured fat, most commonly limited to the lower extremities. Usually occurs in women, beginning in adolescence. Bruising is common and involved areas are tender to palpation.	Bilateral and symmetrical. No ulcerations	Legs and buttocks; feet not involved	Weight loss; reduction of size by surgery is done in some centers but not enough evidence to determine long-term effect

CEAP CLASSIFICATION

Most commonly, LEVD is classified by clinical manifestations, etiologic factors, anatomic distribution of the disease, and underlying pathophysiologic findings attributable to LEVD using the CEAP (Clinical–Etiology–Anatomy–Pathophysiology) system (Eklof et al., 2004; Gloviczki et al., 2011; Rabe & Pannier, 2012). Many clinicians use the "C" section of the 6 classes of clinical manifestations when documenting the severity of disease as follows:

- Class 0/C0: No visible or palpable signs of venous disease
- Class 1/C1: Telangiectases or reticular veins
- Class 2/C2: Varicose veins (distinguished from reticular veins by a diameter ≥3 mm)
- Class 3/C3: Edema due to venous disease
- Class 4/C4: Skin changes due to venous disease:
  - Class 4a/C4a: Pigmentation and/or eczema
  - Class 4b/C4b: Lipodermatosclerosis and/or atrophie blanche
- Class 5/C5: Healed venous ulcer
- Class 6/C6: Active venous ulcer

It should be noted that the term "chronic venous insufficiency" (CVI) is reserved for use with C4–C6 disease. Thus, varicose veins alone without skin changes do not indicate LEVD.

WOUND ASSESSMENT

Assessment of the wound should include onset, duration, location, dimensions, tissue type, bleeding, status of wound edges, periwound skin, odor, and volume and character of drainage. The classic VLU location is superior to the medial malleolus; however, ulcers may occur anywhere on the lower leg or dorsum of the foot. The wound bed is usually shallow, moist, and ruddy red color in color, and a loose or adherent yellow biofilm may be present (**Fig. 24-4** for classic venous ulcer presentation). Tunneling and undermining are atypical. The periwound skin is often macerated; crusts, scales, and hyperpigmentation (hemosiderosis/hemosiderin staining) are common. Exudate is typically moderate to heavy, and odor and bleeding may or may not be present. Monitoring of weekly wound measurements helps predict healing (WOCN, 2019).

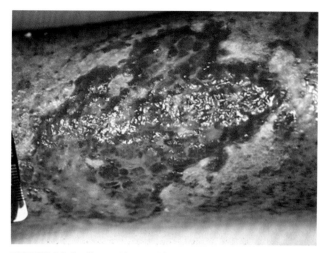

FIGURE 24-4. Classic Venous Ulcer with Periwound Maceration and Dermatitis.

DIAGNOSTIC STUDIES

Vascular studies assist in determining the presence and severity of venous disease and confirm adequate arterial flow for healing in addition to guiding appropriate compression. Venous duplex ultrasound is the most reliable noninvasive test to identify anatomic and hemodynamic abnormalities (Gloviczki et al., 2011; Zygmunt, 2014). Other noninvasive tests include air plethysmography (APG) and photoplethysmography (PPG). Plethysmography is recommended to assess calf muscle pump function or outflow obstruction if duplex scan outcomes are questionable; PPG can be performed relatively quickly and provides a reading of the overall venous refill time (normal is about 20 seconds) (Gloviczki et al., 2011). Venography is useful for patients with VTE/DVT, postthrombotic syndrome, or prior to surgical intervention (Gloviczki et al., 2011).

As previously noted, ABI measurement is critical to assessment and appropriate treatment; thus, a handheld Doppler is an essential diagnostic tool (Bonham et al., 2016). The handheld Doppler may also be helpful when edema makes palpation of pedal pulses difficult.

PRIMARY PREVENTION

Early identification and treatment of LEVD (CEAP levels C1–C3) is essential to minimize symptoms and prevent VLUs. Patients with known risk factors (**Table 24-3**) or early signs of LEVD should wear compression garments (stockings/hosiery) consistently to prevent venous edema and ulceration (Rabe et al., 2018; WOCN, 2019). Weekly calf and ankle circumference measurements may be used to monitor edema reduction (Protz et al., 2016).

In addition to compression, other preventive strategies include weight management, exercise/physical activity, treatment of varicosities, and patient education. Obesity is a strong risk factor for LEVD; thus, all efforts to

TABLE 24-3 RISK FACTORS FOR LOWER EXTREMITY VENOUS DISEASE

• Family history of venous disease	• Sedentary lifestyle and occupation
• Pregnancy (multiple or close together)	• Prolonged sitting and/or standing
• Leg trauma, surgery, or fracture	• Surgery/trauma to the foot/ankle/leg
• Thrombophilia (protein S or protein C deficiency)	• Altered gait
• Systemic inflammation	• Paralysis
• Varicose veins	• Impairment of calf muscle pump
• Venous thromboembolism (VTE)/phlebitis/pulmonary embolism (PE)	• Restricted range of motion of the ankle including inversion and eversion
• Obesity—high body mass index (BMI)	• Older age
• Injection drug use	• Female sex
	• Tobacco use

Adapted from Wound, Ostomy, and Continence Nurses Society (WOCN). (2019). *Guideline for management of wounds in patients with lower-extremity venous disease*. Mount Laurel, NJ: WOCN.

attain and maintain a healthy weight should be considered including dietary alterations, counseling, drug therapy, and weight loss surgery (WOCN, 2019). Because the calf muscle pump plays a critical role in normal function and in the pathophysiology of LEVD, exercise programs aimed at improving function have been shown to be helpful (Couch et al., 2017; Franks et al., 2016; O'Donnell et al., 2014). Physical therapy may be needed to improve range of motion and/or gait (O'Brien et al., 2013, 2017). Interventional treatment of varicosities, such as endovenous laser ablation, radiofrequency ablation, and other approaches to repair veins and valves, have proven to prevent the progression of venous disease and the development of ulcerations (Eberhardt & Raffetto, 2014; Gloviczki et al., 2011). Patients should be educated about the disease process, the need for lifelong compression, and the need to avoid crossing legs and wearing constrictive garments (Baquerizo Nole et al., 2015; Bobridge et al., 2011; Gonzalez, 2014, 2017; Kapp & Miller, 2015; O'Donnell et al., 2014; Van Hecke et al., 2011).

 MANAGEMENT OF LEVD

Management of LEVD, with or without ulceration, involves compression therapy, leg elevation, selected use of pharmaceuticals, and surgical intervention for selected patients.

COMPRESSION THERAPY

Compression and elevation have long been considered to be essential elements of a comprehensive VLU management program (WOCN, 2019). Both help to reduce edema and improve venous return. Compression therapy remains the mainstream approach for both treatment and prevention and "works" mechanically by partially compressing the distended superficial veins. This external pressure reduces the diameter of the vessels and supports the calf muscle pump, which reduces venous hypertension by promoting venous return through enhanced ejection fraction. The normal ejection fraction of the calf muscle pump is approximately 65% (Black, 2014; Lattimer, 2018). Compression therapy also increases the level of pressure in the interstitial space, which reduces edema by preventing leakage of fluid out of the capillary bed and by promoting return of edema fluid to the lymphatic system and capillary bed. While the primary effects of compression therapy are reduction of venous hypertension and control of edema, recent studies suggest that there may be benefits to compression therapy that contribute to venous ulcer healing through reduction in pain, and improvement in QOL and sleep (Konschake et al., 2016; Ozdemir et al., 2016).

Long-term compression therapy has been demonstrated in numerous randomized clinical trials to be beneficial in management of edema and VLUs and remains the gold standard of VLU therapy, despite the fact that there are no internationally accepted performance standards (Rabe et al., 2018). The most recent WOCN LEVD guidelines (2019), which are composed of a systematic review and those of the 2012 Cochrane review (O'Meara et al., 2012), summarize the current evidence regarding the various approaches to compression therapy as follows:

1. Compression increases healing rates when compared with no compression.
2. Multicomponent systems are more effective than single-component systems.
3. Multicomponent systems with an elastic bandage component appear to be more effective than those mainly made up of inelastic components.
4. Two-component bandages appear to perform as well as four-layer bandages (4LB) and inelastic bandages.
5. 4LB systems (including those with an elastic bandage) heal ulcers faster than does the short-stretch bandage (SSB), a type of bandage with very minimal stretch.
6. High-compression stocking systems heal more patients than does SSB.
7. Contraindications to any type of compression include arterial occlusive disease, heart failure, and ABI < 0.50 (Andriessen et al., 2017).
8. Consider using the WOCN Society's algorithm, *Compression for Primary Prevention, Treatment, and Prevention of Recurrence of Venous Leg Ulcers: An Evidence- and Consensus-Based Algorithm for Care across the Continuum* (http://vlu.wocn.org), to identify the appropriate type and level of compression for adults (Ratliff et al., 2016).

The goals of compression therapy are to improve symptoms, reduce edema, and heal VLUs. Compression can be provided by wraps, garments, bandages, or devices and is available in both static devices and intermittent pneumatic compression (IPC) devices.

Static Compression

Static compression therapy involves application of constant gradient pressure to the lower extremity, with highest pressures exerted distally (at the ankle) and lowest pressures exerted proximally (usually at the knee). Therapeutic compression is generally considered to be 30 to 40 mm Hg at the ankle (Attaran & Ochoa Chaar, 2017; Johnson et al., 2016). Examples of static therapy are compression bandages, adjustable devices with Velcro straps, and compression hosiery. While compression bandages can be composed of both elastic and inelastic materials, hosiery by necessity is elastic (WOCN, 2019) (**Table 24-4**). Static compression is considered first-line therapy for most individuals with LEVD; however, static compression is contraindicated for individuals with uncompensated (symptomatic) heart failure, occlusive arterial disease, or severe arterial disease (ABI ≤ 0.5, ankle pressure <70 mm Hg, toe pressure <50 mm Hg) (Bonham et al., 2016; WOCN, 2019). For individuals with moderately severe LEAD (ABI ≥ 0.5 to ≤0.8), modified compression is recommended (23 to 30 mm Hg compression at the ankle) (see Chapter 25 for detailed discussion of compression therapy for patients with mixed arterial–venous disease). Compression may be used with venous eczema/dermatitis (Morton & Phillips, 2013) and may be trialed cautiously in the presence of acute cellulitis (Hanson et al., 2015).

Therapeutic-level compression is contraindicated in patients with uncompensated heart failure, occlusive arterial disease, and ABI < 0.5 (Andriessen et al., 2017). For individuals with moderate arterial disease (ABI > 0.5 to <0.8), closely monitored, lower compression 23 to 30 mm Hg is indicated (Bonham et al., 2016; Ratliff et al., 2016; WOCN, 2019). In the case of revascularization, reevaluation for compression may be warranted (Georgopoulos et al., 2013).

Risks of compression include discomfort, contact allergy or skin irritation, and constriction or pressure damage to skin or nerves (Andriessen et al., 2016). Most risks may be avoided with interventions delivered by skilled clinicians, and thorough assessment and patient education (Andriessen et al., 2016).

Compression Stockings

Prescription compression stockings are widely used for primary and secondary prevention of VLUs. Also known as hosiery and garments, stockings must be sized to fit the leg and are intended for daily, lifelong use. Thus, compression wraps are typically used initially to decrease edema, and then the patient is transitioned to compression hosiery or an alternative device.

Compression stockings are designed to provide a pressure gradient across the length of the stocking, with the greatest pressure exerted at the ankle and the least pressure proximally at the calf. It is generally accepted that an external pressure of 35 to 40 mm Hg at the ankle is necessary to prevent leakage from capillaries affected by LEVD; however, the optimal level of pressure needed to overcome the underlying venous hypertension has not been determined.

Hosiery is available in a variety of lengths: knee-high, thigh-high, chaps (unilateral waist high), standard pantyhose, and maternity pantyhose. Knee-high stockings are sufficient for most patients and are generally well tolerated; however, thigh-high stockings are often prescribed following venous surgery. It is important to instruct the patient to pull the thigh-high stockings up on the thigh so they do not wrinkle at the knee to avoid binding and discomfort.

Stockings are available in five pressure gradients (<20, 20 to 30, 30 to 40, 40 to 50, and >50 mm Hg). To be effective, compression stockings need to exert a minimum of 20 to 30 mm Hg pressure at the ankle. The antiembolism stockings (AES) used in the hospital exert only 8 to 10 mm Hg at the ankle and are ineffective for treatment of LEVD. Patients should be provided with a prescription that specifies length of stocking and level of compression and must be correctly fitted, typically either by a wound care nurse or by trained staff at the supply center. Effective therapy includes appropriately sized, therapeutic level compression stockings and collaboration with the patient to assure appropriate application and consistent use.

A common problem reported by patients wearing compression hosiery is difficulty with application; this is an even greater problem for obese individuals, those who cannot bend over, and those with limited hand strength and dexterity. Fortunately, there are a number of hosiery options and application devices that make it easier to don the stockings. For example, patients with foot deformities typically find it easier and more comfortable to use open-toe stockings. Zippered or layered

TABLE 24-4 COMPRESSION STOCKING CLASSIFICATIONS BETWEEN UNITED STATES AND UNITED KINGDOM

US CLASS	DESCRIPTOR	ANKLE PRESSURE
Class 1	Light support	20–30 mm Hg
Class 2	Medium support	30–40 mm Hg
Class 3	Strong support	40–50 mm Hg
Class 4	Very strong support	50–60 mm Hg

UK CLASS	DESCRIPTOR	ANKLE PRESSURE
Class 1	Light support	14–17 mm Hg
Class 2	Medium support	18–24 mm Hg
Class 3	Strong support	25–35 mm Hg

Adapted from Neumann et al. (2016); O'Meara et al. (2012).

stockings may be beneficial for patients who lack the mobility and hand strength to don regular compression stockings. In addition, stocking butlers and silken liners may ease application. All patients should be advised to apply the stockings in the morning when edema is minimal. If there is a delay before donning the stockings, the patient should elevate the legs for 20 to 30 minutes prior to application. Patients should be advised that it is safer to don the stockings while sitting in a chair with a firm back, rather than sitting on the edge of the bed. It is critical for the wound care nurse to become knowledgeable regarding the available stocking options and donning devices and to work with the patient to find a stocking and application technique that work effectively for that individual. For patients who are unable to don stockings, even with assistive devices, an adjustable compression device might be appropriate. This device is easily applied, is secured with overlapping bands that provide inelastic compression, and can be adjusted when edema fluctuates. It also permits easy removal for bathing and wound care. These devices must be correctly fitted, and the patient must be instructed in their use.

Care of hosiery is important since improper laundering can reduce the strength of compression and thereby compromise therapy. The following points should be included when teaching patients how to care for their stockings:

- Wash new stockings according to instructions before wearing to reduce stiffness.
- Hand wash or machine wash on delicate cycle after each use and hang to dry.
- Moisturize the skin in the evening before going to bed as stockings absorb skin oils.
- Purchase two pairs if possible and alternate wearing.
- Replace at least every 6 months or when stockings no longer have adequate compression.

Compression Bandages

Compression bandaging systems are commonly used in the initial treatment of LEVD and VLUs; they are typically applied by a health care professional at 3- to 7-day intervals, with the specific frequency determined by volume of exudate and degree of edema. Compression wraps can be classified as elastic and/or inelastic and as single layer (one component) or multilayer (two to four components). Classification of compression systems should be based on components rather than layers, since multilayer wraps can have both elastic and inelastic components and since even single-layer wraps overlap, create two layers (O'Meara et al., 2012). Therefore, the terms multicomponent and single component should be used to describe compression bandages, rather than multilayer and single layer. The terms elastic and inelastic refer to the degree of "stretch" of the wrap. Sometimes clinicians use the terms elastic and long stretch (maximum extensibility >100%) interchangeably, to indicate wraps that exhibit high resting pressures and low working (walking) pressures. Inelastic and short stretch (maximum extensibility of <100%) are also used interchangeably to denote products that exhibit high working (walking) pressures and low resting pressures (WOCN, 2019).

Compression bandaging systems are usually the best choice for initial treatment and until edema has been eliminated. Data indicate that elastic systems provide better results than do inelastic and that systems with at least two components provide better results than do single-component systems.

Inelastic Compression

An inelastic system has no "give"; it exerts high "working" pressures (e.g., when the person is ambulating and the calf muscle is contracting) but is unable to tighten to provide continued support when the leg is at rest. In addition, inelastic systems cannot adapt to any changes in leg volume, such as increased edema with dependency or reduced edema resulting from leg elevation or due to the compression bandage itself. Inelastic systems are typically changed every 3 to 7 days and, as with all compression wrap systems, should be applied by trained personnel. The most commonly used inelastic compression system is the Unna's boot, an inexpensive and readily available compression product named after its inventor, German dermatologist Dr. Paul Unna (1850–1929). Today's paste or impregnated bandages, generally made of gauze, come in different widths (common size is 4 inches width and 10 feet length) and can be impregnated with several different products including zinc paste, glycerin, gelatin, and calamine lotion. The goal in applying the impregnated layer is to achieve a smooth conformable "boot" that supports the calf muscle pump; flat "pleats" are usually needed to assure a smooth fit over the foot and ankle. In most settings, the impregnated layer is covered by a cohesive self-adherent bandage, which provides additional compression. Advantages of this inelastic bandage system include its ability to provide high working pressure during walking, its relatively low cost, and its ready availability. The bandage is relatively thin, which usually permits the patient to wear shoes, with noted beneficial effects of the impregnated gauze on venous dermatitis. In addition, because the bandage is inelastic, it may be better tolerated by patients who feel that elastic bandages are "too tight." However, impregnated bandages are no longer considered "optimal" for most patients due to the following disadvantages: inability to adapt to any change in leg volume, inability to provide sustained compression (loss of sub-bandage pressure over time), potential allergic reactions to selected components (e.g., bandages containing calamine), high skill level needed for accurate application, and the need for frequent changes/reapplication when there is significant exudate.

More recent advances are the advent of adjustable compression, defined as removable, reusable, inelastic garments, which provide compression ranging from 20 to 50 mm Hg. This is achieved via an understocking and an outer component with hook and loop (Velcro®) straps that may be adjusted to provide the desired level of compression.

Elastic Wraps

As there is always overlap when wrapping and therefore multiple layers, terminology is moving toward the use of "components" rather than "layers" (O'Donnell et al., 2014; O'Meara et al., 2012). The category of elastic compression includes two-, three-, and four-component disposable wraps. These provide therapeutic or modified compression and both walking and resting support (Johnson et al., 2016). Absorption of exudate is another advantage of the multicomponent wrap. Skill is required to apply the wraps correctly, so they provide therapeutic compression.

If a protocol requires frequent dressing changes, a single-component wrap may be useful. However, the bandage tends to stretch with ambulation, which means that frequent rewrapping may be required. This wrap is most effective for the patient with minimal edema and small ulcers.

The multicomponent wraps with three and four components usually contain the following: (1) base layer: absorbent padding or cast padding that pads and protects the bony prominences and can be layered to assure a circumference of at least 18 cm at the ankle; (2) cotton crepe layer that smooths the padding layer and provides better conformability for the active compression layers (layers three and/or four); (3) elastic conformable bandage that provides 18 to 25 cm of compression; and (4) cohesive self-adherent bandage that brings total compressive force to 40 mm Hg when applied as directed per manufacturer's instructions. Two-component wraps include a base layer that provides padding and protection and is typically applied in a spiral fashion from the base of the toes to 1 inch below the knee, with the heel left out; the second layer is the active compression layer and is typically made of a modified cohesive material that provides therapeutic level compression when applied at full stretch (with the heel included). The advantage of the two-component wrap is the thinner profile, which typically allows the patient to wear her or his own shoes. A multicenter randomized controlled trial (RCT) comparing two-component to four-component compression dressings found that the two-component system was easier to use, well tolerated, and effective with 48% of patients in the two-component group healed within 12 weeks compared to 38% in the four-component group (Lazareth et al., 2012).

The advantages of multicomponent wraps include the following: sustained compression and edema control for up to 1 week (so long as the patient does not require more frequent dressing changes), absorption of moderate-to-large volumes of exudate, and the ability to modify the level of compression by modifying the layers and amount of padding used. Disadvantages include that they cannot be reused and are often bulky, which means the patients cannot wear their shoes. In addition, patients sometimes complain they feel "hot and tight." Accurate application of the compression wrap is essential to therapeutic outcomes; clinicians should utilize the following general guidelines and follow the manufacturer's guidelines for the specific wrap.

1. Clean the leg with warm water, avoiding the use of soap. Dry well.
2. Moisturize the intact skin with a fragrance-free ointment such as petrolatum.
3. Position the ankle in a neutral position at a right angle.
4. Pad with cotton cast padding or similar material to equalize pressure.
5. Wrap each layer starting at the base of the toes; wrap to the patellar notch just distal to the knee.
6. Include the heel in the wrap unless instructed otherwise by manufacturer.

Dynamic Compression

Dynamic (intermittent) compression therapy or IPC does not involve bandaging and may benefit patients who cannot tolerate static compression. It is especially useful for immobile patients or those needing higher pressures than can be obtained with stockings, bandages, or wraps. Studies have indicated that IPC facilitates healing when compared with no compression, but there is a lack of research to support improvement in healing rates when paired with compression wraps or when used instead of compression wraps (Nelson et al., 2014). IPC is contraindicated in patients with uncompensated (symptomatic) heart failure, acute cellulitis, and acute venous thrombosis.

The IPC device involves use of a pump and a single-chamber sleeve that is inflated intermittently, or a sleeve with multiple compartments that inflate sequentially, providing a "milking" action (from distal to proximal). Patients are usually instructed to use the pump one to two times daily, for 1 to 2 hours per treatment session. Benefits include mobilization of interstitial fluid back into the circulation and the ability to enhance venous return without impairing arterial blood flow, which provides safe therapy for the patient with LEVD complicated by moderately severe arterial disease (Bonham et al., 2016). Disadvantages include the requirement that patients must be immobile during therapy, and potential difficulty with self-application and removal for the patient who lives alone. Reimbursement through Medicare, Medicaid, and some private insurers is limited to patients who have "failed" 6 months of conservative therapy (static compression).

ELEVATION

Leg elevation is a simple, practical way to improve venous return using gravitational forces. While few formal studies have demonstrated its effectiveness in preventing or treating LEVD and VLUs, elevation is recommended in almost all standards of care and clinical guidelines (Ratliff et al., 2016). The most common recommendation is to elevate the feet to at least the level of the heart for 30 minutes three to four times per day. Symptoms of mild LEVD may be relieved by this practice alone, but in more severe cases, this will likely be inadequate. Elevation below the level of the heart is ineffective (Alguire & Mathes, 2014). While helpful, many patients find this intervention difficult to consistently perform due to the inability to lie flat or time requirements to spend up to 2 hours each day to perform elevation.

PHARMACOLOGIC THERAPY

A variety of medications and supplements have been used to treat LEVD with varying success and levels of evidence. The most commonly used agents in the United States include pentoxifylline and horse chestnut seed extract. Pentoxifylline (Trental) has been shown in a number of studies to be effective alone and in addition to compression therapy (Jull et al., 2012; Ratliff et al., 2016), specifically through its beneficial effects on the microcirculation; mechanisms of action include its fibrinolytic properties, antiplatelet effects, and ability to reduce adhesion of leukocytes to the endothelium. Dosages of 400 mg three times per day have been shown to accelerate healing and are recommended for ulcers that are slow to heal. However, the potential benefits must be weighed against the cost and side effects, which are commonly GI related.

No phlebotropic or venoactive drugs have been shown to be superior to others in symptom management or VLU healing (Chudek et al., 2016). Multiple studies have shown horse chestnut seed extract (escin/aescin) to be beneficial in controlling pain and pruritus and in reducing edema and leg circumference in patients with LEVD. It works by stimulating the release of prostaglandins (e.g., PGF2-alpha), which induce venoconstriction and reduce the permeability of vessel walls to low molecular proteins, water, and electrolytes (Pittler & Ernst, 2012). The suggested dose is 300 mg, containing 50 mg of the active ingredient aescin, taken twice daily for 12 weeks. It is available over the counter in the United States as an herbal supplement; therefore, purity and standardization of dose is not guaranteed. While it is generally considered safe, it may be toxic in high doses.

While not available in the United States, the phlebotropic drug known as micronized purified flavonoid fraction (MPFF) has been shown to improve outcomes for patients with LEVD and VLUs and is used in Europe and other countries. MPFF used in combination with standard therapy has been shown to improve healing

rates compared to standard therapy alone or to placebo. Its side effect profile is similar to placebo, and cost analysis studies have demonstrated a significant reduction in cost of healing. It has also been shown to improve QOL in patients with LEVD. Hydroxyethylrutoside is another flavonoid compound that has been used extensively in Europe but is not available in the United States. It has been shown to be effective in reducing leg volume, edema, and symptoms of LEVD (Alguire & Mathes, 2014).

Diuretics are sometimes used to treat edema from other conditions, but they have no effect on venous edema or the underlying pathology of LEVD. This is because the edema in LEVD is caused by venous hypertension, which is a mechanical issue and unrelated to fluid overload. In addition, diuretic use can lead to hypovolemia and metabolic complications, particularly in older adults; thus, diuretics should be used cautiously and only when indicated for systemic conditions causing edema (Alguire & Mathes, 2014).

Simvastatin 40 mg daily for 10 weeks in conjunction with compression was shown to significantly decrease time to healing and overall healing rate (Evangelista et al., 2014). Sulodexide (SDX) has demonstrated effectiveness in symptom management, and decreasing time to healing (Andreozzi, 2012; Coccheri & Mannello, 2013; Wu et al., 2016). SDX is antithrombotic and fibrinolytic but the risk of bleeding is lower compared to heparin (Andreozzi, 2012). Further research regarding dose and treatment is recommended (Wu et al., 2016). When combined with diosmin and hesperidin, SDX used in conjunction with compression was shown to speed healing time and improve lipodermatosclerosis (Gonzalez Ochoa, 2017). Limited evidence exists to support aspirin to improve healing time with VLUs (del Rio Sola et al., 2012). Doxycycline used with compression may be helpful by way of decreasing inflammation, but the mechanism is unclear and further study is indicated (Sadler et al., 2012; Serra et al., 2013).

Pycnogenol (a pine bark extract herbal supplement) compared to diosmin/hesperidin (phlebotropic medication) has been shown to stimulate VLU healing and decrease lower extremity edema (Toledo et al., 2017). There is limited or mixed evidence regarding the use of multiple other agents, including granulocyte–macrophage colony-stimulating factor (GM-CSF), defibrotide, stanozolol, solcoseryl, iloprost, and topical growth factors. Other pharmacologic agents are not readily available despite demonstrated efficacy, including sulodexide and hydroxyethylrutoside (Andreozzi, 2012; Coccheri & Mannello, 2013; Wu et al., 2016).

Insufficient evidence exists to support the use of zinc or fish oil supplementation although fish oil may be useful in modulating polymorphonuclear leukocyte levels (McDaniel et al., 2017; Wilkinson, 2014). There is no good evidence to support oral zinc supplementation

(Wilkinson, 2014). There is no current research to support mesoglycan use (WOCN, 2019). Further research is needed to examine the potential effect of eicosapentaenoic acid (EPA) plus docosahexaenoic acid (DHA) supplements on VLU healing by way of polymorphonuclear leukocytes (PMN) modulation.

SURGICAL INTERVENTIONS

Evidence is mixed on the effectiveness of surgical/endovascular interventions to improve healing rates for VLUs. Surgical intervention has been shown to be effective in reducing venous hypertension and preventing VLU recurrence. Most researchers agree that venous surgery for correction of underlying disease in addition to compression remains effective in healing and preventing ulcer recurrence (Malas et al., 2014). Whether surgical interventions compared to conservative treatments are better to improve healing and prevent ulcer recurrence requires additional study. Minimally invasive endovascular ablation of varicose and incompetent perforator veins through techniques such as thermal ablation (radiofrequency, endovascular laser), and nonthermal ablation such as foam sclerotherapy have been shown to promote ulcer healing (de Carvalho, 2015; van Gent & Wittens, 2015) and are associated with lower costs (Belramman et al., 2019; Kelleher et al., 2014) but whether these procedures are as good as or better than surgery remains up for debate (Campos et al., 2015). The subfascial endoscopic perforator surgery (SEPS) procedure and application of skin grafts, biological dressings, and human skin equivalents have also been shown to benefit patients by reducing healing time and should be

considered, especially to reduce recurrence (van Gent & Wittens, 2015) (**Table 24-5**). More recent studies have shown a positive effect on healing rates in addition to reduced recurrence rates using minimally invasive techniques (Alden et al., 2013).

KEY POINT

Surgical procedures to reduce venous hypertension have been shown to reduce the incidence of ulcer recurrence and improve healing rates.

TOPICAL THERAPY GUIDELINES

Dermatitis is common in patients with LEVD. Management requires ongoing attention to prevention, early detection, and prompt intervention. Routine care should include gentle cleansing with a mild nonsoap cleanser with no artificial colors or fragrances (e.g., Dove®, Olay®, Cetaphil®, Neutrogena®) to remove scales, crusts, and bacteria. Emollients such as petrolatum should be applied to the intact periwound skin while it is damp to prevent excessive drying of the skin surface. Emollients with known sensitizing agents such as lanolin should be avoided since patients with VLUs are at high risk for allergic contact dermatitis. In patients with heavy wound exudate, it may be necessary to provide high-level protection of the periwound skin; zinc oxide preparations are commonly used in this situation. When the patient has venous dermatitis/eczema, as evidenced by increased pruritus, erythema, and scaling, topical corticosteroids may be required.

TABLE 24-5 COMMON SURGICAL/INTERVENTIONAL PROCEDURES FOR MANAGEMENT OF LOWER EXTREMITY VENOUS DISEASE

PROCEDURE	METHODS	CONSIDERATIONS
Surgical vein stripping (SVS)	Surgical procedure where the greater saphenous vein (GSV) is ligated at the groin and removed (stripped) to the knee	Surgical procedure requiring general anesthesia Seldom done now that minimally invasive techniques have been developed Used as the "gold standard" to which all subsequent procedures are compared
Endovenous laser ablation (EVLA)	Performed in endovascular suite; a laser fiber is used to produce heat that destroys the vascular endothelium along the GSV, closing the vein	Requires local anesthesia and light sedation Highly effective compared to SVS, verified with multiple studies Fewer complications than SVS with better long-term outcomes
Radiofrequency ablation (RFA)	Thermal energy is delivered using a catheter directly to the GSV walls resulting in closure of the vein	Requires local anesthesia and light sedation Effectiveness has been demonstrated
Ultrasound-guided foam sclerotherapy (USFS)	A sclerosing foam is injected under ultrasound guidance into the GSV—volume depends on length and diameter of vessel	Requires local anesthesia and light sedation Slightly less effective than EVLA and RFA but equal to SVS
Subfascial endoscopic perforator surgery (SEPS)	Surgical procedure done via a scope to close incompetent perforator veins	Used to address perforators when GSV closure was not adequate for symptom relief or ulcer healing

Venous Dermatitis

In order to avoid inappropriate antibiotic use and expensive hospitalizations, it is important to differentiate venous dermatitis from cellulitis (Elwell, 2015). While scant data exist to inform the use of topical corticosteroids, venous dermatitis is typically treated with a mid-potency steroid, such as triamcinolone 0.1% in an ointment form. Once started, the steroid should be continued for at least 2 weeks to clear the dermatitis before switching to a plain emollient. It should be used episodically thereafter for flares (Morton & Phillips, 2013; Ratliff et al., 2016). If ineffective, a dermatology referral may be needed (**Fig. 24-5** for illustration of venous dermatitis).

Patch tests should be performed with prolonged healing or unclear dermatitis diagnosis (Morton & Phillips, 2013). For severe or persistent dermatitis, the use of short-term oral steroids may be indicated (Morton & Phillips, 2013). Limiting edema will assist in decreasing inflammation and drainage.

Topical therapy for VLUs is based on wound characteristics. If biofilm or nonviable tissue is present, debridement should be attempted after ensuring adequate arterial flow (Bianchi et al., 2016). The exception would be a closed wound with dry eschar in a patient with significant arterial compromise. Venous ulcers are typically well perfused, so avascular tissue is usually minimal and is likely to represent biofilm due to high bacterial loads. A topical anesthetic such as EMLA (eutectic mixture of local anesthetics) may be used to reduce discomfort.

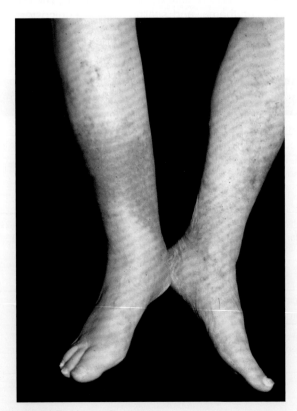

FIGURE 24-5. Venous Dermatitis.

Enzymatic debriding agents have shown little effect. (See Chapter 10 for additional information regarding debridement.)

Routine swab cultures of VLUs are not indicated. Cultures should be performed only when there are clinical signs and symptoms of significant infection as their purpose is to guide systemic antibiotics (WOCN, 2019). Signs of infection that would warrant culture-based antibiotic therapy include the following:

- Local heat and tenderness
- Increasing erythema of the surrounding skin
- Lymphangitis (red streaks up the limb)
- Rapid increase in the size of the ulcer
- Fever

Most VLUs are heavily colonized with both gram-positive and gram-negative bacteria. Topical antibiotics are of little use and, as noted, systemic antibiotics should be used only for signs and symptoms of infection. Topical antimicrobials are frequently used, though there is no evidence to support routine use. Examples include medical grade (Manuka) honey, cadexomer iodine, various silver dressings, and bacteria binding contact layers. Of these agents, medical grade (Manuka) honey and cadexomer iodine have the strongest data. Thyroid function may be affected if cadexomer iodine is used over an extended period (O'Meara et al., 2014). Any of these products can be used if wound healing plateaus and when there is no negative effect on healing or pain (O'Meara et al., 2014).

Most venous ulcers are relatively superficial with significant exudate. When selecting dressings, the wound care nurse should focus on minimizing exposure to potential allergens, protecting the periwound skin from maceration, managing dermatitis, containing exudate, and controlling bioburden. Dressings should be matched to wound characteristics with modifications as the wound changes. Several types of dressings are useful in VLU management, including alginates, hydrofibers, hydroconductive fibers, polyurethane foams, and composite dressings.

Skin grafting has been suggested for ulcers of >12 months' duration or very large ulcers. Types of grafts include autografts, allografts, xenografts, human skin equivalents, or bioengineered skin substitutes (Jones et al., 2013). Split-thickness skin grafts have shown higher rates of closure (92% vs. 12% and 100% vs. 50%) and decreased pain compared to conservative treatment with compression (Reeder et al., 2013; Salome et al., 2014). Less invasive hair follicle containing punch grafts are another treatment option (Martinez et al., 2016). Biologic skin substitutes are categorized as epidermal, dermal, or bilayered. Epidermal substitutes are fragile and have not been shown to be useful in healing VLUs. Dermal substitutes are composed of a bioabsorbable matrix; these "matrix" products may be acellular or may be populated with donor cells, such as fibroblasts.

Products commonly used for VLU treatment include Oasis®, MatriStem®, PriMatrix®, and Endoform®. Bilayered skin substitutes (e.g., Apligraf®) have the strongest evidence and are indicated for VLU treatment in the United States (Jones et al., 2013). Skin substitutes are used in conjunction with compression and should be considered when healing is delayed (Jones et al., 2013; Salome et al., 2014; Serra et al., 2017). New emerging technologies include marine derived products such as omega-3 rich fish skin and shortened fibers of poly-*N*-acetyl glucosamine (pGlcNAc) isolated from microalgae (Kelechi et al., 2012; McDaniel et al., 2017). Other adjuncts to healing, including hyperbaric oxygen, whirlpool, electromagnetic therapy, electrical stimulation, low-level laser therapy (LLLT), and therapeutic ultrasound, have not demonstrated a significant effect on healing of VLUs (Couch et al., 2017; Cullum & Liu, 2017; Kranke et al., 2015; Thakral et al., 2013; Vitse et al., 2017). Whirlpool in particular is not indicated for wound care and should not be used as it may exacerbate edema and could potentially pose an infection hazard. Negative pressure wound therapy (NPWT) has been shown to improve granulation tissue in VLUs, which may be helpful prior to and after skin grafting (Dini et al., 2011; Egemen et al., 2012) however, the effectiveness on healing requires further research. Electromuscular stimulation (EMS) has shown utility in improving QOL by decreasing or eliminating edema and pain through improving calf muscle function (Bogachev et al., 2011), but little is known about the effects on healing.

 ## SECONDARY PREVENTION: PREVENTING RECURRENCE

Ulcer recurrence is high, particularly in patients with a history of a VTE, longer ulcer healing time, higher body mass index, living alone, older age, poor nutrition, failure to elevate legs daily, and physically inactivity (Parker et al., 2015). Educating patients that compression therapy is the hallmark of prevention and will require a lifelong commitment to prevent VLU recurrence is essential. Once a VLU has healed, a compression garment (stocking or wrap) that provides the appropriate amount of compression (highest tolerable level) is worn daily, from the time the patient rises in the morning until bedtime (O'Donnell et al., 2014; Rabe et al., 2018). The prescription for elastic compression stockings includes both the length (calf vs. thigh vs. waist) and the amount of compression. Compression garments should be fitted by trained individuals. In patients with LEVD but without a history of ulcers, those with CEAP class C2 to C3 disease should use compression that provides 20 to 30 mm Hg, CEAP class C4 to C6, 30 to 40 mm Hg, and patients with recurrent ulcers should use products with 40 to 50 mm Hg. Knee length is most commonly used for increased patient adherence so long as symptom relief is adequate (Eberhardt & Raffetto, 2014). Assess the patient's ability

to don and doff the stockings independently or with available assistance. Many aids for donning and doffing stockings are available. Referral to occupational therapy may be needed to determine the best device for the patient. If the patient is unable to use stockings, other methods of compression are available such as tubular elastic bandages or inelastic compression leggings. The goal is to provide the level of compression determined to be most appropriate for the patient's level of disease severity; however, consistent use of lower-level compression provides better outcomes than inconsistent use of higher-level compression.

KEY POINT

Prevention of VLU recurrence requires lifelong adherence to compression therapy. While the goal is to provide the highest level of compression appropriate for the individual, consistent use of lower-level compression provides better outcomes than does inconsistent use of higher-level compression.

Surgical/interventional correction of varicosities and valve dysfunction can also contribute positively to secondary prevention; however, findings from studies remain conflicting on whether surgical intervention is superior to the use of compression to prevent recurrence (Serra et al., 2016). Minimally invasive procedures are emerging as equally effective as surgery to treat varicose veins, but whether they are as effective to enhance healing of VLUs is inconclusive. Additional study is needed to determine outcomes on prevention of VLU recurrence. Data show improved QOL with both minimally invasive and surgical procedures.

All of the measures previously discussed for management of LEVD should be continued such as lifelong exercise programs, weight control, and avoidance of injury. Frequent patient education is paramount to assure adherence. Education should include a practical explanation of venous disease and factors contributing to VLU recurrence, the role of compression, appropriate care and replacement of compression garments, and when to report early symptoms of VLU recurrence.

Medical management may reduce LEVD symptoms (swelling, leg heaviness) through use of phlebotonics/venoactive drugs (e.g., calcium dobesilate, MPFF) and other products/formulations such as horse chestnut seed extract and mesoglycan may also be indicated. Not all of these products are available in the United States. They can also interact with other medications patients may be taking such as anticoagulants. Patients should check with their primary care provider and pharmacist prior to taking any new medication or supplement. Patients should be instructed to practice good skin hygiene including the use of mild soap for cleansing the skin, applying emollients, and avoiding use of known irritants. Physical activity including walking and resistance exercises, in addition to leg elevation, are highly encouraged. The wound care nurse should collaborate with the patient and caregivers to develop a realistic plan for long-term management of LEVD (Kapp & Miller, 2015; Migdalski & Kuzdak, 2015).

 ## MANAGEMENT OF MIXED ARTERIAL–VENOUS DISEASE

Patients with concomitant arterial insufficiency require modifications of their treatment plan. Obtaining an ABI is key to selecting an appropriate level of compression. For patients with an ABI > 0.5 to <0.8, a trial of reduced compression (23 to 30 mm Hg) may be undertaken (Bonham et al., 2016; Ratliff et al., 2016; WOCN, 2014). Educate the patient regarding signs of developing ischemia (numbness, pain, pallor, or cyanosis of toes) and proper response (removal of wrap and notification of wound care clinician). Some patients may tolerate light compression when legs are dependent but will experience pain with elevation to level of the heart. These patients should use a removable compression legging or reusable wrap and should be instructed to remove the wrap or legging at bedtime and reapply in the morning. In addition, these patients may be candidates for a compression pump. Patients with neuropathy should be cautioned to visually inspect the toes to prevent complications from compression (WOCN, 2014, 2019).

Compression is not recommended for individuals with an ABI < 0.5, ankle pressure <70 mm Hg, or toe pressure <50 mm Hg; these individuals should be referred for a vascular workup and possible revascularization. Following revascularization, use of compression should be reevaluated, including use during the postprocedure period when edema may be increased due to a combination of lymphatic and inflammatory processes (WOCN, 2019).

 ## LYMPHEDEMA

Lymphedema is a chronic progressive disease with serious physical, psychosocial, economic, and QOL implications. It is defined as an illness by the International Classification of Diseases from the World Health Organization and is the clinical manifestation of impaired lymphatic circulation or lymphatic insufficiency (Executive Committee, 2016). There is no cure for lymphedema, and the objective for management is to limit disease progression and prevent complications (Grada & Phillips, 2017). Despite advances in lymphology as a science, the disease remains poorly understood (Bernas et al., 2018). Many patients receive inadequate treatment, are unaware that treatment is available, or do not know where to seek help. Patients with long-standing venous disease often develop secondary lymphedema; patients with long-standing venous disease should be evaluated for coexisting lymphedema. Lymphedema requires

lifelong care and maintenance. For cancer patients, specifically, it has been described as a significant survivorship issue (Finnane et al., 2015). The diagnosis and treatment of lymphedema is based on a clear understanding of the lymphatic system. Increased attention to the lymphatic system translates into more accurate diagnoses, improved treatment, and enhanced education for patients with lymphedema.

KEY POINT

Many patients with long-standing venous disease develop secondary lymphedema; lymphedema is also common among individuals after cancer therapy. Unfortunately, lymphedema is frequently underdiagnosed and undertreated.

ANATOMY AND PHYSIOLOGY OF LYMPHATIC SYSTEM

The lymph system is the third component of the circulatory system (Ambroza & Geigle, 2010), and it plays a critical role in the transport of interstitial fluid and molecules back into the circulatory system. Historically, the lymph system and lymphatic pathologies have received much less attention than pathologies associated with venous and arterial diseases.

The normal perfusion cycle involves movement of fluid and molecules out of the arterial capillary bed into the tissues, and most of the fluid and molecules are then returned to the capillary bed on the venous side. However, large molecules (such as plasma proteins) are unable to diffuse back into the venous capillary bed and are trapped in the interstitial space along with limited volumes of fluid. The return of these molecules and fluid to the circulatory system is dependent upon a normally functioning lymphatic system. Approximately 90% of the interstitial fluid is reabsorbed into the blood capillaries and the remaining 10% is handled by the lymphatic system.

The lymphatic system plays a critical role in transport of fluid and molecules out of the tissues and back into the blood stream; the load that the veins are unable to transport. The lymphatic system handles about 10% of the total interstitial fluid load.

Functions

The main functions of the lymph system are as follows:

- To collect and transport excess tissue fluid from the interstitium back to the veins in the blood system (Kunkel, 2010).
- To maintain normal plasma volumes by returning plasma proteins to the bloodstream. The lymphatic vessels absorb 2 to 4 L of protein-rich fluid retained in the interstitial tissue daily due to the venous system's inability to absorb all tissue fluids (Doughty & Holbrook, 2007).

- To prevent edema through its reserve capacity. During times of increased lymphatic load, the capacity for lymph transport is considerably greater than during times of normal lymphatic load (Doughty & Holbrook, 2007).
- To remove toxins from the tissue and protect the body against infection (Doughty & Holbrook, 2007).
- To produce antibodies to help fight disease states (Zuther & Norton, 2013).

Overview of Lymphatic System

The lymphatic system is composed of lymphatic vessels and lymphatic tissue (Lawenda et al., 2009). Lymphatic vessels provide a one-way path for the movement of lymph back into the circulatory system (Kunkel, 2010). As shown in **Figure 24-6**, the lymphatic system is an open system as compared to the closed cardiovascular system; thus, some refer to the lymph system as a transport system rather than as a circulatory system. The lymphatic system also differs from the cardiovascular system in that there is no central pump and lymph transport is interrupted by lymph nodes (Zuther & Norton, 2013).

Lymph is a protein-rich fluid that also contains white blood cells, triglycerides, bacteria, cell debris, water, and salts and has a composition comparable to blood plasma (Sleigh & Manna, 2019). The lymph will appear as clear in color with the exception of the milky white chylous fluid (chyle) found in vessels draining the intestinal system, which contains digested fatty acids. The components

of the lymph fluid are referred to as the lymphatic load (Zuther & Norton, 2013).

The lymphatic vessels run along similar paths as the arteries, veins, and capillaries and are composed of two distinguishable systems, a superficial system and a deep system (Quirion, 2010; Zuther & Norton, 2013). As depicted in **Figure 24-7**, the superficial vessels run close to the skin surface and drain the skin and subcutaneous tissues (Lawenda et al., 2009), while the deep vessels drain the tissues deep to the fascia (Zuther & Norton, 2013). The two systems communicate through perforating vessels that pass through the fascia. In visceral regions, the deep lymphatic system drains organs and provides additional filtration and purification of lymph through the lymph nodes (Zuther & Norton, 2013).

Lymph Capillaries

Lymph flow takes place in a low-pressure system. Uptake begins in the lymphatic capillaries in the interstitial space, the first component of the lymphatic system (Mehrara, 2019). They are open-ended tubes that are in close proximity to the blood capillaries (Kunkel, 2010), and they form a complex dermal network that covers the entire surface of the body. They differ from blood capillaries in that they are larger and more permeable, which allows them to absorb fluids and molecules that are often too large to be reabsorbed into the venous system (Ambroza & Geigle, 2010; Lawenda et al., 2009). Lymph capillaries also have a unique structural support network called "anchoring filaments" that enable the vessels to stay open even when interstitial tissue pressures are elevated; the anchoring filaments act like swinging flaps to open the lymphatic lumen so that interstitial fluid can drain into the capillary (Lawenda et al., 2009). Lymph capillaries do not have valves, so the flow of lymph is controlled by pressure gradients through the process of filtration (Lawenda et al., 2009).

Precollector and Collector Vessels

Lymph flows from the capillaries through precollector vessels to collector vessels (see **Fig. 24-6**). The precollectors contain valves to control the direction of flow; they also have a layer of smooth muscle but do not display any detectable vasomotor activity (Kunkel, 2010). The collector vessels range in diameter from 0.1 to 0.6 mm and are responsible for transporting lymph to the lymph nodes and the lymphatic trunks (Zuther & Norton, 2013). These vessels are histologically similar to veins (though thinner), and they contain paired semilunar valves that prevent retrograde flow (Mehrara, 2019) and assure unidirectional movement of the lymph, from distal to proximal (peripheral to central) (Kunkel, 2010) or toward the systemic circulation (Mehrara, 2019). The interval between valves varies from 6 to 20 mm, and the segment of the collector located between two sets of valves is called a lymphangion. Lymphangions are innervated by the sympathetic nervous system and contract at a frequency of 10 to 12

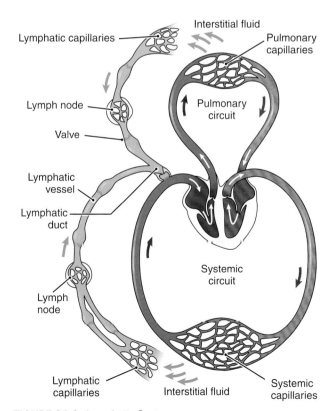

FIGURE 24-6. Lymphatic System.

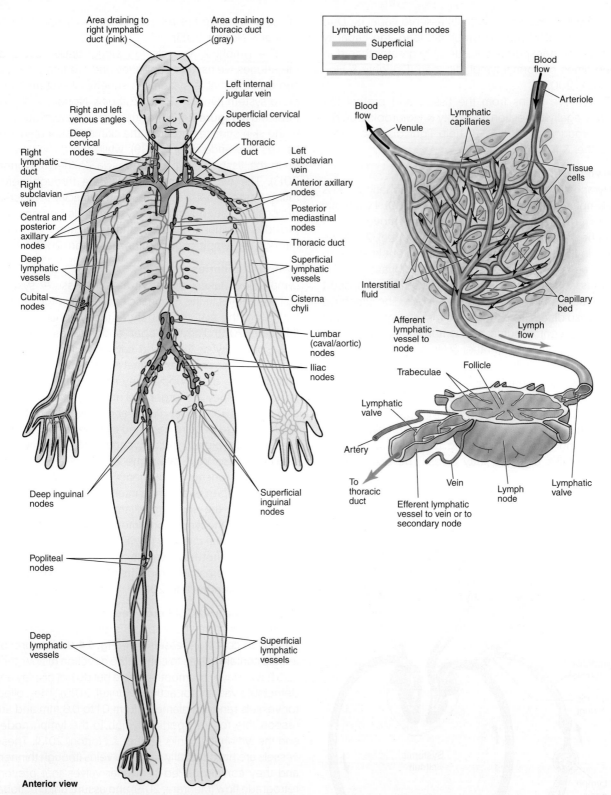

FIGURE 24-7. Lymphatic Vessels (Superficial and Deep System).

contractions per minute at rest. This is known as lymphangiomotoricity or lymphangioactivity (Zuther & Norton, 2013). When a lymphangion contracts, the valve at the distal end of the lymphangion closes and the proximal valve opens to propel lymph proximally (Kunkel, 2010). Lymph collectors react to an increase in lymph formation by increasing contraction frequency. Other factors that influence contraction frequency include external stretch on the wall of the lymphangion (effect of manual lymph drainage [MLD]), temperature, skeletal muscle contraction, movement of joints, diaphragmatic breathing, pulsation of adjacent arteries, and certain tissue hormones (Zuther & Norton, 2013).

Lymphatic Territories

As mentioned earlier, the superficial collectors drain lymph from the skin and subcutaneous tissue toward the lymph nodes; the superficial lymphatic system is subdivided into lymphatic territories. These territories consist of several collectors that all drain the same body area and to the same group of lymph nodes (regional lymph nodes). Watershed (**Fig. 24-8**) is the term used to describe linear, functional divisions of the superficial lymphatic system. Watersheds are characterized by a predictable pattern of lymph flow (Zuther & Norton, 2013). For example, the watershed territories of the right and left head and neck regions drain to the right and left cervical lymph nodes. The right and left upper quadrant watersheds include the upper extremities and upper trunk and drain into the right and left axillary nodes, respectively, while the right and left lower quadrant watersheds include the lower extremities and lower trunk and drain into the right and left inguinal nodes, respectively (Kunkel, 2010). Once lymph drains through a specific watershed territory, it drains into the deeper lymphatic collectors, which run parallel to the larger blood vessels and organ vessels. An understanding of lymph territories and watersheds is very important in the treatment of lymphedema.

Lymphatic Trunks and Ducts

Lymphatic trunks are the next larger classification of lymph vessels. Trunks are formed by the union of efferent lymph vessels (vessels that exit the lymph node) from individual lymph node groups (Kunkel, 2010). They

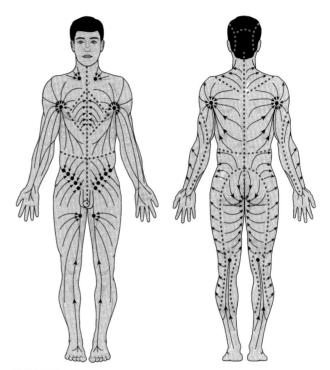

FIGURE 24-8. Lymphatic Watershed.

are similar to lymph collectors in that they are equipped with valves, innervated by the sympathetic nervous system, and contractile (Lawenda et al., 2009). The trunks merge to form ducts. The right lymphatic duct (see **Fig. 24-7**) drains the superficial and deep lymphatics of the right upper limb, thorax, and right side of the head and neck and empties into the right venous angle (right internal jugular and right subclavian veins); this duct returns approximately one quarter of the lymph to the circulation (Zuther & Norton, 2013) (**Fig. 24-9**).

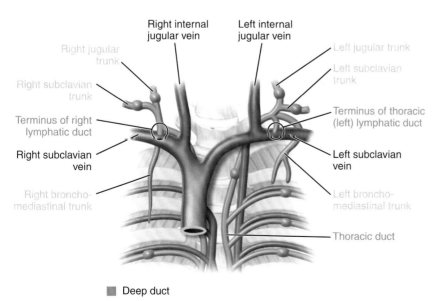

Right internal jugular vein

Left internal jugular vein

Right jugular trunk

Left jugular trunk

Right subclavian trunk

Left subclavian trunk

Terminus of right lymphatic duct

Terminus of thoracic (left) lymphatic duct

Right subclavian vein

Left subclavian vein

Right broncho-mediastinal trunk

Left broncho-mediastinal trunk

Thoracic duct

■ Deep duct

☐ Collecting trunk

FIGURE 24-9. Right and Left Venous Angles.

The thoracic duct is the largest lymph vessel in the body, varying in length from 36 to 45 cm, and perforates the diaphragm (Zuther & Norton, 2013). It empties approximately 3 L of lymph fluid per day directly into the left venous angle (left internal jugular and left subclavian veins). As shown in **Figure 24-7**, the thoracic duct drains the deep lymphatics of the left upper quadrant, left head and neck, and left and right lower quadrants (Lawenda et al., 2009).

Lymph Nodes

Lymph nodes (see **Fig. 24-7**) are a vital part of the lymph system and are arranged in groups or chains. The total number of lymph nodes in the body is estimated to be 600 to 700. Lymph enters the lymph nodes through afferent lymph collectors. Once the lymph is filtered and cleaned, it exits through efferent lymphatics. The main functions of the lymph nodes are as follows:

* To filter out harmful material in the lymph fluid (Zuther & Norton, 2013)
* To generate lymphocytes thus promoting immune function (Zuther & Norton, 2013)
* To thicken the lymph by reabsorbing water—much less lymph exits a lymph node than enters the node (Zuther & Norton, 2013)

EPIDEMIOLOGY

Estimates of the prevalence of lymphedema range widely and depend upon age, gender, and etiology. It is estimated that 250 million people suffer from this condition worldwide (Schulze et al., 2018). The most common cause of lymphedema worldwide is filariasis, due to a parasitic infection by the nematode *Wuchereria bancrofti*, found in certain developing countries, which infiltrates lymph vessels and nodes (Mehrara, 2019). The Centers for Disease Control and Prevention (CDC) considers filariasis to be a neglected tropical disease and the most frequent cause of permanent disability worldwide (Centers for Disease Control and Prevention, 2016) (**Fig. 24-10**). Lymphatic filariasis currently affects over 120 million people in 72 countries and is spread from person to person by mosquitoes living in tropical or subtropical areas found in Asia, Africa, the Western Pacific, part of the Caribbean and South America, Haiti, the Dominican Republic, Guyana, and Brazil. People living with this type of lymphedema are disfigured and frequently shunned.

In the Western world, lymphedema is almost always caused by significant trauma to the lymphatic system and is classified as secondary (acquired) lymphedema. Secondary lymphedema affects approximately 1/1,000 Americans (Sleigh & Manna, 2019). Specific causes of secondary lymphedema include cancer, cancer treatment, inflammatory disorders (arthritis, dermatitis, sarcoidosis) obesity, orthopedic injuries and/or surgeries, severe burns, severe infections, vascular reconstruction, or harvesting of veins for coronary artery bypass procedures. Secondary lymphedema can also be caused

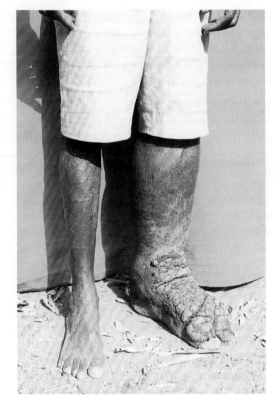

FIGURE 24-10. Lymphatic Filariasis.

by the sequelae of severe CVI, which causes soft tissue fibrosis and disruption of lymphatic structures (Doughty & Holbrook, 2007; Mehrara, 2019) (**Fig. 24-11**).

Cancer-associated lymphedema occurs due to:

* Tumors causing obstruction or infiltration of lymphatic channels and/or nodes
* Removal of lymph nodes at time of surgery (lymphatic dissection/lymphadenectomy)
* Irradiation of regional lymph nodes; can destroy lymphatic channels
* Chemotherapeutic medications

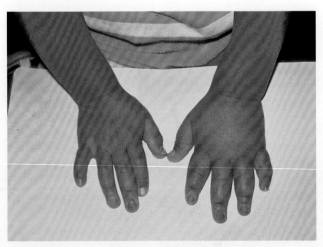

FIGURE 24-11. Secondary Lymphedema in Breast Cancer Patient.

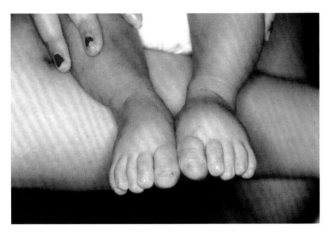

FIGURE 24-12. Congenital Lymphedema in Infant.

The most common cancer related to lymphedema is breast cancer (BCRL). Other malignancies associated with an increased risk of lymphedema include sarcomas, lower extremity melanoma, gynecologic cancer, genitourinary cancer, and head and neck cancer (Mehrara, 2019).

Primary lymphedema is less prevalent. Approximately 1/100,000 will develop primary lymphedema (Sleigh & Manna, 2019). Primary lymphedema is an inherited or congenital condition that causes developmental abnormalities of the lymphatic system most often due to a genetic mutation. Primary lymphedema is divided into three categories: (1) congenital lymphedema, present at birth or recognized within 2 years of birth; (2) lymphedema praecox, occurring at puberty or prior to age 35; or (3) lymphedema tarda, which begins after age 35. The onset for this population is sudden with no apparent cause and can affect one or both extremities (Mehrara, 2019) (**Fig. 24-12**).

Identification of incidence and prevalence of lymphedema is complex. Lymphedema is remarkably prevalent but underreported and underrecognized (Rockson, 2018b). Estimates of the incidence of secondary lymphedema from cancer vary due to the absence of uniform criteria for measuring, defining, and reporting the condition. Available estimates come from the breast cancer registry. Few studies have baseline measurements or long-term follow up (>5 years). The National Cancer Institute (NCI) predicts that there will be more than 4 million breast cancer survivors by the year 2024 and 2 million women with a diagnosis of breast cancer annually worldwide. For this population alone, lymphedema has the potential to become a significant burden to global public health (McLaughlin et al., 2017b).

CLASSIFICATION OF EDEMA

Chronic edema is a broad term encompassing a variety of conditions and etiologies. It is important to conduct a thorough assessment to identify the underlying cause for the edema and an appropriate treatment regimen (Cooper, 2013; Lay-Flurrie, 2011). The word edema means an abnormal accumulation of fluid in the interstitial tissue that is visible and palpable; it develops when the capillary filtration rate overwhelms the lymphatic drainage rate over a period of time (Hampton, 2010). Edema is not a disease, but a symptom associated with a variety of conditions, including congestive heart failure, CVI, immobility, pregnancy, or even pressure from constrictive garments or clothing. Whatever the underlying cause of the edema, the result is the accumulation of fluid in the interstitial space due to either dynamic insufficiency or mechanical insufficiency of the lymphatic system (or a combination of both) (Zuther & Norton, 2013).

Dynamic Insufficiency

Dynamic insufficiency (high-volume insufficiency) is the most common type of problem and occurs whenever the lymphatic load exceeds the transport capacity of the anatomically and functionally intact lymphatic system (Zuther & Norton, 2013). It is also known as high-volume insufficiency or failure. Increased filtration of fluid out of the blood capillaries results in excess interstitial fluid and edema characterized by high fluid and low protein. Examples of dynamic insufficiency–related edema include the edema caused by congestive heart failure, CVI, post-thrombotic syndrome, and dependency. Kidney disease, starvation, severe anemia, and diseases of the liver also result in dynamic insufficiency due to low plasma protein levels (hypoproteinemia) that permit excess movement of fluid out of the vessels into the tissues (also known as third spacing). If dynamic edema persists for a long period of time, the chronic excess workload for the lymph vessels may result in damage to the vessel walls and the lymphatic valvular system (Zuther & Norton, 2013). To avoid secondary damage to the lymphatic system, edema caused by systemic disease should be treated medically. For example, edema due to venous insufficiency (localized edema) should be treated with elevation, compression, and exercise, while edema due to congestive heart failure (generalized edema) usually requires diuretic therapy in addition to treatment of the underlying heart condition (Zuther & Norton, 2013).

Mechanical Insufficiency

Mechanical insufficiency (low-volume insufficiency) occurs as a result of congenital or acquired damage to the lymphatic system that impairs its ability to provide normal transport of lymphatic fluid. Congenital malformation or absence of lymphatic tissue (primary lymphedema) is one cause of low-volume insufficiency; another is damage to the lymphatic system from functional or organic causes that lead to a reduction in the capacity for lymph transport (secondary lymphedema) (Lawenda et al., 2009). Mechanical insufficiency can result from surgery, radiation, trauma, infection, inflammation, and LEVD (organic causes). Functional factors causing mechanical insufficiency include loss of lymphatic contractility due to certain toxins and drugs (Zuther & Norton, 2013). The appropriate treatment of choice for mechanical insufficiency is complete decongestive therapy (CDT).

Combined Insufficiency

Combined insufficiency develops when dynamic and mechanical insufficiencies occur simultaneously. This happens in circumstances in which there is both a reduction in the transport capacity of the lymphatic system and an increase in the lymphatic load (Lawenda et al., 2009). The two primary types of combined insufficiency are hemodynamic insufficiency and lymphovenous edema. Hemodynamic insufficiency causes edema because sustained cardiac insufficiency affects the right side of the heart as well as the left; when the right side of the heart does not empty effectively, there is resistance to venous return and increased volumes of fluid are trapped in the tissues. The persistent congestion of the venous system impairs lymphatic drainage and causes lymphatic overload, resulting in structural damage. MLD and compression therapy are contraindicated in edema caused by cardiac insufficiency due to the risk of cardiac overload (Zuther & Norton, 2013).

Lymphovenous edema is caused by LEVD that results in localized hemodynamic pathology (Lay-Flurrie, 2011). If not diagnosed and treated, the high volumes of fluid leaking into the interstitial space can cause dynamic lymphatic insufficiency and subsequent edema. With LEVD, the dynamic insufficiency can be further complicated by mechanical insufficiency of the lymphatics. The high levels of tissue proteins and chronic inflammation can cause fibrosis of the lymphangion walls and damage to the lymphatic vessels (Zuther & Norton, 2013). As LEVD progresses, there are extensive fibrotic changes to the dermis caused by tissue reaction to the cells and proteins leaking into the soft tissues. These fibrotic changes can damage or obliterate lymphatic channels, leading to obstruction of lymph flow (Doughty & Holbrook, 2007). CDT can be an effective treatment for advanced stages of LEVD (**Table 24-6**) resulting in lymphovenous edema.

PATHOLOGY

Lymphedema due to mechanical insufficiency is defined as an abnormal, generalized, or regional accumulation of protein-rich interstitial fluid resulting in edema formation and change in tissue structure (McLaughlin et al., 2017b). It may be caused by congenital malformations of the lymphatic system (primary lymphedema) or by injury (secondary lymphedema) (Kunkel, 2010). Lymphedema occurs when the lymphatic load exceeds the transport capacity of the impaired lymphatic system and results in an abnormal accumulation of protein-rich fluid in the interstitium. It manifests as swelling of the involved body part; most commonly the extremities are involved, but lymphedema can also involve the trunk, head, neck, and external genitalia.

It is important for clinicians to identify patients at risk for lymphedema (**Table 24-7**) and to educate them regarding measures to reduce the risk. Onset may occur due to a causative event or may be delayed for several decades (Lawenda et al., 2009).

The International Society of Lymphology (ISL) recognizes four stages of lymphedema (McLaughlin et al., 2017a) (**Table 24-8**). Stage 0 (reversible) refers to a latent or subclinical condition not yet evident despite impaired lymph transport. It may exist for months or years before observable edema (Executive Committee, 2016). Stages I (reversible), II (irreversible), and III (irreversible) lymphedema represent progressive changes in the severity of edema and skin and soft tissue changes (Armer et al., 2012). In patients with chronic lymphedema, large amounts of subcutaneous adipose tissue may form. Although not completely understood, this adipocyte proliferation may explain why conservative treatment may not completely reduce the swelling and return the affected area to its usual dimensions (Lymphoedema Framework, 2006).

TABLE 24-6 STAGES OF LEVD AS IT RELATES TO LYMPHATIC FUNCTION

STAGE	STATUS OF LYMPHATIC VESSELS	SYMPTOMS	THERAPEUTIC APPROACH
0	Normal function; normal protein load	None	Compression therapy; elevation; exercise
1	Normal function; increased load	Mild edema	Compression therapy; elevation; exercise
2	High-protein load; morphological changes	Moderate edema with pigmentation, varicosities, pain	CDT
3	Very high-protein load; morphological changes	Severe edema with hypoxia, tissue destruction, pain	CDT with needed wound care

CDT, combined decongestive therapy.
Used with permission from Zuther, J., & Norton, S. (2013). *Lymphedema management: The comprehensive guide for practitioners* (3rd ed.). New York, NY: Thieme.

TABLE 24-7 RISK FACTORS FOR THE DEVELOPMENT OF SECONDARY LYMPHEDEMA

Cancer surgery that involves excision of lymph nodes in the axilla and/or radiation therapy

Postsurgical complications from breast cancer surgery (seroma formation, axillary cording)

Post–breast cancer trauma in the extremity (injection, blood pressure)

Cancer surgery involving excision of inguinal nodes and or pelvic radiation therapy

Advanced cancer

Obesity

Recurrent soft tissue infections

Varicose vein stripping and vein harvesting

Chronic venous insufficiency, stages I and II

Thrombophlebitis and postthrombotic syndrome

Orthopedic injuries and traumas

Burn injuries

Immobility (paralysis)

Sources: Lymphoedema Framework. (2006). *Best practice for the management of lymphoedema. International consensus.* London, UK: MEP Ltd; Wigg, J., & Lee, N. (2014). Redefining essential care in lymphoedema. *British Journal of Community Nursing, 19*(Suppl 4), S20–S27.

DIAGNOSIS

Diagnosis of lymphedema is based on history and clinical findings (Grada & Phillips, 2017). Other conditions such as morbid obesity and LEVD, unrecognized trauma,

TABLE 24-8 INTERNATIONAL SOCIETY OF LYMPHOLOGY—STAGES OF LYMPHEDEMA

Stage 0—Latency (subclinical lymphedema)

Edema is not evident despite impaired lymph transport

Extremity may feel heavy, full, tight, or achy

This stage may exist for months or years before edema is observable

Stage I—Early-onset edema

Edema is observable and measurable

Edema may pit with pressure

Edema resolves with elevation

Tissue feels soft (no fibrosis)

Clothing and jewelry may feel tight and produce constriction

Stage II (May be divided into early and late stage II)

There will be a combination of pitting and nonpitting edema (late stage II)

Edema does not resolve with elevation

Fibrosis present in the tissue (late stage II)

The patient may begin to experience decreased range of motion, difficulty fitting into clothing

Stage III

Significant skin changes present (generalized fibrosis and pitting response is absent)

Hypertrophy of the subcutaneous tissue

Papillomas and warty overgrowths may develop on the skin

Skin folds and lobules begin to develop

Disfigurement of the extremity

Ongoing infections of the tissue likely

Adapted from The International Society of Lymphology. (March 2013). Consensus document on diagnosis and treatment of peripheral lymphedema. *Lymphology*, (1), 1–11.

and repeated infection may complicate the clinical picture. Comorbid conditions such as heart failure may also influence the diagnosis and therapeutic approach (Executive Committee, 2016).

Advanced diagnostics (ultrasound, lymphoscintigraphy, CT, and MRI) may be warranted when the history and physical do not yield a definitive diagnosis or in cases where lymphatic obstruction due to tumor is suspected (Mehrara, 2019). Lymphoscintigraphy is the gold standard, using radiotracers to evaluate the anatomy and function of the lymphatic system (Bernas et al., 2018; Muldoon, 2011). Use of fluorescent imaging with indocyanine green (ICG) is increasing; the contrast agent is not FDA approved and it requires multiple injections (Bernas et al., 2018). Technologies such as photo-acoustics, specific tracer targeting the lymphatic system, may be seen in the future (Chang et al., 2016).

LYMPHEDEMA ASSESSMENT

Lymphedema assessment should be performed at the time of diagnosis and repeated periodically throughout treatment. Assessment should be performed by a practitioner specifically trained in the treatment of lymphedema. The International Lymphedema Framework (ILF) recommends that the following be included in a comprehensive lymphedema assessment (Lymphoedema Framework, 2006).

Measurement of Limb Volume

The most widely used method for measuring limb volume is circumferential limb measurements, which are easy to obtain and cost effective. A reproducible set of measurement points, with the circumference measured at each point (usually every 4 cm) and at fixed time intervals should be used (Balci et al., 2012). A nonelastic tape measure with an attached tensioning device is recommended (Gulick) to ensure the same amount of tension at each measurement (Muldoon, 2011). Software programs exist to determine limb volume (Executive Committee, 2016).

Bioelectrical impedance spectroscopy (BIS) uses a single-frequency low-voltage electrical current passing through the water content of body tissue; this tool can detect alterations in extracellular fluid before clinical signs of edema are present (Muldoon, 2011). Tissue dielectric constant (TDC) estimates water in skin tissues. BIS and TDC are superior methods for reducing false-negative or false-positive results compared to circumferential tape measure (McLaughlin et al., 2017a).

Skin Assessment

The skin should be examined carefully for dryness, color and pigmentation, temperature, scars, wounds, skin folds, fragility, inflammation including cellulitis, and fungal infection. The most common changes resulting from chronic edema are thickened skin, hyperkeratosis, lymphangiectasia, and papillomata. The skin should be assessed for a "pitting" response. In early stages, the skin will pit but as the edema becomes more chronic and inflammatory processes progress, the tissue will become firmer due to fibrosis and adipose tissue deposition. A tonometer is a tool used to assess the resistance of tissue to compression and can aid in determining the extent of fibrosis (Muldoon, 2011). Another assessment parameter is a positive Stemmer sign, which is the inability to pinch or lift the skin fold at the base of the second toe (or middle finger). A negative Stemmer sign does not exclude lymphedema.

Vascular Assessment

Lower extremity arterial disease (LEAD) should be ruled out because it may indicate the need for a modified level of compression. DVT should also be ruled out as a cause of the edema. See Chapter 25 for details of vascular assessment.

Pain Assessment

Pain may be caused by inflammation, infection, distention of the tissue, nerve entrapment, radiation fibrosis, cancer recurrence, or degenerative joint disease. Lymphedema is not associated with a "typical" pain pattern; some patients report no pain, while others report sensations such as aching, tingling, tightness, and weakness. Heavy swollen limbs can cause pain proximal to the edematous limb, that is, hip and back pain with leg edema.

Psychosocial Assessment

Lymphedema may have a negative impact on an individual's QOL. Psychosocial assessment includes evaluating the patient for depression, anxiety, ability to cope, and understanding of the disease process and treatment. The relationship between lymphedema and negative psychological and psychosocial factors has been associated with nonadherence to self-management (Executive Committee, 2016). Other areas of assessment should include the involvement of significant others and their support system, health insurance and finances, and home environment.

Mobility and Functional Assessment

Lymphedema may cause a reduction in mobility and functional status, and affect activities of daily living (ADL). Range of motion in the arms and legs, strength, and ability to lift and move the limbs should be assessed.

Nutritional Assessment

The patient's BMI should be determined, and the patient should be counseled to maintain a healthy body weight. Obesity contributes to the onset of lymphedema and may exacerbate the symptoms of existing lymphedema. Consider referral for weight reduction to facilitate treatment.

Laboratory Tests

There are no routine laboratory tests to diagnose lymphedema. Evaluation of liver and kidney function may be useful to rule out hepatic and renal causes of extremity swelling. If an infection is suspected, a complete blood count should be performed. Blood should be examined for detection of parasites in those who have traveled to endemic areas (Grada & Phillips, 2017).

Genetic Testing

Primary lymphedema has a high degree of genetic heterogeneity. Genetic testing should be considered for individuals with a family history of lymphedema. Infants and children presenting with lymphedema should have a chromosomal karyotyping or targeted variant analysis to test for Turner syndrome. Advances in genomic medicine will play a greater role for screening for syndromes that may be associated with primary lymphedema and in understanding the genetic basis for underlying lymphatic abnormalities (Grada & Phillips, 2017).

> **KEY POINT**
>
> Patients with lymphedema need comprehensive periodic assessment to monitor limb volume and skin status to detect any deterioration in status.

MANAGEMENT

Management of the patient with lymphedema requires a lifelong program of exercise, skin care, massage, and compression garments. Lymphedema centers offer comprehensive interdisciplinary care (Ratliff, 2016).

Prevention

Education on prevention and risk reduction should be provided (**Table 24-9**). Surveillance practices lead to earlier diagnosis and treatment strategies that are more effective and result in lower costs than before the introduction of these practices (Rockson, 2018b). The use of BIS is the most commonly used approach for widespread clinical surveillance. Other approaches include the use of perometry or measurement of the TDC.

> **KEY POINT**
>
> Preventive measures for all at-risk patients includes the importance of maintaining skin integrity and preventing injury and infection to the skin.

Treatment Goals

Lymphedema is an incurable condition because damage to the lymphatics is usually irreversible. It can be effectively managed with the goals of reducing and maintaining limb size, alleviating symptoms, preventing infection, improving limb function, and improving overall psychological well-being (Kunkel, 2010). Intervention should occur as soon as possible following diagnosis to prevent progressive tissue damage. Outcomes are suboptimal when treatment is delayed, increasing the fibrotic changes that occur in the limb (Lawenda et al., 2009).

TABLE 24-9 RISK REDUCTION STRATEGIES FOR PATIENTS AT RISK FOR LYMPHEDEMA
Skin Care
Meticulous care of the skin and nails
Keep the skin clean and dry and well moisturized with low-pH lotions
Avoid trauma and injury to reduce infection risk (including injections and blood draws if possible)
Wear gloves when doing activities that may cause skin injury
Protect exposed skin with sunscreen and insect repellent
Activity and Lifestyle
Maintain an optimal body weight—obesity is a known risk factor for lymphedema
Eat a well-balanced diet
Avoid tight clothing including underwear, watches, and jewelry
Avoid blood pressures in the affected extremity
Avoid carrying a heavy bag or purse on the affected side
Undertake exercise and movement therapy
Avoid extreme temperatures—both heat and cold
Compression Garment
Wear prophylactic compression garments if prescribed
Consider wearing prophylactic compression garment during strenuous exercise and for travel by air to support the extremity at risk

Please note that prevention guidelines are anecdotal and based on clinical experience by experts in the field of lymphology. To see the NLN position papers on prevention, visit lymphnet.org. (Adapted from The National Lymphedema Network.)

Complete Decongestive Therapy

CDT, also known as combined decongestive therapy, comprehensive decongestive therapy, complex physical therapy, and complex decongestive physiotherapy, is the gold standard of lymphedema treatment. CDT is backed by long-standing experience and considered the first-line intervention for both primary and secondary lymphedema in both children and adults (Bernas et al., 2018; Chang et al., 2016; Grada & Phillips, 2017).

History of CDT

The technique of MLD, a component of combined decongestive therapy, was developed in 1932 by Emil Vodder, a PhD from Denmark. This method has evolved into a comprehensive physical therapy approach to management that combines MLD with compression bandaging, skin care, and exercise (Williams, 2010).

Considerations Related to CDT

CDT should be provided by a certified lymphedema health care practitioner (Executive Committee, 2016; Uzkeser, 2012). The components incorporate a multimodality approach including MLD, compression bandaging, compression garments, therapeutic exercises, meticulous skin care, and patient education (Chang et al., 2016; Grada & Phillips, 2017).

CDT consists of two phases. The first phase is the acute intensive (or reductive) phase. In this phase, patients are seen in an outpatient setting for MLD at a frequency of 3 to 5 days a week for 1 to 4 weeks. Length and duration of treatment is determined according to the severity and stage of lymphedema (Korpan et al., 2011). The goal of the first phase of treatment is to reduce the limb to the smallest possible size and to alleviate symptoms such as tightness, discomfort, and decreased range of motion (Fu et al., 2009). The second phase is patient-directed maintenance and home care. This phase is individualized based on the specific needs of the patient and focuses on maintaining limb reduction. Education includes continued skin care and infection prevention, exercises, self-massage, and use of garments and compression aids/devices (Balci et al., 2012; Quirion, 2010). Precautions must be taken with patients with hypertension because CDT can increase central venous blood volume (Lawenda et al., 2009). Caution should also be used in those with compromised sensation, for example, individuals with paralysis or diabetic neuropathies. These patients may not detect pain; improperly placed bandages or garments could result in injury. CDT in patients with bronchial asthma could result in a bronchial asthma attack due to the effects of MLD on the parasympathetic nervous system (Lawenda et al., 2009). Lymphedema affecting the head, neck, trunk, or genitalia can be very challenging and requires a modified CDT approach. Absolute contraindications to CDT include patients with acute infections, symptomatic heart failure, and DVT (Lawenda et al., 2009).

CDT may also be used for palliative care to control secondary lymphedema from tumor-blocked lymphatics (Executive Committee, 2016). The MLD component of CDT reduces edema and may decrease pain and improve QOL.

KEY POINT

CDT is currently accepted as the international gold standard for the treatment of lymphedema; the therapy includes MLD, compression bandaging, compression garments, therapeutic exercises, meticulous skin care, and patient education. CDT should be performed by therapists trained in this method.

CDT Components: Manual Lymph Drainage

MLD is a procedure that involves manual movement and gentle directed stretching of the skin in a circular or spiral motion using very light hand and finger movements (Grada & Phillips, 2017; Rockson, 2018b). It is considered a skin technique and uses low pressure (30 to 40 mm Hg) (Grada & Phillips, 2017). MLD works by promoting lymphatic contractility or flow of lymph through the lymphatic structures located in the subcutaneous tissue. MLD should not be confused with massage therapies, which apply considerable pressure to treat conditions of muscle tissue, tendons, and ligaments. Massage therapy should not be used in the treatment of lymphedema as these techniques can increase vascular flow (which increases lymph formation) (Zuther & Norton, 2013).

MLD enhances the efficiency of the lymph system in several ways. It stretches the smooth muscle sheath of the superficial lymphatic vessels, which increases their pumping rate (lymphangiomotoricity) (Lawenda et al., 2009). MLD redirects lymph flow out of the compromised areas and into healthy functioning areas of the lymphatic system by opening and dilating the collateral vessels that cross lymphatic watersheds; in essence, it "bypasses" the ineffective or damaged lymphatics (Kunkel, 2010). The sequence in which MLD is performed on the body is important and requires an understanding of lymphatic watersheds and patterns of lymphatic drainage. It involves first stimulating the nonaffected areas of the body. Edema fluid is then massaged across the lymphatic watershed toward the functional lymphatic structures and regional lymph nodes. The affected areas are treated last and always from proximal to distal. The benefits of MLD include a reduction in swelling that is produced by decongestion of the impaired lymphatic pathways, reduction in lymphatic load, enhanced development of collateral drainage routes, and stimulation of the functional and patent components of the system (Lymphoedema Framework, 2006). MLD also improves the quality of the tissue by reducing fibrosis.

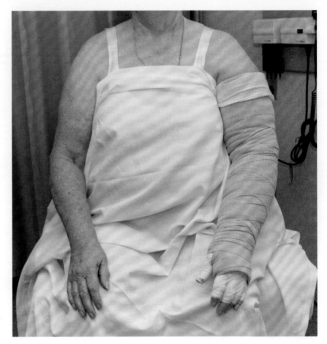

FIGURE 24-13. Short Stretch Multilayer Bandages.

KEY POINT

Manual lymphatic drainage uses very light and strategically directed touch to improve lymphatic flow; it should not be confused with massage, which uses high-pressure touch and is totally contraindicated in the management of lymphedema.

Compression Therapy: Multilayer Compression Bandaging

External compression is the mainstay of management for all stages of lymphedema. The efficacy of compression therapy alone or combined with MLD has been supported by randomized clinical trials (Grada & Phillips, 2017). Compression therapy achieves the following goals (Grada & Phillips, 2017):

- Improvement of lymphatic flow and venous return
- Reduction of accumulated protein and tissue debris
- Facilitating proper shaping of the limb
- Facilitating sustained volume control
- Maintenance of skin integrity
- Protecting the limb from potential trauma

The use of short stretch bandages (SSBs) with low extensibility (inelastic bandages) is indicated for the treatment of lymphedema. SSBs are applied in multiple layers with more layers applied to the distal aspect of the extremity and less applied at the proximal aspect of the extremity (**Fig. 24-13**). Application of bandages in this manner creates a gradient pressure to facilitate lymph flow. The bandages have a high working pressure and a low resting pressure. Muscle contraction facilitates lymph flow due to the antagonistic force between the muscle and the bandage (Uzkeser, 2012). Compression bandages are primarily used during the intensive first phase of treatment to achieve limb reduction. Once the limb has reached maximum reduction in size, the patient is fitted for a compression garment.

KEY POINT

Short-stretch layered bandages are used during the intensive phase of treatment to promote lymphatic flow and to reduce edema; once maximum edema reduction has been obtained, the patient should be fitted for a compression garment.

Compression Therapy: Compression Garments

Compression garments are used in the second phase of therapy and are meant for long-term management of lymphedema. They assist in maintaining edema reduction by accelerating lymph flow. Garments are meant for daytime use as their effect is facilitated by muscle movement. Circular knit garments (ready to wear) have no seams, are made of thinner material, and are cosmetically more acceptable. Flat knit garments (custom-made) have seams and can be adapted to fit the special needs of some patients. Garments come in a variety of pressure strengths (measured as mm Hg) and are determined by the clinician or by the garment fitter in collaboration with the patient and clinician. Generally, the highest compression tolerated by the patient (20 to 60 mm Hg) is likely to be the most beneficial (Executive Committee, 2016). To ensure patient compliance, the garments must be comfortable and fit properly and patient should be well educated in donning and doffing techniques (Grada & Phillips, 2017).

Contraindications to compression garments are LEAD, extreme shape distortion of the limb, deep skin folds, extensive skin damage or ulcerations, acute cardiac failure, and severe peripheral neuropathy (Lymphoedema Framework, 2006). The wearing of compression garments requires a lifelong commitment to maintain edema reduction (Ratliff, 2016).

Therapeutic Exercises

Exercises are meant to enhance lymph flow and should be encouraged by clinicians for patients at risk and with existing lymphedema (Stuiver et al., 2015). There are three main types including aerobic, strength, and flexibility, and they should be customized to the patient's functional ability (Grada & Phillips, 2017). Compression bandages are worn coupled with exercises during the first phase of treatment. Exercises are geared toward increasing muscle strength, flexibility, and range of motion and improving lymphatic circulation (Cheifetz & Haley, 2010). Exercise protocols are established that are easy to learn and perform in order to promote compliance. Exercises are performed while the patient is wearing a compression garment during maintenance therapy (second phase). Water-based exercises (aquatic therapy) may be helpful due to the natural compression of water when exercising (Executive Committee, 2016).

Skin Care

Skin care focuses on optimizing skin health and treating any skin conditions. The skin should be cleansed using a low pH or neutral body wash or soap followed by the application of low pH or neutral lotion. Compression bandages are then applied. Patients are instructed to continue skin care throughout maintenance therapy (Quirion, 2010).

Patient Education

Prior to initiation of any intervention, the patient requires education to attain a thorough understanding of all components of his or her treatment plan (Quirion, 2010). Patients must commit to the lifelong daily regimen of prescribed skin care, exercises, garments, and compression aids (Stuiver et al., 2015). Limitations that may affect compliance include physical challenges in providing self-care, time constraints perceived by the patient, and cost of products (bandages and garments) if not covered by insurance (Fu et al., 2009).

Weight Control and Diet

There is no evidence that a certain diet is beneficial or harmful for patients with lymphedema. Restricted fluid intake has not been proven to be of benefit. Weight reduction is recommended in cases associated with obesity. Failure of treatment is associated with a higher BMI. Obesity is known to cause a worsening of lymphedema due to inflammation and lymphatic vessel damage (Executive Committee, 2016; Grada & Phillips, 2017).

Pharmacotherapy

Medications have limited use in the management of lymphedema.

Diuretics

Lymphedema results in an increase of protein-rich fluid in the interstitial space. Diuretics are not recommended for the management of lymphedema because they worsen the condition by causing an increased concentration of interstitial proteins, facilitating the formation of fibrosis (Grada & Phillips, 2017). Diuretics should be initiated only in cases of cardiac insufficiency resulting in an increase of systemic fluid in the vasculature, or other comorbid conditions or complications (i.e., ascites, hydrothorax, palliative care issues) (Executive Committee, 2016).

Benzopyrones

Coumarin (oral and topical) is a benzopyrone immuno-modulator that aids in increasing local proteolysis in the treatment of lymphedema and filarial elephantiasis. A Cochrane systematic review did not find enough evidence to draw conclusions about the effectiveness of coumarins in the management of lymphedema (Grada & Phillips, 2017). Oral coumarin has been shown to cause hepatotoxicity in some patients.

Antimicrobials

Antibiotics should be administered for infection and related inflammation as in cases of cellulitis, lymphangitis, or erysipelas. Signs and symptoms include erythema, pain, high fever, and possibly septic shock. For fungal skin infections, cleanse with a mild disinfectant and treat with antifungal medications (systemic or topical) (Executive Committee, 2016).

Pneumatic Compression Devices

For patients who cannot complete both phases of CDT, pneumatic devices may increase patient compliance (Executive Committee, 2016). Pneumatic compression devices (PCDs) have long been used for the medical management of swelling. The most recently developed PCDs provide lower pressures and are meant to mimic the therapeutic techniques of MLD. These systems permit variation in the compression patterns to meet individualized needs and apply a light and variable pressure to the affected limb (Ridner et al., 2010; Scheiman, 2011) (**Fig. 24-14**). These advanced PCDs are being used both for accelerating the first treatment phase and for the second treatment phase at home. PCDs can be an adjunctive treatment for appropriate patients but cannot be considered as solo therapy for treatment of lymphedema (Rockson, 2018a). PCDs are contraindicated for patients with heart failure, active infection, or DVT (Balci et al., 2012).

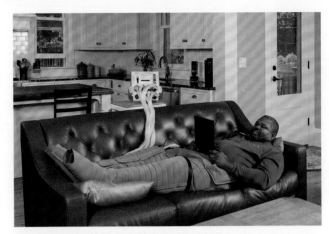

FIGURE 24-14. Pneumatic Compression Device.

Compression Devices

For patients who need ongoing lymphatic drainage during the second phase of lymphedema therapy (maintenance), compressive devices (i.e., ReidSleeve®, JoviPak®, Solaris®) have been developed that can be worn at home while sleeping or during the day if preferred by the patient. These devices are easy to don and can be a beneficial alternative to learning self-bandaging techniques. These devices (sleeves) are composed of convoluted foam with an outer sleeve or straps that can be adjusted to provide the desired compression. Most companies offer both custom-made and ready-to-wear options and work in collaboration with the therapist and patient to achieve the desired outcomes. Some therapists utilize these devices during the first phase of therapy as they facilitate the breakdown and softening of fibrotic tissue.

Compressive Strapping Devices

Several companies have devised a strapping system (e.g., FarrowWrap®, CircAid®) secured with hook and loop (Velcro®) straps that can be used as an alternative to short-stretch compression bandages and garments (**Fig. 24-15**). Indications for use include patients who are intolerant to bandaging or garments, have distorted limb shapes, have hand weakness or back problems, have skin sensitivities, or have compliance issues. These products are available in both standard and custom-made options (Hobday & Wigg, 2013).

Lymphatic Taping

Kinesio tape is a type of medical tape that is applied to the skin to facilitate lymphatic drainage. It has been shown to reduce lymphatic congestion and the sensation of tightness and to improve function and movement. Additionally, it can improve the appearance of scar tissue (Hardy, 2012). Lymph taping is recognized as an effective adjunctive therapy in the management of lymphedema. Lymph taping works by increasing pressure differences within the lymph vessels, promoting opening of the lymphatic capillaries by lifting the skin, and providing a micro-massaging effect. Taping does not replace short-stretch

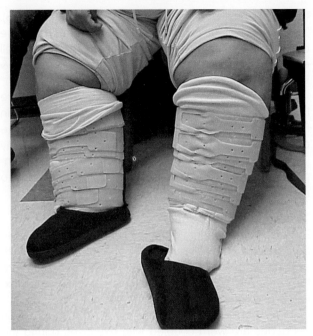

FIGURE 24-15. Hook and Loop (Velcro®) Strapping System.

bandaging and must be applied by someone who has been trained in the application technique. Lymphatic taping can be considered an alternative choice for patients with lymphedema in areas where compression is difficult or impossible to use (Bosman, 2014; Stuiver et al., 2015).

Low-Level Laser Therapy

Research has shown that LLLT can facilitate wound healing; improve lymphatic function; reduce inflammation, pain, and scar tissue; and enhance the effects of MLD (Low Level Laser Therapy, 2011; Wigg & Lee, 2014). LLLT treats the cells by delivering an infrared laser at a wavelength of 904 nm. This wavelength penetrates deeply into the tissue where it is absorbed by cells and converted into energy; the result is a photochemical reaction at the cellular level (Kozanoglu et al., 2009). More studies are needed to confirm findings (Executive Committee, 2016; Finnane et al., 2015; Grada & Phillips, 2017). LLLT should not be used for patients with infection, active cancer, or other medically prohibitive conditions.

Surgical Techniques for Lymphedema

Surgical management of lymphedema is used to alleviate peripheral lymphedema and enhance lymph return. Surgical management techniques are gaining more acceptance. Surgical interventions are aimed at limb volume reduction, prevention of infection, and decreasing the need for compression garments (Executive Committee, 2016; Ratliff, 2016; Williams, 2012).

Excisional Procedures (Reduction of Limb Volume through Resection)

Excisional procedures (debulking procedures) are performed in a staged manner with repeated primary closure. They involve the removal of excess skin and lymphedematous adipose tissue down to the fascia followed by skin grafts and flaps. Removal of the redundant skin folds and subcutaneous tissue reduces the size and weight of the limb (Ratliff, 2016). Many complications can arise from excisional procedures including poor wound healing, extensive scarring, skin ulcerations, nerve damage, poor cosmetic outcomes, and increased edema from damage to residual normal functioning lymphatics (Avraham et al., 2010; Executive Committee, 2016).

Microsurgical Reconstruction

Microsurgical approaches are used to reconstruct lymphatic pathways or bypass damaged lymphatics, augmenting the rate of return of lymph to the blood circulation (Executive Committee, 2016). Techniques for directly reconnecting the lymphatics and restoring lymphatic flow are improving. Experience with these techniques has shown that if performed for early-onset lymphedema, before damage to lymphatic walls and contractility have occurred, outcomes are more durable and long lasting (Executive Committee, 2016). Microsurgery focuses on redirecting lymph flow to the venous circulation at the level of obstruction through lymphatic–venous anastomoses (LVA). LVA procedures have undergone confirmation of long-term patency (>20 years in some cases) and some demonstration of improved lymphatic transport (Executive Committee, 2016). LVAs are indicated when the patient still has functionality of the lymphatic system (Chang et al., 2016).

Reconstructive microsurgery repair focuses on restoring lymphatic flow by bypassing the site of obstruction either directly or with interposition of a vein or a lymphatic graft (Avraham et al., 2010). The techniques involve the use of a lymphatic collector or an interposition vein segment to restore lymphatic continuity in conditions due to a locally interrupted lymphatic system. Autologous lymph vessel transplantation is one reconstructive procedure that aims to mimic normal physiology and has shown long-term patency of more than 10 years. This procedure has been restricted to unilateral lower extremity lymphedema due to the need for one healthy leg to harvest the graft. It has been utilized in bilateral upper extremity lymphedema where two healthy legs are available for graft harvesting (Executive Committee, 2016)

Vascularized Lymph Node Transplantation

Vascularized lymph node transplantation (VLNT) involves transplantation of superficial lymph nodes and lymphatic vessels into areas where the lymphatics are missing or damaged (Chang et al., 2016). This technique has been proposed as both a preventive and therapeutic approach to limb lymphedema (Executive Committee, 2016). There are concerns relating to VLNT including the development of lymphedema in the donor site from lymph node harvesting, especially when harvested from the groin or axilla. Reverse lymphatic mapping may aid in reducing this risk (Chang et al., 2016; McLaughlin et al., 2017a).

Liposuction

Liposuction is a suction-assisted technique that removes subcutaneous fatty tissue from the affected limb. Liposuction has proven effective as an option for reducing limb volume, increasing the blood flow to the limb, and decreasing the incidence of cellulitis (Ratliff, 2016). Liposuction is usually only considered after more conservative methods have been tried (CDT). The patient must maintain any reduction that is achieved with the lifetime use of compression garments. The benefit of liposuction is the complete reduction of nonpitting, nonfibrotic extremity lymphedema that has not responded to conservative therapy in both primary and secondary lymphedema (Munnoch, 2012).

LIPEDEMA

Lipedema (see **Fig. 24-13**) is a chronic condition of unknown etiology that results in the abnormal deposition of fat in the subcutaneous tissue (Hampton, 2010). Many medical practitioners are unfamiliar with this condition, and it is often misdiagnosed as bilateral primary lymphedema or morbid obesity (Zuther & Norton, 2013). It manifests as swelling in the lower extremities but does not involve the feet (foot sparing) (**Fig. 24-16**). Lipedema almost exclusively affects women and is thought to possibly be related to a hormonal disorder. It often starts at times of hormonal changes such as puberty or pregnancy (Lymphoedema Framework, 2006). Lipedema complicated by weight gain can lead to the development

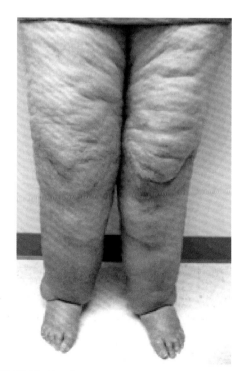

FIGURE 24-16. Lipedema.

of lymphedema (lipolymphedema). Characteristics of lipedema include the following:

- The swelling is bilateral and symmetrical but does not involve the feet (foot-sparing).
- Stemmer sign is negative.
- The tissue is often tender to palpation.
- Bruising is common.
- Hard nodules may be palpated in the tissue.
- Nonpitting edema.
- There is often a family history of lipedema.

Lipedema is also known as "painful fat syndrome"; it involves abnormal deposition of fat in the lower extremities with sparing of the feet. CDT and compression garments may provide some benefit.

Treatment for lipedema includes the following: nutritional guidance if the lipedema is associated with obesity, instruction in routine exercise therapy, medical management for any hormonal imbalance, CDT, and compression garments. The results obtained with CDT are typically slower and less dramatic than those obtained with lymphedema patients, and patients usually require custom-made compression garments. Liposuction is sometimes listed as a treatment option but must be used with extreme caution due to the risk of lymphatic damage.

SKIN/WOUND CARE AND LYMPHEDEMA

Patients with lymphedema are prone to skin issues that can progress to the development of open wounds. Skin care education should include daily cleansing with low-pH soaps or soap substitutes followed by application of emollients. Skin folds should be kept clean and dry. Common skin conditions for those with lymphedema include hyperkeratosis (**Fig. 24-17A**), folliculitis, and fungal infections. Patients with lymphedema are also at risk for recurrent episodes of cellulitis. Prompt recognition and treatment of cellulitis is essential to prevent further soft tissue and lymphatic damage, which would predispose the patient to worsening disease and recurrent episodes.

Advanced skin conditions such as lymphangiectasia (fluid-filled projections from dilation of lymphatic vessels)

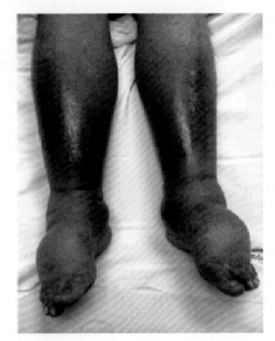

FIGURE 24-18. LEVD and Lymphedema.

and papillomatosis (raised projections on the skin due to dilation of lymphatic vessels and fibrosis, **Fig. 24-17B**) require management by a lymphedema specialist. In cases where lymph is leaking from the skin surface (lymphorrhea), the surrounding skin should be protected with a moisture barrier cream and/or a nonadherent absorbent dressing to avoid maceration of the skin (Lymphoedema Framework, 2006). Patients with lymphedema may develop skin tears and open wounds related to the poorly functioning lymphatic system or as a result of other comorbid conditions. Wounds can also result from trauma, allergies, or therapeutic procedures (e.g., surgery and radiation therapy). Wounds resulting from excessive accumulation of interstitial fluid (LEVD and lymphedema, see **Fig. 24-18**) may be treated with CDT. Open wounds should be treated based on the principles of wound care discussed in Chapter 8. Advanced wound care products designed to manage large volumes of fluid should be used to control exudate and to facilitate debridement. Vascular status must be evaluated prior to initiation of compression therapy (Zuther & Norton, 2013).

REFERRAL FOR LYMPHEDEMA SERVICES

Lymphedema services are provided in the outpatient clinic setting through the physical therapy/occupational therapy department. Wound care nurses should recognize the signs and symptoms of lymphedema and identify local resources for lymphedema therapy. The National Lymphedema Network (www.lymphnet.org) and the Lymphology Association of North America (LANA) (www.clt-lana.org) maintain a database of lymphedema practitioners.

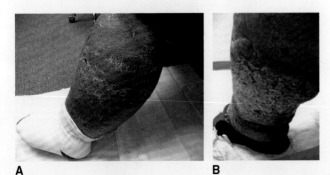

A　　　　　　**B**

FIGURE 24-17. A. Hyperkeratosis. **B.** Stage III lymphedema with papillomatosis.

KEY POINT

The wound care nurse may be the first person to recognize the symptoms of lymphedema in a patient. See **Table 24-10** for lymphedema resources.

 ## CONCLUSION

The venous and lymphatic systems are intricately connected by the capillary system at the tissue level in order to transport venous blood and lymph fluid out of the tissue and back into the systemic circulation. The systems function in a complementary fashion when both are functioning normally. When either of the systems is compromised by pathology (i.e., LEVD or lymphedema), the interdependence creates an additional burden or load on the other system. Understanding this unique relationship is important to the management of patients with LEVD and/or lymphedema. Early diagnosis and intervention are key in both conditions, and wound care nurses are in an optimal position to recognize the problems and provide guidance in treatment.

TABLE 24-10 LYMPHEDEMA RESOURCES

American Cancer Society; Web site has good comprehensive information for patients
American Lymphedema Framework Project (ALFP)
International Lymphedema Framework (ILF)
International Society of Lymphology (ISL)
Lymphology Association of North American (LANA)
Lymph Notes—online Web site for patients and professionals
Lymphatic Education and Research Network (LERN)
Lymphedema Resources, Inc.
Lymphoedema Support Network (LSN)—A British Lymphedema Society
Lymphedema Treatment Act (Legislative Organization)
Medicine Wheel and Lymphedema Impact on the Spirit
National Cancer Institute's PDQs for health care professionals
National Cancer Institute's PDQs for patients
National Lymphedema Network (NLN)
National Organization of Vascular Anomalies (NOVA)
Native American Cancer Research
North American Lymphedema Education Association (NALEA)
Oncology Nursing Society's Putting Evidence into Practice Lymphedema Resources

CASE STUDIES

CASE STUDY: LYMPHEDEMA

The patient is a 42-year-old male with a >10-year history of bilateral lower extremity lymphedema R > L. The edema began following a crush injury of the right thigh on a construction site. Patient's history also includes morbid obesity. He has had repeated episodes of cel-lulitis to the right thigh for which hospitalization was required. The patient presented with significant palpable fibrosis involving both lower extremities. Prior to the initiation of CDT, the patient was counseled on nutrition and lost 35 pounds. The patient was treated with CDT five times a week for 4 weeks. Compression

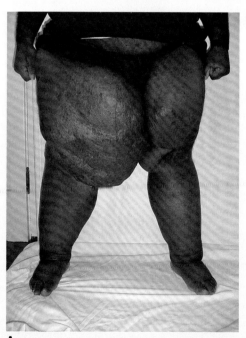
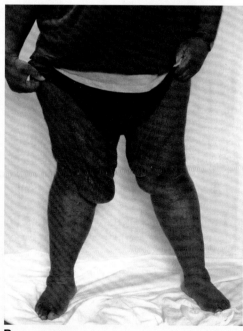

A. Stage III lymphedema. **B.** After treatment.

therapy included the use of convoluted foam sleeves under SSBs used to soften fibrosis. Skin care included daily cleansing and application of an emollient. Following therapy, the patient had redundant skin folds on the medial thighs, which were surgically excised. Complications after surgery included dehiscence of the suture line to the right thigh. This required an additional 2 weeks of treatment with MLD and SSBs until the suture line was healed. He was then fit with compression garments providing 40 to 50 mm Hg.

CASE STUDY: LYMPHEDEMA WITH LEVD AND WOUND

The patient is a 68-year-old female with a 12-year history of LEVD and lymphedema. She sustained a laceration to her right anterior lower leg after falling into a pipe that was protruding through a city street.

The patient also has a history of type 2 diabetes. The wound was unhealed after 2 months due to lymphorrhea. Topical care included daily cleansing, application of triple antibiotic ointment, and a protective cover dressing. The patient presented with hemosiderin staining of the bilateral lower extremities, palpable fibrotic edema (lipodermatosclerosis) from the ankles to knees, and soft edema from the knees to upper thighs. The periwound skin was dry and cracking. The patient was treated with 2 weeks of daily CDT. Skin care included daily cleansing and application of emollient. Cadexomer iodine dressing was placed over the wound followed by superabsorbent dressing and changed daily. The patient had a 35% reduction in affected limb size. The wound healed, and skin condition improved with a palpable softening of fibrosis.

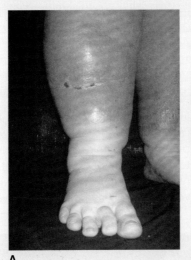 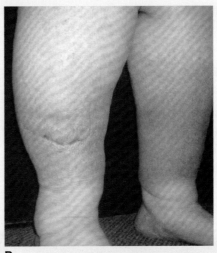

A. LEVD with lymphedema and wound. **B.** After treatment.

CASE STUDY: LEVD

The patient is a 75-year-old retired flight attendant who presents to the outpatient wound clinic with a history of chronic lower extremity edema and a medial left lower extremity ulcer, superior to the ankle, which drains a moderate to large amount of serosanguinous fluid. The ulcer has been present for 1 month and has been getting larger. Pain is rated as 5/10 and is improved with leg elevation. The wound is tender when cleansed and dressed during which time the pain increases to 7/10; the wound measures 3.2 × 4.1 × 0.2 cm and has a ruddy red base with irregular wound edges. The periwound skin is intact but hyperpigmented in the gaiter area and varicose veins are noted. Pedal pulses are difficult to palpate due to edema, skin is warm to the touch, and sensation was intact when tested with a 5.07 monofilament.

Medical history includes degenerative joint disease in the both knees, hypertension, and dyslipidemia. History shows smoking approximately 1 pack per day for 10 years but stopped smoking 20 years ago. BMI is 31. The patient denies any previous ulcer history or trauma to the affected leg. There is a family history of leg ulcers in several female relatives.

Medications include multivitamins, naproxen, atenolol, and simvastatin.

ABI measurement revealed ABI 0.88 on the right and 0.80 on the left.

Compression therapy to the left leg was initiated with a two-component dressing providing therapeutic compression. The left leg was initially wrapped as well to reduce the edema in order to obtain measurements for therapeutic compression stockings. After the edema was reduced, a 30 to 40 mm Hg compression stocking was prescribed for the right leg to prevent VLU in the intact limb. The patient was instructed to elevate legs above the level of the heart for 30 to 45 minutes twice daily and to perform "ankle pump exercises" every 2 hours during the day. The periwound skin was cleansed and then protected from maceration with petrolatum, and the wound was dressed with an antimicrobial alginate dressing followed by a poly-urethane foam for additional absorption under therapeutic compression.

Upon return, the patient reported reduced pain, and a marked reduction in edema was noted; the ulcer had reduced in size to 1.8 × 2.6 × 0.2 cm. Therapy was continued, and the ulcer healed within 8 weeks, at which point the patient was instructed in use of compression stockings providing 30 to 40 mm Hg compression at the ankle.

REFERENCES

Alavi, A., Sibbald, R. G., Phillips, T. J., et al. (2016). What's new: Management of venous leg ulcers. Approach to venous leg ulcers. *Journal of the American Academy of Dermatology, 74*(4), 627–640. doi: 10.1016/j.jaad.2014.10.048.

Alden, P. B., Lips, E. M., Zimmerman, K. P., et al. (2013). Chronic venous ulcer: Minimally invasive treatment of superficial axial and perforator vein reflux speeds healing and reduces recurrence. *Annals of Vascular Surgery, 27*(1), 75–83.

Alguire, P. C., & Mathes, B. M. (2014). Medical management of lower extremity chronic venous disease. In T. W. Post (Ed.), *UpToDate*®. Waltham, MA: Wolters Kluwer Health.

Ambroza, C., & Geigle, P. R. (2010). Aquatic exercise as a management tool for breast cancer-related lymphedema. *Topics in Geriatric Rehabilitation, 26*(2), 120–127.

Andreozzi, G. M. (2012). Sulodexide in the treatment of chronic venous disease. *American Journal of Cardiovascular Drugs, 12*(2), 73–81. doi: 10.2165/11599360-000000000-00000.

Andriessen, A., Apelqvist, J., Mosti, G., et al. (2017). Compression therapy for venous leg ulcers: Risk factors for adverse events and complications, contraindications—A review of present guidelines. *Journal of the European Academy of Dermatology and Venerology, 31*(9), 1562–1568. doi: 10.1111/jdv.14390.

Andriessen, A., Mosti, G., Partsch, H., et al. (2016). *Contraindications, risk factors, adverse events in venous leg ulcer compression therapy—Review of clinical practice guidelines.* Retrieved November 30, 2019, from http://www.tagungsmanagement.org/comp/images/PDF/poster_lr_2016.pdf

Armer, J. M., Stewart, B. R., Wanchai, A., et al. (2012). Rehabilitation concepts among aging survivors living with and at risk for lymphedema. *Topics in Geriatric Rehabilitation, 28*(4), 260–268.

Attaran, R. R., & Ochoa Chaar, C. I. (2017). Compression therapy for venous disease. *Phlebology, 32*(2), 81–88. doi: 10.1177/0268355516633382.

Avraham, T., Daluvoy, S. V., Kueberuwa, E., et al. (2010). Anatomical and surgical concepts in lymphatic regeneration. *Breast Journal, 16*(6), 639–643.

Balci, F. L., DeGore, L., & Soran, A. (2012). Breast cancer-related lymphedema in elderly patients. *Topics in Geriatric Rehabilitation, 28*(4), 243–253.

BaquerizoNole, K. L., Yim, E., Van Driessche, F., et al. (2015). Educational interventions in venous leg ulcer patients. *Wound Repair and Regeneration, 23*(1), 137–140. doi: 10.1111/wrr.12247.

Belramman, A., Bootun, R., Lane, T. R. A., et al. (2019). Endovenous management of varicose veins. *Angiology, 70*(5), 388–396. doi: 10.1177/0003319718780049.

Bernas, M., Thiadens, S. R. J., Smoot, B., et al. (2018). Lymphedema following cancer therapy: overview and options. *Clinical & Experimental Metastasis, 35*(5–6), 547–551. doi: 10.1007/s10585-018-9899-5.

Bianchi, T., Wolcott, R. D., Peghetti, A., et al. (2016). Recommendations for the management of biofilm: A consensus document. *Journal of Wound Care, 25*(6), 305–317. doi: 10.12968/jowc.2016.25.6.305.

Black, C. M. (2014). Anatomy and physiology of the lower-extremity deep and superficial veins. *Techniques in Vascular and Interventional Radiology, 17*(2), 68–73. doi: http://dx.doi.org/10.1053/j.tvir.2014.02.002.

Bobridge, A., Sandison, S., Paterson, J., et al. (2011). A pilot study of the development and implementation of a 'best practice' patient information booklet for patients with chronic venous insufficiency. *Phlebology, 26*(8), 338–343. doi: 10.1258/phleb.2010.010082.

Bogachev, V. Y., Golovanova, O. V., Kuznetsov, A. N., et al. (2011). Electromuscular stimulation with VEINOPLUS(R) for the treatment of chronic venous edema. *International Angiology, 30*(6), 567–590.

Bonham, P. A., Flemister, B. G., Droste, L. R., et al. (2016). 2014 Guideline for management of wounds in patients with lower-extremity arterial disease (LEAD): An executive summary. *Journal of Wound, Ostomy and Continence Nursing, 43*(1), 23–31. doi: 10.1097/WON.0000000000000193.

Bosman, J. (2014). Lymphtaping for lymphoedema: An overview of the treatment and its uses. *British Journal of Community Nursing, 19*(Suppl 4), S12–S18.

Branisteanu, D. E., Feodor, T., Baila, S., et al. (2019). Impact of chronic venous disease on quality of life: Results of the vein alarm study. *Experimental and Therapeutic Medicine, 17*(2), 1091–1096. doi: 10.3892.etm.2018.7054.

Campos, W., Jr., Torres, I. O., da Silva, E. S., et al. (2015). A prospective randomized study comparing polidocanol foam sclerotherapy with surgical treatment of patients with primary chronic venous insufficiency and ulcer. *Annals of Vascular Surgery, 29*(6), 1128–1135. doi: 10.1016/j.avsg.2015.01.031.

Centers for Disease Control and Prevention. (2016). *Parasites-lymphatic filariasis.* Retrieved from http://www.cdc.gov/parasites/lymphaticfilariasis/

Chang, D. W., Masia, J., Garza, R., et al. (2016). Lymphedema: Surgical and medical therapy. *Plastic and Reconstructive Surgery, 138*(3 Suppl), 209S–218S. doi: https://doi.org/10.1097/PRS.0000000000002683.

Cheifetz, O., & Haley, L. (2010). Management of secondary lymphedema related to breast cancer. *Canadian Family Physician, 56*(12), 1277–1284.

Chi, Y-W., & Raffetto, J. D. (2015). Venous leg ulceration pathophysiology and evidence based treatment. *Vascular Medicine, 20*(2), 168–181. doi: 10.1177/1358863X14568677.

Chudek, J., Mikosinski, J., Kobielski, A., et al. (2016). Patients' satisfaction with therapy methods of advanced chronic venous disease. *International Angiology, 35*(1), 98–107.

Coccheri, S., & Mannello, F. (2013). Development and use of sulodexide in vascular diseases: Implications for treatment. *Drug Design, Development and Therapy, 8*, 49–65. doi: 10.2147/DDDT.S6762.

Cooper, G. (2013). Compression therapy in oedema and lymphoedema. *British Journal of Cardiac Nursing, 8*(11), 547–551.

Couch, K. S., Corbett, L., Gould, L., et al. (2017). The international consolidated venous ulcer guideline update 2015: Process improvement, evidence analysis, and future goals. *Ostomy Wound Management, 63*(5), 42–46.

Cullum, N., & Liu, Z. (2017). Therapeutic ultrasound for venous leg ulcers. *Cochrane Database of Systematic Reviews*, (5), CD001180. doi: 10.1002/14651858.CD001180.pub4.

de Carvalho, M. R. (2015). Comparison of outcomes in patients with venous leg ulcers treated with compression therapy alone versus combination of surgery and compression therapy: A systematic review. *Journal of Wound, Ostomy and Continence Nursing, 42*(1), 42–46. doi: 10.1097/WON.0000000000000079.

del Rio Sola, M. L., Antonio, J., Fajardo, G., et al. (2012). Influence of aspirin therapy in the ulcer associated with chronic venous insufficiency. *Annals of Vascular Surgery, 26*(5), 620–629. doi: 10.1016/j.avsg.2011.02.051.

Dini, V., Miteva, M., Romanelli, P., et al. (2011). Immunohistochemical evaluation of venous leg ulcers before and after negative pressure wound therapy. *Wounds, 23*(9), 257–266.

Doughty, D., & Holbrook, R. (2007). Lower extremity ulcers of vascular etiology. In R. A. Bryant & D. P. Nix (Eds.), *Acute and chronic wounds* (3rd ed., pp. 298–303). St. Louis, MO: Elsevier.

Eberhardt, R. T., & Raffetto, J. D. (2014). Chronic venous insufficiency. *Circulation, 130*(4), 333–346. doi: 10.1161/CIRCULATIONAHA.113.006898.

Edwards, H., Finlayson, K., Skerman, H., et al. (2014). Identification of symptom clusters in patients with chronic venous leg ulcers. *Journal of Pain and Symptom Management, 47*(5), 867–875. doi: 10.1016/j.jpainsymman.2013.06.003.

Egemen, O., Ozkaya, O., Ozturk, M. B., et al. (2012). Effective use of negative pressure wound therapy provides quick wound-bed preparation and complete graft take in the management of chronic venous ulcers. *International Wound Journal, 9*(2), 199–205. doi: 10.1111/j.1742-481X.2011.00876.x.

Eklof, B., Rutherford, R. B., Bergan, J. J., et al. (2004). Revision of the CEAP classification for chronic venous disorders: Consensus statement. *Journal of Vascular Surgery, 40*(6), 1248–1252. doi: 10.1016/j.jvs.2004.09.027.

Elwell, R. (2015). Developing a nurse-led 'red legs' service. *Nursing Older People, 27*(10), 23–27. doi: 10.7748/nop.27.10.23.s20.

Evangelista, M. T., Casintahan, M. F., & Villafuerte, L. L. (2014). Simvastatin as a novel therapeutic agent for venous ulcers: A randomized, double-blind, placebo-controlled trial. *British Journal of Dermatology, 170*(5), 1151–1157. doi: 10.1111/bjd.12883.

Executive Committee. (2016). The diagnosis and treatment of peripheral lymphedema: 2016 consensus document of the international society of lymphology. *Lymphology, 49*(4), 170–184.

Finlayson, K., Miaskowski, C., Alexander, K., et al. (2017). Distinct wound healing and quality-of-life outcomes in subgroups of patients with venous leg ulcers with different symptom cluster experiences. *Journal of Pain and Symptom Management, 53*(5), 871–879. doi: 10.1016/j.jpainsymman.2016.12.336.

Finlayson, K., Wu, M. L., & Edwards, H. E. (2015). Identifying risk factors and protective factors for venous leg ulcer recurrence using a theoretical approach: A longitudinal study. *International Journal of Nursing Studies, 52*(6), 1042–1051. doi: 10.1016/j.ijnurstu.2015.02.016.

Finnane, A., Janda, M., & Hayes, S. C. (2015). Review of the evidence of lymphedema treatment effect. *American Journal of Physical Medicine & Rehabilitation, 94*(6), 483–498. doi: 10.1097/PHM.0000000000000246.

Franks, P. J., Barker, J., Collier, M., et al. (2016). Management of patients with venous leg ulcers: Challenges and current best practice. *Journal of Wound Care, 25*(Suppl 6), S1–S67. doi: 10.12968/jowc.2016.25.Sup6.S1.

Fu, M. R., Ridner, S. H., & Armer, J. (2009). Post-breast cancer lymphedema: Part 2. *American Journal of Nursing, 109*(8), 34–42.

Georgopoulos, S., Kouvelos, G. N., Koutsoumpelis, A., et al. (2013). The effect of revascularization procedures on healing of mixed arterial and venous leg ulcers. *International Angiology, 32*(4), 368–374.

Gloviczki, P., Comerota, A. J., Dalsing, M. C., et al. (2011). The care of patients with varicose veins and associated chronic venous diseases: Clinical practice guidelines of the Society for Vascular Surgery and the American Venous Forum. *Journal of Vascular Surgery, 53*(Suppl 5), 2S–48S. doi: 10.1016/j.jvs.2011.01.079.

Gonzalez, A. (2014). Education project to improve venous stasis self-management knowledge. *Journal of Wound, Ostomy and Continence Nursing, 41*(6), 556–559. doi: 10.1097/WON.0000000000000088.

Gonzalez, A. (2017). The effect of a patient education intervention on knowledge and venous ulcer recurrence: Results of a prospective intervention and retrospective analysis. *Ostomy Wound Management, 63*(6), 16–28.

Gonzalez Ochoa, A. (2017). Sulodexide and phlebotonics in the treatment of venous ulcer. *International Angiology, 36*(1), 82–87. doi: 10.23736/S0392-9590.16.03718-4.

Grada, A. A., & Phillips, T. J. (2017). Lymphedema: Diagnostic workup and management. *Journal of the American Academy of Dermatology, 77*(6), 995–1006. doi: 10.1016/j.jaad.2017.03.021.

Hamdan, A. (2012). Management of varicose veins and venous insufficiency. *Journal of the American Medical Association, 308*, 2612–2621.

Hampton, S. (2010). Chronic oedema and lymphoedema of the lower limb. *British Journal of Community Nursing, 15*(Suppl 6), S4–S12.

Hanson, D., Langemo, D., Thompson, P., et al. (2015). Providing evidence-based care for patients with lower-extremity cellulitis. *Wound Care Advisor, 4*(3). Retrieved November 30, 2019, from https://woundcareadvisor.com/providing-evidence-based-care-for-patients-vol4-no3/

Hardy, D. (2012). Management of a patient with secondary lymphedema. *Cancer Nursing Practice, 11*(2), 21–26.

Hobday, A., & Wigg, J. (2013). FarrowWrap: Innovative and creative patient treatment for lymphoedema. *British Journal of Community Nursing, 18*(10), S24–S31.

International Society of Lymphology. (2013). The diagnosis and treatment of peripheral lymphedema: 2013 consensus document. *Lymphology, 46*, 1–11.

Johnson, J., Yates, S. S., & Burgess, J. L. (2016). Venous insufficiency, venous ulcers, and lymphedema. In D. B. Doughty & L. L. McNichol (Eds.), *Wound, Ostomy and Continence Nurses Society core curriculum: Wound management* (pp. 384–419). Philadelphia, PA: Wolters Kluwer.

Jones, J. E., Nelson, E. A., & Al-Hity, A. (2013). Skin grafting for venous leg ulcers. *Cochrane Database of Systematic Reviews*, (1), CD001737. doi: 10.1002/14651858.CD001737.pub4.

Jull, A. B., Arroll, B., Parag, V., et al. (2012). Pentoxifylline for treating venous leg ulcers. *Cochrane Database of Systematic Reviews*, (12), CD001733. doi: 10.1002/14651858.CD001733.pub3.

Kapp, S., & Miller, C. (2015). The experience of self-management following venous leg ulcer healing. *Journal of Clinical Nursing, 24*(9–10), 1300–1309. doi: 10.1111/jocn.12730.

Kelechi, T. J., Dooley, M. J., Mueller, M., et al. (2018). Clinically meaningful differences on symptoms associated with chronic venous disease in response to a cooling treatment compared to placebo: A randomized clinical trial. *Journal of Wound Ostomy and Continence Nursing, 45*(4), 301–309. doi: 10.1097WON.0000000000000441.

Kelechi, T. J., Johnson, J. J., & Yates, S. (2015). Chronic venous disease and venous leg ulcers: An evidence-based update. *Journal of Vascular Nursing, 33*(2), 36–46. doi: 10.1016/j.jvn.2015.01.003.

Kelechi, T. J., Mueller, M., Hankin, C. S., et al. (2012). A randomized, investigator-blinded, controlled pilot study to evaluate the safety and efficacy of a poly-N-acetyl glucosamine-derived membrane material in patients with venous leg ulcers. *Journal of the American Academy of Dermatology, 66*(6), e209–e215. doi: 10.1016/j.jaad.2011.01.031.

Kelleher, D., Lane, T. R., Franklin, I. J., et al. (2014). Socio-economic impact of endovenous thermal ablation techniques. *Lasers in Medical Science, 29*(2), 493–499. doi: 10.1007/s10103-013-1453-8.

Kim, T. I., Forbang, N. I., Criqui, M. H., et al. (2015). Association of foot and ankle characteristics with progression of venous disease. *Vascular Medicine, 20*(2), 105–111. doi: 10.1177/1358863X14568443.

Konschake, W., Riebe, H., Pediaditi, P., et al. (2016). Compression in the treatment of chronic venous insufficiency: Efficacy depending on the length of the stocking. *Clinical Hemorheology and Microcirculation, 64*(3), 425–434. doi: 10.3233/CH-168122.

Korpan, M. I., Crevenna, R., & Fialka-Moser, V. (2011). Lymphedema: A therapeutic approach in the treatment and rehabilitation of cancer patients. *American Journal of Physical Medicine & Rehabilitation, 90*(5), S69–S75.

Kozanoglu, E., Basaram, S., Paydas, S., et al. (2009). Efficacy of pneumatic compression and low-level laser therapy in the treatment of postmastectomy lymphedema: A randomized controlled trial. *Clinical Rehabilitation, 23*(2), 117–124.

Kranke, P., Bennett, M. H., Martyn-St James, M., et al. (2015). Hyperbaric oxygen therapy for chronic wounds. *Cochrane Database of Systematic Reviews*, (6), CD004123. doi: 10.1002/14651858.CD004123.pub4.

Kunkel, K. R. (2010). Identification and impact of standard treatment protocols on the impairments and activity limitations related to lower extremity lymphedema (Doctoral dissertation). Open Access Dissertations. Paper 403. Retrieved from http://scholarlyrepository. miami.edu/oa_dissertations/403

Lattimer, C. R. (2018). Optimizing calf muscle pump function. *Phlebology, 33*(5), 353–360.

Lawenda, B. D., Mondry, T. E., & Johnstone, P. A. (2009). Lymphedema: A primer on the identification and management of a chronic condition in oncologic treatment. *Cancer Journal for Clinicians, 59*(1), 8–24.

Lay-Flurrie, K. (2011). Use of compression hosiery in chronic oedema and lymphoedema. *British Journal of Nursing, 20*(7), 418–422.

Lazareth, I., Moffatt, C., Dissemond, J., et al. (2012). Efficacy of two compression systems in the management of VLUs: Results of a European RCT. *Journal of Wound Care, 21*(11), 553–554, 556, 558 passim. doi: 10.12968/jowc.2012.21.11.553.

Low Level Laser Therapy. (2011). Retrieved July 25, 2014, from http://www.lymphnotes.com/article.php/id/370/

Lymphoedema Framework. (2006). *Best practice for the management of lymphoedema. International consensus*. London, UK: MEP Ltd.

Malas, M. B., Qazi, U., Lazarus, G., et al. (2014). Comparative effectiveness of surgical interventions aimed at treating underlying venous pathology in patients with chronic venous ulcer. *Journal of Vascular Surgery: Venous and Lymphatic Disorders, 2*(2), 212–225. doi: 10.1016/j.jvsv.2013.10.002.

Martinez, M-L., Escario, E., Poblet, E., et al. (2016). Hair follicle-containing punch grafts accelerate chronic ulcer healing: A randomized controlled trial. *Journal of the American Academy of Dermatology, 75*(5), 1007–1014. doi: 10.1016/j.jaad.2016.02.1161.

Matic, M., Matic, A., Djuran, V., et al. (2016). Frequency of peripheral arterial disease in patients with chronic venous insufficiency. *Iranian Red Crescent Medical Journal, 18*(1), e20781.

McDaniel, J. C., Szalacha, L., Sales, M., et al. (2017). EPA + DHA supplementation reduces PMN activation in microenvironment of chronic venous leg ulcers: A randomized, double-blind, controlled study. *Wound Repair and Regeneration, 25*(4), 680–690. doi: 10.1111/wrr.12558.

McLaughlin, S. A., DeSnyder, S. M., Klimberg, S., et al. (2017a). Considerations for clinicians in the diagnosis, prevention, and treatment of breast cancer-related lymphedema: Recommendations from an expert panel: Part 2: Preventive and therapeutic options. *Annals of Surgical Oncology, 24*(10), 2827–2835. doi: https://doi.org/10.1245/s10434-017-5964-6.

McLaughlin, S. A., Staley, A. C., Vicini, F., et al. (2017b). Considerations for clinicians in the diagnosis, prevention, and treatment of breast cancer-related lymphedema: Recommendations from a Multidisciplinary Expert ASBrS Panel: Part 1: Definitions, assessments, education, and future directions. *Annals of Surgical Oncology, 24*(10), 2818–2826. doi: https://doi.org/10.1245/s10434-017-5982-4.

Mehrara, B. (2019). Clinical features and diagnosis of peripheral lymphedema. In J. F. Eidt, J. L. Mills, & Burstein, H. J. (Eds.), *UpToDate*. Waltham, MA: UpToDate Inc. Retrieved December 1, 2019, from https://www.uptodate.com/contents/clinical-features-and-diagnosis-of-peripheral-lymphedema.

Migdalski, L., & Kuzdak, K. (2015). The use of the VEINES-QOL/Sym Questionnaire in patients operated for varicose veins. *Polish Journal of Surgery, 87*(10), 491–498. doi: 10.1515/pjs-2015-0094.

Morton, L. M., & Phillips, T. J. (2013). Venous eczema and lipodermatosclerosis. *Seminars in Cutaneous Medicine and Surgery, 32*(3), 169–176.

Muldoon, J. (2011). Assessment and monitoring of oedema. *Journal of Community Nursing, 25*(6), 26–28.

Munnoch, A. (2012). Liposuction for chronic lymphoedema—NICE251 (online article). Retrieved from http://www.lymphoedema.org/news/Story73.asp

Nelson, E. A., & Adderly, U. (2016). Venous leg ulcers. *BMJ Clinical Evidence, 2016*, 1902. Retrieved August 3, 2017, from https://www.ncbi.nlm.nih.gov/pmc/articles/PMC4714578/

Nelson, E. A., Hillman, A., & Thomas, K. (2014). Intermittent pneumatic compression for treating venous leg ulcers. *Cochrane Database of Systematic Reviews*, (5), CD001899. doi: 10.1002/14651858.CD001899.pub4.

Neumann, H. A. M., Partsch, H., Mosti, G., et al. (2016). Classification of compression stockings: Report of the meeting of the International Compression Club, Copenhagen. *International Angiology, 35*(2), 122–128.

Nicolaides, A., Kakkos, S., Eklof, B., et al. (2014). Management of chronic venous disorders of the lower limbs. Guidelines according to scientific evidence. *International Angiology, 33*(2), 87–208.

O'Brien, J., Edwards, H., Stewart, I., et al. (2013). A home-based progressive resistance exercise programme for patients with venous leg ulcers: A feasibility study. *International Wound Journal, 10*(4), 389–396. doi: 10.1111/j.1742-481X.2012.00995.x.

O'Brien, J., Finlayson, K., Kerr, G., et al. (2017). Evaluating the effectiveness of a self-management exercise intervention on wound healing, functional ability and health-related quality of life outcomes in adults with venous leg ulcers: A randomised controlled trial. *International Wound Journal, 14*(1), 130–137. doi: 10.1111/iwj.12571.

O'Donnell, T. F., Jr., Passman, M. A., Marston, W. A., et al. (2014). Management of venous leg ulcers: Clinical practice guidelines of the Society for Vascular Surgery and the American Venous Forum. *Journal of Vascular Surgery, 60*(Suppl 2), 3S–59S. doi: 10.1016/j.jvs.2014.04.049.

O'Meara, S., Al-Kurdi, D., Ologun, Y., et al. (2014). Antibiotics and antiseptics for venous leg ulcers. *Cochrane Database of Systematic Reviews*, (1), CD003557. doi: 10.1002/14651858.CD003557.pub5.

O'Meara, S., Cullum, N., Nelson, E. A., et al. (2012). Compression for venous leg ulcers. *Cochrane Database of Systematic Reviews, 11*, CD000265. doi: 10.1002/14651858.CD000265.pub3.

Ozdemir, O. C., Sevim, S., Duygu, E., et al. (2016). The effects of short-term use of compression stockings on health related quality of life in patients with chronic venous insufficiency. *Journal of Physical Therapy Science, 28*(7), 1988–1992. doi: 10.1589/jpts.28.1988.

Parker, C. N., Finlayson, K. J., & Edwards, H. E. (2016). Ulcer area reduction at 2 weeks predicts failure to heal by 24 weeks in the venous leg ulcers of patients living alone. *Journal of Wound Care, 25*(11), 626–634. doi: 10.12968/jowc.2016.25.11.626.

Parker, C. N., Finlayson, K. J., Shuter, P., et al. (2015). Risk factors for delayed healing in venous leg ulcers: A review of the literature. *International Journal of Clinical Practice, 69*(9), 1029–1030. doi: 10.1111/ijcp.12677.

Pieper, B., & Templin, T. N. (2015). A cross-sectional pilot study to examine food sufficiency and assess nutrition among low income patients with injection-related venous ulcers. *Ostomy Wound Management, 61*(4), 32–42.

Pittler, M. H., & Ernst, E. (2012). Horse chestnut seed extract for chronic venous insufficiency. *Cochrane Database of Systematic Reviews, 11*, CD003230. doi: 10.1002/14651858.CD003230.pub4.

Pocock, E. S., Alsaigh, T., Mazor, F., et al. (2014). Cellular and molecular basis of venous insufficiency. *Vascular Cell, 6*(1), 24. doi: 10.1186/s13221-014-0024-5.

Protz, K., Heyer, K., Dissemond, J., et al. (2016). Compression therapy-current practice of care: Level of knowledge in patients with venous leg ulcers. *Journal der Deutschen Dermatologischen Gesellschaft, 14*(12), 1273–1282. doi: 10.1111/ddg.12938.

Quirion, E. (2010). Recognizing and treating upper extremity lymphedema in postmastectomy/lumpectomy patients: A guide for primary care providers. *Journal of the American Academy of Nurse Practitioners, 22*(9), 450–459.

Rabe, E., & Pannier, F. (2012). Clinical, aetiological, anatomical, and pathological classification (CEAP): Gold standard and limits. *Phlebology, 27*(Suppl 1), 114–118. doi: 10.1258/phleb.2012.012S19.

Rabe, E., Partsch, H., Hafner, J., et al. (2018). Indications for medical compression stockings in venous and lymphatic disorders: An evidence-based consensus statement. *Phlebology, 33*(3), 163–184. doi: 10.1177/0268355516689631.

Ratliff, C. R. (2016). Lymphedema. In R. Bryant & D. Nix (Eds.), *Acute and chronic wounds: Current management concepts* (5th ed., pp. 227–238). St. Louis, MO: Elsevier.

Ratliff, C. R., Yates, S., McNichol, L., et al. (2016). Compression for primary prevention, treatment, and prevention of recurrence of venous leg ulcers: An evidence- and consensus-based algorithm for care across the continuum. *Journal of Wound, Ostomy and Continence Nursing, 43*(4), 347–364. doi: 10.1097/WON.0000000000000242.

Reeder, S., de Roos, K. P., de Maeseneer, M., et al. (2013). Ulcer recurrence after in-hospital treatment for recalcitrant venous leg ulceration. *British Journal of Dermatology, 168*(5), 999–1002. doi: 10.1111/bjd.12164.

Rice, J. B., Desai, U., Cummings, A. K., et al. (2014). Burden of venous leg ulcers in the United States. *Journal of Medical Economics, 17*(5), 347–356. doi: 10.3111/13696998.2014.903258.

Ridner, S. H., Murphy, B., Deng, J., et al. (2010). Advanced pneumatic therapy in self-care of chronic lymphedema of the trunk. *Lymphatic Research and Biology, 8*(4), 209–215.

Rockson, S. G. (2018a). Intermittent pneumatic compression therapy. In B. B. Lee, S. Rockson, & J. Bergan (Eds.), *Lymphedema: A concise compendium of theory and practice* (2nd ed.). Cham: Springer. Retrieved from https://link.springer.com/book/10.1007%2F978-3-319-52423-8

Rockson, S. G. (2018b). Lymphedema after breast cancer treatment. *The New England Journal of Medicine, 379*(20), 1937–1944. doi: 10.1056/NEJMcp1803290.

Sadler, G. M., Wallace, H. J., & Stacey, M. C. (2012). Oral doxycycline for the treatment of chronic leg ulceration. *Archives of Dermatological Research, 304*(6), 487–493. doi: 10.1007/s00403-011-1201-5.

Salome, G. M., de Almeida, S. A., & Ferreira, L. M. (2014). Evaluation of pain in patients with venous ulcers after skin grafting. *Journal of Tissue Viability, 23*(3), 115–120. doi: 10.1016/j.jtv.2014.04.004.

Scheiman, N. (2011). To pump or not to pump: Is newer technology solving pumping issues in lymphedema? *Advance for Occupational Therapy Practitioners, 27*(4), 8–9.

Schulze, H., Nacke, M., Gutenbrunner, C., et al. (2018). Worldwide assessment of healthcare personnel dealing with lymphoedema. *Health Economics Review, 8*(1), 10. doi: 10.1186/s13561-018-0194-6.

Scotton, M. F., Miot, H. A., & Abbade, L. P. (2014). Factors that influence healing of chronic venous leg ulcers: A retrospective cohort. *Anais Brasileiros de Dermatologia, 89*(3), 414–422. doi: 10.1590/abd1806-4841.20142687.

Serra, R., Amato, B., Butrico, L., et al. (2016). Study on the efficacy of surgery of the superficial venous system and of compression therapy at early stages of chronic venous disease for the prevention of chronic venous ulceration. *International Wound Journal, 13*(6), 1385–1388. doi: 10.1111/iwj.12618.

Serra, R., Buffone, G., Falcone, D., et al. (2013). Chronic venous leg ulcers are associated with high levels of metalloproteinases-9 and neutrophil gelatinase-associated lipocalin. *Wound Repair and Regeneration, 21*(3), 395–401. doi: 10.1111/wrr.12035.

Serra, R., Rizzuto, A., Rossi, A., et al. (2017). Skin grafting for the treatment of chronic leg ulcers: A systematic review in evidence-based medicine. *International Wound Journal, 14*(1), 149–157. doi: 10.1111/iwj.12575.

Sleigh, B. C., & Manna, B. (2019). Lymphedema. In *StatPearls* [Internet]. Treasure Island, FL: StatPearls Publishing. Retrieved from https://www.ncbi.nlm.nih.gov/books/NBK537239/

Stuiver, M. M., ten Tusscher, M. R., Agasi-Idenburg, C. S., et al. (2015). Conservative interventions for preventing clinically detectable upper-limb lymphoedema in patients who are at risk of developing lymphoedema after breast cancer therapy. *Cochrane Database of Systematic Reviews*, (2), CD009765. doi: 10.1002/14651858.CD009765.pub2.

Thakral, G., La Fontaine, J., Najafi, B., et al. (2013). Electrical stimulation to accelerate wound healing. *Diabetic Foot & Ankle, 4*(1). doi: 10.3402/dfa.v4i0.22081.

Toledo, R. R., Santos, M., & Schnaider, T. B. (2017). Effect of pycnogenol on the healing of venous ulcers. *Annals of Vascular Surgery, 38*, 212–219. doi: 10.1016/j.avsg.2016.04.014.

Uzkeser, H. (2012). Assessment of postmastectomy lymphedema and current treatment approaches. *European Journal of General Medicine, 9*(2), 130–134.

van Gent, W. B., & Wittens, C. H. A. (2015). Influence of perforating vein surgery in patients with venous ulceration. *Phlebology, 30*(2), 127–132. doi: 10.1177/0268355513517685.

Van Hecke, A., Grypdonck, M., Beele, H., et al. (2011). Adherence to leg ulcer lifestyle advice: Qualitative and quantitative outcomes associated with a nurse-led intervention. *Journal of Clinical Nursing, 20*(3–4), 429–443. doi: 10.1111/j.1365-2702.2010.03546.x.

Vitse, J., Bekara, F., Byun, S., et al. (2017). A double-blind, placebo-controlled randomized evaluation of the effect of low-level laser therapy on venous leg ulcers. *The International Journal of Lower Extremity Wounds, 16*(1), 29–35. doi: 10.1177/1534734617690948.

Vuylsteke, M. E., Thomis, S., Guillaume, G., et al. (2015). Epidemiological study on chronic venous disease in Belgium and Luxembourg: Prevalence, risk factors, and symptomatology. *European Journal of Vascular and Endovascular Surgery, 49*(4), 432–439. doi: 10.1016/j.ejvs.2014.12.031.

Wigg, J., & Lee, N. (2014). Redefining essential care in lymphoedema. *British Journal of Community Nursing, 19*(Suppl 4), S20–S27.

Wilkinson, E. A. (2014). Oral zinc for arterial and venous leg ulcers. *Cochrane Database of Systematic Reviews*, (9), CD001273. doi: 10.1002/14651858.CD001273.pub3.

Williams, A. (2010). Manual lymphatic drainage: Exploring the history and evidence base. *British Journal of Community Nursing, 15*(4), S18–S24.

Williams, A. (2012). Surgery for people with lymphedema. *Journal of Community Nursing, 26*(5), 27–29, 31–33.

WOCN. (2014). *Guideline for management of patients with lower-extremity arterial disease*. WOCN clinical guideline series 1. Mt. Laurel, NJ: Author.

WOCN. (2019). *Guideline for the management of wounds in patients with lower-extremity venous disease*. Mt. Laurel, NJ: Author.

Wu, B., Lu, J., Yang, M., et al. (2016). Sulodexide for treating venous leg ulcers. *Cochrane Database of Systematic Reviews*, (6), CD010694. doi: 10.1002/14651858.CD010694.pub2.

Yim, E., Richmond, N. A., Baquerizo, K., et al. (2014). The effect of ankle range of motion on venous ulcer healing rates. *Wound Repair and Regeneration, 22*(4), 492–496. doi: 10.1111/wrr.12186.

Zuther, J., & Norton, S. (2013). *Lymphedema management: The comprehensive guide for practitioners* (3rd ed.). New York, NY: Thieme.

Zygmunt, J. A. (2014). Duplex ultrasound for chronic venous insufficiency. *The Journal of Invasive Cardiology, 26*(11), e149–e155. Retrieved September 2018, from https://www.invasivecardiology.com/articles/duplex-ultrasound-chronic-venous-insufficiency

QUESTIONS

1. Which risk factor for LEVD is related to calf muscle pump dysfunction?
   A. Altered gait
   B. Pregnancy
   C. Thrombophilia
   D. Obesity

2. The wound care nurse classifies a patient's LEVD as clinical CEAP 2. What condition does this classification represent?
   A. Telangiectasias
   B. Varicose veins
   C. Edema
   D. Lipodermatosclerosis

3. Which of the following represents an essential "mainstream" therapy for all patients with both LEVD and VLUs?
   A. Pharmacologic interventions such as pentoxifylline
   B. Surgical intervention to eliminate venous reflux
   C. Elevation of the leg to the level of the heart for at least 4 hours daily
   D. Compression therapy to improve venous return

4. The wound care nurse is developing a treatment plan for a patient with stage 1 lymphedema and LEVD. What therapeutic approach would the nurse recommend?
   A. Compression therapy, elevation, exercise
   B. Combined decongestive therapy (CDT)
   C. CDT with needed wound care
   D. Surgical intervention

5. The wound care nurse documents stage II lymphedema on a patient chart. What characteristic distinguishes this condition from earlier stages?
   A. Edema is observable and measurable.
   B. Edema resolves with elevation.
   C. Fibrosis is present in the tissue.
   D. Ongoing infections of the tissue are likely.

6. Which condition is the pathological factor responsible for LEVD?
   A. Damage to the endothelial lining of the vessels
   B. Platelet aggregation
   C. Venous hypertension
   D. Activation of white blood cells

7. Which of the following is the most reliable and commonly used noninvasive test for diagnosing LEVD?
   A. Venous duplex ultrasound
   B. Air plethysmography
   C. Photoplethysmography
   D. ABI measurements

8. The wound care nurse recommends therapeutic-level static compression therapy for patients with LEVD. For which patient is this therapy contraindicated?
   A. A patient with diabetes mellitus
   B. A patient with an ABI < 0.8
   C. A patient who has varicose veins
   D. A patient with hypertension

9. Which general guideline for application of compression wrap would the wound care nurse use?
   A. Omit cleansing the leg prior to applying the wrap.
   B. Avoid using moisturizers on the periwound skin.
   C. Exclude the heel when applying the compression wrap.
   D. Position the ankle in a neutral position at a right angle.

10. Which pharmaceutical agent is indicated for patients who fail to progress with standard therapy and also provides additive benefits when used in conjunction with compression therapy?
   A. Pentoxifylline
   B. Horse chestnut seed extract
   C. Steroid ointment
   D. Diuretics

ANSWERS AND RATIONALES

1. A. Rationale: Failure to ambulate with normal heel strike–toe off mechanism (shuffling gait) prevents the calf muscle pump from functioning.

2. B. Rationale: Definition of CEAP 2 includes varicosities.

3. D. Rationale: Compression is the goal standard for treatment of LEVD and VLUs.

4. A. Rationale: Stage 1 lymphedema is reversible, and both conditions respond to the interventions listed.

5. C. Rationale: Edema is seen in all levels of lymphedema. Edema does not resolve with elevation, and infections risk is not increased in stage II.

6. C. Rationale: Venous hypertension occurs when the venous system does not empty effectively and is the primary etiologic factor for LEVD.

7. A. Rationale: ABI measures arterial blood flow; airplethysmography and photoplethysmography are not first-line tests and require more technical expertise. They are used when venous duplex ultrasound is inconclusive. Venous duplex ultrasound has a high degree of accuracy and is the preferred test.

8. B. Rationale: ABI lower than 0.9 indicates LEAD, which prevents use of therapeutic-level compression.

9. D. Rationale: Maintaining the ankle in neutral position during compression wrap application avoids injury from the wrap and allows normal gait.

10. A. Rationale: Pentoxifylline has beneficial effects on the microcirculation.

CHAPTER 25

ASSESSMENT AND MANAGEMENT OF PATIENTS WITH WOUNDS DUE TO LOWER EXTREMITY ARTERIAL DISEASE (LEAD)

Phyllis Bonham

OBJECTIVES

1. Describe critical parameters to be included in assessment of the individual with a lower extremity wounds due to arterial disease.

2. Describe the procedure for ankle brachial index (ABI) testing.

3. Interpret findings from
   a. Ankle brachial index (ABI) testing
   b. Toe brachial index (TBI) testing
   c. Transcutaneous oxygen tension ($TcPO_2$) testing
   d. Sensory testing with Semmes-Weinstein monofilaments

4. Use assessment data to determine causative and contributing factors for a lower extremity ulcer and to develop individualized management plans that are evidence based.

5. Differentiate acute from chronic limb ischemia.

6. Describe the impact of lifestyle modifications, pharmacologic options, revascularization options, and adjunctive therapy on improving lower extremity perfusion in the patient with an arterial ulcer.

7. Explain why debridement is contraindicated in a noninfected ischemic ulcer covered with dry eschar.

8. Describe indications for referral to a vascular surgeon.

TOPIC OUTLINE

INTRODUCTION

Lower extremity arterial disease (LEAD) is often unrecognized and an underdiagnosed manifestation of atherosclerosis (Campia et al., 2019). LEAD is also known as peripheral arterial occlusive disease, peripheral vascular disease, peripheral arterial disease or peripheral artery disease, and arteriosclerosis obliterans (Campia et al., 2019).

LEAD is not the most common cause of lower extremity wounds, but its presence complicates the healing of lower extremity wounds, and it can be limb threatening due to ischemia. Other nonatherosclerotic causes of ischemic lower extremity ulcers include, but

are not limited to, sickle cell disease, embolism, clotting disorders, thromboangiitis obliterans (Buerger disease), vasculitis, scleroderma, diabetic microangiopathy, and vasospastic diseases such as Raynaud disease (Gerhard-Herman et al., 2017; WOCN, 2014).

KEY POINT

LEAD is not the most common cause of lower extremity wounds, but its presence complicates the healing of wounds caused by other etiologic factors, and wounds caused by LEAD can be limb threatening.

A thorough assessment is essential to determine the correct etiology of a wound as a basis for an accurate diagnosis and appropriate management (Gerhard-Herman et al., 2017; WOCN, 2014). All patients with leg wounds should be carefully examined to determine the presence or absence of LEAD, which is often asymptomatic (Campia et al., 2019; WOCN, 2014). Lower extremity wounds present complex problems and require collaborative, multidisciplinary, and holistic care and management.

PREVALENCE, INCIDENCE, AND SIGNIFICANCE OF LEAD

The prevalence of LEAD is commonly defined by an ankle brachial index (ABI) of 0.90 or less (Criqui & Aboyans, 2015). LEAD is estimated to affect 8.5 million Americans 40 years of age and older, and globally, 202 million adults are reported to have LEAD (Mozaffarian et al., 2015). The highest prevalence of LEAD has been observed among older people, non-Hispanic Blacks, and women (Mozaffarian et al., 2015). LEAD is uncommon in younger people (<50 years of age), but the prevalence rises sharply after age 65 and reaches approximately 20% by 80 years of age (Criqui & Aboyans, 2015).

The incidence of LEAD has not been well documented. Based on a 5-year sample (2003–2008) of insurance claims of adults ≥40 years of age in the United States, the annual incidence and prevalence of LEAD was 2.76% and 2.29%, respectively (Mozaffarian et al., 2015). In Europe, incidence data are also scarce. At age 60, the annual incidence rates of LEAD, based on the presence of intermittent claudication, varied from 0.2% in Iceland to 1% in Israel (Aboyans et al., 2018). In the Netherlands, the overall incidence of asymptomatic LEAD was 9.9 per 1,000 person-years at risk, and for symptomatic LEAD, the overall incidence was 1.0 per 1,000 person-years at risk (Aboyans et al., 2018). LEAD is a manifestation of systemic atherosclerosis, and it is associated with a high risk for morbidity and mortality from coronary artery or cerebrovascular disease including myocardial infarction (MI), ischemic stroke, and vascular death (Campia et al., 2019).

KEY POINT

LEAD can be asymptomatic until late in the disease process, and it has been reported that up to 80% of patients with LEAD are undiagnosed and untreated or undertreated.

LEAD has socioeconomic implications for individuals and the overall health care system. There are high costs for treating LEAD due primarily to expenses for hospitalization and surgical care (e.g., bypass, angioplasty, amputation). Based on an evaluation of 286,160 hospitalizations for patients with LEAD, the median hospital length of stay was 5 days and costs were $15,755, which resulted in an annual cost of $6.31 billion (Kohn et al., 2019). LEAD also impacts the quality of life for patients due to functional limitations and leg-related symptoms (Mozaffarian et al., 2015).

PATHOPHYSIOLOGY/ETIOLOGY OF LEAD AND ISCHEMIC WOUNDS

LEAD is a chronic and progressive disease due to atherosclerosis, which is a systemic condition (Criqui & Aboyans, 2015). **Figure 25-1** illustrates common sites of atherosclerotic obstruction. Atherosclerosis is a dynamic disorder that involves both endothelial dysfunction and inflammation (Abdolmaleki et al., 2019; Mitrovic, 2019). In the lower extremity arteries, atherosclerosis primarily affects the intimal layer, causing plaque formation and endothelial damage that results in stenosis; the injury to the vessel also triggers inflammation, which causes progressive fibrosis and hardening of the arterial walls (Bell, 2013; Mitrovic, 2019). Atherosclerosis and plaque formation can be characterized as developing in the following four stages (Bell, 2013; Mitrovic, 2019):

- Initial lesion develops: Endothelial damage causes white blood cells (macrophages) to migrate into the area and become activated.
- Fatty streaks form: Fatty streaks, which are collections of lipid-filled macrophages, develop in the inner artery and trigger replacement of the smooth endothelial cells in the intimal layer with muscle cells from the medial layer.
- Atheroma develops: An atheroma, which contains large numbers of smooth muscle cells filled with lipids, forms from the fatty streaks.
- Advanced lesion develops: The atheromatous lesion, which contains endothelial cells, smooth muscle cells, and inflammatory cells, continues to develop and is characterized by a lipid core covered by a fibrous cap. Disruption of the fibrous cap exposes the "prothrombotic" necrotic lipid core and subendothelial tissue, which can result in thrombus formation and an acute occlusive arterial event.

As atherosclerosis progresses, the narrowed lumen and increased rigidity of the arterial walls prevent dilatation in response to tissue demands for increased blood and oxygen (**Fig. 25-2**); clinically this is manifest as progressive pain with activity, such as walking, that is relieved only by rest (i.e., intermittent claudication). Advanced disease can severely impair tissue perfusion and can result in ischemic wounds.

SYMPTOMATIC AND ASYMPTOMATIC LEAD

LEAD has varying clinical presentations. Although intermittent claudication is considered the most typical symptom of LEAD, most patients are asymptomatic (Aboyans

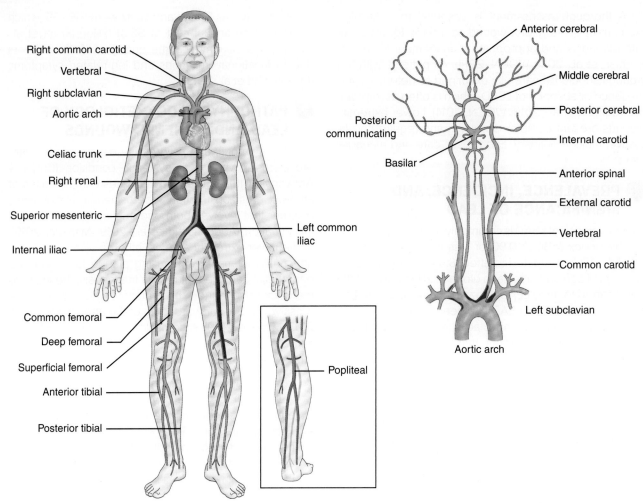

FIGURE 25-1. Example of Common Sites of Atherosclerotic Obstruction in Major Arteries in the Body: Cerebral, Coronary, and Lower Extremities.

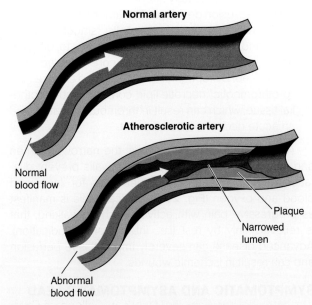

FIGURE 25-2. Example of Impaired Blood Flow in an Atherosclerotic Artery. (Adapted from NHLBI Atherosclerosis homepage; http://www.nhlbi.nih.gov/health/health-topics/topics/atherosclerosis/)

et al., 2018). Only about 10% of individuals with LEAD have the classic symptoms of intermittent claudication; others may have atypical leg symptoms or are asymptomatic (Alahdab et al., 2015). Atypical leg symptoms related to LEAD can include pain or discomfort that starts at rest and worsens with exertion but is not relieved within 10 minutes of rest (Gerhard-Herman et al., 2017), or the atypical symptoms may reflect other pathologies such as neuropathy, arthritis, and lumbar spine disease (Conte et al., 2015).

Asymptomatic LEAD may be detected by a low resting ABI (<0.90) and/or absence of pedal pulses (Aboyans et al., 2018). A subset of individuals with asymptomatic LEAD might have "masked LEAD" without symptoms, which can be due to an incapacity to walk enough to reveal symptoms such as with heart failure and/or reduced pain sensitivity secondary to diabetic neuropathy (Aboyans et al., 2018). Asymptomatic and masked LEAD are associated with an increased risk of cardiovascular and cerebrovascular morbidity and mortality that is similar to symptomatic LEAD (Aboyans et al., 2018; Alahdab et al., 2015).

RISK AND CONTRIBUTING FACTORS

All patients with LEAD should undergo risk assessment to guide primary and secondary preventive interventions. The risk factors for LEAD parallel those for systemic atherosclerotic conditions such as coronary and cerebrovascular disease (Campia et al., 2019). Smoking tobacco, diabetes mellitus, dyslipidemia, hypertension, advanced age, and chronic kidney disease (CKD) are primary risk factors for LEAD (Aboyans et al., 2018; Arinze et al., 2019; Criqui & Aboyans, 2015; Song et al., 2019). Additional, potential contributing factors include elevated homocysteine levels, family history of cardiovascular disease, ethnicity, inflammation, infection, hypercoagulable states, and vessel calcification (Criqui & Aboyans, 2015; Song et al., 2019; WOCN, 2014). Due to heterogeneity in studies, it is unclear if there are differences in the risk or prevalence of LEAD according to gender (Criqui & Aboyans, 2015; Song et al., 2019). Some risk and contributing factors are modifiable (e.g., smoking, diabetes, abnormal lipids, hypertension), and others are nonmodifiable (e.g., age, family history, ethnicity). Comprehensive management for the patient with LEAD includes attention to modifiable risk factors.

KEY POINT

Primary risk factors for LEAD parallel those for cerebrovascular and cardiovascular disease and include tobacco use, diabetes mellitus, dyslipidemia, hypertension, advanced age, and chronic kidney disease.

SMOKING TOBACCO

Smoking tobacco is associated with a 2- to 4-fold increased risk of LEAD; risk increases with smoking intensity and duration (Campia et al., 2019; Criqui & Aboyans, 2015). Evidence has suggested that exposure to smoking accelerates oxidative stress, vascular inflammation, platelet reactivity, and endothelial dysfunction; it contributes to detrimental effects on the cardiovascular system (Ma et al., 2019). Past and current smoking and exposure to passive/secondhand smoking are associated with increased risks for LEAD and other manifestations of cardiovascular disease (Aboyans et al., 2018). The association between smoking and the risk of LEAD persists even after cessation (Aboyans et al., 2018; Ding et al., 2019). Based on a review of 13,355 partici-

pants followed for up to 30 years (median 26 years), 492 patients developed LEAD, and compared to never smokers, those who smoked for 40 or more pack-years had a 4-fold increased risk for LEAD (Ding et al., 2019). Compared to current smokers, the risk was 80% lower after smoking cessation for 30 or more years; however, compared to never smokers, the elevated risk of LEAD was sustained for 30 years after smoking cessation.

DIABETES MELLITUS (DIABETES)

Diabetes accelerates the natural course and distribution of atherosclerosis with a 2- to 4-fold increased risk for LEAD (Aboyans et al., 2018; Campia et al., 2019; Criqui & Aboyans, 2015). Factors increasing the risk of LEAD in patients with diabetes include duration of diabetes, poor glycemic control, and use of insulin (Criqui & Aboyans, 2015).

KEY POINT

Diabetes accelerates the natural course of atherosclerosis and is associated with a 2- to 4-fold increase in risk for LEAD.

The pathogenesis of diabetes-related atherosclerosis is complex and multifactorial. Compared to patients without diabetes, those with diabetes have more disease in distal arteries, experience worse outcomes and have greater morbidity, are five times more likely to have an amputation, and have three times greater odds of mortality (Aboyans et al., 2018; Criqui & Aboyans, 2015). The presence of neuropathy and greater risk of infection increase the risk of amputations in these patients (Aboyans et al., 2018; Criqui & Aboyans, 2015; Miyata et al., 2019).

DYSLIPIDEMIA

Abnormal lipid levels (i.e., elevated total cholesterol; low-density lipoprotein cholesterol [LDL-C]; decreased high-density lipoprotein cholesterol [HDL-C]) play an important role in atherosclerosis and LEAD (Aboyans et al., 2018; Campia et al., 2019; Criqui & Aboyans, 2015; Song et al., 2019). HDL-C has been shown to be protective in large epidemiological studies (Aboyans et al., 2018; Criqui & Aboyans, 2015), whereas lipoprotein(a) is associated with LEAD and its progression (Aboyans et al., 2018). Although triglycerides seem to be associated with LEAD, it is unclear if they are independent risk factors (Aboyans et al., 2018; Criqui & Aboyans, 2015). Patients with LEAD should have their serum LDL-C reduced (<70 mg/dL) or decreased by 50% or more if their LDL-C level is between 70 and 135 mg/dL (Aboyans et al., 2018). According to recent guidelines from the American College of Cardiology and the American Heart Association (ACC/AHA) (Grundy et al., 2019), findings from population studies in the United States suggest that optimal total cholesterol levels are about 150 mg/dL, which corresponds to an LDL-C level of about 100 mg/dL, and adults with cholesterol concentrations in that range have low rates of arteriosclerotic cardiovascular disease (ASCVD). Grundy et al. further reported that lowering cholesterol in high-risk patients lowers the incidence of ASCVD and supports the principle that lower levels of LDL-C are better.

HYPERTENSION

Hypertension is associated with increased odds ratios for LEAD of 1.5 to 2.2 (Aboyans et al., 2018; Campia et al., 2019; Criqui & Aboyans, 2015). The 2017 ACC/AHA blood pressure (BP) guidelines classified hypertension as a BP ≥ 130/80 mm Hg and recommended a target BP < 130/80 mm Hg for all patients with hypertension, including those with LEAD and diabetes, to reduce overall cardiovascular risk (Whelton et al., 2018). Whereas, international guidelines for patients with LEAD and limb-threatening ischemia define hypertension as ≥140/90 mm Hg and recommended a target BP < 140/90 mm Hg (Aboyans et al., 2018; Conte et al., 2019), except for patients with diabetes in whom a diastolic BP < 85 mm Hg was advised (Aboyans et al., 2018).

Although a high prevalence of hypertension has been shown in patients with LEAD, evidence is lacking regarding the specific benefits of BP reduction on LEAD. Some experts question whether lowering BP could affect the perfusion to the distal extremities and exacerbate symptoms of LEAD such as claudication, rest pain, or thrombosis (Aboyans et al., 2018; Itoga et al., 2018). In a secondary analysis of data from 33,357 patients with hypertension who were at high risk for cardiovascular disease, the findings revealed that systolic BP < 120 mm Hg and >160 mm Hg, and diastolic BPs (<70 mm Hg) were associated with increased rates of LEAD-related events such as hospitalizations, surgeries/amputations, outpatient medical treatments, and death (Itoga et al., 2018). Therefore, caution is indicated when lowering BP, and patients should be carefully monitored for tolerance (Aboyans et al., 2018).

AGE

The risk of LEAD increases with age (Song et al., 2019). LEAD is uncommon before the age of 50, but by the age of 80, the prevalence rate is 20% or higher (Aboyans et al., 2018; Campia et al., 2019; Criqui & Aboyans, 2015).

CHRONIC KIDNEY DISEASE

The prevalence of LEAD is three times higher in patients with CKD compared to the general population (Arinze et al., 2019). Prevalence rates of LEAD in patients on dialysis range from 23% to 35.7% (Arinze et al., 2019). Increasing severity of CKD is associated with higher rates of LEAD, which results in increased complications, risk of limb-threatening ischemia, poor limb-salvage rates, and mortality (Arinze et al., 2019; Criqui & Aboyans, 2015; Miyata et al., 2019).

OTHER CONTRIBUTING FACTORS

A variety of other potential risks and contributing factors for LEAD have been examined such as homocysteine, genetic factors, ethnicity, inflammation, and infection. Although studies have shown that patients with LEAD have increased plasma levels of homocysteine compared to controls, there has not been any evidence that lowering homocysteine levels improves clinical outcomes (Criqui & Aboyans, 2015; Gerhard-Herman et al., 2017).

The specific role of genetic factors in the development and progression of LEAD is uncertain due to limited data and is an ongoing area of investigation (Criqui & Aboyans, 2015; Hazarika & Annex, 2017). Wassel et al. (2011) reported an almost 2-fold increased risk of LEAD for individuals with a family history of cardiovascular disease. Also, results from a study of identical twins found that an individual who had an identical twin with LEAD had a 3-fold higher risk of LEAD than nonidentical twins (Wahlgren & Magnusson, 2011). Data on race and ethnicity are also limited. Some studies suggest that African American/Black persons have a higher risk of LEAD compared to White/non-Hispanic persons (Aboyans et al., 2012; WOCN, 2014).

Inflammation and Infection

Chronic inflammation and infection are believed to contribute to the development of atherosclerosis. However, the specific role of infectious and inflammatory agents and the benefits of treatment remain uncertain.

Chlamydia pneumoniae

Chronic infection has been associated with an increased risk of LEAD such as infections due to *Chlamydia pneumoniae* (*C. pneumoniae*) and periodontal disease/infection. Some older studies have reported an association between *C. pneumoniae* and LEAD with contradictory reports regarding the benefit of treatment (Berger et al., 2011; Watson & Alp, 2008). In a recent study that examined the prevalence of *C. pneumoniae* in patients with cardiovascular disease (*N* = 115; 54% with LEAD), *C. pneumoniae* was detected in 61% (70/115) of blood samples and in 86% (31/36) of tissue samples from atheroma plaques (Yazouli et al., 2018). The femoral artery was the most highly affected with 55% (18.36) cases positive for *C. pneumoniae*.

Periodontal Disease

An association between periodontal disease and atherosclerotic vascular disease has been demonstrated, but a causal relationship or benefits of periodontal interventions have not been demonstrated (Soto-Barreras et al., 2013). In a recent systematic review and meta-analysis of seven studies (*N* = 4,307), the results revealed a significant increased risk of periodontitis in patients with LEAD (n = 493) compared to patients (n =3,814) without LEAD (RR = 1.70, 95% CI [1.25, 2.29], p = 0.01; Yang et al., 2018). Therefore, limited data suggest an association between inflammation and chronic infections such as *C. pneumoniae* and periodontitis. However, further research is needed to determine if a causal relationship exists between inflammation and infection and LEAD, and whether treatment is effective in preventing or diminishing the development or progression of atherosclerosis.

KEY POINT

Chronic inflammation and infection are believed to contribute to the development of atherosclerotic disease, although the specific role remains unclear.

Biomarkers of Inflammation, Hypercoagulability, and Vascular Calcification

Elevated levels of several markers of inflammation (e.g., high-sensitivity C-reactive protein [hs-CRP], fibrinogen, interleukin-6 [IL-6]) have been associated with an increased risk for the development, progression, and complications of LEAD (Aboyans et al., 2018; Criqui & Aboyans, 2015; WOCN, 2014). Although these inflammatory markers have shown an association with LEAD, a causal role has not been established (Hazarika & Annex, 2017).

Thrombogenic markers such as D-dimer and fibrinogen may also be associated with LEAD and an increased risk for arterial thrombotic events (Hazarika & Annex, 2017; Kleinegris et al., 2013). Compared to patients without LEAD, higher levels of D-dimer and fibrinogen in patients with LEAD have been associated with increased cardiovascular events and mortality (Hazarika & Annex, 2017; Kleinegris et al., 2013).

Markers of vascular calcification (glycoproteins osteoprotegerin and fetuin-A) have also been associated with LEAD (Mogelvang et al., 2012), particularly in patients with diabetes and LEAD (Demkova et al., 2018; Esteghamati et al., 2015). High concentrations of osteoprotegerin have been associated with increased risk and severity of LEAD, coronary artery atherosclerosis, and hypertension (Demkova et al., 2018; Esteghamati et al., 2015; Mogel vang et al., 2012).

Clinical Implications of Biomarkers

There is considerable diversity in the clinical manifestations and progression of LEAD among individuals, and there is no specific ideal biomarker to screen for LEAD, stratify risk among patients, or to monitor response to revascularization or other therapies (Hazarika & Annex, 2017). Therefore, the specific clinical implications of biomarkers for screening and/or treatment of LEAD remain unclear, and routine measurement of these biomarkers is not currently recommended. Further studies are necessary to determine whether there are biomarkers that can provide additional prognostic information over the traditional measures of risks such as lipid levels.

ASSESSMENT AND DIAGNOSIS

HISTORY

It is essential to identify the presence/absence of LEAD for any patient with a lower extremity wound to guide treatment, evaluate the potential for healing; and determine the need for referrals for additional vascular testing, surgical interventions, or adjunctive therapies (WOCN, 2014). Patients with/or at risk for LEAD should undergo a comprehensive review of their medical history and symptoms. It is important to differentiate wounds due to LEAD from other common etiologies such as venous disease or peripheral neuropathy, which require different management strategies. A number of other pathologic conditions can cause nonhealing leg wounds that may be confused with wounds due to LEAD such as sickle cell disease, vasculitis, pyoderma gangrenosum, malignancy, etc. (Gerhard-Herman et al., 2017). These atypical ulcers are discussed further in Chapter 27. Risks, contributing factors, and coexisting problems that may complicate the care and management of the patient should be identified including a history of smoking tobacco, diabetes, hypertension, and hypercholesterolemia. Due to the systemic effects of atherosclerosis, a history of cardiovascular or cerebrovascular disease or surgeries should be determined. LEAD is associated with high risks for coronary artery disease and cerebrovascular disease, which are the most common causes of death in patients with LEAD accounting for 40% to 60% and 10% to 20% mortality, respectively (Campia et al., 2019).

Several other diseases and conditions have been shown to coexist or be associated with LEAD such as inflammatory polyarthropathy/spondylopathy disorders (Aguero et al., 2015). In a study of 90 patients with rheumatoid arthritis (mean age 58.4 ± 11.3 years), 10 (11%) of patients had LEAD (Kurt et al., 2015). Also, obesity (body mass index [BMI] > 30 kg/m^2; Song et al., 2019) and metabolic syndrome have been associated with LEAD (Vasheghani-Farahani et al., 2017). However, a consistent, independent association between obesity and LEAD has not been demonstrated (Criqui & Aboyans, 2015), and data are currently lacking regarding the effects of weight/BMI reduction on LEAD.

Symptomatic LEAD has been associated with decreased physical and functional capacity with poor walking endurance (Cornelis et al., 2019). Also, limited exercise capacity in patients with LEAD has been associated with increased mortality (Leeper et al., 2013). Therefore, the history should include a review of the patient's functional ability, limitations in ambulation and physical activity, and whether walking aids are required. Ischemia can negatively affect lower extremity nerves and impair muscle function; thus, the patient should be queried regarding signs and symptoms of neuropathy (e.g., decreased sensation, weakness of the ankles or feet, gait abnormalities, foot drop/foot drag).

Additionally, it is important to obtain a history of all pre-scribed and over-the-counter medications. The review should include previous and current medication use (e.g., vasodilators, anticoagulants, antiplatelets, statins, analgesics, diuretics, herbal products). A history of alcohol use should also be determined. Although there has been some evidence that light-to-moderate alcohol consumption may be protective for coronary heart disease (CHD), the risks or benefits of alcohol consumption for LEAD are uncertain (Criqui & Aboyans, 2015).

> **KEY POINT**
>
> Ischemia can negatively affect nerve function; therefore, patients with LEAD should be screened for evidence of neuropathy.

PAIN HISTORY

A detailed pain history is essential and should include the location, type, and characteristics of pain; exacerbating and alleviating factors; onset and duration; and use and effectiveness of analgesics. Also, it is important to determine if a painful wound is present.

The location of pain may indicate the location of stenosis or occlusion; pain typically occurs one joint below the site of the stenosis or occlusion (Rumwell & McPharlin, 2017). For example, pain in the buttock indicates aortoiliac disease and suggests iliofemoral disease if the symptoms are unilateral (Rumwell & McPharlin, 2017). Pain in the thigh indicates distal external iliac/common femoral disease. Pain in the calf indicates femoral/popliteal disease, and pain localized to the foot indicates infrapopliteal disease (Rumwell & McPharlin, 2017).

Intermittent Claudication

The classic type of pain associated with LEAD is intermittent claudication (Campia et al., 2019; Criqui & Aboyans, 2015; Gerhard-Herman et al., 2017). Intermittent claudication is defined as reproducible pain that is consistently brought on by exercise such as walking and is consistently relieved within 10 minutes of rest (Gerhard-Herman et al., 2017). Claudication may be described as fatigue, discomfort, or cramping in the muscles of the lower extremities (Gerhard-Herman et al., 2017). Although the calf muscles are the most often affected, any leg muscle group can be affected such as those in the thigh or buttock (Conte et al., 2015). As previously discussed, only about 10% of individuals with LEAD have the classic symptoms of intermittent claudication (Alahdab et al., 2015). Therefore, it is important for health care providers to understand that persons with LEAD may not recognize and report the classic symptoms of claudication because they might limit their ambulation or activities to avoid leg pain, or they may have other comorbid conditions that limit their activities. Some individuals mistakenly believe their symptoms are due to aging. Also, the symptoms of claudication can be confused with pain due to other conditions such as osteoarthritis, spinal stenosis, or chronic venous disease (Campia et al., 2019; Gerhard-Herman et al., 2017). Finally, patients with impaired sensation due to neuropathy might not experience the classic claudication symptoms (Aboyans et al., 2018).

> **KEY POINT**
>
> The type of pain most often associated with LEAD is intermittent claudication, which is defined as reproducible pain that is consistently brought on by walking or similar activity and consistently relieved within 10 minutes of rest.

Positional and Rest Pain

As the severity of LEAD progresses, patients may experience positional or resting pain in the absence of walking or activity. Positional pain occurs when the legs are elevated and diminishes when the legs are placed in a dependent position (WOCN, 2014). Ischemic rest pain occurs in the absence of activity, most typically at night when the patient is supine or in bed, and the legs are not in a dependent position (Rumwell & McPharlin, 2017). Ischemic rest pain is a sign of more severe vessel occlusion that occurs in the forefoot, heel, and toes, but not in the calf (Rumwell & McPharlin, 2017). Often, patients will dangle their leg(s) over the side of the bed or sit up in a chair in an effort to relieve ischemic pain; many patients report routinely sleeping in a recliner with their legs down. With very advanced LEAD, the pain can become continuous even with the legs in a dependent position.

> **KEY POINT**
>
> Advanced LEAD is manifested by positional pain (pain with elevation) and eventually by pain that persists even when the leg is dependent (rest pain); rest pain is associated with severe vessel occlusion.

DIFFERENTIATION OF ACUTE VERSUS CHRONIC LIMB ISCHEMIA

Assessment of the onset and duration of pain is necessary to differentiate acute from chronic limb ischemia.

Acute Limb Ischemia

Acute limb ischemia (<2 weeks) is severe hypoperfusion of the limb due to a sudden occlusion from arterial disease progression, thrombus/graft thrombosis, embolism, popliteal artery entrapment, hypercoagulable states, trauma, or other causes (Aboyans et al., 2018; Gerhard-Herman et al., 2017; Rumwell & McPharlin, 2017). The hallmark sign of an acute limb-threatening occlusion is the sudden onset of the six "Ps": pulselessness, pain, pallor, paresthesia, paralysis, and polar/coldness (Gerhard-Herman et al., 2017; Rumwell & McPharlin, 2017; WOCN, 2014). Rumwell and McPharlin (2017) suggest including a seventh "P" for the purplish, cyanotic color seen in patients with acute occlusions. Findings should be compared to the contralateral limb. An immediate referral for a vascular surgical evaluation and intervention is indicated for patients with signs and symptoms of acute limb ischemia; irreparable damage can occur within 4 to 6 hours (Aboyans et al., 2018; Chioncel et al., 2019; Gerhard-Herman et al., 2017; Rumwell & McPharlin, 2017). The limb viability and potential for limb salvage should be rapidly evaluated by a vascular specialist (Gerhard-Herman et al., 2017). Acute limb ischemia can be classified into three categories of viability (Aboyans et al., 2018; Chioncel et al., 2019; Gerhard-Herman et al., 2017):

- Grade I. Viable: limb not immediately threatened; no sensory loss or muscle weakness; audible arterial and venous Doppler signals.
- Grade II. Threatened.
    - IIA. Marginally threatened: none to mild sensory loss of toes; no motor deficit; limb salvageable with prompt treatment.
    - IIB. Immediately threatened: sensory loss of more than toes; mild to moderate motor deficit; absence of arterial Doppler signals; limb salvageable if promptly revascularized.
- Grade III. Irreversible: profound sensory loss/anesthetic limb; profound paralysis (rigor); absence of both arterial and venous Doppler signals; major tissue loss and/or permanent nerve damage are inevitable.

Specific intervention for acute limb ischemia depends on limb viability; neurological deficit; etiology, duration, extent of ischemia, and area involved (artery, graft); comorbidities; and therapy-related risks and benefits (Aboyans et al., 2018; Chioncel et al., 2019; Gerhard-Herman et al., 2017). After the diagnosis is established, analgesia and treatment with unfractionated heparin are initiated for grades I and IIA, unless contraindicated; for grade IIB, immediate revascularization is indicated (Chioncel et al., 2019). Treatment techniques include mechanical recanalization with percutaneous aspiration thrombectomy or percutaneous mechanical thrombectomy, pharmacological recanalization by percutaneous catheter-directed thrombolysis, and/or surgery with thrombectomy/embolectomy or bypass (Aboyans et al., 2018; Chioncel et al., 2019). Endovascular percutaneous options are often the first option, particularly in patients with severe comorbidities. Thrombus extraction,

thromboaspiration, and surgical thrombectomy are indicated for patients with severe neurological deficits, and catheter-directed thrombolytic therapy is more appropriate for less severe cases without neurological deficits. If the limb is unsalvageable or fails treatment, amputation may be performed (Gerhard-Herman et al., 2017). Despite advances in treatment of acute limb ischemia, the rate of limb loss is approximately 30%, and the mortality rate as high as 20% (Chioncel et al., 2019). Therefore, early detection, diagnosis, and treatment are essential for management of this severe, high-risk condition.

KEY POINT

The hallmark sign of an acute limb-threatening occlusion is the sudden onset of the six "Ps": pulselessness, pain, pallor, paresthesia, paralysis, and polar (coldness).

Chronic Limb Ischemia

For over 30 years, critical limb ischemia (CLI) has been described as chronic limb ischemia (Mills et al., 2014). CLI has been defined as a chronic condition ($\geq$2 weeks) with objectively proven arterial occlusive disease and ischemic rest pain, nonhealing wounds/ulcers, or gangrene in one or both legs (Campia et al., 2019; Gerhard-Herman et al., 2017). In 2013, the Society for Vascular Surgery (SVS) developed a new framework to classify threatened lower limbs and eliminated the term "critical" from CLI (Mills et al., 2014). Subsequently, two international vascular guidelines endorsed the SVS framework and replaced the nomenclature of CLI with "chronic limb-threatening ischemia" (CLTI) (Aboyans et al., 2018; Conte et al., 2019). The rationale for changing the terminology and definition was that the term "critical" implies urgent treatment is necessary to avoid limb loss, some patients do not suffer limb loss or require revascularization, and ischemia is not the only cause of limb loss (Aboyans et al., 2018; Mills et al., 2014). In addition to ischemia, the risk of amputation depends on the presence/severity of a wound or gangrene and infection (Aboyans et al., 2018; Mills et al., 2014). Also, the existing classification framework for CLI was not intended to include patients with diabetes, and there are increasing numbers of patients with diabetes that have ischemia and neuropathy, accounting for 50% to 70% of patient with CLTI (Chioncel et al., 2019).

CLTI is defined as LEAD that is objectively documented with hemodynamic tests (i.e., ABI < 0.40, ankle pressure <50 mm Hg, toe pressure or transcutaneous oxygen tension [$TCPO_2$] <30 mm Hg), plus the presence of any of the following: ischemic rest pain, nonhealing limb or foot ulcer $\geq$2 weeks, diabetic foot ulcer, or gangrene of a limb or foot (Aboyans et al., 2018; Conte et al., 2019). Because the term CLTI is not universally reflected in the literature, the joint term and abbreviations for CLI/CLTI are used in this chapter.

A small proportion of patients with LEAD progress to CLI/CLTI, which is usually the result of multisegmental disease with impaired blood flow in peripheral and distal tissues (Uccioli et al., 2018). It is estimated that at 5 years, 21% of patients with intermittent claudication progress to CLI/CLTI (Aboyans et al., 2018). The prevalence of CLI/CLTI is reported at 0.4%, and the estimated annual incidence ranges from 500 to 1,000 new cases per million with higher rates in patients with diabetes (Aboyans et al., 2018). CLI/CLTI is associated with a high risk for tissue loss, amputation, cardiovascular events, and mortality (Campia et al., 2019; Uccioli et al., 2018). The annual incidence of major amputations ranges between 120 and 500 million (Aboyans et al., 2018). Six months after diagnosis of CLI/CLTI, the amputation rate is 20% to 40%, and the mortality rate is 20%; after 5 years, the mortality rate is 50% (Uccioli et al., 2018). Due to the high morbidity and mortality, timely referral to a vascular surgical specialist is required for patients with signs and symptoms of CLTI (WOCN, 2014).

WOUND HISTORY

The history of a current or previous wound should include a description of the onset and precipitating factors, course (e.g., improvement/regression), duration, and prior treatment regimens and their effectiveness. Ischemia should be suspected in patients with lower extremity wounds that do not heal despite proper management.

LABORATORY TESTS

A review of available laboratory tests can provide relevant information about risk factors for LEAD and the effectiveness of current interventions such as a fasting plasma glucose and serum lipid profile, serum creatinine and creatinine clearance, and urinalysis (Aboyans et al., 2018). While not specific to LEAD, other tests such as hemoglobin and hematocrit, prothrombin time, and international normalized ratio (INR) for patients on anticoagulants (e.g., warfarin) provide valuable information for patient management (WOCN, 2014). Although the values can be affected by numerous conditions, assessment of albumin or prealbumin may provide information about nutritional deficiencies that contribute to impaired wound healing. Routine monitoring of hemoglobin A1c (HbA$_{1c}$) and blood sugar levels is also indicated for individuals with LEAD and diabetes (Aboyans et al., 2018; WOCN, 2014). If nonhealing wounds are present and infection is suspected, a white blood cell count is warranted.

PSYCHOLOGICAL, SOCIOLOGICAL, AND ENVIRONMENTAL FACTORS

It is important for health care providers to determine the psychological, sociological, and environmental factors that affect patients and their quality of life (e.g., emotional well-being, self-care ability, availability of caretakers, length of illness, employment, recreational activity). Anxiety, depression, job-related stress, and difficulty coping with job-related conflicts are among some of the issues associated with LEAD and decreased lower extremity functioning (Criqui & Aboyans, 2015). In a study of 117 patients with LEAD, Hernandez et al. (2018) found that 55/47% of patients had mild (n = 33) to moderate/severe (n = 22) depression. In addition, they found that the severity of depression symptoms was independently associated with greater inflammation in LEAD. Patients with depression had a higher total inflammatory score compared to patients without depression (p = 0.04). Analysis of individual inflammatory markers found IL-6 levels were significantly higher in the group with moderate/severe symptoms of depression (p = 0.006) compared to the group without symptoms (n = 62), and hs-CRP and soluble intracellular adhesion molecule-1 (ICAM-1) trended upward with increasing depression severity.

LOWER EXTREMITY ASSESSMENT

A comprehensive examination of both lower extremities should be performed on any patient with/or at risk for wounds due to LEAD to determine skin and tissue integrity, sensation, and peripheral circulatory status. It is necessary to examine both limbs because LEAD is often asymptomatic and may not be confined to one limb. A thorough assessment provides the foundational data required for correctly managing the patient and evaluating the effectiveness of therapeutic interventions.

Status of Skin and Tissue

After removing the patient's shoes and any hosiery or compression devices, the nurse should carefully examine the lower limbs and feet (i.e., toes and skin between the toes, nails, and heels) for signs of ischemia, injury, or wounds; findings from each limb should then be compared. Footwear should also be assessed for fit. See **Table 25-1** for common clinical characteristics and skin changes in ischemic limbs.

Individuals with LEAD are at increased risk for developing pressure injuries (PrIs) involving the heels or malleoli due to decreased perfusion; thus, individuals with limited mobility (e.g., bed/chair bound) should be assessed frequently and regularly for evidence of early ischemic damage involving the heel or other bony prominences of the foot. The heel is at particular risk for injury due to the limited subcutaneous tissue and muscle and the limited blood supply to the skin (Lumbers, 2018). In a case control study (N = 30), Twilley and Jones (2016) compared 15 patients with heel PrIs (stages 2 to 4) to 15 patients without PrIs and found that 12 of the patients with PrIs had previously undiagnosed LEAD (ABI < 0.90 or >1.30) compared to four in the control group (OR = 11, 95% CI [1.99, 60.57]). LEAD is also associated with poor healing. In a study of 140 patients with 183 heel PrIs, the investigators

TABLE 25-1 COMMON CLINICAL CHARACTERISTICS AND SKIN CHANGES IN ISCHEMIC LIMBS

CLINICAL CHARACTERISTIC	COMMON SKIN AND LIMB CHANGES IN ISCHEMIA
Color	• Pallor on elevation of legs • Rubor (purplish red color) in dependent position
Temperature	• Skin feels cool to touch
Texture/turgor	• Shiny, taut, and dry skin • Thin, fragile skin • Atrophy of skin, subcutaneous tissue, and muscle
Capillary refill	• Delayed capillary refill (i.e., more than 3 s), which can be affected by environmental temperature
Venous refill	• Prolonged venous refill time (i.e., more than 20 s)
Nails	• Abnormal nails (thin and ridged)
Hair	• Minimal or absent hair
Sensation	• Paresthesia

Adapted with permission from Wound, Ostomy and Continence Nurses Society. (2014). *Guideline for management of wounds in patients with lower extremity arterial disease. WOCN clinical practice guideline series1* (p. 46). Mt. Laurel, NJ: Author.

found that only 70 (38%) of the wounds were on a limb with an adequate arterial supply (ABI ≥ 0.80; McGinnis et al., 2014). McGinnis et al. reported that the presence of LEAD was a significant factor in reducing the probability of wound healing (HR = 0.42, 95% CI [0.21, 0.83], p = 0.010). Because LEAD can be a significant factor that contributes to the development of heel PrIs and poor wound healing, vascular assessment (i.e., examination of pedal pulses and ABI) is indicated for individuals with PrIs on the heel, foot, or lower limb (Twilley & Jones, 2016).

KEY POINT

Individuals with LEAD and limited mobility are at increased risk for pressure injuries involving the heels and malleoli.

Sensory Status

The sensory status of both limbs should be assessed using simple noninvasive tests (WOCN, 2014). Patients with LEAD may have neuropathy due to the impact of ischemia on peripheral nerve function. Although neuropathy is commonly associated with diabetes, it also occurs in individuals without diabetes (Baldereschi et al., 2013). Baldereschi et al. examined 2,512 individuals without diabetes and found that LEAD was an independent predictor of distal symmetric neuropathy (HR = 2.45, 95% CI [1.01, 5.91], p = 0.02). Therefore, patients with LEAD should be screened for loss of protective sensation (LOPS) in the feet (Aboyans et al., 2018; Conte et al., 2019). LOPS can

be quickly determined by testing the feet with a 5.07/10 g Semmes-Weinstein monofilament, assessing vibratory sensation with a tuning fork (128 Hz), and testing ankle reflexes (Conte et al., 2019; WOCN, 2014). The inability to feel the pressure of the monofilament on one or more anatomic sites on the plantar and dorsal surfaces of the foot indicates a LOPS. Four to ten sites should be tested including the first, third, and fifth distal toes and metatarsal heads; medial and lateral plantar surfaces of the foot; and dorsal surface between the great toe and second toe (Varnado, 2016). It is recommended to test the vibratory sensation over the base of the great toe at the first metatarsal bone; an abnormal response is when the patient loses the vibratory sensation while it is still felt by the examiner (Varnado, 2016). Deep tendon reflexes can be tested on the ankle by stretching the Achilles tendon until the foot is in a neutral position and striking the tendon with a percussion hammer, which should result in plantar flexion of the foot. Total absence of the ankle reflex is an abnormal result indicating impaired motor nerve function (Varnado, 2016).

Pulses

The most common approach to assessment of perfusion status is pulse palpation, which includes palpation of the femoral, popliteal, dorsalis pedis on the dorsum of each foot, and the posterior tibial pulse on the medial aspect of the limb behind the ankle (Gerhard-Herman et al., 2017). See **Figure 25-3** for location of pedal pulses. It is important to keep the room warm during pulse palpation to prevent vasoconstriction. It is recommended to assess and record the intensity of the pulse as: 0—absent, 1—diminished, 2—normal, and 3—bounding (Gerhard-Herman et al., 2017; WOCN, 2014). It is important to recognize that the presence of palpable pulses does not rule out arterial disease, because a palpable pulse does not provide an

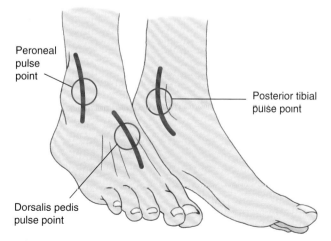

FIGURE 25-3. Location of Pedal Pulses: Peroneal, Dorsalis Pedis, and Posterior Tibial. (Reprinted with permission from Weber, J., & Kelley, J. (2003). *Health assessment in nursing* (2nd ed.). Philadelphia, PA: Lippincott Williams & Wilkins.)

accurate indication of vessel health and volume of blood flow. (In addition, clinicians may actually be feeling their own pulses rather than the pedal pulse of the patient.) Similarly, an absent pulse, alone, is not a sensitive indicator of LEAD because the dorsalis pedis pulse may be congenitally absent in up to 12% of healthy individuals (Criqui et al., 1985; Gerhard-Herman et al., 2017). The importance of conducting a comprehensive assessment and not relying simply on pulse palpation is underscored by the findings of Bozkurt et al. (2011) who evaluated 530 individuals with both pulse assessment and ABI. The investigators reported that 6.5% of the individuals were determined to have LEAD when absence of palpable pulses was the only diagnostic criterion, whereas the true prevalence was 20% when confirmed by an ABI.

Femoral and popliteal arteries can be auscultated for bruits using the bell of a stethoscope; bruits are indicative of turbulent blood flow through stenotic vessels (Rumwell & McPharlin, 2017). However, bruits are low-frequency sounds and may not always be detected.

Noninvasive Assessment/Diagnostic Techniques

Because of the unreliability of pulse palpation and a history of claudication, additional tests using noninvasive techniques are needed to detect the presence and severity of LEAD. Several noninvasive, portable testing methods are available that can be used at the bedside to assess perfusion status including the ABI, toe pressures or toe–brachial index (TBI), and TcPO$_2$.

Ankle Brachial Index

One of the most commonly used noninvasive tests is the ABI, which provides an indirect assessment of arterial blood flow in the lower limbs by comparing the brachial systolic pressure to the systolic pressure at the ankle. ABI is recommended as a first-line, noninvasive test to establish a diagnosis in individuals at high risk or suspected of having LEAD such as individuals who have leg pain with walking, rest pain, or nonhealing wounds; are ≥65 years of age; or are ≥50 years of age with a history of smoking, diabetes, hyperlipidemia, hypertension, a family history of LEAD, or atherosclerotic disease in another vascular bed; and/or have abnormal pulses or physical findings (Gerhard-Herman et al., 2017).

KEY POINT

ABI is recommended as a first-line noninvasive test for individuals at risk for/or suspected of having LEAD.

Measurement of ABI Using Continuous-Wave Doppler

The ABI should be tested bilaterally because LEAD may not develop or progress in the same manner in both limbs. An ABI is obtained by measuring the brachial systolic pressures in both arms and the dorsalis pedis and posterior tibial arteries in both ankles (**Fig. 25-4**). Doppler technique is the preferred method for measuring the arm

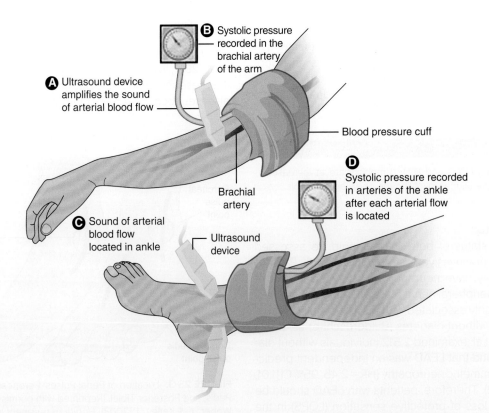

FIGURE 25-4. Use of a Doppler for Measuring ABI. (From National Heart, Lung and Blood Institute as part of the National Institutes of Health and the U.S. Department of Health and Human Services. Retrieved from www.nhlbi.nih.gov/health/dci/Diseases/pad/paddiagnsis.html)

and ankle pressures for the ABI (Aboyans et al., 2018; Gerhard-Herman et al., 2017; WOCN, 2014), because it is more accurate in measurement of low blood pressures at the ankle than other methods such as automated/oscillometric devices, stethoscope, or pulse palpation (Aboyans et al., 2018; Davies et al., 2014; Herraiz-Adillo et al., 2017; Rac-Albu et al., 2014; WOCN, 2014).

Doppler ultrasound waveforms reflect the velocity of red blood cells (RBCs) passing through the vessel (Rumwell & McPharlin, 2017). Blood flow through a normal pedal vessel produces a triphasic waveform and a pressure comparable to brachial pressures, but if the pedal artery is stenosed or occluded, fewer RBCs pass through and the wave form is blunted (either biphasic or monophasic) depending on the severity of occlusion (Rumwell & McPharlin, 2017). Pressures obtained from damaged vessels are typically lower than the brachial pressures. The exception is a vessel that is rigid and poorly compressible or noncompressible; these vessels generate pressures that are higher than the brachial pressures (Rumwell & McPharlin, 2017).

Although values differ according to the methodology used to measure the ABI (e.g., equipment, procedures, expertise/experience of the operator), the ABI has good validity as a first-line test to diagnose LEAD with sensitivities ranging from 68% to 84% and specificities from 84% to 99% (Gerhard-Herman et al., 2017). Results from two studies showed that ABIs measured with portable Dopplers were interchangeable with ABIs measured in the vascular laboratory (Bonham et al., 2007; Nicolai et al., 2008). See **Table 25-2** for the recommended procedure for measuring and calculating the ABI with a continuous-wave Doppler.

The ABI is a ratio calculated by dividing the higher of the ankle systolic pressures (dorsalis pedis or posterior tibial) for each leg by the higher of the brachial systolic pressures from the right or left arm (Aboyans et al., 2018; Rumwell & McPharlin, 2017; WOCN, 2014). If there is a difference in brachial pressures of >20 mm Hg, the patient should be evaluated for subclavian stenosis (Rumwell & McPharlin, 2017). When calculating an ABI, the higher of the ankle pressures is preferred to minimize the overdiagnosis of LEAD in healthy individuals (Aboyans et al., 2012).

ABI Limitations

The ABI is an indirect test for large vessel arterial disease, and it cannot be used to determine the precise anatomic location of a stenotic/occlusive lesion (Rumwell & McPharlin, 2017). In addition, severe vessel calcification renders the ABI ineffective, and elevated (>1.30 to 1.50 or higher) readings are obtained when the vessels are

---

TABLE 25-2 PROCEDURE FOR MEASURING AND CALCULATING THE ANKLE–BRACHIAL INDEX (ABI)	
ACTION	PROCEDURE

Prepare equipment and supplies	1. Gather equipment and supplies for the ABI.
	   a. Portable continuous-wave Doppler with 8- to 10-MHz probe (5 MHz if a large amount of edema is present at the ankle)
	   b. Aneroid sphygmomanometer and pressure cuff
	   c. Ultrasound transmission gel
	   d. Alcohol pads to clean the Doppler and gauze, tissue, or pads to remove the transmission gel from the patient's skin
	   e. Towels, sheets, or blankets to cover the trunk and extremities
	   f. Paper and pen for recording test results; calculator
	2. Inspect the equipment and check the batteries if a battery-operated Doppler is used and replace equipment that is damaged or not calibrated.
	3. Pressure cuffs for arms and ankles should be long enough to fully encircle the limb. The width of the cuff's bladder should be 40% of the limb's circumference and the length sufficient to cover 80% of the limb's circumference.
	   a. Typically, 12-cm-wide cuffs are used for arms and 10-cm-wide cuffs at the ankles.
	   b. Extra-large adult cuffs might be needed (14 cm).

Prepare patient and environment	1. Inquire about recent use of tobacco, caffeine, or alcohol; recent heavy activity; and presence of pain. *Note:* When possible, advise the patient to avoid stimulants or heavy exercise for an hour prior to the test. 2. Perform the ABI in a quiet, warm environment (21°C–23°C ± 1°C) to prevent vasoconstriction of the arteries. 3. The best ABI results are obtained when the patient is relaxed, comfortable, and has an empty bladder. 4. Explain the procedure to the patient. 5. Remove shoes, socks, and tight clothing to permit placement of the pressure cuff and access to the pulse sites by the Doppler probe. 6. Place the patient in a flat, supine position. Place one small pillow behind the patient's head for comfort. 7. Cover the trunk and extremities to prevent cooling. 8. Ensure the patient is comfortable and have the patient rest for a minimum of 10 min prior to the test to allow pressures to normalize. 9. After the rest period, measure the arm and ankle pressures.

(Continued)

TABLE 25-2 PROCEDURE FOR MEASURING AND CALCULATING THE ANKLE–BRACHIAL INDEX (ABI) (*Continued*)

ACTION	PROCEDURE
Measure brachial pressures with Doppler	1. The arm should be relaxed, supported, and at heart level. 2. Prior to placement of the cuff, apply a protective barrier (e.g., plastic wrap) on the extremity if any wounds or alterations in skin integrity are present. 3. Place the pressure cuff with the bottom of the cuff ~2–3 cm above the cubital fossa on the arm. 4. The cuff should be wrapped without wrinkles and placed securely to prevent slipping and movement during the test. 5. Palpate the brachial pulse to determine the location to obtain an audible pulse. 6. Apply transmission gel over the pulse site. 7. Place the tip of the Doppler probe at a 45 degrees angle pointed toward the patient's head until an audible pulse signal is obtained. 8. Inflate the pressure cuff 20–30 mm Hg above the point where the pulse is no longer audible. 9. Deflate the pressure cuff at a rate of 2–3 mm Hg/s, noting the manometer reading at which the first pulse signal is heard and record that systolic value. 10. Cleanse/remove gel from the pulse site. 11. Repeat the procedure to measure the pressure on the other arm. 12. If a pressure needs to be repeated, wait 1 min before re-inflating the cuff. 13. Use the higher of the brachial pressures from the right or left arm to calculate the ABI for both legs.
Measure ankle pressures with Doppler	1. Prior to placing the cuff, apply a protective barrier (e.g., plastic wrap) on the extremity if there are any wounds or alterations in skin integrity. 2. Place the cuff on the patient's lower leg with the bottom of the cuff ~2–3 cm above the malleolus. 3. The cuff should be wrapped without wrinkles and placed securely to prevent slipping and movement during the test. 4. Measure both dorsalis pedis and posterior tibial pulses on each leg. 5. Locate the pulses by palpation or with the Doppler probe. 6. Apply transmission gel to the pulse site. 7. Place the tip of the Doppler probe at a 45-degree angle pointed toward the patient's knee until an audible pulse signal is obtained. 8. Inflate the pressure cuff 20–30 mm Hg above the point where the pulse is no longer audible. 9. Deflate the cuff slowly at a rate of 2–3 mm Hg/s noting the manometer reading at which the first pulse signal is heard, and record that systolic value. 10. Cleanse/remove gel from the pulse site. 11. Repeat the procedure to measure pressures on the other ankle. 12. If a pressure needs to be repeated, wait 1 min before re-inflating the cuff. 13. Use the higher of the ankle pressures of each leg to calculate the ABI for each leg.
Calculate the ABI	1. Divide the higher of the dorsalis pedis or posterior tibial systolic pressure for each ankle by the higher of the right or left brachial pressures to obtain the ABI for each leg. $$ABI = \frac{\text{Higher of either the dorsalispedis or posterior tibial pressures}}{\text{Higher of the brachial pressures}}$$ 2. Interpret and compare the ABI values from each leg (see Table 25-3). 3. Refer the patient for further testing and evaluation if the ABI is <0.90, >1.30, or unmeasurable due to noncompressible vessels and/or if the patient's clinical symptoms and ABI are inconsistent. 4. Document findings, follow-up plans, and referrals.

Adapted with permission from Wound, Ostomy and Continence Nurses Society. (2017). *Ankle brachial index: Procedure for measuring and calculating the ABI.* Mt. Laurel, NJ: Author.

rigid and calcified (Rumwell & McPharlin, 2017). If the vessels are extremely rigid, it is impossible to compress the vessels enough to obtain a systolic pressure measurement. Conditions in which vessel calcification is common include diabetes and advanced kidney disease (Aboyans et al., 2018; Gerhard-Herman et al., 2017; Rumwell & McPharlin, 2017). There is also concern that in patients with some degree of calcification, the ABI may underestimate LEAD due to the possibility that mild to moderate calcification may affect the pressure measurement even though the artery can be compressed and the systolic

blood pressure can be measured (Aerden et al., 2011). It is important to recognize high ABI levels because an ABI > 1.30 to 1.40 is associated with an increased risk for cardiovascular events and mortality with similar strength to an ABI < 0.90 (Aboyans et al., 2018; Alves-Cabratosa et al., 2019; Gu et al., 2019; Rac-Albu et al., 2014).

Currently there is not a universal consensus on the cutoff value for an elevated or high ABI. In a systematic review of 14 guidelines (published 2003–2018), five considered that the range for a normal ABI was 0.90 to 1.30 (Chen et al., 2019), which contrasts with recent guidelines that consider a normal ABI range is 1.00 to 1.40 (Aboyans et al., 2018; Conte et al., 2019; Gerhard-Herman et al., 2017). These differences are highlighted in a recent systematic review of 18 research studies in which 9 investigators defined a high ABI as ≥1.30, and 9 defined a high ABI as ≥1.40 (Gu et al., 2019). In addition, there are various definitions of noncompressible arteries. An ABI > 1.40 has been described as poorly compressible or noncompressible (Campia et al., 2019; Gerhard-Herman et al., 2017). Other experts consider an ABI > 1.30 to be elevated or abnormal due to calcified, noncompressible arteries (Alves-Cabratosa et al., 2019; Rumwell & McPharlin, 2017; Scissons et al., 2019; Uccioli et al., 2018).

We lack the data to identify a specific level of arterial calcification that correlates definitively with vessel rigidity, occlusion, stenosis, or ABI values. The distinction between an elevated ABI and noncompressible vessels (i.e., an unmeasurable ABI) has not been clearly differentiated in most studies, and it is unclear if the two findings have equivalent clinical significance. For example, if the pulse signal can be obliterated with inflation of the pressure cuff and the return of the pulse signal detected upon deflation of the cuff, the ABI may be high but is measurable. In contrast, if the pulse signal cannot be obliterated at high cuff pressures (>250 mm Hg) or detected with cuff deflation, the ABI is unmeasurable due to noncompressible arteries (Criqui et al., 2010; Spreen et al., 2018).

It is important to realize that some individuals have claudication symptoms with activity but a normal ABI at rest; those individuals should be referred to a vascular laboratory for exercise testing (Gerhard-Herman et al., 2017; Rumwell & McPharlin, 2017). Ankle pressures and/or ABI should be obtained at baseline and repeated following exercise. Treadmill testing is the preferred method of exercise testing, but walking a predetermined distance or toe stands can be used if treadmill testing is not available; however, toe stands are limited in their ability to provide meaningful information (Rumwell & McPharlin, 2017). A decrease in ABI of more than 20% after exercise is considered significant for LEAD (Aboyans et al., 2018; Chioncel et al., 2019; Sibley et al., 2017). Ankle pressures that are low or unrecordable immediately after exercise and then increase to resting levels in 2 to 6 minutes suggest a single level obstruction, and pressures that remain reduced or unrecordable for more than 6 minutes suggest multilevel obstructions (Rumwell & McPharlin, 2017).

ABI Interpretation

If arterial blood flow is normal, the pressure in the ankle should be equal to/or only slightly higher than that in the arm with an ABI ratio of 1.00 or higher (Rumwell & McPharlin, 2017; WOCN, 2014). An ABI ≤ 0.90 indicates LEAD (Aboyans et al., 2018; Gerhard-Herman et al., 2017; WOCN, 2014). When interpreting the ABI, clinical

TABLE 25-3 INTERPRETATION OF ANKLE–BRACHIAL INDEX

ABI	INTERPRETATION
Unable to obliterate the pulse signal at cuff pressure >250 mm Hg	Noncompressible arteries (associated with vessel calcification)
>1.30	Elevated
≥1.00	Normal
≤0.90	LEAD
≤0.60–0.80	Borderline perfusion
≤0.50	Severe ischemia
≤0.40	CLI/CLTI (limb threatened)

Reprinted with permission from Wound, Ostomy and Continence Nurses Society. (2014). *Guideline for management of wounds in patients with lower extremity arterial disease. WOCN clinical practice guideline series 1* (p. 60). Mt. Laurel, NJ: Author.

judgment is necessary, taking into consideration the overall findings from the comprehensive lower extremity examination and other vascular assessment findings, and patient management should not be based only on the ABI (Casey et al., 2019). See **Table 25-3** for interpretation of the ABI.

In addition to interpreting the ABI, printouts of the Doppler waveform can be used for further analysis of Doppler signals. Normal lower extremity arterial signals are triphasic with a rapid upstroke, sharp peaked systolic component, rapid downstroke, a short peak below the baseline representing reverse diastolic flow, and resumption of forward diastolic flow above the baseline (Rumwell & McPharlin, 2017). Abnormal signals are biphasic, monophasic, nonpulsatile, or absent (Rumwell & McPharlin, 2017). The degree of obstruction cannot be determined on the basis of waveforms alone because blood flow distal to an obstruction can be affected by the development of collateral circulation (Rumwell & McPharlin, 2017).

Frequency of ABI testing

ABI measurement is recommended for patients with/or at high risk for LEAD (Gerhard-Herman et al., 2017; WOCN, 2014) to facilitate preventive care and timely referrals for further vascular testing or surgical evaluation, and it is a key element of assessment for patients with lower extremity wounds prior to planning care. Patients with nonhealing lower extremity wounds and LEAD should have the ABI rechecked every 3 months (WOCN, 2014, 2019b). ABI can also be used to monitor patients for restenosis following revascularization, but it should not be used as a stand-alone measure of perfusion (Aboyans et al., 2018; Conte et al., 2019; Gerhard-Herman et al., 2017). Routine ABI testing is not recommended for patients who do not have an increased risk of LEAD, are asymptomatic, and/or do not have a history or physical findings suggestive of LEAD (Gerhard-Herman et al., 2017; Skelly & Cifu, 2016).

Toe Pressures and Toe Brachial Index

Toe pressures and/or TBI are recommended for individuals with noncompressible ankle arteries or when the ABI is elevated, inconclusive, or unmeasurable due to presence of a wound (Aboyans et al., 2018; Gerhard-Herman et al., 2017; WOCN, 2014); this is because digital (toe) arteries are usually less affected by calcification than ankle arteries (Gerhard-Herman et al., 2017). A systolic toe pressure <30 mm Hg indicates CLI/CLTI and is predictive of nonhealing wounds (Aboyans et al., 2018; Campia et al., 2019; Gerhard-Herman et al., 2017; WOCN, 2014). In a study of symptomatic patients with LEAD (N = 732), Wickstrom et al. (2017) found that toe pressures <30 mm Hg were significantly associated with cardiovascular mortality (HR = 2.84, 95% CI [1.75, 4.61], $p < 0.001$) and amputation or death (HR = 2.13, 95% CI [1.52, 2.98], $p < 0.001$).

Similar to the diversity in definitions of high or elevated ABI values, the cutoff value for TBI varies substantially in guidelines, clinical settings, and studies. The variation in diagnostic limits is likely due to different equipment, techniques, and procedures for measuring TBI. However, in a review of results from seven studies, despite differences in diagnostic cutoff limits, TBI sensitivity (90% to 100%) and specificity (65% to 100%) were high to detect LEAD (Hoyer et al., 2013). TBI cutoff values for LEAD have included <0.60 (Rumwell & McPharlin, 2017; Sibley et al., 2017); <0.64 (WOCN, 2014); and <0.70 (Aboyans et al., 2018; Campia et al., 2019; Conte et al., 2019; Gerhard-Herman et al., 2017). According to several early studies, a TBI < 0.64, as confirmed by angiography, indicated LEAD and has been a commonly cited cutoff value for LEAD (Carter, 1993; Carter & Lezack, 1971; Hoyer et al., 2013; Lezack & Carter, 1973; Makisalo et al., 1998).

KEY POINT

Toe pressures or TBI measurements are recommended for individuals with noncompressible arteries or high ABI readings (i.e., >1.30), because toe arteries are less affected by calcification than ankle arteries.

Toe Pressure/TBI Technique

The toe pressure is measured on the digital artery of the first (great) toe or second toe using a small digital pressure cuff. A TBI is derived by dividing the toe pressure by the higher of the two brachial systolic pressures. Toe pressures and TBI are most commonly obtained in a vascular laboratory with photoplethysmography (PPG), which detects pulsatile cutaneous blood flow from a transducer attached to the skin of the distal toe pad. Also, portable PPG equipment is available for use outside the vascular

laboratory for measuring toe pressures/TBI that has shown good sensitivity (79%) and high specificity (95%) for detection of LEAD (Bonham et al., 2010). Use of continuous-wave Doppler to measure toe pressures is not recommended because the Doppler is unable to detect the flow of RBCs through constricted arteries when the toes are cold or there is vasospastic disease, and studies have shown that Doppler-derived toe pressures are not equivalent to those obtained in the vascular lab with PPG (Bonham et al., 2007; Kroger et al., 2003). If clinicians do not have the equipment or skill to perform a toe pressure/TBI measurement with specialized equipment such as PPG, patients should be referred to a vascular laboratory.

Transcutaneous Oxygen Tension

$TcPO_2$ measures oxygen levels in the periwound tissues and is indicated when a lower extremity wound is not healing, or if an accurate ABI or TBI cannot be obtained (Aboyans et al., 2018; Gerhard-Herman et al., 2017; WOCN, 2014). A $TcPO_2$ level <40 mm Hg indicates tissue hypoxia (Rumwell & McPharlin, 2017). $TcPO_2 > 40$ mm Hg has been associated with good healing after minor amputations (Aboyans et al., 2018). $TcPO_2 < 30$ mm Hg is consistent with CLI/CLTI and failure to heal (Aboyans et al., 2018; Conte et al., 2019; Gerhard-Herman et al., 2017; Uccioli et al., 2018; Vemulapalli et al., 2015).

If an ABI, toe pressure/TBI, or $TcPO_2$ is inconclusive, inconsistent, or unmeasurable, patients should be referred for further vascular testing. Vascular laboratories can provide additional noninvasive studies to confirm or diagnose LEAD.

Segmental Pressures

Segmental pressures can be used to determine the general anatomic location of stenosis or occlusion but cannot differentiate between stenosis and occlusion, and interpretation can be difficult in multilevel disease (Rumwell & McPharlin, 2017). Consecutive and contralateral levels of pressures (i.e., high thigh, low thigh above knee, below knee, and ankle) are measured with pressure cuffs and a continuous-wave Doppler, and the measurements and limbs are compared. A decrease in pressure >20 to 30 mm Hg between two consecutive levels on the same leg indicates stenosis or occlusion, and a 20 to 30 mm Hg difference in pressure between the two legs at the same location indicates obstructive disease in the leg with the lower pressure (Rumwell & McPharlin, 2017). See **Figure 25-5** for an example of segmental pressures, ABI, and waveforms.

Skin Perfusion Pressure

Skin perfusion pressure (SPP) is measured with a laser Doppler probe enclosed in a pressure cuff placed on the forefoot and can be used to assess blood flow in the microvasculature; it is helpful when calcification prevents accurate ABI measurement or when skin lesions or toe

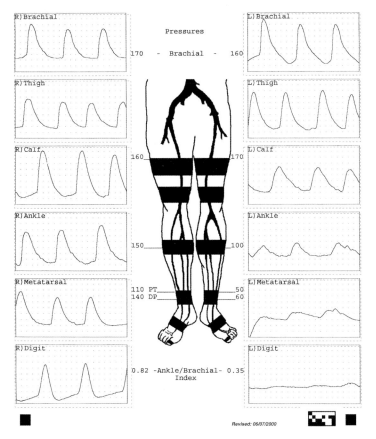

FIGURE 25-5. Segmental Pressures Including ABI and Pulse Volume Recording (PVR). Right ABI is slightly reduced at 0.82 and left ABI of 0.35 indicates critical ischemia. PVR tracings on the left show diminution in amplitude at the calf and ankle, and the digit PVR tracing is flat suggesting severe small vessel disease in the left foot.

amputations prevent toe pressure measurements. SPP < 30 mm Hg indicates failure to heal (Rumwell & McPharlin, 2017), and SPP ≥ 30 to 50 mm Hg is associated with increased likelihood of wound healing (Gerhard-Herman et al., 2017).

Pulse Volume Recording

Pulse volume recordings (PVRs) provide qualitative and quantitative information about limb perfusion; plethysmography is used to measure changes in the volume of the lower limb throughout the cardiac cycle, which is a reflection of arterial inflow (Rumwell & McPharlin, 2017). PVRs can be used to establish an initial diagnosis of LEAD for patients with noncompressible arteries or an elevated ABI, and to monitor patients following lower extremity revascularization. Normal PVRs have a clearly defined sharp upward stroke during peak systole followed by a prolonged downstroke during diastole and a dicrotic notch about halfway through the downstroke, which represents reversed blood flow in early diastole (Rumwell & McPharlin, 2017; Sibley et al., 2017). In the presence of LEAD, the dicrotic notch is diminished or absent, and the amplitude of the waveform decreases (Rumwell & McPharlin, 2017). See **Figure 25-5** for examples of PVR wave forms.

Duplex Ultrasound Scanning

Duplex ultrasound scanning (DUS) produces images of blood flow through vessels and is used to identify the precise anatomic location and severity of stenosis

or occlusion when planning surgery and/or to monitor patency after surgery (Aboyans et al., 2018; Gerhard-Herman et al., 2017; Rumwell & McPharlin, 2017). DUS has 85% to 95% sensitivity and >95% specificity for detection of stenosis (Aboyans et al., 2018). DUS provides less spatial resolution than magnetic resonance angiography (MRA) and computed tomographic angiography (CTA) with calcified arteries (Gerhard-Herman et al., 2017).

Magnetic Resonance Angiography

MRA is used to identify candidates for endovascular procedures or surgical revascularization and to plan treatment. Gadolinium-enhanced MRA provides highly accurate detection of stenosis and occlusion of the arteries in the lower extremity with 95% sensitivity and specificity (Aboyans et al., 2018; Gerhard-Herman et al., 2017). Because of the strong magnets in the machine, MRA cannot be used on patients with pacemakers; defibrillators; metallic stents, clips, or coils; and gadolinium should be avoided in individuals who have kidney failure or are on dialysis (Gerhard-Herman et al., 2017). Other limitations of MRA are that it does not reliably detect calcifications and can overestimate stenosis (Aboyans et al., 2018).

Computed Tomographic Angiography

Modern multidetector-CTA is a fast, noninvasive modality that provides high-resolution, contrast-enhanced images that can be viewed in multiple planes or three-dimensional reconstructions for accurate identification of the anatomic location and degree of stenosis in arterial disease (Aboyans et al., 2018; Conte et al., 2019; Gerhard-Herman et al., 2017). Disadvantages of CTA are that it does not provide functional or hemodynamic data, involves radiation exposure, and uses iodinated contrast agents (Aboyans et al., 2018; Conte et al., 2019). CTA is less invasive than digital subtraction, faster than MRA, and can be used for patients with pacemakers or other devices that prohibit use of MRA. However, its accuracy is limited if extensive calcification is present, and its use is limited in patients with CKD due to the iodine-based contrast agent (Aboyans et al., 2018; Conte et al. 2019; Gerhard-Herman et al., 2017). Suggestions for limiting contrast-induced nephrotoxicity include using a smaller volume of the contrast agent and ensuring adequate hydration before and after the procedure (Aboyans et al., 2018; Iezzi et al., 2012; Vlachopoulos et al., 2018).

Digital subtraction angiography

Arteriography or angiography remains the definitive method to determine the exact level of arterial occlusion and to define vascular anatomy before selecting an appropriate intervention (Rasmussen et al., 2019; WOCN, 2014). The angiogram or arteriogram involves percutaneously inserting a thin flexible catheter into an artery in the leg usually through the groin, and injecting contrast material making the arteries visible on X-rays. Digital subtraction angiography (DSA) is a fluoroscopic technique used extensively in interventional radiology by interventional radiologists and vascular surgeons for visualizing blood vessels. It has historically been considered the gold standard for diagnosis of LEAD because it provides good visualization of patent distal arteries for bypass surgery and can be used simultaneously with minimally invasive percutaneous peripheral interventions (Aboyans et al., 2018; Conte et al., 2019; Meyersohn et al., 2015). However, solely diagnostic DSA is becoming less frequent with improved imaging techniques (i.e., duplex ultrasound, CTA, MRA) (Rasmussen et al., 2019). However, it may be still used for planning surgical interventions or for patients in whom CTA or MRA are contraindicated or inconclusive, particularly for evaluation of below-the-knee arteries (Meyersohn et al., 2015; Vlachopoulos et al., 2018). Renal insufficiency and hypersensitivity to iodinated contrast dye are relative contraindications of DSA. Some centers use carbon dioxide as a contrast agent for these patients (Varcoe, 2019).

WOUND ASSESSMENT

A thorough assessment of the wound along with consideration of the history, etiology, and other clinical findings is essential as a basis for planning care. Assessment of the wound includes location, shape, size (e.g., length, width, depth, tunneling, undermining), appearance of the wound base (e.g., presence or absence of necrosis, slough, granulation or epithelialization), wound edges (e.g., rolled, punched out, smooth, undermined), periwound skin and tissue (e.g., presence or absence of erythema, induration, increased warmth, local edema, sensitivity to palpation, fluctuant or boggy tissue), and exudate (e.g., color, amount, odor, consistency). In addition to the initial assessment, measurement and reassessment of wounds are needed on an ongoing basis. Also, it is important to assess for complications such as infection, cellulitis, gangrene, or osteomyelitis. See **Table 25-4** for common characteristics of lower extremity ischemic wounds and **Figure 25-6** for an example of leg wounds due to arterial insufficiency.

KEY POINT

"Classic" assessment findings for wounds caused by LEAD include the following: location either on distal foot and toes or a nonhealing traumatic injury; ulcer bed is commonly necrotic or pale with no granulation tissue; minimal exudate; and infection is common, but signs of infection are frequently muted.

CLASSIFICATION OF LEAD

Based on clinical findings, LEAD can be classified according to Fontaine's stages or Rutherford's categories (Aboyans et al., 2018; WOCN, 2014). Fontaine's stages are as follows: I—asymptomatic, IIa—mild claudication, IIb—moderate to severe claudication, III—ischemic rest pain, and IV—ulcerations or gangrene. Rutherford's categories are as follows: 0—asymptomatic, I—mild claudication, II—moderate claudication, III—severe claudication, IV—ischemic rest pain, V—minor tissue loss, and VI—ulceration or gangrene.

The lower extremity classification system proposed by the SVS is intended for the initial assessment of patients with ischemic rest pain confirmed with hemodynamic studies; a nonhealing lower extremity wound or diabetic foot ulcer >2 weeks; or gangrene of the lower extremity in order to determine the severity of the condition and stratify the risk of an amputation (Aboyans et al., 2018; Conte et al., 2019; Mills et al., 2014). The SVS classification system as described by Mills et al. (2014) is based on three factors that impact the risk of amputation and clinical management: wound, ischemia, and foot infection (WIfI). Each factor is graded on a scale of 0 to 3 (none to severe). Wound characteristics are graded based on size, depth, and severity (i.e., involvement of deeper structures; presence/absence gangrene). Degree of ischemia is graded according to hemodynamic measures (i.e., ABI, ankle systolic pressures, toe pressure, or $TCPO_2$). Extent of infection is graded

TABLE 25-4 COMMON CHARACTERISTICS OF LOWER EXTREMITY, ISCHEMIC WOUNDS	
ASSESSMENT PARAMETER	**COMMON CHARACTERISTICS**
Location	• If LEAD primary etiology: distal foot and toes; nonhealing traumatic wounds over lower leg or foot • If LEAD contributing factor: over areas exposed to pressure or repetitive trauma (heels, phalangeal heads, malleoli)
Pain	• Often painful; pain usually worsened by activity or elevation
Size and shape	• Often small • Shape and depth vary—can be deep • Tunneling and undermining may be present
Wound edges	• Well-defined, smooth edges; punched-out appearance
Wound base	• Minimal or no granulation tissue • Often appears desiccated • Necrosis • Eschar • Wet or dry gangrene
Color	• Pale, nonviable; gray
Exudate	• Usually minimal
Periwound skin and tissue	• Edema is *not* typical of arterial wounds, and if present is generally due to other systemic conditions or diseases such as chronic heart failure, chronic kidney failure, or venous disease • Localized edema may indicate infection
Possible complications	• Infection/cellulitis: Erythema, induration, warmth, fluctuation, pain, or tenderness with palpation may be present. Often signs of infection are subtle with only a faint halo of erythema around the wound • Gangrene • Osteomyelitis

Adapted with permission from Wound, Ostomy and Continence Nurses Society. (2014). *Guideline for management of wounds in patients with lower extremity arterial disease. WOCN clinical practice guideline series 1* (pp. 44–45). Mt. Laurel, NJ: Author.

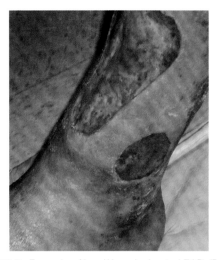

FIGURE 25-6. Example of Leg Wounds due to LEAD. (Reprinted with permission from Berg, D., & Worzala, K. (2006). *Atlas of Adult physical diagnosis.* Philadelphia, PA: Lippincott Williams & Wilkins.)

according to presence/absence of symptoms/signs of infection, depth/extent of infections (i.e., localized to skin and subcutaneous tissue; infection extended to surrounding tissues or deeper structures), and the presence/absence of systemic inflammatory response signs. The grades for the three factors are combined to create a WIfI spectrum score. Potential WIfI spectrum scores are displayed on a grid depicting the risk of amputa-

tion for each score. The risk category of the WIfI score determines the clinical stage of disease and the risk of amputation. Clinical stages range from clinical stage 1 (very low risk) to clinical stage 5 (an unsalvageable foot). Two studies evaluated the WIfI classification system, and the investigators reported that it correlated with risk of amputation, limb salvage rates, and wound healing (Cull et al., 2014; Zhan et al., 2015). The WIfI classification system is not intended as a stand-alone guide for clinical decision-making. However, it may provide a valuable resource to help vascular surgeons evaluate patients with CLI/CLTI for possible revascularization, and it can be used to more effectively classify patients and compare outcomes in clinical trials (Cull et al., 2014; Mills et al., 2014).

INDICATIONS FOR REFERRAL

If a wound is atypical in appearance or location or does not respond to 2 to 4 weeks of appropriate therapy, a referral is warranted for further testing and/or a surgical evaluation and biopsy to determine other etiological factors. See **Table 25-5** for a summary of complications or findings from vascular tests warranting a referral.

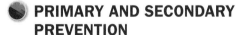 ## PRIMARY AND SECONDARY PREVENTION

Primary prevention deals with delaying or preventing the onset of a disease, and secondary prevention is used after the disease has occurred to prevent further progression of the disease (Karunathilake & Ganegoda, 2018). The goals and interventions for primary and secondary prevention of LEAD are essentially the same.

TABLE 25-5 INDICATIONS FOR REFERRAL: COMPLICATIONS AND/OR FINDINGS FROM VASCULAR TESTS

COMPLICATIONS	FINDINGS FROM VASCULAR TESTS
• Signs or symptoms of infection or cellulitis • Gangrene—urgent referral • Suspected osteomyelitis (exposed bone) • Atypical wounds • Nonhealing wounds: wounds that deteriorate, or fail to improve after 2–4 wk of appropriate therapy • Intractable pain: rest pain or intermittent claudication that interferes with activities of daily living, work, or quality of life	• Absence of both dorsalis pedis and posterior tibial pulses • Inconclusive vascular tests • ABI ≤ 0.90 *plus* a nonhealing wound, intermittent claudication, and/or severe pain • Toe pressure <30 mm Hg (<50 mm Hg with diabetes) • TBI < 0.64 • Ankle pressure <50 mm Hg • ABI ≤ 0.50 • ABI ≤ 0.40 (urgent referral) • ABI > 1.30 or noncompressible vessels

Adapted with permission from Wound, Ostomy and Continence Nurses Society. (2014). *Guideline for management of wounds in patients with lower extremity arterial disease. WOCN clinical practice guideline series 1* (p. 71). Mt. Laurel, NJ: Author.

A clinical priority for patients with LEAD is secondary prevention aimed at reducing the risks for adverse cardiovascular events, progression of atherosclerosis, and mortality. The success of secondary prevention relies on early detection of LEAD and implementation of interventions to prevent progression of the disease rather than waiting until patients develop severe ischemia (Karunathilake & Ganegoda, 2018).

GENERAL MEASURES

Secondary preventive measures involve lifestyle modifications and therapies (e.g., exercise, dietary modifications, pharmacologic interventions) to address major risk factors, which include aggressive management of diabetes, dyslipidemia, and hypertension; weight control or reduction if needed; and tobacco cessation (Chioncel et al., 2019; Firnhaber & Powell, 2019; Karunathilake & Ganegoda, 2018). Diabetes is a significant contributor to the morbidity and mortality in patients with LEAD, and glucose control is essential (Aboyans et al., 2018; Gerhard-Herman et al., 2017). The American Diabetes Association (ADA) recommends keeping HbA$_{1c}$ at a target level <7% for most individuals (ADA, 2019). A more stringent HbA$_{1c}$ goal (<6.5%) may be indicated in selected individuals such as those with CLI/CLTI to reduce limb-related outcomes if it can be achieved without adverse effects

(ADA, 2019; Gerhard-Herman et al., 2017). Numerous factors should be considered when setting glycemic targets, and targets should be individualized based on the patient's risks and characteristics, tolerance, and preferences (ADA, 2019). In addition, a lipid profile should be assessed and dyslipidemia treated with an appropriate level of statin therapy to reduce cardiovascular events (Aboyans et al., 2018; Gerhard-Herman et al., 2017; Jones et al., 2018).

Current guidelines from the ACC/AHA recommend maintaining blood pressure at <130/80 mm Hg for individuals with LEAD (Whelton et al., 2018), and international guidelines recommend a target BP < 140/90 mm Hg, except in patients with diabetes for whom the target diastolic BP is <85 mm Hg (Aboyans et al., 2018; Conte et al., 2019). Angiotensin-converting enzyme (ACE) inhibitors, angiotensin receptor blockers (ARBs), beta-blockers, calcium antagonists, and thiazide diuretics can be utilized to manage hypertension and reduce cardiovascular events for patients with LEAD (Aboyans et al., 2018; Chioncel et al., 2019; Firnhaber & Powell, 2019; Gerhard-Herman et al., 2017). Antiplatelet therapy has been recommended to reduce the risk of MI, stroke, or vascular death in asymptomatic (Firnhaber & Powell, 2019; Gerhard-Herman et al., 2017; Jones et al., 2018) and symptomatic individuals with LEAD (Aboyans et al., 2018; Campia et al., 2019; Chioncel et al., 2019; Firnhaber & Powell, 2019; Gerhard-Herman et al., 2017). A more detailed discussion of medications used for LEAD is included under the section for primary management/interventions.

TOBACCO CESSATION

Cigarette smoking is a major modifiable risk for LEAD and cardiovascular disease, and tobacco cessation is of paramount importance for patients with LEAD (Aboyans et al., 2018; Campia et al., 2019; Ding et al., 2019; Gerhard-Herman et al., 2017; Jones et al., 2018). Smoking cessation is associated with improved cardiovascular, limb, and surgical outcomes; and with lower rates of bypass graft failure, amputations, and death in patients with LEAD (Aboyans et al., 2018; Campia et al., 2019; Gerhard-Herman et al., 2017). In a large study of patients (N = 13,555) who were tobacco smokers that were followed for up to 30 years, there were 492 cases of LEAD, 1,798 cases of CHD cases, and 1,106 stroke cases (Ding et al., 2019). A longer period of smoking cessation was consistently related to lower risks of LEAD, CHD, and stroke. Ding et al. found a lower risk of LEAD, CHD, and stroke within 5 years of tobacco cessation; however, there was an elevated risk of LEAD that persisted up to 30 years after cessation for LEAD and 20 years for CHD.

In a study of patients (N = 693) who underwent lower extremity revascularization for LEAD, 41% were active smokers at the time of surgery (Young et al., 2019).

Compared to patients who smoked one or less packs per day, patients who smoked more than one pack per day had a 48% increase in major adverse limb events, a higher incidence of amputation (12.72% vs. 10.69%), and more than double the risk of death within 1 year after the surgery. Therefore, given the relationship between active smoking and failure of revascularization, Young et al. concluded it was advisable for surgeons to consider waiting to offer an elective revascularization until a patient had sufficient cessation attempts.

In another recent study (N = 2,469), smoking was an independent predictor for postoperative complications (Quan et al., 2019). Quan et al. found that compared with nonsmokers (n = 1,413), smokers (n = 1,056) had significantly higher overall postoperative complications (11.3% vs. 7.5%, p = 0.001), and in particular more pulmonary problems. Greater than 20 pack-years of tobacco use significantly increased the risk of complications, and smokers who stopped smoking ≥4 weeks before surgery had fewer pulmonary problems than those with a shorter period of smoking cessation. Therefore, preoperative smoking cessation (≥4 weeks before surgery) should be encouraged to reduce postoperative wound healing and pulmonary complications (Barua et al., 2018).

Nurses can play an important role in helping patients quit tobacco use, and nurses have been encouraged to include tobacco prevention and cessation counseling in their nursing practice. Based on a systematic review of 58 clinical trials for the Cochrane Library, moderate-quality evidence indicated that advice and support from nurses could increase the success of tobacco cessation for adults whether hospitalized or in the community setting (Rice et al., 2017).

KEY POINT

The wound nurse should educate the patient regarding the relationship between tobacco use and LEAD and should assist the patient to make and implement a plan for quitting (to include medications and nicotine replacement therapy [NRT] when indicated).

It is recommended that health care providers use brief interventions at every visit to encourage tobacco cessation such as the 5 As and 5 Rs (Jones et al., 2018; WOCN, 2014). The 5 As include asking about current tobacco use every visit, advising to quit, assessing the extent of addiction and the readiness to quit, assisting in selecting and agreeing on a quit plan (e.g., behavioral counseling, nicotine replacement therapy [NRT], pharmacotherapy), and arranging a follow-up plan (Barua et al., 2018; Jones et al., 2018; WOCN, 2014). If patients are unwilling to quit tobacco, health care providers can help motivate the patient with a discussion of the 5 Rs:

relevance of quitting to personal health, risks of continued tobacco use, rewards for quitting, roadblocks that interfere with quitting, and repetition of these factors with each encounter (WOCN, 2014).

Smoking cessation interventions include pharmacological, nonpharmacological, and behavioral approaches such as one-to-one, group, or telephone counseling; web-based support; cognitive behavioral skills training; motivational interviewing; incentives; self-help materials, etc. (Barua et al., 2018; Verbiest et al., 2017). Pharmacological approaches such as varenicline, bupropion, and NRT can be used alone or in combination to increase smoking cessation (Barua et al., 2018; Gerhard-Herman et al., 2017; Jones et al., 2018; Verbiest et al., 2017). Several tobacco cessation aids are available without prescription. Commercially available forms of NRT include gum, transdermal patches, nasal sprays, inhalers, and sublingual tablets/lozenges (Jones et al., 2018). It is also recommended that patients with LEAD be advised to avoid passive/second-hand exposure to environmental tobacco smoke at work, home, and in public places (Aboyans et al., 2018; Barua et al., 2018; Gerhard-Herman et al., 2017; Jones et al., 2018). Data are uncertain regarding any benefit of electronic cigarettes on smoking cessation rates, and they are not currently approved by the FDA as effective cessation aids (Barua et al., 2018; Gerhard-Herman et al., 2017).

WOUND MANAGEMENT

Assessment data are used to establish wound management goals and provide baseline information to evaluate the progress and effectiveness of interventions. Systemic support and appropriate topical therapy are necessary to maintain intact skin and promote healing. Strategies that create an environment that facilitates cellular repair and eliminates or diminishes impediments are essential to healing.

Basic principles of wound management serve as a guide for management of ischemic wounds: identification and treatment of infection, removal of necrotic tissue, insulation and protection of the wound, exudate control, maintenance of a moist wound environment, filling dead space, protection of the periwound skin, and treatment of closed wound edges. However, interventions must be tailored to the specific needs of the individual by consideration of the characteristics of the wound and degree of ischemia. For example, certain interventions such as debridement may be contraindicated depending on the nature of the wound and the perfusion status. Also, ischemic wounds should be protected from pressure (Vemulapalli et al., 2015). To determine appropriate treatments, the adequacy of perfusion must be considered (WOCN, 2014, 2019a, 2019b). See **Table 25-6** for wound management based on interpretation of the ABI.

TABLE 25-6 WOUND MANAGEMENT BASED ON ABI INTERPRETATION

ABI	INTERPRETATION	WOUND MANAGEMENT
Unable to obliterate the pulse signal at cuff pressure >250 mm Hg	Noncompressible arteries	• Assess toe pressure/TBI; refer for further vascular testing/ evaluation.
>1.30	Elevated	• Assess toe pressure/TBI; refer for further vascular testing/ evaluation.
≥1.00	Normal: Blood flow is sufficient for healing	• Provide topical therapy according to established principles of topical therapy.
≤0.90	LEAD	• Provide conservative therapy (i.e., wound management that addresses all principles of care including nutrition, pressure relief, local and systemic factors). • Refer for a vascular/surgical evaluation if the wound deteriorates, or there is no response after 2–4 wk of conservative wound care.
≤0.60 to 0.80	Borderline perfusion	• Check TcPO$_2$ if equipment available. • Evaluate the need for adjunctive therapy. • Monitor the wound frequently. • Provide conservative therapy. • Refer for a vascular/surgical evaluation if the wound deteriorates, or there is no response after 2–4 wk of conservative wound care.
≤0.50	Severe ischemia	• Refer for a vascular/surgical evaluation. • Maintain stable, dry, black eschar.
≤0.40	CLI/CLTI	• Refer immediately for an urgent vascular/surgical evaluation. • Maintain stable, dry, black eschar.

Reprinted with permission from Wound, Ostomy and Continence Nurses Society. (2014). *Guideline for management of wounds in patients with lower extremity arterial disease. WOCN clinical practice guideline series 1* (p. 72). Mt. Laurel, NJ: Author.

TOPICAL THERAPY/DRESSINGS

Research has not determined if any specific dressing or topical product promotes the healing of arterial leg wounds (Forster & Pagnamenta, 2015). It is important to avoid cytotoxic cleansing or dressing agents (WOCN, 2014).

Some experts have reported concern about the use of occlusive dressings such as hydrocolloids for ischemic wounds, although no studies are available to either support or refute this concern (Bryant & Nix, 2016; WOCN, 2014). Occlusive or semiocclusive dressings such as hydrocolloids are not recommended for infected wounds (WOCN, 2014). Signs of infection are frequently subtle in wounds caused by LEAD; therefore, dressings that permit frequent visualization and inspection of the wound are generally recommended as opposed to opaque occlusive dressings (Bryant & Nix, 2016; Doughty, 2016; WOCN, 2014). If the ischemic wound is open and draining, has soft slough, necrotic material, or has exposed bones or tendons, moisture-retentive, absorbent dressings are generally of benefit; the goal is to manage exudate while preventing desiccation (Doughty, 2016; WOCN, 2014). It is also recommended to avoid constrictive wraps and creams and ointments containing vasoconstrictive agents on ischemic limbs (WOCN, 2014).

Careful attention to the periwound skin is needed during dressing changes to prevent skin stripping from medical adhesive–related skin injury (MARSI) and maceration from exudate or wet dressings. Nonadherent dressings, skin sealants, or moisture barriers may be necessary to protect fragile periwound skin (Doughty, 2016). Regardless of the type of dressing, individuals with ischemic wounds require careful monitoring to assess the response to the topical therapy and the development of any complications.

INFECTION CONTROL

Patients with ischemic wounds need careful and frequent monitoring because ischemic wounds are at increased risk for infection (Doughty, 2016; International Wound Infection Institute [IWII], 2016). Signs of infection may include increased pain and/or edema, necrosis, or periwound fluctuance. However, clinical manifestations of infection may be subtle due to reduced blood flow with only a faint halo of erythema around the wound (Doughty, 2016).

Infected wounds and/or cellulitis in patients with LEAD or CLI/CLTI are limb-threatening complications that require immediate referral to an appropriate specialist for evaluation, culture-based systemic antibiotic therapy, assessment of vascular perfusion, and determination of the need for surgical intervention (Doughty, 2016; WOCN, 2014). Osteomyelitis is a concern for nonhealing wounds with exposed bone; magnetic resonance imaging (MRI) or a bone biopsy is needed for a definitive diagnosis (Stotts, 2016).

Wound Cultures

Cultures are warranted when there are clinical indications of infection to identify the type and number of infecting organisms and guide selection of antibiotics (IWII, 2016; Stotts, 2016; WOCN, 2014). Blood cultures are also indicated if there are signs of systemic infection (IWII, 2016). Options and guidelines for obtaining an accurate wound culture are covered in Chapter 11, as are guidelines for appropriate management of local and invasive wound infections.

Antiseptics and Antibiotics

The use of topical antiseptics in open wounds is controversial because of concern over the nonselective cytotoxicity of antiseptics, especially at higher concentrations, but dilute or lower strength antiseptics are sometimes used for short periods (e.g., 2 weeks) for localized wound infection (IWII, 2016; Stotts, 2016). In case of a spreading, localized wound infection or a wound with systemic infection, antiseptic dressings may be used in conjunction with culture-guided systemic antibiotics rather than topical antibiotics (IWII, 2016; Stotts, 2016). A consideration in treating patients with LEAD is that higher doses of antibiotics may be required to effectively eliminate the bacteria, because the diminished perfusion results in inadequate absorption (Stotts, 2016). Topical treatment options are discussed in more detail in Chapter 11.

KEY POINT

Culture-based systemic antibiotic therapy is recommended for an ischemic wound with a spreading localized infection or a systemic infection; higher antibiotic doses may be required due to diminished tissue perfusion.

Debridement

For patients with LEAD, the clinician must determine if the goals of care, condition of the wound, perfusion status, and the condition of the patient warrant debridement (WOCN, 2014). Debridement should be avoided in uninfected necrotic wounds until it is determined that the wound has an adequate blood supply for healing (Doughty, 2016; WOCN, 2014). Debriding or increasing moisture in ischemic lesions can convert dry gangrene to wet gangrene and precipitate a life threatening infection or amputation, and removal of eschar converts a closed wound to an open wound at increased risk for infection (Doughty, 2016; WOCN, 2014). Thus, clinical experts recommend keeping stable eschars intact on ischemic wounds that are dry, noninfected, and closed with fixed edges, while protecting and completely relieving pressure from the site (Doughty, 2016; WOCN, 2014). Some clinicians routinely apply an antiseptic (e.g., povidone iodine 10% solution) to the eschar and allow it to dry, with the goal of decreasing the bioburden and maintaining a dry, stable wound; however, evidence is lacking

regarding its effectiveness (Doughty, 2016; WOCN, 2014). Intact, stable blisters should be maintained and monitored closely for infection or rupture (WOCN, 2014).

KEY POINT

Clinical experts recommend maintaining stable eschar on ischemic wounds that are dry, noninfected, and closed with fixed edges.

Infected and necrotic ischemic wounds are limb threatening, and revascularization with surgical debridement is the treatment of choice in this situation (Doughty, 2016; WOCN, 2014). Debridement may also be indicated for wounds in which sufficient blood supply has been established. There are multiple options for debridement and a number of factors to consider in selecting the best approach for a specific patient; issues, considerations, and guidelines are discussed in detail in Chapter 10.

PREVENTION/MANAGEMENT OF HEEL WOUNDS

Bed and/or chair bound patients with LEAD are at high risk for heel PrIs and should have their heels offloaded with products that eliminate heel pressure (EPUAP/NPIAP/PPPIA, 2019; WOCN, 2014, 2016). Ideally, off-loading devices should completely elevate/float the heel without creating pressure in another location, reduce friction and shear, protect from foot drop and rotation of the leg, allow for ambulation, be easy to clean, remain in place while the patient moves, decrease heat to the heel, and be cost-effective (WOCN, 2014). If pillows are used to elevate the heels, they should be placed longitudinally underneath the calf with the heel completely suspended in the air (EPUAP/NPIAP/PPPIA, 2019; Lumbers, 2018; WOCN, 2014, 2016). Frequent monitoring is required to ensure that the pillows are positioned properly to completely suspend the heel. In addition, the heels should be assessed two to three times daily for any sign of an impending PrI (WOCN, 2014). Also, other measures such as the application of prophylactic dressings to heels in conjunction with other evidence-based pressure preventive measures have been recommended to reduce PrIs on the heel (EPUAP/NPIAP/PPPIA, 2019; Ramundo et al., 2018). Dressings should be selected according to their ability to manage microclimate, ease of application and removal, and ability to allow frequent visualization of the wound and periwound (WOCN, 2016). The dressing and wound should be monitored frequently.

KEY POINT

Consistent heel elevation/offloading is an essential element of care for patients with LEAD who are immobile.

MEDICATIONS

Multiple medications are used for patients with LEAD in an attempt to improve arterial blood flow, walking capacity, and reduce pain. Additionally, pharmacotherapy is used to prevent progression of ASCVD and cerebrovascular morbidity and mortality in patients with LEAD, including the following types of drugs: statins, angiotensin-converting enzyme inhibitors (ACEIs), ARBs, thiazide diuretics, calcium antagonists, antiplatelets (Aboyans et al., 2018; Campia et al., 2019; Gerhard-Herman et al., 2017; Whelton et al., 2018), and oral anticoagulants (Anand et al., 2018a; Campia et al., 2019; Kaplovitch et al., 2019; Nicholls & Nelson, 2019).

STATINS

Statin therapy is recommended for all patients with LEAD to lower cholesterol and improve cardiovascular and limb outcomes (Aboyans et al., 2018; Gerhard-Herman et al., 2017; Uccioli et al., 2018). In a randomized controlled trial (RCT) by Stoekenbroek et al. (2015), a high-dose statin (atorvastatin, 80 mg/day), compared to a low-dose statin (simvastatin 20 to 40 mg/day), significantly reduced overall cardiovascular (p = 0.046) and coronary events (p = 0.004), and coronary revascularizations (p = 0.007) in patients with LEAD (N = 374). Parmar et al. (2019) recently examined statin use in patients with LEAD (N = 488) who underwent surgical or endovascular intervention. Parmar et al. found that compared with nonstatin users, statin users had improved overall survival (log-rank p < 0.0001) at 30 days (99.5% vs. 95.4%), 1 year (95.9% vs. 83.4%), and 5 years (88.8% vs. 77.5%) and improved limb salvage (log-rank p = 0.002) at 30 days (98.4% vs. 96.4%), 1 year (95.9% vs. 89.9%), and 5 years (90.7% vs. 79.3%). Statin users had a 69% decrease in the amputation rate (HR = 0.31, 95% CI [0.14, 0.68], p = 0.002).

Current guidelines from the ACC/AHA recommend using the maximum tolerated level of statin therapy for secondary prevention in individuals with ASCVD and LEAD to lower LDL-C levels by ≥50%, rather than treating to achieve a specific LDL-C level (Grundy et al., 2019). According to the ACC/AHA, high-intensity statin therapy is recommended for individuals with ASCVD/LEAD who are 75 years of age or less. In patients who are older than 75 years of age with ASCVD/LEAD, moderate- or high-intensity statin therapy is reasonable to consider after an evaluation of the potential for risk reduction, adverse drug effects or interactions, patient frailty, and patient preferences. Moderate-intensity therapy is recommended for individuals who have contraindications or cannot tolerate high-intensity therapy. High-intensity statin therapy is a daily dose that lowers LDL-C (≥50%) with drugs such as atorvastatin 40 to 80 mg or rosuvastatin 20 to 40 mg. Moderate-intensity statin therapy is a daily dose that lowers LDL-C (30% to 49%) with drugs such as atorvastatin 10 to 20 mg, rosuvastatin 5 to 10

mg, simvastatin 20 to 40 mg, pravastatin 40 to 80 mg, lovastatin 40 to 80 mg, fluvastatin 80 mg, or pitavastatin 1 to 4 mg.

For patients who are taking maximally tolerated statin therapy and still have an LDL-C ≥ 70 mg/dL, a nonstatin drug such as ezetimibe might be added, which lowers LDL-C levels 13% to 20% and has a low incidence of side effects (Grundy et al., 2019). Also, use of a drug to inhibit proprotein convertase subtilisin/kexin type 9 (PCSK9), which is a regulatory protein that affects LDL receptors, is a reasonable option if LDL-C remains ≥70 mg/dL or non-HDL-C is ≥100 mg/dL (Grundy et al., 2019).

> **KEY POINT**
>
> Current guidelines from the ACC/AHA recommend using the maximum tolerated dose of statins as opposed to treating to a certain LDL level.

ANGIOTENSIN-CONVERTING ENZYME INHIBITORS AND ANGIOTENSIN RECEPTOR BLOCKERS

ACEIs and ARBs are cost-effective drugs used to reduce the risk of cardiovascular events and increase pain-free walking distances in patients with LEAD and hypertension (Aboyans et al., 2018; Firnhaber & Powell, 2019; Gerhard-Herman et al., 2017). Ramipril, an ACEI, has been associated with a reduced rate of cardiovascular ischemic events in patients with symptomatic LEAD and asymptomatic patients with a low ABI (Gerhard-Herman et al., 2017). The efficacy of ARBs has not been studied in patients with asymptomatic LEAD (Gerhard-Herman et al., 2017).

ANTIPLATELETS

Antiplatelet therapy with aspirin alone (75 to 325 mg/day) or clopidogrel alone (75 mg/day) is recommended to decrease the risk of MI, stroke, and vascular death in patients with symptomatic LEAD (Firnhaber & Powell, 2019; Gerhard-Herman et al., 2017). The usefulness of antiplatelet therapy in patients with asymptomatic LEAD (ABI ≤ 0.90) or borderline ABI (0.91 to 0.99) is uncertain (Aboyans et al., 2018; Gerhard-Herman et al., 2017; Kaplovitch et al., 2019). Aboyans et al. indicated that clopidogrel is the preferred antiplatelet drug for patients with symptomatic LEAD. Dual antiplatelet therapy with both aspirin and clopidogrel may reduce the risk of adverse, limb-related events in patients with symptomatic LEAD after lower extremity revascularization (Gerhard-Herman et al., 2017). According to a systematic review of 15 RCTs (N = 33,970) for the Cochrane Library, the use of clopidogrel plus aspirin in people at high risk of/or with cardiovascular disease (including LEAD and those without a coronary stent) was associated with a reduction in the risk of MI and ischemic stroke, but it also increased the risk of major and minor bleeding, compared with aspirin alone (Squizzato et al., 2017). Therefore, the usefulness of antiplatelet therapy with aspirin and/or clopidogrel must be weighed against the side effects, especially if patients are at high risk of bleeding (Gerhard-Herman et al., 2017).

Cilostazol is a vasodilator with antiplatelet activity that is an effective therapy to improve symptoms and walking distances for patients with claudication (Bedenis et al., 2014; Firnhaber & Powell, 2019; Gerhard-Herman et al., 2017). In a systematic review for the Cochrane Library, effective dosages of cilostazol ranged from 50 to 150 mg/day (Bedenis et al., 2015). However, the usefulness of the drug is limited by its adverse effects (e.g., dizziness, gastrointestinal symptoms, headache, palpitations), and it is contraindicated in patients with heart failure (Firnhaber & Powell, 2019; Gerhard-Herman et al., 2017). Due to its antiplatelet effects, caution is advised about combining cilostazol with other anticoagulants or antiplatelets (Aboyans et al., 2018).

KEY POINT

Aspirin and clopidogrel, singly or in combination, are effective drugs that reduce the risk of MI, ischemic stroke, or vascular death in individuals with symptomatic LEAD who are not at a high risk of bleeding.

ANTICOAGULANT THERAPY

LEAD is associated with a high risk of systemic atherothrombotic events for major adverse cardiovascular events (MACE) including MI, stroke, and cardiovascular death and major adverse limb events (MALE) such as acute ischemia, CLI/CLTI, and amputation (Anand et al., 2018b; Campia et al., 2019; Kaplovitch et al., 2019; Nicholls & Nelson, 2019). In a recent analysis of 6,391 patients with LEAD who were enrolled in the Cardiovascular Outcomes for People Using Anticoagulant Strategies (COMPASS) RCT, a low-dose direct-acting anticoagulant (rivaroxaban alone or in combination with aspirin) was compared to aspirin alone on the incidence of MALE (Anand et al., 2018b). Compared with aspirin alone (100 mg, once per day), the combination of rivaroxaban (2.5 mg, twice daily) plus aspirin (100 mg once per day) significantly lowered the overall incidence of MALE (43%, p = 0.01), total and major vascular amputations (58%, p = 0.01), peripheral vascular interventions (24%, p = 0.03), and all adverse peripheral vascular outcomes (24%, p = 0.02). In the original COMPASS trial that included patients with carotid artery disease and/or LEAD (N = 7,740), the low-dose rivaroxaban plus aspirin compared to aspirin alone significantly decreased MALE (1% vs. 2%; HR = 0.54, 95% CI [0.35, 0.82], p = 0.004) and also significantly reduced the incidence of MACE (5% vs. 7%; HR = 0.72,

95% CI [0.57, 0.90], p = 0.005; Anand et al., 2018a). However, the combination of low-dose rivaroxaban plus aspirin compared to aspirin only was associated with a significant increase in the risk of bleeding (HR = 1.61, 95% CI [1.12, 2.31], p = 0.009); the most common site of bleeding was gastrointestinal (Anand et al., 2018a). The investigators concluded that the combination therapy of low-dose rivaroxaban and aspirin was an option to improve cardiovascular and limb outcomes in patients with coronary artery disease and/or LEAD who do not have a high risk of bleeding (Anand et al., 2018a, 2018b).

PROSTANOIDS

There is limited evidence regarding the benefits of prostaglandins (such as iloprost) in the treatment of patients with LEAD and intermittent claudication due to variability in the trials, inconsistent results, and adverse reactions (Aboyans et al., 2018). A systematic review and meta-analysis for the Cochrane Library concluded that prostanoids might have some benefit for pain relief and wound healing in patients with CLI/CLTI, but there were no statistically significant differences in amputations or mortality (Vietto et al., 2018). In addition, prostaglandins were associated with significantly higher rates (p < 0.00001) of side effects such as headache, flushing, dizziness, nausea, vomiting, diarrhea, low BP, chest pain, and abnormal cardiac rhythms (Vietto et al., 2018).

PENTOXIFYLLINE

There is insufficient evidence to recommend pentoxifylline for treatment of patients with LEAD and intermittent claudication (Aboyans et al., 2018; Gerhard-Herman et al., 2017). In a systematic review of 24 studies (N = 3,377) for the Cochrane Library, due to the poor quality of the studies and large heterogeneity in the interventions and results, the benefit of pentoxifylline for treatment of intermittent claudication could not be determined (Salhiyyah et al., 2015).

HORMONE THERAPY

Recent evidence of the risks or benefits of hormone therapy for primary or secondary prevention of cardiovascular disease in patients with LEAD is lacking. In a 2015 systematic review and meta-analysis for the Cochrane Library, 19 trials of postmenopausal women (N = 40,410) on oral hormone therapy (estrogen with or without progestogen) were reviewed (Boardman et al., 2015). Boardman et al. concluded that overall, compared to placebo or no treatment, hormone therapy in postmenopausal women had little if any benefit for primary or secondary prevention of cardiovascular disease events, but it increased the risk of stroke and venous thromboembolism (VTE). In a subgroup analysis, they found that women who started hormone therapy <10 years after menopause had lower mortality and CHD, but they were at increased risk of VTE, compared to placebo or no treatment. However, for women who started hormone therapy more than 10 years after menopause, there was an increased risk of stroke and VTE.

NUTRITION

Adequate nutrition and hydration are necessary to maintain overall health, maintain skin integrity, and promote healing if wounds are present. Diet modification may be necessary to control or reduce weight, control lipids, and control blood sugar if the patient has diabetes. Nutritional counseling by a registered dietician is warranted for patients who have nutritional deficits.

Studies have shown that individuals with LEAD and claudication had poor nutrition with diets that were high in saturated fat, sodium, and cholesterol and low in fiber, vitamins E, B_6, and B_{12}, and folate (de Ceniga et al., 2011; Delaney et al., 2014; Gardner et al., 2011). Therefore, the patients with LEAD had a high intake of proatherogenic food and low intake of potentially anti-inflammatory and antioxidant foods (Delaney et al., 2019).

Ogilvie et al. (2017) examined the relationship between dietary intake and the incidence of LEAD in individuals ($N = 14,082$) who were enrolled in the Atherosclerosis Risk in Communities (ARIC) study and followed for up to 20 years. During the follow-up period, 1,569 participants developed LEAD. Ogilvie et al. found that higher meat consumption was associated with an increased risk of LEAD (HR = 1.66, 95% CI [1.36, 2.03], $p < 0.001$). Compared to those who drank no alcohol, those with moderate alcohol consumption (1 to 6 drinks per week) had a lower risk of LEAD (HR = 0.78, 95% CI [0.68, 0.89], $p < 0.024$). In addition, compared to no coffee intake, those with higher coffee intake (≥ 4 cups per day) had lower risk of LEAD (HR = 0.84, 95% CI [0.75, 1.00], $p < 0.014$). There was no association between LEAD and consumption of other food groups: fish/seafood, poultry, dairy, fruits vegetables, whole and refined grains, and nuts.

Low levels of vitamin D (<30 ng/mL) have been associated with an increased prevalence of LEAD and cardiovascular risks, and an increased risk of amputation in patients with LEAD (Gaddipati et al., 2011; Melamed et al., 2008; van de Luijtgaarden et al., 2012). Based on a recent systematic review and meta-analysis of 16 studies, vitamin D deficiency and insufficiency were associated with an increased prevalence of LEAD (Iannuzzo et al., 2018). The prevalence of LEAD was higher in patients with vitamin D <20 ng/mL (OR = 1.098, 95% CI [1.100, 1.195], $p = 0.029$) and with vitamin D <30 ng/mL (OR = 1.484, 95% CI [1.348, 1.635], $p < 0.001$). Another recent study of patients with type 2 diabetes ($N = 1,108$) found that vitamin D deficiency was associated with an increased risk of LEAD (Yuan et al., 2019). Compared to patients without LEAD, vitamin D levels were significantly lower in patients with LEAD (14.81 ± 8.43 ng/mL vs. 11.55 ± 5.65 ng/mL, $p < 0.001$).

NUTRITIONAL SUPPLEMENTS

The specific role of individual nutrients and supplements on LEAD and clinical outcomes is uncertain. Research has not demonstrated a significant clinical benefit for patients with LEAD from supplements including alpha-lipoic acid, garlic, *Ginkgo biloba*, L-arginine, omega-3 fatty acids (fish oil, olive oil), vitamins B_6, B_9 (folic acid/folate), B_{12}, C, or E, and zinc (Aboyans et al., 2018; Gerhard-Herman et al., 2017; Marti-Carvajal et al., 2017; Naqvi et al., 2014; WOCN, 2014). Some studies have shown that vitamins B_6, B_9 (folic acid/folate), and B_{12} were effective in reducing plasma homocysteine levels; however, a systematic review of 15 RCTs ($N = 71,422$) for the Cochrane Library found there was no evidence that the reduction of homocysteine prevented heart attacks or reduced death rates in persons with/or at risk of cardiovascular disease/LEAD (Marti-Carvajal et al., 2017). In addition, although vitamin D deficiency has been associated with LEAD, the role of supplementation is unclear (Nosova et al., 2015).

MEDITERRANEAN DIET

Individuals with LEAD should be encouraged to consider the benefits of a Mediterranean diet (Mattioli et al., 2017; Nosova et al., 2015; WOCN, 2014). A multicenter RCT ($N = 7,435$) compared individuals who consumed a Mediterranean diet supplemented with extra-virgin olive oil (group 1, $n = 2,539$) or nuts (group 2, $n = 2,452$) to a control group (group 3, $n = 2,444$), who were only counseled on a low-fat diet (Ruiz-Canela et al., 2014). Compared to the control group, the risk of LEAD was 66% lower in group 1 and 50% lower in group 2.

KEY POINT

A Mediterranean diet supplemented with extra-virgin olive oil has been shown to reduce the risk of LEAD.

Overall, the role of dietary therapy for risk modification, prevention, and treatment of LEAD is poorly understood and continues to evolve (Delaney et al., 2019). Due to the association of inflammation with LEAD, some experts advocate a diet that is rich in anti-inflammatory and antioxidant properties (Nosova et al., 2015). These findings underscore the importance of nutritional assessment and intervention for any patient with/or at risk for LEAD and especially those with ischemic wounds. In addition, research is needed that focuses specifically on the effects of dietary intake and nutritional supplementation on LEAD.

PAIN MANAGEMENT

For patients with positional pain, keeping legs in a neutral (not elevated) or dependent position may help relieve ischemic pain (WOCN, 2014, 2019b). Medications such as cilostazol might improve symptoms and increase walking distances for patients with claudication (Aboyans et al., 2018; Bedenis et al., 2014; Gerhard-Herman et al., 2017). Prostanoids might benefit some patients with rest pain and CLI/CLTI (Vietto et al., 2018).

EXERCISE

Exercise therapy is beneficial for individuals with LEAD and intermittent claudication to increase pain-free walking and maximal walking distance (Aboyans et al., 2018; Gerhard-Herman et al., 2017; Lane et al., 2017). A systematic review and meta-analysis of nine RCTs (N = 391) for the Cochrane Library by Lane et al. (2017) found that supervised exercise programs (SEPs) compared to no exercise significantly improved pain-free walking distance (p < 0.00001) and maximum walking distance (p < 0.0007) for patients with intermittent claudication. A recent systematic review and meta-analysis of 15 trials (N = 752) had similar findings that SEPs with a median duration of 12 weeks significantly (p < 0.001) improved pain-free and maximum walking distance of patients with intermittent claudication (Cornelis et al., 2019). Supervised exercise for 30 to 45 minutes, three times per week for a minimum of 12 weeks is recommended to improve symptoms of claudication (Gerhard-Herman et al., 2017). Some experts recommend considering an SEP for treatment of intermittent claudication prior to revascularization (Gerhard-Herman et al., 2017). In a systematic review and meta-analysis of eight systematic reviews and 12 trials to assess the effects of exercise therapy, surgery, and endovascular therapy (EVT) on intermittent claudication, all three treatments were found to be superior to medical management in terms of walking distance, pain, and claudication (Malgor et al., 2015). Although the evidence did not clearly identify one treatment as superior to the others, Malgor et al. reported that the combination of an SEP and invasive revascularization was superior to exercise alone. There are also limited data from two RCTs that suggest supervised exercise might be as beneficial as angioplasty for treatment of patients with intermittent claudication (Mazari et al., 2012; Murphy et al., 2015). Supervised exercise therapy provided comparable benefits in walking and quality of life from 12 to 18 months and was less costly (Mazari et al., 2012; Murphy et al., 2015).

In the absence of available SEPs, organized community or home-based exercise programs are more effective in improving functional capacity and quality of life than simply advising individuals to "go home and walk" (Aboyans et al., 2018; Gerhard-Herman et al., 2017). If individuals are not willing or able to participate in supervised walking programs, they should be encouraged to engage in any self-directed walking program (Aboyans et al., 2018).

> **KEY POINT**
>
> Structured exercise programs have demonstrated effectiveness to improve pain, walking distances, and quality of life for patients with intermittent claudication; limited evidence indicates that the benefits of exercise are comparable to angioplasty for up to 18 months.

ANALGESICS

If individuals have severe pain, analgesics may be of some benefit. Recent vascular guidelines for management of patients with CLI/CLTI have recommended the following: Prescribe analgesics of appropriate strength for patients with ischemic rest pain of a lower extremity and foot until pain resolves after revascularization, and for patients with chronic severe pain, use paracetamol (acetaminophen) in combination with opioids for pain control (Conte et al., 2019).

Wounds due to LEAD are often painful, and it is important to assess the need for premedication prior to wound care. In cases of intractable pain that is not controlled with exercise or medications, patients who are surgical candidates should be referred for a vascular surgical evaluation, and those who are not suitable surgical candidates referred to pain specialists for management.

ADJUNCTIVE PAIN MANAGEMENT

According to international guidelines, spinal cord stimulation (SCS) might improve limb salvage and pain relief in selected patients with CLI/CLTI who are not good candidates for revascularization (Aboyans et al., 2018; Conte et al., 2019). SCS is provided by a percutaneous electrode or spinal cord implant. A meta-analysis of patients with CLI/CLTI for the Cochrane Library found that patients treated with SCS had prominent pain relief, increased $TcPO_2$, and higher rates of limb salvage than patients who received conservative care without SCS (Ubbink & Vermeulen, 2013). A 17% risk of complications occurred with SCS that included difficulty with implantation, need for reintervention to change the stimulation, and infection. Therefore, it is important to weigh the benefits of SCS against the additional cost and risk of complications. Prior to treating a patient with an implanted device to deliver SCS, it is recommended to provide a trial period of SCS with an external device to determine if there are improvements in the $TcPO_2$ level and pain control (Aboyans et al., 2018; WOCN, 2014).

Overall, data are quite limited regarding the benefits of lumbar sympathectomy or peridural analgesia for treatment of severe ischemic pain. It remains unclear whether a lumbar sympathectomy can improve pain control or wound healing in patients with CLI/CLTI. In a recent guideline, Conte et al. (2019) recommended against using lumbar sympathectomy for limb salvage in patients with CLI/CLTI.

REVASCULARIZATION FOR INTERMITTENT CLAUDICATION

In carefully selected cases, revascularization may be a reasonable treatment option for patients with severe, lifestyle-limiting claudication, despite guideline-directed medical therapy including supervised exercise (Aboyans et al., 2018; Gerhard-Herman et al., 2017). For patients with intermittent claudication, the goal is improvement in symptoms, functional status, and quality of life; the intervention that is chosen should provide durable relief of symptoms. Endovascular techniques (e.g., angioplasty, stents, atherectomy) may be an option for patients with hemodynamically significant aortoiliac occlusive or femoropopliteal disease, but their effectiveness for infrapopliteal disease is uncertain (Gerhard-Herman et al., 2017). The choice of procedure (endovascular or surgical bypass) for revascularization depends on the characteristics of the lesion such as location, length, and extent of calcification (Gerhard-Herman et al., 2017). Surgical bypass may provide better long-term patency than endovascular techniques in cases with a long or extensive occlusion/stenosis (Aboyans et al., 2018; Gerhard-Herman et al., 2017). In selecting a revascularization strategy for intermittent claudication, there should be a >50% likelihood that the clinical improvement will be sustained for at least 2 years (Conte et al., 2015). Prophylactic surgery is not recommended for patients with asymptomatic LEAD (Gerhard-Herman et al., 2017).

EDEMA MANAGEMENT FOR PATIENT WITH MIXED ARTERIAL–VENOUS DISEASE

Management of individuals with LEAD and edema due to venous disease is challenging. It is estimated that 10% to 18% of patients with lower extremity venous disease also have arterial insufficiency (Matic et al., 2016). Compression is the gold standard for managing wounds and edema due to venous disease (Ratliff et al., 2016; WOCN, 2019b). However, sustained high-level compression (>30 to 40 mm Hg) is not recommended for patients with an ABI < 0.80 due to concerns over the risk of causing increased ischemia and possible tissue necrosis (O'Donnell et al., 2014; WOCN, 2014, 2019a). Therefore, prior to use of compression, patients should be screened for arterial disease with a Doppler measurement of the ABI by suitably trained staff (Bonham et al., 2016; WOCN, 2014, 2019a).

REDUCED COMPRESSION VERSUS NO COMPRESSION

For patients with mixed arterial and venous disease (ABI > 0.50 to <0.80) who have wounds and edema, reduced levels of compression applied with 23 to 30 mm Hg at the ankle can promote healing without complications (Ratliff et al., 2016, WOCN, 2014, 2019a, 2019b). Padding

over bony prominences underneath the compression device is recommended to minimize the risk of injury (Marston, 2011). If a patient's ABI is <0.50, ankle pressure is <70 mm Hg, or toe pressure is <50 mm Hg, sustained compression should be avoided, and the patient should be evaluated for revascularization (WOCN, 2014, 2019a). If the patient is revascularized, compression can then be considered to manage the edema from the venous disease (WOCN, 2014, 2019b).

In a study by Georgopoulos et al. (2013) of patients with mixed arterial and venous leg ulcers (N = 20/20 legs), 11 out of 17 legs (64.7%) with moderate arterial disease (ABI 0.50 to ≤0.75) showed significant healing progress after modified compression (30 mm Hg) and healed at an average time of 24.7 weeks. Six legs with moderate arterial disease (35.3%) failed to improve, underwent revascularization, and subsequently healed at an average time of 16 weeks. Three legs with severe arterial disease (ABI < 0.50) underwent revascularization and healed at an average of 17 weeks.

KEY POINT

For individuals with mixed arterial–venous disease and whose ABI is >0.50 to <0.80, a reduced level of compression (23 to 30 mm Hg at the ankle) can reduce edema without causing ischemic complications.

To determine the appropriate method of compression, a careful assessment (i.e., patient, history, limb, and wound) is necessary. Compression systems and stockings are commercially available that provide reduced levels of compression. Compression wraps should be applied according to the specific manufacturer's recommendations to achieve the desired level of pressure. Patients with mixed arterial and venous disease who are being treated with compression require close monitoring for complications or failure to heal. When compression is initiated, it may be necessary to change the compression more frequently to assess for complications and the patient's tolerance, particularly for patients who have neuropathy and are unable to sense pain or discomfort from the compression. Patients who fail to respond to compression therapy or who develop problems should be promptly referred for a vascular surgical evaluation.

MANAGEMENT POSTOPERATIVE EDEMA

Another circumstance in which compression along with leg elevation may be needed is for management of edema following revascularization/bypass surgery (Georgopoulos et al., 2013; Hedayati et al., 2015; teSlaa et al., 2014; Vartanian & Conte, 2015). According to teSlaa et al. (2014), edema of the lower limb occurs in 40% to 100% of patients after femoropopliteal bypass surgery. Compression is beneficial to prevent breakdown of the incision, which can cause limb-threatening wound complications, but there have been long-standing concerns about using compression after lower extremity bypass grafts. In the previously discussed study of patients with mixed arterial and venous leg ulcers by Georgopoulos et al. (2013), compression with multicomponent wraps was resumed after the revascularization when the ABI was >0.75. When the ulcers healed, patients were evaluated for compression garments (30 to 40 mm Hg).

In an RCT by teSlaa et al. (2014), following femoropopliteal bypass surgery, patients (*N* = 57) were randomized to intermittent pneumatic compression (IPC) of the foot for seven nights or to a class I compression stocking (18 mm Hg) worn day and night for a week. The investigators found that compared to the IPC, postoperative edema of the lower limb was less with use of the compression stockings on days 1, 4, and 7; they concluded that compression stockings were an effective postoperative strategy.

ANTIEMBOLISM STOCKINGS

An area of concern and controversy is the use of antiembolism stockings (AES) for prevention of deep vein thrombosis (DVT) in the presence of LEAD. AES provide a low level of graduated pressure with a higher pressure at the ankle and reduced pressures toward the knee and thigh, and they are often used to prevent DVT in immobile patients after surgery (Wade et al., 2016). AES are considered contraindicated in patients who have LEAD due to the potential for skin and tissue damage in ischemic and neuropathic limbs (Jones, 2013; Lim & Davies, 2014; Robertson & Roche, 2013). However, studies have not specifically investigated the safety and effectiveness of AES to prevent DVT in patients with LEAD. Therefore, if DVT prophylaxis is indicated for a patient with LEAD, careful consideration of the risks and consultation with the primary health care provider are needed to determine what method is appropriate and safe for the patient. Also, AES should not be relied on for control of edema in patients with mixed arterial and venous disease because they provide a low level of pressure (≤20 mm Hg), are designed for bedridden patients, and do not meet the specifications for ambulatory patients (Lim & Davies, 2014; WOCN, 2019a).

● CRITICAL LIMB ISCHEMIA/CHRONIC LIMB-THREATENING ISCHEMIA MANAGEMENT

The primary goal in treating individuals with CLI/CLTI is restoration of blood flow, which may be accomplished by surgical or endovascular interventions (Aboyans et al., 2018; Conte et al., 2019; Gerhard-Herman et al., 2017; Uccioli et al., 2018). However, multiple factors beyond correction of the macrovascular disease are important to consider, and not all individuals are candidates for surgery. Management of individuals with CLI/CLTI includes interventions to reduce the risk of cardiovascular disease, relieve pain, improve function, prevent tissue loss, promote wound healing, prevent amputations (e.g., pressure relief, aggressive treatment of infection, wound care), enhance quality of life, and promote survival (Uccioli et al., 2018).

SURGICAL INTERVENTION AIMED AT LIMB SALVAGE

Surgery is indicated for patients with severe CLI/CLTI who have failed medical treatment and have tissue loss, ischemic rest pain that is objectively confirmed with hemodynamic studies, infected or nonhealing wounds (including diabetic foot ulcers), or gangrene (Aboyans et al., 2018; Chioncel et al., 2019; Conte et al., 2019). Current guidelines recommend referring all patients with suspected CLI/CLTI to a vascular specialist for an evaluation and consideration of limb salvage options (Conte et al., 2019). Health care providers and patients considering surgery for CLI/CLTI should carefully consider the short-term and long-term benefits compared to the risks.

For patients with CLI/CLTI who are able to tolerate surgery, revascularization with bypass surgery, endovascular intervention, or a combination of open surgery and EVT known as hybrid therapy are referred for limb salvage (Aboyans et al., 2018; Chioncel et al., 2019; Conte et al., 2019; Gerhard-Herman et al., 2017; Uccioli et al., 2018). The choice of the type of revascularization and the specific technique should be based on a careful assessment of multiple clinical and anatomical data: pattern of occlusive disease and specific anatomic considerations, extent of tissue loss, presence of infection, previous failed procedures, comorbid conditions, anesthesia risks, risks and durability of the intervention, life expectancy, and goals and preferences of the patient (Conte et al., 2019; Gerhard-Herman et al., 2017; Uccioli et al., 2018; Vartanian & Conte, 2015). For infrainguinal bypass surgery, use of autologous vein grafts is recommended (Aboyans et al., 2018; Conte et al., 2019; Gerhard-Herman et al., 2017). In some selected patients with significant wounds of the midfoot or hindfoot, angiosome-guided revascularization to specifically target the area of ischemic tissue may be a reasonable option (Aboyans et al., 2018; Conte et al., 2019; Gerhard-Herman et al., 2017). In cases of stenosis and short occlusions or high surgical risk, EVT might be the preferred option; whereas, if there are long occlusions, open surgical bypass might provide better patency and limb salvage (Chioncel et al., 2019).

The use of EVT continues to increase and evolve in treatment of CLI/CLTI and complex lesions. EVT includes balloon angioplasty with or without stents (Aboyans et al., 2018). The main advantages of endovascular interventions are reduced morbidity with the procedures and shorter hospital stays; however, these advantages may be offset by less hemodynamic gain and poorer long-term durability compared with bypass surgery (Vartanian & Conte, 2015). Therefore, EVT may be an option for patients who are high-risk surgical candidates with significant comorbidities (Antoniou et al., 2017). Because restenosis occurs frequently in lower-limb arteries, stenting is often performed to prevent restenosis and improve long-term patency (Aboyans et al., 2018). To improve the results of EVT, drug-eluting stents and balloons have been used, which decrease hyperplasia within the arteries (Aboyans et al., 2018; Conte et al., 2019). However, the U.S. Food and Drug Administration (FDA) recently issued a safety warning for paclitaxel-eluting devices and has urged caution in the use of the devices due to an association of the products with increased mortality in long-term follow-up at 5 years (Conte et al., 2019; U.S. Food and Administration, 2019). Other alternative techniques in EVT include use of atherectomy catheters and devices for crossing chronic total occlusions, but evidence is limited regarding their efficacy (Aboyans et al., 2018; Conte et al., 2019; Uccioli et al., 2018). According to two systematic reviews for the Cochrane Library, evidence is insufficient to support the use of other techniques that have been used in addition to EVT to improve vessel patency such as brachytherapy/intravascular radiation based on eight RCTs with 1,090 participants (Andras et al., 2014) and cryoplasty/cooling based on a review of seven RCTs with 478 participants (McCaslin et al., 2013).

Overall, there is insufficient evidence to support open surgery over angioplasty (Antoniou et al., 2017; Uccioli et al., 2018). Based on a review of 11 RCTs for the Cochrane Library (N = 1,486), there was no evidence that bypass surgery was superior to angioplasty in terms of the effects on death, improvement of symptoms, amputation rate, need for additional procedures, or long-term mortality (Antoniou et al., 2017). There was evidence that compared to angioplasty, bypass surgery was associated with longer hospital stays and was more technically successful with a higher patency rate 1 year after the procedure, but the difference in patency disappeared after 4 years. See **Figure 25-7** for examples of vein bypass grafts.

SURGICAL SITE INFECTION

Surgical site infection (SSI) is the primary complication associated with surgical intervention, particularly lower extremity bypass surgery. SSIs are associated with significant morbidity including graft failure, limb loss, reoperations, and increased length of hospital stays, hospital

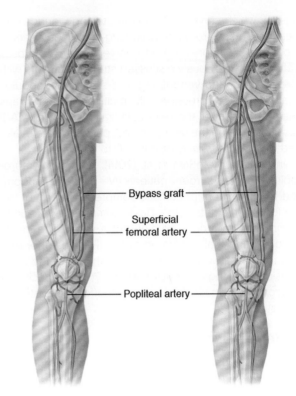

FIGURE 25-7. Examples of Bypass Grafts. *Right leg*: Common femoral to popliteal. *Left leg*: Common femoral to tibioperoneal.

readmissions, costs, and mortality (Aicher et al., 2017; Davis et al., 2017). The reported incidence of SSIs associated with bypass surgery varies from 4.8% to 22.8% (Davis et al., 2017). Multiple variables have been associated with an increased risk of SSI including patient-related factors (i.e., female gender, advanced age, obesity, dialysis, diabetes, hyperglycemia, hypoxia, chronic obstructive pulmonary disease, tobacco use, skin decontamination with povidone iodine, preoperative hair removal) and perioperative factors such as length of surgery and blood transfusions during surgery (Aicher et al., 2017; Davis et al., 2017). Also, postoperative hematoma and serotoma formation are complications of vascular surgery and are associated with wound infection (Aicher et al., 2017; Kuy et al., 2014). In a study of 106 patients who underwent lower extremity revascularization of the femoral artery with a groin incision, 22% (n = 24) developed a serotoma or hematoma, and 31% (n =33) developed an SSI (Kuy et al., 2014). Kuy et al. reported that SSIs were significantly associated with blood transfusion, postoperative serotoma or hematoma, dyslipidemia, and statin usage (p < 0.05). Davis et al. (2017) assessed the risk of SSI after femoral bypass open surgery (N = 3,033), and SSIs occurred in 320 patients (10.6%). Davis et al. found that significant predictors of SSI were dialysis, hypertension, BMI ≥ 25 kg/m², duration of surgery >240 minutes, and iodine skin preparation (p values <0.05). Davis et al. also reported that patients with SSIs were significantly at risk for other postoperative complications within 30 days of the surgery such as requiring a transfusion, major amputation, and revision of the bypass ($p < 0.01$).

Recommended strategies from national guidelines to prevent SSIs include, but are not limited to, the following: administer prophylactic antibiotics (i.e., cefazolin, clindamycin, or vancomycin) within 60 minutes before the incision; select the appropriate antibiotic based on the most common pathogens associated with the procedure; do not remove hair at the operative site unless it interferes with the surgery; control blood glucose; maintain normothermia; optimize tissue oxygenation with supplemental oxygen; and use an alcohol-containing agent for preoperative skin preparation, if not contraindicated (Anderson et al., 2014; Bratzler et al., 2013; Heuer et al., 2017).

THROMBOLYSIS

Thrombolysis, the use of drugs or enzymes to dissolve blood clots, may be an alternative to surgery for acute limb ischemia in carefully selected patients. Compared to surgery, there have been no significant differences in limb salvage, amputation, or death using thrombolytic agents to manage acute limb ischemia, but more complications have occurred with thrombolysis such as hemorrhage, stroke, or distal embolization (Darwood et al., 2018).

FOLLOW-UP THERAPY AFTER REVASCULARIZATION

All patients with CLI/CLTI who have undergone revascularization should continue best medical therapy, including use of antiplatelets and statins and smoking cessation, to slow the impact of atherosclerosis and minimize adverse effects of risk factors (Conte et al., 2019). Although it is uncertain if antiplatelets specifically enhance patency of lower extremity vein grafts, the use of antiplatelets have been shown to enhance patency with prosthetic bypass grafts (Conte et al., 2019). Based on a systematic review of 16 RCTs for the Cochrane Library, antiplatelet therapy with aspirin or with aspirin plus other drugs (i.e., dipyridamole [6 RCTs]; clopidogrel [1 RCT]) had a beneficial effect on bypass grafts with a greater benefit for prosthetic grafts (Bedenis et al., 2015). However, there was increased bleeding in the group taking clopidogrel plus aspirin, compared to aspirin alone.

In recent guidelines, dual antiplatelet therapy (aspirin plus clopidogrel) is recommended for 6 to 24 months after infrainguinal prosthetic bypass, 1 month after infrainguinal endovascular intervention, and 1 to 6 months after repeated catheter-based interventions if the patients have low risk of bleeding. In addition, patients who have had revascularization (surgical or EVT) should have long-term surveillance with clinical follow-up and assessment, ABI, and toe pressures, and DUS for vein grafts (Conte et al., 2019; Gerhard-Herman et al., 2017). If there is a decrease in the ABI $\geq$ 0.15, a recurrence of symptoms, or a change in pulse status in patients with vein grafts, DUS imaging should be performed; if the DUS test reveals >70% stenosis, revision should be considered (Conte et al., 2019).

> **KEY POINT**
>
> Dual antiplatelet therapy (aspirin plus clopidogrel) is recommended after infrainguinal prosthetic bypass, endovascular intervention, and after repeated catheter-based interventions if the patients are low bleeding risks.

INDICATIONS FOR AMPUTATION

Patients with CLI/CLTI have a reduced life expectancy and a high risk of amputation, particularly with major tissue loss (Conte et al., 2019). Conte et al. reported that patients with ischemic tissue loss have a major amputation rate up to 35% at 1 year compared to $\leq$ 10% in patients with rest pain. Even after revascularization, rates of major amputation have been reported as high as 20% (Gabel et al., 2018). It is estimated that 1.5 million individuals in the United States have lower extremity limb loss with 82% due to LEAD, which particularly affects patients with diabetes (Chopra et al., 2018).

An amputation may be required for patients with intractable pain, tissue loss, infection, or gangrene with limb- or life-threatening sepsis. Individuals with CLI/CLTI and the following conditions should be evaluated for a primary amputation rather than revascularization: nonreconstructible arterial disease or multiple surgical procedures are needed to restore a viable limb; significant necrosis on the weight-bearing portions of the foot (if ambulatory); uncorrectable flexion contractures; paralysis of the extremity; refractory ischemic rest pain; sepsis; and/or a limited life expectancy due to comorbid factors (Aboyans et al., 2018; Conte et al., 2019; Elsayed & Clavijo, 2015). For individuals with one or more failed attempts at revascularization and the chance of a success with another intervention is limited or no longer possible, a secondary amputation should be considered (Aboyans et al., 2018; Conte et al., 2019). In a review of 2,939 patients who underwent major lower extremity amputations, Gabel et al. (2018) found that the indications for an amputation were ischemic rest pain, ischemic tissue loss, uncontrolled infection, acute ischemia, and neuropathic tissue loss. Forty-three percent of patients had a prior revascularization; mean ABI was 0.78 and 22%/n = 625 had ABIs < 0.60; and the primary comorbidities included diabetes, coronary artery disease, end-stage renal disease, and chronic obstructive pulmonary disease. Compared to below-knee amputations, patients undergoing above-knee amputations were older, had lower ABIs and lower rates of 30-day complications, but also had higher 30-day mortality rates.

Preoperative Planning

Selecting the level of amputation that will heal is a critical factor for successful rehabilitation, use of prosthetics, and functional mobility (Conte et al., 2019). When planning an amputation, assessment of tissue perfusion with techniques such as $TcPO_2$ and toe pressure measurements can help determine an amputation level that will provide the best chance of healing (Aboyans et al., 2018; Conte et al., 2019; WOCN, 2014). If $TcPO_2$ is >40 mm Hg, the capacity for wound healing is good after a minor amputation; if it is <10 mm Hg, wound healing is unlikely (Aboyans et al., 2018; Arsenault et al., 2012). If the values are between 10 and 40 mm Hg, a challenge test can be utilized to determine if the value rises while the patient breathes 60% oxygen in the supine position (Aboyans et al., 2018). There is a greater chance for healing if there is an increase in the $TcPO_2$ > 10 mm Hg or $\geq$50% from baseline while the patient is breathing oxygen, or a decrease <10 mm Hg when the leg is elevated (Aboyans et al., 2018).

An amputation can be minor or major. Minor amputations include the toes, forefoot, and midfoot; major amputations are generally defined as those performed above the ankle such as transtibial, transfemoral, or knee or hip disarticulations (de Jesus-Silva et al., 2017). The 1 and 5-year mortality rates after minor amputations are reported at 16% and 25%, respectively, and the 5-year mortality after a major amputation varies from 30% to 70% at 5 years (Conte et al., 2019). Overall, mortality rates are higher for individuals with diabetes, above-knee amputations versus below-knee amputations, and bilateral amputations; the risk of a contralateral amputation after an initial limb loss varies from 2.2% to 44% (Conte et al., 2019). Therefore, an amputation is a high-risk surgery, and it is necessary to optimize the patient's condition by managing comorbid conditions such as diabetes, cardiovascular or cardiopulmonary disease, hypertension, or renal disease.

Successful rehabilitation after a lower-limb amputation is influenced by many factors such as the level of amputation, comorbidities, physical condition, cognitive impairment, psychological factors, and social support (Department of Veterans Affairs [VA] & Department of Defense [DoD], 2017). The overall goals of rehabilitation are to optimize the patient's health status, functional independence, and quality of life (VA & DoD, 2017). Whenever possible, prior to an amputation, the patient, caregiver, surgeon, and rehabilitation team should engage in shared decision-making to determine the residual limb's length, amputation level, and rehabilitation goals (Klarich & Brueckner, 2014; VA & DoD, 2017; Webster et al., 2019). In addition, it is helpful if the patient can meet with a certified visitor who has an amputation for peer support (VA & DoD, 2017).

In determining the level of amputation for a patient, it is important to assess status of the limb and strength and range of motion of all joints, current mobility and activity level, overall physical condition, presence of coexisting diseases, cognitive and psychological abilities, psychological and social support, vocation and avocation needs, and the potential for successfully undergoing rehabilitation (Devinuwara et al., 2018; Ertl & Panchbhavi, 2019; Klarich & Brueckner, 2014). The level of amputation impacts prosthetic fitting and the patient's mobility and gait performance. A higher level of amputation requires a greater expenditure of energy to ambulate (Conte et al., 2019; Devinuwara et al., 2018). Consequently, individual risks and comorbid factors must be weighed when considering and planning an amputation. Considerations to insure a successful residual limb and prosthetic fit include, but are not limited to, the following:

- Individuals with severe ischemic heart disease might be unable to walk with a prosthesis due to the extra energy required, and they might have improved mobility using a wheelchair (Devinuwara et al., 2018).
- An above-knee or through-knee amputation might be preferable for patients who are bedbound or chairbound and/or have severe flexion contractures (Conte et al., 2019).
- Surgical techniques that provide an adequate length and construction of the residual limb (also referred to as the stump) are essential to accommodate a good prosthetic fit (Devinuwara et al., 2018).

Current guidelines indicate there is insufficient evidence to recommend one level of surgical amputation over another (VA & DoD, 2017; Webster et al., 2019). Common amputation levels and their rates for primary healing, ambulation, and perioperative mortality include the following (Conte et al., 2019; Devinuwara et al., 2018):

- Transtibial amputation: A common level of amputation that offers good prognosis for mobility; 30% to 92% primary healing; 40% to 80% ambulation; 4% to 10% perioperative mortality.
- Transfemoral amputation: Level chosen when the blood supply is insufficient for healing at a lower level, or the knee joint is not salvageable; has the highest primary healing rates but low ambulation rates; 60% to 95% primary healing; 20% to 40% ambulation; 10% to 20% perioperative mortality.
- Knee disarticulation: Provides a weight-bearing residual limb with preservation of thigh muscles, but has poor cosmetic appearance; generally considered for patients who are nonambulatory prior to amputation; 60% to 81% primary healing; 57% to 70% ambulation; 1% to 17% perioperative mortality.

In a retrospective study of 206 patients that underwent 256 major lower extremity amputations (90.9% below-knee; 1.3% through-knee; 7.8% above-knee), at 1-year follow-up after the amputation, only 46.1% of patients were ambulatory (Chopra et al., 2018). Compared to ambulatory patients, nonambulatory patients had higher BMIs; lower preoperative hematocrits; greater frailty and dependence preoperatively; more chronic alcoholism and illegal drug use; were less likely to be married and lacked family support; were more likely to have an above-knee amputation; and were more likely to have dementia (p values <0.05).

Postoperative Care and Management

Recovery and rehabilitation after an amputation is a lengthy and multifaceted process that requires a specialized, multidisciplinary team (VA & DoD, 2017; Webster et al., 2019). Rehabilitation for an amputation includes the perioperative, preprosthetic, prosthetic training, and life-long care phases (VA & DoD, 2017; Webster et al., 2019).

Pain management is essential after an amputation, and pain management specialists may be needed to guide the treatment of postoperative wound pain and phantom pain. Patients may experience three types of pain or sensations following an amputation (Devinuwara et al., 2018; Ertl & Panchbhavi, 2019; Klarich & Brueckner, 2014; VA & DoD, 2017):

- Phantom limb pain—a painful burning sensation in the missing limb that improves over time.
- Phantom limb sensation—a sensation that the amputated limb is still present that tends to decrease over time.
- Residual limb pain—pain in the remaining part of the limb.

Analgesics such as opioids, local anesthetics, and nonsteroidal, anti-inflammatory drugs are utilized for pain control following amputation. Standard pain medications such as opioids are effective for immediate postoperative pain, but they are not recommended for long-term use (Devinuwara et al., 2018; VA & DoD, 2017). Medications used to treat neuropathic pain such as pregabalin may be effective for treating phantom limb pain (Uustal & Meier, 2014). Other nonpharmacological and noninvasive modalities that may be effective to decrease pain include, but are not limited to, the following: edema control, desensitization techniques, massage, ultrasound, transcutaneous electrical stimulation, and exercise (Klarich & Brueckner, 2014; Uustal & Meier, 2014; VA & DoD, 2017). If pain relief is not achieved with conservative therapies and a localized lesion/neuroma is identified that is contributing to the pain, more invasive approaches may be appropriate such as injections of a steroid and/or local anesthetic, a sympathetic nerve block, or revision of the residual limb and resection of the neuroma (Devinuwara et al., 2018; Uustal & Meier, 2014).

Complications and Care of the Residual Limb

Common complications that may affect the residual limb, in addition to pain and phantom limb sensations, include edema, hematoma, wound dehiscence and/or skin breakdown, flap necrosis, wound or bone infection, joint contractures, formation of neuromas, and trauma due to falls (Ertl & Panchbhavi, 2019; Guest et al., 2018; Monaro et al., 2017). In addition, other postoperative complications include PrIs; cardiac, renal, and respiratory complications; delirium; and depression and psychological problems related to the limb loss (Guest et al., 2018; Monaro et al., 2017). In a retrospective review of patients (N = 106) who underwent major limb amputations due to CLI/CLTI, the overall wound complication rate (i.e., SSI, wound dehiscence) was 13.3% (Morisaki et al., 2018). The complication rate was higher in patients with below-knee amputations (19.5%) compared to above-knee amputations (10.4%). Female sex (HR = 4.66, 95% CI [1.40, 17.3], p = 0.01) and below-knee amputations (HR = 4.36, 95% CI [1.20, 17.6], p = 0.03) were significant risk factors for complications. The 30-day mortality rate was 7.6% due to pneumonia, sepsis, and cardiac disease. Multivariate analysis showed that hypoalbuminemia was a significant risk factor for 30-day mortality (HR = 3.87, 95% CI [1.12, 16.3], p = 0.03).

Multidisciplinary care and interdisciplinary coordination and collaboration are necessary to achieve the best rehabilitative outcomes for patients with lower-limb amputations, and occupational and physical therapists play key roles. Goals for postoperative care and management to maintain integrity of the residual limb and facilitate prosthetic fitting include (VA & DoD, 2017; Webster, 2019)

- Healing and primary wound closure
- Control of edema and shaping the residual limb
- Protection from injury or trauma
- Maintaining and improving range of motion and strength
- Pain management
- Desensitization and preparation for prosthetic fitting

Occupational therapists (OTs) can help patients regain their independence in activities of daily living such as bathing, meal preparation, and toileting. An OT can assess the home environment and determine equipment needed to facilitate self-care and independence.

Physical therapy is essential postoperatively to prevent contractures, limit edema, and facilitate mobility in and out of bed. The patient's level of function and mobility prior to the amputation are important to consider in establishing goals for rehabilitation (Klarich & Brueckner, 2014; Webster, 2019). Under supervision of physical therapy, exercise, transfer training, limb positioning, ambulation, and gait retraining are started early and progressively advanced using appropriate walking aids.

A variety of dressings have been used after amputation to protect the residual limb from injury, control edema, promote wound healing and pain control, and shape/mold the residual limb, which facilitates early prosthetic fitting and rehabilitation (VA & DoD, 2017; Webster et al., 2019). There is a lack of consensus whether rigid (removable and nonremovable plaster casts or fiberglass dressings), semirigid (zinc paste wrap), or soft dressings (e.g., elastic wraps; shrinker socks) are best (Kwah et al., 2019; VA & DoD, 2017).

For transtibial amputations, rigid and semirigid dressings versus soft dressings have been associated with improved wound healing, volume control, and protection from trauma and with reductions in knee contractures, length of hospital stays, and time to prosthetic fitting (VA & DoD, 2017; Webster, 2019). If limb protection is a high priority, rigid postoperative dressings are recommended (VA & DoD, 2017; Webster, 2019). Based on a recent systematic review of nine RCTs (N = 436; 441 limbs) for the Cochrane Library, the conclusion was that evidence was insufficient to determine the benefits and harms of rigid dressings compared with soft dressings for patients who had transtibial amputations (Kwah et al., 2019). Therefore, the selection of soft, rigid, or semirigid dressings should be individualized based on the specific needs of the patient including protection of the limb, risk of infection, need to inspect the incision and skin, etc. (VA & DoD, 2017). Patients with amputations have specialized and lifelong needs for prostheses, orthoses, and equipment (i.e., artificial limbs, mobility assistive devices, durable medical equipment). The specific and individualized prosthetic prescription, fabrication, and fitting are determined by amputee rehabilitation specialists/prosthetists (Webster, 2019). There are multiple technological developments and advances in the designs and features of prosthetics and their components; the selection should be based on the unique needs, goals, and abilities of each individual patient (Keszler et al., 2019; Webster, 2019). A variety of prosthetics are available depending on the type and level of amputation. Additionally, there are prosthetics designed specifically for athletic sports and activities such as golfing, running, and swimming (Keszler et al., 2019; Webster, 2019).

Nurses play a vital role in the care of patients after a lower-limb amputation including providing pain management, encouragement, emotional support, and education to the patient and family as they adjust to the impact of limb loss. Also, patient safety, fall prevention, and prevention of PrIs are key measures for nurses to address. Due to progressive ischemia and other comorbid factors such as diabetes and renal disease, the risk of an amputation in the contralateral limb after an initial limb loss varies from 2.2% to 44% (Conte et al., 2019). Patients must be educated to monitor the remaining limb and promptly report problems to their health care provider and instructed in measures to protect the limb and prevent trauma or injury. In addition, some patients may need psychiatric or psychological counseling to help manage the emotional problems and depression that are common after an amputation including anxiety and grief over loss of the limb, perceived loss of independence, and changes in body image (Uustal & Meier, 2014; VA & DoD, 2017).

KEY POINT

After an initial amputation, the risk of a contralateral limb amputation can be as high as 44%; thus, it is critical to educate the patient regarding ongoing monitoring and protective care of the remaining limb.

CONSERVATIVE THERAPY

For individuals who refuse surgery or are not good surgical candidates, conservative medical care can sometimes be as effective as surgical intervention to promote pain relief, wound healing, and limb salvage. In a recent study of patients with CLI/CLTI, those (n = 35) who did not have revascularization due to contraindications were treated conservatively and were compared to a group (n= 136) that underwent revascularization (Akagi et al., 2018). Findings revealed that limb salvage and survival rates were not significantly different between the two groups. At the 2-year follow-up, the limb salvage rate in the conservative care group was 89% and 92% in the revascularized group; the survival rate was 77% for the conservative care group and 78% in the revascularized group (p values >0.05). In addition, 20% of patients in the conservative care group survived longer than 2 years, and 30% of the patients' wounds improved with medical treatment and proper wound care. The investigators concluded that unless urgent revascularization is needed, conservative care should be attempted prior to revascularization and should also be considered as a treatment option for patients with CLI/CLTI whose prognosis for survival is less than a year.

KEY POINT

For the patient with CLI/CLTI who is not a surgical candidate, conservative care and adjunctive therapies are sometimes as effective as surgery in promoting pain relief, wound healing, and limb salvage.

ADJUNCTIVE THERAPY

Adjunctive therapy may be indicated for patients with LEAD or CLI/CLTI and recalcitrant wounds who have undergone vascular evaluation, and it has been determined that they are not candidates for revascularization, or for patients with nonhealing wounds after revascularization. Adjunctive therapies that may benefit such patients include IPC and negative pressure wound therapy (NPWT).

Intermittent Pneumatic Compression

IPC therapy, also known as circulatory assist or arterial flow augmentation, may benefit patients with CLI/CLTI who are not surgical candidates (Conte et al., 2019; Elsayed & Clavijo, 2015; Gerhard-Herman et al., 2017). IPC devices provide intermittent compression of the calf and/or foot, which forcefully propels blood out of the foot and calf; the end result is an increase in the arteriovenous pressure gradient, which stimulates endothelial vasodilators and growth of collateral vessels and increases the arterial flow, volume, and velocity (Conte et al., 2019). Some IPC devices are cardiosynchronous and deliver compression at the end of diastole. IPC is usually provided three to four times per day for 45 to

60 minutes, and it may be provided in the home or clinic setting as well as acute care (WOCN, 2014).

Conclusions from two systematic reviews were that IPC might be associated with improved limb salvage, wound healing, and pain management for patients with CLI/CLTI, but the authors indicated that the findings were based on low-quality evidence with a high risk of bias (Abu Dabrh et al., 2015; Moran et al., 2015). Conclusions from Abu Dabrh et al. were based on meta-analysis of 13 RCTs and four nonrandomized studies, which had 2,779 enrolled patients. The conclusions from Moran et al. were based on a systematic review of six case series and two controlled before-and-after studies with a total of 433 patients. In a retrospective study, Zaki et al. (2016) compared limb salvage and amputation-free survival in patients with CLI/CLTI who received IPC therapy for 4 months (n = 153) to patients who did not receive IPC (n = 34). The investigators found that there was not a significant difference between the groups in limb salvage; however, there was a significant improvement in rest pain (p < 0.0001), reduction in minor amputation (p = 0.023), and amputation-free survival (p = 0.01) in the patients who received IPC therapy. Recommendations from recent guidelines are to consider IPC therapy for selected patients with CLI/CLTI (e.g., rest pain, minor tissue loss) who are not candidates for revascularization (Conte et al., 2019).

Negative Pressure Wound Therapy

Limited evidence from a few small, older, noncontrolled studies have suggested that NPWT may promote healing in patients with CLI/CLTI with infected, nonhealing wounds who are not candidates for surgery or have infected wounds after revascularization (Acosta & Monsen, 2012; Horch et al., 2008; Nordmyr et al., 2009). In a systematic review of one RCT (N = 60) for the Cochrane Library, the authors concluded there was limited, low-quality evidence that leg ulcers treated with punch grafts and NPWT (n = 30) healed more quickly or became ready for grafting earlier compared to those treated with grafts and standard care (n =30; dressings, compression); however, there was no difference in the healing rate (29 of 30 in each group) between the two groups (Dumville et al., 2016). The patients' wounds were of mixed etiology (43% arterial, 13% mixed venous and arterial, 43% venous), and Dumville et al. reported that there was no RCT evidence of the effectiveness of NPWT as a primary treatment for leg ulcers.

A recent RCT examined the effect of NPWT versus gauze dressings on SSIs in patients (N = 102) with closed groin wounds after revascularization (Lee et al., 2017). Forty-nine patients were in the dressing group and 53 in the NPWT group. The 30-day SSI rate was lower in the NPWT group compared to the dressing group, but the difference was not statistically significant (11% vs. 19%, p = 0.24). The length of stay in the hospital was significantly shorter in the NPWT group than the dressing group (6.4 vs. 8.9 days, p = 0.01). In a recent retrospective study of 161 patients (54% with CLI/CLTI or claudication) who were

treated with NPWT for groin SSIs after vascular surgery (n = 106 reconstructions with grafts), the overall rate of graft preservation was 81% (Andersson et al., 2018). For synthetic grafts, the preservation rate was lower at 64%. The overall healing rate at 120 days was 78.8% with 21.2% treatment failures that were associated with synthetic grafts, bleeding, and pseudoaneurysms.

Other Adjunctive Options with Insufficient Evidence

Due to the lack of studies and the low quality of available evidence, there are insufficient data to support the use of hyperbaric oxygen therapy (HBOT), gene and stem cell therapy, and ultrasound or electrotherapy to promote healing of wounds due to LEAD or CLI/CLTI. The effectiveness of HBOT on wound healing in patients with CLI/CLTI is unknown (Conte et al., 2019). Studies are lacking in patients with LEAD and nonreconstructible CLI/CLTI (Gerhard-Herman et al., 2017). Current recommendations do not support the use of HBOT to promote limb salvage in cases of severe, uncorrected ischemia, or as an alternative to revascularization because it does not prevent major limb amputation (Conte et al., 2019). In a 2015 systematic review of the effectiveness of HBOT on chronic wounds for the Cochrane Library, there were no studies that included patients with arterial disease (Kranke et al., 2015). Kranke et al. reported that in five RCTs of patients with diabetic foot ulcers treated with HBOT (n = 205), there was an increase in wound healing at 6 weeks, but the effect was not sustained at a longer 1-year follow-up, and there was no significant difference in the major amputation rate. Overall, data are insufficient to support the use of adjunctive HBOT for patients with LEAD or CLI/CLTI.

At present, two international guidelines (Aboyans et al., 2018; Conte et al., 2019) and two systematic reviews for the Cochrane Library (Forster et al., 2018; Gorenoi et al., 2017) indicate there is insufficient evidence to support gene and stem cell therapy for patients with LEAD or CLI/CLTI. Current guidelines recommend that the use of gene therapy (i.e., fibroblast, hepatocyte growth factors) and stem cell therapy should be restricted to patients with CLI/CLTI enrolled in clinical trials (Conte et al., 2019).

In addition, data are insufficient to determine the effectiveness of low-frequency ultrasound or electrotherapy treatment of patients with LEAD or CLI/CLTI. Larger, robust investigations that focus on patients with LEAD or CLI/CLTI are needed before any recommendations can be made.

● PATIENT EDUCATION

A key component in secondary prevention for patients with/or at risk for LEAD and wounds is education about risk reduction, disease management, and measures to enhance perfusion, prevent trauma and injuries, manage wounds, and prevent recurrence of wounds (WOCN, 2014). See **Table 25-7** for key points to include in patient education for risk reduction and disease management.

TABLE 25-7 PATIENT EDUCATION FOR RISK REDUCTION AND DISEASE MANAGEMENT

STRATEGIES FOR RISK REDUCTION AND DISEASE MANAGEMENT	PATIENT INSTRUCTIONS

Modify atherosclerotic risks for coronary and cerebrovascular disease.	• Adhere to prescribed medication regimen.
	  • Antiplatelet/antithrombotic drugs
	  • Lipid-lowering drugs
	  • Antihypertensive drugs

Plan for tobacco cessation.	• Develop a plan to quit smoking, including preoperative smoking cessation if surgical interventions are planned. • Avoid secondhand smoke.
Control hyperlipidemia.	• Use the appropriate intensity of statin therapy to reduce ASCVD risks.
Manage diabetes.	• Maintain blood glucose control as demonstrated by $HbA_{1c} < 7\%$. A more stringent HbA_{1c} goal (<6.5%) may be indicated in individuals with CLI/CLTI to reduce limb-related outcomes if it can be achieved without adverse effects.
Control hypertension.	• Maintain BP < 130/80 mm Hg to lower the risk of MI, stroke, chronic heart failure, and cardiovascular death. • Use effective antihypertensive agents, which can include ACEIs, ARBs, beta-blockers, calcium antagonists, and thiazide diuretics.
Maintain adequate nutritional and fluid intake.	• Consider a Mediterranean diet to reduce risk of LEAD. • Drink alcohol in moderation if already consuming alcohol. • Control or reduce weight if obese.
Enhance arterial perfusion.	• Avoid leg elevation. • If there is pain in the supine or recumbent position, place legs in a dependent position. • Avoid exposure to cold. • Avoid garters and constrictive clothes. • Increase walking and exercise (i.e., supervised or self-directed).

Prevent chemical, thermal, and mechanical trauma or injury.	• Avoid medicated corn pads, aggressive tapes and adhesives, hot water bottles, foot soaks, heating pads, and walking on hot surfaces.
	• Perform proper foot care:
	  • Keep feet clean and dry: Wash daily with mild soap and water.
	  • Moisturize, except between toes.
	  • Avoid fragrance or irritants.
	  • File calluses—use pads to protect—no cutting of callus.
	• Protect feet (toes, heels):
	  • Wear well-fitting footwear at all times.
	  • Do not go barefoot, even at home.
	  • Wear socks or stockings with shoes to protect feet: shoes should not rub or cause pressure and should provide good support.
	  • Check and empty shoes before wearing.
	  • If bedbound or chairbound, use pressure redistribution surfaces, products, or devices to offload the heels and protect toes and other bony prominences.

Manage wounds properly.	• Perform wound care as instructed (e.g., dressings, technique, frequency, supplies). • Observe and promptly report symptoms of complications to the health care provider (e.g., signs of infection, new or increased pain, excessive bleeding). • If compression is used for mixed arterial/venous disease, observe for signs that the compression is too tight (e.g., blue, cold, numb or tingling toes; increased pain), and promptly contact the health care provider and/or remove the compression.
Prevent wound recurrence.	• Avoid trauma. • Examine feet daily for blisters, wounds, signs of infection, and skin/nail changes. • Promptly report cuts, breaks, or signs/symptoms of infection to the health care provider. • Obtain routine professional care for toenails, corns, and calluses. • Offload pressure from feet/heels if bedbound or chairbound. • Visit the health care provider on a regular basis.

Adapted with permission from Wound, Ostomy and Continence Nurses Society. (2014). *Guideline for management of wounds in patients with lower extremity arterial disease. WOCN clinical practice guideline series 1* (pp. 120–128). Mt. Laurel, NJ: Author.

CONCLUSION

LEAD is a progressive condition due to atherosclerosis that affects large numbers of individuals in the United States and worldwide. Multiple risks and comorbid conditions are associated with LEAD, many of which are modifiable. Because of the systemic nature of atherosclerosis, individuals with LEAD are also at high risk for cardiovascular and cerebrovascular disease.

Assessment is the foundation for successful management of patients with/or at risk for lower extremity wounds due to LEAD. However, many health care providers utilize unreliable assessment methods to detect LEAD, which is often asymptomatic. Therefore, the majority of individuals with LEAD are unrecognized and/or undertreated. Early detection is the key to secondary prevention of LEAD, and measurement of the ABI is a simple and accurate noninvasive test to detect and monitor LEAD.

Comprehensive care addressing primary and secondary prevention for LEAD requires interventions to reduce the risks for adverse limb, cardiovascular, or cerebrovascular events and the mortality and morbidity associated with LEAD. Key preventive interventions include tobacco cessation; management of diabetes, hypertension, and lipids; increased exercise; and control or reduction of weight for individuals who are obese.

Wounds due to LEAD are challenging and complex with limb- and life-threatening consequences, and care should be guided by a wound care expert. Patients may have mixed disease and multiple problems (e.g., arterial and venous; arterial and diabetes with neuropathy). Wound care must be based on accurate identification of etiology and a thorough and complete examination of the patient, limb, and wound. Preventing wounds and their recurrence is an essential component of care, and patient education is necessary for risk reduction and disease management, including specific education for leg and foot protection.

Collaborative practice and coordinated multidisciplinary care are essential to achieve optimal outcomes for the diverse patients with LEAD and wounds. Multiple health care providers may be needed including vascular surgeons, dermatologists, dieticians, physical or OTs, infection control specialists, pain management specialists, mental health specialists, social services, and in some instances, prosthetists.

CASE STUDY

LEAD CASE STUDY

Case

Patient admitted to home health services for a nonhealing wound on the left leg.

PATIENT PROFILE

History/Risk Factors

Patient was a 96-year-old male who was a poor historian and had recently moved to live with his granddaughter. Patient/family reported a history of hypertension controlled with medication and a stroke 2 years prior to admission. The patient smoked tobacco for many years but quit smoking 30 years ago. The patient was on a regular diet, took a daily multivitamin, and his weight and albumin and protein levels were within normal limits. Other lab tests were normal (i.e., white and RBC counts, hemoglobin/hematocrit). The patient was afebrile, and his blood pressure, pulse, and respirations were within normal limits.

Pain History

The patient denied pain in his legs or feet. He ambulated with a cane in the house and did not walk outside except for physician appointments. He sat up in a chair most all day and denied nocturnal pain or pain with ambulation.

Wound History

The patient had an open, draining wound on the shin of his left leg of unknown etiology and duration. The wound had been treated by the family physician with a week of oral Keflex and twice-a-day dressings (i.e., cleansed with full-strength hydrogen peroxide, applied silver sulfadiazine cream, and left open to air). After 2 1/2 months of treatment with no improvement in the wound, the physician referred the case to home health and requested a consult by the agency's wound care nurse.

INITIAL ASSESSMENT

Perfusion Status/Noninvasive Testing

On the left leg, the dorsalis pedis and posterior tibial pulses were palpable but diminished, capillary refill was 10 seconds, and venous refill was 26 seconds. On the right leg, pulses were palpable with normal capillary and venous refill. The left leg felt cool to touch. An ABI was performed at the bedside by the wound care nurse with a portable Doppler: ABI for the left leg was 0.56 and 0.94 on the right leg. Screening with a 10-g 5.07, Semmes-Weinstein monofilament revealed adequate protective sensation on both feet.

Ischemic Skin/Limb Changes

On both legs, there was little subcutaneous tissue; the skin was shiny, taut, and thin; hair was absent on the toes and legs; and toenails were thin. The patient visited a podiatrist for nail care. The patient used a moisturizer on the feet and legs, and he was instructed to omit the moisturizer between his toes and dry well between the toes. Footwear was well fitting.

Wound and Periwound Characteristics

The patient had an open wound on the lower shin of his left leg. Wound measurements were 1.7 cm length, 1.1 cm width, and 0.5 cm depth, and the wound was undermined 0.3 cm at the 12 o'clock position and 0.4 cm at the 9 o'clock position. The wound had a punched-out appearance with rolled edges (epibole), and the wound base was covered with 100% dense, yellow devitalized tissue. There was a scant amount of serous drainage, no odor, no purulence, and no pain or tenderness of the wound. The periwound skin was intact. There were no signs of induration, erythema, or cellulitis; no exposed bones or tendons. There was no pitting edema, and the ankle and calf measured 19.9 and 27.3 cm in diameter, respectively.

Key Wound Problems Identified

1. Borderline perfusion to the left leg as indicated by ABI of 0.56; diminished pulses; delayed capillary refill; and prolonged venous refill.
2. Impaired skin integrity due to a nonhealing wound on the left shin; wound 100% covered with devitalized tissue with scant drainage.

Initial Wound Goals

Wound free of devitalized tissue within 2 weeks; 50% to 60% red, granulation tissue in 4 weeks; wound free of signs and symptoms of infection; maintain intact periwound skin.

NURSING MANAGEMENT/TREATMENT

Topical Therapy

After consultation with the physician, the devitalized tissue was carefully scored by the wound care nurse, and silver nitrate was applied to the epibole. Daily dressings with an enzymatic debriding agent were instituted, and the patient's granddaughter was instructed how to perform daily dressing changes.

Follow-Up Plans

Home health nursing visits were planned three times per week to assess and measure the wound, and a follow-up visit by the wound care nurse was scheduled in 2 weeks. At the 2-week follow-up by the wound care nurse, the epibole was resolved; wound measurements were 1.7 cm length, 1.1 cm width, and 0.5 cm depth, and wound was undermined 0.4 cm at the 12 o'clock position and 0.5 cm at the 9 o'clock position. The wound base was covered with 95% yellow, devitalized tissue with 5% pink tissue and had a small amount of serosanguineous exudate.

Referrals/Vascular Consult

Due to the limited response of the wound, the patient was referred for further vascular studies and evaluation by a vascular surgeon. Doppler studies with segmental limb pressures and PVRs were performed in the vascular laboratory. The surgeon reported that the patient had normal flow to the popliteal level on the left but had tibial stenosis and poor digital PVRs. Enzymatic dressings were continued, and the surgeon referred the patient for HBOT.

The patient received 20 HBOT treatments (TcPO$_2$ values were not available). Upon completion of the HBOT, the wound measurements were 6 cm length, 2.4 cm width, and 1.0 cm depth, and the wound was undermined 1.0 cm from the 10 to 12 o'clock position and 0.5 cm at the 6 o'clock position. The wound base was covered with 90% red and 10% yellow tissue. The wound was free of odor and pain and had moderate serosanguineous drainage. The enzymatic debriding agent was discontinued by the surgeon, and hydrogel dressings were initiated once daily with home care nurses continuing to follow the patient twice a week.

Within 4 weeks after the HBOT was concluded, the wound began to deteriorate, and the wound care nurse was again consulted. The wound measured 7.8 cm length, 3.2 cm width, and 1.1 cm depth and was undermined 1.2 cm from the 10 to 12 o'clock and 0.7 cm at the 6 o'clock position. There was increased odor and purulent exudate; warmth, erythema, and in duration extended 2 to 4 cm around the wound; and the patient complained of pain in his leg. Ankle and calf measurements on the left leg had increased to 22.4 and 27 cm, respectively. The clinical findings were consistent with complications of infection/cellulitis and possible osteomyelitis due to the proximity of the wound to the underlying bone. The wound care nurse immediately consulted the surgeon, and a bone scan was performed, which confirmed osteomyelitis. The patient was hospitalized and referred to an infectious disease (ID) specialist. A central line was placed, and the patient was started on an intravenous antibiotic (piperacillin sodium) and moist saline dressings twice a day. After a week in the hospital, the patient was discharged home and followed by the ID specialist, surgeon, and home health nurses who continued the intravenous piperacillin and dressings. Topical therapy was modified to silver hydrofiber dressings plus gauze and wrap gauze changed every 2 days. After 8 weeks of the intravenous antibiotic therapy and moist wound healing, the wound completely healed, and the patient was discharged from services.

Patient Education/Discharge Planning

The patient and family received instructions regarding the importance of the following:

- Continue adequate nutrition/protein and fluid intake to maintain intact skin.
- Take antihypertensive medication as prescribed.
- Protect feet/limbs: Wash and dry feet well and moisturize except between the toes; inspect the legs and feet daily and promptly notify the physician for swelling, pain, skin breakdown or wounds; wear properly fitted shoes with socks and no bare feet even in the house; check temperature of the bath water and avoid heating pads and foot soaks to prevent risk of burns; and use a pillow at night to lift heels off mattress to prevent pressure.
- Avoid sitting up with legs dependent for prolonged periods of time.
- Continue nail care with the podiatrist.
- Keep regular physician follow-up appointments and have ABI monitored at least annually.

KEY POINT

This case exemplifies the importance of a thorough assessment and value of the ABI to detect LEAD in a patient with a nonhealing, lower extremity wound. The necessity of carefully monitoring a patient's response to care and making timely referrals when a wound fails to respond or deteriorates, despite appropriate care, is demonstrated. The case shows that establishing specific wound care goals can help gauge progress and guide decisions regarding referrals or use of adjunctive therapies. Also, the case is an example of the importance and value of communication and collaboration among health care providers and across care settings to achieve successful outcomes.

REFERENCES

Abdolmaleki, F., Hayat, S. M. G., Bianconi, V., et al. (2019). Atherosclerosis and immunity: A perspective. *Trends in Cardiovascular Medicine, 29,* 363–371. Retrieved from https://doi.org/10.1016/j.tcm.2018.09.017

Aboyans, V., Criqui, M. H., Abraham, P., et al. (2012). Measurement and interpretation of the ankle-brachial index: A scientific statement from the American Heart Association. *Circulation, 126,* 488–492. doi:10.1161/CIR.0b013e318276fbcb.

Aboyans, V., Ricco, J. B., Bartelink, M. E. L., et al. (2018). 2017 ESC Guidelines on the diagnosis and treatment of peripheral arterial diseases, in collaboration with the European Society for Vascular Surgery (ESVS). *European Heart Journal, 39,* 763–821. doi: 10.1093/eurheartj/ehx095.

Abu Dabrh, A. M., Steffen, M. W., Asi, N. et al. (2015). Nonrevascularization-based treatments in patients with severe or critical limb ischemia. *Journal of Vascular Surgery, 62*(5), 1330–1339. doi: 10.1016/j.jvs.2015.07.069.

Acosta, S., & Monsen, C. (2012). Outcome after VAC® therapy for infected bypass grafts in the lower limb. *European Journal of Vascular and Endovascular Surgery, 44,* 294–299. doi: 10.1016/j.ejvs.2012.06.005.

Aerden, D., Massaad, D., vonKemp, K., et al. (2011). The ankle brachial index and the diabetic foot: A troublesome marriage. *Annals of Vascular Surgery, 25,* 770–777. doi: 10.1016/j.avsg.2010.12.025.

Aguero, F., Gonzalez-Zobl, G., Baena-Diez, J. M., et al. (2015). Prevalence of lower extremity peripheral arterial disease in individuals with chronic immune mediated inflammatory disorders. *Atherosclerosis, 242* (1), 1–7. doi: 10.1016/j.atherosclerosis.2015.06.054.

Aicher, B., Curry, P., Croal-Abrahams, L., et al. (2017). Infrainguinal wound infections in vascular surgery: An antiquated challenge without a modern solution. *Journal of Vascular Nursing, 35*(3), 146–156. doi: 10.1016/j.jvn.2017.03.002.

Akagi, D., Hoskina, K., Akai, A., et al. (2018). Outcomes in patients with critical limb ischemia due to arteriosclerosis obliterans who did not undergo arterial reconstruction. *International Heart Journal, 59,* 1041–1046. doi: 10.1536/ihj.17-592.

Alahdab, F., Wang, A. T., Elraiyah, T. A., et al. (2015). A systematic review for the screening for peripheral arterial disease in asymptomatic patients. *Journal of Vascular Surgery, 61*(3S), 42S–53S. doi: 10.1016/j.jvs.2014.12.008.

Alves-Cabratosa, L., Elosua-Bayes, M., Garcia-Gil, M., et al. (2019). Hypertension and high ankle brachial index: The overlooked combination. *Journal of Hypertension, 37,* 92–98. doi: 10.1097/HJH.000000000001861.

American Diabetes Association. (2019). Glycemic targets: Standards of medical care in diabetes—2019. *Diabetes Care, 42*(Suppl 1), S61–S70.

Anand, S. S., Bosch, J., Eikelboom, J. W., et al. (2018a). Rivaroxaban with or without aspirin in patients with stable peripheral or carotid artery disease: An international, randomized, double-blind, placebo-controlled trial. *Lancet, 391*(10117), 219–229. doi: 10.1016/S0140-6736(17)32409-1.

Anand, S. S., Caron, F., Eikelboom, J. W., et al. (2018b). Major adverse limb events and mortality in patients with peripheral artery disease. *Journal of the American College of Cardiology, 71*(20), 2306–2315. doi: 10.1016/j.jacc.2018.03.008.

Anderson, D. J., Podgorny, K., Berrios-Torres, S. I., et al. (2014). Strategies to prevent surgical site infections in acute care hospitals: 2014 update. *Infection Control and Hospital Epidemiology, 35*(6), 605–627. doi: 10.1086/676022.

Andersson, S., Monsen, C., & Acosta, S. (2018). Outcome and complications using negative pressure wound therapy in the groin for perivascular surgical site infections after vascular surgery. *Annals of Vascular Surgery, 48,* 104–110. doi: 10.1016/j.avsg.2017.10.018.

Andras, A., Hansrani, M., Stewart, M., et al. (2014). Intravascular brachytherapy for peripheral vascular disease. *Cochrane Database of Systematic Reviews,* (1), CD003504. doi: 10.1002/14651858.CD003504.pub2.

Antoniou, G. A., Georgiadis, G. S., Antoniou, S. A., et al. (2017). Bypass surgery for chronic lower limb ischemia. *Cochrane Database of Systematic Reviews,* (4), CD002000. doi: 10.1002/14651858.CD002000.pub3.

Arinze, N. V., Gregory, A., Francis, J. M., et al. (2019). Unique aspects of peripheral artery disease in patients with chronic kidney disease. *Vascular Medicine, 24*(3), 251–260. doi: 10.1177/1358863X18824654.

Arsenault, K. A., Al-Otaibi, A., Devereaux, P. J., et al. (2012). The use of transcutaneous oximetry to predict healing complications of lower limb amputations: A systematic review and meta-analysis. *European Journal of Vascular and Endovascular Surgery, 43*, 329–336. doi: 10.1016/j.ejvs.2011.12.004.

Baldereschi, M., Inzitari, M., Di Carlo, A., et al. (2013). Vascular factors predict polyneuropathy in a non-diabetic elderly population. *Neurological Sciences, 34*(6), 955–962. doi: 10.1007/s10072-012-1167-x.

Barua, R. S., Rigotti, N. A., Benowitz, N. L., et al. (2018). ACC expert consensus decision pathway on tobacco cessation treatment. *Journal of the American College of Cardiology, 72*(25), 3332–3365. doi: 10.1016/j.jacc.2018.10.027.

Bedenis, R., Lethaby, A., Maxwell, H., et al. (2015). Antiplatelet agents for preventing thrombosis after peripheral arterial bypass surgery. *Cochrane Database of Systematic Reviews,* (2), CD000535. doi: 10.1002/14651858.CD000535.pub3.

Bedenis, R., Stewart, M., Cleanthis, M., et al. (2014). Cilostazol for intermittent claudication. *Cochrane Database of Systematic Reviews,* (10), CD003748. doi: 10.1002/14651858.CD003748.pub4.

Bell, D. (2013). Peripheral arterial disease overview. *Podiatry Management,* 175–183. Retrieved April 15, 2014, from www.podiatrym.com/cme/CMEJan13.pdf

Berger, J. S., Ballantyne, C. M., Davidson, M. H., et al. (2011). Peripheral artery disease, biomarkers, and darapladib. *American Heart Journal, 161,* 972–978. doi: 10.1016/j.ahj.2011.01.017.

Boardman, H. M. P., Hartley, L., Eisinga, A., et al. (2015). Hormone therapy for preventing cardiovascular disease in post-menopausal women. *Cochrane Database of Systematic Reviews,* (3), CD002229. doi: 10.1002/14651858.CD002229.pub4.

Bonham, P. A., Cappuccio, M., Hulsey, T., et al. (2007). Are ankle and toe brachial indices (ABI-TBI) obtained by a pocket Doppler interchangeable with those obtained by standard laboratory equipment? *Journal of Wound, Ostomy, and Continence Nursing, 34,* 35–44.

Bonham, P. A., Flemister, B. G., Droste, L. R., et al. (2016). 2014 Guideline for management of wounds in patients with lower extremity arterial disease (LEAD): An executive summary. *Journal of Wound, Ostomy, and Continence Nursing, 43*(1), 23–31. doi: 10.1097/WON.0000000000000193.

Bonham, P. A., Kelechi, T., Mueller, M., et al. (2010). Are toe pressures measured by a portable photoplethysmograph equivalent to standard laboratory tests? *Journal of Wound, Ostomy, and Continence Nursing, 375*(5), 475–486. doi: 10.1097/WON.0b013e3181eda0c5.

Bozkurt, A. K., Tasci, I., Tabak, O., et al. (2011). Peripheral artery disease assessed by ankle brachial index in patients with established cardiovascular disease or at least one risk factor for atherothrombosis—CAREFUL study: A national, multi-center, cross-sectional observational study. *BMC Cardiovascular Disorders, 11,* 4. doi: 10.1186/1471-2261-11-4.

Bratzler, D. W., Dellinger, E. P., Olsen, K. M., et al. (2013). Clinical practice guidelines for antimicrobial prophylaxis in surgery. *American Journal of Health-System Pharmacy, 70*(3), 195–283. doi: 10.2146/ajhp120568.

Bryant, R. A., & Nix, D. P. (2016). Principles of wound healing and topical management. In R. A. Bryant, & D. P. Nix (Eds.), *Acute & chronic wounds. Current management concepts* (5th ed., pp. 306–324). St. Louis, MO: Elsevier.

Campia, U., Gerhard-Herman, M., Piazza, G., et al. (2019). Peripheral artery disease: Past, present, and future. *The American Journal of Medicine, 132*(10), 1133–1141, doi: 10.1016/j.amjmed.2019.04.043.

Carter, S. (1993). Role of pressure measurements in vascular disease. In E. F. Bernstein (Ed.), *Vascular Diagnosis* (4th ed., pp. 486–512). St. Louis, MO: CV Mosby.

Carter, S., & Lezack, J. (1971). Digital systolic pressures in the lower limb in arterial disease. *Circulation, 43,* 905–914.

Casey, S., Lanting, S., Oldmeadow, C., et al. (2019). The reliability of the ankle brachial index: A systematic review. *Journal of Foot and Ankle Research, 12,* 39. doi: 10.1186/s13047-019-0350-1.

de Ceniga, M. V., Bravo, E., Izagirre, M., et al. (2011). Anaemia, iron and vitamin deficits in patients with peripheral arterial disease. *European Journal of Vascular and Endovascular Surgery, 41*(6), 828–830. doi: 10.1016/j.ejvs.2011.01.017.

Chen, Q., Li, L., Chen, Q., et al. (2019). Critical appraisal of international guidelines for the screening and treatment of asymptomatic peripheral artery disease: A systematic review. *BMC Cardiovascular Disorders, 19,* 17. doi: 10.1186/s12872-018-0960-8.

Chioncel, V., Brezeanu, R., & Sinescu, C. (2019). New directions in the management of peripheral artery disease. *American Journal of Therapeutics, 26*(2), e248–e293.

Chopra, A., Azarbal, A. F., Jung, E., et al. (2018). Ambulation and functional outcome after major lower extremity amputation. *Journal of Vascular Surgery, 67*(5), 1521–1529. doi: 10.1016/j.jvs.2017.10.051.

Conte, M. S., Bradbury, A. W., Kolh, P., et al. (2019). Global vascular guidelines on the management of chronic limb-threatening ischemia. *Journal of Vascular Surgery, 69*(Suppl 6), 3S–125S.e40. doi: 10.1016/j.jvs.2019.02.016.

Conte, M. S., Pomposelli, F. B., Clair, D. G., et al. (2015). Society for Vascular Surgery practice guidelines for atherosclerotic occlusive disease of the lower extremities: Management of asymptomatic disease and claudication. *Journal of Vascular Surgery, 61*(Suppl 3), 2S–41S. doi: 10.1016/j.jvs.2014.12.009

Cornelis, N., Nassen, J., Buys, R., et al. (2019). The impact of supervised exercise training on traditional cardiovascular risk factors in patients with intermittent claudication. *European Journal of Vascular and Endovascular Surgery, 58*(1), 75–87. doi: 10.1016/j.ejvs.2018.12.014.

Criqui, M. H., & Aboyans, V. (2015). Epidemiology of peripheral artery disease. *Circulation Research, 116,* 1509–1526. doi: 10.1161/CIRCRESAHA.116.303849.

Criqui, M. H., Fronek, A., Klauber, M. R., et al. (1985). The sensitivity, specificity, and predictive value of traditional clinical evaluation of peripheral arterial disease: Results from noninvasive testing in a defined population. *Circulation, 71*(3), 516–522.

Criqui, M. H., McClelland, R. L., McDermott, M. M., et al. (2010). The ankle-brachial index and incident cardiovascular events in the MESA (Multi-ethnic study of atherosclerosis). *Journal of the American College of Cardiology, 56*(18), 1506–1512. doi: 10.1016/j.jacc.2010.04.060

Cull, D. L., Manos, G., Hartley, M. C., et al. (2014). An early validation of the Society for Vascular Surgery lower extremity threatened limb classification system. *Journal of Vascular Surgery, 60*(6), 1535–1542. doi: 10.1016/j.jvs.2014.08.107.

Darwood, R., Berridge, D. C., Kessel, D. O., et al. (2018). Surgery versus thrombolysis for initial management of acute limb ischaemia. *Cochrane Database of Systematic Reviews,* (8), CD002784. doi: 10.1002/14651858.CD002784.pub3.

Davies, J. H., Kenkre, J., & Williams, E. M. (2014). Current utility of the ankle-brachial index (ABI) in general practice: Implications for its use in cardiovascular disease screening. *BMC Family Practice, 15,* 69. doi: 10.1186/1471-2296-15-69.

Davis, F. M., Sutzko, D. C., Grey, S. F., et al. (2017). Predictors of surgical site infection after open lower extremity revascularization *Journal of Vascular Surgery, 65*(6), 1769–1778. doi: 10.1016/j.jvs.2016.11.053.

de Jesus-Silva, S. G., de Oliveira, J. P., Brianezi, M. H. C., et al. (2017). Analysis of risk factors related to minor and major lower limb amputations at a tertiary hospital. *Jornal Vascular Brasileiro, 16*(1), 16–22. doi: 10.1590/1677-5449.008916.

Delaney, C. L., Miller, M. D., Dickinson, K. M., et al. (2014). Change in dietary intake of adults with intermittent claudication undergoing a supervised exercise program and compared to matched controls. *Nutrition Journal, 13,* 1–7. doi: 10.1186/1475-2891-13-100.

Delaney, C. L., Smale, M. K., & Miller, M. D. (2019). Nutritional considerations for peripheral arterial disease: A narrative review. *Nutrients, 11*(6), 1–15. doi: 10.3390/nu11061219.

Demkova, K., Kozarova, M., Malachovska, Z., et al. (2018). Osteoprotegerin concentration is associated with the presence and severity of peripheral arterial disease in type 2 diabetes mellitus. *VASA, 42*(2), 131–135. doi: 10.1024/0301-1526/a000682.

Department of Veterans Affairs and Department of Defense. (2017). VA/DoD clinical practice guideline for rehabilitation of individuals with lower limb amputation. Retrieved October 5, 2019, from https://www.healthquality.va.gov/guidelines/Rehab/amp/VADoDL-LACPG092817.pdf

Devinuwara, K., Dworak-Kula, A., & O'Connor, R. J. (2018). Rehabilitation and prosthetics post amputation. *Orthopaedics and Trauma, 32*(4), 234–240.

Ding, N., Sang, Y., Chen, J., et al. (2019). Cigarette smoking, smoking cessation, and long-term risk of 3 major atherosclerotic diseases. *Journal of the American College of Cardiology, 74*(4), 498–507. doi: 10.1016/j.jacc.2019.05.049.

Doughty, D. B. (2016). Arterial ulcers. Principles of wound healing and topical management. In R. A. Bryant, & D. P. Nix (Eds.), *Acute & chronic wounds. Current management concepts* (5th ed., pp. 186–203). St. Louis, MO: Elsevier.

Dumville, J. C., Land, L., Evans, D., et al. (2016). Negative pressure wound therapy for treating leg ulcers. *Cochrane Database of Systematic Reviews,* (7), CD011354. doi: 10.1002/14651858.CD011354.pub2.

Elsayed, S., & Clavijo, L. C. (2015). Critical limb ischemia. *Cardiology Clinics, 33*(1), 37–47. doi: 10.1016/j.ccl.2014.09.008.

Ertl, J. P., & Panchbhavi, V. K. (2019). Lower extremity amputations. *Medscape.* Retrieved October 6, 2019, from https://emedicine.medscape.com/article/1232102-print

Esteghamati, A., Aflatoonian, M., Rad, M. V., et al. (2015). Association of osteoprotegerin with peripheral artery disease in patients with type 2 diabetes. *Archives of Cardiovascular Diseases, 108*(8–9), 412–419. doi: 10.1016/j.acvd.2015.01.015.

European Pressure Ulcer Advisory Panel, National Pressure Injury Advisory Panel, and Pan Pacific Pressure Injury Alliance [EPUAP/NPIAP/PPPIA]. (2019). In E. Haesler (Ed.), *Prevention and treatment of pressure ulcers/injuries: Clinical Practice Guideline.* The International Guideline.

Firnhaber, J. M., & Powell, C. S. (2019). Lower extremity peripheral artery disease: Diagnosis and treatment. *American Family Physician, 99*(6), 362–369.

U. S. Food and Drug Administration. (2019). August 7, 2019 Update: Treatment of peripheral arterial disease with paclitaxel-coated balloons and paclitaxel-eluting stents potentially associated with increased mortality. Retrieved October 2, 2019, from https://www.fda.gov/medical-devices/letters-health-care-providers/august-7-2019-update-treatment-peripheral-arterial-disease-paclitaxel-coated-balloons-and-paclitaxel

Forster, R., & Pagnamenta, F. (2015). Dressings and topical agents for arterial leg ulcers. *Cochrane Database of Systematic Reviews,* (6), CD001836. doi: 10.1002/14651858.CD001836.pub3.

Forster, R., Liew, A., Bhattacharya, V., et al. (2018). Gene therapy for peripheral arterial disease. *Cochrane Database of Systematic Reviews,* (10), CD012058. doi: 10.1002/14651858.CD012058.pub2.

Gabel, J., Jabo, B., Patel, S., et al. (2018). Analysis of patients undergoing major lower extremity amputation in the vascular quality initiative. *Annals of Vascular Surgery, 46*, 75–82. doi: 10.1016/j.avsg.2017.07.034.

Gaddipati, V. C., Bailey, B. A., Kuriacose, R., et al. (2011). The relationship of vitamin D status to cardiovascular risk factors and amputation risk in veterans with peripheral arterial disease. *Journal of the American Medical Directors Association, 12*, 58–61. doi: 10.1016/j.jamda.2010.02.006.

Gardner, A. W., Bright, B. C., Ort, K. A., et al. (2011). Dietary intake of participants with peripheral artery disease and claudication. *Angiology, 62*(3), 270–275. doi: 10.1177/0003319710384395.

Georgopoulos, S., Kouvelos, G. N., Koutsoumpelis, A., et al. (2013). The effect of revascularization procedures on healing of mixed arterial andvenous leg ulcers. *International Angiology, 32*(4), 368–374.

Gerhard-Herman, M. D., Gornik, H. L., Barrett, C., et al. (2017). 2016 AHA/ACC guideline on the management of patients with lower extremity peripheral artery disease. *Journal of the American College of Cardiology, 69*(11), e71–e126. doi: 10.1016/j.jacc.2016.11.007.

Gorenoi, V., Brehm, M. U., Koch, A., et al. (2017). Growth factors for angiogenesis in peripheral arterial disease. *Cochrane Database of Systematic Reviews,* (6), CD011741. doi: 10.1002/14651858.CD011741.pub2.

Grundy, S. M., Stone, N. J., Bailey, A. L., et al. (2019). AHA/ACC/AACVPR/AAPA/ABC/ACPM/ADA/AGS/APhA/ASPC/NLA/PCNA guideline on the management of blood cholesterol. *Journal of the American College of Cardiology, 73*(24), e285–e350. doi: 10.1016/j.jacc.2018.11.003.

Gu, Z., Man, C., Zhang, H., et al. (2019). High ankle-brachial index and risk of cardiovascular or all-cause mortality: A meta-analysis. *Atherosclerosis, 282*, 29–36.

Guest, F., Marshall, C., & Stansby, G. (2018). Amputation and rehabilitation. *Vascular Surgery, 37*(2), 102–103.

Hazarika, S., & Annex, B. H. (2017). Biomarkers and genetics in peripheral artery disease. *Clinical Chemistry, 63*(1), 236–244. doi: 10.1373/clinchem.2016.263798.

Hedayati, N., Carson, J. G., Chi, Y.- W., et al. (2015). Management of mixed arterial lower extremity ulcerations: A review. *Vascular Medicine, 20*(5), 479–486. doi: 10.1177/1358863x15594683.

Hernandez, N. V. M., Ramirez, J. L., Khetani, S. A., et al. (2018). Depression severity is associated with increased inflammation in veterans with peripheral artery disease. *Vascular Medicine, 23*(5), 445–453. doi: 10.1177/1358863X18787640.

Herraiz-Adillo, A., Cavero-Redondo, I., Alvarez-Bueno, C., et al. (2017). The accuracy of an oscillometric ankle-brachial index in the diagnosis of lower limb peripheral arterial disease. *International Journal of Clinical Practice, 71*, e12994. doi: 10.1111/ijcp.12994.

Heuer, A., Kossick, M. A., Riley, J., et al. (2017). Update on guidelines for perioperative antibiotic selection and administration from the surgical care improvement project (SCIP) and American Society of Health-System Pharmacists. *AANA Journal, 85*(4), 293–299.

Horch, R. E., Dragu, A., Lang, W., et al. (2008). Coverage of exposed bones and joints in critically ill patients: Lower extremity salvage with topical negative pressure therapy. *Journal of Cutaneous Medicine and Surgery, 12*(5), 223–229.

Hoyer, C., Sandermann, J., & Petersen, L. J. (2013). The toe-brachial index in the diagnosis of peripheral arterial disease. *Journal of Vascular Surgery, 58*(1), 231–238. doi:10.1016/j.jvs.2013.03.044.

Iannuzzo, G., Forte, F., Lupoli, R., et al. (2018). Association of vitamin D deficiency with peripheral arterial disease: A meta-analysis of literature studies. *Journal of Clinical Endocrinology and Metabolism, 103*(6), 2107–2115. doi:10.1210/jc.2018-00136.

Iezzi, R., Santoro, M., Marano, R., et al. (2012). Low-dose multidetector CT angiography in the evaluation of infrarenal aorta and peripheral arterial occlusive disease. *Radiology, 263*(1), 287–298. doi: 10.1148/radiol.11110700.

International Wound Infection Institute. (2016). Wound infection in clinical practice. Principles of best practice. *Wounds International.* Retrieved September 11, 2019, from http://www.woundinfection-institute.com/wp-content/uploads/2017/03/IWII-Wound-infection-in-clinical-practice.pdf

Itoga, N. K., Tawfik, D. S., Lee, C. K., et al. (2018). Association of blood pressure measurements with peripheral artery disease event. *Circulation, 138*, 1805–1814. doi: 10.1161/CIRCULATIONAHA.118.033348.

Jones, M. L. (2013). BPS2: Nursing care of patients wearing antiembolic stockings. *British Journal of Healthcare Assistants, 7*(8), 388–390.

Jones, R., Arps, K., Davis, D. M., et al. (2018). Clinician guide to the ABCs of primary and secondary prevention of atherosclerotic cardiovascular disease. Retrieved September 4, 2019, from https://www.acc.org/latest-in-cardiology/articles/2018/03/30/18/34/clinician-guide-to-the-abcs

Kaplovitch, E., Rannelli, L., & Anand, S. S. (2019). Antithrombotics in stable peripheral artery disease. *Vascular Medicine, 24*(2), 132–140. doi: 10.1177/1358863X18820123.

Karunathilake, S. P., & Ganegoda, G. U. (2018). Secondary prevention of cardiovascular diseases and application of technology for early diagnosis. *BioMed Research International, 2018*, 5767864. doi: 10.1155/2018/5767864.

Keszler, M. S., Heckman, J. T., Kaufman, G. E., et al. (2019). Advances in prosthetics and rehabilitation of individuals with limb loss. *Physical Medicine and Rehabilitation Clinics of North America, 30*, 423–437.

Klarich, J., & Brueckner, I. (2014). Amputee rehabilitation and prepro-sthetic care. *Physical Medicine and Rehabilitation Clinics of North America, 25*, 75–91.

Kleinegris, M.- C. F., ten Cate, H., & ten Cate-Hoek, A. (2013). D-Dimer as a marker for cardiovascular and arterial thrombotic events in patients with peripheral arterial disease. A systematic review. *Thrombosis and Haemostasis, 110*(02), 233–243. doi: 10.1160/TH13-01-0032.

Kohn, C. G., Alberts, M. J., Peacock, W. F., et al. (2019). Cost and inpa-tient burden of peripheral artery disease: Findings from the National Inpatient Sample. *Atherosclerosis, 286*, 142–146.

Kranke, P., Bennett, M. H., Martyn-St. James, M., et al. (2015). Hyperbaric oxygen therapy for chronic wounds. *Cochrane Database of Sys-tematic Reviews*, (6), CD004123. doi: 10.1002/14651858.CD004123.pub4.

Kroger, K., Stewen, C., Santosa, F., et al. (2003). Toe pressure measure-ments compared to ankle artery pressure measurements. *Angiol-ogy, 54*(1), 39–44.

Kurt, T., Temiz, A., Gokmen, F., et al. (2015). Can the ankle brachial pres-sure index (ABPI) and carotid intima media thickness (CIMT) be new early stage markers of subclinical atherosclerosis in patients with rheumatoid arthritis? *Wiener Klinische Wochenschrift, 127*, 529–534. doi: 10.1007/s00508-015-0767-x.

Kuy, S., Dua, A., Desai, S., et al. (2014). Surgical site infections after lower extremity revascularization procedures involving groin inci-sions. *Annals of Vascular Surgery, 28*, 53–58.

Kwah, L. K., Webb, M. T., Goh, L., et al. (2019). Rigid dressings versus soft dressings for transtibial amputations. *Cochrane Database of Sys-tematic Reviews*, (6), CD012427. doi: 10.1002/14651858.CD012427.pub2.

Lane, R., Harwood, A., Watson, L., et al. (2017). Exercise for intermit-tent claudication. *Cochrane Database of Systematic Reviews*, (12), CD000990. doi: 10.1002/14651858.CD000990.pub4.

Lee, K., Murphy, P. B., Ingves, M. V., et al. (2017). Randomized clinical trial of negative pressure wound therapy for high-risk groin wounds in lower extremity revascularization. *Journal of Vascular Surgery, 66*, 1814–1819.

Leeper, N. J., Myers, J., Zhou, M., et al. (2013). Exercise capacity is the strongest predictor of mortality in patients with peripheral arterial disease. *Journal of Vascular Surgery, 57*(3), 728–733. doi: 10.1016/j.jvs.2012.07.051.

Lezack, J. D., & Carter, S. A. (1973). The relationship of digital systolic pressures to the clinical and angiographic findings in limbs with arterial occlusive disease. *Scandinavian Journal of Clinical and Laboratory Investigation, 128*, 97–101.

Lim, C. S., & Davies, A. H. (2014). Graduated compression stock-ings. *Canadian Medical Association Journal, 186*(10), e391–e397. doi:10.1503/cmaj.131281.

Lumbers, M. (2018). Pressure ulcer prevention: Heels at a glance. *Brit-ish Journal of Nursing, 27*(Suppl 6), S6–S8.

Ma, W.- Q., Wang, Y., Sun, X.- J., et al. (2019). Impact of smoking on all-cause mortality and cardiovascular events in patients after coro-nary revascularization with a percutaneous coronary intervention or coronary artery bypass graft: A systematic review and meta-analysis. *Coronary Artery Disease, 30*(5), 367–376. doi: 10.1097/MCA.0000000000000711.

Makisalo, H., Lepantalo, M., Halme, L., et al. (1998). Peripheral arte-rial disease as a predictor of outcome after renal transplantation. *Transplant International, 11*(Suppl 1), S140–S143.

Malgor, R. D., Alahdab, F., Elraiyah, T. A., et al. (2015). A system-atic review of treatment of intermittent claudication in the lower extremities. *Journal of Vascular Surgery, 61*(3 Suppl), 54S–73S. doi: 10.1016/j.jvs.2014.12.007.

Marston, W. (2011). Mixed arterial and venous ulcers. *Wounds, 23*(12), 351–356.

Marti-Carvajal, A. J., Sola, I., Lathyris, D., et al. (2017). Homocysteine-lowering interventions for preventing cardiovascular events. *Cochrane Database of Systematic Reviews*, (8), CD006612. doi: 10.1002/14651858.CD006612.pub5.

Matic, M., Matic, A., Djuran, V., et al. (2016). Frequency of peripheral arterial disease in patients with chronic venous insufficiency. *Ira-nian Red Crescent Medical Journal, 18*(1), e20781.

Mattioli, A. V., Palmiero, P., Manfrini, O., et al. (2017). Mediterranean diet impact on cardiovascular diseases: A narrative review. *Jour-nal of Cardiovascular Medicine, 18*(12), 925–935. doi: 10.2459/JCM.0000000000000573.

Mazari, F. A., Khan, J. A., Carradice, D., et al. (2012). Randomized clinical trial of percutaneous transluminal angioplasty, supervised exercise and combined treatment for intermittent claudication due to femo-ropopliteal arterial disease. *British Journal of Surgery, 99*(1), 39–48. doi: 10.1002/bjs.7710.

McCaslin, J. E., Andras, A., & Stansby, G. (2013). Cryoplasty for periph-eral arterial disease. *Cochrane Database of Systematic Reviews*, (8), CD005507. doi: 10.1002/14651858.CD005507.pub3.

McGinnis, E., Greenwood, D. C., Nelson, E. A., et al. (2014). A prospective cohort study of prognostic factors for the healing of heel pressure ulcers. *Age and Ageing, 43*, 267–271. doi: 10.1093/ageing/aft187.

Melamed, M. L., Muntner, P., Michos, E. D., et al. (2008). Serum 25-hydroxyvitamin D levels and the prevalence of peripheral arte-rial disease. *Arteriosclerosis, Thrombosis, and Vascular Biology, 28*, 1179–1185. doi: 10.1161/ATVBAHA.108.165886.

Meyersohn, N. M., Walker, T. G., & Oliveira, G. R. (2015). Advances in axial imaging of peripheral vascular disease. *Current Cardiology Reports, 17*, 87. doi: 10.1007/s11886-015-0644-2.

Mills, J. L., Conte, M. S., Armstrong, D. G., et al. (2014). The Society for Vascu-lar Surgery lower extremity threatened limb classification system: Risk stratification based on wound, ischemia, and foot infection (WIfI). *Jour-nal of Vascular Surgery, 59*(1), 220–234. doi: 10.1016/j.jvs.2013.08.003.

Mitrovic, I. (2019). Cardiovascular disorders: Vascular disease. In G. D. Hammer, & S. J. McPhee (Eds.), *Pathophysiology of Disease: An introduction to clinical medicine* (8th ed.) New York, NY: McGraw-Hill. Retrieved August 18, 2019, from http://accessmedicine.mhmed-ical.com.ezproxy-v.musc.edu/content.aspx?bookid=2468&sectionid=198222009

Miyata, T., Higashi, Y., Shigematsu, H., et al. (2019). Evaluation of risk factors for limb-specific peripheral vascular events in patients with peripheral artery disease: A post-hoc analysis of the SEASON prospective observational study. *Angiology, 70*(6), 506–514. doi: 10.1177/0003319718814351.

Mogelvang, R., Pedersen, S. H., Flyvbjerg, A., et al. (2012). Compari-son of osteoprotegerin to traditional atherosclerotic risk factors and high-sensitivity C-reactive protein for diagnosis of atherosclerosis. *American Journal of Cardiology, 109*(4), 515–520. doi: 10.1016/j.amj-card.2011.09.043.

Monaro, S., West, S., & Gullick, J. (2017). Vascular disease risk factors. Patient outcomes following lower leg major amputations for periph-eral arterial disease: A series review. *Journal of Vascular Nursing, 35*, 49–56. doi: 10.1016/j.jvn.2016.10.003.

Moran, P. S., Teljeur, C., Harrington, P., et al. (2015). A systematic review of intermittent pneumatic compression for critical limb ischaemia. *Vascular Medicine, 20*(1), 41–50.

Morisaki, K., Yamaoka, T., & Iwasa, K., (2018). Risk factors for wound complications and 30-day mortality after major lower limb ampu-tations in patients with peripheral arterial disease. *Vascular, 26*(1), 12–17. doi: 10.1177/1708538117714197.

Mozaffarian, D., Benjamin, E. J., Go, A. S., et al. (2015). Heart disease and stroke statistics—2015 update. A report from the Ameri-can Heart Association. *Circulation, 131*, e29–e322. doi: 10.1161/CIR.0000000000000152.

Murphy, T. P., Cutlip, D. E., Regensteiner, J. G., et al. (2015). Supervised exercise, stent revascularization, or medical therapy for claudica-tion due to aortoiliac peripheral artery disease: A randomized clinical trial. *Journal of the American College of Cardiology, 65*(10), 999–1009. doi: 10.1016/j.jacc.2014.12.043.

Naqvi, A. Z., Davis, R. B., & Mukamal, K. J. (2014). Nutrient intake and peripheral artery disease in adults: Key considerations in cross-sectional studies. *Clinical Nutrition, 33*(3), 443–447. doi: 10.1016/j.clnu.2013.06.011.

Nicholls, S., & Nelson, A. J. (2019). Rivaroxaban with or without aspirin for the secondary prevention of cardiovascular disease: Clinical implications of the COMPASS trial. *American Journal of Cardiovascular Drugs, 19*(4), 343–348. doi: 10.1007/s40256-018-00322-4.

Nicolai, S. P., Kruidenier, L. M., Rouwet, E. V., et al. (2008). Pocket Doppler and vascular laboratory equipment yield comparable results for ankle brachial index measurement. *BMC Cardiovascular Disorders, 8,* 26. doi: 10.1186/1471-2261-8-26.

Nordmyr, J., Svensson, S., Bjorck, M., et al. (2009). Vacuum assisted wound closure in patients with lower extremity arterial disease. *International Angiology, 28*(1), 26–31.

Nosova, E. V., Conte, M. S., & Grenon, S. M. (2015). Advancing beyond the "heart-healthy diet" for peripheral arterial disease. *Journal of Vascular Surgery, 61*(1), 265–274. doi: 10.1016/j.jvs.2014.10.022.

O'Donnell, T. F. Jr, Passman, M. A., Marston, W. A., et al. (2014). Management of venous leg ulcers: Clinical practice guidelines of the Society for Vascular Surgery and the American Venous Forum. *Journal of Vascular Surgery, 60*(Suppl 2), 3S–59S. doi: 10.1016/j.jvs.2014.04.049.

Ogilvie, R. P., Lutsey, P. L., Heiss, G., et al. (2017). Dietary intake and peripheral arterial disease incidence in middle-aged adults: The Atherosclerosis Risk in Communities (ARIC) study. *American Journal of Clinical Nutrition, 105*(3), 651–659. doi: 10.3945/ajcn.116.137497.

Parmar, G. M., Novak, Z., Spangler, E., et al. (2019). Statin use improves limb salvage after intervention for peripheral arterial disease. *Journal of Vascular Surgery, 70*, 539–546. doi: 10.1016/j.jvs.2018.07.089.

Quan, H., Ouyang, L., Zhou, H., et al. (2019). The effect of preoperative smoking cessation and smoking dose on postoperative complications following radical gastrectomy for gastric cancer: A retrospective study of 2,469 patients. *World Journal of Surgical Oncology, 17,* 61. doi: 10.1186/s12957-019-1607-7.

Rac-Albu, M., Iliuta, L., Guberna, S. M., et al. (2014). The role of ankle-brachial index for predicting peripheral artery disease. *Maedica, 9*(3), 295–302.

Ramundo, J., Pike, C., & Pittman, J. (2018). Do prophylactic foam dressings reduce heel pressure injuries? *Journal of Wound, Ostomy, and Continence Nursing, 45*(1), 75–82. doi: 10.1097/WON.0000000000000400.

Rasmussen, T. E., Clouse W. D., Tonnessen, B. H. (Eds). (2019). Indications and preparation for angiography. In *Handbook of Patient Care in Vascular Diseases* (6th ed., pp. 90–102). Philadelphia, PA: Wolters Kluwer.

Ratliff, C. R., Yates, S., McNichol, L., et al. (2016). Compression for primary prevention, treatment, and prevention of recurrence of venous leg ulcers: An evidence-and consensus-based algorithm for care across the continuum. *Journal of Wound, Ostomy, and Continence Nursing, 43*(4), 347–364. doi: 10.1097/WON.0000000000000242.

Rice, V. H., Heath, L., Livingstone-Banks, J., et al. (2017). Nursing interventions for smoking cessation. *Cochrane Database of Systematic Reviews,* (12), CD001188. doi: 10.1002/14651858.CD001188.pub5.

Robertson, L., & Roche, A. (2013). Primary prophylaxis for venous thromboembolism in people undergoing major amputation of the lower extremity. *Cochrane Database of Systematic Reviews,* (12), CD010525. doi: 10.1002/14651858.CD010525.pub2.

Ruiz Canela, M., Estruch, R., Corella, D., et al. (2014). Association of Mediterranean diet with peripheral artery disease: The PREDIMED randomized trial. *Journal of the American Medical Association, 311*(4), 415–417. doi: 10.1001/jama.2013.280618.

Rumwell, C., & McPharlin, M. (2017). *Vascular technology* (5th ed.). Pasadena, CA: Davies Publishing, Inc.

Salhiyyah, K., Forster, R., Senanayake, E., et al. (2015). Pentoxifylline for intermittent claudication. *Cochrane Database of Systematic Reviews,* (9), CD005262. doi: 10.1002/14651858.CD005262.pub3.

Scissons, R. P., Ettaher, A., & Afridi, S. (2019). Likelihood of normal ABI increases with physiologic testing referral from rural primary care physicians. *Journal for Vascular Ultrasound, 43*(3)1–5. doi: 10.1177/1544316719870070.

Sibley III, R. C., Reis, S. P., MacFarlane, J. J., et al. (2017). Noninvasive physiologic vascular studies: A guide to diagnosing peripheral arterial disease. *Radiographics, 37*(1), 346–357.

Skelly, C. L., & Cifu A. S. (2016). Screening, evaluation, and treatment of peripheral arterial disease. *JAMA, 316*(14), 1486–1487.

Song, P., Rudan, D., Zhu, Y., et al. (2019). Global, regional, and national prevalence and risk factors for peripheral artery disease in 2015: An updated systematic review and analysis. *The Lancet Global Health, 7*(8), e1020–e1030.

Soto-Barreras, U., Olvera-Rubio, J. O., Loyola-Rodriguez, J. P., et al. (2013). Peripheral arterial disease associated with caries and periodontal disease. *Journal of Periodontology, 84*(4), 486–494. doi: 10.1902/jop.2012.120051.

Spreen, M. I., Gremmels, H., Teraa, M., et al. (2018). High and immeasurable ankle-brachial index as predictor of poor amputation-free survival in critical limb ischemia. *Journal of Vascular Surgery, 67*(6), 1864–1871. doi: 10.1016/j.jvs.2017.10.061.

Squizzato, A., Bellesini, M., Takeda, A., et al. (2017). Clopidogrel plus aspirin versus aspirin alone for preventing cardiovascular events. *Cochrane Database of Systematic Reviews,* (12), CD005158. doi: 10.1002/14651858.CD005158.pub4.

Stoekenbroek, R. M., Boekholdt, M., Fayaad, R., et al. (2015). High-dose atorvastatin is superior to moderate-dose simvastatin in preventing peripheral arterial disease. *Heart, 101,* 356–362. doi: 10.1136/heartjnl-2014-306906.

Stotts, N. A. (2016). Wound infection: Diagnosis and management. In R. A. Bryant, & D. P. Nix (Eds.), *Acute & chronic wounds. Current management concepts* (5th ed., pp. 283–294). St. Louis, MO: Elsevier.

teSlaa, A., Dolmans, D., Ho, G., et al. (2014). Treatment strategies and clinical aspects of lower limb edema following peripheral bypass surgery. *Phlebology, 29*(1), 18–25. doi: 10.1177/0268355514527689.

Twilley, H., & Jones, S. (2016). Heel ulcers—Pressure ulcers or symptoms of peripheral arterial disease? An exploratory matched case control study. *Journal of Tissue Viability, 25*(2), 150–156. doi: 10.1016/j.jtv.2016.02.007.

Ubbink, D. T., & Vermeulen, H. (2013). Spinal cord stimulation for non-reconstructable chronic critical leg ischaemia. *Cochrane Database of Systematic Reviews,* (2), CD004001. doi: 10.1002/14651858.CD004001.pub3.

Uccioli, L., Meloni, M., Izzo, V., et al. (2018). Critical limb ischemia: Current challenges and future prospects. *Vascular Health and Risk Management, 14*, 63–74.

Uustal, H., & Meier, R. H. III. (2014). Pain issues and treatment of the person with an amputation. *Physical Medicine and Rehabilitation Clinics of North America, 25,* 45–52.

van de Luijtgaarden, K. M., Voute, M. T., Hoeks, S. E., et al. (2012). Vitamin D deficiency may be an independent risk factor for arterial disease. *European Journal of Vascular and Endovascular Surgery, 11*(3), 301–306. doi: 10.1016/j.ejvs.2012.06.017.

Varcoe, R. L. (2019). Intervention for chronic lower limb ischaemia. In I. Loftus, & R. J. Hinchliffe (Eds.), *Vascular and Endovascular Surgery: A Companion to Specialist Surgical Practice* (pp 44–61). St Louis, MO: Elsevier.

Varnado, M. (2016). Lower extremity neuropathic disease. In D. B. Doughty, & L. L. McNichol (Eds.), *Wound Ostomy and Continence Nurses Society core curriculum: Wound management* (pp. 466–507). Philadelphia, PA: Wolters Kluwer.

Vartanian, S. M., & Conte, M. S. (2015). Surgical intervention for peripheral arterial disease. *Circulation Research, 116* (9), 1614–1628. doi: 10.1161/CIRCRESAHA.116.303504.

Vasheghani-Farahani, A., Hosseini, K., Ashraf, H., et al. (2017). Correlation of ankle-brachial index and peripheral artery disease with the status of body fat deposition and metabolic syndrome in asymptomatic premenopausal women. *Diabetes & Metabolic Syndrome 11*(3), 203–209. doi: 10.1016/j.dsx.2016.09.007.

Vemulapalli, S., Patel, M. R., & Jones, W. S. (2015). Limb ischemia: Cardiovascular diagnosis and management from head to toe. *Current Cardiology Reports, 17*(7), 611. doi: 10.1007/s11886-015-0611-y.

Verbiest, M., Brakema, E., van der Kleij, R., et al. (2017). National guidelines for smoking cessation in primary care: A literature review and evidence analysis. *Primary Care Respiratory Medicine, 27*(1), 2. doi: 10.1038/s41533-016-0004-8.

Vietto, V., Franco, J. V. A., Saenz, V., et al. (2018). Prostanoids for critical limb ischaemia. *Cochrane Database of Systematic Reviews, (1)*, CD006544. doi: 10.1002/14651858.CD006544.pub3.

Vlachopoulos, C., Georgakopoulos, C., Koutagiar, I., et al. (2018). Diagnostic modalities in peripheral artery disease. *Current Opinion in Pharmacology, 39*, 68–76.

Wade, R., Paton, F., Rice, S., et al. (2016). Thigh length versus knee length antiembolism stockings for the prevention of deep vein thrombosis in postoperative surgical patients: A systematic review and network meta-analysis. *British Medical Journal, 6*, e009456. doi: 10.1136/bmjopen-2015-009456.

Wahlgren, C. M., & Magnusson, P. K. (2011). Genetic influences on peripheral arterial disease in a twin population. *Arteriosclerosis, Thrombosis, and Vascular Biology, 31*(3), 678–682.

Wassel, C. L., Loomba, R., Ix J. H., et al. (2011). Family history of peripheral artery disease is associated with prevalence and severity of peripheral artery disease: The San Diego population study. *Journal of the American College of Cardiology, 58*(13), 1386–1392. doi: 10.1016/j.jacc.2011.06.023.

Watson, C., & Alp, N. J. (2008). Role of *Chlamydia pneumoniae* in atherosclerosis. *Clinical Science, 114*(8), 509–531. doi: 10.1042/CS20070298.

Webster, J. B. (2019). Lower limb amputation care across the active duty military and veteran populations. *Physical Medicine and Rehabilitation Clinics of North America, 30*, 89–109.

Webster, J. B., Crunkhorn, A., Sall, J., et al. (2019). Clinical practice guidelines for the rehabilitation of lower limb amputation. *American Journal of Physical Medicine & Rehabilitation, 98*(9), 820–829.

Whelton, P. K., Carey, R. M., Aronow, W. S., et al. (2018). 2017 ACC/AHA/AAPA/ABC/ACPM/AGS/APhA/ASH/ASPC/NMA/PCNA guideline for the prevention, detection, evaluation, and management of high blood pressure in adults: A report of the American College of Cardiology/American Heart Association Task Force on Clinical Practice Guidelines. *Hypertension, 71*(6), e13–e115. doi: 10.1161/HYP.0000000000000065.

Wickstrom, J. E., Laivurori, M., Aro, E., et al. (2017). Toe pressure and toe brachial index are predictive of cardiovascular mortality, overall mortality, and amputation free survival in patients with peripheral artery disease. *European Journal Vascular and Endovascular Surgery, 53*, 696–703. doi: 10.1016/j.ejvs.2017.02.012.

Wound, Ostomy and Continence Nurses Society. (2014). *Guideline for management of wounds in patients with lower extremity arterial disease. WOCN clinical practice guideline series 1.* Mt. Laurel, NJ: Author.

Wound, Ostomy and Continence Nurses Society. (2016). *Guideline for prevention and management of pressure ulcers (injuries). WOCN clinical practice guideline series 2.* Mt. Laurel, NJ: Author.

Wound, Ostomy and Continence Nurses Society. (2017). *Ankle brachial index: Procedure for measuring and calculating the ABI.* Mt. Laurel, NJ: Author.

Wound, Ostomy and Continence Nurses Society. (2019a). *Guideline for management of wounds in patients with lower extremity venous disease. WOCN clinical guideline series 4.* Mt. Laurel, NJ: Author.

Wound, Ostomy and Continence Nurses Society. (2019b). *Venous, arterial, and neuropathic lower-extremity wounds: Clinical resource guide.* Mt. Laurel, NJ: Author.

Yang, S., Zhao, L. S., Cai, C., et al. (2018). Association between periodontitis and peripheral artery disease: A systematic review and meta-analysis. *BMC Cardiovascular Disorders, 18*, 141. doi: 10.1186/s12872-018-0879-0.

Yazouli, L. E., Hejaji, H., Elmdaghri, N., et al. (2018). Investigation of *Chlamydia pneumoniae* infection in Moroccan patients suffering from cardiovascular diseases. *Journal of Infection and Public Health, 11*(2), 246–249. doi: 10.1016/j.jiph.2017.07.029.

Young, J. C., Paul, N. J., Kartas, T. B., et al. (2019). Cigarette smoking intensity informs outcomes after open revascularization for peripheral artery disease. *Journal of Vascular Surgery. 70*(6):1973–1983. e5. doi: 10.1016/j.jvs.2019.02.066.

Yuan, J., Jia, P., Hua, L., et al. (2019). Vitamin D deficiency is associated with risk of developing peripheral arterial disease in type 2 diabetic patients. *BMC Cardiovascular Disorders, 19*, 1–7. doi: 10.1186/s12872-019-1125-0.

Zaki, M., Elsherif, M., Tawfick, W., et al. (2016). The role of sequential pneumatic compression in limb salvage in non-reconstructable critical limb ischemia. *European Journal of Vascular and Endovascular Surgery, 51*(4), 565–571. doi: 10.1016/j.ejvs.2015.12.025.

Zhan, L. X., Branco, B. C., Armstrong, D. G., et al. (2015). The Society for Vascular Surgery lower extremity threatened limb classification system based on wound, ischemia, and foot infection (WIfI) correlates with risk of major amputation and time to wound healing. *Journal of Vascular Surgery, 61*(4), 939–944. doi: 10.1016/j.jvs.2014.11.045.

QUESTIONS

1. A wound care nurse is counseling patients with lower extremity arterial disease (LEAD). Which statement accurately describes a characteristic of the condition?

  A. LEAD is an acute disease caused by uncontrolled hypertension.

  B. LEAD is associated with increased risk of MI, stroke, and vascular death.

  C. LEAD causes progressive fibrosis and softening of the arterial walls.

  D. As LEAD progresses, dilation occurs in response to tissue demands.

2. Which of the following conditions increases the risk for LEAD 2- to 4-fold?

  A. Arthritis

  B. Hypertension

  C. Obesity

  D. Diabetes mellitus

3. A patient is diagnosed with infrapopliteal disease. In what area of the body would the wound care nurse expect the patient to complain of pain?

  A. The foot

  B. The buttocks

  C. The calf

  D. The thigh

4. What is the initial classic type of pain that is associated with LEAD?
   A. Positional pain
   B. Intermittent claudication
   C. Resting pain
   D. Continuous pain

5. The wound care nurse is assessing a patient with acute limb ischemia. Which of the following is a hallmark sign of this condition?
   A. Sudden onset of the six "Ps"
   B. Chronic ischemic rest pain
   C. Development of collateral vessels
   D. Bounding pedal pulses

6. The wound care nurse is assessing the limbs of a patient with ischemia. What common clinical characteristic might the nurse document?
   A. Rubor on elevation of legs
   B. Early capillary refill
   C. Moist, dull, loose skin
   D. Prolonged venous refill time

7. The wound care nurse is measuring and calculating the ABI of a patient with LEAD. Which step of the procedure has the nurse performed correctly?
   A. The nurse performs the ABI in a quiet, cool environment on a patient who has a full bladder.
   B. The nurse places the patient in a flat, supine position with one small pillow placed behind the patient's head for comfort.
   C. The nurse places the pressure cuff with the bottom of the cuff approximately 5 to 7 cm above the cubital fossa on the arm.
   D. The nurse divides the lower of the dorsalis pedis or posterior tibial systolic pressure by the higher of the right or left brachial pressures to calculate an ABI.

8. A wound care nurse documents a patient's ABI as 0.90. What is the interpretation of this finding?
   A. Elevated
   B. Normal
   C. LEAD
   D. Borderline perfusion

9. Which of the following interventions is most appropriate for a patient with an ABI of 0.50 and a heel pressure injury that is covered with stable, black, dry eschar?
   A. Apply a topical antibiotic ointment and a moist gauze dressing to the eschar.
   B. Apply a hydrocolloid dressing to the eschar and elevate the leg.
   C. Score the eschar and apply an enzymatic debriding agent to the eschar.
   D. Keep the eschar dry and stable and refer the patient for a vascular/surgical evaluation.

10. Which of the following patients is at the greatest risk of an amputation due to critical limb ischemia/chronic limb-threatening ischemia (CLI/CLTI)?
   A. Patient has a wound on the medial ankle (gaiter area) for 2 weeks; wound base is red with large amount of exudate; has edema of the lower limb; ABI is 0.80; TBI is 0.50.
   B. Patient has a red granulating wound on the plantar foot surface for 3 weeks; ABI is 0.90; toe pressure is 60 mm Hg.
   C. Patient has a nonhealing wound on the lateral calf for 4 weeks; wound is covered with yellow slough; has a 3 cm halo of erythema around the wound; ABI is 0.30; toe pressure is 26 mm Hg.
   D. Patient has a small wound with pale pink tissue on the lateral malleolus for 2 weeks; ABI is 0.60; TBI is 0.58.

ANSWERS AND RATIONALES

1. B. Rationale: Atherosclerosis and plaque formation contribute to LEAD as well as MI and stroke.

2. D. Rationale: Diabetes accelerates the natural course and distribution of atherosclerosis.

3. A. Rationale: The location of pain may indicate the location of stenosis or occlusion. Pain typically occurs one joint below the site of stenosis or occlusion.

4. B. Rationale: Intermittent claudication is defined as reproducible pain that is brought on by walking or similar activity and relieved by rest. Positional, resting and continuous pain are associated with advanced disease.

5. A. Rationale: The hallmark signs of acute limb-threatening occlusion are sudden onset of pulselessness, pain, pallor, paresthesia, paralysis, and polar (cold).

6. D. Rationale: Common clinical characteristics of an ischemic limb are pallor on elevation, delayed capillary refill, shiny, dry taut skin with atrophy, and prolonged venous refill time.

7. B. Rationale: Measurement of the ABI requires a warm, quiet environment and that the patient has an empty bladder. Blood pressure cuff should be placed 2 to 3 cm above the cubital fossa on the arm. Calculation of the ABI involves dividing the higher of either foot pressures by the higher of the brachial pressures.

8. C. Rationale: Less than or equal to 0.90 is considered to be LEAD.

9. D. Rationale: Debridement of stable dry eschar on the foot is contraindicated. The plan of care for a patient with an ischemic limb requires referral to a vascular surgeon.

10. C. Rationale: Significant indicators for amputation in patients with critical limb ischemia/chronic limb-threatening ischemia include infection and low ABI.

CHAPTER 26

LOWER EXTREMITY NEUROPATHIC DISEASE

Jennifer O'Connor and Myra F. Varnado

OBJECTIVES

1. Compare and contrast arterial, venous, neuropathic, and mixed ulcers in terms of risk factors, pathology, clinical presentation, and management guidelines.

2. Describe critical parameters to be included in assessment of the individual with a lower extremity ulcer.

3. Demonstrate the procedure for sensory testing using Semmes-Weinstein monofilament and tuning fork.

4. Interpret findings from sensory testing and identify implications for patient education and management.

5. Use assessment data to determine causative and contributing factors for a lower extremity ulcer and to

develop individualized management plans that are evidence based.

6. Identify options and guidelines for effective off-loading of plantar surface ulcers.

7. Explain why debridement is contraindicated in a noninfected ischemic ulcer covered with dry eschar.

8. Describe clinical characteristics and management options for Charcot fracture.

9. Describe indications for referral to vascular surgeon, podiatrist, orthotist, and orthopedic surgeon.

TOPIC OUTLINE

INTRODUCTION

Lower extremity neuropathic disease (LEND), also known as peripheral neuropathy (PN), is caused by an acquired or inherited disorder that interferes with the normal neurologic function of the lower extremities. LEND involves damage to the peripheral nervous system, the extensive communication network that conveys information between the central nervous system (brain and spinal cord) and other parts of the body, such as the feet. With normal function, any trauma to the feet activates sensory nerves that send a message to the brain and spinal cord, and the brain and spinal cord respond by coordinating movement to withdraw from the painful stimulus (National Institutes of Neurological Disorders [NIH], 2019; WOCN, 2012). The individual with LEND sustains damage to structures within the peripheral nervous system that interfere with this communication system. The neurologic structures typically affected are the axon, cell body, and/or the myelin sheath (NIH, 2019; WOCN, 2012).

> **KEY POINT**
>
> Lower extremity neuropathic disease involves damage to the system that communicates information between the brain and spinal cord and the lower legs and feet.

LEND is a common feature of many systemic diseases and may lead to autonomic dysfunction, motor disability, and a loss of sensation to the lower extremities, especially the feet. Sensory loss, motor damage causing foot deformities, and changes in blood flow related to autonomic dysfunction place the individual at risk for a foot wound, which may go unrecognized for some time due to the lack of pain. Infection and ischemia frequently complicate neuropathy, and neuropathic and neuroischemic ulcers are the most common reasons for foot amputations and the associated morbidity and mortality (Centers for Disease Control and Prevention [CDC], 2017; NIH, 2019; WOCN, 2012).

> **KEY POINT**
>
> Neuropathic and neuroischemic ulcers are the most common reasons for foot amputations and the associated morbidity and mortality.

ETIOLOGY AND PATHOLOGY OF LEND

There are a number of conditions that can cause PN. They are commonly grouped into acquired neuropathic disorders and inherited neuropathic disorders.

ACQUIRED NEUROPATHIC DISORDERS

PN is a condition affecting up to 20% of the general population (Benn, 2020). Acquired peripheral neuropathies are grouped into three categories: those caused by systemic disease, those caused by trauma, and those caused by infectious or autoimmune disorders. Neuropathies with no known cause are classified as idiopathic neuropathies (NIH, 2019; WOCN, 2012).

Systemic Diseases

Systemic diseases affect the entire body and are a common cause of PN. Any disease state that compromises the body's ability to convert nutrients into energy, to adequately perfuse the tissues, to process and eliminate metabolic waste products, and to support tissue repair can cause nerve damage (CDC, 2017; NIH, 2019; WOCN, 2012). Diabetes mellitus, and the associated chronic hyperglycemia, is a leading cause of PN in the United States and is the disease most researched and referenced in regard to LEND and LEND wounds (WOCN, 2012). Diabetes is not the only systemic condition that results in neuropathy. Other systemic conditions include kidney disease, which can result in abnormally high levels of toxic metabolic end products that severely damage nerve tissue (CDC, 2017; NIH, 2019; WOCN, 2012). Hormonal imbalances, such as hypothyroidism or increased production of growth hormone, can also cause PN. The reduced metabolic rate associated with hypothyroidism leads to fluid retention and edema, which exerts pressure on peripheral nerves. Overproduction of growth hormone can lead to acromegaly, a condition characterized by abnormal enlargement of the bones and joints. The nerves running through the affected joints can become mechanically entrapped (NIH, 2019; WOCN, 2012). Another systemic condition resulting in sensory and motor neuropathy is B_{12} deficiency, such as occurs with pernicious anemia. Neurologic symptoms vary and may be nonspecific but commonly include feelings of numbness, tingling, weakness, lack of coordination, and clumsiness. Both sides of the body are typically affected equally, and the legs are affected more than the arms. A severe deficiency can result in more serious neurologic symptoms, such as paralysis (NIH, 2019; WOCN, 2012).

KEY POINT

Diabetes, and the associated hyperglycemia, is a leading cause of neuropathy in the United States, but it is not the only condition that results in neuropathy.

Trauma

Physical trauma is the most common cause of mechanical injury to the peripheral nervous system. Trauma resulting from motor vehicle accidents, falls, or sports-related activities can cause partial or total disruption, compression, crushing, or stretching of the nerves. The most severe example of trauma-related neuropathy is spinal cord injury, which typically results in partial or complete paraplegia or quadriplegia (NIH, 2019; WOCN, 2012).

Infectious or Autoimmune Disorders

Lyme disease, diphtheria, and Hansen disease (leprosy) are bacterial diseases characterized by extensive peripheral nerve damage. Viral infections such as HIV, West Nile virus, Lyme disease and herpes simplex can cause neuropathic symptoms (NIH, 2019). Viral and bacterial infections can also cause indirect nerve damage by provoking autoimmune disorders, in which specialized cells and antibodies of the immune system attack the body's own tissues, including the nervous system (CDC, 2017; NIH, 2019; WOCN, 2012).

Other Causes

Certain cancer drugs and antiretroviral agents used to treat HIV/AIDS are associated with irreversible peripheral nerve damage, as are selected anticonvulsants, antiviral agents, and antibiotics. When medications cause neuropathic symptoms, the decision to continue use of the drug is based upon a benefit-to-risk comparison: the potential for worsening and irreversible neuropathy against the potential risk of disease progression if the medication is discontinued.

Vitamin deficiencies and alcoholism can cause widespread damage to nerve tissue. Vitamins E, B_1 (thiamine), B_6, and B_{12} and niacin are necessary for healthy nerve function. Thiamine deficiency is common among people with alcoholism because these individuals commonly have poor dietary habits, and thiamine deficiency can cause a painful sensory neuropathy involving the extremities. Some neuropathic research indicates that excessive alcohol consumption may contribute directly to nerve damage, a condition referred to as alcoholic neuropathy (CDC, 2017; WOCN, 2012). Excessive alcohol consumption and cigarette smoking are also known to increase the risk of LEND among individuals with diabetes (CDC, 2017; WOCN, 2012).

INHERITED NEUROPATHIC DISORDERS

Inherited neuropathic disorders known as familial neuropathies, are caused by genetic anomalies or genetic mutations. Some genetic errors lead to mild neuropathies with symptoms that begin in early adulthood and result in little, if any, significant impairment. More severe hereditary neuropathies often appear in infancy or childhood and may lead to reduced life expectancy due to wounds, fractures, and other unrecognized health issues (NIH, 2019). Examples of inherited or familial neuropathies are congenital insensitivity to pain and a group of neuropathies collectively known as Charcot-Marie-Tooth disease. These neuropathies result from genetic flaws that cause impairments in the neuron and/or myelin sheath tissue and result in sensory and motor neuropathies, respectively (NIH, 2019; WOCN, 2012).

⬤ PREVALENCE AND INCIDENCE

Of non–diabetes-related causes of PN and neuropathic wounds, Hansen disease (leprosy) is the primary worldwide cause of treatable PN. Worldwide, 1 to 2 million persons are permanently disabled as a result of Hansen disease. While the infection can be treated and individuals receiving antibiotic treatment are considered free of active infection, the nerve damage remains and must be recognized and treated (NIH, 2019; WOCN, 2012).

KEY POINT

Hansen disease (leprosy) is the primary cause of treatable peripheral neuropathy worldwide.

In the United States, 34.2 million people have diabetes or 10.5% of the population 18 years of age or older. Adults who meet laboratory criteria for diabetes but are not aware that they are diabetic make up 7.3 million or 2.8% of all U.S. adults. The percentage of adults with diabetes increases with age, reaching 26.8% among those 65 years of age or older. The prevalence of diabetes by race or ethnicity is non-Hispanic whites (11.9%), Asian (14.9%), non-Hispanic blacks (16.4%), and Hispanic persons (14.7%) (CDC, 2020).

Diabetes-related neuropathy is the most common cause of foot ulceration in the diabetic population. Complications of neuropathy account for more hospitalizations than all other diabetic complications combined (e.g., three times as many patients are admitted to the hospital for neuropathic foot ulceration than for ischemic ulceration). Neuropathy with loss of protective sensation (LOPS) occurs in 30% to 40% of the population with diabetes in industrialized nations (Adams et al., 2019). Fifteen percent of the individuals with neuropathy will develop foot ulceration, and 14% to 24% of those who develop an ulceration will require amputation (CDC, 2017; NIH, 2019; WOCN, 2012). The overall prevalence of lower extremity neuropathy, as reported by the CDC is 2.4 per 100,000 U.S. individuals. The prevalence is highest among older individuals (9 per 100,000) (NIH, 2019; WOCN, 2012).

In the United States, the cost of diabetes care averages $174 billion annually, with $116 billion related to direct care. Management of neuropathic wounds accounts for a substantial component of the direct care costs. According to the CDC, patients with diabetic neuropathy and wounds have a relapse rate of 66% over 5 years, and 12% of neuropathic wounds result in amputation (CDC, 2017; WOCN, 2012).

KEY POINT

Complications of neuropathy account for more hospitalizations than all other diabetic complications combined.

Diabetes complicated by PN is responsible for 50% to 70% of all nontraumatic amputations in the United States, and 85% of these amputations are preceded by a foot ulcer (CDC, 2017; NIH, 2019; WOCN, 2012). In 2014, about 108,000 nontraumatic lower limb amputations were performed in adults aged 20 years or older with diagnosed diabetes. Amputation is particularly common among the African American population, who are up to four times more likely to have an amputation than white Americans, irrespective of age or socioeconomic status (CDC, 2017; NIH, 2019; WOCN, 2012). In 2009, the age-adjusted lower extremity amputation (LEA) rate was highest for toe amputation (1.8 per 1,000 diabetic population), followed by below-the-knee amputation (0.9 per 1,000 diabetic population), foot amputation (0.5 per 1,000 diabetic population), and above-the-knee amputation (0.4 per 1,000 diabetic population) (CDC, 2017; WOCN, 2012). The immediate mortality rate among patients undergoing above-the-knee amputations is 5%; and 50% to 84% will undergo subsequent amputation of the other limb within 2 to 3 years. These figures are significant since the 5-year survival rate for patients with bilateral amputations is <50% (CDC, 2017; NIH, 2019; WOCN, 2012).

KEY POINT

Diabetes complicated by peripheral neuropathy is responsible for 50% to 70% of all nontraumatic amputations in the United States, and 85% of these amputations are preceded by a foot ulcer.

At least 50% of all amputations due to neuropathy are preventable with early intervention (Hicks & Selvin, 2019; NIH, 2019; WOCN, 2012). The focus of this chapter will be on the pathology, prevention, and early management of neuropathic wounds.

KEY POINT

At least 50% of all amputations due to neuropathy are preventable with early intervention.

 ## PATHOLOGY, CLASSIFICATION, AND MANIFESTATIONS OF PERIPHERAL NEUROPATHY

More than 100 specific types of PN have been identified, and each has a characteristic pattern of development, symptomatology, and prognosis. The type and severity of functional impairment and symptoms depend on the type and severity of nerve damage and can be broadly categorized as sensory neuropathy, motor neuropathy, autonomic neuropathy, and mixed neuropathy (NIH, 2019). Sensory neuropathy results in paresthesias and LOPS, motor neuropathy results in foot deformities and abnormal weight bearing, and autonomic neuropathy causes very dry skin and may contribute to osteopenia and fractures of the bones of the foot. Neuropathic changes often result in a foot ulcer, which is frequently complicated by infection and ischemia. These conditions collectively account for the morbidity and amputations associated with neuropathic ulcers (Birke & Sims, 1986; CDC, 2017; NIH, 2019; WOCN, 2012).

KEY POINT

Neuropathic changes often result in a foot ulcer, which is frequently complicated by infection and ischemia. These conditions together account for the morbidity and amputations associated with neuropathic ulcers.

SENSORY NEUROPATHY

Sensory nerves transmit messages related to touch, position, pressure, temperature, and pain such as the feeling of light touch or the pain caused by stepping on a sharp object. Sensory nerve damage causes a complex array of symptoms because sensory nerves have a diverse and highly specialized range of functions from detecting temperature and pain to detecting pressure and foot position. Patients with sensory nerve damage are typically unable to coordinate complex movements like walking or maintaining balance when their eyes are shut and are at increased risk of falling (Benn, 2020; WOCN, 2012).

Paresthesias are a very painful form of sensory neuropathy. The damaged nerves produce exquisite pain that is usually described as tingling, pins and needles, electric shock, burning, or stabbing in nature. Individuals with paresthesias frequently report that the pain is worse at night. They may also report severe itching, increased sensitivity to normally painless stimuli, as in the bed sheets touching the feet (allodynia) or an abnormally exaggerated response to painful stimuli (hyperalgesia) (Armstrong et al., 1997a; NIH, 2019; WOCN, 2012). Patients with paresthesias should be referred to a neurologist for evaluation and treatment, which typically involves anticonvulsant medications such as gabapentin or pregabalin.

KEY POINT

Paresthesias are a very painful form of sensory neuropathy. These patients require referral to a neurologist for evaluation and treatment.

Sensory neuropathy also causes progressive anesthesia and loss of proprioceptive sense, which accounts for most of the neuropathic ulcers and the increased risk of falling. Individuals with progressive anesthesia may report numbness that begins distally and progresses up the foot. The neuropathy typically occurs in a stocking and glove pattern, with patients feeling as though they are wearing stockings and gloves, although they are not. Many patients cannot recognize the shapes of small objects or distinguish among different shapes, just by touching. Individuals with progressive sensory neuropathy lose the ability to recognize minor and eventually major trauma to the feet. For example, the individual with sensory loss would not recognize a poorly fitting shoe or the resultant blister and would not recognize small objects in the shoe, such as a pebble. Individuals with advanced sensory loss may step on a needle or piece of glass without experiencing pain. They continue to walk on the foot, and the object becomes embedded, resulting in a major infection. Individuals with advanced disease can also sustain major burns from hot water without recognition. Loss of proprioceptive sense means the individual does not perceive situations in which the foot is on the edge of a step or on rough terrain and so does not make adjustments in posture, increasing the risk for falls (NIH, 2019; WOCN, 2012) (**Figs. 26-1 and 26-2**).

KEY POINT

Sensory neuropathy causes progressive anesthesia and loss of proprioception, which places the individual at risk for unrecognized trauma and for falls.

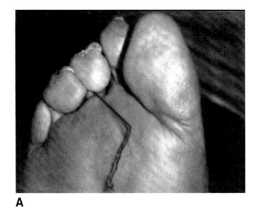
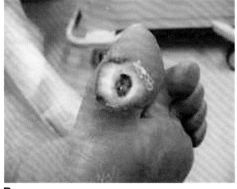

A   **B**

FIGURE 26-1. Injury/Ulceration due to Sensory Neuropathy. **A.** Direct injury from a sewing needle. **B.** Repeated pressure from walking.

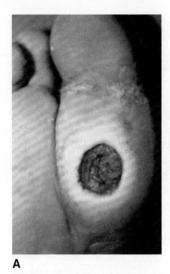

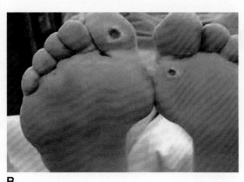

A   **B**

FIGURE 26-2. Injury/Ulceration due to Sensory Neuropathy. **A.** Metatarsal head wound with periwound callus. **B.** IP joint wound of great toe from hallux rigidus.

MOTOR NEUROPATHY

Motor nerves control movement and tone of the foot muscles and affect foot contours, weight bearing, and gait. Damage to the motor nerves altering the contours of the foot resulting in foot deformities, abnormal weight-bearing patterns, and altered gait. For example, abnormal rigidity of the toes and ankles due to atrophy of the intrinsic muscles is a common manifestation of motor neuropathy and causes increased plantar foot pressure when walking. Soft tissue glycosylation can result in shortening of the Achilles tendon, which causes deformities such as abnormally prominent metatarsal heads and claw toes. The abnormal prominence of the metatarsal heads causes abnormal weight bearing and increased exposure of the metatarsal heads to pressure and shear, which is manifest initially by callus formation and eventually by ulcer formation. Damage to the motor nerves can also result in footdrop (Birke & Sims, 1986; NIH, 2019; WOCN, 2012) (**Figs. 26-3 and 26-4** illustrate the effects of motor neuropathy).

> ### KEY POINT
>
> Motor neuropathy alters the contours of the foot, resulting in foot deformities, abnormal weight-bearing patterns, and altered gait.

AUTONOMIC NEUROPATHY

Autonomic nerves regulate biologic activities that are not under conscious control, such as thermal regulation and sweating, and blood vessel tone and diameter. Loss of autonomic control of the sweat glands commonly manifests as severely dry skin (anhidrosis) that may result in partial-thickness or full-thickness fissures. These wounds permit invasion of pathogens that can cause serious soft tissue infections. Autonomic neuropathy can also cause persistent vasodilation of the arterial vessels in the foot (hyperemia), due to loss of sympathetic innervation, which normally provides for partial constriction when the

foot is at rest. Persistent high-volume blood flow is thought to contribute to demineralization of the bones in the foot over time, which produces thin fragile bones (osteopenia) that are vulnerable to fracture. If a fracture is sustained but promptly recognized and appropriately managed with off-loading, the bone normally heals and there is no loss of structure. In many cases, the fracture is unrecognized due to coexisting sensory loss. If the fracture is unrecognized and the individual continues to walk on the damaged foot, additional fractures may occur with progressive damage to the bony structure of the foot.

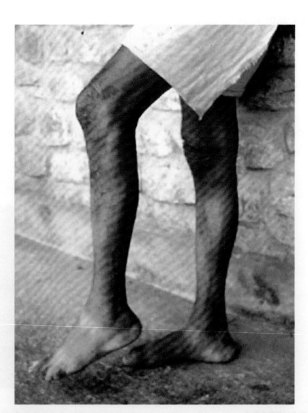

FIGURE 26-3. Changes Characteristic of Motor Neuropathy: Footdrop Related to Loss of Anterior Tibialis Muscle Function.

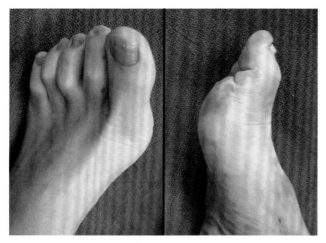

FIGURE 26-4. Changes Characteristic of Motor Neuropathy. Prominent metatarsal heads and claw toe deformity.

The end result may be total collapse of the normal architecture of the foot, with development of a rocker bottom foot that is at high risk for plantar surface ulcerations. This defect is known as Charcot neuroarthropathy. Autonomic involvement may also compromise the function of other body systems, causing complications such as urinary retention due to loss of detrusor contractility, gastroparesis and persistent vomiting due to loss of gastric motility, or lower extremity edema due to cardiovascular compromise (NIH, 2019; WOCN, 2012) (**Figs. 26-5 and 26-6**).

KEY POINT

Autonomic neuropathy causes altered function of the sweat glands, causing very dry feet (anhidrosis). It may also cause high-volume blood flow (hyperemia) that results in osteopenia and increased risk for fractures.

Patients may have a combination of different types of neuropathy concomitantly, such as sensory–autonomic or sensory–motor neuropathy (NIH, 2019; WOCN, 2012). See **Table 26-1** for a comparison of sensory, motor, and autonomic neuropathy.

 DIAGNOSIS OF LEND

Subjective awareness of LEND symptoms is often lacking, as symptoms may be subtle, particularly at the onset of the disease process, with the absence of sensation more difficult to recognize than the occurrence of pain. The diagnosis is also complicated by the fact that symptoms are highly variable.

HISTORY

Prompt diagnosis is dependent on a thorough history and physical exam and the performance of simple noninvasive tests to evaluate sensory, vibratory, and proprioceptive function. The history should include the patient's medical and surgical history, with a focus on chronic conditions known to cause neuropathy, the patient's symptoms, work environment, social habits (including past and current alcohol intake), exposure to toxins, known HIV disease (or risk factors), history of infectious diseases associated with neuropathy, family history of neurologic disease, and past or present use of medications associated with neuropathy (NIH, 2019; WOCN, 2012).

DIAGNOSTIC TESTS

Related diagnostic tests (e.g., CBC, CMP, HbA1c, thyroid profile, B$_{12}$ levels) should be ordered when the cause of the neuropathy is unclear, or for monitoring of a known disease process such as diabetes. Blood tests can be used to diagnose diabetes, vitamin deficiencies, liver or kidney dysfunction, and other hormonal or metabolic disorders and to identify signs of abnormal immune system

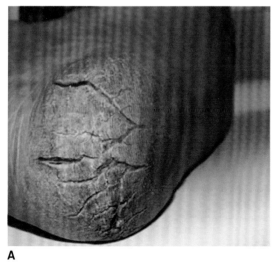

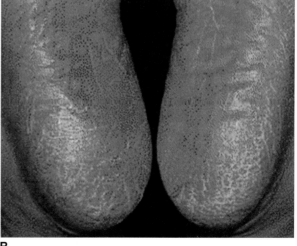

A **B**

FIGURE 26-5. Changes Characteristic of Autonomic Neuropathy: Dry Cracked Feet and Fissures due to Autonomic Neuropathy. **A.** Heel fissures. **B.** Anhidrosis.

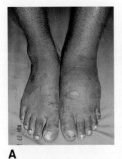 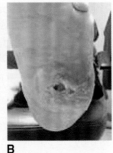 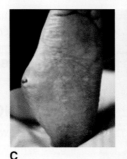 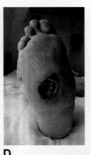 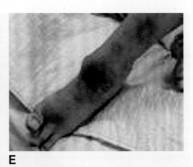

A **B** **C** **D** **E**

FIGURE 26-6. Changes Characteristic of Autonomic Neuropathy. **A.** Forefoot Charcot. **B, C.** Midfoot Charcot. **D.** Hindfoot Charcot. **E.** Ankle Charcot.

activity (CDC, 2017; NIH, 2019; WOCN, 2012). For the patient with diabetes, the HbA1c provides helpful information regarding glycemic control during the 3 months preceding the test.

Based on the results of the patient history, foot exam, tests of peripheral neurologic function, and any previous screening or testing, additional testing, and referral to a neurologist may be required to help determine the nature and extent of the neuropathy and to develop a management plan (NIH, 2019).

COMPREHENSIVE FOOT EXAM

A comprehensive foot exam (CFE) should be performed for at-risk patient populations to promptly identify changes in neurologic or vascular status that increase the risk for neuropathic foot wounds and amputations (Birke & Sims, 1986; CDC, 2017; NIH, 2019; WOCN, 2012). The American Diabetes Association (ADA) includes an annual CFE as a standard of care for individuals with diabetes (ADA, 2019; WOCN, 2012).

KEY POINT

An annual comprehensive foot exam is standard of care for individuals with diabetes.

Overview

The foot exam should be performed on both feet and should include general foot inspection (status of skin, hair,

TABLE 26-1 COMPARISON OF SENSORY, MOTOR, AND AUTONOMIC NEUROPATHY			
NEUROPATHIC COMPONENT	**PATHOPHYSIOLOGY**	**ASSESSMENT TOOLS**	**MANIFESTATION**
Sensory	• Myelin sheath is disrupted by hyperglycemia • Segmental demyelinization causes slowing of nerve conduction and impairment of sensory perception	• Sensory perception testing using a 10-g (5.07 Semmes-Weinstein) monofilament, to identify LOPS • Vibratory perception (using a tuning fork) • Position sense testing	• Loss of protective sensation/ increased risk for painless trauma • Sensory ataxia and increased risk of falls • Insensate lesions • Insensate injury • Charcot neuroarthropathy
Motor	• Atrophy of intrinsic muscles of the foot • Subluxation of metatarsophalangeal joints	• Gait assessment • Range of motion • Muscle testing • Deep tendon reflex testing • Observation for deformities, callus formation	• Callus • Claw/hammer toes • Muscle weakness • Contracture of Achilles tendon
Autonomic	• Loss of vasomotor control • Arterial–venous shunting • Bone blood flow hyperemia • Impaired microvascular skin perfusion	Thorough skin and nail assessment of: • Skin of LE and feet (observe for abnormal dryness and/or fissures) • Interdigital spaces • Evidence of fungal infections • LE hair growth	• Anhidrosis • Callus • Interdigital or plantar surface fissures • Onychomycosis (fungal skin and toenails) • Peripheral edema • Charcot neuroarthropathy

From Birke and Sims (1986), NIH (2019), Pecoraro et al. (1990), WOCN (2012).

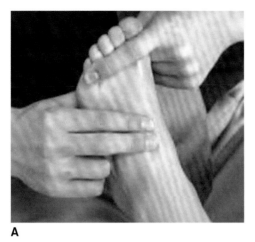 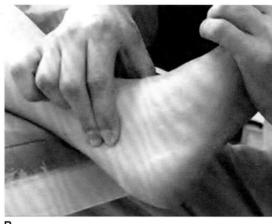

A
B

FIGURE 26-7. Pulse Palpation. **A.** Dorsalis pedis. **B.** Posterior tibialis.

and nails; presence of callus; presence, severity, and distribution of edema), palpation for increased or decreased temperature, assessment of foot pulses (**Fig. 26-7**), assessment of muscle strength at ankles and toes, observation for foot deformities (e.g., claw toes, prominent metatarsal heads, midfoot arch collapse, misshapen foot), testing for LOPS using the 10-g Semmes-Weinstein monofilament, testing for vibratory sense, and testing for position sense (ADA, 2019; Birke & Sims, 1986; Bonham & Kelechi, 2008; WOCN, 2012).

An in-depth assessment provides complete data regarding current foot status and risk factors for development of neuropathy and its complications. In some settings, an in-depth assessment is not feasible. In those settings, a modified assessment can be conducted using validated tools such as Inlow's 60-second Diabetic Foot Screen. This tool has been designed to allow the wound care nurse to screen persons with diabetes for diabetes-related foot ulcers and risk factors for ulceration and other limb-threatening complications. Positive findings on the 60-second Foot Screen mandate follow-up and provide guidance as to needed interventions (**Fig. 26-8**) (Canadian Association of Wound Care [CAWC], 2018).

Sensory Testing with 10-g Monofilament

The 10-g nylon monofilaments are constructed to buckle when a 10-g force is applied. Most monofilament exams call for filament application at 4 to 10 sites: 1st, 3rd, and 5th toes and metatarsal heads; medial and lateral midfoot; and dorsal surface between great toe and 2nd toe. The 10-point exam includes testing of the heel. Many wound care nurses use the 9-point exam, which excludes the heel, due to the high occurrence of false-negative readings at the heel as a result of callus and thickened skin. If the individual has a callus at any of the testing sites, the filament should be applied proximal to the callus.

The inability to detect 10 g of pressure at one or more anatomic sites on the plantar surface of the foot

is considered to be LOPS. LOPS places the individual at high risk for ulceration due to unrecognized repetitive trauma. The risk of ulceration is 9.9 times higher, and the risk of amputation among those with an ulceration is 17 times greater among individuals with LOPS as compared to those with intact sensation. Any individual who fails to respond to all test sites must receive intensive education and counseling regarding foot protection and daily foot inspection (Birke & Sims, 1986; NIH, 2019; Pecoraro et al., 1990; WOCN, 2012). See **Boxes 26-1 to 26-3 and Table 26-2**.

KEY POINT

Sensory function is tested with a 10-g monofilament. Failure to recognize 10 g of pressure represents loss of protective sensation (LOPS), which places the individual at risk for unrecognized repetitive trauma.

Vibratory Sense Testing

While monofilament testing is accepted as the most objective measure of sensory perception, vibratory sense testing is also a reliable and validated indicator of sensory perception. Data suggest that loss of vibratory sense typically occurs prior to LOPS. Vibratory sense testing may enable the wound care nurse to detect neuropathy at an earlier point and to intervene with education and counseling regarding the importance of tight glycemic control. To conduct vibratory sense testing, the wound care nurse uses a 128-Hz tuning fork. The tip of the vibrating fork is placed over the base of the great toe at the first metatarsal bone bilaterally, and the individual is asked to report the point at which vibration ceases. An abnormal response is defined as the individual's loss of vibratory sensation while the examiner still perceives it.

Position Sense Testing

Proprioception is the accurate detection of the foot's spatial position in relation to its environment and the rest

INLOW'S
60-second Diabetic Foot Screen
SCREENING TOOL

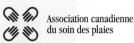

Canadian Association of Wound Care — Association canadienne du soin des plaies
www.cawc.net

Patient Name: _____   Clinician Signature: _____

ID number: _____   Date: _____

Look – 20 seconds	Score Left Foot	Score Right Foot	Care Recommendations
1. Skin 0 = intact and healthy 1 = dry with fungus or light callus 2 = heavy callus buildup 3 = open ulceration or history of previous ulcer			
2. Nails 0 = well-kept 1 = unkempt and ragged 2 = thick, damaged, or infected			
3. Deformity 0 = no deformity 2 = mild deformity 4 = major deformity			
4. Footwear 0 = appropriate 1 = inappropriate 2 = causing trauma			

Touch – 10 seconds	Left Foot	Right Foot	Care Recommendations
5. Temperature – Cold 0 = foot warm 1 = foot is cold			
6. Temperature – Hot 0 = foot is warm 1 = foot is hot			
7. Range of Motion 0 = full range to hallux 1 = hallux limitus 2 = hallux rigidus 3 = hallux amputation			

Assess – 30 seconds	Left Foot	Right Foot	Care Recommendations
8. Sensation – Monofilament Testing 0 = 10 sites detected 2 = 7 to 9 sites detected 4 = 0 to 6 sites detected			
9. Sensation – Ask 4 Questions: i. Are your feet ever numb? ii. Do they ever tingle? iii. Do they ever burn? iv. Do they ever feel like insects are crawling on them? 0 = no to all questions 2 = yes to any of the questions			
10. Pedal Pulses 0 = present 1 = absent			
11. Dependent Rubor 0 = no 1 = yes			
12. Erythema 0 = no 1 = yes			
Score Totals =			

Screening for foot ulcers and/or limb-threatening complications. Use the highest score from left or right foot.
- Score = 0 to 6 ➜ recommend screening yearly
- Score = 13 to 19 ➜ recommend screening every 3 months
- Score = 7 to 12 ➜ recommend screening every 6 months
- Score = 20 to 25 ➜ recommend screening every 1 to 3 months

Comments:

FIGURE 26-8. Inlow 60-Second Screening Tool.

Instructions for Use

General Guidelines: This tool is designed to assist in screening persons with diabetes to prevent or treat diabetes-related foot ulcers and/or limb-threatening complications. The screen should be completed on admission of any person with diabetes and then repeated as directed by risk and clinical judgment. **Do not confuse patient visits with patient screening.** Your patient may require frequent and regular visits for routine care but complete the screening as indicated or as relevant based on clinical judgment.

Specific Instructions:

Step 1: Explain screening to the patients and have them remove their shoes, socks from both feet.

Step 2: Remove any dressings or devices that impair the screening.

Step 3: Review each of the parameters for each foot as listed in the Inlow's 60-second Diabetic Foot Screen and select the appropriate score based on patient's status. (An amputation may affect the score on the affected limb.)

Step 4: Once the screen is completed determine care recommendations based on patient need, available resources and clinical judgement.

Step 5: Use the highest score from either the left or right foot to determine recommended screening intervals.

Step 6: Set up an appointment for the next screening based on screening score and clinical judgement.

Parameter Review

1. Skin

Assess the skin on the foot: top, bottom, and sides including between the toes.

0 = skin is intact and has no signs of trauma. No signs of fungus or callus formation

1 = skin is dry, fungus such as a moccasin foot or interdigital yeast may be present. Some callus buildup may be noted

2 = heavy callus buildup

3 = open skin ulceration present

2. Nails

Assess toenails to determine how well they are being managed either by the patient or professionally.

0 = nails well-kept

1 = nails unkempt and ragged

2 = nails thick, damaged, or infected

3. Deformity

Look for any bony changes that can put the patient at significant risk and prevent the wearing of off-the-shelf footwear

0 = no deformity detected

2 = may have some mild deformities such as dropped metatarsal heads (MTHs) (the bones under the fat pads on the ball of the foot). Each MTH corresponds to the toe distal to it, so there is a 1st MTH at the base of the first toe etc. Bunions/Charcot may also be considered a deformity as well as deformities related to trauma.

4 = Amputation

4. Footwear

Look at the shoes that the patient is wearing and discuss what he or she normally wears.

0 = shoes provide protection, support, and fit the foot. On removal of the footwear there are no reddened areas on the foot

1 = shoes are inappropriate do not provide protection or support for the foot.

2 = shoes are causing trauma (redness or ulceration) to the foot either through a poor fit or a poor style (e.g., cowboy boots).

5. Temperature – cold

Does the foot feel colder than the other foot or is it colder than it should be considering the environment? This can be indicative of arterial disease.

0 = foot is of "normal" temperature for environment.

1 = foot is cold – compared to other foot or compared to the environment

6. Temperature – hot

Does the foot feel hotter than the other foot or is it hotter than it should be considering the environment? This can be indicative of an infection or Charcot changes.

0 = foot is of "normal" temperature for environment

1 = foot is hot – compared to other foot or compared to the environment

7. Range of Motion

Move the first toe back and forth – plantar flex and dorsiflex.

0 = first toe (hallux) is easily moved

1 = hallux has some restricted movement

2 = hallux is rigid and cannot be moved

3 = hallux amputated

8. Sensation – Monofilament testing

Using the 5.07 monofilament, test the sites listed. Do not test over heavy callus.

- digits: 1st, 3rd, 5th
- MTH: 1st, 3rd, 5th
- midfoot: Medial, Lateral
- heel
- top (dorsum) of foot

And then score out of 10:

0 = 10 out of 10 sites detected

2 = 7 to 9 out of 10 sites detected

4 = 0 to 6 out of 10 sites detected

9. Sensation – Questions

Ask the following four questions:

i. Are your feet ever numb?

ii. Do they ever tingle?

iii. Do they ever burn?

iv. Do they ever feel like insects are crawling on them?

0 = answered No to all four questions

2 = answered Yes to one or more of the four questions

10. Pedal pulses

Palpate (feel) the dorsalis pedis pulse located on the top of the foot. If unable to feel the pedal pulse feel for the posterior tibial pulse beneath the medial malleolus.

0 = pulse present

1 = pulse absent

11. Dependent rubor

Pronounced redness of the feet when the feet are down and pallor when the feet are elevated. This can be indicative of arterial disease.

0 = no dependent rubor

1 = dependent rubor present

12. Erythema

Look for redness of the skin that does not change when the foot is elevated. This can be indicative of infection or Charcot changes.

0 = no redness of the skin

1 = redness noted

Reminder: Strategies for the prevention and management of diabetic foot ulcers need to consider more than just the results from a foot screen. It is important that the health care professional completes a holistic assessment that also monitors lipids, hypertension, glucose and patient activity and exercise. **Persons with diabetes who are cognitively impaired or have diseases such as end-stage renal disease are at higher risk and may need more frequent screening than indicated.**

FIGURE 26-8. *(Continued)*

Interpreting Results

Inlow's 60-second Diabetic Foot Screen has been designed to allow the clinician to screen persons with diabetes to prevent or treat diabetes-related foot ulcers and/or limb-threatening complications. By combining the results from different parameters identified with Inlow's 60-second Diabetic Foot Screen, the clinician can identify pathologies and/or care deficits.

Parameters 1	2	3	4	5	6	7	8	9	10	11	12	Indications
												Self-Care Parameters:
■	■		■									High scores in parameters 1, 2 and 4 → indicative of self care deficit.
												Integument Parameters:
			▨			▨						Moderate scores in parameters 4 and 7 → indicative of callus formation.
■					■						■	High scores in parameters 1, 6 and 12 → indicative of infected ulcer.
	■				■						■	High scores in parameters 2, 6 and 12 → indicative of infected nails.
												Arterial Flow Parameters:
				■					■	■		High scores in parameters 5, 10 and 11 → indicative of peripheral arterial disease.
												Sensation Parameters:
							■	■				High scores in parameters 8 and 9 → indicative of loss of protective sensation or neuropathy.
												Boney Changes Parameters:
		■					■	■				High scores in parameters 3, 8 and 9 → indicative of Charcot changes.

Determining Risk

Inlow's 60-second Diabetic Foot Screen can also assist in determining patient risk. By reviewing the results from Inlow's 60-second Diabetic Foot Screen, the clinician can use the International Working Group on the Diabetic Foot (IWGDF) – Risk Classification System to identify a risk category for the patients.

Step 1: Complete Inlow's 60-second Diabetic Foot Screen by assessing both feet on every patient with diabetes.

Step 2: Using the IWGDF Risk Classification System, identify which category your patients falls into.

International Working Group on the Diabetic Foot (IWGDF) —
Risk Classification System (Modified[1])

Risk Category	Criteria
0	Normal—no neuropathy
1	Loss of protective sensation
2a	LOPS and deformity
2b	Peripheral arterial disease
3a	Previous hx of ulceration
3b	Previous hx of amputation

1. Lavery, L., Peters, E., Williams, J., et al. (2008). Reevaluating the way we classify the diabetic foot: Restructuring the diabetic foot risk classification system of the International Working Group on the Diabetic Foot. Diabetes Care, *31*(1), 154–156.

Considerations Based on Clinical Settings

1. **Acute Care:** Due to the high turnover of patients in acute care, clinicians needs to ensure that the initial assessment goes with the patient to the next level of care.

2. **Long Term or Residential Care:** Patients with diabetes may have mobility issues and are in bed or wheelchairs. Feet still may become traumatized by the use of inappropriate footwear even if they are non–weight bearing.

3. **Dialysis Unit:** Some dialysis units may wish to augment this tool with toe pressures and blood work, depending on their clinical support.

4. **Home or Community Care:** Clinicians can use this tool for communication with their patients, each other, or other departments, such as specialized clinics.

5. **Foot Clinic:** Foot clinic standards of assessment will be at a higher standard. However, this document is a good communication tool with other clinicians who may be caring for the person with diabetes.

More Information

For more information on the assessment and management of the diabetic foot, refer to:

1. *Best Practice Recommendations for the Prevention, Diagnosis and Treatment of Diabetic Foot Ulcers*: Update 2010 at www.cawc.net
2. RNAO Best Practice Guideline *Reducing Foot Complications for Persons with Diabetes* at www.rnao.org
3. RNAO Best Practice Guideline *Assessment and Management of Foot Ulcers for People with Diabetes* at www.rnao.org
4. *The International Working Group on the Diabetic Foot* at www.iwgdf.org
5. *Diabetes, Healthy Feet and You* at www.cawc.net/index.php/public/feet/

FIGURE 26-8. (*Continued*)

BOX 26-1 INSTRUCTIONS FOR DIABETES FOOT SCREEN (BOX 26-2)

SECTION 1

The 12 questions can be answered in the "R" (right foot) or "L" (left foot) blank with a "Y" or "N" to indicate a positive or negative finding. Fill in all blanks.

Question 1: Is there a history of foot ulcer?

Question 2: Is there a foot ulcer now?

The purpose of these questions is to determine if the patient currently has or has ever had an ulcer on the foot. History of a foot ulcer places the patient at an increased risk of developing another foot ulcer and increases the potential of future amputation. The patient with a past or present foot ulcer is considered permanently in Risk Category 3.

Question 3: Is there toe deformity?

Question 4: Is there an abnormal shape of the foot?

This is determined by inspecting the general shape of the patient's foot. Conditions to consider include prominent bony areas, partial or complete amputations of the foot or toes, clawed toes, prominent metatarsal heads, bunions, or "Charcot foot."

A Charcot foot is a neuropathic foot that may present with swelling, increased temperature, and *little or no pain*. Advanced cases show progressive signs of deformity into what is referred to as a "rocker bottom" or "boat-shaped" foot. A patient with a Charcot foot is permanently in Risk Category 3.

Question 5: Are the toenails thick or ingrown?

Identify mycotic, significantly hypertrophic, or ingrown nails.

Question 6: Is there callus buildup?

Identify focal and/or heavy callus.

Question 7: Is there swelling?

Swelling may stem from a variety of causes such as a Charcot fracture, infection, venous insufficiency, or CHF.

Question 8: Is there elevated skin temperature?

Elevated, localized skin temperature can indicate excessive mechanical stress, bone fracture, or an infection and requires further evaluation. Skin temperature can be measured by a commercially available thermometer or by touch. A temperature elevation of >2°C on the thermometer or a noticeable difference by touch when compared with the contralateral foot is considered clinically significant.

Question 9: Is there muscle weakness?

A manual muscle test of foot and great toe dorsi- and plantar flexion.

Question 10: Can the patient see the bottom of his/her feet?

Obesity and/or lack of knee and hip flexibility can prevent a patient from seeing his/her feet. Self-inspection and foot care are difficult with these limitations often requiring family or outside assistance.

Question 11: Is the patient wearing improperly fitted shoes? Does the patient wear footwear appropriate for her/his category of risk?

An improperly fitted shoe may create foot pressures that lead to further complications. Patients with sensory loss often wear shoes that are too short and/or narrow resulting in ischemic ulcers on the medial or lateral metatarsal heads or the toes of a foot with claw toe deformity. Properly sized added depth shoes with soft custom-molded insoles are usually indicated for patients with loss of sensation and deformity to prevent ulceration.

Question 12: Is there an absent pedal pulse?

See risk and management categories.

SECTION 2

Examine the foot and record problems identified on the Foot Screen form. Draw calluses, preulcerative lesions (a closed lesion, i.e., blister or hematoma), or open ulcers as accurately as possible using the appropriate "pattern" to indicate what type of condition is present. Label areas that are red as "R," warm "W" (warmer than the other parts of the foot or the opposite foot), dry "D," or macerated "M" (friable, moist, soft tissue) on the corresponding location of the foot drawing provided on the screen form.

A sensory exam using the 10-g monofilament is performed as indicated on the foot drawing. Responses are recorded in the appropriate circles. A positive response is recorded in the corresponding circle with a "+" if the patient is able to feel the filament and a negative response is recorded with a "−" if the patient cannot feel the filament.

SECTION 3

The accurate placement of patients into their respective Risk Category is a key element in the Foot Screen. The higher the Risk Category, the higher the risk a patient has of recurrent foot ulceration, progressive deformity, and, ultimately, amputation of the foot. All patients, regardless of category, should be rescreened annually and should be given basic patient education.

A detailed description of the Risk Category is available in the document "Risk and Management Categories for the Foot."

---

of the body, without the benefit of visual input. Loss of normal proprioception places the individual at increased risk for falls. To test for proprioceptive sense, the person is asked to close the eyes. The wound care nurse then moves the great toe in different directions (up, down, medially, and laterally) and asks the person to tell in which direction the toe is pointing. Inability to consistently identify the direction in which the toe is pointing is considered loss of position sense. Joint position sensing is sensitive and specific enough to help diagnose PN when other testing is not possible (Prabhakar et al., 2019).

KEY POINT

To test for proprioceptive sense, the patient is asked to close the eyes. The wound care nurse then moves the great toe in different directions and asks the patient to state in which direction the toe is pointing.

Reflex Testing

Ankle reflexes can be tested with the patient either kneeling or resting on a couch or/table. The Achilles tendon is stretched until the ankle is in a neutral position. The wound care nurse then strikes the tendon with the reflex hammer and observes for plantar flexion. Total

BOX 26-2   DIABETES FOOT SCREEN INSTRUCTIONS FOR USE IN BOX 26-1

Name (Last, First, MI) _____   Date: ___/___/___

Fill in the following blanks with a "Y" or "N" to indicate findings of the right or left foot

	R	L
Is there a history of a foot ulcer?	_____	_____
Is there a foot ulcer now?	_____	_____
Is there toe deformity?	_____	_____
Is there swelling or an abnormal foot shape?	_____	_____
Are the toenails long, thick, or ingrown?	_____	_____
Is there heavy callus buildup?	_____	_____
Is there swelling?	_____	_____
Is there elevated skin temperature?	_____	_____
Is there foot or ankle muscle weakness?	_____	_____
Can the patient see the bottom of the feet?	_____	_____
Are the shoes appropriate in style and fit?	_____	_____
Is there limited ankle dorsiflexion?	_____	_____
Is there an absent pedal pulse?	_____	_____

Note the level of sensation in the circles:

+ = Can feel the 5.07 filament; **−** = Can't feel the 5.07 filament

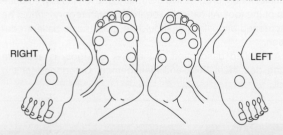

RIGHT   LEFT

Skin conditions on the foot or between the toes:

Draw in: Callous ▤, Preulcer ▦, Ulcer ■ (note length and width in cm)

Label with: **R**, redness; **M**, maceration; **D**, dryness; **T**, tinea

Risk Category:

_____ 0 No loss of protective sensation

_____ 1 Loss of protective sensation

_____ 2 Loss of protective sensation with *either* high pressure (callus/deformity) or poor circulation

_____ 3 History of plantar ulceration, neuropathic fracture (Charcot foot), or amputation

Rev 03/22/12 LSUHSC Diabetes Foot Program Performed by: _____

BOX 26-3   FILAMENT APPLICATION INSTRUCTIONS

Note: The sensory testing device used with the Diabetes Foot Screen is a nylon filament mounted on a holder that has been standardized to deliver a 10-g force when properly applied. Research has shown that a patient who can feel the 10-g filament in the selected sites has "protective sensation" and has a reduced risk of developing plantar ulcers.

1. Use the 10-g filament to test for "protective sensation."
2. Test the sites indicated on the Diabetes Foot Screen.
3. Apply the filament perpendicular to the skin's surface (see diagram **A**).
4. The approach, skin contact, and departure of the filament should be 1½ seconds.
5. Apply sufficient force to cause the filament to bend (see diagram **B**).

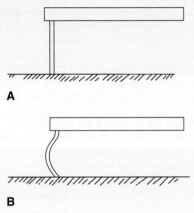

A

B

6. Do not allow the filament to slide across the skin or make repetitive contact at the test site.
7. Randomize the selection of test sites and time between successive tests to reduce patient guessing.
8. Ask the patient to respond "Yes" when the filament is felt and record the response on the Diabetes Foot Screen Form.
9. Apply the filament along the margin of and NOT on an ulcer, callus, scar, or necrotic tissue. DO NOT touch feet with hands-only filament.
10. Have the patient close the eyes while the filament test is being performed.

absence of ankle reflex is regarded as an abnormal result (WOCN, 2012). Abnormal ankle reflexes in conjunction with abnormal vibratory or sensory response is one of the most telling signs of PN (Abraham et al., 2017).

Assessment of Musculoskeletal/Biomechanical Status

Motor neuropathy causes loss of foot muscle strength and shortening of the Achilles tendon. These changes result in altered foot structure and abnormal gait as well as muscle wasting throughout the foot (NIH, 2019; WOCN, 2012). The effects of intrinsic foot muscle deterioration and limited ankle joint mobility have demonstrated significant prominence deformities involving metatarsal heads (Cheuy et al., 2016). Another common change in foot

TABLE 26-2 DIABETES FOOT PROGRAM

RISK CATEGORY	DESCRIPTION
Risk and management categories for the foot	
0	Diabetes, but no loss of protective sensation in feet
1	Diabetes, loss of protective sensation (LOPS) in feet
2	Diabetes, loss of protective sensation in feet with *either* high pressure (callus/deformity) or poor circulation
3	Diabetes, history of plantar ulceration or neuropathic fracture

Note: "loss of protective sensation" is assessed using a 5.07 monofilament at 10 locations on each foot

CATEGORY	MANAGEMENT CATEGORY
Lower extremity amputation prevention program	
0	Education emphasizing disease control, proper shoe fit/design Follow-up yearly for foot screen Follow as needed for skin/callus/nail care or orthoses
1	Education emphasizing disease control, proper shoe fit/design, daily self-inspection, skin/nail care, early reporting of foot injuries Proper fitting/design footwear with soft inserts/soles Routine follow-up 3–6 mo for foot/shoe examination and nail care
2	Education emphasizing disease control, proper shoe fit/design, self-inspection, skin/nail/callus care, early reporting of foot injuries Depth-inlay footwear, molded/modified orthoses; modified shoes as needed Routine follow-up 1–3 mo for foot/activity/footwear evaluation and callus/nail care
3	Education emphasizing disease control, proper fitting footwear, self-inspection, skin/nail/callus care, and early reporting of foot injuries Depth-inlay footwear, molded/modified orthoses; modified/custom footwear, ankle–foot orthoses as needed Routine follow-up 1–12 wk for foot/activity/footwear evaluation and callus/nail care

Diabetes Foot Clinic visit frequency may vary based on individual patient needs.

structure is displacement and thinning of the plantar surface fat pads, due to motor neuropathy, the effects of aging, or both which results in abnormally prominent metatarsal heads (Shirazi et al., 2016; LaBorde, 2009; Maluf et al., 2004). Changes in muscle tone and muscle function can also cause a variety of foot deformities. The claw toe deformity occurs as a result of hyperextension at the metatarsophalangeal joint combined with flexion contractures at the proximal and distal interphalangeal joints. The claw toe deformity usually affects all the toes, though the great toe, 2nd toe, and 3rd toe contractures are typically the most severe. This deformity places the individual at high risk for ulcerations commonly involving the plantar, distal, and dorsal toe surfaces. This is because the hyper-

extension causes the dorsum of the toe to point upward and the flexion contractures cause the distal toe to point downward. The individual will require extra-depth shoes and protection of the distal toe pad. The bony prominences are exposed to repetitive high pressure with every step (CDC, 2017; Cheuy et al., 2016; International Working Group on the Diabetic Foot [IWGDF], 2019; WOCN, 2012).

KEY POINT

To assess for motor neuropathy, the wound care nurse should observe for foot deformities, callus formation, and altered gait and weight bearing and should assess for range of motion, joint flexibility, and muscle strength.

Musculoskeletal assessment includes inspection of the contours of the foot and identification of any deformities. Abnormally prominent metatarsal heads and claw toe deformity are common abnormalities. Other potential deformities include hammer toes, overlapping toes, and forefoot, midfoot and hindfoot deformities, which could be suggestive of a Charcot foot, most commonly seen in the neuropathic or diabetic foot.

Callus formation at the site of the deformity is common, due to repetitive trauma, and can become like a stone or foreign body positioned between the shoe and the underlying bony prominence. The skin and soft tissue over bony deformities are at high risk for ulceration caused by this repetitive exposure to increased pressure and shear stress related to gait abnormality. The cumulative damage is typically unrecognized due to the effects of coexisting sensory neuropathy (Shirazi et al., 2016; WOCN, 2012) (**Fig. 26-9**).

The musculoskeletal assessment should also include muscle strength testing and gait evaluation. To assess muscle strength, the wound care nurse should place his or her hand against the plantar surface and ask the individual to push down against the hand. This should be repeated with the hand on the dorsal surface and the patient should push up. The wound care nurse should also assess range of motion and should be alert to any signs of muscle weakness, such as footdrop or visible atrophy. The wound nurse care should ask the individual to stand and walk and should note any patterned gait abnormalities of the posterior heel aspect, as well as frontal view. The nurse should use a Harris Mat if available to identify abnormalities in patterns of weight bearing.

It is also important to assess footwear for common wear patterns that can indicate gait abnormality and elevated stepping pressure and to observe for callus formation over the plantar surface, since callus formation is indicative of repetitive exposure to friction and superficial shear (Birke & Sims, 1986; Cheuy et al., 2016; IWGDF, 2019; WOCN, 2012; Zimny et al., 2004).

New technologies, known as Smart Shoes, which measure plantar pressure throughout the stepping process are available in the form of insoles. These technologies have

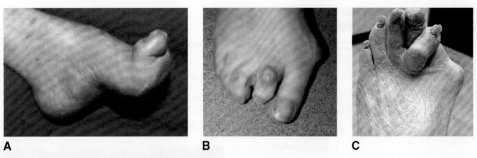

FIGURE 26-9. Common Foot Deformities. **A.** Prominent metatarsal heads. **B.** Bunion deformity and claw toes. **C.** Crossed toes.

sensors that measure and analyze force distribution of stepping on a patient's foot and then transmits these data by smart cellular technology to the provider. A visual representation of specific problem sites is also provided, which can be a teaching tool to use with patients (Hegde et al., 2016; Najafi et al., 2017).

Shoe Condition/Wear Patterns

The wound care nurse should assess the patient's footwear for general condition, wear patterns along the outer soles and heels, and bottomed out areas in the insoles and interior shoe lining. All of these findings are indicative of abnormal pressure points and gait abnormalities. It is also important for the wound care nurse to assess the footwear for appropriateness of fit and design in relation to the size and shape of the patient's foot (Health Resources and Services Administration [HRSA], 2017; WOCN, 2012). Providing patients with a tracing pattern of their feet offers an objective tool to identify appropriateness of shoe design and sizing. The tracing should be made with the patient in a standing position and with weight equally distributed over both feet. The individual's shoes should then be placed over the tracing. If the foot tracing extends beyond the shoe margins, the shoes are not appropriate for that individual to wear (HRSA, 2013; IWGDF, 2019; WOCN, 2012).

> **KEY POINT**
>
> Providing patients with a tracing pattern of their feet offers an objective tool to identify appropriateness of shoe design and sizing.

Pressure mapping is used to identify high pressure points. It is first performed with the patient standing with weight equally distributed and then with a step in motion, which identifies any abnormal pressure points as the patient progresses through the gait cycle. Pressure mapping capability is now available in commercial settings such as local pharmacies and shoe stores that offer over-the-counter insoles and shoes without a prescription. It is also used by orthotists or pedorthotists to identify insoles that provide even weight distribution (WOCN, 2012) (**Fig. 26-10**).

Vascular Assessment

Lower extremity vascular assessment is a key element of neuropathic foot workup, because 30% of patients with neuropathic disease have coexisting arterial disease, which has a profound impact on management and prognosis (Causey et al., 2016). The important elements of vascular assessment include general inspection of the skin, hair, and nails to identify atrophic changes, assessment of pedal pulses and capillary refill, and measurement of ankle–brachial index (ABI) or pulse volume recording (PVR). For a detailed description of the parameters and processes included in a comprehensive vascular exam, please refer to Chapter 25.

> **KEY POINT**
>
> Vascular assessment is a critical element of the comprehensive foot exam. Thirty percent of patients with neuropathic disease also have lower extremity arterial disease or neuroischemia, which can have a profound effect on management and prognosis.

Dermal Temperature Assessment for Soft Tissue Inflammation

Dermal temperature measurement with an infrared, noncontact thermometer is identified by the IWGDF as one of the most valuable technological developments for the objective measurement of inflammation. An increase in temperature of >2°C at a particular plantar foot site, as compared to the same site on the contralateral foot or to nonaffected areas of the same foot, is considered to be positive for inflammation (Armstrong & Lavery, 1997; Armstrong et al., 2007; IWGDF, 2019; Lavery et al., 2004; WOCN, 2012). Dermal temperature assessments are performed at sites of bony deformity and at sites of previous ulceration. This simple measurement can be a powerful addition to the comprehensive foot assessment and can also be used to assess the efficacy of off-loading measures throughout and following healing. Data indicate that 82% of neuropathic foot wounds are preceded by inflammation and callus, which means that the observation of either callus formation or temperature elevation should prompt the wound care nurse to implement preventive care such as assessing adequacy of plantar pressure redistribution and frequent monitoring of the involved area (Armstrong et al., 2007; IWGDF, 2019; Lavery et al., 1997, 2007; Sage et al., 2001; WOCN, 2012). Infrared dermal thermometers are

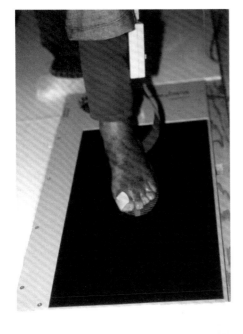

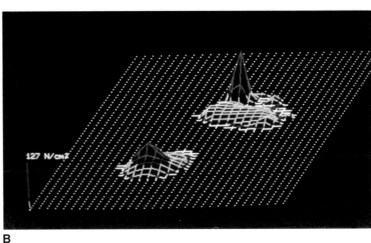

A   **B**

FIGURE 26-10. A, B. Pressure Mapping.

currently available from a variety of retail sources and medical equipment providers with prices ranging from $20 to $800. In a study comparing nine commercially available infrared thermometer options, the lesser priced options performed as well as the higher priced options, in terms of detecting a temperature difference (Foto et al., 2009) **(Fig. 26-11)**.

A variety of new technologies that use Smart device, wireless cell connectivity have emerged that provide temperature readings of specific foot locations. These are of particular benefit for patients with visual impairment or other debilitating conditions. Some of the technologies are wearables, such as socks or insoles, that provide continuous monitoring as frequently as every 2 minutes, and others are episodic, such as shoe insoles and mats, that collect data at predetermined and on-demand intervals (Hegde et al., 2016; Najafi et al., 2017). All of the systems provide data to the prescribing provider, and some provide data for patients. Some also provide color-sensitive thermograms that highlight hot spots (Abbott et al., 2019; IWGDF, 2019; Killeen et al., 2020) **(Fig. 26-12)**.

In a mat study, 129 participants' plantar temperatures were monitored on a daily basis. A total of 37 (28.7%) presented with 53 DFU (0.62 DFU/participant/year). Using the standard threshold of 2.2°C asymmetry of specific healed and at-risk foot sites using contralateral foot measurements, the system correctly predicted 97% of subsequent DFU, with an average lead time of 37 days (Frykberg et al., 2017).

Another recent mat study of 129 patients already amputated of one LE, was performed to identify comparisons among ipsilateral (same foot) foot temperatures. Using this approach, monitoring a single foot was found to predict 91% of impending nonacute plantar foot ulcers on average 41 days before clinical presentation (Lavery et al., 2019) **(Fig. 26-13)**.

KEY POINT

Dermal temperature measurement can be used to detect inflammation, which is indicated by an increase in temperature of >2°C at any site as compared to an unaffected area of the same foot or on a symmetrical area of the contralateral foot.

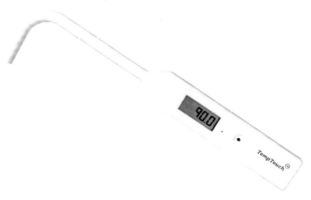

FIGURE 26-11. TempTouch Dermal Thermometer.

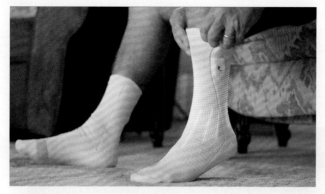

FIGURE 26-12. Smart Socks Technology.

Skin, Nail, and Soft Tissue Assessment

The wound care nurse should assess the skin for color, texture, and turgor, with particular attention to the presence, location, and distribution of any calluses, and skin hydration and the presence of fissures. A callus is a thickened area of skin that occurs in response to repeated exposure to friction, shear, and pressure. Calluses develop over sites of abnormally high pressures associated with altered foot contours and gait (**Fig. 26-14**). Callus development is supported by elevated blood glucose levels, which cause the tissue to become rigid, inflexible, and more resistant to collagenase digestion. Calluses can be generalized, as is seen over the heel,

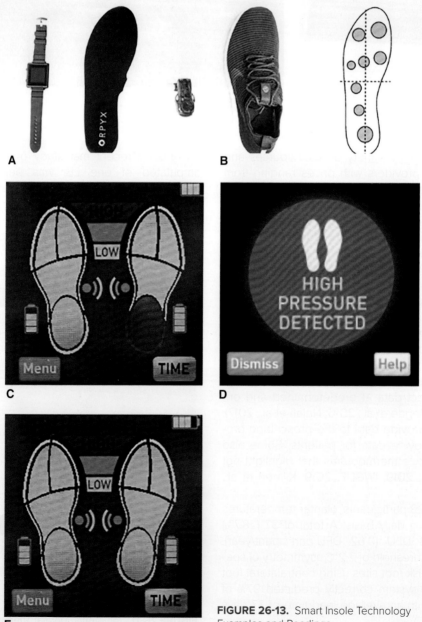

FIGURE 26-13. Smart Insole Technology Examples and Readings.

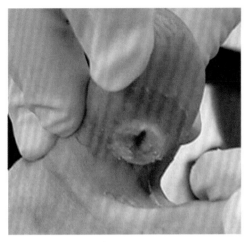

FIGURE 26-14. Interdigital Callus.

or focal, as is frequently seen over the metatarsal heads. Focal calluses are unyielding and particularly destructive lesions because the callus itself increases the pressure and shear exerted on the underlying tissue during walking. A common scenario includes abnormal gait and weight bearing leading to callus formation, further leading to development of an ulcer of the tissue beneath the callus. Because the individual frequently has sensory as well as motor neuropathy, there is typically no discomfort associated with either the callus or the ulcer. The ulcer may go unrecognized for a period of time, especially if the patient does not practice daily foot self-care. Hemorrhage into a callus is a heralding sign of ulceration beneath the callus (IWGDF, 2019; Sage et al., 2001; WOCN, 2012).

In conducting the foot examination, the wound care nurse should observe for and palpate any calluses and should intervene, especially for rigid focal calluses located over bony prominences. Interventions include paring of the callus and providing recommendations regarding pressure redistributing footwear and insoles.

Focal calluses are particularly destructive lesions because the callus itself increases the pressure and shear exerted on the underlying tissues during walking. It is important to ensure proper off-loading after debridement and paring of any plantar callus sites, especially over bony deformities, as the likelihood of developing a wound with weight bearing is increased if pressure is not addressed.

Skin hydration is another critical assessment parameter. Autonomic neuropathy adversely affects the function of the sweat glands, and the most common outcome is very dry skin known as anhidrosis, which may result in fissure formation, typically over the heels and lateral foot aspect. Overhydration of the skin occasionally occurs, and also increases the risk for fissure formation. Fissure formation due to overhydration usually involves the interdigital spaces as well as the skin fold at the base

of the toes on the plantar foot surface. The wound care nurse should assess for either overly dry or overly moist skin and for fissure formation. In assessing the skin, the wound care nurse should also be alert to any lesions and any evidence of fungal infections, which are common among the diabetic population. Tinea pedis is the most common fungal infection involving the foot, with differing clinical presentations based on the specific organism involved. Tinea may manifest as very dry, scaly, circular lesions on the plantar surface, with no itching or pain, or as an acute infection involving the dorsal surface, with erythema, blistering, and pain. Tinea infections can also cause interdigital fissures (IWGDF, 2019; Sage et al., 2001; WOCN, 2012) (**Fig. 26-15**).

The wound care nurse should also assess the nails with emphasis on the presence of ingrown nails (onychocryptosis), cuticle infections (paronychia), or fungal infections of the nails (onychomycosis) with the appearance of thickened, discolored, or abnormally crumbly nails (WOCN, 2012).

The wound care nurse should assess for lower extremity edema, noting the type and severity and whether the edema is unilateral or bilateral. Edema may be related to comorbid conditions such as heart failure, nephropathy, or venous insufficiency. Unilateral edema may be a heralding sign of Charcot deformity (i.e., neuropathic fracture), especially if the edema is accompanied by increased warmth and bounding pulses (IWGDF, 2019; Seidel, 2006; WOCN, 2012). A detailed description of venous insufficiency and lymphedema is provided in Chapter 24.

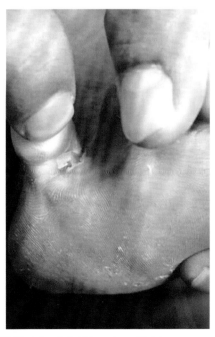

FIGURE 26-15. Interdigital Tinea from Moisture.

TABLE 26-3 CLINICAL CHARACTERISTICS OF NEUROPATHIC ULCERS

WOUND FEATURE	DESCRIPTION
Shape	Usually are rounded or oblong and found over bony prominence May initially be covered with callus tissue May resemble laceration, puncture, or blister, if from direct trauma, shearing, or heat
Wound base	May be necrotic, pink, or pale Depth varies from partial thickness to deep bone involvement
Wound edge	Typically well-defined and smooth edges May or may not have undermining
Periwound	Callus formation around the wound is common when the individual is walking/weight bearing on wound Continued development of callus after serial debridement may indicate inadequate off-loading of pressure Erythema and induration may indicate infection and/or cellulitis Maceration may be present
Exudate	Drainage is usually small to moderate in amount Large amounts of exudate may indicate complicating factors, including venous insufficiency, heart failure, renal failure or insufficiency, or infection Color is usually serous or clear Foul odor and purulence are common indicators of infection
Location	The majority of neuropathic/diabetic foot wounds are located at pressure points and bony deformities on the plantar surface of the forefoot Most common sites are the interphalangeal joint of the great toe and 1st and 5th metatarsal heads

From Falanga (2005), Pecoraro et al. (1990), Sage et al. (2001), Weir (2010), WOCN (2012), Zimny et al. (2004).

ASSESSMENT AND CLASSIFICATION OF NEUROPATHIC FOOT ULCER

If the individual presents with a foot ulcer, the wound care nurse should conduct a comprehensive assessment of wound status (IWGDF, 2019; Seidel, 2006; WOCN, 2012). See Chapter 4 for parameters to be included in wound assessment and see **Table 26-3** for clinical characteristics of neuropathic ulcers.

Several wound classification systems have been developed to assist the wound care nurse in classifying and synthesizing assessment data related to foot ulcers in the diabetic population. Classification systems provide a consistent approach and a common language for health care professionals to describe neuropathic foot ulcers, which directs treatment and reimbursement for care. The IWGDF has analyzed the classification systems to recommend which classification system to use for particular guidance. They recommend (1) for communication among health professionals the use of the SINBAD system (that includes Site, Ischemia, Neuropathy, Bacterial Infection, and Depth) (**Box 26-4**); (2) no existing classification for predicting outcome of an individual ulcer; (3) the Infectious

BOX 26-4   THE SINBAD CLASSIFICATION SYSTEM FOR FOOT ULCERS

CATEGORY	DEFINITION	SINBAD SCORE	EQUIVALENT S(AD)SAD CATEGORIES
Site	Forefoot	0	—
	Midfoot and hindfoot	1	—
Ischemia	Pedal blood flow intact: at least one pulse palpable	0	0–1
	Clinical evidence of reduced pedal blood flow	1	2–3
Neuropathy	Protective sensation intact	0	0–1
	Protective sensation lost	1	2–3
Bacterial infection	None	0	0–1
	Present	1	2–3
Area	Ulcer <1 cm^2	0	0–1
	Ulcer ≥1 cm^2	1	2–3
Depth	Ulcer confined to skin and subcutaneous tissue	0	0–1
	Ulcer reaching muscle, tendon, or deeper	1	2–3
Total possible score		6	—

Source: Ince, P., Abbas, Z. G., Lutale, J. K., et al. (2008). Use of the SINBAD classification system and score in comparing outcome of foot ulcer management on three continents. *Diabetes Care, 31*(5), 964–967.

BOX 26-5 WAGNER CLASSIFICATION SYSTEM

0: At-risk foot, preulcer, no open lesions, skin intact; may have deformities, callus, or cellulitis
1: Superficial ulcer with partial- or full-thickness tissue loss
2: Probing to ligament, tendon, or joint capsule with soft tissue infection
3: Deep ulcer with abscess, osteomyelitis, or joint sepsis
4: Gangrene localized to toes or forefoot
5: Ulcer with gangrene involving entire foot, beyond salvage

BOX 26-6 UNIVERSITY OF TEXAS DIABETIC FOOT CLASSIFICATION SYSTEM

Grading
0: Pre- or postulcer with epithelization
1: Superficial wound not involving tendon, bone, or capsule
2: Ulcer penetrates to tendon or capsule
3: Ulcer penetrates to bone or joint

Staging
A: Neuropathic wound: noninfected/nonischemic
B: Acute Charcot joint: infection present
C: Infected diabetic foot with ischemia
D: Ischemic limb with infection

Diseases Society of America/IWGDF (IDSA/IWGDF) classification for assessment of infection; (4) the WIfl (Wound, Ischemia, and foot Infection) system for the assessment of perfusion and the likely benefit of revascularization; and (5) the SINBAD classification for the audit of outcome of populations (Monteiro-Soares et al., 2020) (**Box 26-4**). Other systems are required for reimbursement for certain treatments. Common systems are reviewed briefly. Additional information can be found at https://iwgdfguidelines.org/.

WAGNER CLASSIFICATION SYSTEM

The Wagner Classification System was originally developed as a treatment guideline, to provide direction for level of surgical intervention (IWGDF, 2019; Wagner, 1981; WOCN, 2012) (**Box 26-5**). It is also used to objectively identify wounds for which treatment with hyperbaric oxygen therapy (HBOT) would be appropriate. A Wagner Grade 3 diabetic foot ulcer qualifies for HBOT. Limitations of this system include limited focus on perfusion status and the presence and severity of neuropathy.

KEY POINT

Several classification systems for foot ulcers in the diabetic population are available including the Wagner Classification System and the University of Texas Diabetic Foot Classification System.

UNIVERSITY OF TEXAS DIABETIC FOOT CLASSIFICATION SYSTEM

The University of Texas Diabetic Foot Classification System (**Box 26-6**) classifies the wound by grade and by stage. Grade captures the depth of the wound and staging captures complications affecting healing, specifically infection and ischemia (Lavery et al., 1996; WOCN, 2012). The classification system has been validated through a retrospective analysis of 360 diabetic patients in an outpatient diabetic foot clinic. The validation study demonstrated that wound outcomes deteriorated as the grade and stage of wounds increased. Healing time has been shown to correlate positively with grade of ulcer. There is a direct relationship between higher stage and greater time to healing and increased risk of amputation (Lavery

et al., 1996). One advantage of this system is its predictive value.

A classification system used with patients having neuroischemic feet was devised by the Society for Vascular Surgery, categorizing and grading the three major risk factors leading to amputation: wound, ischemia, and foot infection. Termed the WIfl Classification System, it merges existing classification systems, including the IDSA classification for diabetic foot infections, into a single concise system. After grading each category, one can then clinically stage the affected limb to estimate risk of amputation at one year, using a smart device calculator (Causey et al., 2016; Cull et al., 2014; Darling et al., 2016; Mills et al., 2014; Zhan et al., 2015). **Figure 26-16** outlines the WIfl system and **Figure 26-17** the IWGDF/IDSA System.

⬤ MANAGEMENT OF NEUROPATHIC ULCERS

Wound management for neuropathic foot wounds includes a focus on basic wound bed preparation tenets as well as management of systemic conditions affecting wound healing (tight glycemic management) and correction of neuropathic wound etiology, which is mainly related to gait abnormalities and off-loading, which is the relief of repetitive pressure and shear stress.

KEY POINT

Management of neuropathic wounds must also include tight glycemic management, and basic wound bed preparation tenets.

NEUROPATHIC FOOT AND WOUND OFF-LOADING

Routine activities, such as walking, can result in repetitive stress and pressure over bony prominences, especially when there are foot deformities and limitations in joint mobility that result in altered gait and abnormal

WIfI Classification System—The Society for Vascular Surgery Lower Extremity Guidelines Committee published a classification system for threatened lower limbs, categorizing and grading (03) the three major risk factors leading to amputation: wound, ischemia, and foot infection (WIfI). The WIfI classification system has been validated to accurately assess amputation risk at one year from initial pathology.

Amputation risk is calculated from input of the assessment components below via digital calculator (app)

Wound Grade	DFU	Gangrene
0	No ulcer *Clinical description: minor tissue loss*	No gangrene
1	Small, shallow ulcer(s) on distal LE or foot; no exposed bone (unless most distal toe aspect) *Clinical description: Salvageable with simple digital amputation with skin coverage*	No gangrene
2	Deeper ulcer with exposed bone, joint, or tendon; generally does not involve the heel Shallow heel ulcer without calcaneal involvement *Clinical description: major tissue loss, salvageable with multiple (≥3) digital amputations or standard transmetatarsal amputation (TMA), may not have skin coverage*	Gangrenous changes limited to digits
3	Extensive, deep ulcer involving the forefoot and/or midfoot; deep, full-thickness heel ulcer with calcaneal involvement *Clinical description: Extensive tissue loss salvageable only with complex foot reconstruction or nontraditional TMA; skin flap coverage or complex wound management needed for large soft tissue defect*	Extensive gangrene involving forefoot and/or midfoot; full-thickness heel necrosis with calcaneal involvement

Ischemia Grade	Ankle–Brachial Index	Ankle Systolic Pressure (mm Hg)	Toe Pressure, Transcutaneous Oxygen Pressure
0	≥0.80	>100	≥60
1	0.6–0.79	70–100	40–59
2	0.4–0.59	50–70	30–39
3	≤0.39	<50	<30

FIGURE 26-16. WIfI Classification System. (From Beropoulis et al., 2016; Causey et al., 2016; Cull et al., 2014; Darling et al., 2016; Mills et al., 2014; Zhan et al., 2015.)

weight bearing. This repetitive stress is a significant component in the pathway to ulcerations in the neuropathic foot. Once an ulcer develops, the continued exposure to pressure and shear prevents healing and contributes to wound deterioration, sometimes to bone. Effective off-loading is a key component of a comprehensive prevention program and an important element of a comprehensive neuropathic wound management plan (Caselli et al., 2002; IWGDF, 2019; WOCN, 2012).

Off-loading is defined as the removal of focal pressure from a specific foot site or area with subsequent redistribution of that pressure over the larger foot surface. The practice of off-loading is a key intervention utilized throughout all phases of the neuropathic diabetic foot unless the deformity is surgically corrected (HRSA, 2017; IWGDF, 2019).

KEY POINT

Routine activities, such as walking, can result in repetitive stress and pressure over bony prominences, especially in patients with altered gait and abnormal weight bearing. Once an ulcer develops, continued exposure to pressure and shear prevents healing and contributes to deterioration.

Effective off-loading is not typically accomplished with use of off-the-shelf self-selected shoes or therapeutic diabetic shoes. Inexpensive Med-Surg shoes do optimize off-loading and promote wound healing. These shoes are designed to permit customization and accommodation of the patient's foot wound and for any site (from toes to heel and either dorsal or plantar surface). An available, reasonably priced, off-the-shelf Med-

IWGDF/IDSA System PEDIS Guideline*

Clinical Manifestations	Infection Severity	Pedis Grade
Wound lacking purulence or manifestations of inflammation	Uninfected	1
Presence of ≥2 manifestations of inflammation (purulence or erythema, tenderness, warmth or induration), but any cellulitis/erythema extends ≤2cm around the ulcer, and infection is limited to the skin or superficial subcutaneous tissues; no other local complications or systemic illness	Mild	2
Infection (as above) in a patient who is systemically well and metabolically stable, but which has ≥1 of the following characteristics: cellulitis extending >2cm, lymphangitic streaking, spread beneath the superficial fascia, deep-tissue abscess, gangrene, and involvement of muscle, tendon, joint, or bone	Moderate	3
Infection in a patient with systemic toxicity or metabolic instability (e.g., fever, chills, tachycardia, hypotension, confusion, vomiting, leukocytosis, acidosis, severe hyperglycemia, or azotemia)	Severe	4

*IWGDF- International Working Group on the Diabetic Foot
*IDSA- Infectious Diseases Society of America
*PEDIS- Perfusion, extent(size) depth (tissue loss), infection, sensation (neuropathy)

Note: Infection refers to any part of the foot, not just of a wound or an ulcer. In any direction, from the rim of the wound. The presence of clinically significant foot ischemia makes both diagnosis and treatment of infection considerably more difficult. If osteomyelitis is demonstrated in the absence of ≥2 signs/symptoms of local or systemic inflammation, classify the foot as grade 3. This guideline is to guide assessment and identification.

FIGURE 26-17. IWGDF/IDSA System PEDIS Guideline.

Surg shoe system with foot in motion pressure mapping data is made and distributed by Darco International. The Darco system for providing customized pressure relief involves the following steps: a transparent film dressing is placed over the wound and the wound site is marked with lipstick; the patient is then asked to step onto the insole, which transfers the marked site onto the insole; the clinician then removes pegs from the insole in the marked area to create off-loading of the wound site during weight bearing. Additional accommodative shoe options are available for forefoot ulcers (Ortho wedge); forefoot, midfoot, and some Charcot foot ulcers (DARCO wound healing shoe); and heel ulcers (heel wedge) (Birke et al., 2000, 2002; IWGDF, 2019; WOCN, 2012). All of these options have simple customization procedures and simple instructions (**Figs. 26-18 and 26-19**).

KEY POINT

Off-loading is defined as the removal of focal pressure from a specific foot site or area and subsequent redistribution of that pressure over the larger foot surface.

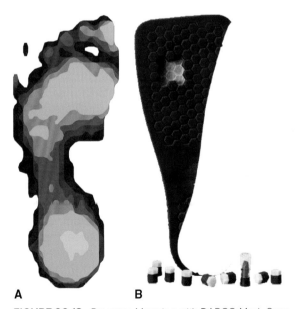

A   **B**

FIGURE 26-18. Pressure Mapping with DARCO Med–Surg Shoe with Peg-Assist Insole. **A.** Pressure mapping. **B.** Pegs can be removed in areas of high pressure or ulceration to provide off-loading. (Courtesy Darco International. http://www.darcointernational.com.)

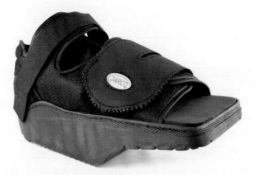

FIGURE 26-19. DARCO OrthoWedge. (Courtesy Darco International. http://www.darcointernational.com.)

Off-Loading and Soft Tissue Management

Off-loading provides for tissue load management of the foot, just as a support surface provides for effective tissue load management across the resting surface of the body. The goal of tissue load management is to maintain soft tissue viability, support the bony architecture, and promote wound healing by protecting the affected site(s) against pressure and shear. Off-loading devices used for prevention are designed to eliminate peak pressures by providing even pressure distribution. Off-loading devices used for treatment are designed to eliminate shear and pressure in the affected area to optimize healing.

Products that provide even distribution of plantar surface pressures (such as customized insoles) can be used for prevention of neuropathic ulcers. Treatment of plantar surface ulcers requires use of products that completely off-load the ulcerated area such as a total contact cast (TCC).

Effective off-loading requires an understanding of plantar surface biomechanics and the complex nature of foot-to-ground interactions. The two mechanical forces that contribute most significantly to neuropathic ulcerations are pressure and shear. Peak plantar pressures are highest in the forefoot and midfoot, compared with the rear or hindfoot. When the metatarsal heads are abnormally prominent, the forefoot pressures are further increased. Charcot foot deformity also causes a marked increase in plantar surface pressures, commonly in mid- and forefoot pressures. Shear forces are affected by friction exerted against the plantar foot surface during walking and related gait velocity and muscle strength. Studies are ongoing in regard to the relative roles played by pressure and shear, with the goal of developing a clinical model that can be used to develop footwear that provides better protection against plantar surface ulceration (IWGDF, 2019; WOCN, 2012; Yavuz et al., 2007, 2008).

Gait abnormalities are common among individuals with neuropathy. These abnormalities play a major role in development of plantar surface ulcers. For example, patients frequently exhibit a conservative gait strategy characterized by slower walking speed and wider gait base, which results in prolonged foot support (increased

pressure) and increased shearing of plantar soft tissue during walking. Glycosylation of soft tissues associated with hyperglycemia causes shortening of the plantar surface tendons. This causes reduced flexibility of ankle, subtalar, and first metatarsophalangeal joints, which has been shown to result in high focal plantar surface pressures and increased risk of ulceration. Motor neuropathy can cause loss of anterior tibialis muscle strength and tone, which results in footdrop and further derangement in gait and pressure distribution. Assistive devices such as ankle–foot orthotics (AFOs) and braces can provide at least partial correction of footdrop and resultant gait abnormalities. Physical therapists should be routinely consulted for evaluation and management of gait abnormalities. All prefabricated off-loading devices must be carefully assessed to provide effective accommodation for the size and shape of the patient's foot with even pressure distribution, and reduction in shear force (Birke et al., 2000, 2002; WOCN, 2012).

Off-Loading Modalities for Treatment of Neuropathic Ulcers

TCC has been considered the gold standard for off-loading neuropathic foot wounds. Studies of the TCC have demonstrated healing rates as high as 95% at 12 weeks (Lewis & Lipp, 2013). Newer data support that any properly fitting nonremovable knee-high off-loading devices such as TCCs and removable walkers that are knee-high that can be rendered to be nonremovable with a strap or wrap, are equally effective and considered the gold standard (IWGDF, 2019). A TCC is minimally padded and molded carefully to the shape of the foot. A rocker bottom walking plate is then attached to allow limited ambulation while completely off-loading the forefoot until the ulcer heals (**Fig. 26-20**). The TCC is closed at the distal foot (toes) to provide protection. It is initially changed every 5 to 7 days, but once the ulcer stabilizes and the

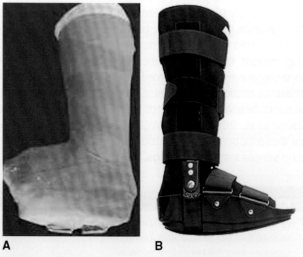

A   **B**

FIGURE 26-20. A. Total contact cast. **B.** Removable cast walker.

exudate and edema are controlled, it can be changed every 1 to 2 weeks.

Total contact casting (TCC) is considered the gold standard for off-loading neuropathic foot wounds and is associated with healing rates as high as 95% at 12 weeks.

TCCs have fixed ankle support and a rigid rocker sole (typically). This prevents forward motion of the tibia during mid-stance, limits forward propulsion during stepping, and redistributes some of the pressure and shear forces to the device. The rocker bottom sole prevents focal pressure during stepping and allows the foot to glide through the stepping phases, totally protecting the forefoot. Ankle high TCCs are not recommended as they do not provide enough casting material and support to transfer pressure and shear forces to the cast. Not all patients with diabetes and foot ulcers are good candidates for TCC. Contraindications for TCC include documented LEAD, active wound infection or a sinus tract with deep extension into the foot that requires daily access for wound care, unstable gait, fluctuating edema, active skin disease, restless leg syndrome, cast claustrophobia or known nonadherence to treatment plan, and lack of adequately trained staff to apply the TCC (Armstrong et al., 2005; IWGDF, 2019; Lewis & Lipp, 2013; WOCN, 2012).

Effective application of a TCC requires a skilled provider. Inappropriate application creates the risk of acquiring device-related pressure injury that goes unrecognized, due to sensory neuropathy, until the cast is changed. Products are being developed that provide for simplified application (e.g., Total Contact Cast EZ®). Another approach is to place the patient in a removable cast walker (RCW) and then to wrap the RCW with cast material to render it nonremovable, which is known as instant total contact cast (iTCC). Some clinicians use the iTCC until the wound is 50% healed and then omit the cast wrapping, converting the device back to an RCW. If healing stalls (likely due to incomplete adherence to off-loading), the clinician can reinstitute the iTCC. Limitations of the iTCC and RCW involve the application of a prefabricated, fixed device to feet that may be misshapen and are typically insensate. Care must be taken to ensure that the fixed device will accommodate the size (especially width) and shape of the patient's foot and will not cause pressure injury in the absence of sensation (Armstrong et al., 2005; IWGDF, 2019; Nabuurs-Franssen et al., 2005; WOCN, 2012).

The TCC and other nonremovable devices are associated with the highest healing rates because they eliminate the issue of patient adherence encountered when using a removable device. Modification of a standard

RCW to increase patient adherence to off-loading (iTCC) may increase both the proportion of ulcers that heal and the rate of healing for diabetic neuropathic wounds (Armstrong et al., 2005; Nabuurs-Franssen et al., 2005; WOCN, 2012).

The TCC and other nonremovable devices are associated with the highest healing rates because they eliminate the problem of patient nonadherence often encountered with removable devices.

Monitoring technologies that identify patient adherence to wearing removable devices are available that can be easily placed within the TCC, iTCC without interfering with off-loading and without patient knowledge (IWGDF, 2019).

There are a variety of off-loading options referenced, but none provide the same rate and degree of healing as the irremovable TCC and iTCC (Armstrong et al., 2005). In clinical situations when expertise applying TCC or iTCC is not available, or when the wound and neuropathic issues (e.g., deformity, gait issues) are minimal, other off-loading options may be feasible. For example, selected systems are commercially available that are relatively inexpensive and that allow for customization for elimination of pressure at the specific wound sites (e.g., DARCO Peg Assist System). Another option is to use accommodative dressings, such as adhesive felt pads and toe crests in combination with off-loading shoes (Birke et al., 2002; IWGDF, 2019; Katz et al., 2005; WOCN, 2012).

One simple and inexpensive approach to off-loading that can be used for patients with plantar metatarsal head ulcers involves use of adhesive felt pads. The adhesive felt is cut to the shape of the foot with a cutout that accommodates the wound site; the felt is then applied directly to the skin surface and secured with a conformable gauze dressing. The patient is then placed in a Med-Surg shoe that accommodates the dressing. The pad remains on the foot at all times and is changed at least weekly by the wound care nurse. This approach has demonstrated excellent off-loading of plantar surface wounds over metatarsal heads (**Fig. 26-21**).

Devices such as crest pads can be used to reduce pressure on the distal toes for patients with claw toes. These devices are made of rolled gauze covered with moleskin, with a cutout in the moleskin for toe placement (Beuker et al., 2005; Birke et al., 2002; IWGDF, 2019; WOCN, 2012). See **Figure 26-22**, which illustrates the crest pad procedure. See **Table 26-4** for off-loading options.

An inexpensive dressing that uses routinely available supplies and does not require the skill of a TCC to apply

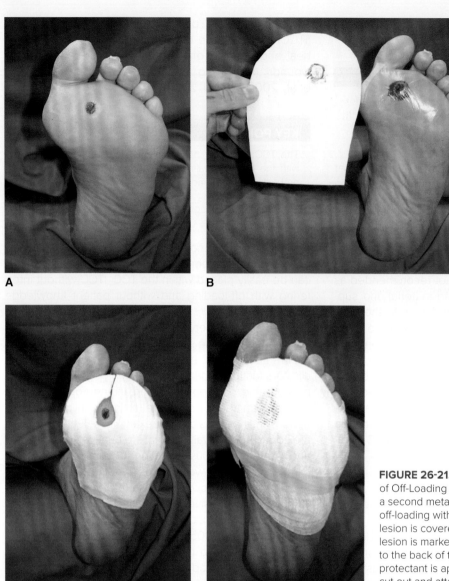

FIGURE 26-21. Steps of Procedure for Construction of Off-Loading Adhesive Felt Pad. **A.** Individual with a second metatarsal head preulceration suitable for off-loading with an adhesive felt relief pad. **B.** The lesion is covered with a transparent dressing and the lesion is marked with lipstick. The mark is transferred to the back of the ¼ inch adhesive felt pad. **C.** Skin protectant is applied to the foot, and the felt pad is cut out and attached insuring that the relief hole is directly over the lesion area. **D.** The pad is wrapped with a roll gauze dressing and secured with tape.

is the Football Dressing. This dressing is used for Grade 3 or 4 Wagner plantar forefoot ulcerations (**Fig. 26-23**; **Box 26-7**).

Assessment of Effective Off-Loading

The wound care nurse managing the patient with a neuropathic ulcer must continually evaluate the effectiveness of the management plan, which includes evaluation of the ability of the off-loading device to sufficiently protect the ulcer from pressure and shear. Specific indicators of off-loading effectiveness include progress in wound healing dimension, improved wound bed tissue quality, minimal recurrence of periwound callus, and absence of localized inflammation as indicated by dermal temperature measurements (i.e., absence of any sites where temperature is > 2°C greater than adjacent or contralateral

sites). In-shoe devices that provide for interface pressure measurements are another option that is gaining recognition in the clinical arena (Abbott et al., 2019; IWGDF, 2019; Lavery et al., 2004; WOCN, 2012).

Off-Loading for Ulcer Prevention

There is limited literature addressing the efficacy of off-loading for prevention of wounds. A Cochrane Review of four off-loading studies for prevention randomized controlled trials (RCTs) found that in-shoe orthotics are of benefit. Other pressure-relieving interventions such as running shoes are widely used but have not been adequately evaluated scientifically, and removable casts or foam inlays do not appear to have been evaluated at all in RCTs (Cavanagh & Bus, 2011; IWGDF, 2019; Spencer, 2000; WOCN, 2012; Yavuz et al., 2008). In identifying

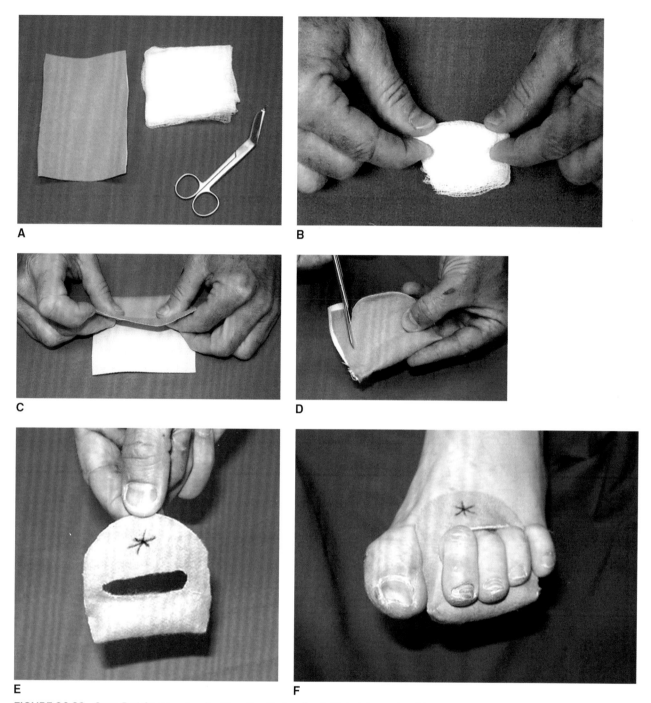

FIGURE 26-22. Crest Pad Construction for Claw Toe Deformity. **A.** Materials used to fabricate a crest pad: moleskin, gauze, scissors. **B.** Cut three to four gauze sponges to size and roll tightly. **C.** Fold moleskin tightly over roll of gauze. **D.** Trim Moleskin as shown. **E.** Finished crest pad with hole cut out for toes. **F.** Crest pad fit to the patient with claw toe deformity and preulcerative callus over the second and third toes.

patients who may benefit from preventive off-loading, the wound care nurse should be aware that risk factors for neuropathic ulceration including the following:

- LOPS demonstrated by a 10-g monofilament exam.
- Bony deformity of toes or foot (claw toes, prominent metatarsal heads, Charcot foot, etc.).
- Rigid interphalangeal and/or ankle joints.

- Compromised arterial perfusion (ABI < 0.9 or > 1.3).
- Focal callus formation.
- History of previous foot ulceration or amputation. Individuals who are unable to visualize the entire foot due to poor eyesight (e.g., due to diabetic retinopathy) or to limited hip/knee joint flexion that makes it difficult to bring the foot within the visual field are also at risk (IWGDF, 2019; NIH, 2019; WOCN, 2012).

TABLE 26-4 OFF-LOADING OPTIONS FOR THE MANAGEMENT OF WOUNDS DUE TO LEND

OFF-LOADING METHOD	ADVANTAGES	DISADVANTAGES	WOUND SITES
Bed rest	• TOTAL non–weight bearing	• Patient adherence is difficult • Presents quality of life issues for patients • Promotes hyperglycemia • Promotes patient debilitation • Increases risk for posterior heel pressures	• All wound sites

Total contact cast	• Gold standard
	• Limits ambulation
	• Irremovable: forces patient compliance
		• Not advisable to use for:
		  • Patients with LEAD
		  • Patients with unstable gait
		  • Infected wounds
		  • Highly exudative wounds
		  • Patients with leg tremors
		  • Claustrophobic patients
		• Requires high clinical skill to apply
			• All wound sites

Walking splints Removable cast shoes	• Provides daily wound surveillance and care • Good option for infected wounds	• Requires strict patient adherence • Requires assistive ambulating device	• All wound sites
Football dressing	• Simple to make • Inexpensive • Ease of use with dressings • Irremovable: forces patient compliance	• May present balance issues	• Forefoot ulcers
Wedge sole shoe with removable off-loading pegs	• Available commercially • May be customized • Inexpensive	• May present balance issues	• Forefoot ulcers
Heel sole shoe with removable off-loading pegs	• Available commercially • May be customized • Inexpensive	• May present balance issues	• Plantar/posterior heel ulcers
Custom modified healing shoe with extra depth toe box	• Provides pressure relief specific to wound location	• Requires specialized equipment • Requires specialized skill to make	• All wound sites
Adhesive felt pad	• Simple to make • Inexpensive • Ease of use with dressings	• Requires at least weekly replacement	• Metatarsal head ulcers
Felted foam pads	• Simple to make • Inexpensive • Ease of use with dressings	• Requires every 3- to 4-day replacement	• Claw toes
Interdigital pads (silicone or foam), lamb's wool padding	• Available commercially • May be used for wound prevention or during healing	• May increase forefoot width	• Crowded toes • Crossed toes • Interdigital wounds
Padded socks	• Available commercially	• May cause local foot ischemia and/or constriction if shoe fit does not allow for increased padding	• Bony deformities
Ball and ring shoe stretcher	• Available commercially • Simple to use • Provides pressure relief on leather shoes at specific sites of bony foot deformity	• Does not work with nonleather shoes	• Bony deformities

Adapted from information in Beuker et al. (2005), Birke et al. (2002), Bus et al. (2008), Cavanagh and Bus (2011), Frykberg et al. (2006), Steed et al. (2006).

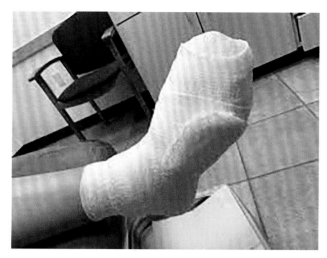

FIGURE 26-23. Football Dressing.

KEY POINT

Individuals at risk for plantar surface ulcerations those with LOPS, LEAD, bony deformities, or history of ulceration require prevention; in-shoe orthotics are of proven benefit, and running shoes are widely used though they have not been scientifically evaluated.

Current recommendations for preventive off-loading in patients with an at-risk foot are as follows:

- Teaching patients to avoid walking barefoot or in stocking feet indoors or outdoors.
- Regular callus removal provided by a skilled health care professional.
- Therapeutic footwear, including a custom-molded insole in a shoe with adequate depth toe box (for individuals at significant risk of ulceration, such as those with foot deformities or history of ulceration); therapeutic footwear should be worn during both indoor and outdoor walking (Cavanagh & Bus, 2011).
- Some off-the-shelf athletic shoe designs are acceptable as a shoe option for patients who do not have severe foot deformities. A shoe list that indicates shoes that can be obtained from local stores can be of great benefit to patients who would benefit from a properly designed off-the-shelf shoe. It is important for wound care nurses to investigate appropriate shoe options within their communities to compile a shoe list to provide patients with a reliable guide to shoes that are both appropriate and available.

COMMERCIALLY AVAILABLE SHOES

Individuals with intact sensation and no deformities can wear commercially available shoes so long as they meet the following criteria for correct fit:

1. Allow for ½ inch space beyond the longest toe.

BOX 26-7   FOOTBALL DRESSING DIRECTIONS FOR FOREFOOT ULCERS

The football dressing consists of: (1) Liquid skin protectant; (2) ¼ inch Adhesive felt; (3) 3 rolls of 4 inch cast padding; (4) 1 roll of 4 inch gauze; (5) 1 roll of 4 inch self-adherent wrap.

APPLICATION DIRECTIONS
1. Apply skin protectant to the periwound.
2. Cut adhesive felt to the shape of the forefoot—cut out a relief at the site of the wound.
3. Apply primary wound dressing over the felt—absorbent foam is a good option based on drainage.
4. The initial layer of cast padding is fan folded and applied in a longitudinal fashion.
5. A second layer is then applied circumferentially about the forefoot.
6. The final layer is applied from the forefoot proximally to the lower leg.
7. A layer of 4 inch gauze is then applied over the entire dressing and is covered by a layer of self-adherent elastic wrap applied without tension.
8. A standard postoperative shoe was dispensed for ambulation on the dressing.

From Rader, A. J., & Barry, T. P. (2008). The football: An intuitive dressing for offloading neuropathic plantar forefoot ulcerations. *International Wound Journal, 5*(1), 69–73. doi: 10.1111/j.1742-481X.2007.00364.x.

2. Allow adequate width and depth to accommodate for toe spread and clearance.
3. Ensure adequate width at the ball of the foot.
4. Assure adequate fit from heel to ball of foot.
5. Assure that the shape of the shoe matches the shape of the foot.

When purchasing shoes, individuals should be counseled to adhere to the following guidelines:

- Size and purchase shoes in the afternoon to accommodate foot edema.
- Stand and walk when sizing and purchasing new shoes.
- Wear socks or stockings that would normally be worn with the shoes during sizing and fitting of new shoes.
- Measure both feet and size shoes to fit the larger foot
- Gradually increase wear time for new shoes, that is, by 2-hour increments each day, with routine foot inspection following each wearing.

THERAPEUTIC FOOTWEAR

- All individuals with any degree of LOPS should have their footwear professionally fitted, because their sensory deficits preclude recognition of problems with the fit of their shoes. Appropriately fitting footwear is critical for indoor as well as outdoor use for all individuals, and especially those who lack normal protective sensation. Individuals with LOPS and foot deformities, callus, impaired perfusion, or history of ulceration or amputation require therapeutic, customized shoes that are sized correctly, effectively accommodate any deformities, and provide even pressure distribution. Therapeutic footwear is a benefit allowed by many insurers in the United States for individuals with diabetes who meet established criteria. At the time of this writing, this benefit does not apply to individuals with neuropathy caused by disease processes other than diabetes. Criteria that qualify patients for therapeutic footwear include the following: Signed and dated Certifying Physician Statement (physician managing the beneficiary's systemic diabetes condition) that specifies the BENEFICIARY MEETS ALL THE CRITERIA LISTED BELOW (CMS, 2018):

- Certifying Physician is an MD (Medical Doctor) or DO (Doctor of Osteopathy)
- Has diabetes
- Has one of the following conditions:
    a. Previous amputation of the other foot, or part of either foot, or
    b. History of previous foot ulceration of either foot, or
    c. History of preulcerative calluses of either foot, or
    d. Peripheral neuropathy with evidence of callus formation of either foot, or
    e. Foot deformity of either foot, or
    f. Poor circulation in either foot is being treated under a comprehensive plan of care for diabetes and needs diabetic shoes
- The certification statement was signed on or after the date of the in-person visit and within 3 months prior to delivery of the shoes/inserts and meets CMS Signature Requirements
- Clinical evaluation documenting the management of the patient's diabetes
    - Evaluation was performed by the Certifying Physician;
    - Visit occurred within 6 months prior to delivery; and
    - Signature meets CMS Signature Requirements
- **Supplier in-person evaluation** conducted prior to or at the time of selection of items includes at least the following:
    - An examination of the patient's feet with a description of the abnormalities that will need to be accommodated by the shoes/inserts/modifications
    - Measurements of the patient's feet; and
    - For custom molded shoes and inserts, information regarding taking impressions, making casts,

or obtaining CAD-CAM images of the patient's feet that will be used in creating positive models of the feet
- **In-person visit, at the time of delivery**, which assesses the fit of the shoes and inserts with the patient wearing them

KEY POINT

Individuals with LOPS and foot deformities, callus, impaired perfusion, or history of ulceration or amputation require therapeutic customized footwear that accommodate any deformities and provide even distribution of plantar surface pressures.

Therapeutic footwear include the following features: (1) extra depth toe box; (2) constructed of leather or suede (preferably); (3) cushioned outer soles; (4) customizable insole cushioning that provides pressure redistribution/relief of pressure at common pressure points, in addition to shear reduction; and (5) option to customize as needed with rocker bottom soles or heel flares. Rocker bottom soles prevent focal pressure to plantar surface sites because they allow the foot to glide through the step without pressure at any point during stepping. Shoes with flared heels provide extra stability for people who strike the ground at midfoot or forefoot (HRSA, 2017; IWGDF, 2019; WOCN, 2012).

Customizable insoles that provide even pressure redistribution and shear reduction are an important feature of therapeutic footwear. Pressure mapping is being increasingly used by orthotists and pedorthists to identify high-pressure areas as a basis for insole customization. A study evaluated the ability of custom insoles designed to match the patient's foot and weight-bearing patterns to reduce plantar surface pressures. Twenty patients with 70 high-pressure areas were evaluated, and pressure was effectively reduced in 64 out of 70 sites. The investigators concluded that use of pressure mapping to develop custom insoles provides positive outcomes in the majority of cases (IWGDF, 2019; Owings et al., 2008).

Another study compared a shear-reducing insole with standard therapy (i.e., extra depth shoes with molded insoles designed to reduce vertical pressure) in the management of 299 diabetic patients with severe neuropathy or a history of previous ulcer or amputation. Patients received podiatrist evaluation, sensorimotor and vascular assessment, and diabetes education. The shear-reducing insole was constructed of two viscoelastic layers, with two intervening thin sheets of a low friction material. This design was shown to reduce peak shear force (but not vertical pressure) by 57%, as compared to three other multilayer viscoelastic insoles that did not have the intervening layers. Among those with a previous ulcer, there was a relative 90% reduction in ulcers (13 out of 38 vs. 1 out of 40). At least in patients with a history of a foot ulcer, reducing shear stress in addition to standard reduction of vertical forces resulted in 90% reduction in foot ulcer recurrence. No benefit was found in patients without a previous plantar foot ulcer (Lavery et al., 2005).

Evidence suggests that insoles with bidirectional fabric coverings that are designed to reduce shear force may be beneficial in reducing the incidence of recurrent ulceration in individuals who have a history of plantar surface ulcers. Additionally, smart insoles are available that can measure both increasing plantar dermal temperature as well as plantar pressure (Abbott et al., 2019).

TOPICAL WOUND CARE

Topical therapy and dressing selection for management of neuropathic ulcers are based on the principles of moist wound healing, specifically exudate management, maintenance of a moist wound bed, and protection of the periwound skin. These principles and guidelines have been addressed in detail in Chapters 8 and 9. The discussion in this chapter will be limited to considerations and evidence unique to neuropathic ulcers.

Dressings

Dressings must be compatible with the off-loading devices in use. Patients being off-loaded with a TCC require dressings that are designed for weekly dressing changes. Dressings with lower moisture vapor transmission rates (MVTR) have been associated with faster healing than those with higher MVTR. In a study involving 36 diabetic patients and 10 Hansen disease patients, 80% healed in 10 weeks with consistent off-loading using a TCC and moisture-retentive dressings (Bolton, 2007).

Any dressings and particularly dressing material used to secure leg and foot dressings should be conformable and accommodating to edema, as the neuropathic patient may not have the ability to identify issues caused by tightening dressings (HRSA, 2017).

A study reviewing clinical literature to identify optimal dressings and topical options for DFU management noted that most of the differences between dressings were not significant. According to the analysis of the nine dressing types, amniotic membrane and hydrogel dressings are the most advantageous in terms of promoting DFU healing. The most suitable dressing should be selected taking into consideration exudate control, comfort, and cost (Zhang et al., 2018). The IWGDF also recommend that dressings are selected principally on the basis of exudate control, comfort, and cost. They recommend not using dressings containing surface antimicrobial agents with the sole aim of accelerating the healing of an ulcer (IWGDF, 2019).

The IWGDF also recommends consideration of the use of negative pressure wound therapy (NPWT) to reduce wound size in patients with diabetes and a postoperative surgical wound on the foot. Since NPWT has not been shown to be superior to heal a nonsurgical diabetic foot ulcer, they suggest preference for best standard wound care (IWGDF, 2019).

Accommodative dressings are designed to provide topical therapy while also providing off-loading of pressure. When using accommodative dressings, it is important to avoid adding other topical dressings that will interfere with the off-loading benefit (IWGDF, 2019). Examples of accommodative dressings include adhesive felt pads for plantar metatarsal head ulcers, football dressings for plantar forefoot ulcers, and crest pads for claw toe deformity ulcers.

Advanced Wound Therapies

Biologic wound dressings, categorized as skin substitutes and dermal cellular tissue replacements, are available for use with diabetic foot wounds and have demonstrated accelerated wound healing when used in combination with adequate wound off-loading. These biologic dressings provide a matrix or scaffolding that promotes cell migration and cellular activities associated with wound healing. They also provide a variety of growth factors, stem cells, and other substances that promote healing and are typically missing in the chronic wound environment.

Definitive comparisons regarding efficacy of one skin substitute type to another is lacking. In a technical paper by the AHRQ, literature regarding 74 commercially available skin substitutes and cellular and tissue-based products to treat chronic wounds were reviewed. Twenty-five of the skin substitutes are specific to DFU. The majority of the skin substitutes are acellular and are derived from human amniotic membrane (the inner layer of the placenta), animal tissue, or human cadaver skin. Available published studies rarely reported whether wounds recurred after initial healing and rarely reported outcomes important to patients, such as return of function and pain relief. Further review is ongoing (Snyder et al., 2020). Biologic dressings are intended for use during the proliferative phase of repair and should not be used until the wound bed is completely clean and infection has been controlled.

Management Bacterial Loads

Heavy bacterial loads prolong the inflammatory phase and prevent the proliferative processes required for wound healing. Individuals with diabetes are at high risk for infectious complications, especially if their glucose levels are poorly controlled and they have coexisting ischemic disease. *Staphylococcus aureus* is the predominant pathogen in diabetic foot infections, but the microbiology of diabetic foot infections includes increased incidence of multidrug-resistant organism (MDRO) infections, such as MRSA, and MSSA has been associated with a higher rate of treatment failure.

Predisposing factors to MDRO infections include prolonged duration of the wound, previous hospitalizations, chronic kidney disease, and nasal colonization with MRSA. Foot wounds with ischemia or gangrene may have anaerobic pathogens. Effective management of the patient with a neuropathic wound includes monitoring for indicators of wound infection and prompt treatment of any infection that occurs to reduce the risk of serious infections progressing to limb loss. There is no evidence to support the use of prophylactic antibiotic therapy. See Chapter 11 for additional information on infection.

> ### KEY POINT
>
> Effective management of the patient with a neuropathic wound includes monitoring for indicators of wound infection and effective management of any infection that does occur to reduce the risk of serious infections progressing to limb loss.

The wound care nurse must be aware that the signs of infection may be subtle in the diabetic patient, especially when there is coexisting ischemia and sensory neuropathy. The wound care nurse must be alert to mild erythema and limited induration with or without complaints of pain or tenderness. The wound care nurse must also be aware that surface infection (colonization) manifests primarily as deterioration in the quality and quantity of granulation tissue, failure to progress, and indicators of persistent inflammation (such as persistent high-volume exudate).

> ### KEY POINT
>
> The diagnosis of wound infection is typically made clinically. The wound care nurse must be aware that signs of infection may be subtle in the diabetic patient, especially if there is coexisting ischemia and sensory neuropathy.

Aggressive intervention is required for infections characterized by deep abscess, extensive bone or joint involvement, crepitus, gangrene, or necrotizing fasciitis. An infectious disease consult may be indicated, in addition to systemic antibiotic therapy and surgical debridement of all necrotic tissue. Severe infections will progress to necrosis without aggressive treatment. They often require intravenous antibiotics and surgical debridement. A foot complicated by ischemia also requires vascular reconstruction.

> ### KEY POINT
>
> Aggressive intervention with infectious disease consult and systemic antibiotic therapy is indicated for deep abscesses, extensive bone or joint involvement, crepitus, substantial necrosis, or necrotizing fasciitis.

Systemic antibiotic therapy is an important element of management for infection involving the periwound tissues, bones, or joints. To assure the use of the appropriate antibiotic, a wound culture should be obtained prior to the initiation of antibiotic therapy whenever there is viable tissue exposed in the wound bed. Tissue obtained by biopsy, ulcer curettage, or aspiration is preferable to wound swab specimens and is considered the gold standard for confirming a diagnosis of infection in diabetic, neuropathic ulcers. Transcutaneous bone biopsies are considered the most accurate approach to diagnosis of osteomyelitis. While tissue culture is ideal, in many settings, this is not an option and the wound care nurse must obtain a swab culture. In this case, the culture should be obtained using the Levine technique. This technique is described in detail in Chapter 11.

Surface infection can usually be managed with topical antimicrobial agents (antiseptics and/or antibiotics). In the patient with diabetes and increased risk of limb-threatening sepsis, systemic antibiotic therapy may be required in addition to topical agents to prevent progression to invasive infection. Topical mupirocin may be used short term (typically <2 weeks) in conjunction with systemic antibiotics. Use of topical antibiotics should be based upon culture results as each has a defined bactericidal spectrum.

There is lack of consensus about the use of topical antimicrobial therapy in addition to systemic antibiotic therapy for infected neuropathic ulcers, especially those complicated by ischemia. Topical agents may help to eradicate MDROs and to promote healing and should generally be considered for at least a 2-week trial in wounds that are responding poorly to systemic agents alone. Topical treatments may also be helpful in the removal of biofilms, which have been implicated in persistent infections. Another approach to delivery of antibiotics is local implantation of antibiotic beads and gels following surgical debridement of necrotic tissue. These agents have proven useful in promoting wound cleansing, limb salvage, and earlier surgical closure.

> ### KEY POINT
>
> A 2-week trial of adjuvant topical antimicrobial therapy should be considered for wounds responding poorly to systemic antibiotics alone.

Evaluation of the neuropathic foot with a wound should involve a thorough examination of the extremity for clinical signs of infection, along with laboratory and imaging studies. (See **Table 26-5** for laboratory and imaging indicators of infection.) In patients with foot ulcers and diabetes, laboratory markers may or may not be elevated in the presence of infection. Normal lab results do not preclude infection. Invasive infection requires culture-based antibiotic therapy and prompt removal of any necrotic tissue. An infectious disease

TABLE 26-5 LABORATORY AND RADIOLOGIC INDICATORS OF INFECTION

IMAGING STUDY	BENEFITS	COMMENTS
Useful imaging studies for diagnosing wound infection		
Plain x-rays	Can detect foot abnormalities such as osteomyelitis, fractures, Charcot foot, soft tissue gas, foreign bodies or structural foot deformity	The sensitivity of plain x-rays is variable and may be attributable to timing of the radiograph in relation to the chronicity of the ulcer
Magnetic resonance imaging (MRI)	Considered the gold standard in diagnosing osteomyelitis	Selective for soft tissue lesions with good sensitivity and specificity: sensitivity 90% and specificity 79%
Technetium-99 phosphate bone scan	Demonstrates moderate accuracy for diagnosis of infection in the toes and forefoot	
Indium-111 (leukocyte scan)	Demonstrates moderately good discrimination characteristics for diagnosing infection and has a low-to-moderate accuracy for osteomyelitis	Usually available in most facilities and at a lower cost than MRI/CT
Positron emission tomography (PET)	PET scans can demonstrate the difference between Charcot foot and florid osteomyelitis	Other more cost-effective options are available, such as plain x-rays

consult may be required and, when there is bone or joint involvement, an orthopedic consult may also be needed. Surface infection can usually be managed with topical antibacterial agents (WOCN, 2012).

OSTEOMYELITIS

Osteomyelitis is an infectious complication of particular importance in the management of diabetic foot ulcers because there are multiple bones in each foot with little soft tissue. Surface infection can rapidly progress to deep soft tissue and bone infection. Diabetes is associated with three comorbid conditions that increase the risk of bone infection: immunocompromised, neuropathy, and arterial disease. *Staphylococcus aureus* is the predominant pathogen, but streptococcal infections are also common, and either pathogen can result in necrotizing fasciitis. Osteomyelitis should be suspected with any tunneling wound and any wound with exposed bone and must be ruled out when there is evidence of Charcot osteoarthropathy. MRI has demonstrated the highest sensitivity and specificity for evaluating soft tissue and bone pathology in patients with diabetes and foot ulcers. Granulocyte scanning is also utilized and is helpful in differentiating between osteoarthropathy and bone infection. When osteomyelitis is determined to be present, bone biopsy with culture is recognized as the gold standard for determining the specific pathogen and its sensitivities. Resection of necrotic bone and long-term systemic antibiotic therapy are required for treatment. Limited evidence suggests that oral agents may be as effective as parenteral antibiotics (IWGDF, 2019; WOCN, 2012).

KEY POINT

Osteomyelitis is a significant complication in the management of diabetic ulcers. Resection of necrotic bone and long-term systemic antibiotic therapy are required for treatment.

Osteomyelitis that persists or recurs after appropriate interventions have been performed or where acute osteomyelitis has not responded to accepted management techniques is considered to be refractory. Osteomyelitis is an indication for HBOT, according to the Undersea Hyperbaric Medical Society (UHMS).

ADJUNCTIVE THERAPIES

Neuropathic ulcers that fail to heal with standard therapy may require the use of adjunctive therapies. Biologic wound dressings, HBOT, NPWT, monochromatic infrared energy, and electrical stimulation have been shown to be of potential benefit in the management of these wounds.

Hyperbaric Oxygen Therapy

HBOT has been shown to reduce the number of major amputations in people with diabetes and chronic foot ulcers. There is a need for high-quality RCTs that demonstrate the benefits of HBOT for this patient population, especially since HBOT is a costly therapy. The IWGDF also recommends consideration of the use of HBOT as an adjunctive treatment in nonhealing ischemic diabetic foot ulcers despite best standard of care. They do not recommend using topical oxygen therapy as a primary or adjunctive intervention in diabetic foot ulcers including those that are difficult to heal.

Negative Pressure Wound Therapy

In a well-designed RCT comparing NPWT to advanced moist wound therapy (AMWT) in the treatment of 342 patients with diabetes and foot ulcers, there was a statistically significant improvement in healing rates among individuals receiving NPWT. NPWT was associated with significantly faster closure. There was no significant difference between the groups in rates of infection, cellulitis, or osteomyelitis (Blume et al., 2008). The IWGDF recommends consideration of use of NPWT to reduce wound size in patients with diabetes and a postoperative foot wound (IWGDF, 2019).

IWGDF recommends avoiding use of agents reported to have an effect on wound healing through alteration of the physical environment including the use of electricity, magnetism, ultrasound, and shockwaves in preference to best standard of care. Current evidence does not support any of these adjunctive measures in lieu of current best care standards (IWGDF, 2019).

Ultrasound Therapy

Ennis et al. (2005) demonstrated in a double-blind, randomized, controlled, multicenter study that therapeutic ultrasound increased the rate of healing of recalcitrant diabetic foot ulcers. However, further study is needed before definitive recommendations can be made.

Monochromatic Infrared Energy (Nitric Oxide)

Nitric oxide (NO) is produced by monochromatic infrared energy therapy (MIRE) and has been shown to improve sensory perception temporarily, in patients with diabetes. In a retrospective study of 2,239 diabetic patients with established neuropathy, MIRE was shown to reduce both LOPS and neuropathic pain. Ninety-three percent demonstrated LOPS prior to treatment, as compared to 53% posttreatment, and neuropathic pain was reduced by 67% (Harkless et al., 2006). MIRE is also thought to potentially enhance wound healing due to the cellular effects of NO. Boykin (2010) suggests that inadequate levels of NO contribute to the impaired healing seen in many diabetic foot wounds, and preliminary studies indicate that NO levels in wound fluid may predict wound healing. Further study is needed to determine the potential role of NO and MIRE in diabetic wound management (Boykin, 2010; IWGDF, 2019).

Electrical Stimulation

In a small study of patients with wounds, patients with and without diabetes were treated with biphasic electrical stimulation for 30 minutes, three times per week. Blood flow increased in the diabetes group at the periphery of the wound, and the healing rate in the diabetes group over 4 weeks was 70%. The evidence suggested that the use of electrical stimulation in a warm room significantly increased healing and skin blood flow. More study is needed since this was a small study with no control arm. Studies have failed to demonstrate any benefit of electrical stimulation in the treatment of diabetic PN (Lawson & Petrofsky, 2007; Petrofsky et al., 2007).

● SURGICAL INTERVENTION

Multiple surgical procedures have been developed to treat diabetic neuropathic and neuroischemic ulcers with varying levels of success. Goals of surgery are to achieve limb salvage, prevent ulceration and reulceration, and promote functionality of the lower extremity. True RCTs comparing operative procedures and techniques are not available.

PROCEDURES TO CORRECT STRUCTURAL DEFORMITIES

Surgical procedures of benefit in the management of the diabetic foot are those designed to correct deformities, which eliminate high-pressure areas and reduce the risk of ulcer development or promote repair of existing ulcers. Tenotomy and exostectomy are the procedures most commonly performed. Claw toe corrections and arthrodesis are less commonly performed.

Tenotomy known as tendon release, tendon lengthening, and heel cord release involves lengthening of the Achilles tendon, which reduces forefoot pressures in patients with limited dorsiflexion, and may promote healing of ulcers involving the metatarsal heads and toes (Laborde, 2009).

Exostectomy involves removal of bony deformities that cause pain, prevent functional shoe fitting, and contribute to ulceration of the soft tissue by increasing pressure and shear forces during walking. It is important to retain enough of the bone to maintain stability of the joint and to immobilize the foot with a cast for at least 6 to 8 weeks postoperatively (IWGDF, 2019; WOCN, 2012).

Arthrodesis (fusion) involves surgical reconstruction of Charcot foot. This procedure is recommended only when there is significant deformity or ulceration that prevents effective off-loading with orthotic devices and is performed in <25% of individuals with Charcot osteoarthropathy. The goals of surgery are to resect and smooth bony prominences, correct deformity, and achieve a stable and level foot that can be appropriately fitted with shoes and protected by accommodative footwear that supports ambulation. Because the bones are soft and fragmented, fusion of one or more joints is usually required. The chronic inflammation of the bone makes this a very difficult procedure with potential for multiple complications. With proper patient selection, 65% to 70% of patients heal with a stable foot. Surgery is delayed until any plantar surface ulcers have healed (Paola et al., 2007; Sayner & Rosenblum, 2005; Sohn et al., 2010; Wang, 2003; Zgonis et al., 2008). Positive outcomes may be further supported by the adjunctive use of an implantable bone growth stimulator (Hockenbury et al., 2007).

NERVE DECOMPRESSION PROCEDURES

> **KEY POINT**
>
> Unrecognized nerve entrapment may coexist with peripheral neuropathy in diabetic patients with foot ulcers.

Surgical decompression of lower extremity nerves is a surgical option with the expectation of releasing compressed nerves that are responsible for some peripheral neuropathies. Decompression has had mixed reviews, and high-quality studies are lacking. New surgical techniques have made the procedure less invasive, rendering it an outpatient procedure with minimal rates of documented complications, including inpatient admission and infection. Studies are ongoing.

SURGICAL CORRECTION OF LEAD

Adequate perfusion is obviously critical to wound healing. The patient with advanced LEAD may require endovascular procedures or bypass to promote repair. It is important to consider the risks versus short-term and long-term benefits. Short-term outcomes may be better in a surgically treated patient, but these effects may not be sustained long term. Surgical options for revascularization include angioplasty with or without stent placement and bypass grafting. There is no evidence to support bypass over angioplasty or other treatments in terms of the effects on walking distance, disease progression, amputation rates, complications, or death. While there may be multiple occlusions involving the vessels supplying the foot, treating the most occluded vessel may improve blood flow sufficiently to promote ulcer healing. See Chapter 25 for more information about surgical treatment of LEAD.

AMPUTATION

The outlook for the patient with a high-level amputation is poor. Various studies have reported a 5-year mortality rate of 40% to 70%. This can be partly attributed to changes in the patient's lifestyle, which becomes more sedentary and restricted, adversely affecting overall health, as well as concomitant diabetes-related macrovascular heart failure. There are situations in which amputation is needed, either to prevent spread of infection and salvage unaffected tissue or to provide for relief of ischemic pain and improved quality of life. When amputation is required, all efforts should be made to carry out the lowest-level amputation possible so that the patient can walk with or without a prosthesis. Partial foot amputation is preferable to below-the-knee amputation. The most commonly performed partial foot amputations are ray amputations, transmetatarsal amputation, and Syme amputation (amputation of the foot through the articulation of the ankle with removal of the malleoli of the tibia and fibula). Ray amputation is performed when necrosis has spread through the base of the toes. Transmetatarsal amputation is necessary when the forefoot is involved. Removal of the metatarsals alters weight bearing of the forefoot and increases the risk for development of ulcers under the remaining metatarsals. Therapeutic footwear is very important for these individuals. Ninety percent of patients with partial foot amputations will be able to use a prosthesis and remain mobile, compared to 75% of those with below-the-knee amputations and only 25% of those requiring above-the-knee amputations (Caputo, 2008; IWGDF, 2019).

CHARCOT NEUROPATHIC OSTEOARTHROPATHY

Any condition that causes sensory and autonomic neuropathy can lead to a Charcot joint, known as neuropathic osteoarthropathy or Charcot foot. This pathology in the United States is commonly due to diabetes, but it can also be caused by syphilis, chronic alcoholism, Hansen disease, spinal cord injury, renal failure and dialysis, and congenital insensitivity to pain. The most common pathology worldwide is Hansen disease (HRSA, 2017; IWGDF, 2019; WOCN, 2012). Charcot foot deformity is caused by an insidious, noninfectious destruction of the bones and joints of the foot, which results in pathologic fractures, joint dislocations, and loss of normal foot structure. Predisposing factors for Charcot foot include bone hyperemia, osteopenia, joint instability, and sensorimotor deficits. Charcot foot deformity increases the risk for plantar surface ulceration and significantly increases the risk for amputation (Armstrong et al., 1997b; Nielsn & Armstrong, 2008; Sella, 2009; Verity et al., 2008).

PATHOLOGY

There are two theories as to the pathology of Charcot foot deformity.

The first theory is the neurotraumatic theory, which suggests that sensory neuropathy leaves the individual unable to recognize traumatic injury and that recurrent unrelieved mechanical stress results in progressive destruction of the bones and joints of the foot. The second theory is the neurovascular theory, which states that autonomic neuropathy results in loss of sympathetic tone to the vessels, which in turn causes persistent dilatation of the vessels supplying the soft tissues and bony structures. The resulting hyperemia causes osteopenia, which leaves the bones much more susceptible to fracture and trauma from walking (Armstrong & Peters, 2002; Jude & Boulton, 2002; Nielson & Armstrong, 2008). In many cases, the damage is probably caused by some combination of unrecognized trauma and increased blood flow (see **Fig. 26-6**).

Factors Leading to Charcot Foot

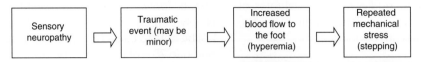

a. Loss of protective sensation (sensory neuropathy).

b. Traumatic event: May simply be a misstep (misplaced or awkward step) or twisting of the foot and/or the ankle causing inflammation.

c. Increased blood flow (hyperemia) related to inflammatory response and arterio venous shunting (autonomic neuropathy) leads to osteopenia and demineralization of bony foot structures resulting in weaker bones

d. Unperceived injury/repeated mechanical stress: Continued ambulation on injured foot (continued, repeated high pressures) leads to collapse of foot architecture.

FIGURE 26-24. Factors Leading to Charcot Foot.

CLINICAL PRESENTATION

Prevention of Charcot foot deformity requires recognition of the initial injury and inflammation, which is manifested by unilateral swelling, increased local skin temperature (3°C to 7°C) as compared to adjacent unaffected sites, erythema, bounding pulses, and possibly complaints of mild pain, which is disproportionate to the severity of the underlying injury. During this acute inflammatory stage, it is sometimes difficult to differentiate between fracture, cellulitis, and osteomyelitis, and laboratory studies commonly used to diagnose infection (e.g., WBC count, sedimentation rate) may also be misleading since they will rise in response to the acute inflammatory process. Plain radiographs (AP, lateral, and oblique views) do provide a definitive diagnosis once bony involvement has occurred. MRI provides detection of Charcot foot in the early stages when it is not yet identifiable on x-ray. MRI also provides definitive diagnosis of osteomyelitis (Armstrong & Peters, 2002; HRSA, 2017; IWGDF, 2019; Nielson & Armstrong, 2008; Nube et al., 2002). Late stages of Charcot foot are manifested as foot deformity, which most commonly involves the forefoot (45%) or midfoot (35%). Specific changes include unusual bony prominences, unstable joints, collapse of the midfoot structures, and development of a rocker bottom foot (Armstrong & Peters, 2002; Nielson & Armstrong, 2008; Nube et al., 2002; Saunders & Mrdjencovich, 1991). See **Figure 26-24**.

KEY POINT

Prevention of Charcot foot requires prompt recognition and appropriate management of any injury. Appropriate management involves off-loading and total non–weight bearing until inflammation subsides, as detected by infrared dermal thermometer, and bony healing has occurred.

PHASES

Charcot foot development progresses through several phases, which include the acute inflammatory phase, the subacute coalescence phase, and the resolution (consolidation) phase (**Table 26-6**). The acute phase represents the phase immediately postinjury and is characterized by severe inflammation. The coalescence phase represents early healing and beginning formation of bone callus; and the consolidation phase represents final healing with stabilization and remodeling of the bone.

TABLE 26-6 EICHENHOLTZ CLASSIFICATION OF CHARCOT FOOT HEALING: CLINICAL PRESENTATION AND PHASES

CLINICAL PRESENTATION	DISSOLUTION PHASE	COALESCENCE PHASE	CONSOLIDATION PHASE
Edema	May be profound	Decreased	Decreased
Erythema	May be severe	Generally absent	Generally absent
Temperature (compare affected site to unaffected site with dermal thermometer)	May be 3°C–7°C increased	Generally >2°C increased	Generally <2°C increased
X-ray image	May demonstrate fractures, dislocations, and subluxations *May NOT show abnormality during the earliest, acute phase of injury*	May demonstrate early consolidation, formation of bone callus	Demonstrates bone consolidation, stability

Adapted from information in Eichenholtz (1966), McCrory et al. (1998).

Indicators of injury include increased local skin temperature (3°C to 7°C) as compared to adjacent unaffected sites; erythema, bounding pulses, and possibly complaints of mild pain, which is disproportionate to the severity of the underlying injury.

IMPACT

Sohn et al. (2010) performed a retrospective review of VA patients with Charcot arthropathy and diabetic foot ulcer. Among the patients with Charcot foot, 59% (538) were treated for foot ulcers during the 5-year period following development of Charcot foot; 66% (354) of those developed a foot ulcer immediately before or at the time of development of Charcot arthropathy, and the remaining 34% developed the ulcer as a complication of Charcot deformity. Individuals with ulcers but no Charcot deformity were seven times more likely to require amputation than those who had Charcot deformity but no ulcers. Those over 65 years of age who had both an ulcer and Charcot deformity had 12 times higher risk of amputation than those with Charcot deformity only. The results of this study suggest that Charcot deformity does not pose a serious amputation risk but it is the development of plantar surface ulceration that causes increased risk of amputation. Prevention of ulceration is of paramount importance in the management of these individuals (Sohn et al., 2010).

MANAGEMENT

Nonsurgical management during the acute phase of Charcot foot is focused on reducing inflammation through non–weight bearing, usually with a TCC or walking splint that is changed every 1 to 2 weeks. Non–weight bearing should be continued until the temperature of the affected foot is within 2°C of the temperature of the unaffected foot, and bone callus consolidation is visible on x-ray. Dermal thermometry assessment should be conducted with every office visit, and serial x-rays should be obtained monthly (Armstrong & Lavery, 1997; Jude & Boulton, 2002; McGill et al., 2000). If the patient is unable to adhere to total non–weight bearing, partial weight bearing with use of an assistive walker or crutches is acceptable in moderation. Surgery is never considered during the acute phase due to the impaired integrity of the bony tissue (Armstrong & Peters, 2002; Edmonds, 2006).

Once the acute inflammation has resolved, the cast can be removed, but the patient should wear a brace to protect the foot. Examples of braces include patellar tendon-bearing brace, accommodative footwear with a modified AFO, a Charcot restraint orthotic walker (CROW), or double metal upright AFO (HRSA, 2017; IWGDF, 2019; Verity et al., 2008).

A Charcot foot can be a progressive deformity causing ongoing foot architecture destruction if there are repeated and extended episodes of increased foot inflammation. This would typically occur related to shoe wear no longer accommodating the deformity or the individual walking barefoot. Long-term management must include lifelong protection and monitoring for the involved limb as well as optimal diabetes management. Specific measures include appropriately fitted footwear. The patient with bony deformities should have custom shoes and orthoses fitted by a certified pedorthist (C-Ped). Management also includes professional foot care on a routine and as-needed basis and patient education. Patients should be educated on Charcot deformity with increased risk for ulceration and amputation, the importance of daily foot inspection and patient self-monitoring of dermal temperature, and prompt reporting of problems to health care professional. They should also be instructed on limiting ambulation, changing to healing shoe or customized walking splint, continued monitoring of dermal temperature, and access to diabetic foot clinic (Armstrong et al., 2007; HRSA, 2017; Jude & Boulton, 2002; Lavery et al., 2004). Surgery is performed in fewer than 25% of patients with Charcot deformity (Armstrong & Peters, 2002; Edmonds, 2006).

Long-term management of the patient with Charcot osteoarthropathy includes protection and monitoring for the involved limb as well as optimal diabetes management.

FUNGAL SKIN AND NAIL INFECTIONS

An infectious complication for the diabetic population is fungal skin and nail infections. Skin infections are of concern, since they can result in blistering or fissures that permit bacterial entry, which can lead to lymphangitis or cellulitis. Clinical presentation, diagnosis, and management of fungal infections (Kelechi & Lukacs, 1997; Singal & Khanna, 2011) are discussed in detail in Chapter 28.

Instructions important to the diabetic patient with a fungal infection include the following:

- Dry feet well after bathing, especially between toes.
- Apply an antifungal powder or cream (e.g., miconazole 2% powder) to the feet daily until symptoms are gone.
- Utilize toe spacers to prevent interdigital crowding and maceration.
- Wear cotton blended socks for moisture wicking.

NUTRITIONAL MANAGEMENT

Basic principles of nutritional management for the patient with diabetes mellitus (i.e., control of serum glucose, hyperlipidemia, and hypertension) should be applied to the patient who has developed a neuropathic foot ulcer. Nutrition therapy should be individualized with consideration given to usual food and eating habits, metabolic profile, treatment goals, and desired outcomes. Nutritional assessment and management have been discussed in detail in Chapter 7. This discussion will be limited to factors of particular importance to the diabetic patient.

GLYCEMIC CONTROL

Tight glycemic control is very important as hyperglycemia is known to adversely affect all phases of wound repair. The most recent ADA treatment guidelines (2019) state that HbA1c should be maintained at <7% in order to reduce the risk of microvascular damage. Glycemic control requires consistent commitment from the patient. The patient should be counseled on the importance of glycemic management and should discuss and agree on treatment goals. Goals should be set that are consistent with the patient's comorbid conditions, preferences, and ability to manage the treatment regime, and HbA1c goals must be individualized for each patient. The ADA suggests less stringent goals for individuals with limited life expectancy, multiple comorbidities, and a history of severe hypoglycemia. More stringent goals, such as <6.5, may be appropriate for those who are newly diagnosed with diabetes, have no cardiovascular issues, and can be controlled with lifestyle or metformin only (ADA, 2019).

KEY POINT

Nutritional management of the patient with diabetes and neuropathy includes tight glycemic control (HbA1c < 7.0%). There is increasing evidence that supplementation with alpha-lipoic acid (ALA) may slow progression or even partially reverse the symptoms of neuropathy.

ALPHA-LIPOIC ACID SUPPLEMENTATION

There is increasing evidence that supplementation with the micronutrient alpha-lipoic acid (ALA) may slow the progression of neuropathy or even partially reverse the symptoms of neuropathy. In an RCT comparing outcomes for 233 diabetic patients who received ALA once daily for 4 years compared to 227 diabetic patients who received placebo, the individuals receiving ALA showed clinical improvement and nonprogression of neuropathic symptoms. These results are consistent with the results of a meta-analysis of 4 RCTs involving 1,258 patients, in which 600-mg ALA per day (given IV) significantly reduced symptoms of neuropathy and improved neuropathic deficits (Ziegler et al., 2011). The Symptomatic Diabetic Neuropathy 2 trial demonstrated significant improvement in neuropathic symptoms and deficits in 181 diabetic patients treated with variable dosages of ALA (Casellini & Vinik, 2007). Garcia-Alcala and colleagues (2015) found that after receiving high-dose ALA for 16 weeks, patients on lower dose therapy needed less pain medication than did those who stopped treatment altogether (Garcia-Alcala et al., 2015). The Sidney 2 trial evaluated the results of variable dosages of ALA (600 mg vs. 1,200 mg

vs. 1,800 mg daily) compared to placebo over 5 weeks and found significant reduction in neuropathic pain in all ALA groups. They also found a dose-dependent increase in side effects and concluded that 600 mg/day offers the best risk/benefit balance (Agathos et al., 2018). In addition to slowing the progression of neuropathy, ALA has also been shown to decrease fasting glucose, HbA1c levels, and triglyceride levels (Akbari et al., 2018).

OTHER MICRONUTRIENT SUPPLEMENTS

One small study compared L-arginine (a precursor to endothelial-derived NO) to placebo and found no effect on endothelial dysfunction, $TcPO_2$ levels, or clinical indicators of neuropathy (Jude et al., 2010).

Thirteen RTCs have addressed the potential benefits of vitamin B_1 (thiamine) on symptoms of diabetic or alcoholic neuropathy, but the trials were small and the overall evidence suggests that vitamin B_1 is less effective than ALA, cilostazol, or cytidine triphosphate in providing short-term improvement in clinical outcomes and nerve conduction (Ang et al., 2008).

One study evaluated the potential benefits of vitamin B_{12} (cobalamin) supplementation in community-dwelling diabetic patients found to have B_{12} deficiency (as determined by methylmalonic acid [MMA] levels and cobalamin levels) and demonstrated improved MMA levels and reduced neuropathy in 88% of the subjects (Solomon, 2011). Combining vitamin B_{12} with prostaglandins has been shown to have greater effects on neuropathy than either medication alone (Jiang et al., 2018).

Vitamin D deficiency, characterized as <30 ng/mL, is associated with self-reported PN symptoms after adjusting for demographic factors, obesity, comorbidities, use of medications for neuropathy, and diabetes duration and control. Vitamin D deficiency has been correlated with symptoms of PN including LOPS (Abdelsadek et al., 2018; Fan et al., 2018; Soderstrom et al., 2012). This suggests that testing for vitamin D deficiency and providing supplementation when indicated may help prevent or improve neuropathy in some individuals (Alam et al., 2017; Soderstrom et al., 2012). Diabetic patients with autonomic neuropathy frequently exhibit reduced bone quality. Individuals who have additional fracture risks should receive aggressive treatment for osteoporosis (Okazaki, 2011).

⬤ NEUROPATHIC PAIN MANAGEMENT

Approximately 20% of the diabetic population suffers from disabling pain due to neuropathy (Luana et al., 2017). The pain can be severe, have a significant impact on quality of life and activities of daily living, and be difficult to treat particularly if complicated by a neuropathic wound. Depression, anxiety, sleep disturbances, and other adverse effects of neuropathic pain should be monitored. Appropriate referrals should be made to assure optimal management (Bates et al., 2019; Dworkin et al., 2007) (**Table 26-7**).

TABLE 26-7 SUGGESTED PHARMACOLOGICAL INTERVENTIONS FOR THE TREATMENT OF NEUROPATHIC PAIN IN PATIENTS WITH LEND

PAIN DESCRIPTION	MEDICATION	COMMENTS
Dysesthesia described as a "burning sensation," "sunburn-like," or "skin tingles;" allodynia	Capsaicin cream (Topical)	Dose: 0.025% and 0.075% topically applied very sparingly 3–4 times per day, in mapped areas (indicating sites of greatest neuropathic pain) May provide pain relief in those who fail to respond to other therapies. Skin irritation may lead to nonadherence. Systemic effects are rare
	Gabapentin (oral) (Neurontin)	Dose: High dosing of 1,200–3,600 mg in divided doses over 24 h may be necessary. Low doses may not be effective Provides high-level pain relief in 1/3 of those with painful neuropathic pain Adverse advents include dizziness, somnolence, edema, and gait disturbance
	Pregabalin (oral) (Lyrica)	Pregabalin dose: 100 mg 3 times daily. Increase gradually to maximum of 600 mg daily. Demonstrated effectiveness in patients with painful diabetic neuropathy. Individual, personalized treatment is needed to maximize pain relief and minimize adverse events.
	Selective serotonin reuptake inhibitors (SSRIs): fluoxetine, paroxetine (oral)	Dose: 20 to 40 mg/day; increase and taper doses gradually SSRIs may be better tolerated by patients but limited evidence for relief in neuropathic pain, and more high-quality studies are required
	Serotonin and noradrenergic reuptake inhibitors (SSNaRI): Duloxetine (Cymbalta) Venlafaxine (oral)	Duloxetine, (Cymbalta) (oral) Dose: 60–120 mg/day; increase and taper doses gradually Six trials ($N = 2,220$) demonstrated effects of duloxetine on diabetic neuropathic pain with 50% pain improvement at 12 wk at a dose of 60 and 120 mg daily. Minor side effects are common at therapeutic doses. Serious side effects are rare. Direct comparisons of duloxetine to other drugs shown to be effective in neuropathic pain are needed 58 patients received duloxetine and amitriptyline in a randomized, double-blind crossover, active-control trial. Significant improvement in pain was achieved with both treatments compared to baseline values ($p < 0.001$ for both) Venlafaxine dose: 75–150 mg/day Evidence supports similar effectiveness to tricyclic antidepressants
Paresthesia described as "pins and needles," "electric-like," "numb aching feet," or "as if my feet have been in ice water," "knife-like," shooting pains, or lancinating pains	Tricyclic antidepressants: imipramine, amitriptyline (oral)	Dose: 50 mg qhs; may be increased to 150 mg by mouth, with lower dosing for elderly Tricyclic antidepressants are effective for moderate pain relief in neuropathic pain, except HIV neuropathy Antidepressants, including tricyclics, duloxetine, and venlafaxine, should be considered for the treatment of patients with painful DPN
	Analgesics (opioids) Tramadol (Ultram) (oral)	Tramadol dose: 100–400 mg q6h Tramadol is an effective symptomatic treatment for peripheral neuropathic pain, particularly for paresthesia, allodynia, and touch-evoked pain.
	Opioids	Short-term studies provided mixed results in effectiveness of opioids for neuropathic pain Intermediate-term studies demonstrate that opioids are effective for any etiology of neuropathic pain over placebo. Further randomized controlled trials are needed to establish long-term efficacy, safety, and effects on quality of life Opiate analgesia in combination with gabapentin should be considered for the treatment of patients with painful DPN, which cannot be controlled with monotherapy
Other pharmacological interventions	Analgesics (systemic administration of local anesthetic agents: intravenous lidocaine, mexiletine, lidocaine plus mexiletine, mexiletine, tocainide, and flecainide) (oral analogs)	32 RCTs demonstrated parenteral lidocaine and its oral analogs (i.e., mexiletine, tocainide, flecainide) were safe and superior to placebo in decreasing the intensity of neuropathic pain. Limited data showed there were no differences in efficacy or adverse effects of lidocaine or its analogs compared to carbamazepine, amantadine, gabapentin, or morphine
	Lidoderm patch (topical)	A Lidoderm patch (lidocaine 5%) can reduce the intensity of common neuropathic pain. The patch is applied topically to the wound site or affected neuropathic area for 12 h. The patch should be left off for 12 h before reapplying to reduce risk of toxicity

EXERCISE PROGRAMS AND HEALTH PROMOTION

Patients should be encouraged to participate in regular exercise programs, with modifications to accommodate any comorbidities and ulcerations. Patients should be instructed to obtain medical advice and clearance before beginning any routine exercise. This is particularly important for individuals who exhibit resting tachycardia and lack of heart rate variability during deep breathing or exercise, since these findings may be indicative of autonomic neuropathy and high risk of coronary artery disease. Individuals with neuropathic ulcers should be instructed to avoid weight-bearing exercises and to focus instead on non–weight-bearing exercises such as swimming, water aerobics, bicycling, rowing, chair, and upper body exercises. Individuals with neuropathy but no active ulcers may pursue weight-bearing exercises with medical clearance but must be educated to wear well-fitting shoes and socks (WOCN, 2012).

The overall goal of management for any individual is improved overall health status. Key elements of health maintenance for the diabetic include management of modifiable risk factors: smoking cessation, weight loss, blood pressure control, and limited intake of alcohol.

Appropriate goals for glucose control should be established based on the individual's comorbidities, life expectancy, and self-care goals. Appropriate education and counseling should be provided to assist the individual in meeting those goals. The individual who is considering smoking cessation, weight loss, or other lifestyle modifications should be provided with education, support, and referrals as indicated. Vitamin B_{12} levels should be monitored routinely with supplementation as indicated. All individuals should be provided with specific education regarding preventive foot care and the importance of daily foot inspection and skin temperature monitoring. Individuals who smoke, have LOPS and foot deformities, or have a history of ulceration or other lower extremity complications should be referred to foot specialists for ongoing preventive care and lifelong surveillance.

PREVENTION OF RECURRENT ULCERATION

Primary and secondary prevention are key areas of focus for the wound care nurse. An analysis of the cost-effectiveness of foot care based on published guidelines found that preventive care can improve survival, reduce ulceration and amputation rates, is cost-effective, and can even save on long-term costs when compared with standard care. Available technologies that provide early detection of pressure and temperature are readily available for patients' home use and are reasonably priced (HRSA, 2017).

Neuropathic ulcer prevention begins with identification of at-risk individuals. Major risk factors for neuropathic ulceration include LOPS, lower extremity arterial disease (LEAD), a history of previous ulceration or amputation, gait abnormalities and high plantar surface pressures, rigid foot deformities, poor glycemic control (as evidenced by HbA1c > 9%), long-standing diabetes (>10 years), diabetic nephropathy (especially individuals on dialysis), smoking, and visual disturbances (Lavery et al., 1998).

The wound care nurse can use the individual's risk profile to develop an individualized program for preventive foot care and surveillance based on their risk level (Table 26-2). Patients who smoke, have LOPS and structural abnormalities, or have a history of lower extremity complications should be referred to foot care specialists for ongoing preventive care and lifelong surveillance. A multidisciplinary approach is recommended for optimal management of these high-risk individuals.

All at-risk individuals should receive periodic foot screening to identify neuropathic changes, deformities, areas of impending ulceration, and indications of vascular compromise. Education and referrals should be based on the findings. The Lower Extremity Amputation Prevention (LEAP) program includes five major prevention interventions: (1) foot screening; (2) patient education; (3) appropriate footwear selection; (4) daily foot inspection by the patient; and (5) management of simple foot problems (to prevent deterioration into more significant problems).

The patient and family are the individuals responsible for daily foot care, foot protection, and foot inspection. Individualized patient education programs are integral to prevention of neuropathic ulcers. A 2010 Cochrane Review found that educating patients about preventive foot care seemed to improve their foot care knowledge and behavior short term. One RCT involving patients with previous diabetic foot disease suggested that education may be effective in preventing recurrent ulceration or amputation. Further study is needed to determine whether education alone, without additional preventive measures, is sufficient to reduce the incidence of ulcers and amputations. Education is considered one element of a comprehensive prevention program with periodic surveillance based on level of risk (Hoogeveen et al., 2015; HRSA, 2017; IWGDF, 2019).

Patient education should include instruction regarding the individual's risk factors and interventions to help ameliorate their specific risk factors, such as therapeutic footwear for individuals with deformities. All patients must be instructed in the following:

- Routine self-care measures (e.g., never going barefoot, inspecting feet daily, breaking shoes in gradually)
- Early recognition and prompt reporting of potential foot problems
- Routine foot surveillance by health care providers
- Individual footwear requirements

In addition, all individuals with neuropathy should have ready access to specialized foot care whenever they detect a potential problem.

Current evidence also supports incorporation of routine skin temperature testing into standard preventive care. One study compared outcomes for diabetic patients in risk categories 2 and 3 (neuropathy and foot deformity, or previous history of ulceration or partial, complete foot amputation) who were randomized to either standard therapy or enhanced therapy. Standard therapy included therapeutic footwear, diabetic foot education, and regular evaluation by a podiatrist. The enhanced therapy also included skin temperature testing at pressure points or previous problematic areas with a dermal thermometer morning and night. Any sites with elevated temperature (>4°F or >2.2°C) were considered to be inflamed, and subjects were instructed to reduce activity and contact the study nurse. Over the 6-month study period, the enhanced therapy group had significantly fewer diabetic foot complications (enhanced therapy group 2% vs. standard therapy group 20%; 7 ulcers and 2 Charcot fractures among standard therapy patients vs. 1 ulcer in the enhanced therapy group) (Lavery et al., 2004).

Another 15-month multicenter study compared individuals with a prior history of diabetic foot ulceration assigned to one of three groups: standard care, standard care + structured foot examination, and enhanced therapy. All subjects received therapeutic footwear, diabetes foot education, and regular foot and nail care. Subjects in the standard care + structured exam group performed a structured foot inspection daily and recorded their findings in a logbook. Subjects in the enhanced therapy group measured skin temperature at 6-foot sites each day. Individuals in the standard therapy and the standard

care + structured exam groups were instructed to contact the study nurse immediately for any identified foot abnormalities, and subjects in the enhanced therapy group were instructed to report temperature differences and to reduce activity until temperatures returned to normal. Subjects in the enhanced therapy group had fewer foot ulcers than did those in the standard therapy and standard therapy + structured foot examination groups (8.5% in enhanced therapy group vs. 29.3% in the standard therapy group and 30.4% in the standard therapy + structured foot examination group) (Armstrong et al., 2007).

Consistent use of properly fitted footwear is an important element of preventive care for the individual with neuropathy. Shoes that are correctly fitted and that have appropriate insoles provide protection against traumatic injury and can also normalize gait and pressure distribution, reducing the size of calluses and preventing new callus formation. One study (n = 78) demonstrated a reduction in callus size that was directly proportional to the amount of time spent wearing running shoes (Singh et al., 2005).

Commercially available shoes are generally appropriate for patients who do not have bony deformities (e.g., prominent metatarsal heads, inflexible great toe [hallux rigidus], or Charcot foot deformity) or LOPS. These shoes are ideally selected according to the following criteria: (1) constructed of natural materials (e.g., leather or suede); (2) shape and size of shoe matches shape and size of foot (rounded or squared toe box); (3) outer soles are cushioned and inner soles are removable; (4) the toe box has sufficient depth to permit the individual to pinch up the exterior shoe material at the toe box; and (5) shoes are secured with Velcro or laces. Individuals should be taught to use their foot tracings to assure that the shoes accommodate their feet.

Individuals with LOPS require professionally fitted footwear since they will be unable to recognize any problems with fit, such as abnormally tight shoes or shoes that rub. Individuals with foot deformities, history of ulceration, or partial foot amputations require custom fit therapeutic footwear and insoles and should be routinely referred to an orthotist or pedorthist.

In teaching individuals with LOPS or ischemia about appropriate use of protective footwear, the wound care nurse should emphasize the importance of wearing protective footwear at all times when out of bed and the importance of shaking the shoes out before donning to assure that there are no foreign bodies.

⬤ CONCLUSION

LEND and wounds associated with LEND continue to be the most significant precedent for nontraumatic LEA in the United States. Direct and indirect health care costs associated with LEND and LEND wounds consume nearly $200 billion annually. LEND results in long-term disability and high mortality within 5 years of incident amputation.

The goal in management of the diabetic patient with neuropathy is prevention of ulceration and amputation, which requires appropriate footwear, daily foot care, and daily foot inspection. In addition, current evidence strongly supports the benefit of skin temperature checks with a dermal infrared thermometer to promptly identify areas of inflammation, coupled with off-loading measures and professional evaluation. Effective management of neuropathic ulcers requires attention to off-loading, glycemic control, aggressive debridement to eliminate necrotic tissue, and systemic and topical therapies to control bacterial loads.

Patient education and patient involvement is critical to success in management and requires mutual goal setting and ongoing patient involvement.

REFERENCES

Abbott, C. A., Chatwin, K. E., Foden, P., et al. (2019). Innovative intelligent insole system reduces diabetic foot ulcer recurrence at plantar sites: A prospective, randomised, proof-of-concept study. *The Lancet Digital Health, 1*(6), e308–e318.

Abdelsadek, S. E., El Saghier, E. O., & Abdel Raheem, S. I. (2018). Serum 25(OH) vitamin D level and its relation to diabetic peripheral neuropathy in Egyptian patients with type 2 diabetes mellitus. *The Egyptian Journal of Neurology, Psychiatry and Neurosurgery, 54*(1), 36. doi: 10.1186/s41983-018-0036-9.

Abraham, A., Alabdali, M., Alsulaiman, A., et al. (2017). The sensitivity and specificity of the neurological examination in polyneuropathy patients with clinical and electrophysiological correlations. *PLOS One, 12*(3), e0171597. doi: 10.1371/journal.pone.0171597.

Adams, O. P., Herbert, J. R., Howitt, C., et al. (2019). The prevalence of peripheral neuropathy severe enough to cause a loss of protective sensation in a population-based sample of people with known and newly detected diabetes in Barbados: A cross-sectional study. *Diabetic Medicine, 36*(12), 1629–1636. doi: 10.1111/dme.13989.

Agathos, E., Tentolouris, A., Eleftheriadou, I., et al. (2018). Effect of α-lipoic acid on symptoms and quality of life in patients with painful diabetic neuropathy. *The Journal of International Medical Research, 46*(5), 1779–1790. doi: 10.1177/0300060518756540.

Akbari, M., Ostadmohammadi, V., Lankarani, K. B., et al. (2018). The effects of alpha-lipoic acid supplementation on glucose control and lipid profiles among patients with metabolic diseases: A systematic review and meta-analysis of randomized controlled trials. *Metabolism, 87*, 56–69. doi: 10.1016/j.metabol.2018.07.002.

Alam, U., Fawwad, A., Shaheen, F., et al. (2017). Improvement in neuropathy specific quality of life in patients with diabetes after vitamin D supplementation. *Journal of Diabetes Research, 2017*, 7928083. doi: 10.1155/2017/7928083.

American Diabetes Association. (2019). Standards of medical care in diabetes—2019. *Diabetes Care, 42*(Suppl 1), s124–s138. doi: 10.2337/dc19-S011.

Ang, C. D., ALviar, M. J. M., Dans, A. L., et al. (2008). Vitamin B for treating peripheral neuropathy. *Cochrane Database of Systematic Reviews,* (3), CD004573. doi: 10.1002//14651858.CD004573.pub2.

Armstrong, D. G., Holtz-Neiderer, K., Wendel, C., et al. (2007). Skin temperature monitoring reduces the risk for diabetic foot ulceration in high-risk patients. *American Journal of Medicine, 120*(12), 1042–1046.

Armstrong, D. G., & Lavery, L. A. (1997). Monitoring healing of acute Charcot's arthropathy with infrared dermal thermometry. *Journal of Rehabilitation Research and Development, 34*(3), 317–321.

Armstrong, D. G., Lavery, L. A., Fletschrit, J., et al. (1997a). Is electrical stimulation effective in reducing neuropathic pain in patients with diabetes? *Journal of Foot and Ankle Surgery, 36*(4), 260–263.

Armstrong, D. G., Lavery, L. A., Wu, S., et al. (2005). Evaluation of removable and irremovable cast walkers in the healing of diabetic foot wounds: A randomized controlled trial. *Diabetes Care, 28*, 551–554.

Armstrong, D. G., & Peters, E. J. (2002). Charcot's arthropathy of the foot. *Journal of the American Podiatric Medical Association, 92*(7), 390.

Armstrong, D. G., Todd, W. F., Lavery, L. A., et al. (1997b). The natural history of acute Charcot's arthropathy in a diabetic foot specialty clinic. *Journal of American Podiatric Medical Association, 87*(6), 272–278.

Bates, D., Schultheis, B. C., Hanes, M. C., et al. (2019). A comprehensive algorithm for management of neuropathic pain. *Pain Medicine, 20*(Suppl 1), S2–S12. doi: 10.1093/pm/pnz075.

Benn, M. (2020). Peripheral neuropathy—Time for better biomarkers? *Clinical Chemistry, 66*(5), 638–640. doi: 10.1093/clinchem/hvaa075.

Beropoulis, E., Stavroulakis, K., Schwindt, A., et al. (2016). Validation of the Wound, Ischemia, foot Infection (WIfI) classification system in nondiabetic patients treated by endovascular means for critical limb ischemia. *Journal of Vascular Surgery, 64*(1), 95–103.

Beuker, B., VanDeursen, R. W., Price, P., et al. (2005). Plantar pressure in off-loading devices used in diabetic ulcer treatment. *Wound Repair and Regeneration, 13*, 537–542.

Birke, J. A., Patout C. A. Jr., & Foto, J. G. (2000). Factors associated with ulceration and amputation in the neuropathic foot. *Journal of Orthopaedic and Sports Physical Therapy, 30*(2), 91–97.

Birke, J. A., Pavich, M. A., Patout, C. A., et al. (2002). Comparison of forefoot ulcer healing using alternative offloading methods in patients with diabetes mellitus. *Advances in Skin & Wound Care, 15*, 210–215.

Birke, J. A., & Sims, D. S. (1986). Plantar sensory threshold in the ulcerated foot. *Leprosy Review, 57*(3), 261–267.

Blume, P. A., Walters, J., Payne, W., et al. (2008). Comparison of negative pressure wound therapy using vacuum-assisted closure with advanced moist wound therapy in the treatment of diabetic foot ulcers. *Diabetes Care, 31*, 631–636.

Bolton, L. (2007). Operational definition of moist wound healing. *Journal of Wound, Ostomy, and Continence Nursing, 34*(1), 23–29.

Bonham, P., & Kelechi, T. (2008). Evaluation of lower extremity arterial circulation and implications for nursing practice. *Journal of Cardiovascular Nursing, 23*(2), 144–152.

Boykin, J. V. Jr. (2010). Wound nitric oxide bioactivity: A promising diagnostic indicator for diabetic foot ulcer management. *Journal of Wound, Ostomy, and Continence Nursing, 37*(1), 25–32.

Bus, S. A., Valk, G. D., van Deursen, R. W., et al. (2008). Specific guidelines on footwear and offloading. *Diabetes/Metabolism Research Reviews, 24*(Suppl 1), S192–S193.

Canadian Association of Wound Care (CAWC). (2018). Inlow's 60 second diabetic foot exam. Retrieved from https://www.diabetes.ca/DiabetesCanadaWebsite/media/Health-care-providers/2018%20Clinical%20Practice%20Guidelines/Inlows-60-second-diabetic-foot-screen-Wounds-Canada.pdf?ext=.pdf

Caputo, W. (2008). Surgical management of the diabetic foot. *Wounds, 20*(3), 74–83.

Caselli, A., Pham, H., Giurini, J. M., et al. (2002). The forefoot-to-rearfoot plantar pressure ratio is increased in severe diabetic neuropathy and can predict foot ulceration. *Diabetes Care, 25*(6), 1006.

Casellini, C., & Vinik, A. (2007). Clinical manifestations and current treatment options for diabetic neuropathies. *Endocrine Practice, 13*(5), 550–566.

Causey, M. W., Ahmed, A., Wu, B., et al. (2016). Society for Vascular Surgery limb stage and patient risk correlate with outcomes in an amputation prevention program. *Journal of Vascular Surgery, 63*(6), 1563–1573.

Cavanagh, P. R., & Bus, S. A. (2011). Offloading the diabetic foot for ulcer prevention and healing. *Plastic and Reconstructive Surgery, 127*(Suppl 1), 248S–256S.

Centers for Disease Control and Prevention (CDC). (2017). National diabetes statistics report, 2017. Retrieved from https://www.cdc.gov/diabetes/pdfs/data/statistics/national-diabetes-statistics-report.pdf

Centers for Disease Control and Prevention (CDC). (2020). *National diabetes statistics report, 2020*. Atlanta, GA: Centers for Disease Control and Prevention, U.S. Department of Health and Human Services.

Centers for Medicare and Medicaid Services (CMS). (2018). Therapeutic shoes for persons with diabetes statement of certifying physician template guidance. Retrieved from www.medicare.gov/

Cheuy, V. A., Hastings, M. K., Commean, P. K., et al. (2016). Muscle and joint factors associated with forefoot deformity in the diabetic neuropathic foot. *Foot & Ankle International, 37*(5), 514–521.

Cull, D. L., Manos, G., Hartley, M. C., et al. (2014). An early validation of the Society for Vascular Surgery lower extremity threatened limb classification system. *Journal of Vascular Surgery, 60*(6), 1535–1542.

Darling, J. D., McCallum, J. C., Soden, P. A., et al. (2016). Predictive ability of the Society for Vascular Surgery Wound, Ischemia, and foot Infection (WIfI) classification system following infra-popliteal endovascular interventions for critical limb ischemia. *Journal of Vascular Surgery, 64*(3), 616–622.

Dworkin, R. H., O'Connor, A. B., Backonja, M., et al. (2007). Pharmacologic management of neuropathic pain: Evidence-based recommendations. *Pain, 132*(3), 237–251.

Edmonds, M. (2006). Diabetic foot ulcers: Practical treatment recommendations. *Drugs, 66*(7), 913–929.

Eichenholtz, S. N. (1966). *Charcot joints* (Vol. 227). Springfield, IL: Charles C. Thomas.

Ennis, W., Foremann, P., Mozen, N., et al. (2005). Ultrasound therapy for recalcitrant diabetic foot ulcers: A randomized, double-blind, controlled, multicenter study. *Ostomy and Wound Management, 51*(9), 14.

Falanga, V. (2005). Wound healing and its impairment on the diabetic foot. *The Lancet, 366*(9498), 1736–1743.

Fan, L., Zhang, Y., Zhu, J., et al. (2018) Association of vitamin D deficiency with diabetic peripheral neuropathy in Tianjin, China. *Asia Pacific Journal of Clinical Nutrition, 27*(3), 599–606. doi: 10.6133/apjcn.062017.11.

Foto, J., Brasseaux, D., Hupp, D., et al. (2009). A comparison of different handheld infrared thermometers for measuring dermal skin temperature. *Diabetes, 58*, A290.

Frykberg, R. G., Gordon, I. L., Reyzelman, A. M., et al. (2017). Feasibility and efficacy of a smart mat technology to predict development of diabetic plantar ulcers. *Diabetes Care, 40*(7), 973–980.

Frykberg, R. G., Zgonis, T., Armstrong D. G., et al. (2006). Diabetic foot disorders: A clinical practice guideline (2006 revision). *Journal of Foot and Ankle Surgery, 45*(5 Suppl), S1–S66.

Garcia-Alcala, H., Santos Vichido, C. I., Islas Macedo, S., et al. (2015). Treatment with α-Lipoic acid over 16 weeks in type 2 diabetic patients with symptomatic polyneuropathy who responded to initial 4-week high-dose loading. *Journal of Diabetes Research, 2015*, 189857. doi: 10.1155/2015/189857.

Harkless, L. B., de Lellis, S., Carnegie, D. H., et al. (2006). Improved foot sensitivity and pain reduction in patients with peripheral neuropathy after treatment with monochromatic infrared photo energy—MIRE. *Journal of Diabetes and its Complications, 20*(2), 81–87.

Health Resources and Services Administration (HRSA). (2013). Foot care for a lifetime. Retrieved from https://www.hrsa.gov/sites/default/files/hansensdisease/leap/footcareforalifetime.pdf

Health Resources and Services Administration (HRSA). (2017). *LEAP resources*. Retrieved October 30, 2019, from http://www.hrsa.gov/hansensdisease/leap/index.htm

Hegde, N., Melanson, E., & Sazonov, E. (2016, August). Development of a real time activity monitoring Android application utilizing SmartStep. *Annual International Conference of the IEEE Engineering in Medicine and Biology Society, 2016*, 1886–1889.

Hicks, C. W., & Selvin, E. (2019). Epidemiology of peripheral neuropathy and lower extremity disease in diabetes. *Current Diabetes Reports, 19*(10), 86. doi: 10.1007/s11892-019-1212-8.

Hockenbury, R. T., Gruttadauria, M., & McKinney, I. (2007). Use of implantable bone growth stimulation in Charcot ankle arthrodesis. *Foot and Ankle International, 28*(9), 971–976.

Hoogeveen, R. C., Dorresteijn, J. A., Kriegsman, D. M., et al. (2015). Complex interventions for preventing diabetic foot ulceration. *Cochrane Database of Systematic Reviews*, (8), CD007610.

Ince, P., Abbas, Z. G., Lutale, J. K., et al. (2008). Use of the SINBAD classification system and score in comparing outcome of foot ulcer management on three continents. *Diabetes Care, 31*(5), 964–967.

International Working Group on the Diabetic Foot (IWGDF) Editorial Board. (2019). *IWGDF guidelines*. Retrieved from https://iwgdf-guidelines.org/definitions-criteria

Jiang, D. Q., Zhao, S. H., Li, M. X., et al. (2018). Prostaglandin E1 plus methylcobalamin combination therapy versus prostaglandin E1 monotherapy for patients with diabetic peripheral neuropathy: A meta-analysis of randomized controlled trials. *Medicine, 97*(44), e13020. doi: 10.1097/MD.0000000000013020.

Jude, E. B., & Boulton, A. J. (2002). Medical treatment of Charcot's arthropathy. *Journal of the American Podiatric Medical Association, 92*(7), 381.

Jude, E. B., Dang, C., & Boulton, A. J. (2010). Effect of L-arginine on the microcirculation in the neuropathic diabetic foot in type 2 diabetes mellitus: A double blind, placebo-controlled study. *Diabetic Medicine, 27*(1), 113–116.

Katz, I., Harlan, A., Miranda-Polma, B., et al. (2005). A randomized trial of two irremovable off-loading devices in management of plantar neuropathic diabetic foot ulcers. *Diabetes Care, 28*, 555–559.

Kelechi, T. J., & Lukacs, K. S. (1997). Patient with dystrophic toenails, calluses, and heel fissures. *Journal of Wound Ostomy & Continence Nursing, 24*(4), 237–242.

Killeen, A. L., Brock, K. M., Dancho, J. F., et al. (2020). Remote temperature monitoring in patients with visual impairment due to diabetes mellitus: A proposed improvement to current standard of care for prevention of diabetic foot ulcers. *Journal of Diabetes Science and Technology, 14*(1), 37–45. https://doi.org/10.1177/1932296819848769

Laborde, M. (2009). Midfoot ulcers treated with gastrocnemius–soleus recession. *Foot and Ankle International, 30*(9), 842–846.

Lavery, L. A., Armstrong, D. G., & Harkless, L. B. (1996). Classification of diabetic foot wounds. *Journal of Foot and Ankle Surgery, 35*, 528–531.

Lavery, L. A., Armstrong, D. G., Vela, S., et al. (1998). Practical criteria for screening patients at high risk for diabetic foot ulceration. *Archives of Internal Medicine, 158*(2), 157–162.

Lavery, L. A., Armstrong, D. G., & Walker, S. C. (1997). Healing rates of diabetic foot ulcers associated with midfoot fracture due to Charcot's arthropathy. *Diabetic Medicine, 14*(1), 46–49.

Lavery, L. A., Higgins, K. R., Lanctot, D. R., et al. (2004). Home monitoring of foot skin temperatures to prevent ulceration. *Diabetes Care, 27*(11), 2642–2647.

Lavery, L. A., Lanctot, D., Constantinides, G., et al. (2005). Wear and biomechanical characteristics of a novel shear-reducing insole with implications for high-risk persons with diabetes. *Diabetes Technology & Therapeutics, 7*(4), 638–646.

Lavery, L. A., Petersen, B. J., Linders, D. R., et al. (2019). Unilateral remote temperature monitoring to predict future ulceration for the diabetic foot in remission. *BMJ Open Diabetes Research and Care, 7*, e000696. doi: 10.1136/bmjdrc-2019-000696.

Lawson, D., & Petrofsky, J. S. (2007). A randomized control study on the effect of biphasic electrical stimulation in a warm room on skin blood flow and healing rates in chronic wounds of patients with and without diabetes. *Medical Science Monitor, 13*(6), CR258–CR263.

Lewis, J., & Lipp, A. (2013). Pressure-relieving interventions for treating diabetic foot ulcers. *Cochrane Database of Systematic Reviews*, (3), CD002302. doi: 10.1002/14651858.CD002302.pub2.

Luana, C., Taylor, L., Didier, B., et al. (2017). Neuropathic pain. *Nature Reviews. Disease Primers, 3*, 17.

Maluf, K. S., Mueller, M. J., Strube, M. J., et al. (2004). Tendon Achilles lengthening for the treatment of neuropathic ulcers causes a temporary reduction in forefoot pressure associated with changes in plantar flexor power rather than ankle motion during gait. *Journal of Biomechanics, 37*, 897–906.

McCrory, J., Morag, E., Norkitis, A., et al. (1998). Healing of Charcot fractures: Skin temperature and radiographic correlates. *The Foot, 8*, 158–165.

McGill, M., Molyneaux, L., Bolton, T., et al. (2000). Response of Charcot's arthropathy to contact casting: Assessment by quantitative techniques. *Diabetologia, 43*(4), 481–484.

Mills, J. L. Sr, Conte, M. S., Armstrong, D. G., et al.; Society for Vascular Surgery Lower Extremity Guidelines Committee. (2014). The Society for Vascular Surgery lower extremity threatened limb classification system: Risk stratification based on wound, ischemia, and foot infection (WIfI). *Journal of Vascular Surgery, 59*(1), 220–234.

Monteiro-Soares, M., Russell, D., Boyko, E. J., et al.; International Working Group on the Diabetic Foot (IWGDF). (2020). Guidelines on the classification of diabetic foot ulcers (IWGDF 2019). *Diabetes/Metabolism Research and Reviews, 36*(S1), e3273. doi: 10.1002/dmrr.3273.

Nabuurs-Franssen, M. H., Sleegers, R., Huijberts, M. S., et al. (2005). Total contact casting of the diabetic foot in daily practice: A prospective follow-up study. *Diabetes Care, 28*, 243–247.

Najafi, B., Ron, E., Enriquez, A., et al. (2017). Smarter sole survival: Will neuropathic patients at high risk for ulceration use a smart insole-based foot protection system? *Journal of Diabetes Science and Technology, 11*(4), 702–713. https://doi.org/10.1177/1932296816689105

National Institutes of Neurological Disorders and Stroke. (2019). Peripheral neuropathy fact sheet. Retrieved from https://www.ninds.nih.gov/Disorders/Patient-Caregiver-Education/Fact-Sheets/Peripheral-Neuropathy-Fact-Sheet

Nielson, D. L., & Armstrong, D. G. (2008). The natural history of Charcot's neuroarthropathy. *Clinics in Podiatric Medicine and Surgery, 25*(1), 53–62.

Nube, V. L., McGill, M., Molyneaux, L., et al. (2002). From acute to chronic: Monitoring the progress of Charcot's arthropathy. *Journal of the American Podiatric Medical Association, 92*(7), 384.

Okazaki, R. (2011). Diabetes mellitus and bone metabolism. *Clinical Calcium, 21*(5), 669–675.

Owings, T. M., Woerner, J. L., Frampton, J. D., et al. (2008). Custom therapeutic insoles based on both foot shape and plantar pressure measurement provide enhanced pressure relief. *Diabetes Care, 31*(5), 839–844.

Paola, L. D., Volpe, A., Varotto, D., et al. (2007). Use of a retrograde nail for ankle arthrodesis in Charcot neuroarthropathy: A limb salvage procedure. *Foot & Ankle International, 28*(9), 967–970. doi: 10.3113/FAI.2007.0967.

Pecoraro, R. E., Reiber, G. E., & Burgess, E. M. (1990). Pathways to diabetic limb amputation: Basis for prevention. *Diabetes Care, 13*, 513–521.

Petrofsky, J. S., Schwab, E., Lo, T., et al. (2007). The thermal effect on the blood flow response to electrical stimulation. *Medical Science Monitor, 13*(11), 498–504.

Prabhakar, A. T., Suresh, T., Kurian, D. S., et al. (2019). Timed vibration sense and joint position sense testing in the diagnosis of distal sensory polyneuropathy. *Journal of Neurosciences in Rural Practice, 10*(2), 273–277. doi: 10.4103/jnrp.jnrp24118.

Rader, A. J., & Barry, T. P. (2008). The football: An intuitive dressing for offloading neuropathic plantar forefoot ulcerations. *International Wound Journal, 5*(1), 69–73. doi: 10.1111/j.1742-481X.2007.00364.x.

Sage, R. A., Webster, J. K., & Fisher, S. G. (2001). Outpatient care and morbidity reduction in diabetic foot ulcers associated with chronic pressure callus. *Journal of the American Podiatric Medical Association, 91*(6), 275–279.

Saunders, L. J., & Mrdjencovich, D. (1991). Anatomical patterns of bone and joint destruction in neuropathic diabetics. *Diabetes, 40*, 529A.

Sayner, L. R., & Rosenblum, B. I. (2005). External fixation for Charcot foot reconstruction. *Current Surgery, 62*(6), 618–623.

Seidel, H. M. (2006). Blood vessels. In H. M. Seidel (Ed.), *Mosby's guide to physical examination* (6th ed.). St. Louis, MO: Mosby, Elsevier Science.

Sella, E. J. (2009). Current concepts review: Diagnostic imaging of the diabetic foot. *Foot and Ankle International, 30*(6), 568–576.

Shirazi, A. A., Nasiri, M., & Yazdanpanah, L. (2016). Dermatological and musculoskeletal assessment of diabetic foot: A narrative review. *Diabetes & Metabolic Syndrome: Clinical Research & Reviews, 10*(2), S158–S164.

Singal, A., & Khanna, D. (2011). Onychomycosis: Diagnosis and management. *Indian Journal of Dermatology, 77*(6), 659–672.

Singh, N., Armstrong, D. H., & Lipsky, B. (2005). Preventing foot ulcers in patients with diabetes. *JAMA, 293*(2), 217–228.

Snyder, D., Sullivan, N., Margolis, D., et al. (2020). *Technology assessment: Skin substitutes for treating chronic wounds* [Internet]. Rockville, MD: Agency for Healthcare Research and Quality (AHRQ) (US). Retrieved from https://www.ncbi.nlm.nih.gov/books/NBK554220/. Accessed April 25, 2020.

Soderstrom, L. H., Johnson, S. P., Diaz, V. A., et al. (2012). Association between vitamin D and diabetic neuropathy in a nationally representative sample: Results from 2001–2004 NHANES. *Diabetic Medicine, 29*(1), 50–55.

Sohn, M. W., Stuck, R. M., Pinzur, M., et al. (2010). Lower-extremity amputation risk after charcot arthropathy and diabetic foot ulcer. *Diabetes Care, 33*(1), 98–100.

Solomon, L. R. (2011). Diabetes as a cause of clinically significant functional cobalamin deficiency. *Diabetes Care, 34*(5), 1077–1080.

Spencer, S. A. (2000). Pressure relieving interventions for preventing and treating diabetic foot ulcers. *Cochrane Database of Systematic Reviews,* (3), CD002302. doi: 10.1002/14651858.CD002302.

Steed, D. L., Attinger, C., Colaizzi, T., et al. (2006). Guidelines for the treatment of diabetic ulcers. *Wound Repair and Regeneration, 14*(6), 680–692.

Verity, S., Sochocki, M., Embil, J. M., et al. (2008). Treatment of Charcot foot and ankle with a prefabricated removable walker brace and custom insole. *Foot and Ankle Surgery, 14*(1), 26–31.

Wagner, F. W. (1981). The dysvascular foot: A system for diagnosis and treatment. *Foot & Ankle, 2*(2), 64–122.

Wang, J. C. (2003). Use of external fixation in the reconstruction of the Charcot foot and ankle. *Clinics in Podiatric Medicine and Surgery, 20*(1), 97–117.

Weir, G. (2010). Diabetic foot ulcers—Evidence-based wound management. *Continuing Medical Education, 28*(40), 76–80.

Wound, Ostomy and Continence Nurses Society (WOCN). (2012). *Guideline for management of wounds in patients with lower-extremity neuropathic disease.* Mt. Laurel, NJ: Author.

Yavuz, M., Erdemir, A., Botek, G., et al. (2007). Peak plantar pressure and shear locations: Relevance to diabetic patients. *Diabetes Care, 30*(10), 2643–2645.

Yavuz, M., Tajaddini, A., Botek, G., et al. (2008). Temporal characteristics of plantar shear distribution: Relevance to diabetic patients. *Journal of Biomechanics, 41*(3), 556–559.

Zgonis, T., Stapleton, J. J., Jeffries, L. C., et al. (2008). Surgical treatment of Charcot neuroarthropathy. *AORN Journal, 87*(5), 971–990.

Zhan, L. X., Branco, B. C., Armstrong, D. G., et al. (2015). The Society for Vascular Surgery lower extremity threatened limb classification system based on Wound, Ischemia, and foot Infection (WIfI) correlates with risk of major amputation and time to wound healing. *Journal of Vascular Surgery, 61*(4), 939–944.

Zhang, X., Sun, D., & Jiang, G. (2018). Comparative efficacy of nine different dressings in healing diabetic foot ulcers: A Bayesian network analysis. *Journal of Diabetes, 11*(6), 418–426. doi: 10.1111/1753-0407.12871.

Ziegler, D., Low, P. A., Litchy, W. J., et al. (2011). Efficacy and safety of antioxidant treatment with a α-lipoic acid over 4 years in diabetic polyneuropathy: The NATHAN 1 trial. *Diabetes Care, 34*(9), 2054–2060.

Zimny, S., Schatz, H., & Pfohl, M. (2004). The role of limited joint mobility in diabetic patients with an at-risk foot. *Diabetes Care, 27*, 942–946.

QUESTIONS

1. The wound care nurse is assessing a patient who has developed a rocker bottom foot with plantar surface ulcerations. What condition would the nurse document?
   A. Charcot neuroarthropathy
   B. Footdrop
   C. Progressive anesthesia and loss of proprioception
   D. Paresthesia

2. The wound care nurse provides testing of lower extremity sensory function for patients at risk for lower extremity neuropathic disease (LEND). Which statement accurately describes this testing?
   A. 5-g monofilament should be used to test for sensory function and loss of protective sensation.
   B. Loss of vibratory sense typically occurs after LOPS. Therefore, vibratory sense testing is not as reliable a test as monofilament testing.
   C. Inability to consistently identify the direction in which the toe is pointing is considered loss of position sense.
   D. Foot deformities such as hammer toes are indicative of sensory neuropathy.

3. The wound care nurse palpates a callus on the heel of a diabetic patient. What interventions would the nurse recommend?
   A. Off-loading involving bed rest
   B. Paring of the callus
   C. Skin hydration
   D. Removing shoes in the home setting

4. The wound care nurse documents a patient's wound risk category as 2 as outlined in the Diabetes Foot Program guidelines. Along with education emphasizing disease control and proper shoe fit, what follow-up schedule would be recommended for this patient?
   A. Yearly for foot screen
   B. 3 to 6 months for foot/shoe examination and nail care
   C. 1 to 3 months for foot/activity/footwear examination and nail care
   D. 1 to 12 weeks for foot/activity/footwear evaluation and callus/nail care

5. The wound care nurse is conducting a filament test using the diabetes foot screen. Which step of the procedure is performed accurately?
   A. The filament is applied perpendicular to the skin's surface.

   B. The approach, skin contact, and departure of the filament is 5 seconds.
   C. The filament is slid across the skin to achieve repetitive contact at test site.
   D. The filament is applied directly on an ulcer, callus, scar, or necrotic tissue.

6. The wound care nurse is classifying a diabetic foot ulcer using the Wagner Classification System. What number would the nurse use to document a deep ulcer with joint sepsis?
   A. 1
   B. 2
   C. 3
   D. 4

7. Which off-loading option is considered to be the "gold standard" for management of plantar surface ulcers in the diabetic patient?
   A. Removable cast walker with rocker bottom
   B. Total contact cast
   C. Customized diabetic shoe
   D. Heel sole shoe with removable off-loading pegs

8. Which imaging study is the gold standard in diagnosing osteomyelitis?
   A. Plain x-rays
   B. Magnetic resonance imaging (MRI)
   C. Technetium-99 phosphate bone scan
   D. Positron emission tomography (PET)

9. Which pharmacological intervention would the wound care nurse typically recommend for a patient with pain described as "dysesthesia"?
   A. Capsaicin cream
   B. Tricyclic antidepressant
   C. Analgesics
   D. Opioids

10. The wound care nurse is teaching a patient with intact foot sensation how to purchase and wear commercial shoes to lower the risk of skin damage. Which of the following is a recommended guideline?
   A. Allow for ¼ inch space beyond the longest toe.
   B. Size and purchase shoes in the morning before edema sets in.
   C. Measure both feet and size shoes to the smaller foot.
   D. Gradually increase wear time for new shoes by 2-hour increments daily.

ANSWERS AND RATIONALES

1. A. Rationale: If the individual continues to walk on the damaged foot, additional fractures may occur with progressive damage to the bony structure of the foot. The end result may be total collapse of the normal architecture of the foot, with development of a rocker bottom foot that is at high risk for plantar surface ulcerations. This defect is known as Charcot neuroarthropathy.

2. C. Rationale: To test for proprioceptive sense, the person is asked to close the eyes. The wound care nurse then moves the great toe in different directions (up, down, medially, and laterally) and asks the person to tell in which direction the toe is pointing. Inability to consistently identify the direction in which the toe is pointing is considered loss of position sense.

3. B. Rationale: The wound care nurse should observe for and palpate any calluses and should intervene, especially for rigid focal calluses located over bony prominences. Interventions include paring of the callus and providing recommendations regarding pressure-redistributing footwear and insoles.

4. C. Rationale: From Table 26-2—Depth-inlay footwear, molded/modified orthoses; modified shoes as needed; routine follow-up 1 to 3 months for foot/activity/footwear evaluation and callus/nail care.

5. A. Rationale: From Box 26-3—3. Apply the filament perpendicular to the skin's surface (see diagram **A**).

6. C. Rationale: From Box 26-5—Wagner Classification System—3: Deep ulcer with abscess, osteomyelitis, or joint sepsis

7. B. Rationale: Total contact casting (TCC) has been considered the gold standard for off-loading neuropathic foot wounds.

8. B. Rationale: MRI provides detection of Charcot foot in the early stages when it is not yet identifiable on x-ray. MRI also provides definitive diagnosis of osteomyelitis.

9. A. Rationale: From Table 26-7—Capsaicin cream—(Topical) Dose: 0.025% and 0.075% topically applied very sparingly three to four times per day, in mapped areas (indicating sites of greatest neuropathic pain).

10. D. Rationale: Individuals with intact sensation and no deformities can wear commercially available shoes. They should be instructed to gradually increase wear time for new shoes, that is, by 2-hour increments each day, with routine foot inspection following each wearing.

CHAPTER 27

ATYPICAL LOWER EXTREMITY WOUNDS

Barbara A. Pieper

OBJECTIVES

1. Describe critical parameters to be included in the assessment of an individual with an atypical lower extremity ulcer.

2. Use assessment data to determine causative and contributing factors for an atypical lower extremity ulcer and to develop individualized management plans that are evidence based.

3. Identify indications that a lower extremity ulcer is "atypical" and requires additional diagnostic workup and/or medical–surgical intervention.

4. Describe pathology, clinical presentation, and management for each of the following: vasculitic ulcers, pyoderma gangrenosum, calciphylaxis, sickle cell ulcer, basal cell carcinoma, squamous cell carcinoma, factitious ulcers and warfarin-induced skin necrosis.

TOPIC OUTLINE

INTRODUCTION

As discussed in previous chapters, the most common types of lower extremity ulcers are venous ulcers, neuropathic ulcers, and arterial (ischemic) ulcers. However, there are several other pathologic conditions that can result in lower extremity ulcers, and the most common of those conditions are the focus of this chapter, that is, vasculitis, sickle cell disease, pyoderma gangrenosum (PG), calciphylaxis, squamous and basal cell carcinoma (BCC), and factitious ulcers. While these ulcers are often considered less common, Tang et al. (2012) examined 350 wound biopsies sent for diagnoses to a wound pathology service and found that 29.7% were "atypical" causes. The majority of the specimens were neoplasms with the most common being squamous cell carcinoma; neoplasms were followed by PG and vasculitis (Tang et al., 2012). Shanmugam et al. (2017) reported 20% to 23% of nonhealing wounds that are refractory to vascular interventions have other causes such as the ones in this chapter. Effective management of the wounds presented in this chapter primarily involves treatment of the underlying condition versus specific dressings used for wound care; thus, the focus is on the pathology, clinical presentation, diagnosis, and management of the underlying pathology.

A number of lower extremity ulcers are caused by pathologies other than venous, arterial, and neuropathic disease; thus, the wound nurse must always be alert to indicators of atypical wounds and must complete a thorough assessment in order to identify etiology.

 VASCULITIS AND ULCERATION

PREVALENCE AND INCIDENCE

Vasculitis is an autoimmune connective tissue disease that leads to inflammation and potential damage to vital organs (Lakdawala & Fedeles, 2017) and is characterized by damage or destruction of blood vessels of any size. Cutaneous and systemic vasculitides are uncommon, and there are limited epidemiologic data. The estimated annual incidence of cutaneous vasculitis is reported as 38.6 cases per million (de Araujo & Kirsner, 2001). Papi and Papi (2016) approximated 3% to 5% of skin ulcers may be caused by vasculitic disorders. Some authors state that it is more common in women (de Araujo & Kirsner, 2001); others say it appears more commonly in men than in women, although women are diagnosed at a younger age (Brown, 2012). Authors agree that vasculitis is more common among adults with a mean age of 47 years (Shavit et al., 2018). Although rare, vasculitis can occur in children (mean age 7 years) and tends to have a self-limiting course (Lakdawala & Fedeles, 2017; Shavit et al., 2018).

The nomenclature for vasculitis can be confusing. Vasculitis is defined as an autoimmune connective tissue inflammatory disease that targets blood vessels. In contrast, vasculopathy is a noninflammatory condition characterized by excessive thrombus formation in the microcirculation (Kerk & Goerge, 2013a, 2013b). In some conditions, the terms are used interchangeably; for example, livedoid vasculopathy, also called livedoid vasculitis, is characterized by painful purpuric lesions of the lower extremities that frequently ulcerate and leave white, stellate atrophic scars (atrophie blanche) with dyspigmentation and telangiectasia (de Araujo & Kirsner, 2001; Kerk & Goerge, 2013a, 2013b). Although livedoid vasculitis clinically resembles a vasculitis, it is a vasculopathy, not a vasculitis; namely, it is a thrombotic phenomenon without inflammation. Definitions for vasculitides were adopted by the 2012 International Chapel Hill Consensus Conference on the Nomenclature of Vasculitides (Jennette et al., 2013).

PATHOLOGY

The etiology of vasculitis is most likely multifactorial, with a combination of predisposing factors and triggering factors. Predisposing factors include genetic makeup, ethnicity, environmental exposure, and gender (de Araujo & Kirsner, 2001), while triggering factors include infectious causes (most common), drugs (about 10% of cases), malignancy (less common and most likely to involve lymphoproliferative malignancies), connective tissue diseases, and cryoprotein disorders, among others. In some patients, the definitive etiologic agent for cutaneous vasculitis cannot be identified. An infectious cause that needs to be considered due to its occurrence is hepatitis C virus (Monti et al., 2019)

Vasculitis may be recurrent or intermittent with new lesions appearing over time (Brown, 2012; de Araujo & Kirsner, 2001). Because of similarities to other clinical conditions, histologic confirmation is essential to confirm a diagnosis and its classification (de Araujo & Kirsner, 2001; Shavit et al., 2018). Shavit et al. recommend biopsy of a lesion within 48 hours of occurrence, if feasible. de Araujo and Kirsner (2001) note that cutaneous vasculitis involves the postcapillary venules and is characterized by the following: endothelial cell swelling, neutrophilic invasion of blood vessel walls, presence of disrupted neutrophils (often called leukocytoclasia), extravasation of red blood cells (RBCs), and fibrinoid necrosis of the blood vessel walls. This constellation of findings is known as cutaneous necrotizing vasculitis.

For further information on the etiology and pathology of vasculitis, the reader is referred to the American College of Rheumatology Web site dated 2019 with content for practitioners and patients (http://www.rheumatology.org/Practice/Clinical/Patients/Diseases_And_Conditions/Vasculitis/) as well as the British Society for Rheumatology (BSR) and British Health Professionals in

Rheumatology (BHPR) Guideline for the Management of Adults with Antineutrophil cytoplasmic antibodies (ANCA)-associated Vasculitis (Ntatsaki et al., 2014).

CLINICAL PRESENTATION

Vasculitis commonly presents as palpable purpura (raised areas of nonblanchable erythema), which signifies extravasation of RBCs outside of the blood vessel into the surrounding tissue (de Araujo & Kirsner, 2001). The clinical presentation varies and may include red macules, wheals, papules, nodules, ulcers, vesicles, and blisters (Papi & Papi, 2016; Shavit et al., 2018). The size of the blood vessel affected determines the clinical picture; for example, if large vessels are affected, the lesions may be widespread. The lesions are most commonly located on the lower legs and are symmetrical but can occur anywhere on the body. Some cutaneous lesions may heal quickly (in 1 to 4 weeks), but ulcerative lesions frequently have a prolonged healing course. Scarring and hyperpigmentation may occur (de Araujo & Kirsner, 2001). **Figure 27-1** shows a vasculitic ulcer on the lower extremity with purpura and necrosis.

The severity of the disease process can be assessed with the Birmingham Vasculitis Activity Score (BVAS) (http://www.epsnetwork.co.uk/BVAS/bvas_flow.html); currently in use is version 3 (Suppiah et al., 2011). The scale is divided into sections reflecting new-onset or worsening disease in nine organ systems: general, cutaneous, mucous membrane/eyes, ENT, chest, and the cardiovascular, abdominal, renal, and nervous systems. A total score is calculated and is used to guide treatment decisions and other disease activity assessments (Mukhtyar et al., 2009).

DIAGNOSIS

Diagnosis of vasculitis lesions begins by eliminating other causes/conditions, namely with a thorough history, physical examination, and laboratory data (Papi &

Papi, 2016; Shanmugam et al., 2017; Shavit et al., 2018). The aim is to identify the triggering factor if possible and to determine the presence and severity of organ system involvement. Some of the laboratory tests include antinuclear antibodies, complement levels, cryoglobulins, antistreptolysin O antibodies, Hemoccult testing, and antibodies for viral hepatitis, rheumatoid factor, and urinalysis to assess for renal involvement. Various radiographs may be done to diagnose respiratory tract or neurologic disease. A biopsy of the lesion for histological evaluation is crucial. Even if the patient is known to have a condition associated with vasculitis, the clinician cannot assume that the ulcer is due to vasculitis; a thorough workup and histologic evaluation must always be performed. For example, Seitz et al. (2010) examined the causative factors for leg ulcers in 36 persons with rheumatoid arthritis and found the following: 3 patients had necrotizing vasculitis, 2 had PG, 8 had venous ulcers, 4 had arterial ulcers, 3 had combined venous/arterial ulcers, 5 had pressure ulcers, and 11 were due to other causes. These findings underscore the fact that vasculitic ulcers are less common and that a thorough workup is necessary to determine the cause of the patient's wound.

KEY POINT

Vasculitic ulcers are acutely painful wounds that require treatment with anti-inflammatory medications; diagnosis is based on clinical assessment, laboratory studies, and biopsy.

MANAGEMENT

If a triggering factor for vasculitis is identified, initial management should focus on management of that disease process or triggering agent. If the disease process involves multiple organ systems, the management approach must address all involved systems. Disease limited to the skin may require only treatment of the skin lesions and is based on the characteristics of the lesions. Shavit et al. (2018) recommended that treatment of cutaneous small vessel vasculitis be based on the clinical experience with primary goals of therapy to prevent extensive cutaneous infarction, comfort, and control of symptoms. For example, therapy may include bed rest, warming, elevation of lower extremities, nonsteroidal anti-inflammatory drugs (NSAIDs), analgesics, and antihistamines to control burning and itching. Care must be taken with NSAIDs since NSAIDs may be an incriminating drug causing vasculitis. Lower extremity lesions accompanied by edema may necessitate compression in addition to topical therapy. If the disease process and/or lesions are widespread, systemic corticosteroids may be used; the dose of corticosteroids is determined by the severity of the disease activity. Sometimes

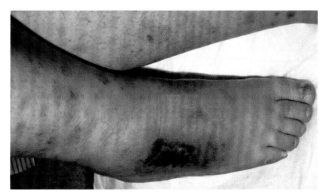

FIGURE 27-1. A Vasculitic Ulceration that Has Occurred in a Patient Who Has Leukocytoclastic Vasculitis. (Reprinted with permission from Goodheart, H. P. (2003). *Goodheart's photoguide of common skin disorders* (2nd ed.). Philadelphia, PA: Lippincott Williams & Wilkins.)

corticosteroids are combined with other immunosuppressive agents (such as cyclophosphamide). Other immunosuppressive therapies may be used depending upon the number of organ systems involved, relapse rates, and side effect profile (Brown, 2012). Examples of other drugs reported in the literature include colchicine, dapsone, pentoxifylline, and hydroxychloroquine (Papi & Papi, 2016; Shavit et al., 2018).

In discussing vasculitis in general, Brown (2012) presented the following as priorities for nursing management: (1) general patient education and information about vasculitis; (2) information and discussion regarding medication regimens; (3) discussion of side effects of medications and implications for monitoring and reporting; (4) assessment for complications of drug therapy, to include blood work monitoring; (5) provision of information about patient support groups; (6) advice regarding self-care such as regular exercise, rest, and positive life style choices; (7) informed consent and patient agreement to adhere to complex drug regimens; (8) involvement of family and friends in care if the patient desires; (9) if vasculitis affects work, advice regarding how to inform the work environment; (10) measures to promote quality of life; and (11) advice as to when the patient should seek advice and support. If the person with vasculitis has open wounds, the dressing should be selected to fit the area of the body involved, to manage any exudate and maintain a moist surface, and to prevent traumatic removal by limiting the application of adhesive to the skin. The dressing should be one that the patient can apply, and the patient's insurance coverage for the dressing needs to be considered. Some patients experience marked pain with vasculitis. Pain should be treated with appropriate analgesics taking into consideration the patient's overall health status, prescribed medications, and incriminating drugs for vasculitis. Topical anesthetics may improve pain symptoms (Shavit et al., 2018).

⬤ SICKLE CELL ULCERS

PREVALENCE AND INCIDENCE

Sickle cell disease is a single amino acid molecular disorder of hemoglobin that leads to several pathological changes; these include changes in the shape and rigidity of the RBC that cause obstruction of the microcirculation with subsequent tissue ischemia and infarction (Kato et al., 2009; Minniti et al., 2010). Sickle cell disease is the most common inherited hematologic disorder and is chronic (Jenerette et al., 2014). It affects about 100,000 persons in the United States with most of them being African American (Centers for Disease Control and Prevention, 2019). In the 21st century, the majority of patients with sickle cell disease reach adulthood (Minniti & Kato, 2016). Leg ulcers are a common and often disabling

complication of sickle cell disease; interestingly, the first patient described with sickle cell disease in the United States in 1910 had leg ulcers (Minniti et al., 2010). Senet et al. (2017) noted the prevalence of lower extremity ulcers in sickle cell disease depends on genotype, geographical location, age of the population, and social environment. The prevalence of leg ulcers varies, but they are uncommon in children <10 years of age (Minniti et al., 2010). There is insufficient evidence to link sickle cell trait with leg ulcers (Tsaras et al., 2009).

PATHOLOGY

As noted, sickle cell disease is a genetic disorder involving abnormal hemoglobin. A child born with sickle cell disease has two genes for hemoglobin S, one from each parent. The abnormal hemoglobin causes RBCs to develop a crescent (sickle) shape and to become stiff and sticky; these altered RBCs are unable to pass normally through the smaller blood vessels and instead obstruct the blood vessels, thus causing acute ischemia of the involved tissues or organs. In contrast to sickle cell disease (designated as HbSS to indicate two genes for hemoglobin S), the child born with sickle cell trait has only one abnormal gene; the other hemoglobin gene is normal (HbAS). These children do not develop sickle cell disease, but they can pass the sickle cell gene on to their children. There is also a condition known as HbSC, which is a more common and milder sickling disorder associated with lower incidence of complications such as leg ulcers (Madu et al., 2013).

The pathology of sickle cell anemia is marked by repeated episodes of vascular occlusion, reperfusion injury, hypoxemia, and vascular inflammation (Jenerette et al., 2014). This process results in unpredictable episodes of "sickle cell crisis"; these episodes are acutely painful and may result in organ or tissue damage due to the ischemic nature of the underlying pathology. Leg ulcers are more common in patients with homozygous sickle cell disease (HbSS) and less common in those with the milder HbSC disease (Delaney et al., 2013; Minniti et al., 2010). Estimates of sickle cell ulcers are 14% to 18% in the United States and Europe, and 29.5% in Jamaica (Senet et al., 2017).

The pathogenesis of leg ulcers in sickle cell disease is complex and includes a combination of factors: vascular obstruction by dense sickled red cells, venous incompetence, bacterial infections, excessive vasoconstriction when in a dependent position, in situ thrombosis, anemia resulting in decreased oxygen carrying capacity, and decreased nitric acid bioavailability (Minniti et al., 2010; Senet et al., 2017). Nitric oxide (NO) is produced by the endothelium and is a critical regulator of normal vascular function and vasodilation (Kato et al., 2009). Intravascular hemolysis, such as occurs during sickle cell crises, releases hemoglobin into the plasma, and hemoglobin acts as a potent scavenger of NO. Chronic NO depletion may contribute to vasoconstriction and further tissue ischemia (Kato et al., 2009; Morris, 2008). Sickle cell ulcers may be caused by an acute ischemic episode or by minor trauma to chronically ischemic tissues; any break in the skin is then vulnerable to secondary infection. The mechanisms of the ulcers remain largely unexplained (Aractingi, 2017).

Minniti et al. (2014) examined the microcirculation of the tissues in and around sickle cell leg ulcers. They found the highest blood flow within the ulcer bed with reduced blood flow in the immediate periwound area. They also found evidence of venous stasis, inflammation, and thrombotic changes that were consistent with the pathology of chronic venous ulcers in non–sickle cell disease individuals.

CLINICAL PRESENTATION

Sickle cell ulcers usually occur in areas with minimal subcutaneous tissue, thin skin, and decreased blood flow. The most common sites are the medial and lateral malleoli of the lower leg (Minniti et al., 2010) (**Fig. 27-2**). Less common sites include the anterior tibia, dorsum of the foot, and Achilles tendon. The ulcers are typically painful, indolent, intractable, very slow to heal, prone to recurrence, and commonly associated with venous insufficiency. Having a sickle cell leg ulcer is also associated with priapism and pulmonary hypertension, and all are markers of advanced sickle vasculopathy (Minniti et al., 2010).

Halabi-Tawi et al. (2008) presented a 20-case series of patients with sickle cell anemia and current or past leg ulcers; they completed chart reviews, interviewed

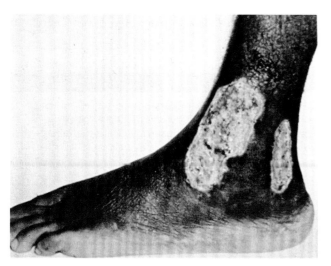

FIGURE 27-2. Chronic Leg Ulcers in an Adult Patient with Sickle Cell Anemia (SCA). (Reprinted with permission from Greer, J. P., et al. (2013). *Wintrobe's clinical hematology* (13th ed.). Philadelphia, PA: Wolters Kluwer Health.)

the patients, and conducted clinical examinations. The clinical features they identified included the following: median ulcer area was 12 cm^2; median ulcer time was 29.5 months; 85% had local/regional infection; 50% had ankle stiffness; 85% had mood disorders; and median age of ulcer onset was 21 years. These patients had many additional physical conditions such as priapism in 50% of males; acute chest syndrome, 50%; proteinuria, 35%; retinopathy, 30%; osteonecrosis, 30%; pulmonary hypertension, 22%; and stroke, 10%. Senet and colleagues (2017) examined factors predictive of leg ulcer healing in sickle cell disease (*N* = 98). Multivariate analyses showed ulcer area of <8 cm^2 and <9 weeks ulcer duration as independently associated with healing at week 24; no sickle cell disease characteristics were found associated with healing. At 24 weeks, 47% of leg ulcers were healed. Factors independently associated with recurrence were not identified.

DIAGNOSIS

The diagnosis is generally made based on the history of sickle cell disease and the clinical presentation (Madu et al., 2013). As with any ulceration, a biopsy may be done to rule out other causes.

MANAGEMENT

Management involves treatment of the underlying disease process, pain control, and topical therapy based on ulcer characteristics. Systemic treatment commonly involves either hydroxyurea, which increases the production of fetal (normal) hemoglobin, or blood transfusions to temporarily correct anemia and provide normal RBCs (Delaney et al., 2013). Hydroxyurea has also been noted to promote ulcers in patients with sickle cell disease (Minniti & Kato, 2016). NO-based therapies are reported as beneficial in the early and late phases of wound healing. NO increases extracellular matrix production, modulates immunologic response to the wound, stimulates keratinocyte proliferation and angiogenesis, is antiplatelet, and has bactericidal properties (Minniti & Kato, 2016). There are only anecdotal reports of blood transfusions' effectiveness in stimulating ulcer healing; thus, decisions to use them need to be made case by case (Minniti & Kato, 2016; Senet et al., 2017). Current data indicate that pain is an issue for most patients. Halabi-Tawi and colleagues (2008) found that 90% of patients needed analgesics for management of ulcer pain, and many used more than one type of analgesic. Comfortable shoes should be encouraged. Topical therapy is based on the principles addressed throughout this text: establishment of a clean wound bed, management of exudate, maintenance of a moist wound bed, and protection from infection and trauma. Because venous insufficiency is common in patients with sickle cell ulcers, compression wraps are commonly indicated. Debridement is essential if there is necrotic tissue, and osteomyelitis should be ruled out whenever a wound is slow to heal. Studies indicate that systemic infection, amputation, and death due to leg ulcers are uncommon in patients with sickle cell disease (Minniti et al., 2010).

Wound management for sickle cell ulcers is not yet standardized (Senet et al., 2017). A variety of treatment strategies have been suggested for nonhealing sickle cell ulcers, including skin grafts, hyperbaric oxygen therapy, arginine butyrate, growth factor therapy, zinc sulfate, and herbal agents; however, Minniti et al. (2010) concluded that there has been little improvement in the efficacy of management and clinical outcome in leg ulcers related to sickle cell disease over the last 100 years and that care is fragmented and inadequate. Similarly, Marti-Carvajal et al. (2014) performed a Cochrane review of six randomized controlled trials including 198 participants with 250 ulcers related to sickle cell disease. Study treatments included topical agents to the ulcer and systemic medications. The authors concluded that the evidence for use of interventions to treat people with sickle cell ulcers is not strong and all trials had a high risk of bias.

Obviously, a primary goal of management for individuals with sickle cell disease is ulcer prevention. This involves overall disease management, to reduce the incidence of vasoocclusive episodes, and prevention of trauma, which is commonly the precipitating factor for ulcer development. Prevention strategies include use of protective wraps, shin guards, or orthotic devices, especially during activities that could cause injury to the lower leg; strict avoidance of venipunctures to the lower extremity; and management of venous insufficiency and edema (Minniti et al., 2010; Minniti & Kato, 2016).

⬤ PYODERMA GANGRENOSUM

PREVALENCE AND INCIDENCE

PG is a rare chronic inflammatory skin disease that affects 3 to 10 patients per million population per year. It typically begins with an acutely painful nodule or pustule that breaks down to form a progressively enlarging ulcer (Lemos et al., 2017). It most commonly occurs between 20 and 50 years of age and is slightly more common among women than among men. Pediatric cases have been diagnosed. About 50% of patients have coexisting systemic inflammatory diseases, with the most common being inflammatory bowel disease (ulcerative colitis and Crohn disease); about 2% to 12% of patients with PG also have IBD. Other inflammatory conditions that have been associated with PG include arthritis (seronegative arthritis, spondylitis of inflammatory bowel disease, and rheumatoid arthritis) and lymphoproliferative disorders (myelogenous leukemia, hairy cell leukemia,

myelofibrosis, and monoclonal gammopathy) (Kridin et al., 2018; Lemos et al., 2017; Pompeo, 2016). The mortality rate for PG can be as high as 30%; negative prognostic indicators include male gender, advanced age at onset, and bullous PG associated with malignant hematologic conditions.

PATHOLOGY

Although the etiology is unknown and the pathogenesis not well understood, PG does not appear to be an infectious process as was theorized in 1930 and is not associated with lymphangitis or lymphadenopathy (Ruocco et al., 2009). Because it is associated with systemic conditions with a suspected autoimmune pathogenesis, the most commonly held theory is that it represents an autoimmune process targeting the skin. Another theory suggests that PG is caused by a dysfunction of the neutrophils and is included in neutrophilic dermatosis (Vallini et al., 2017). However, the disease is idiopathic in 25% to 50% of patients, underscoring the fact that we do not yet understand either the etiology or the pathology of PG, but advances have been made (Ahn et al., 2018; Vallini et al., 2017). Several types/variant forms of PG have been described in the literature: classic or ulcerative (most common), pustular, bullous or pemphigoid, vegetative, peristomal, genital, infantile, and extracutaneous (Lemos et al., 2017; Vallini et al., 2017).

CLINICAL PRESENTATION

The hallmark of PG is an ulcer with a raised dusty red or violaceous (purplish) border that is inflamed and frequently undermined and a boggy, necrotic base (Lemos et al., 2017; Pompeo, 2016) (**Fig. 27-3**). The base may appear perforated, and light pressure frequently produces purulent drainage. There is typically a bright halo of erythema extending about 2 cm from the ulcer border.

KEY POINT

Pyoderma gangrenosum ulcers are caused by an autoimmune process that causes full-thickness skin loss; the ulcers are painful and may exhibit pathergy (acute exacerbation in response to minor trauma).

The ulcer starts as a deep, painful nodule or a superficial hemorrhagic pustule; it may develop spontaneously or in response to minimal trauma (Lemos et al., 2017; Vallini et al., 2017). Ulcers often expand rapidly in one direction and slowly in another resulting in a serpiginous pattern. Ulcers can enlarge through extension of the undermined border or through development of new hemorrhagic pustules, either singular or multiple. PG ulcers can be confined to the dermis but often extend

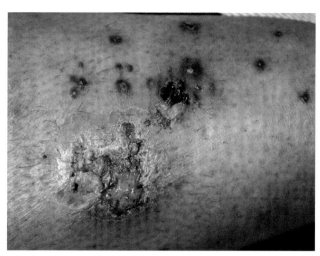

FIGURE 27-3. Pyoderma Gangrenosum, with Early Pustules and Ulcerations on the Shin. (Reprinted with permission from Gorroll, A. H., & Mulley, A. G. (2009). *Primary care medicine* (6th ed.). Philadelphia, PA: Wolters Kluwer Health.)

into the fat or fascia. Although they can develop on any area of the body, the ulcers most commonly occur on the lower extremities or trunk (**Fig. 27-4**).

The progression and long-term outcome of PG are unpredictable. The clinical course may involve an explosive onset and rapid spread of the lesions or an indolent progression with gradually spreading ulcers. In the explosive version, the individual usually experiences pain, fever, hemorrhagic blisters with purulent drainage, extensive necrosis, and a soggy ulcer border with a marked inflammatory halo. The indolent version is characterized by slowly enlarging and acutely painful ulcers that frequently exhibit granulation tissue within the ulcer bed and crusting and hyperkeratosis at the border

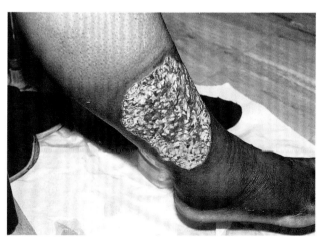

FIGURE 27-4. This Large Pyoderma Gangrenosum Ulceration Is Located on the Lower Extremity and Shows Beginning Healing with a Crater-Like (Cribriform) Scar. (Reprinted with permission from Goodheart, H. P. (2003). *Goodheart's photoguide of common skin disorders* (2nd ed.). Philadelphia, PA: Lippincott Williams & Wilkins.)

(Lemos et al., 2017; Pompeo, 2016; Vallini et al., 2017). The ulcers may heal in one area, only to recur in the same area or at another site. Trauma, either accidental trauma or surgical trauma, may precipitate ulcer development; this is known as Koebner phenomenon. In addition, even minor trauma can precipitate an exacerbation of existing lesions, a phenomenon known as pathergy.

PG has variant forms, one of which is peristomal and is classified as a rare subset, accounting for 0.6% of peristomal skin problems (Hanley, 2011; Lemos et al., 2017). Patients with ulcerative colitis or Crohn disease who have undergone ileostomy or colostomy are potentially at risk for peristomal PG. The lesions appear in the peristomal area 2 months to 25 years after the surgery and may be triggered or worsened by trauma to the skin from leakage of stool or adhesive trauma caused by repetitive removal of the appliance.

DIAGNOSIS

The diagnosis is based primarily on the history and clinical presentation. A detailed history is important to rule out other potential causes of the skin lesions and to determine if there is a treatable associated systemic disorder. A biopsy is typically done for differential diagnostic causes such as malignancy, vasculitis, and infection. The histopathologic findings are nonspecific and include an undermined ulcer border with edema, neutrophilic inflammation, and engorgement and thrombosis of small and medium blood vessels; neutrophilic inflammation is the cytologic hallmark (Lemos et al., 2017; Ratnagobal & Sinha, 2013). Other studies may be indicated to rule out associated systemic disorders; for example, laboratory studies may be done to rule out hematologic malignancies and arthritis syndromes, and colonoscopy should be done for the patient who has signs and symptoms of inflammatory bowel disease.

MANAGEMENT

Treatment is empiric since the etiology and pathology of PG are not well understood (Ruocco et al., 2009). Treatment is dependent upon the severity of the lesions, associated diseases, overall health status of the patient, and risk of prolonged treatment. Goals of care are to (1) reduce inflammation and promote healing; (2) reduce pain; and (3) control any underlying disease process, while minimizing adverse effects (Ruocco et al., 2009). Systemic corticosteroids and cyclosporine are effective, but the severity of the PG lesions must justify the risks of using these medications. Effective treatment of the underlying systemic disease (when present) usually results in healing or improvement of the ulcers.

Surgical debridement can be done to remove necrotic tissue for infection control (Lemos et al., 2017). Aggressive surgical debridement should be avoided because the inflammatory response in the surgical wound can act as a trigger for PG (Lemos et al., 2017; Vallini et al., 2017). Autolytic or enzymatic debridement is a much safer approach for these patients. Should surgery be required for a patient with a history of PG, the surgeon should always be made aware so that he or she can limit the size of incisions and can make every attempt to minimize tissue trauma. Some surgeons use prophylactic systemic corticosteroids or cyclosporine perioperatively to reduce the risk of development of PG ulcers.

Systemic treatment is usually needed to control the inflammatory process, and corticosteroids are often considered the gold standard in treatment (Lemos et al., 2017; Pompeo, 2016; Vallini et al., 2017). Doses may be initially high (e.g., 100 to 200 mg/day of prednisone) in order to establish remission; pulsed therapy with methylprednisone 1 g/day for 5 consecutive days is another approach that is frequently used. The rarity of PG has not allowed trials for therapy, but there is consensus on systemic and topical corticosteroids (Lemos et al., 2017). Once the inflammation is under control, the dose can be tapered. Any patient being treated with corticosteroids must be monitored and treated for the side effects of steroid therapy. Alternatives to corticosteroid therapy include other anti-inflammatory drugs, such as sulfasalazine, dapsone, and sulfapyridine; these drugs may be given as solo therapy or may be given in combination with corticosteroids. Other systemic agents mentioned in the literature include steroid-sparing immunosuppressives, cyclosporine, methotrexate, intravenous immunoglobulins, and infliximab (Lemos et al., 2017; Vallini et al., 2017).

Local therapy includes dressings to manage the exudate and maintain a moist wound bed; antimicrobial dressings are sometimes used to control bacterial loads and reduce inflammation. Because pain is a major issue for these patients, dressings should provide for atraumatic removal; around-the-clock analgesics may be needed as well. Foam dressings have been suggested because they are nonadherent and absorbent (Pompeo, 2016; Vallini et al., 2017). Topical and intralesional corticosteroids have also been used (Vallini et al., 2017). When PG lesions are located adjacent to a stoma, the wound ostomy continence (WOC) nurse needs to consider both treatment of the ulcers and fit of the ostomy pouching system. Topical agents should provide for exudate management and should be applied in accordance with manufacturers' recommendations. Although a convex appliance may improve the pouch seal and help to prevent leakage of effluent, the associated peristomal pressure may exacerbate the peristomal PG; thus, a flexible version may be needed as opposed to a rigid product (Hanley, 2011). The contracted, cribriform scarring that results from healing of peristomal PG necessitates careful appliance selection (Hanley, 2011).

● CALCIPHYLAXIS (CALCIFIC UREMIC ARTERIOLOPATHY)

PREVALENCE AND INCIDENCE

Calciphylaxis, also called calcific uremic arteriolopathy, occurs most commonly in patients with end-stage renal disease, though it has also been reported in nonuremic individuals. The incidence is higher in patients treated with peritoneal than hemodialysis (Nigwekar et al., 2018). The reported annual incidence among individuals undergoing hemodialysis in the United States is 35 cases per 10,000 patients, but there are concerns that these numbers may rise as a result of the increasing prevalence of chronic kidney disease in the United States (Nigwekar et al., 2018). Calciphylaxis is more common in women and Caucasians; obesity, diabetes, hypercoagulability, warfarin therapy, hyperparathyroidism, hypoalbuminemia, and trauma are additional risk factors (Chang, 2019; Nigwekar et al., 2018). The mean age of patients at diagnosis is 50 to 70 years (Nigwekar et al., 2018), and the disease is associated with severe pain and a generally poor prognosis of <1 year (Nigwekar et al., 2018). Risk of mortality is affected by the site of the calciphylaxis lesions; proximal disease (lesions affecting the abdomen, thighs, and buttocks) is associated with a higher mortality rate than distal disease (lesions affecting the lower limbs) (Vedvyas et al., 2012).

PATHOLOGY

The pathogenesis of calciphylaxis is unclear (Nigwekar, 2017). Microvascular calcification and thrombosis are believed to be key processes (Chang, 2019; Nigwekar, 2017). Contributing factors seem to include hypercalcemia, hyperphosphatemia, and high calcium–phosphate product levels, and these findings have led to recommendations that patients with end stage renal disease may benefit from low-calcium dialysate and careful attention to both calcium and phosphorus levels. Histopathologic findings in patients with active disease include intimal proliferation, medial calcification, and thrombosis of the small vessels in the dermis and subcutaneous tissue and calcium deposits in the soft tissues; these pathologic changes cause progressive tissue ischemia and subcutaneous tissue necrosis (Chang, 2019; Nigwekar et al., 2018).

CLINICAL PRESENTATION

As noted, calciphylaxis is characterized by thrombosis of the small vessels in the dermis and subcutaneous fat leading to cutaneous ischemia, tissue infarction, and necrosis (Chang, 2019). The lesions are described as violaceous (purple-hued) reticulated plaques progressing to nonhealing, deep, stellate (star-shaped) ulcers that usually become gangrenous (Seethapathy et al., 2019) (**Fig. 27-5**). They are extremely painful, and pain management may be the patient's greatest concern. Pain may be unresponsive to high-dose opioids, and opioid

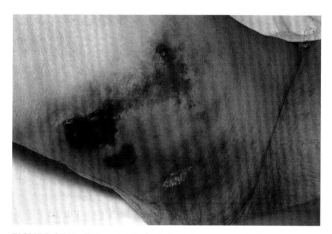

FIGURE 27-5. This calciphylaxis leg ulcer presented on an elderly female with end-stage renal disease and elevated parathyroid hormone level; she developed widespread induration of the lower extremities, which led to purpuric and necrotic ulcerations.

toxicity may develop (Nigwekar et al., 2018). Multiple pain treatment modalities may be needed. The most common location is the lower leg, but lesions can also occur on the abdomen, buttocks, thighs, pannus, breasts, and penis; there may be internal organ involvement as well. Lesions are usually multiple. There are no approved therapies for calciphylaxis (Nigwekar et al., 2018), but countermeasures to stop vascular calcification are being used (Chang, 2019). The ulcers predispose the patient to secondary infection and sepsis, which are contributing factors to the high mortality rate associated with this disease (Meissner et al., 2006).

KEY POINT

Calciphylaxis is commonly seen in patients with end-stage renal disease; effective management requires treatment of the underlying disease process, measures to prevent and manage infection, and pain control.

DIAGNOSIS

There is no single definitive diagnostic study for calciphylaxis; the diagnosis is based primarily on the patient's history and clinical manifestations and supported by laboratory values (e.g., elevated calcium, phosphorus, and calcium–phosphorus product levels) (Chang, 2019). The differential diagnosis must rule out other conditions that result in painful necrotic skin ulcers, such as diabetic gangrene, skin necrosis due to heparin-induced thrombocytopenia, warfarin skin necrosis, scleroderma, and PG (Nigwekar et al., 2018). Hayashi (2013) proposed diagnosis based on the following: on hemodialysis for chronic kidney disease or glomerular filtration rate (GFR) of <15 mL/min/173 m^2 and the presence of painful, non-treatable skin ulcers with concomitant painful purpura. Chang (2019) noted that bone scan may prove to be a

reliable, noninvasive diagnostic test for calciphylaxis. Imaging studies are not routinely recommended for diagnosis (Nigwekar et al., 2018). Although skin biopsy is the standard method for confirmation of clinically suspected calciphylaxis, its role in practice is debated because of provoking new, nonhealing ulcers (Nigwekar et al., 2018). When biopsy is done, a punch biopsy with a double trephine technique is the preferred method. This punch biopsy will obtain more subcutaneous tissue (Chang, 2019). Biopsy findings include (1) calcific deposits in the medial layer of small to medium blood vessels of the reticular dermis and subcutaneous fat, (2) intramural fibrin thrombi in the dermis and subcutaneous tissue, and (3) lobular fat necrosis with increased neutrophils, lymphocytes, and foamy histiocytes (Markova et al., 2012; Ong & Coulson, 2012).

MANAGEMENT

There are few effective treatments, and at present, care is primarily supportive. Chang (2019) identified four goals of prevention and treatment: stopping vascular occlusion, decalcification of calcified vessels to restore blood flow, wound care, and pain management. Stopping vascular occlusion often includes longer and/or more frequent dialysis sessions, converting to hemodialysis from peritoneal dialysis, dietary phosphate restriction, correcting hypercalcemia, correcting hyperparathyroidism, stopping vitamin D, and discontinuing warfarin (Chang, 2019; Nigwekar et al., 2018; Seethapathy et al., 2019).

Strategies to promote decalcification of the blood vessel include sodium thiosulfate (STS) and vitamin K. STS is generally considered the standard of therapy (Chang, 2019). The standard of care is to give it intravenously during the last hour of hemodialysis. Chang noted the minimum duration of STS treatment is 3 months with the total around 6 months or until the lesions heal. STS can also be injected directly around the border of the ulcer or into its center (Chang, 2019). It appears to work by binding calcium ions with resulting complexes eliminated in the urine or by dialysis and neutralizing reactive species that promote inflammation, thrombosis, and vasoconstriction. Vitamin K is considered investigational but may be a decalcifying agent (Chang, 2019; Nigwekar et al., 2018). Some references mention bisphosphonates. Mechanisms of action for bisphosphonates include inhibition of osteoclast activity, mobilization of intravascular calcium, and suppression of inflammatory cytokines, which is thought to be the primary mechanism underlying the rapid pain relief reported by some patients (Nigwekar et al., 2018; Seethapathy et al., 2019). Data about bisphosphonates need further investigation.

Wound care and pain management strategies vary. Wound dressings should focus on moisture control and comfort. Surgical debridement can be considered for infected wounds to prevent systemic infection and when there is purulent exudate (Chang, 2019). Antibiotics should be avoided unless there are clear signs of infection (Seethapathy et al., 2019). Severe pain can limit debridement. Severe hypoxia can result in poor healing of debrided areas. Hyperbaric oxygen therapy has been used on a small number of individuals (Chang, 2019; Nigwekar et al., 2018). Pain management is a challenge. Morphine and hydromorphone are discouraged because of active metabolites that accumulate in renal failure and cause respiratory depression and mental status changes (Chang, 2019; Seethapathy et al., 2019). Methadone and fentanyl are preferred (Seethapathy et al., 2019). Other classes of medication that have been used for pain management include neuropathic agents and regional anesthetics (Seethapathy et al., 2019). A pain management practitioner involved in the plan of care is highly encouraged.

 ## MALIGNANT WOUNDS: SQUAMOUS CELL CARCINOMA AND BASAL CELL CARCINOMA

PREVALENCE AND INCIDENCE

Skin cancer is the most common type of cancer in the United States affecting about 1 in 5 Americans in their lifetime (Higgins et al., 2018). Nonmelanoma skin cancer (i.e., keratinocyte carcinoma) affects more than 3.3 million persons annually in the United States (Bichakjian et al., 2018). BCC is stated to be about 80% of keratinocyte carcinoma and squamous cell carcinoma about 20% but the number of cutaneous squamous cell carcinoma (cSSC) is increasing (Bichakjian et al., 2018; Cameron et al., 2019a). When malignant melanoma and nonmelanoma skin cancers are examined by racial groups, they have a 40% incidence in Caucasians, 5% in Hispanics, 4% in Asians, and 2% in African Americans (Higgins et al., 2018). Awareness is growing in patients with skin of color who are also at risk but often the skin cancers are in areas not exposed to the sun (Alam et al., 2018). Sun exposure, especially in childhood and youth, is a critical variable in development of both basal cell and squamous cell carcinoma (Alam et al., 2018). Other risk factors identified include living near the equator, personal or family history of skin cancer, and use of tanning beds and photosensitizing drugs (Dokic et al., 2019). There is a growing concern about nonmelanoma skin cancers in the elderly because of the increasing numbers of older adults, greater longevity, and the impact of lifetime sun exposure. Other groups at risk for squamous cell carcinoma are immunosuppressed patients, especially those who have received a transplant, and cigarette smokers (Alam et al., 2018).

Squamous and basal cell skin cancers can also occur in chronic leg ulcers. Performing punch biopsies on 144 patients with 154 chronic leg ulcers, Senet et al. (2012) reported a 10.4% skin cancer frequency in chronic leg ulcers; of the 16 skin cancers, 9 were squamous cell and 5 were basal cell. In this study, factors associated with skin cancer were older age, abnormal excessive granulation tissue at the wound edge, high clinical suspicion of cancer, and number of biopsies (Senet et al., 2012). Chronic wounds can undergo malignant transformation, and these wounds are known as Marjolin ulcers; while malignant transformation of a leg ulcer remains rare (Schnirring-Judge & Belpedio, 2010), the diagnosis should be considered whenever an ulcer presents as a vegetating lesion, an ulcer with an irregular base or margin, excessive granulation tissue, and an increased size despite appropriate therapy (Choa et al., 2015). Factors that increase the risk for malignant transformation of a chronic wound include exposure to the cytotoxic by-products of chronic inflammation, impairments in the cell reproduction (mitotic) cycle, epidermal implantation resulting in a dermal foreign body reaction, immunologic factors, and epithelial cell mutations (Bazalinski et al., 2017). Combemale et al. (2007) examined malignant transformation in leg ulcers, 80% of which were venous ulcers. Important findings were abnormal granulation tissue, absence of healing, and unusual patterns of ulcer enlargement/extension. Pathology revealed that 98% of the tumors were squamous cell carcinoma and 82% were very well or well differentiated. The overall death rate was 32% and was higher among patients with lymph node or visceral metastases (Combemale et al., 2007).

PATHOLOGY

National Comprehensive Cancer Network (NCCN) system stratifies low- versus high-risk cSCC (Alam et al., 2018). This system is divided into clinical and pathologic parameters; it is recommended for clinical practice. The Brigham and Women's Hospital (BWH) tumor classification system is used to obtain the most accurate prognostication of the patient with cSCC (Alam et al., 2018). Alam and colleagues (2018) also outlined pathology report elements. Bichakjian and colleagues (2018) present recommendations for clinical information and pathology report for BCC.

CLINICAL PRESENTATION

Figure 27-6 provides a comparison of BCC, cSCC, and malignant melanoma. BCC often appears as a non-healing sore or a pearly pink papule with a rolled, well-rounded border and adjacent crusting (Dokic et al., 2019). The lesion most typically occurs in a sun-exposed area but can also occur in an area of minimal exposure. BCC has four subtypes: superficial multifocal, nodular (most common type), morpheaform (without defined borders)/infiltrative, and basosquamous (metatypical) (**Fig. 27-7**).

KEY POINT

SCC and BCC can be mistaken for chronic wounds; a biopsy is indicated for any wound that fails to respond to appropriate therapy.

Cancer

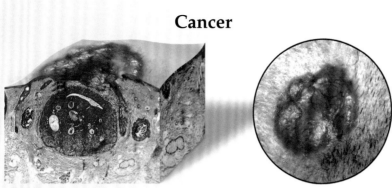

Basal cell carcinoma, the most common skin cancer, begins as a papule, enlarges, and develops a central crater. This cancer usually only spreads locally.

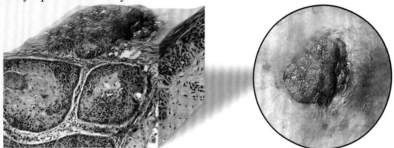

Squamous cell carcinoma begins as a firm, red nodule or scaly, crusted flat lesion. If not treated, this cancer can spread.

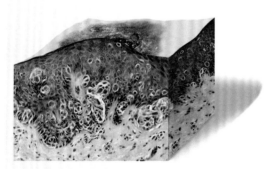

Malignant melanoma can arise on normal skin or from an existing mole. If not treated promptly, it can spread downward into other areas of the skin, lymph nodes, or internal organs.

FIGURE 27-6. Comparison of Basal Cell, Squamous Cell, and Malignant Melanoma. (Courtesy Anatomical Chart Company.)

Actinic keratosis is a known precursor to cSCC; these lesions appear as scaly pink plaque or nodule, commonly on the head, face, and dorsal hands/forearms (Dokic et al., 2019) (**Fig. 27-8**). Davies (2009) stated that patients typically describe the lesions as starting as a pimple and increasing in size to a thickened lesion (see **Fig. 27-8**). On the lip and genitalia, the squamous cell lesion presents as a fissure or small erosion that bleeds, fails to heal, and may be tender (Davies, 2009). Invasive squamous cell carcinoma presents as a nonhealing or wart-like growth. These lesions tend to develop where there is evidence of sun damage, such as thickened, wrinkled skin; hyperkeratotic skin; telangiectasia; and irregular pigmentation (Davies, 2009). Metastasis is more likely for cSCC versus BCC. The 5-year metastatic rate of smaller cSCC lesions is 5%; for lesions >2 cm, it is 30% (Dokic et al., 2019; Potenza et al., 2018).

DIAGNOSIS

Tissue biopsy is the gold standard for diagnosis. Schniring-Judge and Belpedio (2010) stated that the biopsy should be taken from the proximal or leading edge of

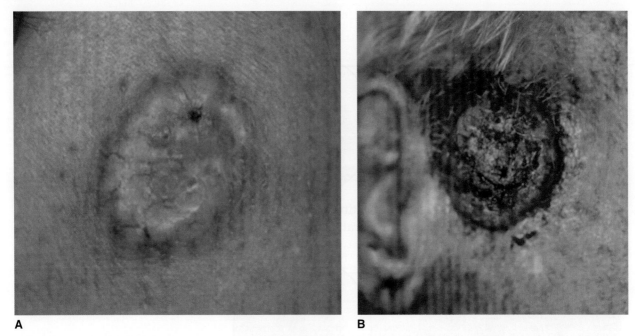

A   **B**

FIGURE 27-7. Nodular Basal Cell Carcinoma. **A.** A *red*, translucent nodule with rolled border, as seen here, is a classic presentation of nodular basal cell carcinoma. **B.** Nodular basal cell carcinoma demonstrating ulceration. (Reprinted with permission from DeVita, V. T., Lawrence, T. S., & Rosenberg, S. A. (2008). *DeVita, Hellman, and Rosenberg's cancer principles & practice of oncology* (8th ed.). Philadelphia, PA: Wolters Kluwer Health.)

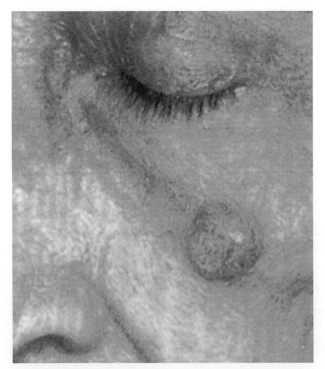

FIGURE 27-8. Squamous Cell Carcinoma Usually Appears on Sun-Exposed Skin of Fair-Skinned Adults over 60. It may develop in an actinic keratosis. The face and the back of the hand are often affected, as shown here. (Reprinted with permission from Hall, J. C. (2000). *Sauer's manual of skin diseases* (8th ed.). Philadelphia, PA: Lippincott Williams & Wilkins.)

the wound and should include 50% of wound and 50% adjacent tissue. This is done so the interface between the pathology and surrounding tissue can be described. A second specimen should be taken in the middle of the wound. Specimens need to be carefully labeled and described. Alam et al. (2018) in the guideline noted the literature does not identify a single optimal biopsy technique for cSCC but that specimen size and depth must be adequate to provide accurate diagnosis. The biopsy provides information about the histopathological subtype, degree of differentiation, histologic grade, and presence or absence of perineural vascular or lymphatic invasion (Momen & Al-Niaimi, 2013). Nonmelanoma skin cancers are staged according to the TNM staging system. Imaging with magnetic resonance imaging (MRI) or computed tomography (CT) is used to assess the anatomical degree of invasion (Momen & Al-Niaimi, 2013).

The differential diagnosis of cSCC includes BCC, malignant melanoma, actinic keratosis, pyogenic granulomas, seborrheic warts, warts, and other wounds (Momen & Al-Niaimi, 2013). Kricker et al. (2014) examined growth rates and patterns for basal and squamous cell carcinomas. BCC increased in size over time; there was no consistent evidence that cSCC demonstrated progressive enlargement. Larger BCC were independently associated with older age, male gender, no skin checks by a physician, aggressive tumor type, ulceration, and lesions associated with scar tissue, whereas cSCC was associated with male gender, location on an extremity, and skin checks by a physician (Cameron et al., 2019b; Kricker et al., 2014).

MANAGEMENT

The aim of treatment is to remove the primary tumor and any metastases (if possible) while preserving function and aesthetic appearance (Momen & Al-Niaimi, 2013; Potenza et al., 2018); some advanced tumors cannot be removed. Surgical excision of nonmelanoma skin cancers is the primary method of treatment; Mohs micrographic surgery may be selected because it allows preservation of normal tissue and complete resection of the tumor. Excision of BCC has a cure rate of 95% (Council, 2013). cSCCis most effectively treated by surgery (Alam et al., 2018). Cure rates for cSCC are reported by extensiveness and treatment, that is, metastatic cSCC has a 5-year cure rate at 34%; Mohs surgery, 95%; and radiotherapy, 90% (Momen & Al-Niaimi, 2013).

Cryotherapy is commonly used to treat actinic keratosis. Imiquimod (applied five times weekly for 6 weeks) and 5-fluorouracil (applied twice daily for 6 to 12 weeks) are topical therapies used for precancerous actinic keratosis and FDA approved for treatment of BCC (Council, 2013). Bath-Hextall et al. (2014) reported results from a randomized controlled trial that indicated imiquimod was inferior to surgery for BCC; however, it may still be an option for small low-risk superficial or nodular BCC. Available data do not support use of topical modalities for treatment of cSCC (Alam et al., 2018). Radiation therapy is used to treat advanced, inoperable basal and squamous cell carcinomas, and definitive radiation may also be recommended for curative intent in patients who are not candidates for surgical treatment (Alam et al., 2018; Fecher, 2013). For BCC that is unresectable, cisplatin-based chemotherapy has shown the most activity alone and in combination with other cytotoxic agents; many therapies are in development (Fecher, 2013; Potenza et al., 2018).

Patient teaching in terms of safe sun exposure is important for prevention. This teaching may include avoiding/minimizing sun exposure from 10 AM to 4 PM, which is the time for peak UVB; sunscreen with a solar protection factor (SPF) of 30 or higher; protective clothing, hats, and sunglasses; and avoidance of tanning beds (1.5 times greater risk of BCC and 2.5 times greater risk of cSCC) (Davies, 2009; Dokic et al., 2019; Firnhaber, 2012; Momen & Al-Niaimi, 2013).

It is important to consider the patient's quality of life when providing education and counseling. Mathias et al. (2014) examined quality of life in persons with advanced BCC. The most commonly reported and problematic symptoms were hair loss (79%), loss of taste (79%), bleeding (57%), and oozing or open wounds (50%). They reported feeling anxious, depressed, unable to concentrate, and worried about future surgery and procedures.

After diagnosis and treatment, patients need to be regularly followed. The follow-up period for screening for new skin cancers is once per year adjusting frequency on the patient's risk (Alam et al., 2018; Bichakjian et al., 2018). A patient with at least 1 BCC or cSCC is at risk for additional BCC or cSCC as well as other skin cancers (Alam et al., 2018; Bichakjian et al., 2018). The American Academy of Dermatology presented guidelines for basal cell and squamous cell carcinomas (Alam et al, 2018; Bichakjian et al., 2018).

● FACTITIOUS ULCERS: DERMATITIS ARTEFACTA

PREVALENCE AND INCIDENCE

Factitious means artificially created or developed. Factitious disorder refers to a mental disorder in which a person deliberately produces, feigns, or exaggerates symptoms as if having a physical or mental illness when, in fact, the person has consciously created his or her symptoms. Within factitious disorders, dermatitis artefacta is a psychocutaneous condition where the person creates skin lesions to satisfy a conscious or unconscious desire to assume the sick role (Gupta & Gupta, 2019; Lavery et al., 2018). The person is fully aware of the actions (Holt et al., 2013). Unconscious motivating factors (bereavement, divorce, unemployment, debt, bullying, and abuse) are often responsible for this self-destructive behavior (Holt et al., 2013). The highest incidence occurs in late adolescence to early adulthood; most affected are women (female–male ratios range from 3:1 to 20:1) who have a personality disorder (Lavery et al., 2018; Rodriguez Pichardo & Garcia Bravo, 2013). It is considered a rare condition. The incidence is not known, but the prevalence is 33% in patients diagnosed with anorexia and bulimia (Gattu et al., 2009; Koblenzer, 2000). Self-induced dermatoses account for about 2% of dermatology patient visits (Gupta & Gupta, 2019).

PATHOLOGY

The pathology relates to the source of the ulcers as they can be caused by any mechanical or irritant factors (**Fig. 27-9**). For example, one woman placed cotton threads and needles under the skin to cause keloids and other changes (Choudhary et al., 2009). Cohen and Vardy (2006) reported a case series of 14 soldiers with acute contact dermatitis with systemic symptoms, that is, acute erythematous rash with numerous papules and pustules in a linear pattern (arms, abdomen, and thighs), fever, malaise, and headache. All were dissatisfied with military service but denied intentionally inflicting the skin lesions; eight admitted to exposure to inflicting agents such as plants or blankets. Besides ulcers, other clinical features are excoriation, blisters, panniculitis, localized crusting, eczematous lesions, edema, purpura, and bruises (Rodriguez Pichardo & Garcia Bravo, 2013).

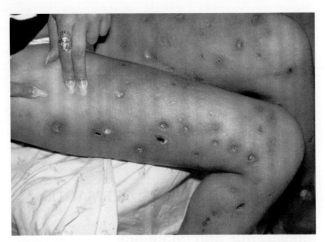

FIGURE 27-9. Neurotic Excoriations (Factitia). The self-induced ulcers are seen in a patient convinced that she was infested with lice. (Reprinted with permission from Goodheart, H. P. (2003). *Goodheart's photoguide of common skin disorders* (2nd ed.). Philadelphia, PA: Lippincott Williams & Wilkins.)

Histopathology of the ulcer may rule out organic causes. The diagnosis must be carefully made in order to avoid missing significant pathology. The morphology of the lesion, patient's personality, and the medical and mental health histories need to be examined (Gupta & Gupta, 2019; Lavery et al., 2018; Rodriguez Pichardo & Garcia Bravo, 2013). For example, a 20-year-old woman presented with itchy, edematous, purple crusted lesions on the right upper extremity, which were diagnosed as dermatitis artefacta. The histopathologic, immunohisto-chemical staining, and other studies revealed a rare sub-cutaneous panniculitis-like T-cell lymphoma (Soylu et al., 2010).

CLINICAL PRESENTATION

The ulcers/wounds are located on body locations that are easily reached by the dominant hand (Gregurek-Novak et al., 2005; Motherway et al., 2008). The ulcers or skin lesions are produced through mechanical means (fingernails, sharp or blunt objects, etc.) (See **Fig. 27-9**) or the application of irritants (chemicals, burning cigarettes, etc.) (Choudhary et al., 2009; Cohen & Vardy, 2006). The person typically denies the self-inflicted cause (Choudhary et al., 2009). The prognosis for cure is poor, and the condition tends to wax and wane with life circumstances and events (Rodriguez Pichardo & Garcia Bravo, 2013).

Factitial dermatoses can occur in children; in this population, the most common manifestations are trichotillomania (compulsive urge to pull out one's hair), neurotic excoriations (repetitive scratching), and acne excoriee (picking acne) (Shah & Fried, 2006).

DIAGNOSIS

Dermatitis artefacta is difficult to diagnosis by clinical findings. Diagnostic clues include denial, amnesia, or indifference to the symptoms or how the lesions occurred (Choudhary et al., 2009). The diagnosis is usually made by exclusion or when the person is discovered inflicting the lesion. Lesions do not conform to known dermatoses, are located on easily reached body locations, and have bizarre, clear-cut, or linear morphological features (Choudhary et al., 2009; Cohen & Vardy, 2006; Gregurek-Novak et al., 2005). Examples of locations may include the inguinal region, under the breasts, face, arms, and legs (Gregurek-Novak et al., 2005).

MANAGEMENT

The wound care/dermatology practitioner needs to work closely with the mental health provider. The mental disorder needs to be treated. Medications such as selective serotonin reuptake inhibitors, low-dose antipsychotic medications, and antidepressant medications have been used (Gupta & Gupta, 2019; Jones et al., 2018). For example, Kwon et al. (2006) and Motherway et al. (2008) presented case studies of women with recurrent skin lesions and abscesses; treatment of the mental health problem markedly improved the skin disease. The person may deny psychiatric distress and have negative feelings toward the provider for raising such an issue. Creating an accepting, empathic, and nonjudgmental relationship is important. Even after the lesions have healed, it is sometimes helpful to continue to see the patient for supervision and to offer support (Koblenzer, 2000). The lesions tend to heal when covered. Therefore, selection of a dressing that fits the location and characteristics of the ulcers/lesions and that provides coverage is appropriate.

Children's treatment needs are similar to that of the adult. The treatment includes a nonjudgmental care provider, avoiding accusations and blame, observation of the parent–child interaction, screening for other psychiatric conditions, and psychotherapy if necessary (Shah & Fried, 2006). Although antidepressants are beneficial for the adult, they must be carefully considered in children in terms of the potential for short- and long-term side effects and safety (Shah & Fried, 2006).

⬤ WARFARIN-INDUCED SKIN NECROSIS

Warfarin-induced skin necrosis (WISN) is an infrequent complication of warfarin treatment. WISN incidence has been estimated between 0.01% and 0.1% (Bakoyiannis et al., 2016). The exact pathogenesis is not clear but it appears to be associated with a decrease in vitamin K–dependent clotting factors (e.g., protein C) or deficiencies of protein S, factor V Leiden, and antithrombin III, which may cause microthrombi to impede blood flow to the skin causing necrosis (Bakoyiannis et al., 2016). It is more common in obese women >50 with the areas of the body most affected being the breast, buttocks, abdomen, thighs, and calves, which is probably from reduced blood supply to adipose tissue. It is usually seen with international normalized ratio (INR) above 4. In the past, it has been treated with surgical debridement. However, with the recent administration of novel oral anticoagulant

(NOAC) medications and decreased usage of warfarin, this phenomenon may be seen even less frequently.

 CONCLUSION

Although often considered lesser diagnosed wounds, atypical lower extremity ulcers need to be considered when examining wounds on the lower extremities. Although this chapter focused on the lower extremity, many of these wounds can occur on other areas of the body. Vasculitis, PG, sickle cell anemia, calciphylaxis, squamous and basal cell carcinomas, and factitious ulcers are examples of atypical ulcers. The assessment of these ulcers includes a detailed history and possibly a wound biopsy. Although the wound dressing is an important aspect of care, generally the underlying pathology is the crucial focus of treatment. These wounds can be excruciatingly painful and result in deformities/scarring of the skin. Thus, pain needs to be managed and quality of life and psychosocial issues dealt with. Patient/family teaching is critical due to the long-term follow-up and intensive treatment required.

REFERENCES

Ahn, C., Negus, D., & Huang, W. (2018). Pyoderma gangrenosum: A review of pathogenesis and treatment. *Expert Review of Clinical Immunology, 14*(3), 225–233.

Alam, M., Armstrong, A., Baum, C. et al. (2018). Guidelines of care for the management of cutaneous squamous cell carcinoma. *Journal of the American Academy of Dermatology, 78*(3), 560–578.

American College of Rheumatology. (2019). Vasculitis. Retrieved from http://www.rheumatology.org/Practice/Clinical/Patients/Diseases_And_Conditions/Vasculitis/ Last Accessed October 11, 2019.

Aractingi, S. (2017). To learn more about sickle cell ulcers. *British Journal of Dermatology, 177*, 177–178.

Bakoyiannis, C., Karaolanis, G., Patelis, N., et al. (2016). Dabigatran in the treatment of warfarin-induced skin necrosis: A new hope. *Case Reports in Dermatological Medicine, 2016*, Article ID 3121469, 3 pages. doi: 10.1155/2016/3121469.

Bath-Hextall, F., Ozolins, M., Armstrong, S. J., et al.; on behalf of the Surgery versus Imiquimod for Nodular and Superficial Basal Cell Carcinoma (SINS) Study Group. (2014). Surgical excision versus imiquimod 5% cream for nodular and superficial basal-cell carcinoma (SINS): A multicentre, non-inferiority, randomized controlled trial. *Lancet Oncology, 15*, 96–105.

Bazalinski, D., Przybek-Mita, J., Baranska, B., et al. (2017). Marjolin's ulcer in chronic wounds—review of available literature. *Contemporary Oncology, 21*(3), 197–202.

Bichakjian, C., Armstrong, A., Baum, C., et al. (2018). Guidelines of care for the management of basal cell carcinoma. *Journal of the American Academy of Dermatology, 78*(3), 540–559.

Birmingham Vasculitis Activity Score (version 3). Retrieved from http://www.epsnetwork.co.uk/BVAS/bvas_flow.html. Last Accessed October 11, 2019.

Brown, S. (2012). Vasculitis: Pathophysiology, diagnosis and treatment. *Nursing Standard, 27*(12), 50–57.

Cameron, M. C., Lee, E., Hibler, B. C., et al. (2019a). Basal cell carcinoma. Epidemiology; pathophysiology; clinical and histological subtypes; and disease associations. *Journal of the American Academy of Dermatology, 80*(2), 303–317.

Cameron, M. C., Lee, E., Hibler, B. C., et al. (2019b). Basal cell carcinoma. Contemporary approaches to diagnosis, treatment, and

prevention. *Journal of the American Academy of Dermatology, 80*(2), 321–339.

Centers for Disease Control and Prevention. (2019). Data & statistics on sickle cell disease. Retrieved from https://www.cdc.gov/ncbddd/sicklecell/data.html. Last Accessed October 11, 2019.

Chang, J. J. (2019). Calciphylaxis: Diagnosis, pathogenesis, and treatment. *Advances in Skin & Wound Care, 32*(5), 205–215.

Choa, R., Rayatt, S., & Mahtani, K. (2015). Marjolin's ulcer. *British Medical Journal, 351*:h3997. doi: 10.1136/bmj.h3997.

Choudhary, S., Khairkar, P., Singh, A., et al. (2009). Dermatitis artefacta: Keloids and foreign body granuloma due to overvalued ideation of acupuncture. *Indian Journal of Dermatology, Venereology and Leprology, 75*(6), 606–608.

Cohen, A. D., & Vardy, D. A. (2006). Dermatitis artefacta in soldiers. *Military Medicine, 171*(6), 497–499.

Combemale, P., Bousquet, M., Kanitakis, J.; The Angiodermatology Group of the French Society of Dermatology. (2007). Malignant transformation of leg ulcers: A retrospective study of 85 cases. *Journal of the European Academy of Dermatology and Venereology, 21*(7), 935–941.

Council, M. L. (2013). Common skin cancers in older adults: Approach to diagnosis and management. *Clinics in Geriatric Medicine, 29*(2013), 361–372.

Davies, A. (2009). The effective management of squamous cell carcinoma. *British Journal of Nursing, 18*(9), 539–543.

de Araujo, T. S., & Kirsner, R. S. (2001). Vasculitis. *Wounds, 13*(3), 99–112.

Delaney, K. M., Axelrod, K. C., Buscetta, A., et al. (2013). Leg ulcers in sickle cell disease: Current patterns and practices. *Hemoglobin, 37*(4), 325–332.

Dokic, Y., Boyd, M. E., & Rizk, C. (2019). Small, friable lesion. *The Clinical Advisor, 22*(7), 27–32. Retrieved on December 2, 2020, from https://issuu.com/clinicaladvisor/docs/clinicaladvisor_july-august_2019_digital

Fecher, L. A. (2013). Systemic therapy for inoperable and metastatic basal cell cancer. *Current Treatment Options in Oncology, 14*(2), 237–248.

Firnhaber, J. M. (2012). Diagnosis and treatment of basal cell and squamous cell carcinoma. *American Family Physician, 86*(2), 161–168.

Gattu, S., Rashid, R. M., & Khachemoune, A. (2009). Self-induced skin lesions: A review of dermatitis artefacta. *Cutis, 84*(5), 247–251.

Gregurek-Novak, T., Novak-Bilic, G., & Vucic, M. (2005). Dermatitis artefacta: Unusual appearance in an older woman. *Journal of the European Academy of Dermatology and Venereology, 19*(2), 223–225.

Gupta, M. A., & Gupta, A. K. (2019). Self-induced dermatoses: A great imitator. *Clinics in Dermatology, 37*, 268–277.

Halabi-Tawi, M., Lionnet, F., Girot, R., et al. (2008). Sickle cell leg ulcers: A frequently disabling complication and a marker of severity. *British Journal of Dermatology, 158*, 339–344.

Hanley, J. (2011). Effective management of peristomal pyoderma gangrenosum. *British Journal of Nursing, 20*(7), S12–S17.

Hayashi, M. (2013). Calciphylaxis: Diagnosis and clinical features. *Clinical and Experimental Nephrology, 17*(4), 498–503.

Higgins, S., Nazemi, A., Chow, M., et al. (2018). Review of nonmelanoma skin cancer in African Americans, Hispanics, and Asians. *Dermatologic Surgery, 44*(7), 903–910.

Holt, P., El-Dars, L., Kenny, A., et al. (2013). Serial photography and Wood's light examination as an aid to the clinical diagnosis of dermatitis artefacta. *Journal of Visual Communication in Medicine, 36*(1–2), 31–34.

Jenerette, G. M., Brewer, C. A., Edwards, L. J., et al. (2014). An intervention to decrease stigma in young adults with sickle cell disease. *Western Journal of Nursing Research, 36*(5), 599–619.

Jennette, J. C., Falk, P. A., Bacon, N., et al. (2013). 2012 revised International Chapel Hill Consensus Conference Nomenclature of Vasculitides. *Arthritis & Rheumatism, 65*(1), 1–11.

Jones, G., Keuthen, N., & Greenberg, E. (2018). Assessment and treatment of trichotillomania (hair pulling disorder) and excoriation (skin picking) disorder. *Clinics in Dermatology, 36*, 728–736.

Kato, G. J., Hebbel, R. P., Steinberg, M. H., et al. (2009). Vasculopathy in sickle cell disease: Biology, pathophysiology, genetics, translational medicine, and new research directions. *American Journal of Hematology, 84*(9), 618–625.

Kerk, N., & Goerge, T. (2013a). Livedoid vasculopathy—Current aspects of diagnosis and treatment of cutaneous infarction. *Journal of the German Society of Dermatology, 11*, 407–410.

Kerk, N., & Goerge, T. (2013b). Livedoid vasculopathy—A thrombotic disease. *VASA, 42*, 317–322.

Koblenzer, C. S. (2000). Dermatitis artefacta. Clinical features and approaches to treatment. *American Journal of Clinical Dermatology, 1*(1), 47–55.

Kricker, A., Armstrong, B., Hansen, V., et al. (2014). Basal cell carcinoma and squamous cell carcinoma growth rates and determinants of size in community patients. *Journal of the American Academy of Dermatology, 70*(3), 456–464.

Kridin, K, Cohen, A. D., & Amber, K. T. (2018). Underlying systemic disease in pyoderma gangrenosum: A systematic review and meta-analysis. *American Journal of Clinical Dermatology, 19*(4), 479–487.

Kwon, E., Dans, M., Koblenzer, C., et al. (2006). Dermatitis artefacta. *Journal of Cutaneous Medicine and Surgery, 10*(2), 108–113.

Lakdawala, N., & Fedeles, F. (2017). Vasculitis: Kids are not just little people. *Clinics in Dermatology, 35*, 530–540.

Lavery, M. J., Stull, C., McCaw, I., et al. (2018). Dermatitis artefacta. *Clinics in Dermatology, 36*(6), 719–722.

Lemos, A. C., Aveiro, D., Santos, N., et al. (2017). Pyoderma gangrenosum: An uncommon case report and review of the literature. *Wounds, 29*(9), E61–E69.

Madu, A. J., Ubesie, A., Madu, K. A., et al. (2013). Evaluation of clinical and laboratory correlates of sickle leg ulcers. *Wound Repair and Regeneration, 21*(6), 808–812.

Markova, A., Lester, J., Wang, J., et al. (2012). Diagnosis of common dermopathies in dialysis patients: A review and update. *Seminars in Dialysis, 25*(4), 408–418.

Marti-Carvajal, A. J., Knight-Madden, J. M., & Martinez-Zapata, M. J. (2014). Interventions for treating leg ulcers in people with sickle cell disease (review). *Cochrane Database of Systematic Reviews*, (12), CD008394. doi: 10.1002/14651858.CD008394.pub3.

Mathias, S. D., Chren, M. M., Colwell, H. H., et al. (2014). Assessing health-related quality of life for advanced basal cell carcinoma and basal cell carcinoma nevus syndrome: Development of the first disease-specific patient-reported outcome questionnaire. *JAMA Dermatology, 150*(2), 169–176.

Meissner, M., Gille, J., & Kaufmann, R. (2006). Calciphylaxis: No therapeutic concepts for a poorly understood syndrome? *JDDG: Journal der Deutschen Dermatologischen Gesellschaft, 4*, 1037–1044.

Minniti, C. P., & Kato, G. J. (2016). How we treat sickle cell patients with leg ulcers. *American Journal of Hematology, 91*, 22–30.

Minniti, C. P., Delaney, K. M., Gorbach, A. M., et al. (2014). Vasculopathy, inflammation, and blood flow in leg ulcers of patients with sickle cell anemia, *American Journal of Hematology, 89*(1), 1–6.

Minniti, C. P., Eckman, J., Sebastiani, P., et al. (2010). Leg ulcers in sickle cell disease. *American Journal of Hematology, 85*(10), 831–833.

Momen, S., & Al-Niaimi, F. (2013). Squamous cell carcinoma—Aetiology, presentation and treatment options. *Dermatological Nursing, 12*(2), 14–20.

Monti, S., Bond, M., Felicetti, M., et al. (2019). One year in review 2019: Vasculitis. *Clinical and Experimental Rheumatology, 37*(Suppl 117), S3–S19.

Morris, C. R. (2008). Mechanisms of vasculopathy in sickle cell disease and thalassemia. *Hematology, 2008*(1), 177–185. doi: 10.1182/asheducation-2008.1.177.

Motherway, L., Gallagher, D., Guerandel, A., et al. (2008). Dermatitis artefacta: An unusual diagnosis in psychodermaology. *Irish Journal of Psychological Medicine, 25*(2), 71–72.

Mukhtyar, C., Lee, R., Brown, D., et al. (2009). Modification and validation of the Birmingham Vasculitis Activity Score (version 3). *Annals of the Rheumatic Diseases, 68*(12), 1827–1832.

Nigwekar, S. U. (2017). Calciphylaxis. *Current Opinion in Nephrology and Hypertension, 26*, 276–281.

Nigwekar, S. U., Thadhani, R., & Brandenburg, V. M. (2018). Calciphylaxis. *New England Journal of Medicine, 378*, 1704–1714.

Ntatsaki, E., Carruthers, D., Chakravarty, K., et al. (2014). BSR and BHPR guideline for the management of adults with ANCA-associated vasculitis. *Rheumatology (Oxford), 53*, 2306–2309. doi: 10.1093/rheumatology/ket445.

Ong, S., & Coulson, I. H. (2012). Diagnosis and treatment of calciphylaxis. *Skinmed, 10*(3), 166–170.

Papi, M., & Papi, C. (2016). Vasculitic ulcers. *The International Journal of Lower Extremity Wounds, 15*(1), 6–16.

Pompeo, M. Q. (2016). Pyoderma gangrenosum: Recognition and management. *Wounds, 28*(1), 7–13.

Potenza, C., Bernardini, N., Balduzzi, V., et al. (2018). A review of the literature of surgical and nonsurgical treatments of invasive squamous cells carcinoma. *BioMedical Research International, 2018*, Article ID 9489163, 1–9. doi: 10.1155/2018/9489163.

Ratnagobal, S., & Sinha, S. (2013). Pyoderma gangrenosum: Guideline for wound practitioners. *Journal of Wound Care, 22*(2), 68–72.

Rodriguez Pichardo, A., & Garcia Bravo, B. (2013). Dermatitis artefacta: A review. *Actas Dermo-Sifiliográficas, 104*(10), 854–866.

Ruocco, E., Sangiuliano, S., Gravina, A. G., et al. (2009). Pyoderma gangrenosum: An updated review. *Journal of the European Academy of Dermatology and Venereology, 23*, 1008–1017.

Schnirring-Judge, M., & Belpedio, D. (2010). Malignant transformation of a chronic venous stasis ulcer to basal cell carcinoma in a diabetic patient: Case study and review of pathophysiology. *Journal of Foot and Ankle Surgery, 49*(2010), 75–79.

Seethapathy, H., Brandenburg, V. M., Sinha, S., et al. (2019). Review: Update on the management of calciphylaxis. *QJM: An International Journal of Medicine, 112*(1), 29–34.

Seitz, C. S., Berens, N., Brocker, E. B., et al. (2010). Leg ulceration in rheumatoid arthritis—An underreported multicausal complication with considerable morbidity: Analysis of thirty-six patients and review of the literature. *Dermatology, 220*(3), 268–273.

Senet, P., Blas-Chatelain, C., Levy P., et al. (2017). Factors predictive of leg-ulcer healing in sickle cell disease: A multicenter, prospective cohort study. *British Journal of Dermatology, 177*, 206–211.

Senet, P., Combemale, P., Debure, C., et al.; for the Angio-Dermatology Group of the French Society of Dermatology. (2012). Malignancy and chronic leg ulcers. *Archives of Dermatology, 148*(6), 704–708.

Shah, K. N., & Fried, F. G. (2006). Factitial dermatoses in children. *Current Opinion in Pediatrics, 18*(4), 403–409.

Shanmugam, V. K., Angra, D., Rahimi, H., & McNish, S. (2017). Vasculitic and autoimmune wounds. *Journal of Vascular Surgery. Venous and Lymphatic Disorders, 5*(2), 280–292.

Shavit, E., Alavi, A., & Sibbald, R. G. (2018). Vasculitis—What do we have to know? A review of literature. *The International Journal of Lower Extremity Wounds, 17*(4), 218–226.

Soylu, S., Gul, U., Kilic, A., et al. (2010). A case with an indolent course of subcutaneous panniculitis-like T-cell lymphoma demonstrating Epstein-Barr virus positivity and simulating dermatitis artefacta. *American Journal of Clinical Dermatology, 11*(2), 147–150.

Suppiah, R., Mukhtyar, C., Flossmann, O., et al. (2011). A cross-sectional study of the Birmingham Vasculitis Activity Score version 3 in systemic vasculitis. *Rheumatology, 50*(5), 899–905.

Tang, J. C., Vivas, A., Rey, A., et al. (2012). Atypical ulcers: Wound biopsy results from a university wound pathology service. *Ostomy and Wound Management, 58*(6), 20–29.

Tsaras, G., Owusu-Ansah, A., Boateng, F. O., et al. (2009). Complications associated with sickle cell trait: A brief narrative review. *American Journal of Medicine, 122*(6), 507–512.

Vallini, V., Andreini, R. A., & Bonadio, A. (2017). Pyoderma gangrenosum: A current problem as much as an unknown one. *The International Journal of Lower Extremity Wounds, 16*(3), 191–201.

Vedvyas, C., Winterfield, L. S., & Vleugels, R. A. (2012). Calciphylaxis: A systematic review of existing and emerging therapies. *Journal of the American Academy of Dermatology, 67*(6), e253–e260. doi: 10.1016/j.jaad.2011.06.009.

QUESTIONS

1. From what data would a definitive diagnosis of vasculitis be derived?
   A. Patient history
   B. Presence of comorbid conditions
   C. Blood testing
   D. Histologic evaluation of the lesion

2. A patient presents with sickle cell ulcers. On what site are these ulcers most commonly seen?
   A. Medial and lateral malleoli
   B. Anterior tibia
   C. Dorsum of the foot
   D. Achilles tendon

3. A wound nurse is managing the leg ulcers of a patient with sickle cell disease. Which intervention is NOT normally recommended as therapy?
   A. Use of hydroxyurea to increase production of fetal hemoglobin
   B. Blood transfusions to provide normal RBCs
   C. IV morphine for pain management
   D. Compression wraps to prevent venous insufficiency

4. Which patient would the wound nurse consider to be at higher risk for the development of pyoderma gangrenosum?
   A. A patient with diabetes mellitus
   B. A patient with Crohn disease
   C. A patient with sickle cell anemia
   D. A patient with lupus

5. A patient presents with a leg ulcer that is characterized by thrombosis of the small vessels in the dermis and subcutaneous fat, leading to cutaneous ischemia, tissue infarction, and necrosis. Which type of atypical leg ulcer would the wound nurse suspect?
   A. Sickle cell
   B. Calciphylaxis
   C. Vasculitis
   D. Pyoderma gangrenosum

6. The wound nurse is assessing a patient with calciphylaxis. What management regimen would the nurse recommend?
   A. Use of conservative sharp debridement
   B. Skin grafts, hyperbaric oxygen therapy, and zinc sulfate

   C. Corticosteroids combined with other immunosuppressive agents
   D. Supportive care until underlying disease process is under control

7. A patient presents with a skin lesion that appears as a scaly pink papule on the leg, which according to the patient, "started as a bump and got bigger and more firm over time." What underlying diagnosis would the wound nurse suspect?
   A. Pyoderma gangrenosum
   B. Squamous cell carcinoma
   C. Vasculitis
   D. Dermatitis artefacta

8. A patient is scheduled for a tissue biopsy to diagnose squamous cell carcinoma. What is a step in the procedure for obtaining these specimens?
   A. The biopsy should be taken from the proximal edge of the wound.
   B. The biopsy should include 25% of wound and 25% of adjacent tissue.
   C. A second specimen should be taken from the lateral side of the wound.
   D. A third specimen should be taken from the skin adjacent to the wound.

9. A patient is diagnosed with actinic keratosis. What type of therapy is commonly used to treat this condition?
   A. Surgical excision of the lesions
   B. Mohs micrographic surgery
   C. Cryotherapy
   D. Use of selective serotonin reuptake inhibitors

10. The wound nurse is assessing an adolescent patient who is diagnosed with dermatitis artefacta on her arms. What is a diagnostic characteristic of these lesions?
   A. Unexplained clear-cut or linear morphological features
   B. Nonhealing pearly pink papules
   C. Cutaneous ischemia, tissue infarction, and necrosis
   D. Palpable purpura (raised areas of nonblanchable erythema)

ANSWERS AND RATIONALES

1. D. Rationale: Skin biopsy is the gold standard for the diagnosis of vasculitis, which is then used to confirm clinical findings.

2. A. Rationale: Microvascular vaso-occlusion is the common clinical manifestation of sickle cell disease. Smaller vessels near the ankle are commonly affected.

3. C. Rationale: The other three choices are recommended therapies for management of sickle cell leg ulcers.

4. B. Rationale: About 50% of patients have coexisting systemic inflammatory disease with the most common being inflammatory bowel disease.

5. B. Rationale: Calciphylaxis is characterized by intimal proliferation, medial calcification, and thrombosis of the small vessels of the dermis and subcutaneous.

6. D. Rationale: There are few effective treatments for calciphylaxis, and care is primarily supportive.

7. B. Rationale: Squamous cell carcinoma presents as a scaly pink papule.

8. A. Rationale: Biopsy is taken from the proximal or leading edge of the wound and should include 50% of the wound and 50% of the adjacent tissue.

9. C. Rationale: Cryotherapy is commonly used and is a minimally invasive method to treat precancerous lesions.

10. A. Rationale: Factitious lesions do not conform to other known dermatological conditions.

CHAPTER 28

FOOT AND NAIL CARE

Tara Beuscher

OBJECTIVES

1. Identify goals and objectives for a structured comprehensive foot and nail program.

2. Describe factors to be included in a comprehensive lower extremity assessment, to include client history, vascular assessment, sensorimotor assessment, skin and nail assessment, wound assessment, and pain assessment.

3. Describe common pathologic conditions affecting the foot and nails, and implications for the foot and nail care nurse.

4. Outline guidelines for foot and nail care, to include the following: management of hypertrophic nails, management of hypertrophic skin and cuticles, management of corns and calluses, and prevention and management of ingrown nails.

5. Describe infection control issues and implications for the foot care nurse.

6. Discuss the role of the foot care nurse in patient education and appropriate referrals.

TOPIC OUTLINE

● INTRODUCTION

The primary goal for wound care nurses is to prevent skin and tissue breakdown when possible and to promote healing when wounds occur. This is important when caring for individuals with lower extremity arterial disease (LEAD) or lower extremity neuropathic disease (LEND), since they are high risk for ulceration, impaired healing, and amputation. The incidence of amputation increases with age with most amputations occurring in those over the age of 65 (Steinberg et al., 2019). One in 190 Americans are currently living with an amputation with the number projected to double by 2050 (Ziegler-Graham et al., 2008). There are over one hundred thousand limbs amputated each year in the United States, which equates to over 2,000 limbs amputated per week. Amputation renders the individual vulnerable to fear and anxiety, depression, limited mobility, and increased risk of mortality (Barshes et al., 2013; McDonald, et al., 2014). The International Diabetes Federation estimated that 1 in every 11 adults (451 million) had diabetes in 2017, and 1 in 10 (693 million) will have diabetes by 2045. Diabetes-related lower extremity complications (DRLECs) typically first present as neuropathy. Neuropathy is the critical risk factor for developing foot ulceration, and foot ulceration is the critical risk factor for foot infection and amputation. It is estimated that up to 50% of people with diabetes have neuropathy, up to 34% will develop a foot ulcer in their lifetime, and 50% of those ulcers will become infected and 20% amputated. DRLECs account for up to 80% of global lower extremity amputations and are a leading cause of hospitalization (Zhang et al., 2020). The total medical cost for the management of diabetic foot disease in the United States ranges from $9 to $13 billion in addition to the cost of management of DM alone (Rice et al., 2014).

Many amputations may be avoided through attention to self-care and clinical care practices to manage risk factors, including glycemic control and cardiovascular disease risk factors, and through early detection and appropriate treatment of foot ulcers. Increasing rates of NLEAs, particularly minor amputations, suggest either early prevention practices (e.g., self-management education, appropriate footwear, foot examinations, and identification of high-risk feet) might not be optimally performed to prevent foot ulcers or there may be delays in timely treatment of ulcers (Geiss et al., 2019). The International Working Group on the Diabetic Foot (IWGDF) has determined that 75% of foot ulcers are preventable and have called for a renewed emphasis on prevention (Bus & van Netten, 2016). There is an opportunity for improvement in the frequency of foot examinations by health care providers for adults with diabetes (Peraj et al., 2019). Foot and nail care, screening, and education are key responsibilities for the certified wound care nurse (CWCN) and certified foot and nail care nurse (CFCN) (Ellefson et al., 2016). Both specialty certifications are offered through the Wound, Ostomy and Continence Nursing Certification Board (WOCNCB). Three out of four Americans experience serious foot problems in their lifetime, and foot care nurses are prepared to assist with prevention and management (Crawford & Fields-Varnado, 2013; Gallagher, 2012).

The foot and wound care nurse may play a key role in reducing the complications and cost of care for people with diabetes and LEAD, specifically by preventing injuries and wounds, assuring appropriate footwear, providing education, and initiating prompt and appropriate referrals (WOCN, 2012, 2014).

Research has shown that implementation of a foot care program incorporating effective assessment tools and evidence-based procedures for foot and nail care reduces foot-related pain, injury, and reduces the number of amputations (Fujiwara et al., 2011; Sheridan, 2012; Musuuza et al., 2019). The CFCN can establish an independent practice as an entrepreneur or incorporate skills into their present practice as an intrapreneur. The foot and nail care nurse can reduce complications and cost for individuals with diabetes and LEND or LEAD by preventing injuries and wounds, assuring appropriate footwear, providing education, and initiating prompt and appropriate referrals. Patient education may have a dramatic effect on the quality of life for individuals with a diabetic foot ulcer (Sonal Sekhar et al., 2019).

The purpose of this chapter is to provide guidelines for foot and nail assessment, vascular and sensorimotor screening, basic foot and nail care, and appropriate and timely referrals. The specific objectives of a comprehensive foot and nail care program are listed in **Box 28-1**.

Appropriate foot and nail care has a significant impact on quality of life, specifically by promoting mobility, maintaining comfort, and preventing wounds, amputations, and falls (Lavery et al., 2013). Painful corns, calluses, and deformities increase the risk of falls in the older population (Menz et al., 2018), and toenails that have not been trimmed appropriately or in a timely manner increase the risk for injury in both older and neuropathic individuals (Reich & Szepietowski, 2011). Raynaud disease, arthritis, gout, diabetes with LEND, lower extremity venous disease (LEVD), LEAD, and end-stage renal disease (ESRD) are common conditions that compromise the individual's ability to safely care for the feet and nails (Harding et al., 2019; Khan et al., 2018). Chronic wounds and amputations lead to depression, limited mobility, pain, morbidity, and increased risk of mortality (Alvarsson et al., 2012; Kimmel & Robin, 2013).

FOOT AND NAIL CARE: OVERVIEW

One responsibility of the foot care nurse is to conduct a comprehensive lower extremity assessment, to include vascular status, sensorimotor status, skin and nail status, presence and status of any wounds, ability to heal, and appropriateness of footwear and foot care (Beuscher, 2019). The objective is to promptly identify any individual with or at risk for ulceration and to intervene appropriately to prevent injury and/or to promote healing and prevent amputation (Peraj et al., 2019).

The risk of ulceration is highest among people with LEND and loss of protective sensation (LOPS) (WOCN, 2012). Peripheral polyneuropathy is common among people with diabetes, Hansen disease, alcoholism, and those with a spinal cord injury or multiple sclerosis. LOPS creates risk for unrecognized injury. The injury initiates an inflammatory response but, because there is no pain, the person does not recognize the injury and fails to provide appropriate care. Wounds may go unnoticed for days or weeks and are often recognized only when infection has developed. At that point, there is a marked reduction in the potential for healing and a significant increase in the risk for amputation (Lipsky et al., 2012).

Vascular assessment is a component of lower limb assessment because adequacy of perfusion is the determining factor in wound healing outcomes. Those with adequate perfusion are generally able to heal, while those with poor perfusion are at high risk for failure to heal with resultant amputation. The risk of amputation is highest among people with LEAD (Kohlman-Trigoboff, 2013; Mills et al., 2014; WOCN, 2014). Diminished or absent blood flow significantly compromises the ability to heal and increases the risk of infection and may result in amputation. Chronic limb ischemia worsens over time, but signs and symptoms are frequently insidious and unrecognized until a wound is sustained that fails to heal and/or deteriorates rapidly (Khan et al., 2018).

BOX 28-1   OBJECTIVES OF FOOT AND NAIL CARE PROGRAM

- Conduct comprehensive foot and nail assessments.
- Develop individual plans of care based on findings.
- Prevent or minimize development or progression of foot deformities.
- Reduce injuries and ulcerations that may lead to amputation.
- Compensate for existing deformities through appropriate footwear modifications.
- Facilitate proper use of footwear and compression stockings.
- Identify high-risk individuals and refer appropriately.
- Educate patients regarding importance of foot care.
- Increase patient satisfaction.
- Reduce hospital admissions and emergent care visits.

KEY POINT

Adequacy of perfusion is the determining factor for any individual with a wound. Those with adequate perfusion are generally able to heal, while those with poor perfusion are at high risk for failure to heal with resultant amputation.

Prevention of unrecognized trauma and amputation in the high-risk individual requires skilled foot and nail care provided by professionals. Patient education and referrals are recommended to maximize perfusion, minimize sensorimotor loss, and assure appropriate protective footwear (Wexler, 2019; Wu et al., 2014). With the aging population and increasing incidence of obesity and diabetes, foot and nail care should be incorporated as a standard component of health care in every setting

(Amaeshi, 2012; Beuscher, 2019; Brechow et al., 2013; Gallagher, 2012; Moakes, 2012).

⬤ ANATOMY AND PHYSIOLOGY OF THE FOOT AND NAILS

The anatomy and function of the feet change over time, and these changes are accelerated by age, pregnancy, and trauma. The bony prominences of the plantar surface are prone to stress fractures, the fat pads on the plantar surface gradually thin, the feet get longer and wider, and the arch has a tendency to flatten. The joints and skin undergo structural and physiological degeneration with age. These are all normal age-related changes in the feet. There are 26 bones, 33 joints, 107 ligaments, and 19 muscles in each foot. There are three anatomical sections of the foot: forefoot, midfoot, and hindfoot (**Fig. 28-1**).

The multiple bones, joints, ligaments, nerves, and muscles work together to enable weight bearing and locomotion throughout the activities of daily living. Normal structure and function of the bones, muscles, joints, and connective tissue are essential for normal gait and for protection against abnormal pressure and shear forces. The skin provides protection against bacterial and fungal invasion, and maintenance of intact skin is a concern for the foot care nurse. The nails function to protect the distal digits. The nail unit consists of the nail matrix, nail bed, hyponychium, and proximal and lateral nail folds (**Fig. 28-2**).

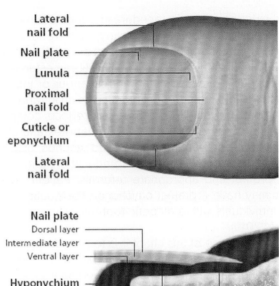

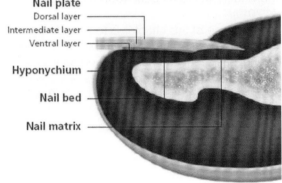

FIGURE 28-2. Nail Unit.

KEY POINT

Normal structure and function of the bones, muscles, joints, and connective tissue are essential for normal gait and for protection against abnormal pressure and shear forces.

The nail plate (toenail) is composed of three overlapping layers of keratinized epithelial cells. The nail plate functions to protect the distal digit against friction and pressure. The water content of the nail plate is normally 10% to 30%; lower water content results in brittle nails, and higher water content results in nails that are soft and prone to splitting. The nail bed refers to the epithelium that lies directly beneath the nail plate and interlocks with the nail plate to provide tight adherence. The nail matrix is the reproductive layer of the nail bed and the source of new nail. It extends from a point about 8 mm proximal to the cuticle to the distal edge of the lunula (the white crescent-shaped area at the base of the nail). Normal time frame for development of a new toenail is 12 to 18 months. The nail folds are the folds of skin adjacent to the nail. The proximal nail fold is continuous with the cuticle, which seals and protects the nail bed against microorganisms. The hyponychium is the junction between the free nail border (distal nail that is not attached to the nail bed) and the adherent nail (nail plate attached to the underlying epithelium). It is sometimes referred to as the "quick."

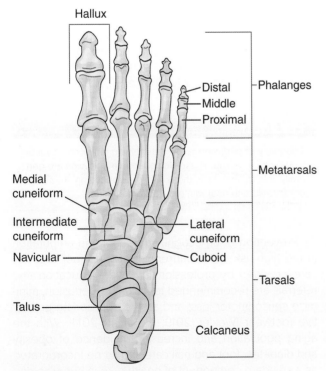

FIGURE 28-1. Anatomical Sections of the Feet.

In providing foot and nail care, the foot or wound care nurse must be cognizant of systemic conditions affecting perfusion and sensorimotor function that affect the feet and nails. The most common pathologic conditions of the legs, feet, toes, and nails are related to LEAD, LEND, and LEVD. These conditions have been covered in detail in previous chapters (Chapters 24, 25, and 26). Fungal skin infections involving the skin and nails are common. Conditions unique to the foot include bony deformities, stress fractures, and neuromas. Common pathologic conditions unique to the nail and surrounding skin include onychomycosis, onychogryphosis, subungual hemorrhage, paronychia, and onychocryptosis.

ASSESSMENT GUIDELINES

Effective foot and nail care requires a focused health and medication history and physical examination (Gallagher, 2012).

PATIENT HISTORY

A history is conducted to determine the social, familial, and health history and to assess cognitive and functional status. The medication history should be obtained prior to conducting any clinical intervention. It provides insight into conditions, diseases, and symptoms that may not have been reported during the history and highlights medications that would affect foot and nail care (such as anticoagulants or chemotherapeutic agents). The history should also include lifestyle issues such as smoking and current patterns of tobacco use, exercise, foot hygiene, weight, body mass index, and nutritional intake (WOCN, 2012).

Social History

It is important to learn as much as possible about the individual's daily routines and resources. Appropriate questions to ask include the following: Where do you live (home, apartment, assisted living facility, car, etc.) (Muirhead et al., 2011)? Do you live alone and provide your own care, or do you have a caregiver? Are you on a fixed income? Can you afford to purchase new shoes and other care items? Do you drive yourself, or do you have someone who can take you to the doctor's office or to other appointments? How do you manage foot and nail care at present, and what concerns do you have about your foot and nail care? How is your vision, and can you see your feet? Can you put on and take off your shoes and socks? When asking these questions, the wound care nurse should also assess the individual's affect, any indicators of depression or hopelessness, and quality of their support system (Gallagher, 2012). Living situation is particularly important as homeless individuals are more likely to have foot problems including tinea pedis, foot pain, functional limitations with walking, and improperly fitting shoes when compared to housed individuals (To et al., 2016).

Family History

A brief family history is helpful in assessing the individual's risk for LEAD, LEVD, and LEND. The wound care nurse should ask the individual as to whether or not they have any immediate relatives with early-onset cardiovascular disease, diabetes, leg ulcers caused by LEAD or LEVD, or other circulatory problems (Kimmel & Robin, 2013; Kohlman-Trigoboff, 2013; Wellborn & Moceri, 2014; WOCN, 2012, 2014, 2019).

Health History

The wound care nurse should ask the individual about any medical problems or surgical history. Most individuals over the age of 50 have one or more comorbidities that may affect perfusion, mobility, or sensorimotor status. Specific questions regarding arthritis, diabetes, cardiovascular disease, and nerve damage/neuropathy are relevant (Boulton, 2013). For the individual with diabetes, it is important to ask about usual management, blood glucose levels, and the last HbA1c results. The individual should be asked about foot and leg pain and, if present, should be queried further in regard to characteristics, severity, and exacerbating and relieving factors. The individual should also be asked about recent changes in the feet or nails and any problems with footwear or foot care.

KEY POINT

Most individuals over the age of 50 have one or more comorbidities that may affect perfusion, mobility, or sensorimotor status.

Medication History

It is important to ask about medications and allergies, which provides insight to existing health issues and potential side effects. This is particularly important when assessing an older individual, since polypharmacy is common for older individuals to take 10 or more medications each day (Golchin et al., 2015).

KEY POINT

Medication history provides additional insights to existing health issues and potential side effects.

Functional Status and Mobility

Normal structure and function of the feet is important to gait, mobility, and functional status. Abnormalities in either the bony structure or sensorimotor function of the foot place the individual at risk for functional disability (reduced mobility and ability to carry out activities of daily living). Foot weakness, compromised balance, and the presence of foot pain are risk factors for mobility issues and falls. Three quarters of active older adults complain of foot pain, and loss of mobility is a frequently verbalized concern for these individuals. Functional disability is common among individuals with poor foot health or foot pain, including an increased incidence of falls (Neville et al., 2020). Normal balance is vital to activities of daily living, such as getting out of a chair or bending over to put on shoes. The ability to maintain balance is a complex process requiring accurate sensory input regarding the body's position, normal cerebrocortical ability to process this information, and normal function of the muscles and joints that coordinate movement and maintain balance. Gait abnormalities and balance disorders often result in falls and fractures (Neville et al., 2020). In assessing for functional ability, the wound care nurse should ask about the client's mobility and ambulatory stability (e.g., ability to rise from a chair and walk to another point [Timed Up and Go Test]), ability to lift the feet and legs and climb stairs, ability to stand erect with correct posture, visual acuity (ability to see the feet), cognitive function, and independence in activities of daily living (Benavent-Caballer et al., 2016; Osoba et al., 2019).

PHYSICAL ASSESSMENT

In addition to a focused history and assessment of functional status, the foot care nurse must conduct a limited physical examination. The specific areas to be addressed include vascular status, sensorimotor function, musculoskeletal issues, and status of the skin and nails. Primary (screening) assessment is accomplished through the use of visual inspection, palpation, and evaluation of vascular and sensory status using noninvasive tools (Beuscher, 2019). The goal is to identify risk factors for lower extremity ulceration and amputation and to use the assessment data to construct an individualized plan of care for education and management that promotes limb preservation (Jones et al., 2013). (See **Fig. 28-3** for sample screening form.)

Research has shown that implementation of a foot care program using effective assessment tools, policies, and procedures reduces pain and injuries among people at risk for limb loss (Sibbald et al., 2012; Musuuza et al., 2019).

Vascular Assessment

Diminished blood flow is the single most significant risk factor for amputation (Kohlman-Trigoboff, 2013; WOCN, 2014). Blood flow to the lower extremity can be classified as normal, diminished, or absent and symmetric versus asymmetric or 0 (absent), 1+ (diminished), 2+ (normal), 3+ (prominent) suggesting local aneurysm (Rasmussen et al., 2019). Early detection of compromised blood flow allows for prompt medical treatment and less invasive surgical procedures to eradicate blockages (Burland, 2012; Kohlman-Trigoboff, 2013; WOCN, 2019).

The foot care nurse should conduct a noninvasive vascular assessment of the lower extremity to detect indicators of arterial or venous disease that require referral. Assessment parameters include the following:

- General inspection of the skin, hair, and nails to determine the presence of atrophic changes such as thin shiny skin, diminished or absent hair growth, and/or thinning and ridging of the nails (WOCN, 2014). Visible muscle atrophy is another potential indicator of arterial insufficiency, as is clubbing (ends of the fingers and toes enlarge and the nails curve.)
- Assessment for color changes in the lower extremity with elevation and dependency. The patient should be placed in the supine position, and the leg should be raised above the level of the heart for 10 to 20 seconds. The foot care nurse should observe for color changes, such as development of pallor (light skin) or a cyanotic or gray tone (dark skin). The individual should then be placed in a sitting position with the foot and leg hanging down, and the foot care nurse should observe for dependent rubor (a purple red discoloration of the distal leg and foot) (WOCN, 2014).
- Palpation of lower extremity pulses, both the posterior tibialis and the dorsalis pedis. A handheld Doppler can be used to auscultate the pulses; this is important when the pulses are difficult to palpate or nonpalpable.
- Palpation of the legs and feet for temperature changes, using the back of the hand and comparing the temperature of one foot and leg to the contralateral foot and leg and temperature of the distal leg and foot to the proximal leg. Findings should be recorded as hot, warm, cool, or cold.
- Assessment of capillary refill. The foot care nurse should apply firm pressure with their thumb to the pad of the great toe for 2 seconds. When pressure is released, the color should return to normal within 2 to 3 seconds. Capillary refill time >3 seconds is an indicator of possible LEAD. (Although capillary refill is commonly evaluated using the nail bed, the nails are often discolored and thickened due to onychomycosis; the toe pad should be used instead of the nail bed.)
- Ankle–brachial index (ABI), also known as ankle–brachial pressure index (ABPI). This is the most objective noninvasive measure of perfusion to the lower extremity and is an element of the vascular assessment (Rasmussen et al., 2019). In order to get valid results, it is important to follow evidence-based guidelines for ABI measurement and interpretation. See Chapter 25 for additional information.

Annual Comprehensive Diabetes Foot Exam Form

Name: _____   Date: _____   ID#: _____

I. Presence of Diabetes Complications
1. Check all that apply.
❑ Peripheral Neuropathy
❑ Nephropathy
❑ Retinopathy
❑ Peripheral Vascular Disease
❑ Cardiovascular Disease
❑ Amputation *(Specify date, side, and level)*
_____

Current ulcer or history of a foot ulcer?
Y____ N____

For Sections II & III, fill in the blanks with "Y" or "N" or with an "R," "L," or "B" for positive findings on the right, left, or both feet.

II. Current History
1. Is there pain in the calf muscles when walking that is relieved by rest?
   Y____ N____

2. Any change in the foot since the last evaluation? Y ____ N____
3. Any shoe problems? Y___ N____
4. Any blood or discharge on socks or hose? Y____ N____
5. Smoking history? Y___N___
6. Most recent hemoglobin A1c result _____% _____ date

III. Foot Exam
1. Skin, Hair, and Nail Condition
   Is the skin thin, fragile, shiny and hairless? Y ___ N___

   Are the nails thick, too long, ingrown, or infected with fungal disease? Y ___ N___

Measure, draw in, and label the patient's skin condition, using the key and the foot diagram below.
C=Callus   U=Ulcer   PU=Pre-Ulcer
F=Fissure M=Maceration R=Redness
S=Swelling W=Warmth D=Dryness

2. Note Musculoskeletal Deformities
   ❑ Toe deformities
   ❑ Bunions (Hallux Valgus)
   ❑ Charcot foot
   ❑ Foot drop
   ❑ Prominent Metatarsal Heads

3. Pedal Pulses Fill in the blanks with a "P" or an "A" to indicate present or absent.
Posterior tibial Left____ Right____
Dorsalis pedis Left____ Right____

4. Sensory Foot Exam *Label sensory level with a "+" in the five circled areas of the foot if the patient can feel the 5.07 (10-g) Semmes-Weinstein nylon monofilament and "-" if the patient cannot feel the filament.*

Notes

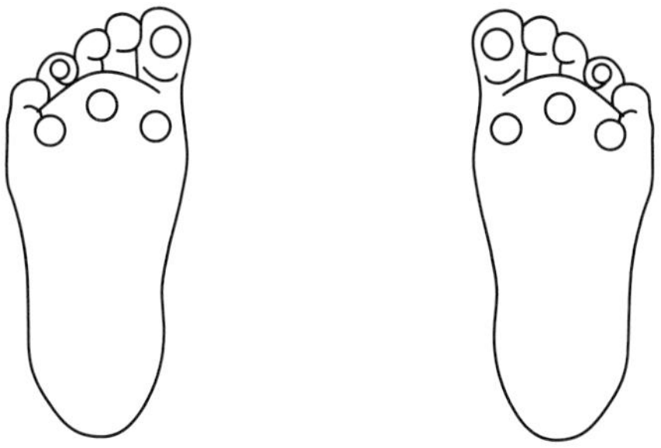

Right Foot

Notes

Left Foot

IV. Risk Categorization *Check appropriate box.*

❑ **Low Risk Patient**
All of the following:
❑ Intact protective sensation
❑ Pedal pulses present
❑ No deformity
❑ No prior foot ulcer
❑ No amputation

❑ **High Risk Patient**
One or more of the following:
❑ Loss of protective sensation
❑ Absent pedal pulses
❑ Foot deformity
❑ History of foot ulcer
❑ Prior amputation

V. Footwear Assessment *Indicate yes or no.*
1. Does the patient wear appropriate shoes? Y___ N ___
2. Does the patient need inserts? Y ___ N ___
3. Should corrective footwear be prescribed? Y ___ N ___

VI. Education *Indicate yes or no.*
1. Has the patient had prior foot care education? Y __N__
2. Can the patient demonstrate appropriate foot care? Y__N__
3. Does the patient need smoking cessation counseling?
   Y__N__
4. Does the patient need education about HbA1c or other diabetes self-care? Y__N__

VII. Management Plan *Check all that apply.*
1. Self-management education:
Provide patient education for preventive foot care. Date: _____
Provide or refer for smoking cessation counseling. Date: _____
Provide patient education about HbA1c or other aspect of self-care. Date: _____
2. Diagnostic studies:
   ❑ Vascular Laboratory
   ❑ Hemoglobin A1c (at least twice per year)
   ❑ Other: _____

3. Footwear recommendations:
   ❑ None
   ❑ Athletic shoes
   ❑ Accommodative inserts
   ❑ Custom shoes
   ❑ Depth shoes

4. Refer to:
   ❑ Primary Care Provider
   ❑ Diabetes Educator
   ❑ Podiatrist
   ❑ RN Foot Specialist
   ❑ Pedorthist
   ❑ Orthotist
   ❑ Endocrinologist
   ❑ Vascular Surgeon
   ❑ Foot Surgeon
   ❑ Rehab. Specialist
   ❑ Other: _____

5. Follow-up Care:
   Schedule follow-up visit. Date: _____

Provider Signature _____

FIGURE 28-3. Screening Form.

- Assessment for edema. Edema can be caused by a number of pathologic conditions, including cardiovascular or renal disease, severe malnutrition, LEVD, lymphatic disorders, and a condition known as lipedema (see Chapter 24). The foot care nurse should note whether the edema is generalized or limited to the legs and feet, whether it is unilateral or bilateral, and whether there are other indicators of venous disease, lymphedema, or lipedema. Individuals with evidence of venous or lymphatic disorders require referral to a vascular specialist or lymphedema specialist, while individuals with generalized edema should be referred to their primary care physician, cardiologist, or nephrologist.
- Assessment for indicators of venous disease. Early indicators of venous disease include pitting edema of variable severity, varicosities, dilated ankle and foot veins, and hemosiderosis (WOCN, 2019). Venous dermatitis is another indicator; this is manifested as dermatitis (dry scaly skin, pruritus, and erythema) involving the lower leg. Manifestations of venous disease are discussed in detail in Chapter 24.

Sensorimotor Assessment

Diabetes is a common comorbid condition among older individuals and those seeking foot care services, and long-standing or poorly controlled diabetes significantly increases the risk for both LEAD and LEND (WOCN, 2012, 2014). There are many conditions other than diabetes that increase the risk for neuropathic disease. Neuropathy places the individual at risk for LOPS resulting in painless trauma, loss of position sense resulting in falls, altered gait resulting in plantar surface ulcers, and Charcot foot deformity. Neuropathy is a major contributing factor for nontraumatic lower limb amputations. The screening assessment for any individual seeking foot care must include assessment for sensory and

motor function. The critical elements of a screening assessment are discussed briefly in this chapter; Chapter 26 provides an in-depth discussion of the pathology, assessment, and management of LEND and neuropathic ulcers.

> ### KEY POINT
>
> Long-standing or poorly controlled diabetes significantly increases the risk for both LEAD and LEND, both of which increase the risk of ulceration and possible amputation.

Monofilament Testing of Sensory Function

This test should be done using the Semmes-Weinstein 5.07 monofilament instrument (Crawford & Fields-Varnado, 2013), a nylon filament (fishing line) mounted on a holder and standardized to deliver 10 g of force when pressed against the skin with enough force to bend the monofilament into a C-shape. This tool is recommended by both the International Diabetes Federation and the World Health Organization (WHO) for screening of sensory function (Atkins, 2010; Beuscher, 2019; Ousey et al., 2018; Plucknette et al., 2012). The wound care nurse asks the patient to close their eyes and to report each time they sense touch on their foot; the nurse tests 4 to 10 sites on the plantar surface and dorsum of the foot. If the patient senses touch at all sites, they have intact protective sensation; inability to sense touch at any site denotes LOPS. LOPS has immediate implications for education and counseling; for example, the patient with any degree of LOPS must be counseled to have footwear professionally fitted since they will be unable to accurately detect discomfort from shoes that are rubbing. (See **Fig. 28-4A and B** for typical neuropathic wounds, i.e., loss of the fifth toe and damage to the great toe due to poorly fitted shoes.) The patient with LOPS must be reminded to wear protective footwear whenever out of bed, to check

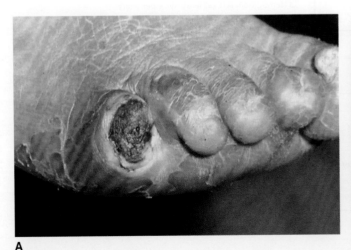

A

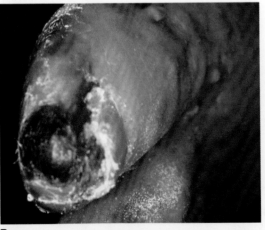

B

FIGURE 28-4. A, B. Neuropathic Wounds (loss of the fifth toe and damage to the great toe due to poorly fitted shoes).

bathwater temperature, and to visually inspect the feet daily. (See Chapter 26 for further information regarding monofilament testing.)

> **KEY POINT**
>
> LOPS has immediate implications for education and counseling. The individual with LOPS must be educated to wear protective footwear, to check bathwater temperature, and to visually inspect the feet every day for evidence of impending or actual ulceration.

Vibratory Sense Testing

The use of a tuning fork delivering 128 Hz is another reliable method of testing for sensory neuropathy (Beuscher, 2019). The wound care nurse strikes the tuning fork on an object or their hand, places the handle of the fork to the base of the great toe or the medial aspect of the first metatarsophalangeal joint, and records the patient's ability to perceive the vibration and point at which the vibration ceases. If the patient cannot accurately report vibratory sense or the point at which the vibration stops (either spontaneously or as a result of the nurse squeezing the prongs of the tuning fork), they are considered to have loss of vibratory sense and early-onset sensory neuropathy.

Position Sense Testing

As noted, patients who lose position sense are at increased risk for falls because they fail to recognize when their foot is at the edge of a step or on rough terrain and fail to compensate by adjusting their posture and gait appropriately (Neville et al., 2020). A simple test for proprioception is to have the patient close their eyes; the wound care nurse moves the great toe up, down, medially, and laterally and asks the patient to report the direction in which the toe has been moved. Inability to reliably report position of the great toe is documented as loss of position sense and requires patient education to hold onto stair rails and to watch their feet when walking.

Inspection for Deformities Caused by Motor Neuropathy

Damage to the motor nerves causes impaired function of the muscles that are responsible for maintenance of normal foot contours, gait, and weight bearing. Motor neuropathy leads to muscle imbalance, anatomic changes, and functional disorders (Kelechi & Johnson, 2012). Deformities caused by motor neuropathy include hammer toes, overlapping toes, foot drop, hallux valgus (deviation of the great toe away from midline, also known as bunion), hallux varus (deviation of the great toe toward midline), displacement of the plantar surface fat pads, abnormally prominent metatarsal heads,

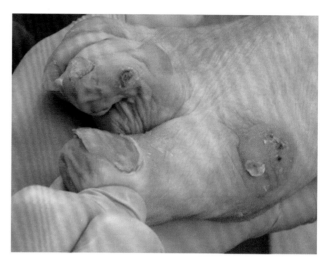

FIGURE 28-5. Corn/Callus.

and an abnormally prominent fifth metatarsophalangeal joint, also known as a tailor bunion or bunionette. These deformities increase the risk of friction damage (e.g., corns and calluses) (**Fig. 28-5**) and ulcers from poorly fitted footwear (**Fig. 28-6**). Other visual indicators of motor neuropathy include signs of abnormal weight bearing (e.g., callus formation and abnormal wear patterns in footwear).

Altered Weight Bearing and Plantar Surface Pressure Points

This is a simple test that provides very helpful information regarding plantar surface pressures during weight bearing; it requires a pressure mapping device such as a Harris Mat or digital imprint device. The patient is asked to stand on the device, and this provides an "ink print" (Harris Mat) or digital imprint that visibly displays any areas of high pressure. The presence of high-pressure areas (also known as "hot spots") mandates referral to an orthotist or pedorthist for fitting with weight redistributing insoles and therapeutic shoes.

Foot Tracing

This allows the wound care nurse and patient to evaluate the fit of the current footwear. The patient stands on a sheet of paper and the nurse traces the outline of each foot while the patient is weight bearing. The patient's shoes are then placed over the tracings; if the shoes do not fit within the lines of the tracings, it provides visual evidence that the footwear is not correctly fitted. A foot tracing also allows a caregiver to purchase shoes for an individual who is homebound.

Assessment of Muscle Strength and Range of Motion

Range of motion is assessed by asking the patient to move the foot up and down and back and forth (active range of motion). Muscle strength is assessed by placing

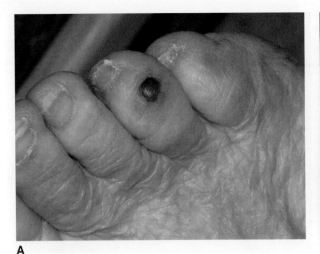

A

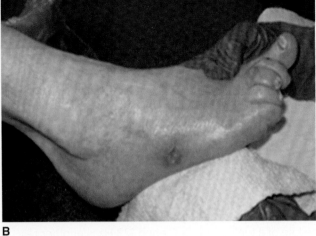

B

FIGURE 28-6. A, B. Injury/Ulcer Due to Poorly Fitted Shoes.

the wound care nurse's hand against the plantar surface of the foot and asking the patient to push the foot down against the nurse's hand. Hand is then placed on the dorsum of the foot, and the patient is asked to pull toes back against the nurse's hand. Both extremities are evaluated, and one side is compared to the other (Bonham et al., 2016; Crawford & Fields-Varnado, 2013). Reduced strength and/or range of motion are indicators of motor neuropathy.

Assessment for Autonomic Neuropathy

Autonomic neuropathy involves damage to the nerves that control sweat gland function and appropriate vasoconstriction of the arteries in the lower extremity. Damage to these nerves is evidenced by dry cracked skin with or without fissure formation, an abnormally warm erythematous foot, and, in severe cases, development of Charcot neuroarthropathy, also known as Charcot foot (**Fig. 28-7**) (Game, 2012; Vopat et al., 2018). Whenever

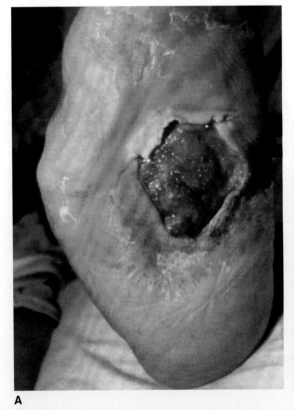

A

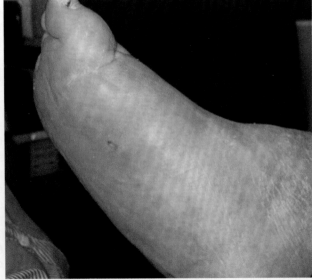

B

FIGURE 28-7. A, B. Examples of Charcot Neuroarthropathy.

a patient presents with an abnormally warm erythematous foot, it is important to rule out an infectious process by assessing for fever, elevated white blood cell (WBC) count, and hyperglycemia (Madan & Pai, 2013; Milne et al., 2013). An x-ray may be needed to rule out an acute fracture and to differentiate among acute arthritic conditions (e.g., gout), chronic arthritis, and early-onset Charcot neuroarthropathy (Milne et al., 2013; WOCN, 2012).

KEY POINT

Whenever a patient presents with an abnormally warm and erythematous foot, it is necessary to rule out Charcot neuro-arthropathy by x-ray and laboratory tests.

Charcot neuroarthropathy (also known as Charcot osteoarthropathy) is a complex complication resulting from a combination of autonomic neuropathy, sensory neuropathy, and possibly motor neuropathy. Autonomic neuropathy results in persistent vasodilation of the pedal arteries, which is thought to cause, over time, demineralization of the small bones in the foot (osteopenia). These fragile bones are at increased risk for fracture as a result of minor trauma. The risk is even greater if the individual also has motor neuropathy resulting in abnormal gait and weight bearing. The architecture of the foot is preserved if the fracture is recognized promptly and the foot is appropriately off-loaded until the fracture heals. Because of sensory neuropathy and LOPS, the fracture(s) may not be recognized and left untreated. The patient continues to walk on the fractured foot, resulting in additional fractures over time with eventual collapse of the normal architecture of the foot (Milne et al., 2013; Pupp & Kolvunen, 2011). This results in a "rocker-bottom foot" with

high midfoot pressures and higher risk of ulceration and possible amputation (Pupp & Kolvunen, 2011) (**Fig. 28-8**). A Charcot joint is most common in the midfoot but can involve the great toe, knee, or other jointed area (Madan & Pai, 2013; Vopat et al., 2018).

Assessment of Skin Status

The condition of the skin of the lower extremity and foot is an indicator of underlying conditions and usual foot care and hygiene. The foot care nurse should carefully inspect the skin of the lower leg, foot, and web spaces for texture, hydration, and cleanliness. The nurse should be alert to the following: thin atrophic skin, excessively dry skin, fissures (especially on the heels), corns and calluses (including interdigital corns), maceration of web spaces and any lesions involving the web spaces, tinea pedis (athlete's foot), which may present as dry scaly lesions on the plantar surface or as moist painful desquamation of the plantar surface and painful fissures between the toes, and plantar warts (Erwin et al., 2013). Plantar warts (verruca plantaris) are caused by the human papillomavirus. The foot care nurse must be aware that there are a myriad of dermatologic conditions that may cause foot lesions, including psoriasis, contact dermatitis, and melanomas (Bristow et al., 2010; Johnson & Taylor, 2012; Zafren & Mechem, 2018). Any suspicious or unknown lesion requires referral to a dermatologist (Johnson & Taylor, 2012; Murphy & Dolan, 2018).

Presence and Characteristics of Any Wounds

Any lesions or wounds on the feet and legs should be noted and appropriate referrals made. If the patient is being managed in a foot and wound care center, the wound care nurse can provide in-depth wound assessment and management and involve other specialists as

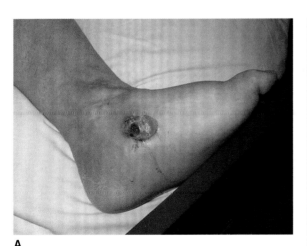

A

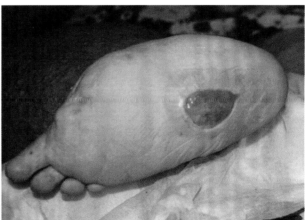

B

FIGURE 28-8. A, B. Rocker-Bottom Foot.

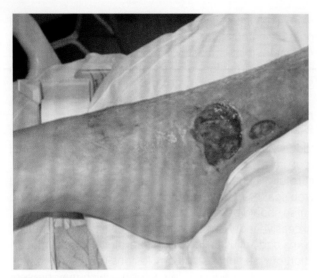

FIGURE 28-9. Arterial Ulcer.

indicated (Snyder et al., 2010). If the patient is being seen in a center limited to foot care, they should be referred to a wound treatment center or the appropriate specialist. See Chapters 24, 25, and 26 for an in-depth discussion of the pathology, presentation, and management of lower extremity wounds caused by LEVD, LEAD, and LEND. (**Figs. 28-9 to 28-11** depict ulcers of arterial, neuropathic, and venous etiology.)

Condition of the Toenails and Cuticles
Toenails should remain relatively the same throughout the life span, though both old and new injuries

may affect the shape, size, and rate of growth of the nail. The cuticle is the hardened skin at the base and edge of the nail that serves to seal and protect the nail matrix from invasion of pathogens (see **Fig. 28-2**). Factors to include in assessment of the nails and cuticles include the following: thickness, color, and brittleness of the nails, nail deformities (e.g., incurvated nails, "ram's horn" nails [onychogryphosis], or thickened deformed nails [onychodystrophy]); fungal infection (onychomycosis), integrity of the cuticle, ingrown nails (onychocryptosis), and inflammation and infection around the toenail (paronychia) (Beuscher & Kelechi, 2019; Erwin et al., 2013; Nevares-Pomales et al., 2018) (**Fig. 28-12A–E**).

KEY POINT

Factors to include in assessment of the nails and cuticles include thickness, color, and brittleness of the nails, nail deformities, evidence of fungal infection, integrity of the cuticle, evidence of ingrown nails, and evidence of inflammation around the nail.

The information gathered during the physical assessment allows the foot care nurse to develop an individualized plan of care for education and counseling that addresses self-protection during activities of daily living and referrals for further evaluation, follow-up, and management.

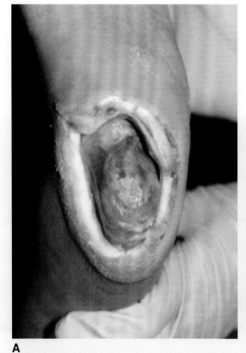

A

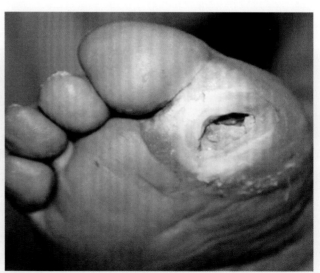

B

FIGURE 28-10. A, B. Neuropathic Ulcers.

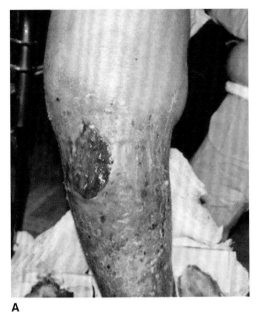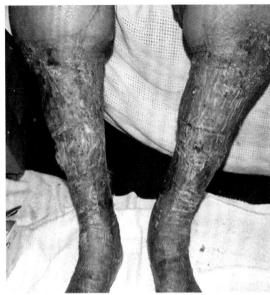

A   **B**

FIGURE 28-11. A, B. Venous Ulcers.

ASSESSMENT OF LOWER EXTREMITY PAIN

Pain has been defined as "An aversive sensory and emotional experience typically caused by, or resembling that caused by, actual or potential tissue injury" (IASP, 2019). Pain is a common symptom of many disorders involving the lower extremities, including LEAD, LEND, LEVD, musculoskeletal conditions (such as arthritis or plantar fasciitis), and nerve damage (such as interdigital neuroma). Pain is subjective, and no confirmatory physical or laboratory examination can substantiate the presence or

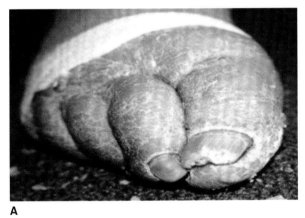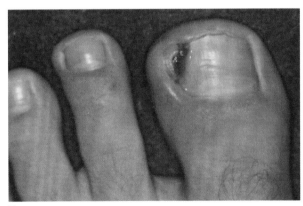

A   **B**

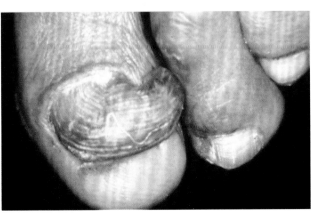

FIGURE 28-12. Abnormalities in the Nails and Cuticles. **A.** Onychomycosis with tinea pedis. **B.** Onychocryptosis with paronychia. **C.** Onychogryphosis.

C

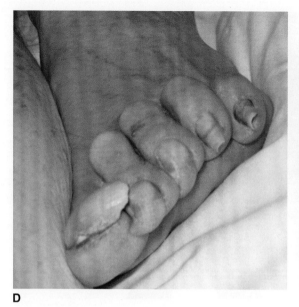

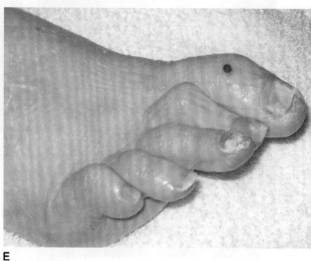

D

E

FIGURE 28-12. (*Continued*) **D.** Thickened elongated nails. **E.** Onychomycosis with onychodystrophia and hammer toe.

severity. Pain assessment involves a history that includes the following: intensity of pain using established pain scale, frequency and time of occurrence, characteristics, and exacerbating and relieving factors (Bonham et al., 2016; Crawford & Fields-Varnado, 2013; Wellborn & Moceri, 2014; WOCN, 2019). (See **Box 28-2** for characteristics of pain associated with arterial, neuropathic, and venous disease.)

BOX 28-2   CHARACTERISTICS OF ARTERIAL, NEUROPATHIC, AND VENOUS PAIN

LEAD (arterial pain)
- Characteristics
  - Intermittent claudication
  - Aching
  - Cramping
  - May occur at night (rest pain)

LEND (neuropathic pain)
- Altered sensation not described as pain
  - Numbness
  - Warm/cool
  - Prickling
  - Tingling
  - "Stocking/glove" pattern
  - Characteristics of pain
  - Burning, itching
  - Shooting, "electrical shock"
  - Paresthesia
  - Unrelenting

LEVD (venous pain)
- Characteristics
  - Throbbing or aching of variable severity
  - May be relieved by leg elevation and compression
  - End of the day—achy leg syndrome—heavy legs

COMMON PATHOLOGIC NAIL CONDITIONS

ONYCHOMYCOSIS

Onychomycosis is a common fungal infection of the nail plate, nail bed, or both and accounts for over 50% of common nail disorders in older adults (**Figs. 28-12A and 28-13**). The most common causative organism is *Trichophyton rubrum*; other organisms are dermatophyte fungi, nondermatophyte fungi, and yeast (Gupta et al., 2011). Toenails are 25 times more likely than fingernails to develop onychomycosis, and the first and second toes are the most susceptible, probably due to repeated trauma that weakens the seal between the nail plate and nail bed, permitting entry of the pathogen

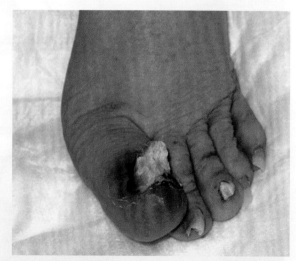

FIGURE 28-13. Onychomycosis with Hypertrophic Nail and C-Shaped Nails.

(Kelechi & Johnson, 2012). The infection easily spreads to other toenails and is a challenge to treat due to the difficulty of medications penetrating the nail (Beuscher & Kelechi, 2019; Elewski & Tosti, 2014).

> **KEY POINT**
>
> Onychomycosis is a common fungal infection that accounts for over 50% of common nail disorders in older adults; it is usually more of an aesthetic issue than health issue.

There is a strong correlation between close quarter living environments (nursing homes, boarding schools, and military living quarters) and transmission of onychomycosis. People of all ages can be affected by onychomycosis, but older and adolescent populations are most at risk (Gazes & Zeichner, 2013). While onychomycosis is in general more of an aesthetic issue than a health issue, evidence suggests that patients with diabetes and onychomycosis are at increased risk for diabetic foot ulcers (Elewski & Tosti, 2014; Takehara et al., 2011).

The signs and symptoms of onychomycosis include (1) discoloration of the nail plate (white, brown, yellow patches or streaks), (2) subungual hyperkeratosis (thickening and deformity of the toenails), (3) onycholysis (separation of nail plate from nail bed), and (4) brittle and crumbly nails. In addition to the cosmetic issues, some individuals with onychomycosis report tenderness and trauma to the lateral skin folds of the affected nail(s).

If systemic treatment is being considered, the diagnosis must be confirmed prior to initiation of therapy (Lipner & Scher, 2019). The diagnosis typically involves examination of nail scrapings obtained from the undersurface of the nail, top of the nail, or nail bed proximal to the affected portion of the nail. Specimens, direct microscopy, and cultures may be performed. There are risks and benefits to systemic intervention.

Systemic treatment and topical solutions are utilized either separately or concurrently. The most common method is a combination of both because systemic treatment is more effective than topical treatment in penetrating hyperkeratotic layers of the nail. The provider must consider the causative organism, potential adverse events, drug interactions, patient compliance, and cost (Lipner & Scher, 2019). Liver toxicity is a potential adverse effect, and it is necessary to monitor liver function at baseline and throughout treatment (Beuscher & Kelechi, 2019). Allylamines and azoles are the most commonly used systemic antifungal agents; reported cure rates range from 35% to 70%, but recurrence is common. Treatment can take up to 1 year because it is difficult for the drugs to penetrate the keratin layers, due to the lack of blood vessels (Westerberg & Voyack, 2013).

Topical antifungals have low incidence of drug–drug interactions and few contraindications; this makes them useful for older patients, especially those taking multiple medications and those for whom oral antifungals are contraindicated (Lipner & Scher, 2019). If <50% of the nail bed is affected, some wound care nurses may opt to use topical therapy alone (Kelechi & Johnson, 2012), even in individuals for whom systemic therapy would be an option. Ciclopirox 8% lacquer is a topical agent that can be applied daily up to 7 days; it should then be removed using nail polish remover.

> **KEY POINT**
>
> Topical antifungals have limited contraindications and drug–drug interactions and are useful for older patients taking multiple medications and those for whom oral agents are contraindicated.

Some clinicians use a 20% to 40% urea compound to reduce hyperkeratosis, either as a solo treatment or followed by nail debridement (Kelechi & Johnson, 2012). Menthol vapor rub and tea tree oil have also been used to treat onychomycosis. Daily application around the cuticle is typically recommended for one full year to allow complete regrowth of the toenail, since these agents primarily affect the developing nail. The mechanism of action remains unclear, but anecdotal outcomes have been good, and these agents are low cost and low risk in addition to being of potential great benefit. Topical agents also serve as a deodorizer.

Up to 50% of individuals with onychomycosis develop recurrent infections within 1 year after treatment (Elewski & Tosti, 2014). It is important for the foot and nail care nurse to educate patients on strategies to reduce the risk of infection or reinfection (Pariser et al., 2013). These include the following:

- Avoid walking barefoot in public places such as pools, spas, gyms, and locker rooms where moisture is abundant and fungal organisms can thrive.
- Bring your own nail clippers and files to the nail salon.
- Wear properly fitting shoes made of natural materials with a toe box high enough to accommodate thickened nails and any toe deformities.
- Trim the nails according to the shape of the end of the toe (either curved or straight across) to avoid nail trauma that could cause breaks in the skin.
- File the nails with a course nail or emery board to smooth the edges after trimming.
- Wash the feet and dry between the toes daily (Kelechi & Johnson, 2012).
- Treat tinea pedis promptly, because fungal skin infections are thought to cause onychomycosis due to the proximity of the skin and nails (Elewski & Tosti, 2014).
- For individuals with onychomycosis, wash or replace shoes and inserts regularly.

ONYCHOCRYPTOSIS

Onychocryptosis (ingrowing or ingrown toenail) affects 20% of the population, with older adults and adolescents being most affected (see **Fig. 28-12B**). Adolescents are at increased risk because their feet are growing at a rapid rate and they perspire more heavily. This creates a moist environment that makes the nails more susceptible to splitting. Older patients who have difficulty caring for their feet and nails due to loss of visual acuity or physical mobility may develop an overgrowth of skin and nails that increases risk for ingrown nails (Mayeaux et al., 2019).

Onychocryptosis occurs when the lateral edge of the nail splinters and invades the periungual space, producing pain and reducing mobility and activity; the resulting inflammation at the site can lead to infection (Mayeaux et al., 2019). The great toe is the most common site, although ingrown toenails can involve any nail (Mayeaux et al., 2019).

Factors contributing to onychocryptosis include improper nail trimming or tearing of the nails, excessive pressure during ambulation, repetitive or accidental trauma, tight shoes, C-shaped pattern of nail growth (incurvated nails), and obesity. These factors can add additional pressure to the nail and increase the risk for toe and nail injury. Proper nail trimming is one element of care in prevention of onychocryptosis (Geizhals & Lipner, 2019).

One conservative treatment of onychocryptosis (ingrown nails) involves placing a narrow strip of an alcohol prep pad between the edge of the nail and the skin/cuticle of the affected area to prevent the nail from growing into the periungual space (Mayeaux et al., 2019). Gutter splint, a surgical intervention, involves partial nail avulsion of the affected lateral edge of the nail bed followed by chemical matricectomy (removal of part or all of the nail).

ONYCHOGRYPHOSIS

Onychogryphosis is described as abnormally thickened nails with the appearance of an oyster shell or ram's horn (see **Fig. 28-12C**). The nail plate can be uneven, thickened, brown, or opaque and may curve toward the other nails. The main risk factor for this condition is inadequate nail care, due to self-neglect or inability to perform nail care due to limited mobility, lack of dexterity, poor eyesight, or insufficient professional nursing services. The older populations are most affected. It is also prevalent in the homeless and cognitively impaired populations. Proper nail trimming and filing is a key preventive measure (Ko & Lipner, 2018). Management requires thinning of the nail followed by appropriate trimming to reduce the height and length of the nail using nippers and a sturdy file.

 ## COMMON SKIN DISORDERS OF THE FOOT AND LOWER EXTREMITY

The older population and people with diabetes are at increased risk for LEAD, LEVD, and LEND. The foot care nurse must be knowledgeable regarding these conditions and must be able to recognize and manage wounds caused by these pathologies (or make appropriate referrals). The foot care nurse must be able to identify and manage common skin conditions, for example, xerosis, fissures, and tinea pedis. The foot care nurse must be alert to indicators of skin malignancies (squamous cell carcinoma, basal cell carcinoma, and melanoma) and assure referral to dermatology for any abnormal lesions or suspected malignancies.

The goal in provision of foot and nail care is to prevent conditions that can be managed and treated. Maintenance of normal nail thickness and length may optimize mobility and comfort and prevent traumatic injuries to the adjacent toes. Identification of early ischemic or neuropathic changes with appropriate referrals and education may prevent ulcerations that could progress to amputation. Appropriate management of an ingrown toenail may reduce pain, infection, and ulceration that could lead to more problems or eventual amputation.

 ## SYSTEMIC CONDITIONS AND IMPLICATIONS FOR FOOT CARE NURSES

Some of the systemic conditions that commonly affect the legs, feet, and nails are osteoarthritis, gout, LEAD, LEND, LEVD, and Raynaud disease.

OSTEOARTHRITIS

Osteoarthritis is the most common type of arthritis, especially among the older population. Rheumatoid arthritis is less common but causes greater morbidity. Osteoarthritis produces pain and stiffness, while rheumatoid arthritis causes deformity and loss of function in addition to pain. Any form of arthritis limits the individual's ability to provide their own foot care. Care goals include relief of pain, improvement in joint function, and enhanced ability to perform activities of daily living (Graham et al., 2017; Riskowki et al., 2011). Interventions include foot care, gentle massage, use of therapeutic shoes, compression stockings, exercises, smoking cessation and weight loss, and orthotics (Riskowki et al., 2011).

GOUT

Gout is a less common form of arthritis that usually affects the joint of the great toe but may also present in the ankles and knees. It is caused by the accumulation of urate crystals in joints; this triggers an acute inflammatory response and severe pain. Gout is more common in males and is triggered by high levels of uric acid. Treatment involves measures to reduce uric acid levels. It is important to avoid alcoholic beverages, lose weight, and consume smaller amounts of purine-rich foods such as asparagus, mushrooms, mussels, and organ meats (Abhishek & Dohertt, 2018). The foot care nurse may assess individuals and assist in diagnosis, intervention, therapeutic foot and nail care, and footwear selection (Rome et al., 2013).

LOWER EXTREMITY ARTERIAL DISEASE

LEAD is manifest by changes in the skin and nails as well as abnormal ABI, diminished pulses, and prolonged capillary refill time. In addition to assuring that the patient is referred to a vascular specialist, the nurse must avoid any trauma to the skin during foot and nail care. Patient education should include measures to improve perfusion (e.g., smoking cessation) and to prevent injury to the leg and foot during activities that increase the risk for trauma (e.g., use of protective footwear and shin guards) (Bonham et al., 2016). Routine foot and nail care is important to monitor disease progression and to prevent wounds that could lead to an amputation.

> **KEY POINT**
>
> The wound care nurse must take every precaution to avoid trauma to the skin during foot and nail care and must educate the patient regarding measures to prevent trauma and improve perfusion.

LOWER EXTREMITY VENOUS DISEASE

LEVD is manifest by edema, hemosiderosis, and/or venous dermatitis (Paul et al., 2011). Calf pump muscle dysfunction is a key contributing factor to LEVD and chronic lower extremity venous ulcers. The foot and nail nurse should assure that the individual is being followed by a vascular specialist and should reinforce the importance of leg elevation, consistent use of compression stockings, and adherence to walking/exercise programs (WOCN, 2019).

> **KEY POINT**
>
> The individual with edema or evidence of LEVD should be educated regarding the importance of leg elevation and routine use of compression stockings.

LOWER EXTREMITY NEUROPATHIC DISEASE

LEND is usually manifest by diminished sensory awareness, foot deformities, altered weight bearing, and dry skin. Some patients report paresthesias (pins and needles sensation, burning pain, and "electric shock" sensations). These individuals require referral to neurology and pain management (WOCN, 2012). Foot care nurses play an important role in management of patients with LEND, specifically in monitoring for changes in sensorimotor status and perfusion status. They are responsible for ongoing education and counseling regarding protective footwear, foot care, and daily foot inspection. Additional responsibilities include providing nail care that maintains the nails at an appropriate length and thickness and intervening for problems such as an ingrown nail or callus (Aalaa et al., 2012). For the individual with diabetes, appropriate care also involves reinforcement of the importance of tight glycemic control (Christman et al., 2011; Sacks & John, 2014).

> **KEY POINT**
>
> Foot care nurses play an important role in management of patients with LEND, monitoring for changes in sensorimotor function and perfusion. They provide ongoing education regarding glycemic control, protective footwear, and routine foot inspection.

RAYNAUD DISEASE

Raynaud disease is a vasoconstrictive condition that results in decreased blood flow to the hands and feet in response to cold or stress (Temprano, 2016). The foot care nurse should intervene by educating the patient to avoid cold and to slowly and gently warm the hands and feet.

COMMON FOOT MALFORMATIONS

The most common malformations and disorders of the foot are hallux valgus (bunion), hallux varus, hallux rigidus/limitus, bunionette (tailor bunion), Charcot foot (neuroarthropathy, osteoarthropathy), neuroma, flat feet (pes planus), high arch (pes cavus), plantar fasciitis, and heel spurs. Malformations of the toes, feet, and ankles lead to an increased risk of corns, calluses, falls, pain, wounds, and amputations.

HALLUX VALGUS

Hallux valgus (bunion) is an abnormal prominence (outgrowth) of the joint between the big toe and the foot (first metatarsophalangeal joint) (**Fig. 28-14A and B**). Hallux

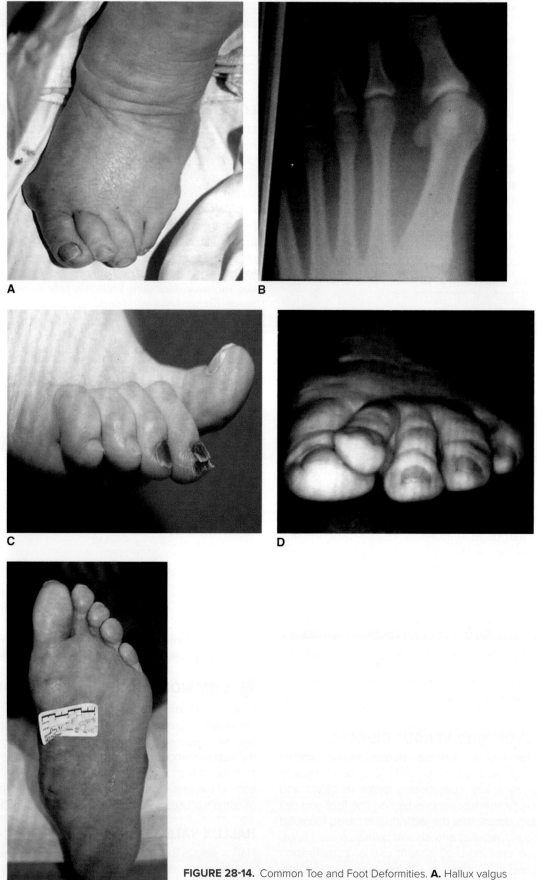

FIGURE 28-14. Common Toe and Foot Deformities. **A.** Hallux valgus (bunion). **B.** X-ray of bunion. **C.** Hallux rigidus with claw toes and subungual hematoma. **D.** Overlapping toes. **E.** Charcot neuroarthropathy.

valgus is a very common deformity. It may or may not cause pain but may cause a serious balance and mobility issue. It may be related to genetics, use of tight, narrow and pointed footwear, and trauma. Clinical presentation includes bulging of the first metatarsophalangeal joint medially and away from the foot. The hallux (great toe) tilts toward the second toe and may move over or under the toe. Calluses may form due to ill-fitting shoes or because of pressure, shear, or friction from the deformity causing an abnormal gait. An x-ray may identify the skeletal changes including changes due to osteoarthritis. Wearing shoes with a wider and deeper toe box to accommodate the deformity may reduce symptoms. It may be helpful to refer the patient to an orthotist or pedorthist for inserts and therapeutic shoes. If the patient has intractable symptoms or is interested in surgical intervention, the foot care nurse should initiate a referral to a podiatric or orthopedic surgeon.

> **KEY POINT**
>
> Corns and calluses form due to ill-fitting shoes or pressure, shear, and friction caused by bony abnormalities and abnormal weight bearing.

HALLUX VARUS

Hallux varus is characterized by a medial deviation of the great toe (hallux) from its straight axis. The toe begins to point toward the other foot. The deformity often develops after a previous surgery for hallux valgus, usually due to overcorrection. Other causes include trauma, rheumatoid arthritis, and psoriasis. Taping the great toe toward the little toe for 3 months may help. Depending on the length of time the deformity has been present and other comorbidities, surgery may be indicated. To prevent injury, the individual should be counseled to wear shoes that have a wider toe box and are made of soft moldable materials.

HALLUX RIGIDUS/HALLUX LIMITUS

Hallux rigidus and hallux limitus are both great toe joint issues in which movement of the hallux becomes restricted (see **Fig. 28-14C**). With hallux limitus, joint movement is restricted during weight bearing but is otherwise normal. This condition is characterized by intact cartilage and little or no arthritis. With hallux rigidus, the great toe becomes arthritic with associated cartilage loss, resulting in bone-on-bone motion and pain. Hallux rigidus/limitus is the result of trauma and hyperglycemia and most commonly occurs in people with diabetes. Clinical presentation includes stiffness of the great toe joint. Pain is caused by excessive flexion of the great toe. It may also occur during standing, due to pronation and rolling of the big toe joint that causes restricted motion. Surgery

is often required to correct the structural problem. Like most foot and toe malformations and conditions, wearing appropriate footwear is essential to prevent pressure, shear, and friction causing calluses and wounds.

BUNIONETTE

Bunionette (tailor bunion) is a bulge caused by an abnormally prominent fifth metatarsal joint. Intervention involves accommodation of the deformity with a wider forefoot toe box. Shoes should be sized to accommodate the width of the foot to alleviate any pressure, shear, and friction, and to off-load any existing wounds. Surgery is rarely indicated. When the deformity cannot be managed with conservative measures, a referral to a podiatrist or orthopedic surgeon is indicated.

CHARCOT FOOT

Charcot foot (osteoarthropathy, neuroarthropathy) is a deformity of the foot directly related to poor glucose control. Nearly 13% of individuals with diabetes who have LOPS and autonomic neuropathy may develop Charcot foot disease (CFD) (Vopat et al., 2018). CFD involves gradual thinning of the bones (osteopenia), fractures, deformities, and abnormalities in weight bearing. The midfoot is the segment most commonly involved, but exacerbations can also involve the forefoot (Game & Jeffcoate, 2013) (see **Fig. 28-14E**). The initial presentation is unilateral swelling and a hot, erythematous foot resulting from an acute fracture. Because these individuals also have LOPS, they are typically unaware of the injury, fail to seek medical care, and continue weight bearing. This creates an environment of continued inflammation, additive damage, and gradual settling of the bones into a chronic Charcot joint. With severe deformity, difficulties in gait and balance become an issue increasing risk for falls. The bony deformities result in abnormal increases in pressure, shear, and friction, leading to calluses, wounds, and increased risk of amputation (Pupp & Kolvunen, 2011). Charcot osteoarthropathy is often missed during the acute phase (following acute fracture); failure to recognize the initial injury results in additional fractures because the individual fails to off-load the injured foot. The patient who monitors the feet for evidence of inflammation and appropriately off-loads the foot in response to evidence of injury may prevent additional injury and deformity. Recognizing the initial presentation and initiating referrals to podiatric or orthopedic surgery is important (Vopat et al., 2018).

> **KEY POINT**
>
> Charcot foot disease (CFD) involves gradual thinning of the bones (osteopenia), fractures, deformities, and abnormalities in weight bearing.

CONDITIONS CAUSING HEEL/ARCH PAIN

Heel or arch pain may be due to thinning of the fat pads, which is normal with aging or can occur as a result of repetitive activity that increases pressure on these areas. Pes planus (flat foot) and pes cavus (high arch foot) should be considered when evaluating symptoms that include pain on the bottom, edge, or back of the heel or foot. Burning or shooting pain that occurs upon standing after sleeping or prolonged sitting is a common symptom of pes planus and pes cavus.

The most common cause of heel pain is an outgrowth of the bone also known as a spur. Plantar fasciitis is another common cause and is caused by inflammation of the plantar fascia and/or Achilles tendon, often due to poor foot mechanics (Weatherford, 2017; Young, 2012). Other causes include tendonitis, which is usually related to repetitive activity, and arthritic conditions such as rheumatoid arthritis or gout. X-rays are important for determining the underlying problem and to rule out stress fractures, osteoarthritis, and other inflammatory or skeletal issues. Treatment is based on the underlying problem. Footwear modifications to support normal foot mechanics can frequently help to reduce pain. Night splints, strapping, orthotics, and padding may be indicated for heel and arch support and can also contribute to symptom control (Hawke & Burns, 2012). Contrast bathing (cold and then hot) and stretches may help to reduce pain, and nonsteroidal anti-inflammatory drugs (NSAIDs) may be recommended. There is no preferred treatment choice among conservative interventions, and a combination of therapies may be needed (Rasenberg et al., 2018). Surgery or injections are additional options for some patients. The foot care nurse should refer any patient with significant or refractory symptoms to a primary care provider, podiatrist, or orthopedic surgeon.

Neuroma is a painful overgrowth of nerve tissue that most often occurs between the third and fourth toes. The overgrowth of nerves is triggered by bony compression that causes irritation and inflammation of the nerve. The bones are pressed together by footwear that is too tight and poorly fitted. Neuromas are common among women who wear high-heeled shoes and people who are on their feet for extended periods of time. The patient reports aching or sharp, burning, shooting pain in the ball of the foot that is triggered or worsened by walking. Other symptoms may include tingling or numbness or the sensation of having a stone in the shoe. Treatment recommendations include footwear modifications and the addition of orthotics. Padding and taping, physical therapy, and medication may be indicated (Matthews et al., 2019). The patient with severe or refractory symptoms should be referred to a podiatrist for steroid injections or surgery.

 ## COMMON TOE DEFORMITIES AND MALFORMATIONS

Hammer toes, claw toes, and mallet toes are deformities caused by contractures of the interphalangeal joints (see **Fig. 28-12E**). A hammer toe is the contracture of the proximal interphalangeal joint, a mallet toe is the contracture of the distal interphalangeal joint, and a claw toe is the contracture of both the proximal and distal interphalangeal joints. All of these deformities cause the interphalangeal joints to protrude upward and the distal toe to point downward. Causative factors include ill-fitting shoes, hyperglycemia, and previous trauma. They present as a deformity that may contribute to the development of corns and calluses that cause pain with ambulation (due to pressure, shear, and friction that occurs with walking). People with toe deformities benefit from footwear with a toe box that is made of flexible material with a wide and deep toe box to accommodate the deformity. Pressure redistribution strategies such as hammertoe cushions, gel pad sleeves, and soft silicone toe spacers may also be helpful. Surgery may be indicated (Malhotra et al., 2016). Other deformities include webbed toes, six toes, and second or third toes that are longer than the first. Any foot or toe deformity must be taken into consideration when providing recommendations, education, or referrals regarding footwear.

KEY POINT

Hammer toes, claw toes, and mallet toes are deformities caused by contractures of the interphalangeal joints. Conservative management involves modifications in footwear to accommodate the deformities. Definitive management requires surgery to correct the deformity.

 ## GUIDELINES FOR FOOT AND NAIL CARE

Foot and nail care must be provided with caution and appropriate equipment. The overall goals of care are to reduce the length and height of the nails to within normal range, maintain intact cuticles, and pare or file corns and calluses. Hygienic care is provided first. For example, briefly bathing the feet in warm water with or without a mild cleanser assures that the feet and nails are clean. Bathing the feet also softens the nails and cuticles facilitating foot care. Soaking feet may cause dry skin, which may contribute to impaired skin integrity and increase risk of infection (Beuscher, 2019).

ASSESSMENT

At the initial visit, a comprehensive lower extremity assessment should be conducted. Follow-up visits require general inspection for evidence of any lesions or ulcers, assessment of dorsalis pedis and posterior tibialis pulses, observation for dependent rubor, and assessment for LOPS. The patient should also be asked about any foot-related pain or concerns.

The feet should be inspected for corns or calluses and for any lesions or maceration of the interdigital spaces. The foot care nurse should use a nail curette, spatula, or orange wood stick to remove debris from beneath the nails and to assess the free nail border (Etnyre et al., 2011; Gallagher, 2012; Schaper et al., 2017). During this process, the nurse also assesses the nails for length and thickness. If there is callus obscuring the distal end of the toe and the free nail border, the callus should be removed either by paring (with a scalpel or rasper) or by filing with an emery board.

MANAGEMENT OF HYPERTROPHIC NAILS

If the nail is abnormally thickened, it should be thinned prior to trimming. This may be done with use of a large coarse grain emery board or with an electric grinder. If an electric grinder is used, the wound care nurse must be aware of the potential for aerosolizing mycotic and bacterial organisms and must implement appropriate Centers for Disease Control and Prevention infection control guidelines (AFCNA, 2018; Etnyre et al., 2011; Ratcliffe, 2017).

Due to concerns regarding aerosolization of organisms, many foot care nurses elect not to use a grinder and use alternative methods for thinning hypertrophic nails. One approach is to apply a 2 × 2 gauze or cotton ball soaked with mineral oil, warm water, or saline to the nail for 5 minutes to soften the nail and then to reduce the nail with a nipper (cutting from top down), followed by filing with a coarse grain emery board. The nail should not be trimmed until it has been adequately thinned and the free nail border has been established. The nail should be trimmed in a side-to-side fashion, and the general rule of thumb is to follow the contours of the nail and toe. The foot care nurse should be careful to trim only the nail beyond the free nail border. The nail should always be filed after trimming to eliminate sharp edges that may cause trauma or predispose the toe to an ingrown nail. Hands on clinical experience in a supervised setting may be helpful in gaining comfort with these skills (Beuscher et al., 2019).

KEY POINT

The nail should not be trimmed until it has been adequately thinned and the free nail border has been established. The nail should be filed after trimming to eliminate sharp edges.

MANAGEMENT OF HYPERTROPHIC SKIN AND CUTICLES

Excessive skin around the nail should be trimmed with caution. It is safer to file rough skin with an emery board or to remove excess skin with a rasper or scalpel. A pterygium blade is an acceptable and safe instrument for reduction of overgrown cuticles. Cuticles should be manipulated with caution, and the foot care nurse should avoid pushing the cuticles back or clipping the skin around the cuticles, as injury to the cuticles increases the risk for bacterial invasion and infection.

MANAGEMENT OF CORNS AND CALLUSES

Corns or calluses should be carefully pared or filed from "top down" using a rasper, scalpel, or file. Some individuals experience acute tenderness if the callus or corn is completely removed. When caring for a patient with corns or calluses, the foot care nurse must determine the source of friction. The patient with plantar surface calluses should be referred to an orthotist for off-loading insoles and may benefit from a protective dressing. The patient with corns needs to be educated regarding the need for a wider and deeper toe box and to use a protective toe sleeve, mole skin, corn pad, or lambswool.

EQUIPMENT AND POLICIES/PROCEDURES

Having the right equipment and established policies and procedures for foot and nail care are important (**Box 28-3**). Nippers, clippers, curettes, orange sticks, pterygium blades, files of a variety of coarseness, and nail raspers are commonly used tools. A list of commonly used pieces of equipment, supplies, and tools is provided in **Box 28-4** and illustrated in **Figure 28-15**. Infection control is important for protection of both the provider and recipient of foot care. Tools and equipment must be effectively disinfected using cold disinfection protocols, disinfecting solutions, steam, or autoclave (**Box 28-5**). It is important for the foot care nurse to use appropriate personal protective equipment (PPE), including mask, gown, gloves, and eye protection. Disinfecting surfaces with appropriate medical grade wipes, sterilizing or disinfecting equipment using approved methods, regular use of sanitizing gel, and handwashing are all important for reducing the risk of cross-contamination.

KEY POINT

Infection control measures are essential for protection of both the provider and recipient of foot care.

 ## EDUCATION, PREVENTION, AND ROUTINE MANAGEMENT

Education and referrals are elements of the foot care nurse role. Patients and caregivers should be taught the basics of foot care, signs and symptoms that require follow-up, and the importance of appropriate footwear and activity (Adiewere et al., 2018). Van Netten et al. (2020) conducted a systematic review regarding six interven-

---

BOX 28-3   YOUR INSTITUTIONAL OR COMPANY NAME

Nursing Practice Manual

Guidelines for Foot and Nail Care to Include Hygiene, Assessment, and Intervention (HAI)

The care of the hands/feet and finger/toenails is part of daily personal hygiene. Assessment of the lower extremity helps in detection of infection, wounds, nail/skin integrity issues, and/or other complications associated with overall health.

Purpose

To guide the practice of certified foot and nail care nurses (CFCNs) who, within their scope of practice and specialty training, incorporate foot and nail care to meet nursing and patient goals of health-promotion, patient education, health risk reduction, and promotion of comfort and safety.

CFCNs provide foot and nail care based on theoretical knowledge of:

1. Anatomy and physiology of the lower extremity
2. Structure and function of the feet and nails
3. Common pathology of the foot and related nursing interventions
4. Normal aging-related changes of the feet and hands

5. Abnormal changes of the feet and hands due to underlying conditions or life style behaviors
6. Lower extremity assessment to include peripheral neuropathy, perfusion, dermatologic conditions, and musculoskeletal deformities
7. Use of nail care instruments
8. Universal precautions and instrument disinfection

Equipment/Supplies

1. Nail and cuticle clipper and nipper
2. Rasper, curettes, and nail files/emery boards
3. Wash cloths and towels
4. Monofilament and Doppler
5. Skin care products, for example, pH balanced cleanser, moisturizer, antifungal powder

Precautions

1. A lower extremity assessment will be conducted specifically for peripheral neuropathy and perfusion prior to intervention.
2. Individuals with diabetes, peripheral vascular disease (PVD), or thickened or otherwise abnormal toenails may be referred to a DPM, PCP, and/or vascular surgeon.

STEPS	KEY POINTS
1. Wash the hands before and after the procedure	1. Standard universal precaution
2. Explain the procedure to the patient	2. Relieve patient anxiety and use as an opportunity to educate
3. Apply nonsterile gloves	3. Universal precautions
4. Provide hand/foot hygiene	4. Basic personal hygiene
5. Dry thoroughly, especially between the toes	5. Moisture between the toes can lead to maceration, irritation, and increased susceptibility to fungus
6. Debride nails—reduce length and height (you may refer to Medicare Codes here for Foot and Nail Care)	6. Nails should extend slightly beyond the end of the fingers or toes. Debride nails according to the shape of the finger or toe
7. Smooth rough edges with a nail file or emery board	7. To prevent further injury
8. Reduce hyperkeratotic lesions with rasper or file	8. Helps to reduce increasing pressure, shear, or friction and possible wound or lesion
9. Apply moisturizer to the feet and hands, may apply antifungal powder to web spaces	9. Keep the skin moist, web spaces dry—reduce maceration
10. Educate and refer as needed for proper foot and nail care for individuals with personal hygiene problems, diabetes, peripheral neuropathy, and vascular disease	10. Use adult learning principles with simple to complex concepts and continuous reinforced instruction and praise

APPROVED BY:	REVIEWED:
EFFECTIVE DATE:	
SUPERSEDES:	
PREPARED BY:	

References:
American Diabetes Association. (2019). 11. Microvascular complications and foot care: Standards of medical care in diabetes-2019. *Diabetes Care, 42*(Suppl 1), S124–S138. Retrieved from https://doi.org/10.2337/dc19-S011
Chan, H., Lee, D., Leung, E., et al. (2012). The effects of a foot and toenail care protocol for older adults. *Geriatric Nursing, 33*(6), 1–9.
Lippincott Procedures. (2019). Procedure for nail care. Retrieved from https://procedures.lww.com/lnp/view.do?pId=3719139&hits=care,nail,nails&a=false&ad=false

---

tions to treat modifiable risk factors for diabetic foot ulceration (i.e., patient education, health care provider education, self-management, preulcer treatment, orthotic interventions, and foot- and mobility-related exercises). They found low quality of evidence for the effectiveness of interventions targeting modifiable risk factors for ulceration in at-risk patients with diabetes. They concluded that structured education may improve behavior of both patients and health care professionals, that callus removal and therapeutic footwear may be effective in reducing mechanical pressure, and that foot- and mobility-related exercises may improve neuropathy symptoms and foot and ankle joint range of motion (Van Netten et al., 2020). Patients should be referred to an orthotist or pedorthist for properly fitted footwear and insoles if indicated (Malemute et al., 2011; Robinson et al., 2015).

BOX 28-4   FOOT AND NAIL CARE EQUIPMENT, SUPPLIES, TOOLS, AND ACCESSORIES

- Basin or no-rinse disposable cloths
- Heavy-duty car wash paper towels
- Nail nippers (4.5- to 5.5-inch spring barrel type)
- Pterygium blade
- Emery boards or files
- Orange sticks
- Curettes—small for dental and nails
- Emollients
- Gloves
- Gauze pads—for flossing toes
- Goggles, gown, mask (refer to institutional policy regarding safety and infection control)
- Disinfectant solution—dimethyl benzyl ammonium chloride—Barbicide/Marvicide—fungicide, bactericide, germicide
- Alcohol prep pads
- Bleach
- Tea tree—antibacterial, antifungal
- Vapor rub
- Variety of corn, callus, toe pads, lambswool for accommodating deformities, etc.
- Instruments for lower extremity assessment—blood pressure cuff, Doppler, Semmes-Weinstein monofilament, tape measure, tuning fork, Plexor

BOX 28-5   DISINFECTION OF FOOT AND NAIL EQUIPMENT

CDC.GOV Guidelines for Sterilization and Disinfecting of Foot and Nail Care Instruments

A. Heat sterilization, including steam or hot air (see manufacturer's recommendations, steam sterilization processing time from 3 to 30 minutes).
B. Glutaraldehyde-based formulations (>2% glutaraldehyde, caution should be exercised with all glutaraldehyde formulations when further in-use dilution is anticipated); glutaraldehyde (1.12%) and 1.93% phenol/phenate. One glutaraldehyde-based product has a high-level disinfection claim of 5 minutes at 35°C.
C. Hydrogen peroxide 7.5% (will corrode copper, zinc, and brass).
D. Hypochlorite, single-use chlorine generated on-site by electrolyzing saline containing >650 to 675 active free chlorine (will corrode metal instruments).
E. Sodium hypochlorite (5.25% to 6.15% household bleach diluted 1:500 provides >100 ppm available chlorine).
F. Phenolic germicidal detergent solution (follow product label for use—dilution).
G. Iodophor germicidal detergent solution (follow product label for use—dilution).

Disinfecting solutions commonly used are Barbicide and Marvicide.

Instruments must be cleaned and disinfected between clients.

From Centers for Disease Control and Prevention at www.cdc.gov

KEY POINT

Walking and other exercise, with or without the use of mobility aids, is important to maintenance of strength, endurance, and independence in activities of daily living.

FOLLOW-UP

Frequency of follow-up is based on the patient's risk status, as determined by the presence or absence of protective sensation and foot deformities, perfusion status, and presence or history of ulcerations or amputations. A base line assessment should be done at the point of entry into the foot care practice. The frequency of in-depth follow-up assessment is based on results of the initial assessment. The Lower Extremity Amputation Prevention (LEAP) program may assist in determining the frequency of follow-up. It prescribes a minimum of an annual foot screening, with patient education and appropriate footwear selection. Daily foot inspection by the patient and management of simple foot problems to prevent deterioration into more significant problems is also suggested (HRSA, 2019). If the individual is high risk, follow-up assessments should be done in 3 to 6 months; an individual at lower risk requires in-depth assessment less frequently (e.g., annually). Limited assessment (to include pulse palpation, inspection for dependent rubor, and inspection of the feet, web spaces, and nails) is performed at each visit. The objective is to monitor the patient closely to identify an injury that could lead to a wound, especially a nonhealing wound due to LEAD or LEND. The foot care nurse should be attentive in assessing individuals over 50 years of age with a history of cardiovascular disease; those over 60 years of age with a history of smoking, cardiovascular disease, or diabetes; and all individuals over 70 years of age (these populations represent individuals at high risk for compromised blood flow or LOPS) (WOCN, 2012). See Chapter 26 for additional information about LEND.

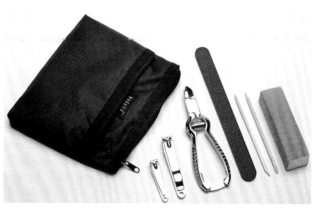

FIGURE 28-15. Foot Care Tools.

OFF-LOADING AND PADDING

Off-loading and padding are important for people with diabetes, over the age of 70, with arthritis, and with foot deformities, calluses, or wounds (Armstrong et al., 2014; Caselli, 2011; Cheskin, 2013). Reduction in plantar surface pressures may be achieved with orthotics, moleskin or pads, or total contact casting (Bus & van Netten, 2016; Bus et al., 2016a, 2016b; Rizzo et al., 2012). Total contact casting is limited to treatment of plantar ulcers and Charcot deformity and is not used for prevention. Patients with significant callus formation or deformities should be referred to an orthotist or pedorthist for construction of custom-molded toe lifts (for patients with hammer toes) or customized insoles for plantar calluses or pressure points (Lavery et al., 2012).

ROUTINE FOOT CARE

Routine foot care includes hygiene, skin care, and nail care. Hygiene should be conducted daily, less often may be appropriate for older individuals or those with dry skin. The patient should be taught to gently lather a cleanser on the skin of the feet and between the toes, to use a cloth to reduce hyperkeratotic lesions and cuticle overgrowth around the nails, and to rinse the feet well prior to drying them. The foot care nurse should emphasize the importance of special attention to web spaces, heels, and cuticles, especially for older patients and those with diabetes, who are at high risk for dry skin (Terrie, 2013; Woodbury et al., 2013). Patients should be taught to moisturize the feet with a small amount of a gentle fragrance-free cream or lotion but to avoid putting cream between the toes. If the web spaces tend to be moist, the foot care nurse should consider recommending use of an over-the-counter antifungal powder, such as miconazole. Remove excess powder between the toes to prevent caking. Patients with calluses or corns should be taught to use a pumice stone to those areas after bathing (Chan et al., 2012). Nail care between provider visits includes use of a file or emery board to smooth the nail edges and observation for injury, ingrown nails, or signs of paronychia (infection in or around the nail).

FOOTWEAR AND FOOT INSPECTION

Proper therapeutic footwear and daily foot inspection are two important interventions in preventing injuries that lead to wounds, pain, and amputations (HRSA, 2019). Additional resources are available at https://www.medicare.gov/coverage/therapeutic-shoes-inserts. Medicare has defined a therapeutic shoe as one that is long enough, wide enough, and high enough to accommodate the foot and any deformities, that has a rubber nonskid sole, and that can be secured with laces or a hook and latch closure (Cheskin, 2013; Schaum, 2018). Since 2005, Medicare coverage has included therapeutic footwear for beneficiaries with diabetes and one other related complication (such as LOPS, compromised blood flow, foot deformity, prior ulcer, or amputation) (Cheskin, 2013). Unfortunately, only 9% of the beneficiaries have taken advantage of this benefit; barriers include lack of awareness of the benefit; difficulty in obtaining the prescription; the time required for fitting, ordering, and refitting the shoes and inserts; and challenges in obtaining reimbursement (Burdette-Taylor, 2015; Janisse, 2013). Footwear should be customized or fit to the individual needs including foot shape and off-loading of high-pressure areas on the plantar surface. Shoes should be worn whenever walking (Bus et al., 2016a, 2016b). In addition to consistent use of therapeutic shoes, the foot care nurse must teach the patient the importance of daily foot inspection to assure that there are no signs of injury or inflammation (HRSA, 2019;

KEY POINT

Proper therapeutic footwear and daily foot inspection are two important interventions in preventing injuries that lead to wounds, pain, and amputations.

Woodbury et al., 2013).

It is common for a person's feet to differ in size; the foot care nurse should teach the patient to purchase shoes based on size of the larger foot (Cheskin, 2013). The patient should be taught to break in new shoes gradually, for example, to increase wear time by 2 hours each day and to inspect the feet carefully for any indicators of pressure or trauma. It is important to instruct patients to wear shoes with socks of appropriate thickness. When shopping for shoes, the patient should wear the socks that they will routinely wear with the shoes and shop at the end of the day when pedal edema is likely to be present (Kimmel & Robin, 2013; WOCN, 2012).

COMPRESSION SOCKS OR STOCKINGS

Patients who have mild edema or lower leg discomfort may be taught to wear light over-the-counter (OTC) graduated compression stockings. The level of compression should be determined by the severity of the edema and the underlying venous insufficiency (Rosales-Velderrain et al., 2013). Light OTC graduated compression socks begin at 12 to 16 mm Hg. Patients with limited edema may obtain satisfactory results with this level or may require socks or stockings with 15 to 20 mm Hg. If light compression stockings do not control the edema, referral for vascular assessment should be considered. Individuals with significant edema due to LEVD typically require at least 20 to 30 mm Hg and may require 30 to 40 mm Hg compression (Clarke-Moloney et al., 2012; Farrow, 2010; WOCN, 2019). Edema and lymphedema are common lower extremity conditions that interfere with activities of daily living and comfort; these conditions also increase the risk for ulceration and impaired healing. See Chapter 24 for additional information about LEVD.

WALKING AND EXERCISE

Walking and other exercise is important to maintain strength, endurance, and independence in activities of daily living (WOCN, 2012, 2014, 2019). Use of mobility aids may be indicated for safe ambulation, and a referral to physical therapy may be indicated to ensure that the individual is using the mobility device correctly (Nagai et al., 2011; Tofthagen et al., 2012). There are various types of exercises that can be incorporated into activities of daily living for improved mobility and quality of life. Activities that enhance endurance, strength, balance, and flexibility are recommended for older patients and those with diabetes. The foot care nurse should be aware that inactivity is a contributing factor to disease. Walking is associated with reduced falls, increased self-esteem, improved posture and balance, and socialization. In a systematic review, Van Netten et al. (2020) found that foot- and mobility-related exercises may improve neuropathy symptoms and foot and ankle joint range of motion. Walking on a regular basis is also associated with weight maintenance and stronger muscles and bones (Kreider et al., 2011; Neville et al., 2020; Taylor, 2014).

Crews et al. (2016) assessed the feasibility of objectively, synchronously, and continuously monitoring physical activity and its location in individuals at-risk and with active DFU. Five at-risk and five active DFU patients were monitored continuously for 72 hours with physical activity and GPS monitors. Active DFU patients' total time (walking, standing, sitting, and lying) away-from-home was only 7.7% (5.5 hours) of 72 hours monitored in contrast to 20.5% (14.8 hours) for at-risk participants. The foot care nurse should encourage patients to incorporate exercise into their daily activities and should consider suggesting that the patient use an exercise tracker to measure activity each day. Tracking exercise is an objective method of helping patients to see results and motivate them to continue (Huebschmann et al., 2011).

KEY POINT

Frequency of follow-up is individualized based on the patient's risk status, which is determined by the presence or absence of protective sensation and foot deformities, perfusion status, and presence or history of ulcerations or amputations.

SMOKING CESSATION

Smoking significantly increases the risk of LEAD and amputation. Smoking cessation is important for healthy feet and prevention of LEAD (Bonham et al., 2016). It constricts the blood vessels throughout the body, causes arterial damage and thickening of the vessel walls, and increases the cardiac workload. The foot care nurse should educate patients regarding the deleterious effects of smoking. Patients committed to smoking cessation may be referred to a comprehensive smoking cessation program.

GLYCEMIC CONTROL

Foot care nurses may play a role in helping patients to manage their diabetes by encouraging and motivating them to adhere to management protocols (Hamdy & Colberg, 2014). Use of adult learning principles, motivational strategies, and a client-centered approach increases the chances that the nurse will be able to assist the client to achieve a higher level of health (Gravely et al., 2011).

 ## MULTIDISCIPLINARY TEAMS

Improved patient outcomes will require a multidisciplinary approach, a commitment to evidence-based practice, and education for all involved. Multidisciplinary teams that include surgeons, nurses, podiatrists, pedorthists, orthotists, diabetes educators, wound and foot care nurses, and dietitians should participate in the development of evidence-based policies, protocols, and algorithms (Musuuza et al., 2019). The foot care nurse plays an important role in the assessment and management of feet.

 ## CONCLUSION

Foot and nail care is an important element of an LEAP program. Foot care nurses are prepared to provide ongoing monitoring of vascular status, sensorimotor status, and foot and nail issues. They provide preventive care, education, and referrals to optimize perfusion and prevent limb loss. Foot care nurses identify common foot and nail pathology, trim hypertrophic nails, pare corns and calluses, and provide referrals for appropriate footwear and foot care.

REFERENCES

Aalaa, M., Malazy, O. T., Sanjari, M., et al. (2012). Nurses' role in diabetic foot prevention and care; a review. *Journal of Diabetes and Metabolic Disorders, 11*(24), 1–6.

Abhishek, A., & Doherty, M. (2018). Education and non-pharmacological approaches for gout. *Rheumatology, 57*, i51–i58.

Adiewere, P., Gillis, R. B., Jiwani, S. I., et al. (2018). A systematic review and meta-analysis of patient education in preventing and reducing the incidence or recurrence of adult diabetes foot ulcers (DFU). *Heliyon, 4*(5), e00614.

AFCNA. (2018). Instrument Disinfection for Foot Care. Retrieved April 5, 2020, from https://footcarenursing.com/2018/12/19/best-practice-guidelines/

Alvarsson, A., Sandgren, B., Wendel, C., et al. (2012). A retrospective analysis of amputation rates in diabetic patients: Can lower extremity amputations be further prevented? *Cardiovascular Diabetology, 11*(18), 1–11.

Amaeshi, I. J. (2012). Exploring the impact of structured foot health education on the rate of lower extremity amputation in adults with type 2 diabetes. A systematic review. *Diabetic Foot Journal (Clinical Review), 15*, 1–8.

Armstrong, D., Adam, I., Bevilacqua, N. J., et al. (2014). Offloading foot wounds in people with diabetes. *Wounds, 26*(1), 13–20.

Atkins, C. (2010). Evidence-based foot care in patients with diabetes. *Lower Extremity Review Magazine.* Retrieved March 5, 2012, from www.lowerextremityreview.com

Barshes, N. R., Sigireddi, M., Wrobel, J. S., et al. (2013). The system of care for the diabetic foot: Objectives, outcomes, and opportunities. *Diabetic Foot and Ankle, 4,* 21847. doi: 10.3402/dfa.v4iO.21847.

Benavent-Caballer, V., Sendín-Magdalena, A., Lisón, J. F., et al. (2016). Physical factors underlying the Timed "Up and Go" test in older adults. *Geriatric Nursing, 37*(2), 122–127.

Beuscher, T. L. (2019). Guidelines for diabetic foot care: A template for the care of all feet. *Journal of Wound Ostomy Continence Nursing, 46*(3), 241–245.

Beuscher, T. L., & Kelechi, T. (2019). Onychomycosis: Diagnosis, treatment, and prevention. *Journal of Wound Ostomy Continence Nursing, 46*(4), 333–335.

Beuscher, T. L., Moe H. L., Stolder, M. E., et al. (2019). Expanding a foot care education program for nurses. *Journal of Wound Ostomy Continence Nursing, 46*(5), 441–445.

Bonham, P. A., Flemister, B. G., Droste, L. R., et al. (2016). 2014 guideline for management of wounds in patients with lower-extremity arterial disease (LEAD): An executive summary. *Journal of Wound Ostomy Continence Nursing, 43*(1), 23–31.

Boulton, A. J. M. (2013). The pathway to foot ulceration in diabetes. *Medical Clinic of North America, 97,* 775–790.

Brechow, A., Slesaczeck, T., Münch, D., et al. (2013). Improving major amputation rates in the multicomplex diabetic foot patient: Focus on the severity of peripheral arterial disease. *Therapeutic Advances in Endocrinology and Metabolism, 4*(3), 83–94.

Bristow, I. R., de Berker, D. A., Acland, K. M., et al. (2010). Clinical guidelines for the recognition of melanoma of the foot and nail unit. *Journal of Foot and Ankle Research, 3*(1), 25.

Burdette-Taylor, M. S. (2015). Prevent wounds by conducting a comprehensive foot examination and intervention. *Healthcare, 3*(3), 586–592.

Burland, P. (2012). Vascular disease and foot assessment in diabetes. *Practice Nursing, 23*(4), 187–193.

Bus, S. A., van Deursen, R. W., Armstrong, D. G., et al. (2016a). Footwear and offloading interventions to prevent and heal foot ulcers and reduce plantar pressure in patients with diabetes: A systematic review. *Diabetes Metabolism Research and Reviews, 32*(S1), 99–118.

Bus, S. A., & van Netten, J. J. (2016). A shift in priority in diabetic foot care and research: 75% of foot ulcers are preventable. *Diabetes Metabolism Research and Reviews, 32*(Suppl 1), 195–200.

Bus, S. A., van Netten, J. J., Laverty, L. A., et al. (2016b). IWGDF guidance on the prevention of foot ulcers in at-risk *patients with diabetes. Diabetes Metabolism Research and Reviews, 32*(Suppl 1), 16–24.

Caselli, M. A. (October, 2011). Prescription shoes for foot pathology. *Podiatry Management,* 165–178.

Chan, H. Y., Lee, D. T., Leung, E. M., et al. (2012). The effects of a foot and toenail care protocol for older adults. *Geriatric Nursing, 33*(6), 446–453.

Cheskin, M. (2013). Sizing up footwear. *Podiatry Management, 32*(8), 109–118.

Christman, A. L., Selvin, E., Margolis, D. J., et al. (2011). Hemoglobin A1c is a predictor of healing rate in diabetic wounds. *Journal of Investigational Dermatology, 131,* 2121–2137.

Clarke-Moloney, M., Keane, N., O'Connor, V., et al. (2012). Randomized controlled trial comparing European standard class 1 to class 2 compression stockings for ulcer recurrence and patient compliance. *International Wound Journal, 11,* 404–408.

Crawford, P. E., & Fields-Varnado, M. (2013). Guideline for the management of wounds in patients with lower-extremity neuropathic disease: an executive summary. *Journal of Wound, Ostomy, and Continence Nursing, 40*(1), 34–45.

Crews, R., Yalla, S., Dhatt, N., et al. (2016). Monitoring location specific physical activity via integration of accelerometry and geotechnology. *Foot and Ankle Surgery, 2*(22), 111–112.

Elewski, B. E., & Tosti, A. (2014). Tavaborole for the treatment of onychomycosis. *Expert Opinion on Pharmacotherapy, 15*(10), 1439–1448.

Ellefson, L. L., Thompson, L. L., & Trelease, J. (2016). Update on eligibility for the foot care examination. *Journal of Wound Ostomy Continence Nursing, 43*(1), 88–90.

Erwin, B. L., Styke, L. T., & Kyle, J. A. (2013). Fungus of the feet and nails. *US Pharmacist, 38*(6), 51–54.

Etnyre, A., Zarate-Abbott, P., Roehrick, L., et al. (2011). The role of certified foot and nail care nurses in prevention of lower extremity amputation. *Journal of Wound Ostomy Continence Nursing, 38*(3), 1–10.

Farrow, W. (2010). Phlebolymphedema—A common underdiagnosed and undertreated problem in the wound care clinic. *Journal of the American College of Certified Wound Specialists, 2,* 14–23.

Fujiwara, Y., Kishida, K., Terao, M., et al. (2011). Beneficial effects of foot care nursing for people with diabetes mellitus: An uncontrolled before and after intervention study. *Journal of Advanced Nursing, 67*(9), 1952–1962.

Gallagher, D. (2012). The certified foot care nurse and the importance of comprehensive foot assessments. *Journal of Wound Ostomy Continence Nursing, 39*(2), 194–196.

Game, F. (2012). Choosing life or limb: Improving survival in the multi complex diabetic foot patient. *Diabetes/Metabolism Research Reviews, 28*(Suppl 1), 97–100.

Game, R., & Jeffcoate, W. (2013). The Charcot foot: Neuropathic osteoarthropathy. *Advances in Skin and Wound Care, 26*(9), 421–428.

Gazes, M. I., & Zeichner, J. (2013). Onychomycosis in close quarter living: Review of the literature. *Mycoses, 56*(6), 610–613.

Geiss, L. S., Li, Y., Hora, I., et al. (2019). Resurgence of diabetes-related nontraumatic lower-extremity amputation in the young and middle-aged adult U.S. population. *Diabetes Care, 42*(1), 50–54. doi: 10.2337/dc18-1380.

Geizhals, S., & Lipner, S. R. (2019). Review of onychocryptosis: Epidemiology, pathogenesis, risk factors, diagnosis and treatment. *Dermatology Online Journal, 25*(9), 1.

Golchin, N., Frank, S. H., Vince, A., et al. (2015). Polypharmacy in the elderly. *Journal of Research in Pharmacy Practice, 4*(2), 85–88.

Graham, A. S., Stephenson, J., & Williams, A. E. (2017). A survey of people with foot problems related to rheumatoid arthritis and their educational needs. *Journal of Foot and Ankle Research, 10,* 12. doi: 10.1186/s13047-0193-6.

Gravely, S. S., Hensley, B. K., & Hagood-Thompson, C. (2011). Comparison of three types of diabetic foot ulcer education plans to determine patient recall of education. *Journal of Vascular Nursing, 29*(3), 1–8.

Gupta, A. K., Drummond-Main, C., Cooper, E. A., et al. (2011). Systematic review of nondermatophyte mold onychomycosis: Diagnosis, clinical types, epidemiology, and treatment. *American Academy of Dermatology, 66*(3), 494–502.

Hamdy, O., & Colberg, S. (2014). 10 keys to long-term weight loss for adults with diabetes. *Diabetes Self-Management, 31,* 64–67.

Harding, J. L., Pavkov, M. E., Gregg, E. W., et al. (2019). Trends of Nontraumatic Lower-Extremity Amputation in End-stage renal disease and diabetes: United States, 2000–2015. *Diabetes Care, 42*(8), 1430–1435.

Hawke, F., & Burns, J. (2012). Brief report: Custom foot orthoses for foot pain: what does the evidence say? *Foot & Ankle International, 33*(12), 1161–1163.

Health Resources & Services Administration (HRSA). (2019). Lower extremity amputation prevention (LEAP). Retrieved March 21, 2020, from https://www.hrsa.gov/hansens-disease/leap

Huebschmann, A. G., Crane, L. A., Belansky, E. S., et al. (2011). Fear of injury with physical activity is greater in adults with diabetes than in adults without diabetes. *Diabetes Care, 34*(8), 1717–1722.

International Association for the Study of Pain (IASP). (2019). IASP's Proposed New Definition of Pain Released for Comment. Retrieved from IASP-pain.org/Publications/NewsDetail.aspx?ItemNumber=9218. Accessed December 1, 2019.

Janisse, D. (2013). Understanding and accessing Medicare's therapeutic shoes for persons with diabetes benefit. *AADE In Practice, 1*(4), 33–35.

Johnson, S. R., & Taylor, M. A. (2012). Identification and management of malignant skin lesions among older adults. *Journal of Nurse Practitioners, 6*(8), 1–8.

Jones, N. J., Chess, J., Cawley, S., et al. (2013). Prevalence of risk factors for foot ulceration in a general haemodialysis population. *International Wound Journal, 10*(6), 683–688. doi: 10.1111/j.1742-481X.2012.01044.x.

Kelechi, T. J., & Johnson, J. J. (2012). Guideline for the management of wounds in patients with lower extremity venous disease. *Journal of Wound Ostomy Continence Nursing, 39*(6), 598–606.

Khan, T., Shin, L., Woelfel, S., et al. (2018). Building a scalable diabetic limb preservation program: four steps to success. *Diabetic Foot & Ankle, 9*(1), 1452513.

Kimmel, H. M., & Robin, A. L. (2013). An evidence-based algorithm for treating venous leg ulcers utilizing the Cochrane database of systematic reviews. *Wounds, 25*(9), 242–250.

Ko, D., & Lipner, S. (2018). Onychogryphosis: Case report and review of the literature. *Skin Appendage Disorders, 4*, 326–330.

Kohlman-Trigoboff, D. (2013). Management of lower extremity peripheral arterial disease interpreting the latest guidelines for nurse practitioners. *Journal of Nurse Practitioners, 9*(10), 653–668.

Kreider, R. B., Serra, M., Beavers, K. M., et al. (2011). A structured diet and exercise program promotes favorable changes in weight loss, body composition, and weight maintenance. *Journal of American Dietetic Association, 111*(6), 828–843.

Lavery, L. A., La Fontaine, J., Higgins, K. R., et al. (2012). Shear-reducing insoles to prevent ulceration in high-risk diabetic patients. *Advances in Skin & Wound Care, 25*(11), 519–524.

Lavery, L. A., La Fontaine, J., & Kim, P. J. (2013). Preventing the first or recurrent ulcers. *Medical Clinics of North America, 97*, 807–820.

Lipsky, B. A., Berendt, A. R., Cornia, P. B., et al. (2012). 2012 Infectious Diseases Society of America clinical practice guideline for the diagnosis and treatment of diabetic foot infections. *Clinical Infectious Diseases, 54*(12), e132–e173.

Lipner, S. R., & Scher, R. K. (2019). Onychomycosis: Treatment and prevention of recurrence. *Journal of the American Academy of Dermatology, 80*(4), 853–867.

Lippincott Procedures. (2019). Procedure for Nail Care. Retrieved April 5, 2020, from https://procedures-lww-com.proxy.lib.duke.edu/lnp/view.do?pId=3181250&hits=nails,foot&a=true&ad=false.

Madan, S. S., & Pai, D. R. (2013). Charcot neuroarthropathy of the foot and ankle. *Orthopaedic Surgery, 5*, 86–93.

Malemute, C. L., Shultz, J. A., Ballejos, M., et al. (2011). Goal setting education and counseling practices of diabetes educators. *The Diabetes Educator, 37*(4), 549–563.

Malhotra, K., Davda, K., & Singh, D. (2016). The pathology and management of lesser toe deformities. *EFORT Open Reviews, 1*(11), 409–419.

Matthews, B. G., Hurn, S. E., Harding, M. P., et al. (2019). The effectiveness of non-surgical interventions for common plantar digital compressive neuropathy (Morton's neuroma): A systematic review and meta-analysis. *Journal of Foot and Ankle Research, 12*, 12. doi: 10.1186/s13047-019-0320-7.

Mayeaux, E. J., Carter, C., & Murphy, T. E. (2019). Ingrown toenail management. *American Family Physician, 100*(3), 158–164.

McDonald, S., Sharpe, L., & Blaszczynski, A. (2014). The psychosocial impact associated with diabetes-related amputation. *Diabetic Medicine, 31*(11), 1424–1430. doi: 10.1111/dme.12474.

Menz, H. B., Auhl, M., & Spink, M. J. (2018). Foot problems as a risk factor for falls in community-dwelling older people: A systematic review and meta-analysis. *Maturitas, 118*, 7–14. doi: 10.1016/j.maturitas.2018.10.001.

Mills, J. L., Sr., Conte, M. S., Armstrong, D. G., et al., & Society for Vascular Surgery Lower Extremity Guidelines Committee. (2014). The Society for Vascular Surgery lower extremity threatened limb classification system: risk stratification based on wound, ischemia, and foot infection (WIfI). *Journal of Vascular Surgery, 59*(1), 220–234.

Milne, T. E., Rogers, J. R., Kinnear, E. M., et al. (2013). Developing an evidence-based clinical pathway for the assessment, diagnosis and management of acute Charcot Neuro-Arthropathy: A systematic review. *Journal of Foot and Ankle Research, 6*(1), 30.

Moakes, H. (2012). An overview of foot ulceration in older people with diabetes. *Nursing Older People, 24*(7), 14–19.

Muirhead, L., Roberson, A. J., & Secrest, J. (2011). Utilization of foot care services among homeless adults: Implications for advanced practice nurses. *Journal of American Academy of Nurse Practitioners, 23*, 209–215.

Murphy, B., & Dolan, O. (2018). Avoiding delay in diagnosing melanoma of the foot. *InnovAiT: Education and Inspiration for General Practice, 11*(3), 133–137.

Musuuza, J., Sutherland, B. L., Kurter, S., et al. (2019). A systematic review of multidisciplinary teams to reduce major amputations for patients with diabetic foot ulcers. *Journal of Vascular Surgery, 71*(4), 1433–1446. doi: 10.1016/j.jvs.2019.08.244.

Nagai, K., Inoue, T., Yamada, Y., et al. (2011). Effects of toe and ankle training in older people: A cross-over study. *Geriatrics & Gerontology International, 11*, 246–255.

Nevares-Pomales, O. W., Sarriera-Lazaro, C. J., Battera-Llaurador, J., et al. (2018). Pigmented lesions of the nail unit. *American Journal of Dermatopathology, 40*(11), 793–804.

Neville, C., Nguyen, H., Ross, K., et al. (2020). Lower-limb factors associated with balance and falls in older adults: A systematic review and clinical synthesis. *Journal of the American Podiatric Medical Association, 110*(5), 1–29. doi: 10.7547/19-143.

Osoba, M. Y., Rao, A. K., Agrawal, S. K., et al. (2019). Balance and gait in the elderly: A contemporary review. *Laryngoscope Investigative Otolaryngology, 4*, 143–153. doi: 10.1002/lio2.252.

Ousey, K., Chadwick, P., Jawien, A., et al. (2018). Identifying and treating foot ulcers in patients with diabetes: saving feet, legs and lives. *Journal of Wound Care, 27*(5 Suppl 5b), S1–S51.

Paul, J. C., Pieper, B., & Templin, T. N. (2011). Itch: Association with chronic venous disease, pain, and quality of life. *Journal of Wound Ostomy Continence Nursing, 38*(1), 46–54.

Pariser, D., Scher, R. K., Elewski, B., et al. (2013). Promoting and maintaining or restoring healthy nails: Practical recommendations for clinicians and patients. *Seminars in Cutaneous Medicine and Surgery, 33*, 19–20.

Peraj, E., Subhani, M. R., Jeong, J., et al. (2019). Characteristics among adult patients with diabetes who received foot exam by a health care provider in the past year: An analysis of NHANES 2011–2016. *Primary Care Diabetes, 13*(3), 242–246.

Plucknette, B. F., Brogan, M. S., Anain, J. M., et al. (2012). Normative values for foot sensation: Challenging the 5.07 monofilament. *Journal of Diabetic Foot Complications, 4*(1), 16–25.

Pupp, G., & Kolvunen, R. (2011). Limb salvage and the Charcot foot: What the evidence shows. *Podiatry Today, 24*(3), 68–74.

Rasenberg, N., Riel, H., Rathleff, M. S., et al. (2018). Efficacy of foot orthoses for the treatment of plantar heel pain: A systematic review and meta-analysis. *British Journal Sports Medicine, 52*, 1040–1046.

Rasmussen, T. E., Clouse, W. D., & Tonnessen, B. H. (2019). *Handbook of patient care in vascular diseases*. Philadelphia, PA: Wolters Kluwer.

Ratcliffe, M. (2017). Nail dust and the use of personal protective equipment—face masks, a review. *Podiatry Review, 74*(1), 26+. Gale Academic OneFile. Accessed December 7, 2019.

Reich, A., & Szepietowski, J. C. (2011). Health-related quality of life in patients with nail disorders. *American Journal of Clinical Dermatology, 12*(5), 313–320.

Rice, J. B., Desal, U., & Cummings, A. K. (2014). Burden of DFUs for Medicare and private insurers. *Diabetes Care, 37*, 651–658.

Riskowki, J., Dufour, A. B., & Hannan, M. T. (2011). Arthritis, foot pain, and shoe wear: Current musculoskeletal research on feet. *Current Opinions in Rheumatology, 23*(2), 148–155.

Rizzo, L., Tedeschi, A., Fallani, E., et al. (2012). Custom-made orthesis and shoes in a structured follow-up program reduces the incidence of neuropathic ulcers in high-risk diabetic foot patients. *International Journal of Lower Extremity Wounds, 11*(1), 59–64.

Robinson, C., Major, M. J., Kuffel, C., et al. (2015). Orthotic management of the neuropathic foot: An interdisciplinary care perspective. *Prosthetics and Orthotics International, 39*(1), 73–81.

Rome, K., Stewart, S., Vandal, A. C., et al. (2013). The effects of commercially available footwear on foot pain and disability in people with gout. *BMC Musculoskeletal Disorders, 14*(278), 1–16.

Rosales-Velderrain, A., Padilla, M., Choe, C. H., et al. (2013). Increased microvascular flow and foot sensation with mild continuous external compression. *Physiological Reports, 1*(7), e00157.

Sacks, D. B., & John, W. G. (2014). Interpretation of hemoglobin A1c values. *JAMA, 311*(22), 2271–2272.

Schaper, N. C., Van Netten, J. J., Apelqvist, J., et al., & International Working Group on the Diabetic Foot. (2017). Prevention and management of foot problems in diabetes: A Summary Guidance for Daily Practice 2015, based on the IWGDF guidance documents. *Diabetes Research and Clinical Practice, 124*, 84–92.

Schaum, K. D. (2018). Orders and documentation are vital to diabetic shoe coverage. *Advances in Skin & Wound Care, 31*(2), 90–92.

Sheridan, S. (2012). The need for a comprehensive foot care model. *Nephrology Nursing Journal, 39*(5), 387–401.

Sibbald, R., Ayello, E., Alavi, A., et al. (2012). Screening for the high-risk diabetic foot: A 60-second tool. *Advances in Skin and Wound Care, 25*(10), 465–476.

Snyder, R. J., Kirsner, R. S., Warriner, R. A., et al. (2010). Consensus recommendations on advancing the standard of care for treating neuropathic foot ulcers in patients with diabetes. *Wounds, 56*(Suppl 4), S1–S24.

Sonal Sekhar, M., Unnikrishnan, M. K., Vijayanarayana, K., et al. (2019). Impact of patient-education on health-related quality of life of diabetic foot ulcer patients: A randomized study. *Clinical Epidemiology and Global Health, 7*(3), 382–388.

Steinberg, N., Gottlieb, A., Siev-Ner, I., et al. (2019). Fall incidence and associated risk factors among people with a lower limb amputation during various stages of recovery—a systematic review. *Disability and Rehabilitation, 41*(15), 1778–1787.

Takehara, K., Oe, M., Tsunemi, Y., et al. (2011). Factors associated with presence and severity of toenail onychomycosis in patients with diabetes: A cross-sectional study. *International Journal of Nursing Studies, 48*, 1101–1108.

Taylor, D. (2014). Physical activity is medicine for older adults. *Postgraduate Medical Journal, 90*, 26–32.

Temprano, K. K. (2016). A review of Raynaud's disease. *Missouri Medicine, 113*(2), 123–126.

Terrie, Y. C. (2013). Diabetic foot care: The importance of routine care. Retrieved December 5, 2013, from www.pharmacytimes.com/publications/issue/2013/October2013/diabetic-foot-care

To, M. J., Brothers, T. D., & Van Zoost, C. (2016). Foot conditions among homeless persons: A systematic review. *PLoS One, 11*(12), e0167463. doi: 10.1371/journal.pone.0167463.

Tofthagen, C., Visovsky, C., & Berry, D. L. (2012). Strength and balance training in adults with peripheral neuropathy and high risk of fall: Current evidence and implications for future research. *Oncology Nursing Forum, 39*(5), E416–E424.

van Netten, J. J., Sacco, I. C., Lavery, L. A., et al. (2020). Treatment of modifiable risk factors for foot ulceration in persons with diabetes: a systematic review. *Diabetes/Metabolism Research and Reviews, 36*, e3271. Retrieved April 5, 2020, from https://onlinelibrary.wiley.com/doi/epdf/10.1002/dmrr.3271

Vopat, M. L., Nentwig, M. J., Chong, A. C. M., et al. (2018). Initial diagnosis and management for acute Charcot neuroarthropathy. *Kansas Journal of Medicine, 11*(4), 114–119.

Weatherford, B. M. (2017). Diseases and conditions: Heel pain. *American Association of Orthopedic Surgeons.* Retrieved March 21, 2020, from https://orthoinfo.aaos.org/en/diseases--conditions/heel-pain/

Wellborn, J., & Moceri, J. T. (2014). The lived experiences of persons with chronic venous insufficiency and lower extremity ulcers. *Journal of Wound Ostomy & Continence Nursing, 41*(2), 122–126.

Westerberg, D. P., & Voyack, M. J. (2013). Onychomycosis: Current trends in diagnosis and treatment. *American Family Physician, 88*(11), 762–770.

Wexler, D. J. (2019). Patient education: Foot care in diabetes (Beyond the Basics), 1–13. *Up to Date.* Retrieved December 12, 2019, from www.uptodate.com

Woodbury, M. G., Botros, M., Kuhnke, J. L., et al. (2013). Evaluation of a peer-led self-management programme PEP talk: Diabetes, healthy feet and you. *International Wound Journal, 10*(6), 703–710.

Wound Ostomy Continence Nurses' Society (WOCN). (2012). *Guideline for management of wounds in patients with lower-extremity neuropathic disease.* WOCN Clinic Practice Guideline Series. Mt. Laurel, NJ: Author.

Wound Ostomy Continence Nurses' Society (WOCN). (2014). *Guideline for management of wounds in patients with lower-extremity arterial disease.* WOCN Clinic Practice Guideline Series. Mt. Laurel, NJ: Author.

Wound Ostomy Continence Nurses' Society (WOCN). (2019). *Guideline for management of wounds in patients with lower-extremity venous disease.* WOCN Clinic Practice Guideline Series. Mt. Laurel, NJ: Author.

Wu, S. F., Tung, H. H., Liang, S. Y., et al. (2014). Differences in perceptions of self-care, health education barriers, and educational needs between diabetes patients and nurses. *Contemporary Nurse, 46*(2), 187–196.

Young, C. (2012). Plantar fasciitis. *Annals of Internal Medicine, 156*(1 Pt 1), ITC1-1.

Zafren, K., & Mechem, C. C. (2018). Frostbite, 1–11. Retrieved December 12, 2019, from www.uptodate.com/contents/frostbite

Zhang, Y., Lazzarini, P. A., McPhail, S. M., et al. (2020). Global disability burdens of diabetes-related lower-extremity complications in 1990 and 2016. *Diabetes Care, 43*, 964–974. doi: 10.2337/dc19-1614.

Ziegler-Graham, K., MacKenzie, E. J., Ephraim, P. L., et al. (2008). Estimating the prevalence of limb loss in the United States: 2005 to 2050. *Archives of Physical Medicine and Rehabilitation, 89*(3), 422–429.

QUESTIONS

1. Onychocryptosis is a term that refers to which of the following conditions?
A. All types of toe pain.
B. A nail that has splintered and invaded the periungual space.
C. Oyster shell appearance of the nail.
D. Fungal infection of the nail.

2. A foot tracing can be used to
A. Ensure that the toe box is high enough to prevent pressure
B. Prevent overlapping toes
C. Purchase shoes for an individual who is homebound
D. Prevent Charcot foot

3. The foot care nurse assesses the toes of a patient and notes a toe with a contracture of the proximal interphalangeal joint. What condition would the nurse document?
A. Claw toe
B. Hammer toe
C. Bunion
D. Mallet toe

4. The hyponychium is
A. Skin adjacent to the lateral nail
B. Epithelium that lies directly beneath the nail plate
C. The reproductive layer of the nail bed
D. The junction between the free nail border and the adherent nail

5. Gout is a form of arthritis which is caused by
A. Traumatic injury
B. Over use of the joint
C. Accumulation of urate crystals
D. An autoimmune disorder

6. What is the most important factor in wearing new therapeutic footwear in preventing ulceration?
A. Appearance of the shoes
B. Alternating between therapeutic shoes and slippers
C. Amount of time shoes are worn
D. Proper use of assistive devices such as cane or walker

7. Hallux valgus is a condition referring to the
A. Lateral deviation of the big toe
B. Medial deviation of the big toe
C. Restriction of movement of the big toe during weight bearing
D. Big toe sticking straight up

8. The foot care nurse refers a patient with onychomycosis for treatment. The nurse counsels the patient regarding which side effect of oral antifungal therapy?
A. Elevated blood glucose levels
B. Liver toxicity
C. Irregular heartbeat
D. Osteoarthritis flair

9. Edema, hemosiderosis, and/or venous dermatitis are hallmark symptoms of which disorder?
A. LEAD
B. LEND
C. LEVD
D. Xerosis

10. Loss of protective sensation (LOPS) is determined with which instrument?
A. 128 Hz tuning fork
B. Semmes-Weinstein monofilament
C. Reflex hammer
D. Doppler

ANSWERS AND RATIONALES

1. B. Rationale: Onychocryptosis occurs when the lateral edge of the nail splinters and invades the periungual space, producing pain and reducing mobility and activity; the resulting inflammation at the site can lead to infection.

2. C. Rationale: A foot tracing allows a caregiver to purchase shoes for an individual who is homebound.

3. B. Rationale: A hammer toe is the contracture of the proximal interphalangeal joint, a mallet toe is the contracture of the distal interphalangeal joint, and a claw toe is the contracture of both the proximal and distal interphalangeal joints.

4. D. Rationale: The hyponychium is the junction between the free nail border (distal nail that is not attached to the nail bed) and the adherent nail (nail plate attached to the underlying epithelium). It is sometimes referred to as the "quick."

5. C. Rationale: Gout is caused by the accumulation of urate crystals in joints; this triggers an acute inflammatory response and severe pain.

6. C. Rationale: The patient should be taught to break in new shoes gradually, for example, to increase wear time by 2 hours each day and to inspect the feet carefully for any indicators of pressure or trauma.

7. A. Rationale: Hallux valgus is the deviation of the great toe away from midline, also known as bunion.

8. B. Rationale: Liver toxicity is a potential adverse effect of systemic antifungals, and it is necessary to monitor liver function at baseline and throughout treatment.

9. C. Rationale: Lower extremity venous disease (LEVD) is manifest by edema, hemosiderosis, and/or venous dermatitis.

10. B. Rationale: Sensory testing should be done using the Semmes-Weinstein 5.07 monofilament instrument, a nylon filament (fishing line) mounted on a holder and standardized to deliver 10 g of force when pressed against the skin with enough force to bend the monofilament into a C-shape.

CHAPTER 29

WOUNDS CAUSED BY INFECTIOUS PROCESSES

Sarah Wolfe

OBJECTIVES

1. Describe the presentation and management of the following microorganisms or infectious manifestations: herpes simplex; varicella-zoster; superficial fungal infections; deep fungal infections; impetigo; ecthyma; ecthyma gangrenosum; hidradenitis suppurativa; cellulitis; erysipelas; necrotizing fasciitis; folliculitis; and nontuberculous mycobacteria infection.

2. Identify indications and contraindications to wound cultures for the patient with cellulitis.

3. Explain the significance of prompt diagnosis of necrotizing fasciitis, and early indicators of the condition.

TOPIC OUTLINE

INTRODUCTION

Though infection is not commonly considered to be a major cause of wounds in the United States, with an aging population and rising numbers of individuals treated with immunosuppressive medications, the susceptibility for infection is rising. Common infections often present to primary care providers. Wound care nurses are expected to recognize when an infection is causing or contributing to persistence of a wound. All health care providers should be familiar with the various infectious pathogens of the skin, including their clinical manifestations and appropriate management options.

Many types of pathogens can contribute to wounds, including viral, fungal, bacterial, and mycobacterial microorganisms. Wounds caused by infectious processes vary in severity from minor, limited skin disease to ulcers and deep infection that can be life threatening. This chapter describes the majority of common infections that cause or contribute to wounds in the United States.

 VIRAL INFECTIONS CAUSING WOUNDS

The human herpesvirus family is composed of a group of eight viruses that cause an array of disease in humans. Following primary infection, these viruses become latent within cells, which means that they are a lifelong threat with the potential to reactivate and cause recurrent disease. These viruses include cytomegalovirus, which can cause congenital birth defects, gastrointestinal infection, and rare skin eruptions, the Epstein-Barr virus, which causes infectious mononucleosis, and human herpesvirus 8, which is implicated in the pathogenesis of Kaposi sarcoma. Two very common human herpesviruses, herpes simplex virus (HSV) and the varicella–zoster virus (VZV), can cause skin wounds consisting of vesicles, erosions, and ulcers and are discussed in greater detail here.

> **KEY POINT**
>
> Herpes viruses become latent within cells following primary infection, meaning they are a lifelong threat with the potential to cause recurrent disease on the skin.

HERPES SIMPLEX VIRUS

One of the most common infections in humans is caused by HSV. The U.S. prevalence of positive antibody serology is around 48% for HSV-1 and about 12% for HSV-2 (McQuillan et al., 2018). Following primary mucocutaneous infection, HSV become latent within adjacent sensory nerve dorsal root ganglia with potential for reactivation on the mucosa and skin. Most infections are subclinical, that is, the majority of those infected do not know they have the disease. When clinical disease does occur, it presents as a prodrome of pain, tingling, or itch

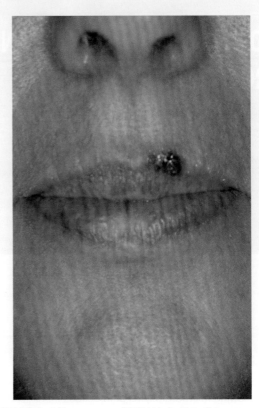

FIGURE 29-1. A Recurrence of HSV-1 Infection, "Herpes Labialis." As shown here, these recurrences tend to be localized to the vermilion border of the lip and are grouped vesicles on an erythematous base.

for 24 hours followed by an outbreak of grouped vesicles and erosions on an erythematous base on the skin or mucous membranes (**Fig. 29-1**) (Spruance et al., 1977). Crusting and resolution occurs then in 2 to 6 weeks.

While HSV-1 is more commonly localized to the orolabial area and HSV-2 has been more commonly attributed to genital herpes, in more recent years, the distribution patterns are less linked and an increasing number of new genital herpes infections are occurring from HSV-1 infection (**Fig. 29-2**) (Bernstein et al., 2013). A primary infection with herpes simplex type 1 (HSV-1) or herpes simplex type 2 (HSV-2) will either be asymptomatic or manifest with a widespread eruption of localized painful vesicles along with systemic findings of fever, lymphadenopathy, and malaise.

Recurrent herpes outbreaks are less severe, more limited in vesicle number and distribution, and last a shorter duration than primary infection. Recurrence of orolabial herpes, also known as cold sores or fever blisters traditionally occurs at the vermillion border (edge of the lip) but can occur at the loose mucosal buccal tissue within the mouth. Vesicles and erosions below the waist may also present outside of the direct genital area on the thighs, buttocks, perineum, or groin (Corey et al., 1983). Since herpes infections are not limited to the orolabial or genital area, it is important to recognize that any eruption

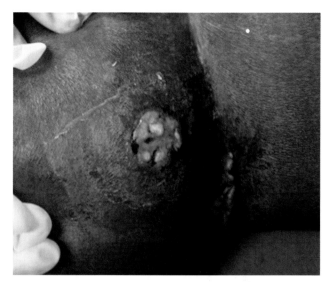

FIGURE 29-2. Anogenital Ulceration Caused by HSV-2.

of painful grouped vesicles or erosions in any location on the body should raise suspicion for HSV infection.

An HSV infection of the finger or nail folds is herpetic whitlow. It can occur via autoinoculation but can also develop in an individual whose finger comes in contact with an active oral lesion of another. Herpes sycosis consists of herpes vesicles involving the hair follicle, most commonly the beard. These tend to present as erosions, and the area of involvement may be extensive. Herpes gladiatorum refers to herpetic lesions involving the lateral neck, forearms, and face that develop in wrestlers after a match with an infected wrestler (Usatine & Tinitigan, 2010). Eczema herpeticum is a unique eruption of more widespread HSV vesicles in a patient with atopic dermatitis, especially those taking immunosuppressive medications for their dermatitis. This eruption consists of an increase in skin pain and vesicles or erosions on a background of atopic dermatitis or similar rash. Prompt treatment with antivirals is needed including intravenous acyclovir treatment in severe cases (Mackool et al., 2012).

Episodes of recurrent outbreaks can occur spontaneously or follow triggers such as stress, illness, fever, ultraviolet light, local tissue damage, or in the setting of immunosuppression (Spruance et al., 1977). In comparing the two types of HSV, recurrence is more common with HSV-2 than with HSV-1. Recurrence is also more common in immunocompromised individuals such as those taking immunosuppressive medications, experiencing hematologic malignancy or in those infected with HIV. Viral shedding with risk of transmission to other intimate contacts can occur even when an individual is asymptomatic without visible herpetic skin changes present (Gupta et al., 2007).

The diagnosis of these conditions is most commonly made on an empiric basis but can be confirmed when vesicles or ulcers are of unclear etiology. The diagnosis of HSV infection is typically based upon confirmation through DNA detection via polymerase chain reaction (PCR) or culture of the virus. HSV PCR is a more sensitive test for HSV detection than viral culture (Ramchandani et al., 2016). Alternatively, the Tzanck smear or direct fluorescent antibody testing performed on a scraping of the base of an ulcer can also be performed in lieu of viral culture as a more rapid test. In many clinical testing sites, it takes days longer to obtain a result from viral culture than from PCR. The technique for obtaining an adequate specimen for HSV PCR or culture is to unroof a vesicle with a sterile swab or needle, then swab the base of the ulcer to isolate surface epidermal cells, which contain HSV. If no intact vesicle roof is present, swabs can be obtained from the base of erosions or ulcers. Serology testing for HSV antibodies is not helpful for diagnosing the etiology of specific skin lesions because HSV antibodies remain positive for life following first exposure and so cannot confirm or deny that a particular skin eruption is caused by HSV.

Treatment

All patients with a first outbreak of genital herpes should be treated with antiviral therapy (Workowski, 2015). For episodes of recurrent outbreaks, treatment should be initiated within the first 72 hours from the time of onset of the prodromal symptoms of pain, tingling, or pruritus. Early treatment aides in reducing the amount of time to the phase of crusting and healing occurs (Reichman et al., 1984). Some patients with mild recurrent outbreaks may choose to forgo antiviral treatment. Antiviral treatment options include oral acyclovir, valacyclovir, and famciclovir, and in severe cases, intravenous acyclovir. Treatment with IV acyclovir should be initiated for treatment of eczema herpeticum, persistent HSV infection in immunocompromised patients, and severe primary infection with HSV. In general, there is no role for topical antiviral therapy due to lack of benefit, especially when compared to oral antivirals which have a high safety profile (Workowski, 2015). Individuals with severe or frequent recurrence of herpes outbreaks greater than six times a year may benefit from chronic suppressive therapy taken each day to reduce the frequency of outbreaks rather than only as needed episodic treatment (Cernik et al., 2008; Mattison et al., 1988). Herpes lesions are partial thickness wounds and should be treated with moist wound healing principles.

KEY POINT

Since herpes infections are not exclusively limited to the orolabial or genital area, it is important to recognize that any eruption of painful grouped vesicles or erosions on any area of the body should raise suspicion for herpes simplex infection.

VARICELLA–ZOSTER VIRUS

VZV is one virus that causes two distinct diseases, varicella (commonly known as chicken pox) and herpes zoster (commonly known as shingles). Before the advent of the varicella vaccine in 1995, varicella was a common self-limiting childhood disease. The virus is spread by aerosolized nasopharyngeal droplets of an actively infected individual and is very contagious. Clinical presentation of varicella includes fever, malaise, pharyngitis, and a widespread eruption of pruritic vesicles on an erythematous base in various stages of healing favoring the face and trunk. Following primary infection, the virus becomes dormant in the sensory nerve ganglia.

When the virus reactivates at a later time and begins to travel down a nerve to the skin, the clinical syndrome that develops is termed herpes zoster. Herpes zoster begins as an area of pain and skin discomfort followed by eruption of grouped or confluent vesicles, papules, or edema with erythema confined to a unilateral dermatomal configuration. The most commonly affected dermatomes are in the thoracic region, but lumbar and sacral dermatomes can also be involved (Yawn et al., 2007). As vesicles rupture, erosions and ulcers then form (**Fig. 29-3**). These wounds can rarely become secondarily infected with bacteria. Once the lesions have entered the crusted phase, they are no longer contagious. The rash typically resolves in 2 to 4 weeks, but pigmentary changes and scarring may persist.

Various complications can occur with herpes zoster. Herpes zoster involvement of the eye, known as herpes zoster ophthalmicus, can result in eye injury and vision loss. Immediate referral to ophthalmology then is imperative when associated eye pain or rash directly around the eye is present. Disseminated zoster is a more widespread eruption and occurs when three or more dermatomes are involved, typically only in those who are immunocompromised. Hospitalization is required for

administration of IV acyclovir in immunocompromised individuals with disseminated zoster (Fehr et al., 2002). The risk for post-herpetic neuralgia (PHN) that consists of chronic, debilitating pain in the affected dermatome months to years following the infection is 10% to 18% (Harpaz et al., 2008). Diagnosis of PHN is made when pain persists beyond 4 months in the same distribution as herpes zoster. Risk factors included advanced age, severe prodromal pain with acute herpes zoster, severe preceding rash, distribution in trigeminal or brachial plexus dermatomes and presence of allodynia. Gabapentin, pregabalin, and tricyclic antidepressants (TCAs) are generally the drugs of first choice for the treatment of PHN (Ortega, 2019).

KEY POINT

VZV is one virus that cause two distinct infections, varicella (chicken pox) and herpes zoster (shingles). The virus is spread by nasopharyngeal droplets or from fluid from vesicles and is very contagious.

Approximately 30% of individuals will develop herpes zoster in their lifetime in the United States (Harpaz et al., 2008). Age is the greatest risk factor for the development of herpes zoster, especially after the age of 50 most likely due to the age-related decrease in cellular immunity, which allows the VZV to replicate and cause disease (Cohen et al., 2013; Yawn et al., 2007). Other risk factors include use of immunosuppression medications or immunocompromise from disease states such as AIDS or malignancy. The risk of developing another outbreak of herpes zoster is low, a rate of up to 6% (Kawai et al., 2014). Individuals with herpes zoster are only contagious to those who have never had varicella or never had the VZV vaccine. The exposed, susceptible individual would then develop varicella for the first time. Covering herpes zoster vesicles and erosions until they crust over will prevent exposure to others who could be susceptible to new infection.

Diagnosis

Varicella and herpes zoster are often diagnosed clinically. Diagnostic testing may be appropriate in the case that a rash presents in an atypical pattern or to help diagnose disseminated zoster in an immunocompromised individual. The diagnosis of zoster involves the same techniques as are used for diagnosing HSV with PCR or viral culture. PCR obtained through swab of the base of vesicles provides a more sensitive result for virus confirmation than viral culture for VZV (Harbecke et al., 2009). Alternatively, the Tzanck smear or direct fluorescent antibody testing performed on a scraping of the base of an ulcer can also be performed in lieu of viral culture as a more rapid test.

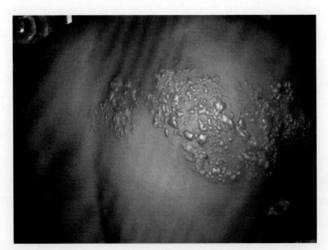

FIGURE 29-3. A Herpes Zoster Outbreak in a T2 Dermatomal Distribution.

Treatment

Treatment of zoster is with a choice of acyclovir, famciclovir, or valacyclovir for 7 days, though treatment is more feasible with valacyclovir or famciclovir than with acyclovir because of a less frequent dosing schedule. Treatment is ideally initiated within 72 hours of the appearance of lesions. Oral analgesia may be needed for associated pain. Local wound care with occlusion and a moist environment is also appropriate. For prevention, the recombinant zoster vaccine is available for individuals 50 years of age or older. This is not a live vaccine. The recombinant zoster vaccine is recommended over the original live attenuated zoster vaccine because of greater efficacy against the development of shingles and against PHN (McGirr et al., 2019).

KEY POINT

Herpes zoster infections should be treated with antivirals and with the principles of moist wound healing. Oral analgesia is frequently needed for associated pain relief.

FUNGAL INFECTIONS CAUSING WOUNDS

Fungal infections are more likely to cause rashes than wounds; however, severe fungal infections may cause areas of erosions and ulceration. In addition, fungal infections commonly occur in the periwound or perineal area where moisture is prevalent so the wound care nurse must be able to recognize and recommend treatment for common fungal infections. The most common superficial fungal infections of the skin include the dermatophytes and *Candida albicans*. Less commonly deep fungal infection can occur with organisms that may present as ulcers or ulcerated nodules due to deeper involvement of the organisms within the tissue. Representative deep fungal infections such as sporotrichosis, coccidioidomycosis, histoplasmosis, and North American blastomycosis are endemic to the United States and can present in localized or disseminated disease patterns on the skin.

KEY POINT

Superficial fungal infections cause rashes that when severe may cause areas of erosion and ulceration. These infections are common in the periwound and perineal area where moisture is prevalent. The wound care nurse must be able to recognize these and provide appropriate treatment recommendations.

DERMATOPHYTES

The dermatophytes are fungi that subsist on keratin, a protein that is found in the superficial skin, nails, and hair.

The diseases that they cause include tinea capitis, tinea barbae, and tinea pedis. These three are discussed in more detail as these forms of tinea can lead to wounds in certain cases.

Tinea Capitis

Commonly known as ringworm of the scalp, tinea capitis is a fairly common childhood disease in the United States. Most cases occur in school age, preadolescent African-American boys. About 90% of cases are caused by *Trichophyton tonsurans*, which invades the hair shaft and causes a scaly, red rash on the involved area of the scalp. The rash is composed of papules in an annular configuration. The hairs in the affected areas break off near the surface of the scalp, leaving areas of alopecia. Diagnosis of tinea capitis requires use of a scalpel to take a scraping of the scalp that includes some hair follicles and scale. The scraping is treated with potassium hydroxide (KOH prep) and is examined for presence of fungal hyphae under the microscope. A minority of cases of tinea capitis are due to *Microsporum* species. These cases can be diagnosed with use of a Wood's lamp (black light), which causes the affected area to fluoresce a greenish yellow color. However, since *Microsporum* is a minor cause of tinea capitis in the United States, a negative Wood's lamp examination does not exclude the diagnosis of tinea capitis (Mirmirani & Tucker, 2013).

KEY POINT

Dermatophytes are fungi that live on keratin. They cause infections such as tinea capitis, tinea cruris (jock itch), tinea barbae (beard), and tinea pedis (athletes' foot).

If the immune response to the fungus is exaggerated, a kerion may form at the affected area, which presents as a painful, boggy, inflamed nodule that is often mistaken for an abscess due to the pustules and crusts on the surface (**Fig. 29-4**). Removal of the crust can help with relief of pain. The erosions revealed by crust removal should be treated with moist wound healing and, in the event of a secondary bacterial infection, with antibiotics. Treatment with an oral antifungal, terbinafine or griseofulvin, is necessary to eliminate the dermatophyte involvement in the hair follicle (Gupta et al., 2018).

Tinea Cruris

Tinea cruris, commonly known as jock itch, is a dermatophyte infection involving the crural folds. It often begins as an itchy, erythematous patch on the medial upper thigh with subsequent enlargement and central clearance. Involvement may spread to the perineum, gluteal cleft, and buttocks, with sparing of the scrotum in males. A slightly elevated border with scalloped edge may help distinguish this from other causes of irritation in the groin

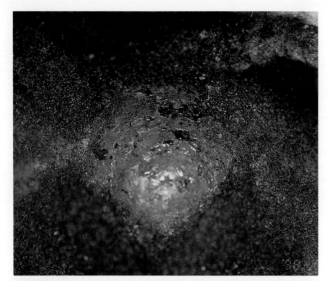

FIGURE 29-4. A Tinea Capitis Infection with Formation of a Painful, Boggy Nodule Known as a Kerion. (Reprinted with permission from Fleisher, G. R., Ludwig, S., & Baskin, M. N. (2004). *Atlas of pediatric emergency medicine*. Philadelphia, PA: Lippincott Williams & Wilkins.)

folds. Infection may occur because of transfer of fungi on clothing from the feet that have tinea pedis. Common causative dermatophytes are *Trichophyton rubrum, Epidermophyton floccosum,* and *Trichophyton mentagrophytes.*

Tinea Barbae

Tinea barbae is another fungal infection that affects the hair follicle. The target organ is the hair of the beard and mustaches of men. The fungi that cause this pathology are the zoonotic fungi *T. mentagrophytes* and *Trichophyton verrucosum.* Cattle and horses are the usual source of the fungus, and the infection is most common in men working in the agricultural business. It usually presents as a very red and highly inflamed kerion-like lesion. Pustules or crusting with erosions may be seen as well. The hairs within the lesion are easily and painlessly removed. These wounds may result in secondary bacterial infections that require systemic antibiotics. The diagnosis and treatment are the same as for tinea capitis, as both infect the hair follicle. The wound care nurse should be aware that oral antifungal therapy is necessary as topical antifungals are nontherapeutic (Furlan et al., 2017).

Tinea Pedis

Fungal infection of the feet, or tinea pedis, is often referred to as athlete's foot. It is very common, affecting about 15% of the population (Bell-Syer et al., 2012). *Trichophyton rubrum* and *T. mentagrophytes* are common causes. Infection can cause a variety of presentations. The commonly seen chronic form of tinea pedis presents as a mildly erythematous background rash with associated scale and a moccasin distribution over the feet. The moccasin distribution means that the rash

covers the areas of the foot covered by a shoe (moccasin) and is due to the tendency of fungal organisms to grow in moist, warm, occluded areas covered by shoes. Another pattern, interdigital tinea pedis, presents as itchy, moist scaling, and erythema between the toes, especially the third and fourth toe web spaces. Associated fissures can be painful. A third pattern, vesiculobullous (inflammatory) tinea pedis, is characterized by an itchy, occasionally painful vesicular and bullous eruption with surrounding erythema located more commonly on the medial instep of the foot. *Trichophyton mentagrophytes* is a common culprit. Infrequently, ulcerative tinea pedis consisting of ulceration between the toes occurs which is associated with concurrent bacterial infection.

Diagnosis involves examination of skin scrapings for fungal elements under the microscope through a KOH prep, as described previously for the diagnosis of other forms of tinea. Presence of onychomycosis, toenail fungal infection, also increases the likelihood of tinea pedis.

Treatment with topical antifungals such as terbinafine, azoles, ciclopirox, or tolnaftate for approximately 4 weeks is appropriate for most cases of tinea cruris or pedis (Crawford & Hollis, 2007). Nystatin, which is a very effective treatment for *Candida* infections, is not effective for dermatophyte infection. Topical steroids will alter the appearance of a fungal infection and may worsen the infection. Oral antifungals such as terbinafine or itraconazole are reserved for extensive or refractory tinea cruris or pedis.

Wound care should follow principles of wound bed preparation. If the patient has diabetes, care should be taken to offload the wounds to prevent chronic ulceration.

KEY POINT

Chronic tinea pedis is manifested by a mildly erythematous scaly rash that causes minimal or no symptoms. Acute tinea pedis is manifested by itchy and painful fissures, bullae or ulcers present in the third and fourth web spaces, or on the instep of the foot in inflammatory cases.

Candida albicans

Although a component of the normal flora for humans, the fungus *C. albicans* can become pathogenic under certain conditions. *Candida* can cause a wide array of human pathology, from minor superficial skin infections to invasive systemic disease in immunocompromised individuals. Superficial infection of the skin is discussed here. Clinically, intertriginous dermatitis (ITD) with superficial infection with *Candida* presents as itchy and painful, beefy-red, macerated and eroded plaques, and patches, often with peripheral scaling and smaller satellite pustules or papules. Commonly affected areas include the inframammary area, area at the base of the pannus, inguinal folds, gluteal cleft, and the scrotum. Predisposing factors for the development of *Candida* infection include diabetes mellitus, hyperhidrosis, occlusion, corticosteroids use, systemic antibiotic use, and immunocompromise (Hay & Ashbee, 2016; Pappas & Ray, 1998). Though clinical presentation when fitting the classic characteristics may be sufficient for diagnosis, a scraping of scale for KOH examination under the microscope can help confirm the diagnosis and help to distinguish candidal intertrigo from skin fold irritation from moisture alone.

Intertrigo, a term used to refer to inflammation in the skin folds, can come from various causes, and candidal intertrigo may superimpose on other underlying causes of intertrigo. It is important to understand the various causes of intertrigo. Other common causes for intertrigo include irritant contact dermatitis, allergic contact dermatitis, and erythrasma. A form of moisture-associated skin damage (MASD), ITD, may occur on exposure to persistent sweat or with exposure to urine or stool in an incontinent individual (Black et al., 2011; Gray et al., 2011). Allergic contact dermatitis can develop from exposure to cleansers, emollients, or materials touching the skin. Erythrasma is a type of intertrigo presenting as an asymptomatic broad pink to brown patch caused by a superficial bacterial infection with *Corynebacterium minutissimum*. When available, a Wood's lamp (black light) is used to diagnose or rule out infection since the area of affected skin will fluoresce a coral-red color when *Corynebacterium* is present. It is important to understand that candidal infection, and even bacterial infection, caused by staph, strep, or *Corynebacterium*, can initiate or aggravate intertrigo, so more than one trigger for inflammation in the skin folds may need to be addressed.

KEY POINT

Candidal superinfection is common in patients with ITD. Diabetes, hyperhidrosis, occlusion, corticosteroids, systemic antibiotics, and immunosuppression can predispose to infection with *Candida*.

For ITD with superficial infection with *Candida*, a moisture wicking fabric with antimicrobial silver (InterDry®) can be used in skin folds to wick away moisture. The fabric is placed between the folds of skin and should extend from the base of the fold to at least 2 inches beyond the fold to allow for wicking and evaporation. The antimicrobial agent is intended to reduce the risk of cutaneous infections including candidiasis. The silver within the textile provides antimicrobial action for up to 5 days. Placement of the low coefficient of friction (CoF) textile provides separation of the body folds and reduces the risk of friction damage. In the past, multiple interventions have been used unsuccessfully, including feminine hygiene products, washcloths, deodorant, powders, and abdominal pads. These products do not wick moisture away from the skin fold. When using the wicking textile, the use of powders and creams should be avoided (Kalra et al., 2014). Treatment should continue until the ITD has resolved. Continued use of the wicking textile may prevent reoccurrence (Gray et al., 2011).

ITD complicated by fungal infection may also be managed with topical antifungals if wicking fabric is not available. Nystatin is effective only for candidal intertrigo. Clotrimazole, ketoconazole, oxiconazole, or econazole may be used for both *Candida* and dermatophyte infections. Topical treatments are applied twice daily until the rash resolves. Fluconazole 100 to 200 mg daily for 7 days is used for resistant fungal infections, although patients who are obese may require an increased dosage. Oral azoles may potentiate the effects of hypoglycemic agents, leading to low blood glucose levels, and patients with diabetes should be instructed to monitor their blood glucose levels with concomitant use of these medications (Kalra et al., 2014). See Chapter 18 for further discussion regarding pathology, prevention, and management of ITD with superficial infection with *Candida*.

DEEP FUNGAL INFECTIONS

Sporotrichosis

Sporotrichosis, a condition caused by the dimorphic fungus, *Sporothrix schenckii*, is a nodular and ulcerative infection of the subcutaneous tissue following an inoculation exposure. Epidemiologically, it is seen most often in South and Central America, but outbreaks and isolated cases are seen all over the world, including in the U.S. *S. schenckii* is a saprophyte found in soil, wood, rose thorns, shrubs, and straw and occasionally on animals such as cats and armadillos (De Araujo et al., 2001). It most commonly causes disease when it is directly inoculated into the skin, classically when the thorn of a rose bush traumatically pierces a gardener's skin. Those with occupational exposure, such as carpenters, landscapers, and gardeners, are at greatest risk of acquiring the condition. Less commonly, the conidia of the fungus can be inhaled with resultant systemic disease, but this is only seen in immunocompromised individuals.

Lymphocutaneous sporotrichosis begins at the site of inoculation as a small indurated papule weeks following exposure, which subsequently grows in size to form a nodule, which frequently ulcerates. The infection spreads through the lymphatics (lymphocutaneous or sporotrichoid spread), and new papules form proximal to the inoculation site along the lymphatic pathway. These new lesions then also progress to nodules and ulcerations. A less common form of this infection is fixed cutaneous sporotrichosis. These lesions present as verrucous plaques or ulcers, but there is no lymphocutaneous spread (De Araujo et al., 2001).

The diagnosis of sporotrichosis is confirmed through skin biopsy culture on sabouraud agar. Histologic examination of skin biopsy tissue alone with stains for fungal organisms may not reveal the causal organism, as they are often low in number. Sporotrichosis is usually treated with systemic medications including itraconazole, amphotericin B, or saturated solution of potassium iodide (Kauffman et al., 2007). Itraconazole is the preferred treatment for lymphocutaneous and fixed cutaneous cases, with few side effects and a high cure rate. Amphotericin B is used in severe or disseminated cases. Oral potassium iodide is a low-cost treatment that is mainly used in developing nations. Alternatively, topically applied heat is a treatment option for those who are intolerant to antifungal medications, as the organism grows at low temperatures (Ramos-e-Silva et al., 2007).

KEY POINT

Deep fungal infections are less common and usually occur when the causative organism is inoculated into the skin via traumatic injury with a contaminated object (e.g., when a rose thorn pierces a gardener's thumb).

Chromoblastomycosis

Chromoblastomycosis is a subcutaneous mycosis that can be caused by numerous different pigmented fungi. Chromoblastomycosis can be chronic and difficult to treat. It is caused most commonly by direct inoculation of the skin with one of the following genera of fungi that are naturally found as saprophytes in the soil and on plants: *Fonsecaea*, *Phialophora*, and *Cladosporium* (Ameen, 2009). It is most common among agricultural workers living in tropical climates. Most cases are in Brazil and Madagascar, though it can be seen in rural areas of North America. Given that chromoblastomycosis is mostly seen in people working in agriculture, it is predominantly seen in middle-aged men.

Clinically, chromoblastomycosis occurs at a site of fungus inoculation months to years after the original trauma, most commonly on the lower extremities. The lesion begins as a small asymptomatic red papule that slowly progresses to a verrucous-appearing nodule that spreads and can create cauliflower-like lesions. Black dots, representing sites of transdermal elimination of the fungus, can be seen on the surface of the lesions. Other clinical morphology patterns beside verrucous type lesions include plaque type, tumoral type, or atrophic-type lesions (Brito & Bittencourt, 2018). The surface can ulcerate and crust, and though rare, neoplastic transformation has been reported. Though the infection remains in the subcutaneous fat, in some cases, elephantiasis may develop due to lymphatic invasion and damage.

Diagnosis of the lesion can be made with a KOH test, which is best performed by taking a sample from an area with a black dot. Microscopically, a signature Medlar body will be seen, which looks like a copper penny and represents fungal cells. Diagnosis can also be made by histology and fungal culture. The disease can be refractory to treatment, and antifungal courses are needed for months to over 1 year. Treatment of small lesions may involve surgical excision in combination with antifungals. Lesions may recur. Itraconazole is the standard first-line therapy with terbinafine following second in frequency of use (Queiroz-Telles et al., 2017). Posaconazole may be used in severe or refractory cases (Chowdhary et al., 2014).

Coccidioidomycosis

Coccidioidomycosis is a systemic mycosis acquired through the inhalation of the pathogenic fungus *Coccidioides immitis* that when disseminated can cause cutaneous lesions. In the United States, *Coccidioides* is endemic to the soil of California's San Joaquin River Valley, and endemic zones include the US southwest, northern Mexico, and Central and South America. While 60% of infections are asymptomatic, following spore inhalation symptoms can consist of a flu-like illness with fever, fatigue, sore throat, and cough (Pappagianis, 1993). This is known as Valley fever and can persist for up to a few weeks. A minority of patients with Valley fever will develop cutaneous hypersensitivity manifestations, such as erythema nodosum or erythema multiforme as a reactive process where organisms are not identified within the lesions (Borchers & Gershwin, 2010).

Though rare, some individuals are at risk for developing disseminated disease to other organs including the skin as the most common site. These individuals include those with immunosuppression related to HIV, hematologic malignancy, inflammatory arthritis, diabetes, and organ transplantation medications (Garcia Garcia et al., 2015). Women who are pregnant are also at higher risk. Dissemination occurs hematogenously and causes granulomatous infection in the bones, skin, and meninges, although virtually any organ can be infected. Skin lesions often appear on the face, classically the nasolabial fold, though they can occur on the extremities as well. They can begin as a verrucous papule or nodule and may eventually ulcerate. Rarely, localized cutaneous disease develops as a result of direct inoculation of the skin. These primary lesions present as a painless nodule that ulcerates and may be complicated by lymphocutaneous spread.

Though rare, coccidioidomycosis must be considered by health care providers when patients present with ulcerations in atypical locations. A detailed medical history and attention to recent travel to endemic locations are important for an accurate diagnosis. To confirm a diagnosis of coccidioidomycosis, culture and histology from skin biopsy should be performed. Treatment for disseminated disease or solitary skin lesions typically involves itraconazole or fluconazole for up to 12 months (Galgiani et al., 2000).

Histoplasmosis

Classically caused by the dimorphic fungus *Histoplasma capsulatum*, histoplasmosis is another infection that is contracted via inhalation of spores. It can be entirely asymptomatic, or it can cause pulmonary disease, with rare dissemination to other organs, including the skin. *H. capsulatum* is endemic to the Mississippi and Ohio River Valley in the United States and is frequently found in bat and bird droppings. Disseminated disease can cause indurated plaques within the oronasopharynx, which may ulcerate. Individuals living with HIV, those immunosuppressed for organ transplantation, and those on anti-TNF-α inhibitor medications are more susceptible to disseminated and potentially fatal infection. When disseminated histoplasmosis occurs in immunocompetent individuals, the most common mucocutaneous presentation is with oral ulcers. In immunocompromised individuals, disseminated histoplasmosis can present with a variety of presentations including mucocutaneous erosions and ulcers as well as crusted diffuse papules or plaques (Vallabhaneni & Chiller, 2016). Primary (direct inoculation) skin infection is exceedingly rare but has been reported as a penile chancre (Chang & Rodas, 2012). Diagnostic options include quick testing blood or urine for the Histoplasma antigen detection enzyme immunoassay as well as skin biopsy for histology and fungal culture. For treatment of disseminated and severe disease, especially in those who are immunocompromised, amphotericin B therapy is recommended (Johnson et al., 2002). Itraconazole can be used in patients with less severe disease.

North American Blastomycosis

Blastomyces dermatitidis is a dimorphic fungus endemic to North America, specifically the Southeast and the Great Lakes area. The fungus is transmitted through inhalation of aerosolized spores of the organism. The lungs are the most common site of the infection, and the skin is the second most common site of involvement (Saccente & Woods, 2010). Affected patients are middle-aged to elderly males, and the immunocompromised. Those with HIV, those on immunosuppression for organ transplantation, and those on anti-TNF-α inhibitor medications are at greater risk for severe lung disease. Skin lesions begin as asymptomatic papules or nodules that evolve into verrucous lesions with irregular but clearly defined borders. The lesions vary in color from gray to violaceous. The lesions may form crusts with underlying erosions. While growth from tissue or sputum culture is the gold standard for diagnosis, skin histology with fungal stains to identify fungal forms can be helpful as well. After a diagnosis is made, itraconazole for 6 months is the recommended therapy (Lopez-Martinez & Mendez-Tovar, 2012). Ulcerated lesions typically resolve as the infection is treated.

BACTERIAL INFECTIONS CAUSING WOUNDS

Though commonly thought of as agents that infect existing wounds, bacteria can also be the primary reason a wound exists. Wounds caused by bacterial infections range in severity from mild to life threatening.

IMPETIGO

Impetigo is a superficial bacterial infection of the topmost layer of skin, the epidermis. It is a common skin infection among children. It is one of the top skin disorders seen by general practitioners in the pediatric population (Mohammedamin et al., 2006). The average age of presentation with impetigo is between 1 and 8 years (Koning et al., 2006). *Staphylococcus aureus* is the main causal pathogen, but it can also be caused by *Streptococcus pyogenes*. Both are gram-positive organisms. The disease usually manifests on areas of the body that are not covered by clothing, such as the face, arms, hands, and neck. Nonbullous impetigo begins as red macules that progress to vesicles that rupture and leave a classic honey-colored crust (**Fig. 29-5**). The crusts are easily removed, leaving erosions. These wounds are infectious. The fluid that forms on them can be transferred to others, to other areas of the body, and to fomites. Existing wounds or skin breaks can also become secondarily infected, or impetiginized, as in the case of impetiginized atopic dermatitis or even impetiginized herpes simplex eruptions (Baddour, 2019).

Bullous impetigo is a more severe variant of impetigo. It is caused by a strain of *S. aureus* that produces an exfoliative toxin, which attacks cell adhesion molecules within the epidermis, separating cell layers, and causing

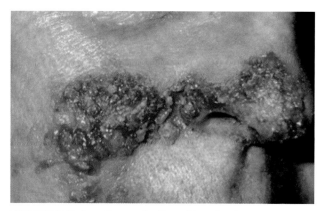

FIGURE 29-5. Impetigo on the Face. Note the characteristic honey-colored crusting.

the formation of bullae. It is usually seen in newborn infants, where it can be life threatening, but adults can develop the condition as well. The trunk is commonly affected, and when the bullae burst, the result is open erosions or crusted lesions.

ECTHYMA

Ecthyma is an ulcerative form of impetigo caused by *S. pyogenes* with infection extending into the dermis. Infection begins as vesicles on a red skin base with development of thicker yellow and hemorrhagic crusts, which, if removed, reveal punched-out ulcers (**Fig. 29-6**). Because the lesions extend into the deep dermis, they usually heal with scarring. It is important to provide proper wound care in addition to treatment of the infection itself. The lesions should be kept moist and occluded to accelerate the healing process. These lesions are most commonly seen in patients with poor hygiene, those who are immunosuppressed, and elderly patients.

In nonbullous impetigo, bullous impetigo, and ecthyma, the diagnosis is made on clinical appearance. For limited, nonbullous disease, topical antibiotics such as mupirocin or retapamulin are sufficient along with removal of crust through washing and wet wraps. In ecthyma, bullous impetigo, and extensive nonbullous impetigo, empiric oral antibiotic therapy should be provided with agents such as cephalexin, dicloxacillin, or clindamycin (Stevens et al., 2014). If the patient does not respond to empiric treatment, the lesions may be cultured with a bacterial swab to determine the causative organism and antibiotic susceptibilities.

> **KEY POINT**
>
> Impetigo, bullous impetigo, and ecthyma are diagnosed clinically and treated empirically, with topical or systemic antibiotics that are effective against *S. aureus* and *S. pyogenes*.

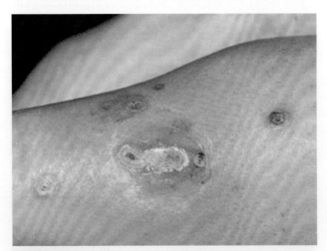

FIGURE 29-6. Ecthyma of the Lower Extremity. Note the *yellow-gray* thick crust. It is harder and thicker than the crust of impetigo.

BACTERIAL FOLLICULITIS

Folliculitis is inflammation of the superficial or deep portion of the hair follicle. It usually begins with trauma or occlusion of the hair follicle that renders the hair follicle vulnerable to pathogen invasion. Folliculitis presents as clusters of multiple small, pruritic, red, papules, and pustules involving the hair follicles where when magnified, hair can be seen piercing within. Certain conditions additionally predispose patients to folliculitis including immunosuppression, existing dermatoses, diabetes mellitus, obesity, use of heavy emollients, and living in a humid climate. Though folliculitis is very common, the true incidence is not known because most cases are minor, resolve quickly, and do not require professional intervention.

While irritation alone from occlusion causes many cases of folliculitis, *S. aureus* is the most common cause when folliculitis is triggered by an infectious microorganism (Laureano et al., 2014). Staphylococcal folliculitis can occur on any hair-bearing area, but the face, buttocks, legs, and axillae are the sites most commonly affected. One of the most important risk factors for bacterial folliculitis is frequent shaving such that folliculitis is often seen in the beard and mustache area of men in a pattern known as sycosis barbae. The associated pustular rash usually starts around the nose and upper lip area and is extremely pruritic. Shaving and facial cleansing can cause the pustules to burst, with resultant spread of the infection. Persistent trauma and deeper infection can eventually lead to scarring and alopecia of the area (Laureano et al., 2014). When several *S. aureus*–infected hair follicles coalesce into a single, inflamed area or nodule, it is known as a carbuncle. If the infection involves the dermis or subcutaneous fat, the entity is termed a furuncle.

> **KEY POINT**
>
> Folliculitis is characterized by a pustular rash with hair protruding from the center of the lesions. Treatment involves use of topical antibacterial agents or oral antibiotics if extensive.

Treatment with topical antibiotics such as mupirocin and topical clindamycin is usually sufficient for mild folliculitis from *S. aureus* (Lopez & Lartchenko, 2006). If infection persists or is more severe, then a 1-week course of antibiotics directed toward MSSA or MRSA is recommended (Laureano et al., 2014).

Gram-negative folliculitis, a rare folliculitis, can be caused by the bacterial species Proteus, Klebsiella, Enterobacter, and Serratia. This is most common in patients who are taking long-term antibiotic therapy (often for acne vulgaris). Because this condition is common in patients with acne, gram-negative folliculitis can be confused for an acne flare. The lesions are usually around the nose and chin. Samples of the drainage from the pustules should be sent for Gram stain and culture to confirm the diagnosis, and the condition should be treated with oral antibiotics and/or isotretinoin (Böni & Nehrhoff, 2003).

Pseudomonas aeruginosa folliculitis is a specific type of gram-negative folliculitis that presents in patients who have recently been in a whirlpool, and it is colloquially known as hot-tub folliculitis. It can also be seen in patients who have worn a wet suit for prolonged periods of time. The lesions are papular and pustular and located around the hair follicles in areas occluded by swimwear. The infection is self-limiting but may leave areas of erosions and hypopigmentation. No treatment is indicated.

ECTHYMA GANGRENOSUM

Not to be confused with ecthyma caused by *S. pyogenes*, ecthyma gangrenosum is a deeper necrotic skin ulcer most commonly caused by the gram-negative bacterium *P. aeruginosa*, though other bacterial, viral, and fungal organisms have been documented to cause the same pattern of skin ulcer (Reich et al., 2004). The lesions develop in immunocompromised individuals due to bacterial invasion of blood vessels and are a sign of *Pseudomonas* bacteremia and impending sepsis. Blood vessel disruption then causes ischemic necrosis of the surrounding skin. The wound then involves necrosis of the epidermis through the deep dermis.

While ecthyma gangrenosum is an uncommon condition, it is more common in individuals with serious chronic health conditions, such as immunodeficiency or malignant disease, and it may be the first sign of a malignancy or HIV. Although it can present at all ages, it is more common in children. The anogenital region, axillae, and limbs are the most common sites of presentation (Sarkar et al., 2016).

Lesions present initially as vesicles surrounded by a pink halo but within 12 hours become indurated, violaceous, and hemorrhagic, and become necrotic. The final lesions are ulcers with central black eschar with an erythematous border (**Fig. 29-7**).

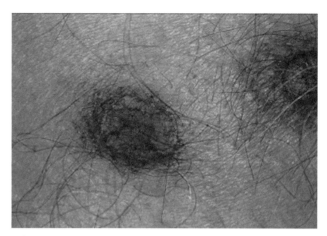

FIGURE 29-7. Ecthyma Gangrenosum. Note the central *gray-black* eschar surrounded by an erythematous halo.

diaper dermatitis where the macerated occlusive environment leads to superficial breaks in the skin that permit *Pseudomonas* inoculation (Goolamali et al., 2009). Any site of trauma in a neutropenic patient can serve as a portal of entry for the pathogen. Oncology patients, especially children, when neutropenic then are at risk for developing ecthyma gangrenosum. Treatment involves prompt administration of empiric intravenous antipseudomonal antibiotics though blood cultures and swab cultures of wounds should be obtained to verify the causative microorganism and antimicrobial susceptibilities. If the lesions do not respond to antibiotic therapy, surgical debridement may be required to prevent further seeding and spread of the bacterium.

HIDRADENITIS SUPPURATIVA

Hidradenitis suppurativa (HS) is characterized by follicular occlusion in areas of the body with apocrine glands, which leads to subsequent inflammation, infection, and abscess formation. The lesions present clinically as painful nodules that occur most commonly in the axillae and inguinal areas. These lesions can become secondarily infected and can also rupture to form shallow erosions and ulcerations. HS progresses to interconnecting sinus tracts and cord-like scarring in affected areas, causing pain, embarrassment, and disfigurement. The exact pathogenesis remains unknown, but studies have suggested that an abnormal immune is responsible. The prevalence of the disease is around 1%. HS is more common in women, smokers, and those who are overweight/obese. It most commonly occurs in adults aged 20 to 40, and the increased androgen levels in this age group are thought to play a potential contributing role.

Treatment begins with addressing lifestyle factors such as smoking, weight loss, and wearing loose clothing to avoid friction to the involved areas. Medical management includes washing the affected areas with antiseptic solutions to reduce commensal bacteria, daily oral

> **KEY POINT**
>
> Ecthyma gangrenosum develops in immunocompromised individuals due to bacterial invasion of blood vessels and is a sign of *Pseudomonas* bacteremia and impending sepsis.

A nonbacteremic form of ecthyma gangrenosum exists that is characterized by development of lesions at the site of *Pseudomonas* inoculation. Though initially a local cutaneous infection, untreated lesions can progress to bacteremia and eventual sepsis. For example, this is sometimes seen in otherwise healthy infants with doxycycline or minocycline, and daily topical clindamycin. If treatment is unsuccessful, or there is scar development, oral clindamycin 300 mg twice daily and oral rifampicin 300 mg twice daily for 10 weeks may be tried. Biologics such as infliximab, adalimumab, and ustekinumab can be considered in severe disease. Isotretinoin can be used for severe disease as well but is less efficacious than when used for treatment of acne. Intralesional corticosteroids can be used for acute flares. Surgery should be reserved for those who have failed lifestyle/medical interventions and is performed to remove active foci of disease or areas of severe scarring/sinus tract formation. Despite therapy, the usual course of disease is chronic, often lasting around 20 years. Routine follow-up with a dermatologist, surgeon, and wound care nurse is recommended (Jemec, 2012).

KEY POINT

Hidradenitis suppurativa is a chronic condition of the hair follicles and apocrine glands (typically in the axillae and perineum) that causes significant pain and scarring. Treatment involves hygienic care, topical and systemic antibiotics and anti-inflammatory agents, and sometimes surgical excision of the involved area.

CELLULITIS AND ERYSIPELAS

Cellulitis is a very common bacterial infection of the skin, involving the deep dermis and subcutaneous fat. It most commonly involves the lower extremity but can occur anywhere on the body. Usually, cellulitis causes local symptoms, but patients can develop systemic symptoms such as fever and chills, indicating bacteremia. Early clinical indicators include erythema, swelling, tenderness, and increased warmth of the affected area. Blistering, erosions, and ulcers may also be present. It is usually caused by *S. pyogenes* (most common) and *S. aureus*. The most common noninfectious mimickers of cellulitis include stasis dermatitis and contact dermatitis (Strazzula et al., 2015). Cellulitis is most often unilateral, and the seeming appearance of bilateral involvement should prompt consideration of alternative diagnoses such as stasis dermatitis (Ratliff et al., 2016; WOCN, 2019).

Multiple conditions predispose to cellulitis especially those that include skin breaks, including preexisting eczema, fungal infections, lymphedema, surgical wounds, traumatic wounds, venous insufficiency, and ulcerations (Phoenix et al., 2012). The diagnosis of cellulitis is made clinically. Taking culture swabs from intact skin is not helpful or recommended (Stevens et al., 2014). In the case that the cellulitis is accompanied by purulence or a fluctuant abscess that can be incised and drained. A bacterial culture swab can be useful in identifying the causative microorganism. Blood cultures are indicated only in the case of severe infection, no previous antibiotic use, presence of signs and symptoms of sepsis, proximal limb involvement, or in those with underlying immunodeficiency or malignancy (Peralta et al., 2006).

Empiric treatment for nonpurulent cellulitis involves systemic antibiotic therapy covering MSSA and beta-hemolytic *Streptococcus*. Antibiotics for cellulitis with associated abscess or purulence should cover MRSA until culture results can verify a causative microorganism and antibiotic susceptibilities. Management includes limb elevation to reduce edema, treating underlying skin abnormalities, moisturizing cream for eczema, and topical therapies for tinea pedis (Stevens et al., 2014). Signs of improvement and medication efficacy include a reduction of pain, erythema, and swelling.

Erysipelas is also a soft tissue infection involving erythema, edema pain, and fever that is differentiated from cellulitis by a more acute onset and sharper ridge-like demarcation in the skin. Common locations are the lower extremity and face. In contrast to cellulitis that involves the deeper dermis and subcutaneous fat, erysipelas involves the upper dermis and superficial lymphatics (Bisno & Stevens, 1996). Lymphedema and chronic cutaneous ulcers are some of the predisposing factors. It is caused by group A streptococci, and empiric antibiotics should be directed toward this microorganism.

KEY POINT

In the case of cellulitis that occurs in the absence of any visible wound or purulent drainage, cultures are of no benefit, and empiric antibiotics should be prescribed that target MSSA and beta-hemolytic *Streptococcus*.

NECROTIZING FASCIITIS

Though uncommon, necrotizing fasciitis (necrotizing soft tissue infection to deeper levels of tissue) is a life-threatening infection that involves rapid spread of inflammation and necrosis throughout the skin, subcutaneous fat, and fascia, resulting in massive tissue loss and very large wounds (**Fig. 29-8**). The incidence is reported to be around 0.3 to 15 per 100,000 (Stevens & Bryant, 2017). Mortality rates are high with rates for infection with group A *Streptococcus* ranging from 15% to 45% (Wong & Stevens, 2013) and for infections with some clostridium species, mortality can range from 70% to 100% (Aldape et al., 2006). The most important factor affecting mortality is the time between onset and debridement of the lesions, so it is important for health

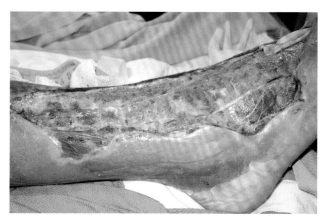

FIGURE 29-8. Necrotizing Fasciitis of the Lower Extremity. There is loss of the epidermis, dermis, and subcutaneous tissue. Note how the fascia is easily visible. (Reprinted with permission from *Wound care: An incredibly visual! pocket guide (Incredibly Easy! Series)*. Philadelphia, PA: Lippincott Williams & Wilkins, 2010.)

care providers to immediately recognize and accurately diagnose this condition (Bellapianta et al., 2009).

Types

Necrotizing fasciitis typically begins after minor or major trauma to the skin that permits bacterial inoculation, such as insect bites, cuts, surgical incisions, ulcers, or burns. Many types of bacteria can cause the infection, and necrotizing fasciitis is divided into major types based on the infecting organism(s). Type I is the most common and is due to a polymicrobial infection, involving as many as 4 to 5 different aerobic and anaerobic organisms. These organisms may include non–group A *Streptococcus*, *Escherichia coli*, *Bacteroides*, *Clostridium* spp., and even opportunistic fungi such as zygomycosis in immunocompromised patients. Type I tends to occur in the elderly or in those with underlying illnesses.

Type II is due to monomicrobial infection most commonly with *S. pyogenes* (Khamnuan et al., 2015), followed by methicillin-resistant *S. aureus* (Cheng et al., 2011) and can occur in any age group without any underlying illness (Stevens et al., 2014). Rare infection occurs with other bacteria including marine bacteria, *Vibrio vulnificus* and *Aeromonas hydrophila*, and others including *P. aeruginosa* or *H. influenzae* type b. Risk factors for necrotizing fasciitis are numerous with the most common including diabetes, obesity, malignancy, burns, AIDS, and other conditions associated with immunosuppression (Kihiczak et al., 2006).

KEY POINT

Necrotizing fasciitis is a life-threatening and rapidly progressing infection that can cause massive tissue loss. Prompt detection and early aggressive debridement are essential for positive outcomes.

Clinical Presentation

The skin findings typically begin as erythematous, painful, edematous areas on the skin that are often mistaken for cellulitis with rapid evolution. The most common site of involvement is an extremity, but perianal lesions and trunk wounds are also common. Head and facial wounds have also been reported. An early clue for necrotizing fasciitis is pain that is out of proportion to the early physical findings. Another major indicator is rapid progression of the area of involvement within 24 to 72 hours. The erythematous border can advance rapidly, while involved skin becomes gray or dusky in color and serosanguinous blisters begin to form. The infection is able to spread so rapidly because fascia has a relatively poor blood supply. The infection damages and destroys the cutaneous nerves as well as the soft tissues and the skin, later resulting in anesthesia of the involved skin and necrosis of the soft tissues in the involved area. Deeper subcutaneous tissue may become firm on palpation. Patients become progressively more toxic as the disease progresses, with fever, chills, unstable vital signs, and eventually vascular collapse and multiorgan failure.

Diagnosis

The diagnosis of necrotizing fasciitis is made initially clinically and requires a high index of suspicion. It is helpful to use a skin marking pen to indicate the area of initial involvement and to closely monitor the site for rapid progression. Lab values will show an elevated WBC count with a left shift, and a normochromic, normocytic anemia may also be seen. The ESR will be high. CT, MRI, or plain radiographs can be used to identify or rule out free air in the tissues. If present, this is an indicator of gas-producing organisms (Stevens & Bryant, 2017).

Treatment

When necrotizing fasciitis is suspected, an urgent surgical consult is required because, as already noted, the most important aspect of treatment is early and aggressive surgical debridement to eliminate all of the infected tissue. It is the only intervention proven to decrease mortality. Broad-spectrum antibiotic therapy should also be instituted after cultures have been obtained; although penetration to the fascia is low due to the poor blood supply, broad spectrum antibiotic therapy does decrease bacterial loads and levels of bacterial toxins and can reduce the risk of multiorgan failure (Bellapianta et al., 2009). Hyperbaric oxygen therapy (HBOT) has also been reported to be of benefit in controlling bacterial loads and is sometimes used as adjunctive therapy in addition to wide surgical debridement and systemic antibiotics. Supportive care is essential and includes IV fluids, vasopressors if indicated, nutritional support, and management of comorbidities. Once a clean wound bed is established, negative pressure wound therapy is initiated to promote rapid ingrowth of healthy granulation tissue. Flaps and grafts are typically required for final wound closure.

Vibrio vulnificus

Vibrio vulnificus, a type of bacteria found in coastal marine environments, can cause a range of infection severity from localized cellulitis to necrotizing fasciitis and septicemia. *Vibrio vulnificus* is endemic in the United States off the Atlantic and Gulf Coast (Horseman & Surani, 2011), and susceptible patients develop infection through either oral ingestion of raw shellfish, such as oysters, or direct inoculation in the skin from new breaks or existing wounds (Dechet et al., 2008). Aside from consumption of contaminated raw shellfish, exposure usually occurs following skin injury during handling of shellfish, water sports, fishing, or boating. In the United States, the majority of reported cases to the Centers for Disease Control (CDC) come from locations near the Gulf Coast followed by the Atlantic Coast (Dechet et al., 2008). Patients with liver disease are especially susceptible to infection and more severe disease. Other associated comorbidities in those with infection include heart disease, diabetes, and excessive alcohol consumption.

In most individuals, cutaneous infection with the organism results in cellulitis and fever. The cellulitis begins to form within days of exposure at the site of inoculation in the case of skin trauma exposure. They also develop in the majority of individuals with septicemia from ingestion of undercooked shellfish. They begin as painful areas of erythema and edema, which can progress to hemorrhagic bullae and broad erosions with rupture. The skin lesions can present anywhere on the body but are usually seen on the lower extremities (**Fig. 29-9**). The lesions associated with systemic *V. vulnificus* can rapidly progress to ulcers and, at worst,

necrotizing fasciitis and septicemia (Horseman & Surani, 2011), especially in susceptible individuals. The mortality rate for sepsis caused by this organism exceeds 50%, with preexisting advanced liver disease portending a worse prognosis.

Both systemic sepsis and severe localized wound infections caused by *V. vulnificus* are treated with a combination of oral minocycline or doxycycline (100 mg twice a day) and intravenous cefotaxime or ceftriaxone (Liu et al., 2006). Minor wound infections in healthy hosts can be treated with oral minocycline or doxycycline and local wound care.

KEY POINT

Vibrio vulnificus, a type of bacteria found in marine environments, can cause serious cellulitis with hemorrhagic bullae and septicemia in certain individuals who eat contaminated raw shellfish or have skin injury exposure to contaminated coastal waters. The diagnosis can be obtained through standard blood cultures or bacterial wound swab culture.

MYCOBACTERIAL INFECTIONS CAUSING WOUNDS

There are numerous species of mycobacteria, and while most are not common causes of infection, because of a rise in nontuberculous (atypical) mycobacterial infections in healthy and immunocompromised individuals, it is important to understand the potential for infection. Mycobacteria are nonmotile acid-fast bacilli that grow slower than traditional bacteria. Nontuberculous (NTM) mycobacteria refer to types of mycobacteria that are not *Mycobacterium leprae* (the cause of leprosy) or *M. tuberculosis* (the cause of tuberculosis). NTM are found in the environment such as rivers and lakes, tap water, soil, vegetation, and dust (Lamb & Dawn, 2014). Tap water comprises the main reservoir for most NTM pathogens. While infection can occur in healthy individuals, the likelihood of infection increases for those who are immunosuppressed. The means of disease entry is through inhalation, mucosa, or percutaneous penetration (Kullavanijaya, 1999). Chronic lesions that develop at sites of trauma or surgical procedures, especially those that do not respond to standard antibiotic therapy, should prompt the consideration of mycobacterial infection. Infections of the skin by NTM are increasingly common among hospital-acquired infections and following cosmetic procedures (Brown-Elliott et al., 2002). Skin lesions can appear as pustules, keratotic plaques, or nodules with or without purulence and draining sinuses. Nodules may develop in a sporotrichoid (lymphocutaneous) pattern which indicates a linear pattern of development in the direction of lymphatic drainage along the limbs. Immunocompromised individuals may develop nodules that are disseminated. Lesions have

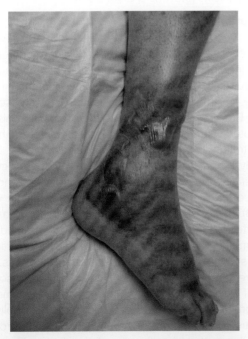

FIGURE 29-9. *Vibrio vulnificus*. Cellulitis with characteristic bullae with hemorrhage.

a variable incubation period ranging from 2 weeks to 9 months depending on the characteristics of the causative *Mycobacterium* and state of immunocompetency of the infected individual (Palenque, 2000). The most common mycobacteria species causing cutaneous NTM disease in the United States and Europe are *Mycobacterium marinum* and the rapidly growing *M. abscessus*, *M. fortuitum*, and *M. chelonae* (Wagner & Young, 2004).

> **KEY POINT**
>
> Chronic lesions that develop at sites of trauma or surgical procedures, especially those that do not respond to standard antibiotic therapy, should prompt the consideration of mycobacterial infection.

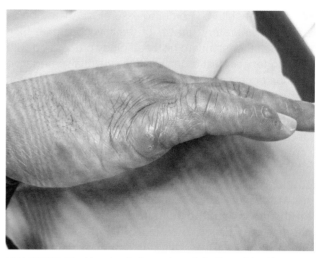

FIGURE 29-10. *Mycobacteria marinum* Infection of the Finger Near the Nail While Fishing with Subsequent Development of Nodules Near the Knuckle and Side of the Hand.

Mycobacterium leprae

Leprosy (also known as Hansen disease) is an infectious disease caused by *M. leprae* and *Mycobacterium lepromatosis* that involves the skin and peripheral nerves. It is rare with only 205 new cases detected in the United States in 2010. Seventy-five percent of new cases are among immigrants. Leprosy is not highly contagious, and very effective treatment is available. Those with immunosuppression are at greatest risk. Infected individuals may develop a broad range of clinical manifestations, which include skin lesions with areas of central anesthesia. Nerve damage is caused by inflammation, causing affected individuals to be more susceptible to injury. In some instances, the nerve damage is due to bacterial infiltration of the nerves. In the United States, this damage is often mistaken for diabetic neuropathy. Diagnosis should be considered in patients with skin lesions and/or enlarged nerve(s) accompanied by sensory loss and requires skin biopsy and PCR testing for *M. leprae*. Treatment of leprosy consists of multiple drug therapy (MDT) with first-line medications including dapsone, rifampin, for a 12-month period for the tuberculoid form and 24 months for the lepromatous form, adding clofazimine in addition (Franco-Paredes et al., 2018).

Mycobacteria marinum

Mycobacteria marinum infection, also known as fish tank granuloma, occurs following trauma and exposure to contaminated water including fresh water, salt water, brackish water, and fish tank water. The infection begins at the site of trauma, often fingers, hands, or arms, as a nodule or verrucous plaque that can emerge as growing nodules in a sporotrichoid or lymphocutaneous pattern (**Fig. 29-10**). Classically this may occur after cleaning an aquarium when the skin was injured. The incubation period from exposure to apparent infection is typically 2 to 3 weeks though can range up to 3 months (Hautmann & Lotti, 1994; Steinbrink et al., 2017).

Rapidly Growing Mycobacteria: *M. abscessus*, *M. fortuitum*, and *M. chelonae*

These organisms are commonly grouped together as the fortuitum complex (Kullavanijaya, 1999) and have similar clinical features including a propensity for skin and soft tissue infection. They are considered mycobacteria rapid growers because their growth on culture is typically faster, often within 1 week, compared to other *Mycobacterium* species that take longer. Infection appears as erythematous or purplish, often nonpainful, nodules at sites of trauma, surgery, or following exposure to surgical instruments. Infection has been reported with these organisms following various procedures including acupuncture, liposuction, tattooing, placement of implants, and after exposure to contaminated water during a pedicure when abscesses formed on the legs (LeBlanc et al., 2012; Winthrop et al., 2002). Contaminated hospital tap water has been implicated as a common source of outbreaks of systemic infection with *M. abscessus* following lung transplantation and cardiac procedures (Baker et al., 2017). When the skin was involved in these outbreaks, sternal wounds were the most common presentation.

Diagnosis

Wound care nurses should have a high level of suspicion for the presence of mycobacteria when wounds or abscesses, especially those following trauma or surgeries, fail to respond to standard antibiotic treatments. For cutaneous infections, identification of the mycobacteria on tissue biopsy culture is important. An alternate means of identification is through skin biopsy samples sent for PCR or 16S ribosomal DNA sequencing. These tests have higher positive detection and identification rates than standard mycobacteria culture, but they do not provide an opportunity to test for antibiotic susceptibilities. It is important for patients to be off of antibiotics at the time of biopsy for culture in order to assure adequate opportunity for laboratory growth of the mycobacteria. Skin biopsy sent for standard histopathology processing with staining for acid-fast organisms may yield false negative findings because of low numbers of organisms present in specimens (Bartralot et al., 2000).

Treatment

Once an organism has been identified and antibiotic susceptibilities have been established, reasonable treatment often involves more than one antibiotic due to the risk of development of resistance. For *M. marinum*, *M. abscessus*, *M. fortuitum*, and *M. chelonae*, empiric treatment with clarithromycin may be reasonable until culture results are received confirming antibiotic susceptibilities. Ideally treatment is not initiated until the susceptibilities are verified. The treatment course includes treating for 1 month beyond clinical clearance which often falls in a 3 to 6 months duration for cutaneous infection. In some cases, treatment may need to be longer. Extensive infection often requires additional intravenous antibiotic treatment. A referral to an infectious disease specialist is typically warranted for appropriate treatment recommendations. Surgical removal can be considered in the case of localized *M. abscessus*, *M. fortuitum*, and *M. chelonae* infection.

 CONCLUSION

Infectious wounds are a common cause of wounds worldwide. Viruses, bacteria, fungi, and mycobacteria can all cause or contribute to wounds. Infections range in severity from common wounds, such as herpes labialis, to severe and life-threatening wounds, such as necrotizing fasciitis. Though many infections do not cause chronic wounds, some infections can cause great damage to the skin and underlying tissues, resulting in lasting morbidity and disability even when the infection has resolved. It is important for the wound care nurse to be aware of the history and physical findings associated with wounds caused by infectious processes and to assure accurate diagnoses. Effective treatment of the underlying infection is the first step in resolving the cutaneous manifestations.

REFERENCES

Aldape, M. J., Bryant, A. E., & Stevens, D. L. (2006). Clostridium sordellii infection: epidemiology, clinical findings, and current perspectives on diagnosis and treatment. *Clinical Infectious Diseases, 43*(11), 1436–1446.

Ameen, M. (2009). Chromoblastomycosis: Clinical presentation and management. *Clinical and Experimental Dermatology, 34*(8), 849–854. doi: 10.1111/j.1365-2230.2009.03415.x.

Baddour, L. M. (2019). Impetigo. In D. J. Sexton, S. L. Kaplan, & T. Rosen (Eds.), *UpToDate*. Waltham, MA: Wolters Kluwer. Accessed April 17, 2020.

Baker, A. W., Lewis, S. S., Alexander, B. D., et al. (2017). Two-phase hospital-associated outbreak of Mycobacterium abscessus: Investigation and mitigation. *Clinical Infectious Diseases, 64*(7), 902–911.

Bartralot, R., Pujol, R. M., Garcnd-Patos, V., et al. (2000). Cutaneous infections due to nontuberculous mycobacteria: Histopathological review of 28 cases. Comparative study between lesions observed in immunosuppressed patients and normal hosts. *Journal of Cutaneous Pathology, 27*(3), 124–129.

Bell-Syer, S. E., Khan, S. M., & Torgerson, D. J. (2012). Oral treatments for fungal infections of the skin of the foot. *Cochrane Database of Systematic Reviews*, (10), CD003584. doi: 10.1002/14651858.CD003584.pub2.

Bellapianta, J. M., Ljungquist, K., Tobin, E., et al. (2009). Necrotizing fasciitis. *Journal of the American Academy of Orthopaedic Surgeons, 17*(3), 174–182.

Bernstein, D. I., Bellamy, A. R., Hook, E. W., III., et al. (2013). Epidemiology, clinical presentation, and antibody response to primary infection with herpes simplex virus type 1 and type 2 in young women. *Clinical Infectious Diseases, 56*(3), 344–351.

Bisno, A. L., & Stevens, D. L. (1996). Streptococcal infections of skin and soft tissues. *New England Journal of Medicine, 334*(4), 240–246.

Black, J. M., Gray, M., Bliss, D. Z., et al. (2011). MASD part 2: Incontinence-associated dermatitis and intertriginous dermatitis. A consensus. *Journal of Wound Ostomy & Continence Nursing, 38*(4), 359–370.

Böni, R., & Nehrhoff, B. (2003). Treatment of gram-negative folliculitis in patients with acne. *American Journal of Clinical Dermatology, 4*(4), 273–276.

Borchers, A. T., & Gershwin, M. E. (2010). The immune response in coccidioidomycosis. *Autoimmunity Reviews, 10*(2), 94–102. doi: 10.1016/j.autrev.2010.08.010.

Brito, A. C. D., & Bittencourt, M. D. J. S. (2018). Chromoblastomycosis: an etiological, epidemiological, clinical, diagnostic, and treatment update. *Anais Brasileiros de Dermatologia, 93*(4), 495–506.

Brown-Elliott, B. A., Griffith, D. E., & Wallace, R. J. (2002). Newly described or emerging human species of nontuberculous mycobacteria. *Infectious Disease Clinics, 16*(1), 187–220.

Cernik, C., Gallina, K., & Brodell, R. T. (2008). The treatment of herpes simplex infections: An evidence-based review. *Archives of Internal Medicine, 168*(11), 1137–1144.

Chang, P., & Rodas, C. (2012). Skin lesions in histoplasmosis. *Clinics in Dermatology, 30*(6), 592–598. doi: 10.1016/j.clindermatol.2012.01.004.

Chowdhary, A., Meis, J. F., Guarro, J., et al. (2014). ESCMID and ECMM joint clinical guidelines for the diagnosis and management of systemic phaeohyphomycosis: Diseases caused by black fungi. *Clinical Microbiology and Infection, 20*, 47–75.

Cheng, N. C., Wang, J. T., Chang, S. C., et al. (2011). Necrotizing fasciitis caused by Staphylococcus aureus: The emergence of methicillin-resistant strains. *Annals of Plastic Surgery, 67*, 632–636.

Cohen, K. R., Salbu, R. L., Frank, J., et al. (2013). Presentation and management of herpes zoster (shingles) in the geriatric population. *Pharmacy and Therapeutics, 38*(4), 217.

Corey, L., Adams, H. G., Brown, Z. A., et al. (1983). Genital herpes simplex virus infections: Clinical manifestations, course, and complications. *Annals of Internal Medicine, 98*(6), 958–972.

Crawford, F., & Hollis, S. (2007). Topical treatments for fungal infections of the skin and nails of the foot. *Cochrane Database of Systematic Reviews*, (3), CD001434.

De Araujo, T., Marques, A. C., & Kerdel, F. (2001). Sporotrichosis. *International Journal of Dermatology, 40*(12), 737–742.

Dechet, A. M., Yu, P. A., Koram, N., et al. (2008). Nonfoodborne Vibrio infections: An important cause of morbidity and mortality in the United States, 1997–2006. *Clinical Infectious Diseases, 46*(7), 970–976.

Fehr, T., Bossart, W., Wahl, C., et al. (2002). Disseminated varicella infection in adult renal allograft recipients: Four cases and a review of the literature. *Transplantation, 73*, 608–611.

Franco-Paredes, C., Marcos, L. A., Henao-Martínez, A. F., et al. (2018). Cutaneous mycobacterial infections. *Clinical Microbiology Reviews, 32*(1), e00069.

Furlan, K. C., Kakizaki, P., Chartuni, J. C. N., et al. (2017). Sycosiform tinea barbae caused by trichophyton rubrum and its association with autoinoculation. *Anais Brasileiros de Dermatologia, 92*(1), 160–161.

Galgiani, J. N., Catanzaro, A., Cloud, G. A., et al. (2000). Comparison of oral fluconazole and itraconazole for progressive, nonmeningeal coccidioidomycosis. A randomized, double-blind trial. Mycoses Study Group. *Annals of Internal Medicine, 133*(9), 676–86.

Garcia Garcia, S. C., Salas Alanis, J. C., Flores, M. G., et al. (2015). Coccidioidomycosis and the skin: A comprehensive review. *Anais Brasileiros de Dermatologia, 90*(5), 610–619. doi: 10.1590/abd1806-4841.20153805.

Goolamali, S. I., Fogo, A., Killian, L., et al. (2009). Ecthyma gangrenosum: An important feature of pseudomonal sepsis in a previously well child. *Clinical and Experimental Dermatology, 34*(5), e180–e182. doi: 10.1111/j.1365-2230.2008.03020.x.

Gray, M., Black, J. M., Baharestani, M. M., et al. (2011). Moisture-associated skin damage: overview and pathophysiology. *Journal of Wound Ostomy & Continence Nursing, 38*(3), 233–241.

Gupta, A. K., Mays, R. R., Versteeg, S. G., et al. (2018). Tinea capitis in children: A systematic review of management. *Journal of European Academy of Dermatology & Venereology, 32*(12), 2264–2274. doi: 10.1111/jdv.15088.

Gupta, R., Warren, T., & Wald, A. (2007). Genital herpes. *The Lancet, 370*(9605), 2127–2137.

Harbecke, R., Oxman, M. N., Arnold, B. A., et al. (2009). A real-time PCR assay to identify and discriminate among wild-type and vaccine strains of varicella-zoster virus and herpes simplex virus in clinical specimens, and comparison with the clinical diagnoses. *Journal of Medical Virology, 81*(7), 1310–1322.

Harpaz, R., Ortega-Sanchez, I. R., & Seward, J. F. (2008). Prevention of herpes zoster: Recommendations of the Advisory Committee on Immunization Practices (ACIP). *Morbidity and Mortality Weekly Report: Recommendations and Reports, 57*(5), 1–30.

Hautmann, G., & Lotti, T. (1994). Atypical mycobacterial infections of the skin. *Dermatologic Clinics, 12*(4), 657–668.

Hay, R. J., & Ashbee, H. R. (2016). Fungal infections. In C. Griffiths, J. Barker, T. Bleiker, et al. (Eds.), *Rook's Textbook of Dermatology* (9th ed., pp. 1–110). Hoboken, NJ: Wiley-Blackwell.

Horseman, M. A., & Surani, S. (2011). A comprehensive review of *Vibrio vulnificus*: An important cause of severe sepsis and skin and soft-tissue infection. *International Journal of Infectious Diseases, 15*(3), e157–e166. doi: 10.1016/j.ijid.2010.11.003.

Jemec, G. B. (2012). Hidradenitis suppurativa. *New England Journal of Medicine, 366*(2), 158–164.

Johnson, P. C., Wheat, L. J., Cloud, G. A., et al. (2002). Safety and efficacy of liposomal amphotericin B compared with conventional amphotericin B for induction therapy of histoplasmosis in patients with AIDS. *Annals of Internal Medicine, 137*(2), 105–109.

Kalra, M. G., Higgins, K. E., & Kinney, B. S. (2014). Intertrigo and secondary skin infections. *American Family Physician, 89*(7), 569–573.

Kauffman, C. A., Bustamante, B., Chapman, S. W., et al. (2007). Clinical practice guidelines for the management of sporotrichosis: 2007 update by the Infectious Diseases Society of America. *Clinical Infectious Diseases, 45*(10), 1255–1265.

Kawai, K., Gebremeskel, B. G., & Acosta, C. J. (2014). Systematic review of incidence and complications of herpes zoster: Towards a global perspective. *BMJ open, 4*(6), e004833.

Khamnuan, P., Chongruksut, W., Jearwattanakanok, K., et al. (2015). Necrotizing fasciitis: Epidemiology and clinical predictors for amputation. *International Journal of General Medicine, 8*, 195.

Kihiczak, G. G., Schwartz, R. A., & Kapila, R. (2006). Necrotizing fasciitis: A deadly infection. *Journal of the European Academy of Dermatology and Venereology, 20*(4), 365–369. doi: 10.1111/j.1468-3083.2006.01487.x.

Koning, S., Mohammedamin, R. S. A., Van Der Wouden, J. C., et al. (2006). Impetigo: Incidence and treatment in Dutch general practice in 1987 and 2001—results from two national surveys.

British Journal of Dermatology, 154(2), 239–243. doi: 10.1111/j.1365-2133.2005.06766.x.

Kullavanijaya, P. (1999). Atypical mycobacterial cutaneous infection. *Clinics in Dermatology, 17*(2), 153–158.

Lamb, R. C., & Dawn, G. (2014). Cutaneous non-tuberculous mycobacterial infections. *International Journal of Dermatology, 53*(10), 1197–1204. doi: 10.1111/ijd.12528.

Laureano, A. C., Schwartz, R. A., & Cohen, P. J. (2014). Facial bacterial infections: Folliculitis. *Clinics in Dermatology, 32*(6), 711–714.

LeBlanc, P. M., Hollinger, K. A., & Klontz, K. C. (2012). Tattoo ink–related infections—awareness, diagnosis, reporting, and prevention. *New England Journal of Medicine, 367*(11), 985–987. doi: 10.1056/NEJMp1206063.

Liu, J. W., Lee, K., Tang, H. J., et al. (2006). Prognostic factors and antibiotics in Vibrio vulnificus septicemia. *Archives of Internal Medicine, 166*(19), 2117–2123.

Lopez, F. A., & Lartchenko, S. (2006). Skin and soft tissue infections. *Infectious Disease Clinics of North America, 20*(4), 759–72.

Lopez-Martinez, R., & Mendez-Tovar, L. J. (2012). Blastomycosis. *Clinics in Dermatology, 30*(6), 565–572. doi: 10.1016/j.clindermatol.2012.01.002.

Mackool, B. T., Goverman, J., & Nazarian, R. M. (2012). Case 14–2012: A 43-year-old woman with fever and a generalized rash. *New England Journal of Medicine, 366*(19), 1825–1834. doi: 10.1056/NEJMcpc1111572.

Mattison, H. R., Reichman, R. C., Benedetti, J., et al. (1988). Double-blind, placebo-controlled trial comparing long-term suppressive with short-term oral acyclovir therapy for management of recurrent genital herpes. *The American Journal of Medicine, 85*(2A), 20–25.

McGirr, A., Widenmaier, R., Curran, D., et al. (2019). The comparative efficacy and safety of herpes zoster vaccines: A network meta-analysis. *Vaccine, 37*(22), 2896–2909.

McQuillan, G. M., Kruszon-Moran, D., Flagg, E. W., et al. (2018). Prevalence of herpes simplex virus type 1 and type 2 in persons aged 14–49: United States, 2015–2016. *NCHS Data Brief*, (304), 1–8. US Department of Health and Human Services, Centers for Disease Control and Prevention, National Center for Health Statistics.

Mirmirani, P., & Tucker, L. Y. (2013). Epidemiologic trends in pediatric tinea capitis: A population-based study from Kaiser Permanente Northern California. *Journal of the American Academy of Dermatology, 69*(6), 916–921. doi: 10.1016/j.jaad.2013.08.031.

Mohammedamin, R. S., van der Wouden, J. C., Koning, S., et al. (2006). Increasing incidence of skin disorders in children? A comparison between 1987 and 2001. *BMC Dermatology, 6*(1), 4. doi: 10.1186/1471-5945-6-4.

Ortega, E. (2019). Postherpetic neuralgia. In J. M. Shefner (Ed.), *UpTo-Date*. Waltham, MA: Wolters Kluwer. Accessed April 17, 2020.

Palenque, E. (2000). Skin disease and nontuberculous atypical mycobacteria. *International Journal of Dermatology, 39*(9), 659–666.

Pappas, A. A., & Ray, T. L. (1998). Cutaneous and disseminated skin manifestations of candidiasis. In B. E. Elewski (Ed.), *Cutaneous fungal infections* (2nd ed.). Boston, MA: Blackwell Science.

Pappagianis, D. (1993). Coccidioidomycosis. *Seminars in Dermatology, 12*(4), 301–309.

Peralta, G., Padron, E., Roiz, M. P., et al. (2006). Risk factors for bacteremia in patients with limb cellulitis. *European Journal of Clinical Microbiology and Infectious Diseases, 25*(10), 619–626.

Phoenix, G., Das, S., & Joshi, M. (2012). Diagnosis and management of cellulitis. *BMJ, 345*, e4955. doi: 10.1136/bmj.e4955.

Queiroz-Telles, F., de Hoog, S., Santos, D. W. C., et al. (2017). Chromoblastomycosis. *Clinical Microbiology Reviews, 30*(1), 233–276.

Ramchandani, M., Kong, M., Tronstein, E., et al. (2016). Herpes simplex virus type 1 shedding in tears, and nasal and oral mucosa of healthy adults. *Sexually Transmitted Diseases, 43*(12), 756.

Ramos-e-Silva, M., Vasconcelos, C., Carneiro, S., et al. (2007). Sporotrichosis. *Clinics in Dermatology, 25*(2), 181–187. doi: 10.1016/j.clindermatol.2006.05.006.

Ratliff, C. R., Yates, S., McNichol, L., et al. (2016). Compression for primary prevention, treatment, and prevention of recurrence of venous leg ulcers: An evidence-and consensus-based algorithm for care across the continuum. *Journal of Wound, Ostomy, and Continence Nursing, 43*(4), 347.

Reich, H. L., Fadeyi, D. W., Naik, N. S., et al. (2004). Nonpseudomonal ecthyma gangrenosum. *Journal of the American Academy of Dermatology, 50*(5), 114–117.

Reichman, R. C., Badger, G. J., Mertz, G. J., et al. (1984). Treatment of recurrent genital herpes simplex infections with oral acyclovir: a controlled trial. *JAMA, 251*(16), 2103–2107.

Saccente, M., & Woods, G. L. (2010). Clinical and laboratory update on blastomycosis. *Clinical Microbiology Reviews, 23*(2), 367–381.

Sarkar, S., Patra, A. K., & Mondal, M. (2016). Ecthyma gangrenosum in the periorbital region in a previously healthy immunocompetent woman without bacteremia. *Indian Dermatology Online Journal, 7*(1), 36–39.

Spruance, S. L., Overall, J. C., Jr., Kern, E. R., et al. (1977). The natural history of recurrent herpes simplex labialis: Implications for antiviral therapy. *New England Journal of Medicine, 297*(2), 69–75.

Steinbrink, J., Alexis, M., Angulo-Thompson, D., et al. (2017). Mycobacterium marinum remains an unrecognized cause of indolent skin infections. *Cutis, 100*(5), 331–336.

Stevens, D. L., Bisno, A. L., Chambers, H. F., et al. (2014). Practice guidelines for the diagnosis and management of skin and soft tissue infections: 2014 update by the Infectious Diseases Society of America. *Clinical Infectious Diseases, 59*(2), e10–e52.

Stevens, D. L., & Bryant, A. E. (2017). Necrotizing soft-tissue infections. *New England Journal of Medicine, 377*(23), 2253–2265.

Strazzula, L., Cotliar, J., Fox, L. P., et al. (2015). Inpatient dermatology consultation aids diagnosis of cellulitis among hospitalized patients: A multi-institutional analysis. *Journal of the American Academy of Dermatology, 73*(1), 70–75. doi: 10.1016/j.jaad.2014.11.012.

Usatine, R., & Tinitigan, R. (2010). Nongenital herpes simplex virus. *American Family Physician, 82*(9), 1075–1082.

Vallabhaneni, S., & Chiller, T. M. (2016). Fungal infections and new biologic therapies. *Current Rheumatology Reports, 18*(5), 29.

Wagner, D., & Young, L. S. (2004). Nontuberculous mycobacterial infections: a clinical review. *Infection, 32*(5), 257–270.

Winthrop, K. L., Abrams, M., Yakrus, M., et al. (2002). An outbreak of mycobacterial furunculosis associated with footbaths at a nail salon. *New England Journal of Medicine, 346*(18), 1366–1371.

Wong, C. J., & Stevens, D. L. (2013). Serious group A streptococcal infections. *Medical Clinics of North America, 97*(4), 721–736.

Workowski, K. A. (2015). Centers for Disease Control and Prevention sexually transmitted diseases treatment guidelines. *Clinical Infectious Diseases, 61*(Suppl 8), S759–S762.

Wound, Ostomy, and Continence Nurses Society (WOCN). (2019). *Guideline for the management of wounds in patients with lower-extremity venous disease.* Mt. Laurel, NJ: Author.

Yawn, B. P., Saddier, P., Wollan, P. C., et al. (November, 2007). A population-based study of the incidence and complication rates of herpes zoster before zoster vaccine introduction. *Mayo Clinic Proceedings, 82*(11), 1341–1349.

QUESTIONS

1. The wound care nurse is devising a treatment plan for a patient diagnosed with their first episode this year of recurrent severe orolabial herpes (HSV-1). Which therapy is recommended?
   A. Topical antiviral agents alone
   B. Systemic antivirals initiated within 72 hours of onset of symptoms
   C. Chronic suppressive therapy
   D. Systemic antivirals and chronic suppressive treatment

2. The wound care nurse is teaching new nurses how to recognize and treat erosions from herpes simplex. Which statement accurately describes this disease process and the recommended treatment?
   A. Herpes lesions are full-thickness wounds that should be kept dry.
   B. Herpes lesions should be treated with moist wound healing principles.
   C. Recurrent episodes of genital herpes tend to be more severe than primary.
   D. Recurrences of genital herpes are more common with HSV-1 infection than with HSV-2.

3. Which patient would the wound care nurse place at higher risk for developing zoster (shingles)?
   A. A 32-year-old patient who has never had chickenpox
   B. A 47-year-old patient who has active genital herpes
   C. A 12-year-old patient who was immunized for varicella–zoster virus
   D. A 79-year-old patient who had chicken pox as a child

4. The wound care nurse is assessing a patient who presents with a red and inflamed kerion-like lesion in the beard area, with hair that is easily removed. The patient states his occupation as cattle farmer. What disease state would the wound care nurse suspect?
   A. Tinea barbae
   B. Tinea pedis
   C. *Candida albicans*
   D. Candidal intertrigo

5. A pediatric nurse is assessing a rash on the face of a 4-year-old patient. The rash contains red macules and vesicles that have ruptured and caused a "honey-colored" crust. What common childhood skin infection would the nurse suspect?
   A. Ecthyma gangrenosum
   B. Impetigo
   C. Tinea capitis
   D. Cellulitis

6. Which skin condition requires immediate recognition by the wound care nurse, as it is usually an indicator of bacteremia and actual or impending sepsis?
A. Ecthyma gangrenosum
B. Gram-negative folliculitis
C. Cellulitis
D. Bullous impetigo in an adult

7. What is the reference standard test for diagnosis of skin infection with nontuberculous mycobacteria?
A. Culture of skin biopsy tissue for mycobacteria
B. Routine swab for culture
C. Appearance of mycobacteria organisms on histology
D. Staining purulent exudate for acid-fast bacilli

8. The wound care nurse is developing a treatment plan for a patient with hidradenitis suppurativa. Which measure is recommended for this chronic condition?

A. Maintaining tight glycemic control
B. Wearing tighter clothing to protect against bacterial invasion
C. Daily oral doxycycline or minocycline
D. Atraumatic hair removal and topical antibacterial and antibiotic agents

9. The wound care nurse is planning treatment for a patient diagnosed with mild cellulitis. Which action is recommended?
A. Taking culture swabs from intact skin
B. Systemic antibiotic therapy with an agent that covers MSSA
C. Ordering blood cultures
D. Surgical debridement of the lesions

10. The wound care nurse documents type 2 necrotizing fasciitis on a patient chart. What is the typical causative factor for this type of infection?
A. Non–group A *Streptococcus*
B. *Streptococcus pyogenes*
C. *Vibrio vulnificus*
D. Methicillin-sensitive *Staphylococcus aureus*

ANSWERS AND RATIONALES

1. B. Rationale: For episodes of recurrent outbreaks of HSV, treatment should be initiated within the first 72 hours from the time of onset of the prodromal symptoms of pain, tingling, or pruritus. In general, there is no role for topical antiviral therapy due to lack benefit.

2. B. Rationale: Herpes lesions are partial-thickness wounds and should be treated with moist wound healing principles.

3. D. Rationale: Age is the greatest risk factor for the development of herpes zoster, especially after the age of 50 most likely due to the age-related decrease in cellular immunity, which allows the VZV to replicate and cause disease.

4. A. Rationale: Cattle and horses are the usual source of the fungi *T. mentagrophytes* and *T. verrucosum*. Tinea barbae infection is most common in men working in the agricultural business.

5. B. Rationale: Nonbullous impetigo begins as red macules that progress to vesicles that rupture and leave a classic honey-colored crust.

6. A. Rationale: Ecthyma gangrenosum develops in immunocompromised individuals due to bacterial invasion of blood vessels and is a sign of *Pseudomonas* bacteremia and impending sepsis.

7. A. Rationale: For cutaneous infections, identification of the mycobacteria on tissue biopsy culture is important.

8. C. Rationale: Medical management of HS includes washing the affected areas with antiseptic solutions to reduce commensal bacteria, daily oral doxycycline or minocycline, and daily topical clindamycin.

9. B. Rationale: In the case of cellulitis that occurs in the absence of any visible wound or purulent drainage, cultures are of no benefit, and empiric antibiotics should be prescribed that target MSSA and beta-hemolytic *Streptococcus*.

10. B. Rationale: Type II necrotizing fasciitis is due to monomicrobial infection most commonly with *Streptococcus pyogenes* followed by methicillin-resistant *Staphylococcus aureus*.

CHAPTER 30

WOUNDS CAUSED BY DERMATOLOGIC CONDITIONS

Danielle Pecone, Ashwin G. Agarwal, and Adela Rambi Cardones

OBJECTIVES

1. Describe the pathology, clinical presentation, and management of blistering skin diseases such as pemphigus vulgaris and bullous pemphigoid.

2. Differentiate between Stevens-Johnson syndrome and toxic epidermal necrolysis and outline management guidelines for both of these conditions.

3. Explain the basic pathology and management of psoriasis.

4. Explain the difference in pathology and presentation of irritant contact dermatitis and allergic contact dermatitis and discuss management guidelines.

TOPIC OUTLINE

INTRODUCTION

Correction of etiologic factors is an important step for effective wound management. Some wounds are caused by dermatologic conditions that cause acute inflammation of the epidermal and dermal layers, or epidermal loss. The wound care nurse needs to be knowledgeable regarding dermatologic conditions that can cause skin and tissue loss and should assure appropriate workup and treatment when there is reason to suspect that dermatologic pathology is causing or contributing to the wound. This chapter focuses on dermatologic conditions associated with skin and tissue loss.

AUTOIMMUNE BLISTERING SKIN DISEASES (PEMPHIGUS VULGARIS AND BULLOUS PEMPHIGOID)

Pemphigus vulgaris (PV) is the most common form of the pemphigus category of cutaneous diseases. It is a potentially life-threatening autoimmune blistering disorder, characterized by the formation of flaccid intraepithelial skin layer blisters (**Fig. 30-1**) and the loss of skin cell adhesion in the epidermal layer of the skin as well as the mucous membranes (**Fig. 30-2**). The underlying pathology involves development of self-antibodies to cell adhesion molecules. This triggers an immune reaction, which causes destruction of cell-to-cell connections and results in separation of cells and cell layers. PV itself is a rare disease, with an incidence reported between 0.1% and 0.5% per 100,000 people per year, although rates are higher among those of Jewish ancestry and those from Southeast Europe, India, and the Middle East (Kneisel & Hertl, 2011). The average age of onset is between 40 and 60 years, with a reported equivalent or close to equivalent sex ratio (Joly & Litrowski, 2011).

KEY POINT

The pathology of blistering pemphigoid skin disorders is development of antibodies to cell adhesion molecules, which causes breakdown of cell-to-cell and skin layer-to-skin layer connections and results in blister formation.

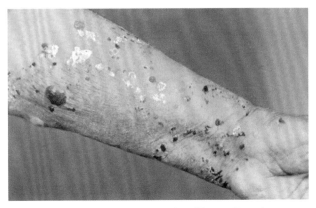

FIGURE 30-1. Pemphigus Vulgaris Skin Blisters. Pemphigus vulgaris blisters on the forearm. (Reprinted with permission from Smeltzer, S., & Bare, B. (2000). *Brunner and Suddarth's textbook of medical-surgical nursing* (9th ed.). Philadelphia, PA: Lippincott Williams & Wilkins.)

Bullous pemphigoid (BP) is another autoimmune blistering skin disease that is characterized by tense subepithelial blisters of the skin and erosive mucous membrane lesions (**Fig. 30-3**). The blisters and erosions are caused by the deposition of autoantibodies within the basement membrane, which is located below the epidermis but above the dermis. The dermal papillae lie just under this membrane (**Fig. 30-2**). Just as with pemphigus, there is a subsequent immune system–mediated activation and destruction of skin cells bound to the antibodies. It is a disease of older adults, usually over the age of

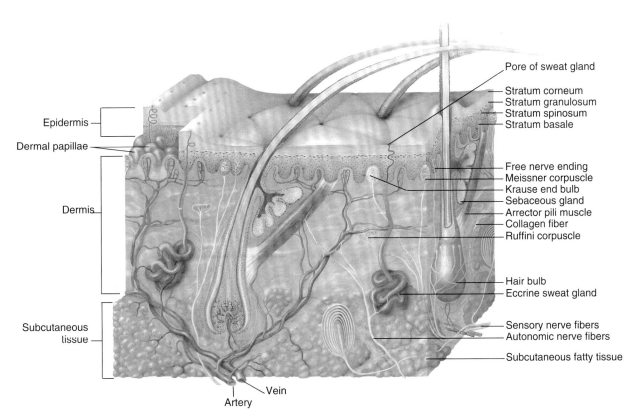

Epidermis

Dermal papillae

Dermis

Subcutaneous tissue

Vein

Artery

Pore of sweat gland

Stratum corneum
Stratum granulosum
Stratum spinosum
Stratum basale

Free nerve ending
Meissner corpuscle
Krause end bulb
Sebaceous gland
Arrector pili muscle
Collagen fiber
Ruffini corpuscle

Hair bulb
Eccrine sweat gland

Sensory nerve fibers
Autonomic nerve fibers

Subcutaneous fatty tissue

FIGURE 30-2. Layers of the Skin Graphic. Layers of the skin (epidermis and dermis), associated adnexa, and underlying subcutaneous tissue.

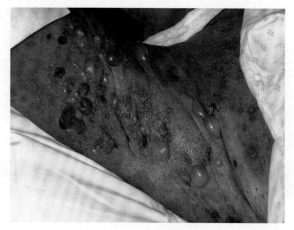

FIGURE 30-3. Bullous Pemphigoid Skin Blisters. Axilla bullae in bullous pemphigoid.

60 years, with incidence rates cited as 4 to 22 cases per million individuals per year (Joly et al., 2012; Marazza et al., 2009). It is the most common autoimmune blistering skin disease in Europe but may be seen more in countries such as Malaysia and Thailand (Kulthanan et al., 2011). Data suggest a slight female predominance in BP, although the reason is unknown (Marazza et al., 2009).

KEY POINT

PV causes destruction of cell-to-cell connections within the epidermis and causes flaccid intraepithelial blisters. BP causes separation between the epidermal and dermal layers and results in formation of tense blisters.

PATHOLOGY

PV is mediated by IgG autoantibodies that target protein components of desmosomes which are important in maintaining epidermal cell-to-cell adhesion and skin integrity with specific targets including the desmoglein-1 (Dsg1) and/or desmoglein-3 (Dsg3) components of desmosomes (Amagai et al., 1999). With BP, the IgG autoantibodies target two major hemidesmosomal proteins: bullous pemphigoid antigen 180 (BP 180) and bullous pemphigoid antigen 230 (BP 230). These proteins normally function to maintain tight adherence between epithelial cells and the underlying basement membrane layer (Kasperkiewicz et al., 2012). Understanding the pathology and the specific proteins targeted by the autoantibodies helps to explain differences in clinical presentation among patients with PV and those with BP. Patients with PV demonstrate flaccid, intraepithelial blisters since the proteins targeted are those that maintain cell-to-cell adhesion of epidermal cells. Patients with BP present with tense, subepithelial blisters because the autoantibodies target the proteins that maintain adhesion between the epidermis and basement membrane layers.

CLINICAL PRESENTATION

Patients with PV present with flaccid bullae, skin erosions, and possibly mucous membrane erosions. Most PV patients do develop mucosal involvement, and these lesions most commonly occur in the oral cavity (**Fig. 30-4**). Other sites include the conjunctivae, nose, esophagus, vulva, vagina, cervix, and anus. There can be significant pain associated with PV lesions, and oral lesions can compromise chewing and swallowing, resulting in poor dietary intake and weight loss. Patients with oral lesions may also complain of hoarseness. Intact PV blisters are flaccid and easily ruptured, and these patients typically have a positive Nikolsky sign, that is, mechanical pressure applied to normal skin or the edge of blisters results in new blister formation or extension of the existing blister and sloughing of the epidermis (Venugopal & Murrell, 2011). The end result is painful erosions that bleed easily.

BP may begin with a prodromal phase of weeks to months preceding blister appearance. This phase is characterized by a pruritic, eczema-like skin rash or urticarial plaques (Kasperkiewicz et al., 2012). The classic blisters are tense bullae on an erythematous or urticarial base. They are numerous, widely distributed, 1 to 3 cm in diameter (see **Fig. 30-3**), and often associated with intense itching. The blisters eventually rupture, resulting in weeping erosions with crust formation. The lesions resolve without scarring (**Fig. 30-5**). The commonly involved areas include the trunk, underarms, and groins, and extremity flexures (Yancey & Egan, 2000). Mucosal erosions are seen in about 10% to 30% of patients with

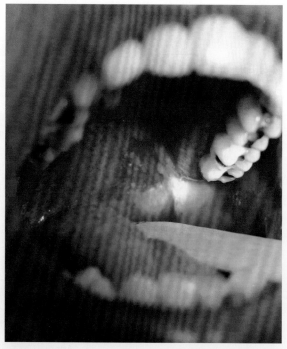

FIGURE 30-4. Pemphigus Vulgaris Oral Lesions. Oral mucosal pemphigus vulgaris lesion.

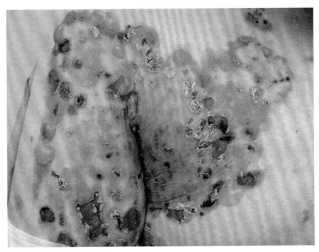

FIGURE 30-5. Bullous Pemphigoid Crusts/Weeping Erosions from Burst Bullae. Bullous pemphigoid lesions seen in various stages of development including tense bullae, weeping erosions, and crusts.

BP (Kneisel & Hertl, 2011) and present as erosive gingivitis or inflammation of the mucosa. Localized forms of BP occur in up to 30% of patients, with lesions found on the lower legs, sites of trauma, or the anogenital region (Tran & Mutasim, 2005).

> **KEY POINT**
>
> Most patients with PV and some patients with BP develop mucosal lesions, commonly oral lesions.

The typical clinical course for both PV and BP is one of chronicity, characterized by recurrent episodes of relapse and remission over months to years, with lesions at varying stages depending on the level of disease control. BP patients have reported remission rates of up to 50% following 3 years of treatment (Venning & Wojnarowska, 1992). Polansky et al. (2019) conducted a retrospective chart review on 20 patients who received at least 1 dose of rituximab therapy, either as initial therapy for severe BP or as therapy for recalcitrant disease after having failed conventional immunotherapies. Seventy-five percent of patients ($n = 15$) achieved remission an average of 169 days following rituximab therapy (Polansky et al., 2019).

> **KEY POINT**
>
> The typical clinical course for both PV and BP is one of chronicity, characterized by recurrent episodes of relapse and remission over months to years.

DIAGNOSIS

The gold standard for diagnosing PV or BP remains direct immunofluorescence (DIF) of the adjacent, unaffected skin. Patients with PV will demonstrate a characteristic interepithelial IgG deposition, whereas patients with BP demonstrate linear IgG and C3 complement in the basement membrane (Jordan et al., 1971). A 4-mm punch biopsy at the edge of a blister or erosion can also aid in the diagnosis. Histologic findings characteristic of PV include detachment of epithelial cells but retention of the basal layer of the epidermis, which resembles a row of tombstones. In contrast, BP is characterized by detachment of the basal epidermal layer from the basement membrane separating the epidermis and dermis. The infiltrate in BP tends to be eosinophil rich, sometimes forming small abscesses. In the urticarial phase, significant dermal edema may also be present (Elder et al., 2009).

MANAGEMENT

PV varies in severity from relatively mild to life threatening, and therapy must be tailored to the severity of the disease as well as the patient's age and comorbidities (Hooten et al., 2014). For mild disease, therapy with topical corticosteroids is usually sufficient. For moderate to severe disease, systemic corticosteroid therapy (prednisone 1 to 1.5 mg/kg/d) is highly effective in controlling active disease. There are significant adverse side effects and risks associated with chronic systemic corticosteroid therapy including high blood pressure, the development of diabetes mellitus, osteoporosis, increased risk of infection, gastrointestinal ulcers, weight gain, and bone necrosis. For this reason, long-term therapy should involve adjuvant or, when possible, primary therapy with steroid-sparing agents such as azathioprine and mycophenolate mofetil (Hooten et al., 2014). Rituximab immunotherapy has been reported to be effective in treating refractory disease (Hooten et al., 2014; Kasperkiewicz et al., 2011; Martin et al., 2011). Rituximab received an FDA indication for the treatment of Pemphigus in 2018 (Kridin et al., 2019). The drug works by down-regulating autoantibody secreting plasma cell precursors and desmoglein-specific CD4+ T-cells (Kridin et al., 2019). A standardized dosing schedule and optimal duration of treatment for rituximab in the treatment of PV has yet to be established. Studies have suggested that rituximab can be used successfully as a first-line agent (Craythorne et al., 2011; Joly et al., 2017).

Similar principles apply to the treatment of BP. First-line therapy for mild to moderate disease is topical therapy, whereas moderate to severe disease often requires systemic immunomodulation. Even in the presence of extensive disease, therapy with high-potency topical steroids (such as clobetasol 0.05% ointment) may be attempted. This may be as effective as systemic corticosteroid therapy, but with fewer associated side effects (Joly et al., 2002). Systemic anti-inflammatory agents, such as tetracyclines, may also be helpful for some patients. Adjuvant long-term steroid-sparing agents, such as azathioprine, mycophenolate mofetil, and methotrexate, are recommended to minimize the risk of adverse effects from chronic steroid therapy. Biologic agents such as rituximab and intravenous immunoglobulin (IVIG) are additional options for treatment of refractory disease.

Evidence-based wound care is important to promote wound healing and to reduce infection risk for patients with either PV or BP. It is appropriate to puncture and drain large blisters in a sterile environment. The epithelial roof should be left intact after drainage to provide wound coverage. Open wounds should be managed with principles of moist wound healing. Dressings should be selected with the goals of managing exudate, maintaining a moist wound bed, and providing atraumatic removal. Adhesive dressings are usually contraindicated due to the potential for further epidermal trauma with removal. Nonadhesive contact layer dressings, foam dressings, or gel dressings are generally preferred and should be secured with wrap gauze, binders, or other alternatives to adhesive securement. Twice-daily application of high-potency topical corticosteroids such as clobetasol propionate ointment or gel may be used as adjunct to systemic therapy and has been shown to promote healing of erosions (Bystryn & Rudolph, 2005). It is important to maintain a clinical index of suspicion for bacterial or viral superinfection of PV wounds, likely due to immunosuppression and often caused by herpes simplex. If superinfection occurs, it should be treated appropriately, either with oral antibiotics or with antiviral therapy, because infection may delay healing and worsen existing lesions (Caldarola et al., 2008).

KEY POINT

Management of blistering skin conditions involves topical and systemic corticosteroids. Open wounds should be managed with principles of moist wound healing, specifically management of exudate, maintenance of a moist wound environment, and avoidance of trauma with dressing removal.

 STEVENS-JOHNSON SYNDROME/ TOXIC EPIDERMAL NECROLYSIS

Stevens-Johnson syndrome (SJS) and toxic epidermal necrolysis (TEN) are severe, life-threatening immune system–mediated skin and mucous membrane disorders characterized by significant epidermal necrosis and detachment and often resulting from a drug reaction. They are considered as two variants of the same skin disease and are differentiated by disease severity and the percentage of body surface area (BSA) affected by the associated erosions and blisters. SJS is characterized by skin fragility, detachment, and denudation involving >10% BSA in addition to widespread macules or flat atypical targetoid lesions. Lesions typically involve the trunk and face. Mucous membrane involvement is present in over 90% of patients. TEN is considered more severe, with a proposed definition of skin detachment involving >30% BSA (Bastuji-Garin et al., 1993). In addition to large areas of epidermal denudation, patients present with widespread erythematous macules or flat targetoid lesions and with mucous membrane involvement. Both SJS and TEN typically cause systemic symptoms that include fever and respiratory distress.

KEY POINT

SJS and TEN are frequently caused by a drug reaction and are characterized by skin fragility, epidermal detachment, and extensive denudation. Mucous membrane involvement is present in >90% of cases. TEN is the more severe form, with >30% BSA involvement.

The estimated incidence of SJS/TEN ranges from 1–2 to 7 cases per million people per year, with SJS being more common. The ratio of SJS to TEN is approximately 3 cases to 1 (Chan et al., 1990; Woolum et al., 2019). These conditions are more than one hundred times more common among HIV-infected individuals as compared to the general population and are also more common in women than men (Mittmann et al., 2012). Mortality rates are estimated to be approximately 10% for SJS and more than 30% for TEN (Sekula et al., 2013).

PATHOLOGY

Although not fully understood, SJS and TEN are thought to be mediated by a T-cell–mediated destruction of skin epithelial cells. Once activated by a particular drug or infection, an inflammatory cascade ensues that leads to epithelial cell death, blistering, and partial to full necrosis of the epidermis (Nassif et al., 2004). Various T-cell protein mediators of cell death are elevated in patients with SJS and TEN, lending further support to the hypothesis that these conditions are autoimmune in origin. For example, the blister fluid level of granulysin, a cytotoxic protein secreted by killer T cells, has been shown to be elevated in these patients and correlates with disease severity (Chung et al., 2008). Soluble Fas ligand, a protein involved in a different cell death pathway, is also found in high concentrations in the blister fluid of these patients (Murata et al., 2008).

CLINICAL PRESENTATION

The prodromal phase is manifested by fever (usually >38°C) and influenza-like symptoms including malaise, muscle pains, and aches. These symptoms occur 1 to 3 days before the onset of skin lesions. During this phase, patients may also complain of visual problems, itching or burning of the eyes, and pain with swallowing. Some patients develop a nonspecific and diffuse red rash prior to appearance of the classic SJS/TEN lesions. It is important to suspect SJS/TEN whenever patients present with fever >38°C, mucosal inflammation, skin tenderness, and blistering (Bircher, 2005). When the reaction is caused by a medication, the cutaneous lesions usually appear within the first 8 weeks of treatment in both children and adults. The most commonly implicated medication is allopurinol. Other drugs commonly associated with SJS/TEN include anticonvulsants (e.g., phenobarbital, carbamazepine, lamotrigine), sulfonamide drugs, nevirapine, and NSAIDs (Halevy et al., 2008). A newer class of anticancer drugs, the checkpoint inhibitors, have been associated with SJS-like reactions (Coleman et al., 2019). These drugs are frequently used in cases of metastatic cancers. Several case reports have associated PD-1 checkpoint inhibitors, nivolumab and pembrolizumab, with SJS/TEN skin eruptions (Logan et al., 2019; Nayar et al., 2016; Robinson et al., 2019; Salati et al., 2018; Shah et al., 2018).

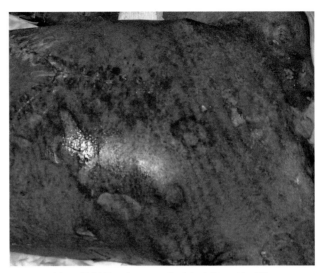

FIGURE 30-7. TEN Skin Lesions. Scalded skin with diffuse redness and sloughing between lesions in this patient with TEN. (Reprinted with permission from Mulholland, M. W., Maier, R. V., et al. (2006). *Greenfield's surgery scientific principles and practice* (4th ed.). Philadelphia, PA: Lippincott Williams & Wilkins.)

KEY POINT

Drugs commonly associated with SJS/TEN include allopurinol, anticonvulsants, sulfonamides, nevirapine, and NSAIDs. The newer class of cancer drugs, PD-1 checkpoint inhibitors (pembrolizumab and nivolumab), have recently been associated with SJS/TEN.

KEY POINT

Early SJS/TEN lesions present as confluent macules or papules or as diffuse erythema and are associated with significant tenderness and pain that is out of proportion to the findings on the skin examination.

The skin lesions initially present either as confluent, red oval macules or as papules with pruritic centers or as diffuse erythema (atypical target lesions) (see **Figs. 30-6 and 30-7**). The lesions are associated with significant tenderness and pain that is out of proportion to the findings on the skin examination. The lesions usually start on the face and trunk and spread symmetrically to other areas. The scalp, palms, and soles are usually spared. More classic target lesions with dusky, dark centers are sometimes seen, followed by formation of vesicles (clear fluid-filled blisters <1 cm in diameter) and bullae (fluid-filled blisters >1 cm in diameter).

Patients with TEN may also experience sudden onset of extensive skin sloughing in the absence of an erythematous rash. The clinical picture often resembles extensive thermal injury (**Fig. 30-8**). These patients also demonstrate a positive Nikolsky sign (Lyell, 1956). The large areas of denudation gradually reepithelialize, but resurfacing may take up to 4 weeks (Jordan et al., 1991; Woolum et al., 2019). Patients with SJS are more likely to

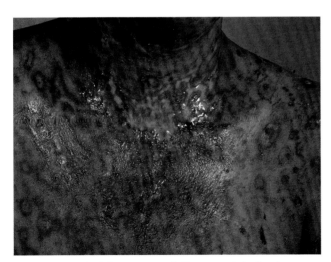

FIGURE 30-6. SJS Skin Lesions. SJS targetoid, dusky plaques with ulceration.

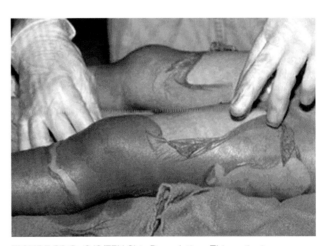

FIGURE 30-8. SJS/TEN Skin Denudation. This patient demonstrates confluent epidermal sloughing, which is easily removed with gentle pressure (the Nikolsky sign).

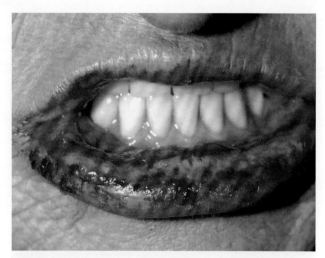

FIGURE 30-9. SJS Mucosal Lesions. Ulcerations on the lower lip mucosal surface in SJS.

experience a morbilliform drug eruption as part of the clinical picture.

Painful ocular, nasal, and oral mucosal erosions and crusts are seen in most patients with SJS/TEN in addition to the skin lesions (see **Fig. 30-9**). Ocular lesions usually involve purulent conjunctivitis, bullae, or corneal ulcerations and are seen in around 80% of patients (Morales et al., 2010). Oral lesions typically present as hemorrhagic erosions with inflammation. In women, vulvovaginal erosions, bullae, or ulcers may be seen along with other pathology.

DIAGNOSIS

A large (>4 mm) punch biopsy or deep shave biopsy is helpful in confirming the diagnosis through histologic analysis. DIF can be used to rule out other immune-mediated blistering disorders. Skin biopsy may reveal subepidermal bullae, complete epidermal necrosis, and T cells in the dermis. Soluble Fas ligand and granulysin proteins are elevated in SJS/TEN. Studies are ongoing regarding their usefulness as diagnostic serum studies (Abe et al., 2009; Murata et al., 2008).

MANAGEMENT

Patients who are thought to have early signs of SJS/TEN should have any suspected culprit drug discontinued immediately. Early discontinuation has been shown to reduce the risk of death. Mortality risk is reduced by 30% for every day preceding development of blisters and erosions (Garcia-Doval et al., 2000). Patients should be admitted to an inpatient facility and to an intensive care or burn unit depending on the extent of skin involvement or other diseases. It is important to monitor for significant fluid loss in patients with extensive skin sloughing. Severe hypovolemia may result in low-volume state shock, systemic infection, and multiorgan dysfunction.

For this reason, care of the patient with TEN should resemble major burn care with ongoing attention to wound management, fluid and electrolyte supplementation, nutritional support, infection monitoring, and pain control. Ophthalmologic consultation should be obtained to monitor for eye inflammation and to assure appropriate ocular care, and gynecologic examination should be performed on all female patients to prevent complications. While the principles of supportive care are clear, definitive treatment for SJS and TEN is not well defined (Worswick & Cotliar, 2011). Some authors recommend high-dose IVIG as standard therapy, but the evidence for this remains controversial (Worswick & Cotliar, 2011). The therapy must be weighed against the risks including acute renal failure, thrombotic complications, volume overload, and hemolysis. The use of systemic steroids is equally controversial. A multicenter study suggested a possible benefit to combining IVIG and systemic steroids versus using either agent alone (Micheletti et al., 2018). Some authors recommend corticosteroids for patients with SJS but not those with TEN. There is some evidence of increased mortality when corticosteroids are used to treat TEN patients. Cyclosporine has shown promise as a systemic agent, with decreased mortality compared to IVIG (Kirchhof et al., 2014). A 2018 meta-analysis of nine studies demonstrated a reduction in observed mortality among SJS/TEN patients when compared to predicted mortality for these patients by SCORTEN (Ng et al., 2018). SCORTEN is a validated scoring system used to determine prognosis in SJS/TEN. Plasmapheresis and antitumor necrosis factor (TNF) monoclonal antibodies are other therapeutic options that have been used. Infliximab (TNF-α monoclonal antibody) and etanercept (TNF-α decoy receptor) are other potential treatments for SJS/TEN. In a randomized, controlled trial (RCT) of TNF-alpha antagonists versus traditional corticosteroids, etanercept demonstrated decreased mortality and improved skin healing time (Wang et al., 2018).

KEY POINT

Patients who are thought to have early signs of SJS/TEN should have any suspected culprit drug discontinued immediately to reduce mortality.

The extent of skin sloughing should be evaluated regularly. Debridement is not recommended, as this results in extensive denudation. Patients who were treated with IVIG and conservative skin management had a dramatically lower mortality rate compared to patients who were treated with aggressive debridement (Stella et al., 2007). Topical therapy should follow the principles of moist wound healing. Dressings should be selected that absorb excess exudate, maintain a moist wound bed, and provide atraumatic removal. Petrolatum and other nonadherent contact layer dressings are commonly used. Nonadherent gauze impregnated with nanocrystalline silver is another commonly used approach. The nanocrystalline silver dressing can be left in place for up to 7 days, which may improve patient comfort and reduce pain associated with dressing changes (Fong & Wood, 2006). Roll gauze and other nonadhesive options should be used to secure the primary contact layer dressing in place to prevent medical adhesive-related skin injury (MARSI).

KEY POINT

Management of the patient with SJS/TEN requires intensive systemic support (fluid and electrolyte replacement, nutritional support, pain management), ophthalmologic and gynecologic consults, infection prevention, and evidence-based wound care.

⬤ PSORIASIS

Psoriasis is a chronic skin disorder characterized most often by well-circumscribed, erythematous plaques with silver scales (**Fig. 30-10**). The incidence of psoriasis is estimated to be around 100 cases per 100,000 individuals, with reported prevalence ranging from 0.91% to 8.5% of the population, and no clear gender bias (Parisi et al., 2013). Psoriasis appears to have two age peaks of onset: one between ages 30 and 39 and a second between the ages of 50 and 59. Genetic predisposition is a major

risk factor. Up to 40% of patients with psoriasis have first-degree relatives with the disorder (Boehncke & Schön, 2015; Gladman et al., 1986). There are also a number of environmental factors that appear to be risk factors for psoriasis including smoking, obesity, and alcohol consumption (Higgins, 2000; Li et al., 2012; Setty et al., 2007).

KEY POINT

Genetic predisposition is a major risk factor for psoriasis. Other risk factors include smoking, obesity, and alcohol consumption.

PATHOLOGY

Psoriasis is currently considered to be an immune system–mediated disease resulting in hyperproliferation and abnormal differentiation of the epidermis, leading to redness and scaling (Nickoloff & Nestle, 2004). Individuals with psoriasis manifest a larger number of epidermal stem cells, more cells undergoing mitosis, and shorter epidermal turnover time.

CLINICAL PRESENTATION

Patients with psoriasis can exhibit different phenotypes (Callen et al., 2003). Up to 80% of adult patients with the disease present with the classic plaque psoriasis (see **Fig. 30-10**). These patients have symmetrically distributed erythematous plaques with silver scale on the scalp, back, and extensor surfaces of the elbows and knees (Tollefson et al., 2010). They may also have lesions involving the intergluteal cleft, external ear canal, and umbilical region. The lesions can be pruritic, although this is not always the case. Psoriasis can also present in an inverse form, affecting the inguinal, perineal, genital, intergluteal, axillary, and inframammary regions. In the inverse form, the plaques may lack the characteristic silvery white scaling and may instead present as well-demarcated erythematous plaques with inverse distribution. Guttate psoriasis is manifest by numerous small (<1 cm), drop-like, red, and scaly papules that are located primarily on the trunk (**Fig. 30-11**). This type of psoriasis is frequently associated with a precipitating factor, such as a recent streptococcal throat infection. Pustular psoriasis is a severe form of the disease that can be life threatening. These patients present with acute widespread erythema, scaling, and sheets of pustules and erosions (**Fig. 30-12**). The cutaneous manifestations may be accompanied by fever, liver dysfunction, and diarrhea. This form of psoriasis is associated with pregnancy, infection, and withdrawal of oral corticosteroid therapy. A subset of patients with psoriasis have limited palmoplantar involvement. Although the actual BSA involved in these cases is limited, the location of the plaques and papules may make

Scales

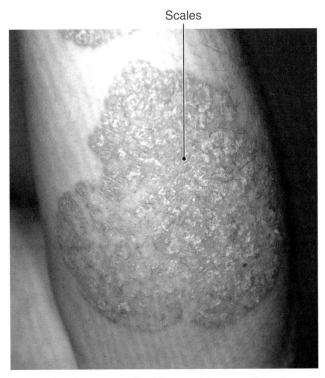

FIGURE 30-10. Psoriasis Skin Plaques. A large, erythematous plaque with secondary silvery scaling in this patient with plaque psoriasis.

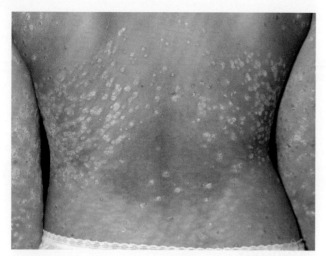

FIGURE 30-11. Guttate Psoriasis Lesions. Small drop-like spots of guttate psoriasis may be seen during different stages of the disease, especially during an acute flare.

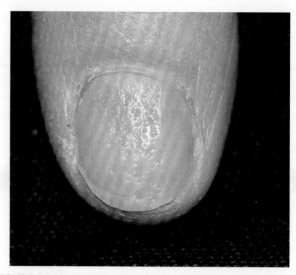

FIGURE 30-13. Psoriasis Nail Pitting. Nail pitting in psoriasis. Onycholysis and "oil spots" (not shown here) can also be seen.

this condition debilitating. Patients with psoriasis can present with erythroderma, or redness and scaling involving > 30% BSA. These patients require supportive treatment to prevent excessive loss of fluid and protein and often require systemic therapy.

KEY POINT

Eighty percent of adult patients present with plaque psoriasis, which most commonly involves the scalp, back, and extensor surfaces of the elbows and knees. Less common forms of psoriasis include inverse psoriasis, guttate psoriasis, and pustular psoriasis, which can be life threatening.

Nail plate involvement can be an important clue in the diagnosis of psoriasis. Nail changes seen with psoriasis include pitting, brown color changes, small hemorrhages, and nail bed thickening (**Fig. 30-13**). Another potential

diagnostic clue is joint pain. From 7% to 48% of patients with psoriasis also have arthritis which can precede or follow onset of the skin manifestations (Reich et al., 2009). Patients with psoriasis are thought to have a higher risk of coronary artery disease (Kaiser et al., 2019).

The wound care nurse caring for the patient with psoriasis should be aware that exacerbating factors include bacterial and viral infections and a number of drugs, including beta-blockers, lithium, antimalarial agents such as hydroxychloroquine, angiotensin converting enzyme (ACE) inhibitors, and NSAIDs.

DIAGNOSIS

The diagnosis of psoriasis is made by a thorough history and characteristic findings on physical examination. A 4-mm punch skin biopsy is helpful in ruling out other pathologic conditions with similar presentations. Histologic findings include psoriasiform hyperplasia or thickening of the epidermis, retention of cell nuclei in the topmost layer of epidermis, neutrophils in the epidermis, and sometimes microabscesses.

MANAGEMENT

Limited, mild to moderate disease (<5% to 10% of BSA) is often managed with emollients, supportive therapy, and topical agents. Topical corticosteroids remain the mainstay of therapy for limited disease. The vehicle and potency of the corticosteroid may be varied depending on the patient's preference, severity of disease, and the location on the body. A liquid solution or foam would be a better choice for the scalp, whereas an ointment or cream would be better for glabrous (hairless) skin. High-potency topical steroids such as clobetasol 0.05% can be used on thick plaques on the trunk, but lower-potency steroids such as hydrocortisone 2.5% would be more

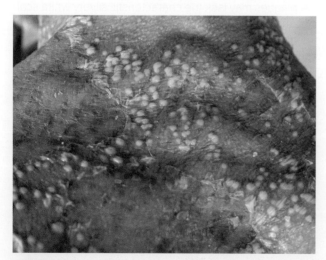

FIGURE 30-12. Pustular Psoriasis Lesions. Pustular psoriasis lesions seen here with lakes of pus.

appropriate for facial or intertriginous involvement. Non-steroidal alternatives, such as calcipotriene and topical tacrolimus or pimecrolimus, can be used as steroid-sparing agents for facial or intertriginous areas to minimize skin atrophy. Other commonly used alternatives are topical retinoids (e.g., once daily tazarotene 0.05% cream). Keratolytics such as topical salicylic acid preparations can also be used to help remove scaling and increase the effectiveness of other topical agents.

> **KEY POINT**
>
> Topical corticosteroids remain the mainstay of therapy for limited psoriatic disease. Phototherapy and biologic agents may be required for more extensive disease.

Phototherapy, most frequently with narrow band ultraviolet B (UVB), may be utilized for more extensive disease. Moderate-to-severe disease necessitates systemic therapies including retinoids, methotrexate, and cyclosporine. Several biologic agents are available as treatment options for moderate-to-severe psoriasis. Anti-TNF agents are effective and safe therapies. There are five FDA-approved anti-TNF medications available in the United States: etanercept, adalimumab, infliximab, certolizumab, and golimumab. Other biologic agents, such as the monoclonal antibody ustekinumab (an IL-12/23 inhibitor) and secukinumab (an IL-17 inhibitor), have been gaining popularity for patients who fail conventional treatment. It is important that the side effects and appropriateness of each therapy be reviewed before therapy is initiated. Any monitoring guidelines need to be addressed as well. Referral to dermatology is recommended when the diagnosis is unclear, initial topical therapy is inadequate, the provider is unfamiliar with treatment modalities, or the patient has widespread disease. Rheumatology referral is important if joint disease is suspected.

IRRITANT AND ALLERGIC DERMATITIS

Irritant contact dermatitis (ICD) is a local inflammatory skin reaction to various chemical or physical agents. It is caused by a direct, irritant-induced cell death effect and is not a primary immune-mediated phenomenon, in contrast to allergic contact dermatitis (ACD). ICD comprises up to 80% of occupation-related contact dermatitis (Clark & Zirwas, 2009) and is commonly seen among professionals in food handling, health care, mechanical, and cleaning industries. Other predisposing factors include age with highest number of reactions found among infants and decreasing reactivity with increasing age, women at greater risk, family history of eczema, and environmental conditions such as warm temperatures and high humidity (Schwindt et al., 1998; Thyssen et al., 2010). Common culprit agents include detergents, solvents (e.g., benzene,

acetone), oxidizing agents (bleach, benzoyl peroxide), acids (sulfuric acid), alkaline agents (soap, soda, cement, ammonia), metals, fiberglass, wood, plants, paper, and soil. These agents act to disrupt the skin barrier causing cell damage (Dickel et al., 2002).

ACD is a T-cell immune system–mediated delayed hypersensitivity reaction to external agents, which leads to a cutaneous reaction. An eczematous dermatitis is the most common reaction. Manifestations include redness, blister formation, itching, and skin thickening at and around the site of contact. The most common inciting stimuli include poison ivy, oak, and sumac, latex materials, nickel, soaps, fragrances, hair care and makeup products, rubber, plastics, cleansers, resins, acrylics, and protective equipment (Davis et al., 2008; Nosbaum et al., 2009). Unlike ICD, the incidence of ACD increases with age.

> **KEY POINT**
>
> ICD is a local skin reaction caused by direct cellular damage from a chemical agent and is the most common form of contact dermatitis. ACD is a T-cell immune system–mediated hypersensitivity reaction.

PATHOLOGY

ICD develops when the top layer of the epidermis (stratum corneum) is disrupted by chemical or physical agents, leading to a loss of the skin barrier and damage to epidermal cells. The damaged cells then release cytokines that attract immune cells such as macrophages to remove the dead and damaged epidermal cells. ACD is characterized by swelling of the epidermal cells and vesicle (blister) formation and histopathologic evidence of lymphocytes and eosinophils within the epidermal skin layer.

CLINICAL PRESENTATION

ICD is characterized by skin redness, dryness, and an eczema-like skin reaction and may result in a chemical burn. Acute ICD can occur from a single exposure to an irritating substance and may present with swelling, vesicles, bullae, oozing, redness, burning, and pain limited to the site of contact (**Fig. 30-14**). Chronic ICD, on the other hand, is caused by repeated exposure to mild- or low-concentration irritants. It is manifested by redness, scaling, thickening of the skin, and fissure formation, typically on the face, fingertips, digit web spaces, and the dorsum of the hands (**Fig. 30-15**). With both ICD and ACD, patients may complain of stinging, itching, and generalized skin discomfort and pain.

Acute ACD lesions are scaly, red, and hardened (**Fig. 30-16**). The initial presentation is the site of contact. The edges of the lesion may be well defined, but they can spread locally or even at a distance (Nosbaum et al.,

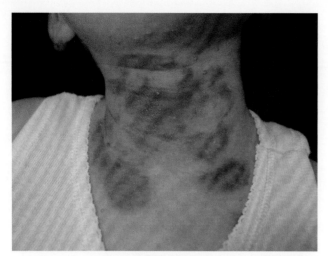

FIGURE 30-14. Acute ICD Rash with Vesicles. This patient demonstrated a localized irritant dermatitis to imiquimod therapy used for molluscum of neck. (Image provided by Stedman's.)

2009). They may also present as weepy vesicles and bullae on an edematous base, especially when the lesions involve the eyelids, lips, or genitalia. Patients may complain of itching, burning, pain, and stinging. In chronic disease resulting from continued exposure, the skin is scaly but thicker, dry, and fissured with swelling and crusting. In both acute and chronic ACD, the lesions are usually surrounding and including sites of contact with the inciting stimulus and are frequently seen on the hands and face. If the allergen is a lotion, detergent, body wash, or other general use product, the lesions may exhibit widespread distribution.

DIAGNOSIS

The diagnosis of ICD or ACD is based on a thorough history and detailed physical examination. The history should focus on any exposure to occupational, chemical,

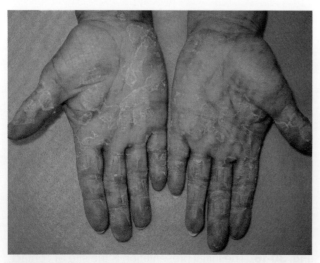

FIGURE 30-15. Chronic Irritant Contact Dermatitis. ICD seen on the hands of this health care worker, with scaling, thickened skin. (Image provided by Stedman's.)

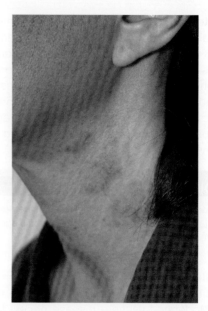

FIGURE 30-16. Allergic Contact Dermatitis. Acute ACD from poison ivy exposure. The patient's dog had rubbed her neck and face.

or physical agents commonly associated with ICD and ACD and specifically on agents to which the involved areas have been exposed. The physical examination involves thorough inspection of the skin and the affected areas, with attention to the location and morphology of the lesions. It is necessary to rule out ACD via patch testing. Patch testing for a specific product may be done by the wound care nurse using a small piece of the product secured with paper tape near the area of intended use. Formal patch testing may be done in conjunction with an outpatient dermatology consultation. A skin biopsy may also be performed to exclude other skin pathologies such as psoriasis or other inflammatory dermatoses. A KOH preparation and culture swabs of scaling may rule out a fungal or bacterial infection (Hamzelou et al., 2014).

MANAGEMENT

The primary goal of therapy for both ICD and ACD is to identify and eliminate contact with the inciting stimulus, followed by treatment of the inflamed skin to allow for healing and reestablishment of the skin barrier. Topical corticosteroid ointments and emollients, such as petrolatum, are used empirically as first-line therapy and act to reduce inflammation and to protect the affected skin (Bourke et al., 2009). For mild ICD, high-potency corticosteroids, such as clobetasol 0.05%, fluocinonide 0.05%, or betamethasone dipropionate 0.05% ointments, are preferred to be used once to twice daily for several weeks. For facial and intertriginous ICD and ACD involvement, low-medium potency corticosteroids are advised, such as hydrocortisone 2.5% ointment once to twice daily for several weeks. For severe acute ICD and ACD or chronic ICD with skin thickening, a high-potency topical corticosteroid can be used such as clobetasol 0.05% ointment. For chronic ACD, medium-potency topical corticosteroids such as triamcinolone 0.1% ointment or cream can be used.

Topical calcineurin inhibitors, such as tacrolimus 0.01% and pimecrolimus 1% twice daily, may be used as an alternative to topical corticosteroids for chronic ACD, localized ACD unresponsive to corticosteroids, and ACD of the face or intertriginous regions. For ACD involving >20% of BSA or for acute ACD affecting the face, hands, feet, and genitalia, oral corticosteroids (e.g., prednisone taper starting at 0.5 to 1 mg/kg/d, maximum 60 mg daily) are first-line therapy for a quick response (Beltrani et al., 2006). Phototherapy can also be used in chronic ACD unresponsive to topical and oral corticosteroids. In limited case reports and small studies, it is unclear whether dupilumab, an FDA-approved monoclonal antibody for the treatment of atopic dermatitis, may actually be beneficial in the treatment of ACD (van der Schaft et al., 2019).

Emollients, moisturizers, and colloidal oatmeal packs are beneficial in the treatment of both ICD and ACD, as they soften the skin, reduce water loss, decrease irritation, and improve skin barrier function. They should be applied multiple times per day. For weeping dermatitis, dermatologists often recommend a drying agent, such as aluminum acetate soaks. Caregivers and patients should be aware that skin barrier recovery may take up to 4 weeks after irritant exposure, while skin hyperreactivity can last for more than 10 weeks (Lee et al., 1997).

CONCLUSION

Common dermatologic conditions are likely to be encountered by the wound care nurse. Blistering conditions, such as autoimmune blistering disorders and severe drug reactions, can be life-threatening and require both supportive and systemic therapy. Because these disorders can result in erosions, appropriate wound care is an integral part of their treatment. Other papulosquamous disorders, such as psoriasis and contact dermatitis, are not associated with the development of ulcerations or wounds. These are conditions commonly encountered in clinical practice, and the wound care nurse should be able to recognize them and make appropriate referrals.

REFERENCES

Abe, R., Yoshioka, N., Murata, J., et al. (2009). Granulysin as a marker for early diagnosis of the Stevens-Johnson syndrome. *Annals of Internal Medicine, 151*(7), 514–515.

Amagai, M., Tsunoda, K., Zillikens, D., et al. (1999). The clinical phenotype of pemphigus is defined by the anti-desmoglein autoantibody profile. *Journal of the American Academy of Dermatology, 40*(2), 167–170.

Bastuji-Garin, S., Rzany, B., Stern, R. S., et al. (1993). Clinical classification of cases of toxic epidermal necrolysis, Stevens-Johnson syndrome, and erythema multiforme. *Archives of Dermatology, 129*(1), 92–96.

Beltrani, V. S., Bernstein, I. L., Cohen, D. E., et al. (2006). Contact dermatitis: A practice parameter. *Annals of Allergy, Asthma, and Immunology, 97*(3 Suppl 2), S1–S38.

Bircher, A. J. (2005). Symptoms and danger signs in acute drug hypersensitivity. *Toxicology, 209*(2), 201–207. doi: 10.1016/j.tox.2004.12.036.

Boehncke, W. H., & Schön, M. P. (2015). Psoriasis. *Lancet, 386*(9997), 983–994. doi: 10.1016/S0140-6736 (14)61909-7.

Bourke, J., Coulson, I., & English, J. (2009). Guidelines for the management of contact dermatitis: An update. *British Journal of Dermatology, 160*(5), 946–954. doi: 10.1111/j.1365-2133.2009.09106.x.

Bystryn, J. C., & Rudolph, J. L. (2005). Pemphigus. *Lancet, 366*(9479), 61–73. doi: 10.1016/s0140-6736(05)66829-8.

Caldarola, G., Kneisel, A., Hertl, M., et al. (2008). Herpes simplex virus infection in pemphigus vulgaris: Clinical and immunological considerations. *European Journal of Dermatology, 18*(4), 440–443. doi: 10.1684/ejd.2008.0439.

Callen, J. P., Krueger, G. G., Lebwohl, M., et al. (2003). AAD consensus statement on psoriasis therapies. *Journal of the American Academy of Dermatology, 49*(5), 897–899. doi: 10.1016/S0190-9622(03)01870-X.

Chan, H. L., Stern, R. S., Arndt, K. A., et al. (1990). The incidence of erythema multiforme, Stevens-Johnson syndrome, and toxic epidermal necrolysis. A population-based study with particular reference to reactions caused by drugs among outpatients. *Archives of Dermatology, 126*(1), 43–47.

Chung, W. H., Hung, S. I., Yang, J. Y., et al. (2008). Granulysin is a key mediator for disseminated keratinocyte death in Stevens-Johnson syndrome and toxic epidermal necrolysis. *Nature Medicine, 14*(12), 1343–1350. doi: 10.1038/nm.1884.

Clark, S. C., & Zirwas, M. J. (2009). Management of occupational dermatitis. *Dermatologic Clinics, 27*(3), 365–383, vii–viii. doi: 10.1016/j.det.2009.05.002.

Coleman, E., Ko, C., Dai, F., et al. (2019). Inflammatory eruptions associated with immune checkpoint inhibitor therapy: A single-institution retrospective analysis with stratification of reactions by toxicity and implications for management. *Journal of the American Academy of Dermatology, 80*(4), 990–997. doi: 10.1016/j.jaad.2018.10.062.

Craythorne, E. E., Mufti, G., & DuVivier, A. W. (2011). Rituximab used as a first-line single agent in the treatment of pemphigus vulgaris. *Journal of the American Academy of Dermatology, 65*(5), 1064–1065. doi: 10.1016/j.jaad.2010.06.033.

Davis, M. D., Scalf, L. A., Yiannias, J. A., et al. (2008). Changing trends and allergens in the patch test standard series: A mayo clinic 5-year retrospective review, January 1, 2001, through December 31, 2005. *Archives of Dermatology, 144*(1), 67–72. doi: 10.1001/archdermatol.2007.2.

Dickel, H., Kuss, O., Schmidt, A., et al. (2002). Importance of irritant contact dermatitis in occupational skin disease. *American Journal of Clinical Dermatology, 3*(4), 283–289.

Elder, D. E., Elenitsas, R., Rosenbach, M., et al. (Eds.) (2009). *Lever's histopathology of the skin* (11th ed.). Philadelphia, PA: Wolters Kluwer Health.

Fong, J., & Wood, F. (2006). Nanocrystalline silver dressings in wound management: A review. *International Journal of Nanomedicine, 1*(4), 441.

Garcia-Doval, I., LeCleach, L., Bocquet, H., et al. (2000). Toxic epidermal necrolysis and Stevens-Johnson syndrome: Does early withdrawal of causative drugs decrease the risk of death? *Archives of Dermatology, 136*(3), 323–327.

Gladman, D. D., Anhorn, K. A., Schachter, R. K., et al. (1986). HLA antigens in psoriatic arthritis. *Journal of Rheumatology, 13*(3), 586–592.

Halevy, S., Ghislain, P. D., Mockenhaupt, M., et al. (2008). Allopurinol is the most common cause of Stevens-Johnson syndrome and toxic epidermal necrolysis in Europe and Israel. *Journal of the American Academy of Dermatology, 58*(1), 25–32.

Hamzelou, S., Jafari, M., Aminizadeh, E., et al. (2014). An 80-year-old man with erythema, scales and pustules on the left ear auricle. *BMJ Case Reports, 2014,* bcr2014203758. doi: 10.1136/bcr-2014-203758.

Higgins, E. (2000). Alcohol, smoking and psoriasis. *Clinical and Experimental Dermatology, 25*(2), 107–110.

Hooten, J. N., Hall III, R. P., & Cardones, A. R. (2014). Updates on the management of autoimmune blistering diseases. *Skin Therapy Letter, 19*(5), 1–6.

Joly, P., Baricault, S., Sparsa, A., et al. (2012). Incidence and mortality of bullous pemphigoid in France. *Journal of Investigative Dermatology, 132*(8), 1998–2004. doi: 10.1038/jid.2012.35.

Joly, P., & Litrowski, N. (2011). Pemphigus group (vulgaris, vegetans, foliaceus, herpetiformis, brasiliensis). *Clinics in Dermatology, 29*(4), 432–436.

Joly, P., Maho-Vaillant, M., Prost-Squarcioni, C., et al. (2017). First-line rituximab combined with short-term prednisone versus prednisone alone for the treatment of pemphigus (Ritux 3): A prospective, multicentre, parallel-group, open-label randomised trial. *Lancet, 389*(10083), 2031–2040. doi: 10.1016/s0140-6736(17)30070-3.

Joly, P., Roujeau, J. C., Benichou, J., et al. (2002). A comparison of oral and topical corticosteroids in patients with bullous pemphigoid. *New England Journal of Medicine, 346*(5), 321–327. doi: 10.1056/NEJMoa011592.

Jordan, M. H., Lewis, M. S., Jeng, J. G., et al. (1991). Treatment of toxic epidermal necrolysis by burn units: Another market or another threat? *The Journal of Burn Care & Rehabilitation, 12*(6), 579–581.

Jordan, R. E., Triftshauser, C. T., & Schroeter, A. L. (1971). Direct immunofluorescent studies of pemphigus and bullous pemphigoid. *Archives of Dermatology, 103*(5), 486–491.

Kaiser, H., Abdulla, J., Henningsen, K. M. A., et al. (2019). Coronary artery disease assessed by computed tomography in patients with psoriasis: A systematic review and meta-analysis. *Dermatology, 235*(6), 478–487. doi: 10.1159/000502138.

Kasperkiewicz, M., Shimanovich, I., Ludwig, R. J., et al. (2011). Rituximab for treatment-refractory pemphigus and pemphigoid: A case series of 17 patients. *Journal of the American Academy of Dermatology, 65*(3), 552–558.

Kasperkiewicz, M., Zillikens, D., & Schmidt, E. (2012). Pemphigoid diseases: Pathogenesis, diagnosis, and treatment. *Autoimmunity, 45*(1), 55–70. doi: 10.3109/08916934.2011.606447.

Kirchhof, M. G., Miliszewski, M. A., Sikora, S., et al. (2014). Retrospective review of Stevens-Johnson syndrome/toxic epidermal necrolysis treatment comparing intravenous immunoglobulin with cyclosporine. *Journal of the American Academy of Dermatology, 71*(5), 941–947. doi: 10.1016/j.jaad.2014.07.016.

Kneisel, A., & Hertl, M. (2011). Autoimmune bullous skin diseases. Part 1: Clinical manifestations. *JDDG: Journal der Deutschen Dermatologischen Gesellschaft, 9*(10), 844–857.

Kridin, K., Ahn, C., Huang, W. C., et al. (2019). Treatment update of autoimmune blistering diseases. *Dermatologic Clinics, 37*(2), 215–228. doi: 10.1016/j.det.2018.12.003.

Kulthanan, K., Chularojanamontri, L., Tuchinda, P., et al. (2011). Prevalence and clinical features of Thai patients with bullous pemphigoid. *Asian Pacific Journal of Allergy and Immunology, 29*(1), 66–72.

Lee, J. Y., Effendy, I., & Maibach, H. I. (1997). Acute irritant contact dermatitis: Recovery time in man. *Contact Dermatitis, 36*(6), 285–290.

Li, W., Han, J., Choi, H. K., et al. (2012). Smoking and risk of incident psoriasis among women and men in the United States: A combined analysis. *American Journal of Epidemiology, 175*(5), 402–413. doi: 10.1093/aje/kwr325.

Logan, I. T., Zaman, S., Hussein, L., et al. (2020). Combination therapy of ipilimumab and nivolumab-associated toxic epidermal necrolysis

(TEN) in a patient with metastatic melanoma: A case report and literature review. *Journal of Immunotherapy, 43*(3), 89–92. doi: 10.1097/cji.0000000000000302.

Lyell, A. (1956). Toxic epidermal necrolysis: An eruption resembling scalding of the skin. *British Journal of Dermatology, 68*(11), 355–361.

Marazza, G., Pham, H. C., Scharer, L., et al. (2009). Incidence of bullous pemphigoid and pemphigus in Switzerland: A 2-year prospective study. *British Journal of Dermatology, 161*(4), 861–868. doi: 10.1111/j.1365-2133.2009.09300.x.

Martin, L. K., Werth, V. P., Villanueva, E. V., et al. (2011). A systematic review of randomized controlled trials for pemphigus vulgaris and pemphigus foliaceus. *Journal of the American Academy of Dermatology, 64*(5), 903–908.

Micheletti, R. G., Chiesa-Fuxench, Z., Noe, M. H., et al. (2018). Stevens-Johnson syndrome/toxic epidermal necrolysis: A multicenter retrospective study of 377 adult patients from the United States. *Journal of Investigative Dermatology, 138*(11), 2315–2321. doi: 10.1016/j.jid.2018.04.027.

Mittmann, N., Knowles, S. R., Koo, M., et al. (2012). Incidence of toxic epidermal necrolysis and Stevens-Johnson Syndrome in an HIV cohort: An observational, retrospective case series study. *American Journal of Clinical Dermatology, 13*(1), 49–54. doi: 10.2165/11593240-000000000-00000.

Morales, M. E., Purdue, G. F., Verity, S. M., et al. (2010). Ophthalmic manifestations of Stevens-Johnson syndrome and toxic epidermal necrolysis and relation to SCORTEN. *American Journal of Ophthalmology, 150*(4), 505–510.e1. doi: 10.1016/j.ajo.2010.04.026.

Murata, J., Abe, R., & Shimizu, H. (2008). Increased soluble Fas ligand levels in patients with Stevens-Johnson syndrome and toxic epidermal necrolysis preceding skin detachment. *Journal of Allergy and Clinical Immunology, 122*(5), 992–1000. doi: 10.1016/j.jaci.2008.06.013.

Nassif, A., Bensussan, A., Boumsell, L., et al. (2004). Toxic epidermal necrolysis: Effector cells are drug-specific cytotoxic T cells. *Journal of Allergy and Clinical Immunology, 114*(5), 1209–1215. doi: 10.1016/j.jaci.2004.07.047.

Nayar, N., Briscoe, K., & Fernandez Penas, P. (2016). Toxic epidermal necrolysis-like reaction with severe satellite cell necrosis associated with nivolumab in a patient With ipilimumab refractory metastatic melanoma. *Journal of Immunotherapy, 39*(3), 149–152. doi: 10.1097/cji.0000000000000112.

Ng, Q. X., De Deyn, M., Venkatanarayanan, N., et al. (2018). A meta-analysis of cyclosporine treatment for Stevens-Johnson syndrome/toxic epidermal necrolysis. *Journal of Inflammation Research, 11,* 135. doi: 10.2147/jir.S160964.

Nickoloff, B. J., & Nestle, F. O. (2004). Recent insights into the immunopathogenesis of psoriasis provide new therapeutic opportunities. *Journal of Clinical Investigation, 113*(12), 1664–1675. doi: 10.1172/jci22147.

Nosbaum, A., Vocanson, M., Rozieres, A., et al. (2009). Allergic and irritant contact dermatitis. *European Journal of Dermatology, 19*(4), 325–332.

Parisi, R., Symmons, D. P., Griffiths, C. E., et al. (2013). Global epidemiology of psoriasis: A systematic review of incidence and prevalence. *Journal of Investigative Dermatology, 133*(2), 377–385. doi: 10.1038/jid.2012.339.

Polansky, M., Eisenstadt, R., DeGrazia, T., et al. (2019). Rituximab therapy in patients with bullous pemphigoid: A retrospective study of 20 patients. *Journal of the American Academy of Dermatology, 81*(1), 179–186. doi: 10.1016/j.jaad.2019.03.049.

Reich, K., Kruger, K., Mossner, R., et al. (2009). Epidemiology and clinical pattern of psoriatic arthritis in Germany: A prospective interdisciplinary epidemiological study of 1511 patients with plaque-type psoriasis. *British Journal of Dermatology, 160*(5), 1040–1047. doi: 10.1111/j.1365-2133.2008.09023.x.

Robinson, S., Saleh, J., Curry, J., et al. (2019). Pembrolizumab-induced Stevens-Johnson syndrome/toxic epidermal necrolysis in a patient with metastatic cervical squamous cell carcinoma: A case report. *The American Journal of Dermatopathology, 42*(4), 292–296. doi: 10.1097/dad.0000000000001527.

Salati, M., Pifferi, M., Baldessari, C., et al. (2018). Stevens-Johnson syndrome during nivolumab treatment of NSCLC. *Annals of Oncology, 29*(1), 283–284. doi: 10.1093/annonc/mdx640.

Schwindt, D. A., Wilhelm, K. P., Miller, D. L., et al. (1998). Cumulative irritation in older and younger skin: A comparison. *Acta Dermato-Venereologica, 78*(4), 279–283.

Sekula, P., Dunant, A., Mockenhaupt, M., et al. (2013). Comprehensive survival analysis of a cohort of patients with Stevens-Johnson syndrome and toxic epidermal necrolysis. *Journal of Investigative Dermatology, 133*(5), 1197–1204. doi: 10.1038/jid.2012.510.

Setty, A. R., Curhan, G., & Choi, H. K. (2007). Obesity, waist circumference, weight change, and the risk of psoriasis in women: Nurses' Health Study II. *Archives of Internal Medicine, 167*(15), 1670–1675. doi: 10.1001/archinte.167.15.1670.

Shah, K. M., Rancour, E. A., Al-Omari, A., et al. (2018). Striking enhancement at the site of radiation for nivolumab-induced Stevens-Johnson syndrome. *Dermatology Online Journal, 24*(6), 13030/qt97g3t63v. Retrieved December 5, 2019, from https://escholarship.org/uc/item/97g3t63v#author

Stella, M., Clemente, A., Bollero, D., et al. (2007). Toxic epidermal necrolysis (TEN) and Stevens–Johnson syndrome (SJS): Experience with high-dose intravenous immunoglobulins and topical conservative approach: A retrospective analysis. *Burns, 33*(4), 452–459.

Thyssen, J. P., Johansen, J. D., Linneberg, A., et al. (2010). The epidemiology of hand eczema in the general population—prevalence and main findings. *Contact Dermatitis, 62*(2), 75–87. doi: 10.1111/j.1600-0536.2009.01669.x.

Tollefson, M. M., Crowson, C. S., McEvoy, M. T., et al. (2010). Incidence of psoriasis in children: A population-based study. *Journal of the American Academy of Dermatology, 62*(6), 979–987. doi: 10.1016/j.jaad.2009.07.029.

Tran, J. T., & Mutasim, D. F. (2005). Localized bullous pemphigoid: A commonly delayed diagnosis. *International Journal of Dermatology, 44*(11), 942–945. doi: 10.1111/j.1365-4632.2004.02288.x.

van der Schaft, J., Thijs, J. L., de Bruin-Weller, M. S., et al. (2019). Dupilumab after the 2017 approval for the treatment of atopic dermatitis: What's new and what's next? *Current Opinion in Allergy and Clinical Immunology, 19*(4), 341–349. doi: 10.1097/aci.0000000000000551.

Venning, V., & Wojnarowska, F. (1992). Lack of predictive factors for the clinical course of bullous pemphigoid. *Journal of the American Academy of Dermatology, 26*(4), 585–589.

Venugopal, S. S., & Murrell, D. F. (2011). Diagnosis and clinical features of pemphigus vulgaris. *Dermatologic Clinics, 29*(3), 373–380.

Wang, C. W., Yang, L. Y., Chen, C. B., et al. (2018). Randomized, controlled trial of TNF-alpha antagonist in CTL-mediated severe cutaneous adverse reactions. *The Journal of Clinical Investigation, 128*(3), 985–996. doi: 10.1172/jci93349.

Woolum, J. A., Bailey, A. M., Baum, R. A., et al. (2019). A review of the management of Stevens-Johnson syndrome and toxic epidermal necrolysis. *Advanced Emergency Nursing Journal, 41*(1), 56–64. doi: 10.1097/TME.0000000000000225.

Worswick, S., & Cotliar, J. (2011). Stevens-Johnson syndrome and toxic epidermal necrolysis: A review of treatment options. *Dermatologic Therapy, 24*(2), 207–218. doi: 10.1111/j.1529-8019.2011.01396.x.

Yancey, K. B., & Egan, C. A. (2000). Pemphigoid: Clinical, histologic, immunopathologic, and therapeutic considerations. *Journal of the American Medical Association, 284*(3), 350–356.

QUESTIONS

1. The wound care nurse differentiates pemphigus vulgaris from bullous pemphigoid when planning care for patients. Which statement accurately describes a characteristic of these diseases?
A. Bullous pemphigoid causes destruction of cell-to-cell connections within the epidermis causing flaccid intraepithelial blisters.
B. Pemphigus vulgaris causes separation between the epidermal and dermal layers of the skin.
C. Patients with bullous pemphigoid present with flaccid bullae, skin erosions, and possibly mucous membrane erosions.
D. Bullous pemphigoid may begin with a prodromal phase of weeks to months characterized by a pruritic, eczema-like skin rash or urticarial plaques.

2. The wound care nurse is preparing a treatment plan for a patient with severe pemphigus vulgaris. Which of the following is a recommended treatment measure?
A. Therapy with topical corticosteroids
B. Systemic corticosteroid therapy
C. Topical corticosteroids plus antibiotic therapy
D. Systemic corticosteroids plus adjuvant therapy with steroid-sparing agents

3. The wound care nurse is planning evidence-based wound care for a patient with bullous pemphigoid. Which intervention is recommended?
A. Puncture and drain large blisters in a sterile environment.
B. Remove the epithelial roof of blisters that have been punctured.
C. Select dressings with the goal of managing bleeding.
D. Select adhesive dressing to manage exudate.

4. What is the most frequent etiology for Steven-Johnson syndrome (SJS) and toxic epidermal necrolysis (TEN)?
A. Burns
B. Electric shock
C. Drug reactions
D. Influenza

5. The wound care nurse is assessing a patient who presents with fever (38.5°C), visual disturbances, itching of the eyes, and pain upon swallowing. The patient is currently taking allopurinol for chronic gout. What skin condition would the nurse suspect?
  A. Bullous pemphigoid
  B. Pemphigus vulgaris
  C. Steven-Johnson syndrome
  D. Psoriasis

6. What should be the focus of care management for a patient with severe SJS/TEN?
  A. Continuing current medication regimen
  B. Care resembling major burn care
  C. Therapy with topical corticosteroids
  D. Use of surgical debridement

7. Psoriasis is considered to be an immune system–mediated disease. Which of the following is a characteristic of psoriasis?
  A. Large number of epidermal stem cells
  B. Fewer cells undergoing mitosis
  C. Longer epidermal turnover time
  D. Asymmetrical ulcer development on scalp, back, elbows, and knees

8. The wound care nurse is assessing the skin of a patient presenting with numerous small (<1 cm), drop-like, red, and scaly papules that are located primarily on the trunk. The patient states that she had recently been diagnosed with a streptococcal throat infection. What form of psoriasis would the nurse suspect?
  A. Plaque psoriasis
  B. Inverse psoriasis
  C. Guttate psoriasis
  D. Pustular psoriasis

9. Which of the following is a mainstay of therapy for limited psoriatic disease?
  A. Topical corticosteroids
  B. Phototherapy
  C. Biologic agents
  D. Immunosuppressant therapy

10. A patient presents with skin redness, dryness, an eczema-like skin reaction, and a resultant chemical burn. The patient states that the rash occurred after he used a new cleanser to clean his bathroom. What type of skin infection would the nurse suspect?
  A. Psoriasis
  B. Allergic dermatitis
  C. Pemphigus vulgaris
  D. Contact dermatitis

ANSWERS AND RATIONALES

1. D. Rationale: BP may begin with a prodromal phase of weeks to months preceding blister appearance. This phase is characterized by a pruritic, eczema-like skin rash or urticarial plaques.

2. D. Rationale: For severe PV disease, systemic corticosteroid therapy is highly effective. Treatment may include adjuvant therapy with steroid-sparing agents such as azathioprine and mycophenolate mofetil.

3. A. Rationale: It is appropriate to puncture and drain large blisters in a sterile environment. The epithelial roof should be left intact after drainage to provide wound coverage.

4. C. Rationale: Stevens-Johnson syndrome (SJS) and toxic epidermal necrolysis (TEN) are severe, life-threatening immune system–mediated skin and mucous membrane disorders characterized by significant epidermal necrosis and detachment and often resulting from a drug reaction.

5. C. Rationale: For SJS/TED, the most commonly implicated medication is allopurinol.

6. B. Rationale: Care of the patient with TEN should resemble major burn care with ongoing attention to wound management, fluid and electrolyte supplementation, nutritional support, infection monitoring, and pain control.

7. A. Rationale: Individuals with psoriasis manifest a larger number of epidermal stem cells, more cells undergoing mitosis, and shorter epidermal turnover time.

8. C. Rationale: Guttate psoriasis is manifested by numerous small (<1 cm), drop-like, red, and scaly papules that are located primarily on the trunk. This type of psoriasis is frequently associated with a precipitating factor, such as a recent streptococcal throat infection.

9. A. Rationale: Topical corticosteroids remain the mainstay of therapy for limited psoriatic disease. Phototherapy and biologic agents may be required for more extensive disease.

10. D. Rationale: ICD is characterized by skin redness, dryness, and an eczema-like skin reaction and can result in a chemical burn.

CHAPTER 31

ONCOLOGY-RELATED SKIN AND WOUND CARE

Carole Bauer

OBJECTIVES

1. Describe the pathology and presentation of radiodermatitis and current guidelines for prevention and management.

2. Describe common skin reactions associated with targeted chemotherapies and implications for prevention and management.

3. Outline strategies and resources for management of extravasation injuries.

4. Identify common challenges and patient concerns related to malignant fungating wounds and options for management.

5. Describe presentation and management for each of the following: palmar–plantar erythrodysesthesia, cutaneous T-cell lymphoma, and graft versus host disease.

TOPIC OUTLINE

⬤ INTRODUCTION

In 2019, the American Cancer Society reported that there will be an estimated 1.7 million new cases of cancer diagnosed. Based on this estimate, 39 out of 100 men and 38 out of 100 women can expect to develop cancer during their lifetime. There will be 606,880 cancer deaths in the United States. This makes cancer the second most common cause of death in the United States (American Cancer Society, 2019). These statistics emphasize the importance of understanding skin and wound conditions unique to the cancer patient. Wounds in oncology patients can provide challenges to the wound care nurse. Not only must the wound care nurse consider all of the traditional wounds and their causes, but skin disorders related to the cancer itself or to the treatment being provided must also be considered. This chapter will address skin lesions that are manifestations of the malignant process as well as disorders resulting from the effects of treatments to eliminate or control the disease.

⬤ RADIATION DERMATITIS

Radiation therapy is the use of high-energy waves, rays, or particles to shrink or kill cancer cells. There are several types of radiation beams currently used in the treatment of cancer, including gamma rays, x-rays, and proton beams. Radiation therapy can be delivered externally in the form of a beam delivered to the targeted areas through the skin, or internally, via implantation of a radioactive source. Internal radiation therapy, also known as brachytherapy, can be provided in many forms, such as placing the radioactive source into temporary catheters, tubes, or balloons or implanting the radioactive energy into the body in the form of seeds or pellets. Radiation works by altering the DNA structure of the cancer cell, which either kills the cell or prevents the cell from replicating. Radiation also affects normal cells within the radiation field that are reproducing, such as skin cells. For the patient undergoing external beam radiation, skin changes can be expected (American Cancer Society, 2018).

PREVALENCE/INCIDENCE

Radiation therapy is a commonly used modality in the treatment of cancer. It is estimated that at least 50% of patients diagnosed with cancer will receive radiation therapy during the course of their treatment. No true incidence has been recorded for radiation dermatitis. Many authors report that up to 95% of patients who receive radiation will experience some type of skin reaction (Feight et al., 2011; Lucas et al., 2018; Lucey et al., 2017; Russi et al., 2015; Singh et al., 2016).

PATHOLOGY

Radiation therapy delivers high-energy particles to the treatment field. These particles damage the cells' DNA, which disrupts replication and causes cell death. This explains the therapeutic benefit in treatment of cancer. The radiation damages rapidly proliferating tumor cells. Other rapidly proliferating cells in the treatment field, including the skin, are also affected. A number of terms have been used to describe radiation dermatitis, including radiodermatitis, radiation skin reaction, moist desquamation, and even radiation burns. The term radiation burn is no longer used as a description for the skin changes caused by radiation therapy and rather is reserved for those persons who are involved in radiation accidents.

In 1990, Hopewell was the first to describe the radiation-induced changes in the skin. These changes occur over time and are described as: (1) A transient early erythema, seen within a few hours of irradiation, which subsides after 24 to 48 hours; (2) the main erythematous reaction, reflecting indirectly a varying severity of loss of epidermal basal cells; either a dry or moist desquamatory response may be seen after 3 to 6 weeks; (3) a late phase of erythema associated with dermal ischemia and possibly necrosis, seen after 8 to 16 weeks; and (4) the appearance of late skin damage, that is, dermal atrophy (>26 weeks), telangiectasia, and necrosis (>52 weeks) (Hopewell, 1990).

Radiation dermatitis is caused by direct cellular injury to the dermis, epidermis, and vascular structures of the skin, which triggers an inflammatory response. Initially, cells within the radiation field are damaged by the energy from the ionizing radiation with each treatment causing increased cellular death. Damage to the dermis occurs causing erythema due to vessel dilation and release of a histamine-like substance. As the patient has more treatments, there is more damage and the skin attempts to increase the rate of mitosis in the basal keratinocyte cell layer. The rate of turnover is greater than the shedding of old cells, which leads to dry desquamation. If there is a total loss of stem cells in the basal layer of the dermis, moist desquamation will occur. Damage also occurs to the vascular endothelium which causes hypoxia and release of cytokines that cause further cellular damage.

The mechanism for radiation-induced inflammation is not well understood, but there is a cascade release of cytokines and chemokines that result in skin fibrosis; production of matrix metalloproteases, which negatively affect the components of the dermis and the basal cell layer; as well as an up-regulation of adhesion molecules. Transendothelial migration of leukocytes and other immune cells also occur in the inflammatory cascade, which is a hallmark of radiation-induced skin injury (Meghrajani et al., 2013; Singh et al., 2016; Wolf, 2019).

The total dose of radiation prescribed is divided into fractions or smaller portions of the total dose given over a set period of time. Each subsequent exposure results in inflammatory cell recruitment to the radiation field. This results in inhibition of normal granulation tissue, fibrogenesis, and angiogenesis. The damage that occurs is a result of multiple factors including damage to stem cells, endothelial cell changes, inflammation, apoptosis, and necrosis (Hymes et al., 2006).

In addition to the acute damage, radiation therapy can produce late effects in the skin and soft tissue that may become evident months or years following therapy. Late toxicity is defined as those changes that occur beyond 90 days after the completion of radiation therapy and include subcutaneous induration, hyperpigmentation, hypopigmentation, telangiectasia, photosensitivity,

xerosis, atrophy, fibrosis, ulceration, and impaired healing (Russi et al., 2015; Singh et al., 2016; Wolf, 2019). The skin and soft tissue changes seen with late radiation toxicity are the result of progressive changes to the vasculature and the soft tissue, primarily progressive damage to the dermal vessels, loss of normal fibroblasts and collagen, and progressive fibrosis of the soft tissues. These changes make the tissue more vulnerable to breakdown and less likely to heal. Radiation necrosis can be related to several factors including high-dose treatment, acute dermatitis that has never resolved, and dermal ischemia. Management of wounds in previously radiated tissue is difficult due to the persistent dermal ischemia (Russi et al., 2015; Hymes et al., 2006; Singh et al., 2016).

KEY POINT

The skin and soft tissue changes seen with late radiation toxicity are the result of progressive changes to the vasculature and the soft tissue, primarily progressive damage to the dermal vessels, loss of normal fibroblasts and collagen, and progressive fibrosis of the soft tissues. These changes are thought to be the result of the release of cytokines and the effect on the coagulation and inflammatory cascades. These changes make the tissue more vulnerable to breakdown and less likely to heal.

RADIATION RECALL

Radiation recall is defined as a skin reaction that occurs after the administration of certain chemotherapeutic drugs including epidermal growth factor receptor (EGFR) inhibitors, anti-PD-1 monoclonal antibodies, and BRAF tyrosine kinase inhibitors in an area where radiation has previously been administered. Little is known about the treatment, incidence, and pathogenesis, but several theories have been proposed including local vascular injury that affects cellular permeability of certain drugs and epithelial stem cell depletion or mutation (Bahaj et al., 2019; Hack et al., 2018). This leaves health care providers and the patient with only two options: discontinue the chemotherapeutic agent, which may adversely affect overall prognosis, or continue the agent despite the risk of further skin reaction. Symptoms of radiation recall dermatitis are the same as those for radiation dermatitis and include erythema, desquamation, edema, vesiculation, necrosis, ulceration, and hemorrhage (Russi et al., 2015; Wolf, 2019).

KEY POINT

Radiation recall is a skin reaction that occurs after administration of certain chemotherapeutic drugs including EGFR inhibitors, anti-PD-1 monoclonal antibodies, and BRAF tyrosine kinase inhibitors in a previously irradiated area.

RISK FACTORS

Little is known about the specific risk factors related to radiation dermatitis. It is hypothesized that both treatment-related factors and patient-related factors can affect the development of radiation dermatitis. Treatment-related factors have undergone the most scrutiny.

Treatment Factors

The risk of skin damage is related to the total dose as well as the fraction dose, the type of radiation energy used (photon and electrons deliver a higher dose to the skin), and the volume and surface area of skin exposed. If the fraction is >2 Gy per treatment, the time to onset of skin damage is reduced and there is an increased risk for the development of a more severe skin reaction. Radiation therapy is often delivered via linear accelerators or megavoltage units, which are skin sparing. These units deliver the radiation to target the tissues 1.5 to 3 cm below the skin surface. Electron beams, which have a shorter wave length, are often used to deliver what is sometimes called a boost for treatment of lymph nodes that lie close to the skin surface. Electron beam therapy is associated with more severe skin reactions. Cobalt 60, an older type of treatment unit, is used to target tissues only 0.5 cm below the skin surface and is associated with increased risk of skin damage. In addition to the type of energy, fraction dose, and total dose delivered, the duration of therapy also affects the onset and severity of radiation dermatitis. Those patients who undergo a longer treatment course are at greater risk for severe dermatitis as compared to those who have a shorter treatment course. Several other treatment-related factors can affect the development and severity of radiation dermatitis. If the patient's treatment field includes the head and neck region, breast, axilla, perineum, or areas with skin folds, the patient is at risk for earlier onset and greater severity of skin reactions. The size of the treatment field also affects risk; larger treatment areas are associated with earlier onset and greater severity of skin reactions (McQuestion, 2011; Russi et al., 2015; Singh et al., 2016).

KEY POINT

The risk of skin damage is related to the total radiation dose, fraction dose, type of radiation used, the volume and surface area of exposed skin, skin integrity at baseline, skin care provided during therapy, and whether or not the involved area involves body folds resulting in skin-to-skin contact.

If a tangential field is used or a bolus is given, the patient is at greater risk for significant radiation dermatitis. With a bolus (boost) dose, overlapping fields may receive increased radiation at the skin level. Tissue expanders such as those used with breast cancer patients also present a unique problem related to the development of radiation dermatitis because of the thin skin over the area of the tissue expander. Patients undergoing concurrent chemotherapy, immunotherapy, or targeted therapy are at increased risk for radiation dermatitis (Russi et al., 2015; Singh et al., 2016).

Patient Factors

Several patient-specific factors also affect the risk for radiation dermatitis. These factors are similar to those known to result in impaired wound healing and include smoking, poor nutritional status, older age, obesity, race, comorbid conditions (e.g., diabetes, renal failure), and problems with skin integrity prior to initiation of radiation therapy. Previous sun exposure and normal skin care routines (e.g., use of harsh soaps, perfumed soap, or lotions or scrubbing the skin) can also affect the risk for radiation dermatitis. If the patient is receiving treatment to an area where there is skin-to-skin contact such as in the axilla, under the breast, or in the perineal area, there is an increased risk for the development of radiation dermatitis (Russi et al., 2015; Singh et al., 2016). Patients who are receiving chemotherapy concurrently, including traditional therapy as well as targeted therapy, are at an increased risk to develop radiation dermatitis (Wolf, 2019).

Genetic factors were previously thought to affect risk for development of radiation dermatitis based on small studies and case reports. Data from large case series and a few case–control studies do not support this idea (Parker et al., 2017; Wolf, 2019).

CLINICAL PRESENTATION

Transient erythema frequently develops following the first treatment and typically disappears within a few hours but returns following subsequent treatments. Persistent erythema, warmth, and a rash-like appearance to the skin may develop during the first 2 weeks of therapy, assuming 1.8 to 2 Gy per treatment (single-dose fraction). Hyperpigmentation may develop at weeks 2 to 4 due to overactivity of the melanocytes. When the total dose reaches 20 Gy or more, dryness, pruritus, flaking, and dry desquamation may occur. Moist desquamation may develop once the total dose reaches 45 to 60 Gy (**Fig. 31-1**). Moist desquamation results in partial-thickness skin loss with exposure of the dermis; the involved areas are moist, red, and painful. The volume of exudate is variable; if the lesions are exposed to air and the exudate is allowed to dry on the surface of the wound, there is crusting (**Fig. 31-2**) (Hegedus et al., 2017; McQuestion, 2011; Wolf, 2019).

Patients may complain of sensations of skin tightness, dryness, pruritus, pain, general distress, and negative impact on activities of daily living (ADL) and quality of life. If symptoms are severe, patients may have difficulty with self-care activities. The patient may experience financial burden related to radiation dermatitis if he or she is unable to work or must purchase wound care supplies (Beamer & Grant, 2018; Feight et al., 2011).

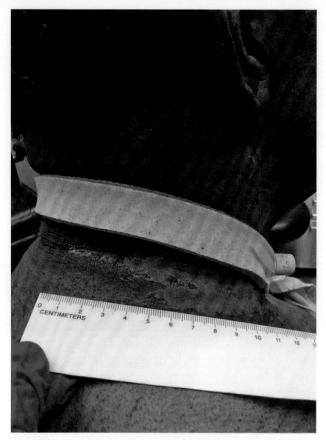

FIGURE 31-1. Radiodermatitis with Moist Desquamation.

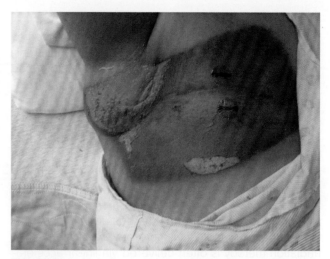

FIGURE 31-2. Moist Desquamation with Crusting.

Severe skin reactions may cause the patient to discontinue therapy.

There are several scales that are used for assessment and classification of radiation dermatitis, but no standard tool has been adopted. The most widely used are the Common Terminology Criteria for Adverse Events (CTCAE) (**Table 31-1**) and the Radiation Therapy Oncology Group (RTOG)/European Organization for Research and Treatment of Cancer (EORTC) scale or Late Effects Normal Tissue Task Force/Subjective, Objective, Management, and Analytic (LENT/SOMA) scale. Although

these are the scales most often used, few reliability or validity data have been published, and the scales remain highly subjective.

Due to the lack of reliability and validity and large increments between the levels of the current grading scales, several other scales have been developed that have narrower increments. Several objective methods such as Doppler perfusion imaging, quantitative ultrasound, spectrophotometry, and digital photography have been utilized in studies to more accurately demonstrate radiation dermatitis. These advanced technologies remain in use for research purposes only (Singh et al., 2016; Wolf, 2019).

DIAGNOSIS

Diagnosis of radiation dermatitis is based on thorough history and physical exam and is typically straightforward. However, the examining clinician should consider the following in the differential diagnosis: skin infection, contact dermatitis, eczema, and cutaneous hypersensitivity syndromes. If the cause of the skin reaction is not clear based on physical exam and history, the patient should be referred to a dermatologist.

TABLE 31-1 COMMON TERMINOLOGY CRITERIA FOR ADVERSE EVENTS V4.0: RADIATION DERMATITIS					
ADVERSE EVENT	1	2	3	4	5
Dermatitis, radiation	Faint erythema or dry desquamation	Moderate to brisk erythema; patchy moist desquamation, mostly confined to skin folds and creases; moderate edema	Moist desquamation in areas other than skin folds and creases; bleeding induced by minor trauma or abrasion	Life-threatening consequences; skin necrosis or ulceration of full-thickness dermis; spontaneous bleeding from involved site; skin graft indicated	Death

Used with permission from Chen, A. P., Setser, A., Anadkat, M. J., et al. (2012). Grading dermatologic adverse events of cancer treatments: The common terminology criteria for adverse events version 4.0. *Journal of the American Academy of Dermatology, 67*(5), 1025–1039.

PREVENTION

While it would be preferable for prevention measures to be instituted prior to the development of radiation dermatitis, there is little evidence to support the use of any one product for the prevention of radiation dermatitis (Hegedus et al., 2017; Singh et al., 2016; Wolf, 2019). The Oncology Nursing Society (ONS), among others, supports only general hygiene practices and the use of topical steroids for itching as measures to prevent radiation dermatitis. In 2013, Wong et al. convened an international multidisciplinary group of experts to develop an evidence-based guideline on prevention and treatment of both acute and late toxicities of radiation therapy. This guideline, supported by those of the Skin Toxicity Study Group of the Multinational Association for Supportive Care in Cancer (MASCC), further expounds upon the guideline developed by Feight and colleagues in 2011 for the ONS. The recommendations by both groups include the following:

- Bathing/shampooing with mild soap/shampoo and water was associated with lower incidence and severity of radiation dermatitis (Russi et al., 2015; Singh et al., 2016; Wolf, 2019; Wong et al., 2013). Use of antiperspirants was found to be safe for women undergoing radiation for breast cancer (Lewis et al., 2014; Wolf, 2019; Wong et al., 2013).
- Topical corticosteroids such as mometasone were found to reduce discomfort, burning, and itching. The recommendation is to begin therapy prior to the first treatment (Singh et al., 2016; Wolf, 2019; Wong et al., 2013).
- A weak recommendation was made for use of silver sulfadiazine cream to reduce severity of radiation dermatitis among women receiving radiation for breast cancer (Singh et al., 2016; Wong et al., 2013).

KEY POINT

There is limited evidence-based guidance for prevention of radiodermatitis. Current guidelines endorse routine bathing with gentle cleansers, routine use of antiperspirants, and preventive use of topical corticosteroids to reduce discomfort, burning, and itching.

Other recommendations consist of the following skin care regimen for patients receiving radiation therapy, based primarily on expert opinion:

1. Instruct patients undergoing radiation therapy to clean the skin twice daily with pH-balanced cleansers paying particular attention to areas with skin-to-skin contact. Pat the skin dry; do not rub.
2. Use only an electric razor in the treatment field.
3. Do not apply topical moisturizers, gels, or emulsions before treatment. Moisturizers are recommended twice daily but should be applied after treatment to the treatment field. These moisturizers should be plain, nonscented, lanolin-free, hydrophilic creams.
4. If itching or irritation develops, initiate low-dose corticosteroid creams (if not already in use).
5. Avoid the following:

    - Swimming in lakes and pools and use of hot tubs or saunas.
    - Tapes and adhesives in the treatment field.
    - Use of ice or heating pads.
    - Exposure to sun. The skin should be protected against sunlight and against cold (Hegedus et al., 2017; Wolf, 2019).

There is a recommendation against the use of aloe vera, and trolamine based on current evidence.

The current evidence is too weak or contradictory to permit any recommendations for or against the use of sucralfate and its derivatives, hyaluronic acid or hyaluronic acid–based combinations, silver dressings, ascorbic acid, LED (light-emitting diode lasers), calendula, petroleum-based ointments, Theta-Cream™, dexpanthenol, oral proteolytic enzymes, oral zinc, or oral pentoxifylline (Lucey et al., 2017; Singh et al., 2016).

More studies are needed in the area of prevention of radiation dermatitis that are of better rigor (Singh et al., 2016). With advancing knowledge of the underlying pathophysiology related to radiation dermatitis, studies should focus on this knowledge while including objective measurements and universal outcomes (Singh et al., 2016).

TREATMENT

Wong et al. (2013) conclude, in their published guideline for prevention and treatment of radiation skin reactions, that there is insufficient evidence to support use of any specific products for treatment of radiation dermatitis. The authors reported on studies involving dressings, sucralfate cream, hydrocortisone 1%, honey, and trolamine. In the studies to date, none of these products reduced the time for resolution of radiation dermatitis.

Dry Desquamation

For patients with dry desquamation, the wound care nurse should continue to recommend preventive care including washing with pH-balanced soap, application of fragrance- and dye-free skin moisturizers twice daily, and the use of topical steroids such as mometasone for symptom management of burning, itching, and discomfort.

Moist Desquamation

Little evidence is available to support the use of one dressing over another to promote healing of moist desquamation. The principles of moist wound healing should be used to guide dressing selection based on wound location, volume of exudate, presence or absence of bleeding, and the radiation oncologist's requirements regarding dressing removal for treatments.

Guidelines for the treatment and management of radiation skin reactions do not recommend for or against hydrocolloids, hydrogels, or honey-impregnated dressings (Ferreira et al., 2017; Russi et al., 2015).

KEY POINT

There is insufficient evidence to recommend any specific products for treatment of radiodermatitis. Dry desquamation should be managed with preventive measures (moisturizers and topical corticosteroids), and moist desquamation should be managed according to the principles of moist wound healing.

Late Radiation Toxicity

Wong et al. (2013) provide the only published guideline for late radiation toxicities. The available evidence focuses only on telangiectasia and cutaneous fibrosis. The guideline provides a weak recommendation for the use of pulsed dye laser to improve visual appearance of telangiectasias and states that there is insufficient evidence to support use of pentoxifylline (800 mg/day) and vitamin E (1,000 IU/day) for treatment of fibrosis (Wolf, 2019; Wong et al., 2013). Strategies with limited evidence include the use of advanced wound dressings, negative pressure wound therapy, and hyperbaric oxygen therapy. Therapy is predicted to include use of special dressings, injection of (multipotent) cells, topical administration of active substances, and the use of growth factors (Spalek, 2016).

 EXTRAVASATION

Extravasation has been defined as the accidental leakage of fluid from a vein into the surrounding tissue (Coyle et al., 2014). Better recognition and management of extravasation has contributed to a decreased incidence. Chemotherapy extravasation is now an uncommon event, occurring in only 0.1% to 6% of all patients who receive peripheral IV chemotherapy. The incidence is thought to be even lower among patients who receive chemotherapy via a central venous access device (0.3% to 4.7%) (Coyle et al., 2014; Jackson-Rose et al., 2017).

RISK FACTORS

Risk factors for extravasation can be classified as patient specific and procedure related. Patient-specific risk factors include the following: small, fragile veins; limited vein selection; history of multiple venipunctures; prior therapy with irritating or sclerosing drugs; sensory, cognitive, or communication deficits interfering with ability to report signs and symptoms of extravasation; difficult venous access (e.g., obese patient, prominent but mobile veins); predisposition to bleeding; and impaired perfusion (e.g., Raynaud's, superior vena cava syndrome, atherosclerosis related to advanced diabetes). Procedure-related

risk factors include probing during IV catheter insertion, failure to adequately secure the IV catheter, placement of IV in site with minimal underlying tissue (e.g., dorsum of hand), use of rigid IV needle as opposed to pliable catheter, prolonged infusion, bolus infusion, high-pressure flow, and poorly placed central venous access device (Boulanger et al., 2015; Coyle et al., 2014; Kimmel et al., 2018).

PATHOLOGY

Chemotherapeutic agents are classified as vesicants, irritants, or nonirritants, and the severity of tissue damage is related primarily to the irritant or vesicant properties of the specific agent involved (**Table 31-2**). Vesicant drugs exert damage to tissues in two different ways. The first category of vesicants causes tissue damage by binding to nucleic acids in the DNA of the healthy cells in the involved tissue, causing initial cell death. The damaged and dying cells release complexes that cause further damage and necrosis of the surrounding cells, causing cell death over an extended period of time. Drugs that fall into this category of vesicant include the anthracyclines (i.e., daunorubicin, doxorubicin, epirubicin, idarubicin), dactinomycin, mechlorethamine, and mitomycin. The second category of vesicants includes drugs that do not bind to the cellular DNA. These drugs undergo metabolism and are excreted more quickly compared to the other class of vesicants. The injury does not persist over an extended period of time. Drugs in this category are also more easily neutralized compared to drugs that bind to DNA. Drugs included in this category of vesicants include paclitaxel and the plant alkaloids (vinblastine, vincristine, vindesine, vinorelbine).

Drugs classified as irritants may cause inflammation and irritation to the vein when they are infused peripherally but do not cause significant cell death and tissue damage. At times, drugs that are classified as irritants may have vesicant properties. Drugs in this category include oxaliplatin, vinorelbine, melphalan, brentuximab, and ado-trastuzumab (Kimmel et al., 2018; Onesti et al., 2017).

CLINICAL PRESENTATION

Initial symptoms of extravasation include complaints of burning, tingling, and pain at the infusion site. Visual inspection at this point may reveal discernible swelling at the site. (Some extravasated drugs may not result in symptoms until hours or days later.) Later signs include blistering, necrosis, and ulceration (**Fig. 31-3**). The degree of tissue damage depends upon the specific drug administered, the concentration of the drug, and the amount of drug extravasated. In severe cases, the patient can experience nerve, tendon, and joint damage, loss of limb function, sensory impairment, disfigurement,

TABLE 31-2 CLASSIFICATION OF CHEMOTHERAPY DRUGS ACCORDING TO THEIR ABILITY TO CAUSE LOCAL DAMAGE AFTER EXTRAVASATION

VESICANTS	IRRITANTS	NONVESICANTS
DNA-binding compounds	Alkylating agents	Arsenic trioxide
Alkylating agents	Carmustine	Asparaginase
Mechlorethamine	Ifosfamide	Bleomycin
Bendamustine*	Streptozocin	Bortezomib
Anthracyclines	Dacarbazine	Cladribine
Doxorubicin	Melphalan	Cytarabine
Daunorubicin	Anthracyclines (other)	Etoposide phosphate
Epirubicin	Liposomal doxorubicin	Gemcitabine
Idarubicin	Liposomal daunorubicin	Fludarabine
Others (antibiotics)	Mitoxantrone	Interferons
Dactinomycin	Topoisomerase II inhibitors	Interleukin-2
Mitomycin C	Etoposide	Methotrexate
Mitoxantrone*	Teniposide	Monoclonal antibodies
Non–DNA-binding compounds	Antimetabolites	Pemetrexed
Vinca alkaloids	Fluorouracil	Raltitrexed
Vincristine	Platin salts	Temsirolimus
Vinblastine	Carboplatin	Thiotepa
Vindesine	Cisplatin	Cyclophosphamide
Vinorelbine	Oxaliplatin	
Taxanes	Topoisomerase I inhibitors	
Docetaxel*	Irinotecan	
Paclitaxel	Topotecan	
Others	Others	
Trabectedin	Ixabepilone	

*Single case reports describe both irritant and vesicant properties.
Used with permission from Pérez Fidalgo, J. A., García Fabregat, L., Cerbantes, J., et al. (2012). Management of chemotherapy extravasation: ESMO-EOPNS clinical practice guidelines. *Annals of Oncology, 23*(Suppl 7), vii167–vii173.

and even loss of limb (Kimmel et al., 2018; Onesti et al., 2017).

DIAGNOSTICS

Diagnosis initially is based on history of drug administration and patient complaint during the infusion.

MANAGEMENT

No randomized controlled studies have been conducted on management of extravasation injuries, due to ethical considerations. All recommendations are based on expert opinion and case reports. Whenever extravasation is suspected, the infusion should be stopped

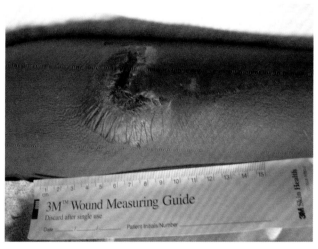
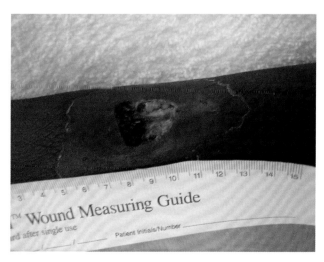

FIGURE 31-3. Extravasation Injuries.

TABLE 31-3 EXTRAVASATION MANAGEMENT

DRUG CLASSIFICATION	IMMEDIATE TOPICAL THERAPY	ANTIDOTE
Alkylating agents	Ice	Sodium thiosulfate
Anthracyclines	Ice	Totect®
Antitumor antibiotics	Ice	No known antidote
Plant alkaloid or microtubular-inhibiting agents	Warm pack	Hyaluronidase
Taxanes	Ice	No known antidote

immediately and the prescribing health care professional should be notified. An attempt to aspirate any residual vesicant from the IV device using a 1- to 3-mL syringe should be attempted, and the IV should then be discontinued. At that point, either ice or heat should be applied, with the specific modality determined by the chemotherapeutic agent involved. Antidotes and treatments per institutional policy should then be administered (Boulanger et al., 2015; Kimmel et al., 2018). (See **Table 31-3** for management recommendations for specific agents.) To manage late side effects, particularly those related to DNA-binding agents, surgical debridement may be indicated although there is no standard procedure for surgical treatment. Signs that surgical debridement is indicated include continued erythema, edema, pain, or unresolved tissue necrosis or skin ulcerations (Boulanger et al., 2015).

The wound care nurse's role in management of extravasation injuries is to recommend topical therapy once initial treatment has been provided. Principles of moist wound healing should be followed, with recommendations based on the characteristics of the wound. No one dressing has been proven to be superior over another. It is common for plastic surgery to be involved and for skin grafting to be indicated in significant extravasation injuries; the wound care nurse should consult plastic surgery whenever the extravasation injury produces a full-thickness wound located over or adjacent to a tendon, bone, or joint.

KEY POINT

The wound care nurse's role in management of extravasation injuries is to recommend topical therapy based on moist wound-healing principles (once initial treatment protocols have been completed) and to initiate a plastic surgery consult if there is full-thickness damage over or adjacent to a tendon, bone, or joint.

 TARGETED CHEMOTHERAPY SKIN REACTIONS

Targeted chemotherapy is the use of drugs or other chemicals that block cellular pathways and processes essential to cell growth and survival; drugs in this class include angiogenesis inhibitors, hormone therapies, signal transduction inhibitors, gene expression modulators, apoptosis inducers, immunotherapies, and toxin delivery molecules (National Cancer Institute, 2019a,b). Specific medications currently available include EGFR inhibitors such as monoclonal antibodies and tyrosine kinase inhibitors, mammalian target inhibitors (mTOR), antiangiogenic agents, cytokines, and KIT and BCR-ABL inhibitors. This is an evolving area of cancer therapy, and new drugs are continually being developed and brought to market. It is beyond the scope of this chapter to list all of the medications in these classes.

KEY POINT

Targeted chemotherapies involve agents that block cellular pathways and processes essential to cell growth. Skin reactions are common with these drugs, and these reactions have been linked to tumor response and overall survival.

Although the mechanism of action is poorly understood, these agents can cause adverse skin and nail effects. The most commonly encountered skin reaction is a papulopustular rash. Hair changes, increased severity of radiation dermatitis, pruritus, fissures, and paronychia are all potential side effects of targeted therapies.

A positive correlation between the development of skin toxicity, including rash, has been linked to tumor response and overall survival. Several theories about this relationship have been advanced, but to date, no data have confirmed a causal relationship (Hofheinz et al., 2017).

PREVALENCE/INCIDENCE

The incidence of skin rash caused by targeted therapies varies based on the specific drug and if the drug is used in combination with traditional chemotherapy. Hofheinz et al. (2017) present pooled data on the use of EGFRi for the treatment of gastrointestinal cancers with the use of cetuximab and panitumumab. They report an incidence of over 85% for those receiving monotherapy and as high as 96% for those receiving combination therapy. Sibaud (2018) reports the incidence of skin rash for patients who are receiving checkpoint inhibitors. He reports an incidence between 24.3% and 14.3% for drugs such as ipilimumab, pembrolizumab, and nivolumab.

RISK FACTORS

Risk factors for skin reactions related to targeted therapies continue to be explored with researchers looking for biomarkers to be used to predict which patients will develop skin reactions (Kubo et al., 2016). Wei et al. (2018) report that the risk factors for developing a skin rash in patients receiving anti–epidermal growth factor receptors for biliary cancer are better performance status, male gender, younger age, and less exposure to smoking. Risk factors for rash continue to be variable depending upon the drug administered.

PATHOLOGY

Targeted therapies are novel agents that block specific pathways affecting cellular function; the different drugs affect different areas of cellular pathways. The antitumor mechanism of these drugs lies in their ability to target erroneously active or overexpression of growth factors in tumors. EGFR inhibitors, for example, target overexpression or aberrantly active EGFR in some tumors such as colorectal cancers. EGFR is essential to normal keratinocyte function, such as the ability to proliferate, differentiate, and migrate. It plays an important role in wound healing as well as carcinogenesis. Inhibition of this pathway causes the characteristic skin changes associated with this drug class (Kubo et al., 2016). Drugs in this class of medications include for example, cetuximab, which binds to the extracellular portion of EGFR, and erlotinib and gefitinib, which bind to the intracellular tyrosine kinase domain of EGFR. In general, the disruption of the cellular pathways results in skin effects that can be problematic.

Research has provided insight into the pathogenesis of the rash and skin changes associated with targeted agents that inhibit EGFR, but the exact pathologic mechanisms remain poorly understood. Inhibition of EGFR prevents epidermal keratinocytes from controlling intercellular signal transduction pathways. Arrested cell growth, migration, apoptosis, and abnormal maturation and differentiation result. There is also an increased release of chemokines as well as cutaneous inflammation, altered immunosuppression, neutrophil accumulation, epidermal keratinocyte proliferation, and erosion of the stratum corneum. This activates an inflammatory response, immunosuppression, and superinfection, which is thought to be responsible for the dermatologic manifestations (Annunziate et al., 2019; Lacouture & Sibaud, 2018).

CLINICAL PRESENTATION

Skin changes associated with targeted therapies include rash, hand–foot skin reaction, xerosis, pruritus, and paronychia.

Rash

The rash associated with targeted therapies has a classic presentation. The rash, which most commonly occurs within the first 2 weeks of therapy, presents as erythem-

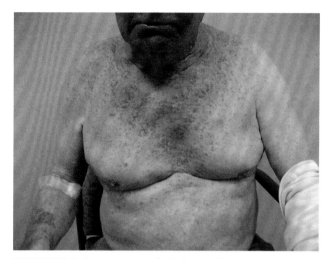

FIGURE 31-4. Papulopustular Rash Due to Targeted Chemotherapy.

atous papules and pustules primarily along the seborrheic-rich areas on the face (nose, cheeks, nasolabial folds, chin, forehead, perioral region), scalp, and upper trunk. It less commonly will extend to the lower trunk, extremities, and buttocks. Initial presentation begins with edema, erythema, and sensory disturbances (pain, burning, and irritation). The next phase is eruption of the papulopustular rash (**Fig. 31-4**). During weeks 3 to 5, the rash is covered with crusts. In the 2nd month, the papulopustular rash resolves, but there is persistent erythema, xerosis, and formation of telangiectasias in the areas previously affected by the rash (Barton-Burke et al., 2017; Hofheinz et al., 2016).

Rash severity varies from patient to patient and typically waxes and wanes during the course of therapy. The rash is expected to resolve completely within 4 weeks following discontinuation of therapy although postinflammatory changes such as erythema and pigmentation changes may remain. Rash severity is typically graded according to the National Cancer Institute's Common Terminology Criteria for Adverse Events (CTCAE) (**Table 31-4**). Researchers believe that no scale is adequately capturing skin reactions. There is a need for more clear definitions as to what classifies each skin reaction as patients may develop severe skin reactions in one area of the body. The CTCAE follows the rule of nines, which would underscore locally severe rashes. The Multinational Association of Supportive Care in Cancer (MASCC) EGFR Inhibitor Skin Toxicity Tool (MESTT©) and Wollenberg tools provide a more accurate assessment of the skin, but neither have been adopted routinely in clinical practice at this time (Hofheinz et al., 2016).

KEY POINT

Specific skin reactions associated with targeted chemotherapies include papulopustular rash, hand–foot skin reaction, xerosis, pruritus, and paronychia.

TABLE 31-4 COMMON TERMINOLOGY CRITERIA FOR ADVERSE EVENTS V4.0: RASH, ACNEIFORM

ADVERSE EVENT	1	2	3	4	5
Rash, acneiform	Papules and/or pustules covering <10% BSA, which may or may not be associated with symptoms of pruritus or tenderness	Papules and/or pustules covering 10%–30% BSA, which may or may not be associated with symptoms of pruritus or tenderness; associated with psychosocial impact; limiting instrumental ADL	Papules and/or pustules covering >30% BSA, which may or may not be associated with symptoms of pruritus or tenderness that limit self-care ADL; associated with local superinfection with oral antibiotics indicated	Papules and/or pustules covering any % BSA, which may or may not be associated with symptoms of pruritus or tenderness and are associated with extensive superinfection with IV antibiotics indicated; life-threatening consequences	Death

Definition: A disorder characterized by an eruption of papules and pustules, typically appearing on the face, scalp, upper chest, and back.
Reprinted from Chen, A. P., Setser, A., Anadkat, M. J., et al. (2012). Grading dermatologic adverse events of cancer treatments: The common terminology criteria for adverse events version 4.0. *Journal of the American Academy of Dermatology, 67*(5), 1025–1039, Used with permission of Elsevier.

Hand–Foot Skin Reaction

Another type of skin reaction that may occur with targeted therapies is known as hand–foot skin reaction. These patients typically experience dysesthesia and paresthesia of the hands and/or feet that begin within the first 6 weeks of therapy, followed by development of tender lesions with or without blisters. The blisters are surrounded by an erythematous rim. The lesions are frequently located on areas subjected to pressure and friction, such as the distal tips of the fingers, the heels, and the skin over the metacarpophalangeal and interphalangeal joints. The lateral aspects of the soles, finger webs, and periungual regions can also be involved. Resolution of the blisters is followed by development of painful hyperkeratotic lesions. Hand–foot skin reaction is a distinct entity despite similar presentations of hand–foot syndrome associated with cytotoxic agents such as doxorubicin, 5-fluorouracil, and capecitabine (McLellan et al., 2015) (**Fig. 31-5**).

Xerosis

Xerosis is a late event that typically follows the rash associated with EGFR inhibitors. It presents as scaly, pruritic skin changes at times described as eczema craquelé. If not treated effectively, the xerosis can progress to chronic xerotic dermatitis, which can lead to increased risk for superinfections. If the xerosis involves the hands and feet, the patient is at risk for development of painful fissures on the tips of the fingers, toes, and dorsal aspects of the interphalangeal joints (Guggina et al., 2017; Valentine et al., 2015).

Pruritus

Although not visible, pruritus is a significant problem for patients receiving targeted therapies. Pruritus often accompanies the rash associated with targeted therapies with some authors stating the pruritus occurs before xerosis and others reporting that the xerosis causes the pruritus. Studies report that pruritus affects the quality of life of patients and can result in dose reduction or discontinuation even if the therapy is effective and lifesaving (Clabbers et al., 2016; Valentine et al., 2015).

Paronychia

Paronychia is a delayed reaction that occurs in 10% to 25% of patients following at least 4 weeks of targeted therapy.

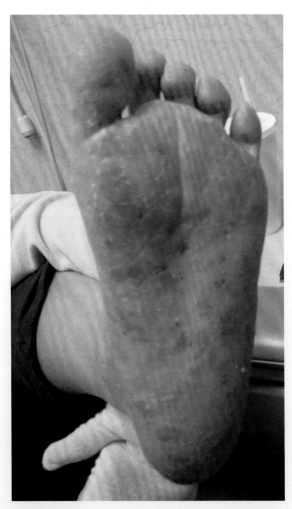

FIGURE 31-5. Hand–Foot Skin Reaction.

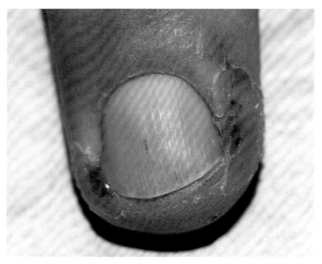

FIGURE 31-6. Paronychia.

It is characterized by tender, edematous inflammation of the periungual folds. Initially, the lesions are aseptic, but superinfections with purulence can occur. The inflammation can progress to a pyogenic granuloma–like lesion that gives the appearance of an infected ingrown nail. This most often affects the toes but can also affect the fingers (**Fig. 31-6**) (Lacouture & Sibaud, 2018).

MANAGEMENT

Strategies to manage the dermatologic side effects of targeted therapies continue to be refined. Based on evidence and consensus, multiple management plans have been proposed with variability being noted from country to country. All of the management plans agree that the dermatologic side effects should not result in dose reduction or discontinuation of therapy. The first clinical practice guidelines that addressed evidence-based interventions for prevention and management of skin reactions to targeted therapies are the Multinational Association of Supportive Care in Cancer (MASCC) Skin Toxicity Study Group (Lacouture et al., 2011) and a French interdisciplinary therapeutic algorithm (Reguiai et al., 2012). Current recommendations build upon these studies, and all stress the importance of routine preventive care unless there are patient-specific contraindications. Adverse skin reactions may occur as soon as 2 days after administration (Annunziate et al., 2019; Hofheinz et al., 2017).

Rash

Prevention strategies focus on good topical skin care including a skin assessment prior to the initiation of therapy and at regular intervals during therapy. Sun exposure should be avoided. Sunscreen of SPF 25 or higher is recommended if patients must go out into the sun. Washing with lukewarm water and a pH-balanced cleanser while avoiding hot showers is recommended. Consistent use of emollient-based moisturizers is especially important. This should be applied to the face, hands, feet, back, and chest in the morning. Hydrocortisone 1% should then be applied to the same areas at bedtime. The use of tetracycline or tetracycline-class antibiotics is recommended. Tetracycline 250 to 500 mg, doxycycline 100 to 200 mg, and minocycline 100 mg are believed to be the most effective for prevention. Minocycline has the least photosensitizing effects and is the most appropriate choice in areas with a high ultraviolet index.

If a grade 1 rash develops, a topical antibiotic should be prescribed along with the preventative regimen. Topical antibiotics include clindamycin 1%, erythromycin 1%, or preparations containing metronidazole. For those patients who develop a grade 2 rash, topical corticosteroids should be added if not already in use or their potency should be increased. Medium- to high-potency topical corticosteroid such as alclometasone 0.05% or fluocinonide 0.05% b.i.d. should be applied topically as well as a topical antibiotic as recommended for grade 1 rash. If the patient is not already on systemic therapy preemptively, then this should be prescribed. If a grade 3 rash develops, dose reduction or temporary discontinuation of the drug may be necessary. At times a short course of oral corticosteroid therapy may be beneficial. Those patients who develop more severe or extensive rash should be referred to a dermatologist. Other interventions supported by the guidelines include cutting the nails straight but not too short, and nonaggressive shaving (Hofheinz et al., 2016, 2017; Lacouture et al., 2018).

> **KEY POINT**
>
> Prevention and management of the rash associated with targeted chemotherapy agents include gentle skin care, moisturizers, sunscreen, topical corticosteroids, and doxycycline or minocycline.

Hand–Foot Skin Reaction

Preventive care for the individual at risk for hand–foot skin reactions includes the following:

- Education regarding symptoms. The patient should know to notify the health care team promptly if symptoms develop.
- Ongoing monitoring via full-body skin exam, with referral to podiatrist or orthotist if indicated.
- Thick cotton socks to help keep soles of feet dry.
- Shoes with padded insoles.
- Avoidance of excessive temperature, pressure, and friction (avoid long walks and constrictive shoes).
- Use of mild soap for bathing.
- Ammonium lactate 12% or heavy moisturizer (e.g., petroleum jelly) b.i.d. for prophylaxis.

Treatment of hand–foot skin reaction depends on the severity (grade) of the reaction. For grade 1 reactions, current recommendations include keratolytics including urea cream 1% to 40% or salicylic acid 5% to 10% on hyperkeratotic areas only. Lidocaine gel or other topical analgesics can help to relieve pain. Topical corticosteroids such as clobetasol 0.05% applied twice daily are recommended with use of thick socks at night. If oozing lesions are present, these may be treated with antiseptic baths. Agents recommended include potassium permanganate, chlorhexidine gluconate, or diluted bleach. For Grade 2 or 3 reactions, recommendations include (1) topical antibiotics for blisters and erosions; (2) topical corticosteroids (clobetasol 0.05% or fluocinonide 0.05%) applied twice daily to areas that are erythematous, inflamed, and painful; (3) topical keratolytic preparations (salicylic acid 6% or urea 20% to 40%) applied twice daily to hyperkeratotic areas only; and (4) pain management with systemic medications. These measures should be used in addition to those already addressed for prevention and management of grade 1 reactions. For grade 3 reactions, treatment should be interrupted until the severity is reduced to grade 0 to 1 (MacDonald et al., 2015; McLellan et al., 2015).

Xerosis

Guidelines for prevention of xerosis are straightforward and include use of tepid water for bathing (with bath oils or mild moisturizing soaps), regular use of moisturizing creams, and avoidance of direct sunlight and extremes in temperature.

Treatment guidelines are less clear but include the following as options:

- Occlusive emollient creams that are fragrance free and alcohol free; these include products that are petrolatum based and those that contain urea or colloidal oatmeal.
- Exfoliant products on scaly areas (e.g., ammonium lactate 12% or lactic acid cream 12%).
- Urea creams (10% to 40%) or salicylic acid (6%).
- Zinc oxide (13% to 40%).
- Severe xerosis: medium- to high-potency steroid creams (triamcinolone acetonide 0.025%, desonide 0.05%, fluticasone propionate 0.05%, alclometasone 0.05%).
- Avoid alcohol-containing lotions, retinoids, and benzoyl peroxide (Barton-Burke et al., 2017; Guggina et al., 2017; Hofheinz et al., 2017; Valentine et al., 2015).

Pruritus

Prevention of pruritus includes the measures already listed for prevention of xerosis, which is a common contributing factor. Patients should be counseled regarding the importance of gentle skin care. Treatment is based on the severity of the pruritus. Classes IV to V steroids in cream or ointment form twice daily are recommended (triamcinolone acetonide 0.025%, desonide 0.05%, fluticasone propionate 0.05%, or alclometasone 0.05%). Topical antipruritic agents are also recommended (menthol-based products *or* pramoxine 0.5% *or* doxepin 1%). If the pruritus is refractory to topical therapy, then systemic agents such as oral antihistamines (cetirizine, hydroxyzine) or gabapentin/pregabalin should be initiated if antihistamines are ineffective. Other agents showing promising results in management of pruritus include doxepin and aprepitant (Barton-Burke et al., 2017; Guggina et al., 2017; Valentine et al., 2015).

Paronychia

Recommendations for prevention of paronychia include the following:

- Dilute bleach soaks (0.005%, i.e., 1/8 to 1/4 cup of 6% bleach to 3 to 5 gallons of water)
- White vinegar soaks (1 part white vinegar to 1 part water)
- Cutting nails straight but not too short
- Use of fragrance-free, dye-free pH-balanced cleansers
- Wearing comfortable shoes
- Wearing gloves for cleaning

Treatment recommendations include culturing the lesion to rule out superinfection, topical corticosteroids and anti-inflammatory dose of tetracycline (e.g., doxycycline 200 mg twice daily until resolution), and electrocautery, silver nitrate, or nail avulsion for excessive granulation tissue (Guggina et al., 2017; Hofheinz et al., 2017; Lacouture et al., 2018; Macdonald et al., 2015).

 PALMAR–PLANTAR ERYTHRODYSESTHESIA (HAND–FOOT SYNDROME)

Palmar–plantar erythrodysesthesia (PPE) is a painful erythematous rash that occurs on the palms of the hands and the soles of the feet. The reaction may progress to desquamation and bullae formation with resultant impairment in function. It is known by several other names including hand–foot syndrome, palmar–plantar erythema, acral erythema, and Burgdorf reaction. It is associated with doxorubicin, capecitabine, docetaxel, cytarabine, and 5-fluorouracil (Huang et al., 2018; Nikolaou et al., 2016).

> **KEY POINT**
>
> Palmar–plantar erythrodysesthesia (PPE) is a painful erythematous skin reaction on the palms of the hands and soles of the feet that may progress to desquamation and bullae formation with resultant impairment in function. Management of any open lesions is based on the principles of moist wound healing.

PREVALENCE/INCIDENCE

The incidence of PPE has been reported to be between 6% and 42% of all patients treated with doxorubicin, capecitabine, docetaxel, cytarabine, 5-fluorouracil, cyclophosphamide, and vinorelbine. Capecitabine is the agent most commonly associated with PPE, with an incidence of 45% to 68% (Kang et al., 2010).

RISK FACTORS

Currently there are no specific risk factors for PPE although several theories have been proposed. A genetic predisposition may be present due to deficiencies in dihydropyrimidine dehydrogenase (DPD), which is an enzyme involved in the metabolism of fluoropyrimidines. This deficiency results in an increased half-life of 5 FU. This deficiency is more apparent in African Americans and other racial groups and less likely with Caucasians. A second theory is that there is a deletion of the allele of rs3215400 in the cytidine deaminase (CDD) gene. This gene plays a role in the metabolism of a number of antitumor cytosine nucleoside analogues, which leads to activation into 5-FU. Both theories require further study to support the role that these genetic predispositions may play in the development of PPE. The appearance of PPE is related to the specific chemotherapeutic agent, the dose, and the schedule of administration although there is no direct association for all patients who develop PPE (Nikolaou et al., 2016).

PATHOLOGY

The pathology of PPE is difficult to determine as it occurs with multiple chemotherapeutic agents with different mechanisms of action. The reaction has common features regardless of the associated chemotherapeutic agent. The areas involved are characterized by temperature gradients, a high concentration of eccrine glands, and exposure to significant friction and trauma.

This supports the idea that local factors, such as pressure, friction, and trauma may play a role in the development of PPE. Several theories of causation have been proposed. One theory is that the drug is transported to the skin surface via the sweat and deposited into the stratum corneum where it generates free radicals that react with the epidermal cells to cause PPE. Another theory related to capecitabine-related PPE proposes causation from damage to deep capillaries. This may be due to enzymes involved in the metabolism of capecitabine leaking resulting in cyclooxygenase (COX) inflammatory-type reactions. A third theory is that PPE may be caused by a reduction in the antioxidative potential of the skin due to intensive radical formation. Further study needs to be done to determine the true pathology of this disorder (Nikolaou et al., 2016).

CLINICAL PRESENTATION

The first symptoms of PPE are tingling, numbness, or pain on the palms of the hands or the soles of the feet. This is followed by bilateral erythematous changes that are sharply demarcated. The erythema may progress to formation of bullae and desquamation. In severe cases, ischemic necrotic lesions can develop in the area of bullae formation. Patients with a dark complexion may present with hyperpigmentation and thickening of the skin that may result in stiffness. The hands and feet are most often affected, but other areas of the body may also be involved, including the axillae, groin, waist, inner surface of knees, posterior elbows, anterior folding lines of the wrists, sacral area, bra line, and other areas exposed to occlusion or friction (**Fig. 31-7**) (Nikolaou et al., 2016).

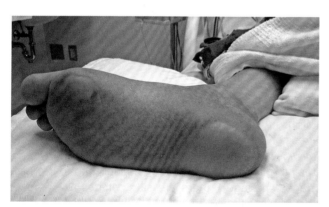

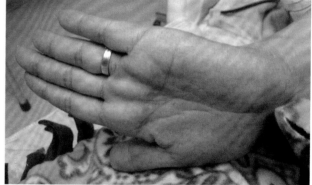

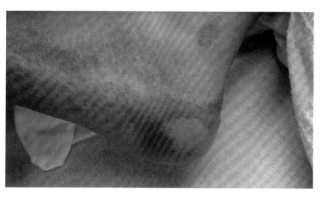

FIGURE 31-7. Palmar–Plantar Erythrodysesthesia.

TABLE 31-5 LIFESTYLE STRATEGIES FOR PREVENTION OF PLANTAR–PALMAR ERYTHRODYSESTHESIA

- Keep areas well lubricated with emollient creams.
- Avoid skin irritants such as perfumes or alcohol.
- Protect the hands and feet with thick cotton socks and gloves.
- Avoid tight or constricting shoes or clothing.
- Avoid adhesives.
- Avoid activities that add pressure to areas at risk.
- Minimize perspiration.
- Wear protective gloves when performing household tasks.
- Pat skin dry; do not rub.
- Avoid direct sun exposure.
- Keep affected limbs elevated.

PREVENTION AND MANAGEMENT

There are no known preventive therapies. In 2018, Huang et al. reviewed the clinical evidence for the prevention of PPE. In their review, a total of 17 studies were included in the meta-analysis. They reported that while pyridoxine was once thought to be effective in prevention of PPE, none of the 10 studies reviewed supported its use. Huang et al. also examined the evidence for celecoxib, urea/lactic acid, silymarin, Fuzheng Jiedusan, and neurotropin. None of these were found to have evidence to support the use of these products. General prevention measures are directed toward maintenance of healthy skin and prevention of skin trauma and are outlined in **Table 31-5** (Huang et al., 2018).

Treatment of PPE primarily involves dose reduction of the offending agent. The patient should be counseled to continue lifestyle prevention strategies, and analgesics should be prescribed as needed to control the pain (Nikolaou et al., 2016). The wound care nurse may be consulted to assist with dressing recommendations for patients who have significant PPE. Dressing selection should be based on the principles of moist wound healing and is affected by the location of the lesions and volume of drainage. Use of a nonadherent dressing (e.g., petrolatum gauze dressing) secured by roll gauze is a reasonable choice in most situations. The dressing should be changed at least twice daily to allow for inspection of the skin.

⬤ CUTANEOUS T-CELL LYMPHOMA (MYCOSIS FUNGOIDES AND SÉZARY SYNDROME)

Cutaneous T-cell lymphoma is a heterogeneous group of non-Hodgkin lymphomas where monoclonal T lymphocytes invade the skin. There is a wide variety of disorders included in this group, with mycosis fungoides (MF) and Sézary syndrome (SS) being identified as common subtypes. MF is the most commonly occurring of the two and is considered indolent. SS is the aggressive leukemic variant. It can present as a progression of MF or can occur as new-onset lesions that progress rapidly (Peterson et al., 2019).

KEY POINT

MF and SS are two subtypes of cutaneous T-cell lymphoma; MF is more common and is usually indolent, while SS is an aggressive leukemic variant.

PREVALENCE/INCIDENCE

Cutaneous lymphomas represent close to 4% of all non-Hodgkin's lymphomas, with 75% of primary cutaneous lymphomas being T-cell derived. Of these, two thirds are classified as MF and SS. The annual age-adjusted incidence is estimated at 4 to 9.6 cases per million in the United States. Older individuals are at greater risk (median age at diagnosis is 55 to 60), and the male to female ratio is 2:1 (Foss & Girardi, 2016; Mahalingam & Reddy, 2015; Peterson et al., 2019; Wilcox, 2017).

RISK FACTORS

Risk factors for MF and SS are not well understood, but certain factors have been explored. These include exposure to agents that cause chronic antigenic stimulation, such as pesticides and other chemicals including other occupational chemical exposure. Both bacterial and viral exposures are also theorized to play a causative role (Foss & Girardi, 2016; Mahalingam & Reddy, 2015).

PATHOLOGY

The cause of MF/SS remains unknown. Several theories have been proposed including chronic antigen stimulation, stimulation by viruses, and ultraviolet irradiation. None of these theories have identified a definitive cause (Peterson et al., 2019; Wilcox, 2017). What is known is that this is a disorder of complex chromosomal abnormalities and genetic instability and mutations that are beyond the scope of this chapter.

CLINICAL PRESENTATION

MF has a classic presentation of patches or plaques on areas of the body that are not sun exposed. These areas may be well defined and pruritic and over time may progress to tumors. The disease is defined into four clinical stages. In stage 1, there are skin patches and plaques that cover either <10% body surface area (stage 1A) or more than 10% body surface area (stage 1B). Stage IIA disease is characterized by lymphadenopathy without nodal infiltration; Stage IIB is characterized by cutaneous tumors. The presence of generalized erythroderma is characteristic of Stage III disease. Pathologically positive lymph nodes are indicative of Stage IVA disease, while visceral disease characterizes Stage IVB.

SS is characterized by the combination of circulating neoplastic T cells and erythroderma, with or without lymphadenopathy. Patients may also suffer from disabling pruritus. SS should be suspected in any patient who has atypical lymphocytes in the blood and an unexplained pruritic erythroderma (**Fig. 31-8**) (PDQ, 2019).

DIAGNOSTICS

At the time of suspected initial diagnosis, the following studies should be performed: CBC with differential, chemistry panel, lactate dehydrogenase, and skin biopsy specimen for dermatopathology, immunophenotyping, and T-cell receptor gene rearrangement studies. In addition, flow cytometry and TCR studies of tissue or blood, Sézary cell count, circulating T-cell subsets and clonality, and immunophenotyping are recommended. MRI, PET/CT scans, and/or lymph node biopsy should be performed for those patients with higher stage disease. The results of these tests are essential for staging and treatment planning (Peterson et al., 2019; Wilcox, 2017).

MANAGEMENT

Management is based on disease stage. The National Comprehensive Cancer Network (NCCN) has developed guidelines for the workup and management of MF/SS (https://www.nccn.org/professionals/physician_gls/default_nojava.aspx#site). The reader is directed to this guideline for additional information.

Treatment for early disease is based on observational studies and case reports and includes the following topical agents: corticosteroids, imiquimod, nitrogen mustard, local radiation, phototherapy, topical retinoids, and total skin electron beam therapy. More advanced disease or disease that fails to respond to topical therapy is treated with systemic therapy. Various forms of chemotherapy, immune therapy, targeted therapies, extracorporeal photopheresis, and, for advanced disease, stem cell transplant are mainstays of therapy (Jawed et al., 2014; NCCN, 2018).

The wound care nurse may be consulted for topical care recommendations as the patient experiences disease progression. In these cases, since the skin changes are due to tumor, the goal of care is palliation of symptoms. The role of the wound care nurse will center on addressing potential complicating factors such as prevention of pressure injury, infection prevention and control, debridement, exudate management, odor control, and appropriate topical care. Little has been written about the topical wound care of MF or SS, and no one dressing or treatment has been established as superior over another.

GRAFT VERSUS HOST DISEASE

Bone marrow transplant (BMT) has been performed since the 1960s with the goal of providing cure for a variety of hematologic and solid tumors. There are several different types of transplants. Allogeneic transplants involve cells from a related donor or an unrelated volunteer. Autologous transplantation involves harvesting the patient's cells prior to the administration of high-dose chemotherapy and then reinfusing the patient's own cells following the high-dose chemotherapy. Syngeneic transplant is the use of cells from an identical twin (Kavand et al., 2017).

Graft versus host disease (GVHD), an immune-mediated reaction is more often associated with allogeneic transplants. GVHD can be divided into two categories, acute and chronic. Acute GVHD usually affects three

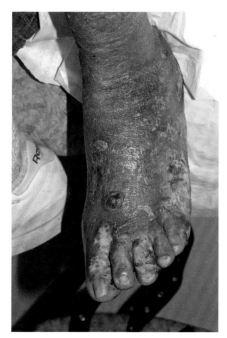
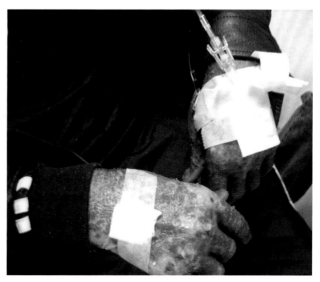

FIGURE 31-8. Sézary Syndrome (Pruritic Erythroderma).

body systems (skin, liver, and gastrointestinal tract) and has been commonly defined as occurring within the first 100 days posttransplant. In 2005, the National Institutes of Health Consensus Project changed the classifications of GVHD. Classic acute GVHD is now defined as reactions occurring before day 100 while persistent, recurrent, or late-onset acute GVHD may occur after day 100. Chronic GVHD occurs after the first 100 days and may involve any tissue, though most commonly the skin, eyes, oral cavity, GI tract, and liver are involved. Overlapping GVHD has symptoms of both acute and chronic GVHD (Kavand et al., 2017; Rodrigues et al., 2018).

KEY POINT

Graft versus host disease is usually associated with allogeneic transplants, may be either acute or chronic, and frequently results in skin pathology. A minority of patients experience severe cutaneous GVHD, which results in extensive moist desquamation.

PREVALENCE/INCIDENCE

Acute GVHD occurs in 40% to 80% of all allogeneic bone marrow transplant recipients. It accounts for 15% of deaths following a transplant; prompt recognition and treatment are essential to recovery. The severity of the acute GVHD is prognostic (Kavand et al., 2017; Villarreal et al., 2016).

Chronic GVHD occurs in approximately 30% to 70% of all patients who undergo an allogeneic transplant and 60% to 80% of the adult survivors of acute GVHD. Median time for presentation is approximately 5 months with 10% presenting with symptoms at >1 year. It is the primary cause of long-term morbidity and mortality (Kavand et al., 2017; Wang et al., 2019).

RISK FACTORS

Risk factors for GVHD vary according to time of onset (acute vs. chronic) (Kavand et al., 2017; Rodrigues et al., 2018). The risk factors are listed in **Table 31-6**.

PATHOLOGY

Acute GVHD is believed to represent an inflammatory response caused by a cytokine storm. One theory proposes a three-phase model that begins with tissue injury during the conditioning regimen, followed by donor T-cell priming and finally an effector phase with target tissue apoptosis from T and natural killer cells and cytokines. Chronic GVHD is most likely the result of dysfunctional donor B and T cells. A defect in B-cell hemostasis results for circulating antibodies against the recipient antigens. Other theories continue to develop, which are examining the role of other antibodies and genetic changes (Kavand et al., 2017; Rodrigues et al., 2018; Villarreal et al., 2016)

TABLE 31-6 RISK FACTORS FOR ACUTE AND CHRONIC GVHD

ACUTE GVHD	CHRONIC GVHD
Age of recipient; age of donor	Acute GVHD
GVHD prophylaxis	Older age
HLA matching between the donor and recipient (mismatched donor)	HLA matching between the donor and recipient (mismatched donor)
Intensity of the conditioning regimen	Donor gender (female donor with male recipient)
Graft composition	Use of peripheral blood as stem cell source
Donor gender (female donor with male recipient) Use of donor lymphocyte infusion Use of total body irradiation (TBI) in the conditioning regimen	Use of donor lymphocyte infusion

CLINICAL PRESENTATION

Acute GVHD

Skin manifestations of GVHD typically present in the first 10 to 14 days posttransplant with a rash that begins acrally but eventually becomes generalized in distribution. The rash may be morbilliform or maculopapular and is generally symmetrical. The back and neck are commonly involved (**Fig. 31-9**). In severe cases, there is diffuse erythroderma and bullae formation with a positive Nikolsky sign (ability to cause peripheral extension of a blister by applying lateral pressure to the border of an intact blister), followed by extensive moist desquamation that resembles toxic epidermal necrolysis (TENS) (**Fig. 31-10**).

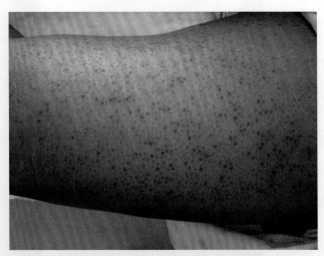

FIGURE 31-9. Rash Secondary to Acute GVHD.

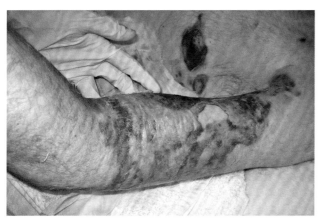

FIGURE 31-10. Extensive Moist Desquamation Secondary to Acute GVHD.

Chronic GVHD

Chronic GVHD has a more subtle onset and variable presentation; possible signs and symptoms include the following (**Fig. 31-11**):

- Xerosis
- Keratosis pilaris–like lesions
- Ichthyosis
- Papulosquamous lesions
- Psoriasiform and pityriasis rosea–like skin changes
- Annular lesions
- Superficial erythema
- Lichenoid lesions
- Sclerotic changes with plaques
- Poikilodermatous changes
- Hair and nail changes (dystrophy, thickening or thinning, vertical ridging of nails, onycholysis, and scarring and nonscarring alopecia) (Kavand et al., 2017; Rodrigues et al., 2018; Villarreal et al., 2016).

Diagnosis of acute GVHD is based on clinical assessment and often verified by skin biopsy, although controversy remains about the utility of a skin biopsy. The diagnosis of chronic GVHD requires at least one clinical feature and one distinctive clinical sign that is confirmed by biopsy. There must also be one laboratory or

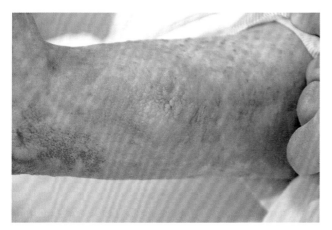

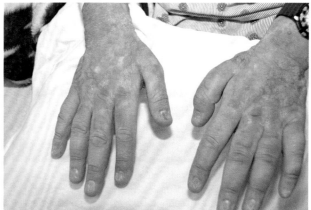

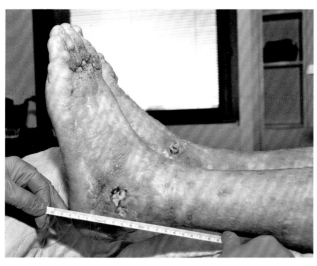

FIGURE 31-11. Skin and Soft Tissue Changes Due to Chronic GVHD.

TABLE 31-7 PREVENTION AND TREATMENT OF ACUTE GVHD

PREVENTION	TREATMENT
Immunosuppression	Glucocorticoids for grades II–IV
Reduced-intensity conditioning regimens	Immune modulators including mycophenolate mofetil, imatinib mesylate, rituximab, rapamycin, methrotrexate
T-cell suppression or depletion in the donor marrow	Skin-targeted therapies: topical corticosteroids, topical calcineurin inhibitors Phototherapy and extracorporeal photopheresis New drugs on the horizon including ibrutinib, ruxolitinib, tofacitinib

radiologic test in the same or another organ to confirm the diagnosis. All other possible diagnoses must also be ruled out (Kavand et al., 2017).

MANAGEMENT OF ACUTE GVHD

Management of acute GVHD is based on systemic therapy. Systemic management principles are listed in **Table 31-7**. The role of the wound care nurse will center on supportive care. Supportive care includes gentle cleansing; use of nonadherent dressings that absorb exudate, inhibit bacterial growth, and maintain a moist wound surface; and support surfaces that provide pressure redistribution, reduce shear and friction, and provide microclimate control.

KEY POINT

Management of acute GVHD includes systemic therapy to control the underlying process, topical therapy based on moist wound healing, and support surfaces that provide pressure redistribution, reduction in shear and friction, and microclimate control.

MANAGEMENT OF CHRONIC GVHD

Systemic therapy is one element of management for chronic GVHD. Supportive care is also important to positive outcomes.

Supportive care includes personal hygiene, use of appropriate antimicrobial agents when indicated, liberal use of emollient agents to keep the skin soft, and use of compression garments to manage venous insufficiency caused by soft tissue fibrosis. Moisturizers that contain 3% to 10% urea or glycerol are best for maintaining skin hydration but may cause irritation (Carpenter et al., 2015; Neumann, 2017; Rodrigues et al., 2018)

The role of the wound care nurse in management of the patient with GVHD also involves dressing selection

for patients with open wounds and recommendations regarding support surfaces. Dressing selections should be made on the basis of moist wound therapy, control of drainage, and prevention of infection. Support surfaces should be selected to provide maximum pressure redistribution in addition to microclimate control. The patient's level of mobility is a critical decision-making factor in support surface selection. Many times, patients with chronic GVHD have significant skin issues but continue to be ambulatory. Surfaces must be chosen that provide pressure redistribution while maintaining the patient's mobility. Compression therapy or compression garments should be considered for all patients with fibrotic changes in the soft tissue as this will lead to venous insufficiency. There are no evidence-based guidelines or standards of care for the management of wounds in the patient with GVHD. This is an area where research is needed.

 ## MALIGNANT FUNGATING WOUNDS

The term malignant fungating wound refers to those wounds that develop because of a malignant process. The National Cancer Institute defines a fungating lesion as a type of skin lesion that is marked by ulcerations (breaks on the skin or surface of an organ) and necrosis (death of living tissue) and that is usually malodorous (National Cancer Institute, n.d.).

Skin metastases are indicative of advanced disease with life expectancy ranging from 6 to 12 months (Tilley et al., 2016; Tsichlakidou et al., 2019). These wounds are very difficult for clinicians, patients, and caregivers to manage. Their presence is a constant reminder of the disease for the patient and family. When caring for patients with malignant fungating wounds, the goal is to manage symptoms rather than to resolve the wounds.

PREVALENCE/INCIDENCE

There are no specific data regarding the incidence and prevalence of malignant fungating wounds, but it is estimated that between 5% and 10% of cancer patients will develop these lesions (Tandler & Stephen-Haynes, 2017; Tsichlakidou et al., 2019). Some cancers are more likely to cause a malignant fungating wound than others. The most common cancers to cause metastasis to the skin include melanoma (45%), breast (30%), nasal sinuses (20%), larynx (16%), oral cavity (12%). These wounds occur commonly on the breast or chest wall (39% to 62%), head and neck (24% to 33.8%), back, trunk or abdomen (1% to 3%), axilla and groin (3% to 7%), and genitals (3% to 5%) (Ramasubbu et al., 2017).

In women, the tumor most likely to result in a malignant fungating wound is breast cancer. It is estimated that approximately 70% of all malignant fungating wounds are of breast origin. The most common sites for malignant fungating wounds resulting from breast cancer are the chest and abdomen, though these lesions may also present on the scalp, neck, upper extremities, and back. Women may also develop malignant fungating wounds from other malignancies, including melanoma (5%), colon cancer (9%), lung cancer (4%), and ovarian cancer (4%). The location of the malignant tumor wound may be indicative of the primary tumor. Melanoma wounds tend to occur on the lower extremities; colon wounds on the abdomen and pelvis; lung wounds on the chest wall, back, and scalp; and ovarian wounds on the abdomen and back.

In men, 13% of all fungating tumor wounds are caused by melanoma, with lesions presenting most commonly on the chest, back, and extremities. Lung cancer accounts for 24% of all malignant fungating wounds in men. These lesions most often present on the chest wall, back, and scalp. Colon cancer accounts for 19% of these wounds, with lesions presenting on the abdomen and pelvis. Squamous cell cancer of the oral cavity accounts for 12% of the wounds with lesions occurring in a localized distribution in the head and neck region (Helm & Elston, 2019).

RISK FACTORS

The only known risk factor for the development of a metastatic skin lesion is a cancer diagnosis, though some cancers are more likely than others to metastasize to the skin. Some cancers present with direct extension to the skin (e.g., Paget disease).

PATHOLOGY

Metastasis is a complex process that is dependent not only on the characteristics of the tumor but also on host response. Metastatic disease follows a specific distribution pattern dependent upon the tumor type.

Initially, a transforming event occurs that stimulates tumor cells to grow and expand. Nutrients are provided to the tumor by simple diffusion. As the tumor cells multiply, proangiogenic factors are secreted by the tumor, which stimulate development of a network of capillaries. This provides the support needed for further tumor growth. Penetration of the lymphatic and blood vessels is then enabled, which allows the tumor cells to enter into circulation. As the tumor cell enters into circulation, it can be deactivated by mechanical trauma or by the immune system. If the tumor cell survives, it will settle into the capillary bed of a selected organ. The site can be random or site specific depending on the tumor of origin. When the tumor cell reaches the capillary bed of the organ, extravasation of tumor cells occurs. The final step in the process occurs when the tumor cells proliferate at the new site and produce a new tumor.

Metastatic distribution can be completed by three processes. It can occur by mechanical tumor stasis, metastatic extension into the surrounding tissue or the lymphatic drainage bed. Mechanical tumor stasis is the most common pattern of metastasis, accounting for 50%

to 60% of all distribution patterns. Metastatic distribution can also occur by site-specific attachment where the tumor cells target a specific organ and other regional areas are bypassed. The presence of a site-specific adhesion molecule dictates this type of metastatic pattern. The third way in which metastasis occurs is through a nonspecific pattern. This is commonly encountered with highly aggressive tumors. These tumors have the ability to adhere to vessel walls and establish themselves in many different sites (Rolz-Cruz & Kim, 2008). There are many genetic pathways under investigation regarding cancer development and metastasis (Turajlic & Swanton, 2016).

CLINICAL PRESENTATION

Malignant skin lesions may present either as ulcerative lesions or as raised nodules. The initial presentation may be painless skin nodules that vary in color from pale pink to purple. The lesion may involve only one nodule or multiple nodules, and the texture of the nodules can be either firm or rubbery. As the tumor proliferates, the lesion progresses to ulceration and cavity formation or to a raised lesion with a cauliflower-like (fungating) appearance (**Fig. 31-12**).

DIAGNOSIS

Definitive diagnosis requires tissue biopsy to prove the presence of tumor cells.

MANAGEMENT

Management of these wounds centers on control of symptoms including exudate management, odor control, pain management, and control of bleeding. Since these wounds are caused by cancerous cells, no topical therapy alone will result in wound closure. For these wounds to resolve, systemic therapy in the form of chemotherapy, targeted therapy, biologic therapy, hormone therapy, or radiation therapy must be administered.

Cleansing

Wound cleansing is an important aspect of care for any wound, including a malignant tumor wound. Wound cleansing should be gentle to avoid causing increased pain or bleeding. Showering is a common and simple approach to cleansing these wounds. If the patient is unable to shower, irrigation with normal saline or warm tap water is also an acceptable method of cleansing. Topical antiseptic solutions may be considered (Tandler & Stephen-Haynes, 2017; Tsichlakidou et al., 2019).

Odor Control

Odor is problematic for patients with malignant wounds, but there is no documented definitive cause of the odor. The odor is hypothesized to be due to some combination of the following: anaerobic bacteria supported by the breakdown of proteins in the necrotic tissue, aerobic bacteria, clinical infection, necrotic tissue, and/or the

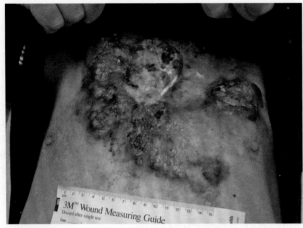
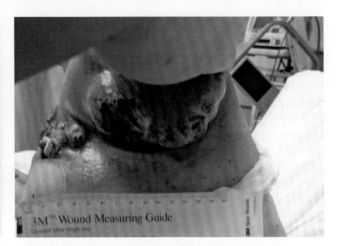

FIGURE 31-12. Malignant Fungating Wounds.

stagnant exudate contained within the dressings (Tandler & Stephen-Haynes, 2017; Villela-Castro et al., 2018).

Control of odor associated with malignant wounds has been accomplished in one of three ways: oral metronidazole, topical metronidazole, and use of advanced dressings or topical antiseptics. There is insufficient evidence to prove that any one approach is superior.

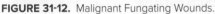

KEY POINT

Common issues with fungating malignant wounds include odor, exudate control, and control of bleeding; strategies shown in limited studies to be beneficial in odor control include topical metronidazole, medical grade honey, polyhexanide, and silver dressings. Anecdotal reports suggest that Dakin solution may also be of benefit.

Metronidazole

Metronidazole is used both systemically and topically to control odor, but there are limited data to support its use. Historically, two studies compared the use of metronidazole to placebo. The first study was conducted in 1984 and compared oral metronidazole to placebo. Six patients were treated in a crossover design, and a significant reduction in odor was noted with metronidazole as compared to placebo. The investigators decided not to do a more in-depth study, because the beneficial effects of metronidazole were so great that they felt it would be unethical to withhold the drug (Ashford et al., 1984). Bower et al. (1992) compared metronidazole gel to placebo. In this study, eleven patients were enrolled, and, in every case, there was a statistically significant reduction in the assessment of odor. The Cochrane review by Adderly and Holt (2014) also failed to identify any evidence to guide practice. Akhmetova et al. (2016) published a comprehensive review of topical odor-controlling treatment options for chronic wounds. In this review, five studies of poor quality were evaluated.

Although all the studies in the review reported a reduction in odor, the author notes that in the United States use of metronidazole is considered off label. In a more recent study, Watanabe et al. (2016) examined the use of topical metronidazole 0.75% with 21 subjects. In this study, the clinical success rate was 95.2% when evaluating odor score. Patient satisfaction was markedly or moderately improved 71.4%. Case reports have reported similar findings regarding the beneficial effects of both topical and oral metronidazole (Costa Santos et al., 2010; George et al., 2017). Topical metronidazole is the preferred route of administration due to the side effect profile of this medication (Alexander, 2009a). Metronidazole is available as a wound gel, which donates moisture to the wound bed and may be the preferred agent for wounds with minimal exudate. Metronidazole tablets have also been crushed and applied directly to the wound bed with improvement in odor being noted (Bauer et al., 2000).

Dakin Solution

Topical dressings have also been used to decrease odor from malignant fungating tumor wounds. The use of Dakin solution either as a cleanser or applied to gauze and placed onto the wound bed twice daily can be effective as a deodorizer. The effect most likely is due to its negative effect on microorganisms. There are no published data on the strength, frequency of application, systemic absorption, or comparison of Dakin solution to other products. More research is needed on the use of Dakin's for odor control with fungating tumor wounds (Tilley et al., 2016)

Polyhexanide

Villela-Castro et al. (2018) examined the use of polyhexanide versus metronidazole for odor control. In a double-blind study (*N* = 29), there was no difference in odor control between the groups. They concluded that polyhexanide is not inferior to metronidazole for odor control. Given that this product is an antiseptic rather than a medication, they conclude that this product is an alternative to metronidazole for clinicians who are not authorized to prescribe medications.

Silver-Impregnated Dressings

One small study (N = 26) has demonstrated a significant reduction in odor with use of silver foam dressings as compared to foam dressings without silver. In this study, there was no increase in odor while standard foam dressings were in use. There was a significant reduction in odor with the silver foam dressing (Kalemikerakis et al., 2012).

Medical Grade Honey

Medical grade honey dressings have also been used for odor control though definitive data regarding benefits are lacking. Lund-Nielsen et al. (2011) randomized 69 patients to either a silver dressing or a honey dressing. In this study, honey and silver dressings were found to be essentially equal in terms of odor control, and no statistical difference in odor between the two groups was noted.

Charcoal Dressings

Although no studies on the use of charcoal dressing have specifically been done with fungating tumor wounds, Akhmetova et al. (2016) report on the use of this type of dressing to absorb or trap volatile organic compounds that product wound odors.

Other Therapies

Other therapies have been proposed to decrease odor of fungating tumor wounds. These include the use of yogurt, buttermilk, various antibiotic combinations, chlorophyllin copper complex, aromatherapy, sugar paste, baking soda, vanilla extract, vinegar, coffee granules, cat litter, chloramphenicol, debridement, and cadexomer iodine. None of these products have demonstrated success in decreasing wound odor. In all cases, the cost of the dressing as well as the effectiveness must also be considered. Interventions should be directed at those that prevent malodor at the source rather than those that will mask the odor (Alexander, 2009a).

Exudate Management

Malignant wounds may produce high volumes of exudate due to the increased capillary permeability caused by the disorganized tumor vasculature that is characteristic of these wounds. Autolysis of necrotic tissue within the wound bed is also responsible for a larger volume of exudate. Inflammation and edema are common with these wounds, which further increases the management challenge. Exudate management is a primary goal of topical therapy. Control of exudate may improve quality of life for the patient. The wound care nurse may be challenged with the cost of advanced dressings with absorptive properties due to restrictions placed on the use of dressings for these types of wounds by third-party reimbursement.

There is no ideal dressing that has been defined for malignant wounds, but certain characteristics of wound dressings should be considered when choosing a wound dressing. These characteristics include nonadherence to the wound bed, conformability, ability to transfer excessive moisture away from the wound bed itself, high absorbency, and aesthetic acceptability (Adderly & Holt, 2014; Alexander, 2009a; Tandler & Stephen-Haynes, 2017; Tilley et al., 2016). For wounds that are slightly exudative, the application of a hydrogel dressing may be recommended. Alternatives would include simple and inexpensive nonadherent dressings such as those impregnated with petrolatum. Since healing is dependent on response to systemic therapy, the focus in topical therapy should be simply to provide coverage of the tumor and management of any exudate. It may be appropriate to leave the minimally exudative wound open to air if there are confounding circumstances such as lack of third-party reimbursement or lack of caregiver support. Wounds that are more exudative may require the use of an alginate or foam dressing to contain the drainage. Other advanced dressings are also available and effective, but the clinician must consider cost and simplicity as well as absorptive capacity when making recommendations. Some authors have recommended the use of pouching systems to manage highly exudative wounds (Cochran & Jakubek, 2010). The complexity of placing a wound pouch in addition to the cost of these systems may make this option cost prohibitive.

Control of Bleeding

Control of bleeding continues to be an important management goal. Malignant fungating wounds tend to bleed easily due to the fragility of the wound bed and erosion of capillaries by the tumor. There may also be impairment of the coagulation cascade due to the disease process and/or the treatments for the cancer (Adderly & Holt, 2014; Tandler & Stephen-Haynes, 2017; Tilley et al., 2016). The primary focus is on patient education to prevent bleeding. Patients and caregivers should be instructed on gentle cleansing. Atraumatic dressing removal is of paramount importance. If the dressing is adherent to the wound bed, it should be moistened prior to removal.

Measures to manage bleeding include the following:

- Direct pressure for 10 to 15 minutes
- Ice packs to the wound
- Use of topical coagulants or hemostatic agents or dressings (e.g., WoundSeal® Powder, Gelfoam®, QuikClot®, Mohs paste [zinc chloride paste], Monsel solution [ferric subsulfate])
- Silver nitrate sticks
- Topical sucralfate suspension (Cochran & Jakubek, 2010)

If bleeding is heavy, patients should be instructed to seek professional assistance. In a controlled setting, antifibrinolytics, vasoconstrictors, ligation, and cauterization may be options to control heavy bleeding (Alexander, 2009b).

Pain Management

The first step in management of wound-related pain is a thorough assessment of the pain including the site, nature, duration, onset, frequency, and severity as well as the impact on the patient's life. Aggravating and alleviating factors should also be determined. Systemic pain medication continues to be the gold standard and should be prescribed. Measures to ensure comfort with dressing changes should be undertaken including medication with short-acting pain medications prior to dressing changes, the use of nonadherent dressings, and decreased frequency of dressing changes. Topical anesthetics have been proposed as a means to improve patient comfort as well as the use of morphine in hydrogel. While there are several case reports on these products with malignant wounds, little evidence exists to support the use of these products in malignant lesions, and their use remains off-label (Cochran & Jakubek, 2010; Tilley et al., 2016).

CONCLUSION

Wound and skin care for the cancer patient is an evolving area of practice as new therapies are implemented to eradicate cancer that affects basic cellular pathways. Many new drugs and therapies are on the horizon that will affect the skin and the way the patient responds to injury. The wound care nurse should assess each patient individually, consult the primary team for the effects of the therapeutic agents, and then address the skin change with evidence-based interventions if available. These wounds and skin changes are a unique challenge for the wound care nurse. By adhering to the basic principles of wound care, the wound care nurse can choose appropriate therapies for this unique population.

REFERENCES

Adderly, U. J., & Holt, I. G. S. (2014). Topical agents and dressings for fungating wounds. *Cochrane Database of Systematic Reviews*, (2), CD003948. doi: 10.1002/14651858.CD003948.

Akhmetova, A., Saliev, T., Allan, I. U., et al. (2016). A comprehensive review of topical odor-controlling treatment options for chronic wounds. *Journal of Wound, Ostomy, and Continence Nursing*, 43(6), 598–609. doi: 10.1097/WON.0000000000000273.

Alexander, S. (2009a). Malignant fungating wounds: Managing malodour and exudate. *Journal of Wound Care*, 18(9), 374–382.

Alexander, S. (2009b). Malignant fungating wounds: Key symptoms and psychosocial. *Journal of Wound Care*, 18(8), 325–329.

American Cancer Society. (2018). Radiation therapy basics. Retrieved September 25, 2019, from http://www.cancer.org/treatment/treatments-and-side-effects/treatment-types/radiation/basics.html

American Cancer Society. (2019). Cancer facts & figures 2019. Retrieved September 24, 2019, from https://www.cancer.org/research/cancer-facts-statistics/all-cancer-facts-figures/cancer-facts-figures-2019.html

Annunziate, M. C., De Stefanno, A., Fabbrocini, G., et al. (2019). Current recommendations and novel strategies for the management of skin toxicities related to anti-EGFR therapies in patients with metastatic colorectal cancer. *Clinical Drug Investigation*, 39, 825–834. doi: 10.1007/s40261-019-00811-7.

Ashford, R., Plant, G., Maher, J., & Teares, L. (1984). Double-blind trial of metronidazole in malodorous ulcerating tumours. *The Lancet*, 323(8388), 1232–1233.

Bahaj, W., Ya'qoub, L., Toor, M., et al. (2019). Radiation recall in a patient with intrahepatic cholangiocarcinoma: Case report and a literature review. *Cureus*, 11(6), e5020. doi: 10.7759/cureus.5020.

Barton-Burke, M., Ciccolini, K., Mekas, M., et al. (2017). Dermatologic reactions to targeted therapy: A focus on epidermal growth factor receptor inhibitors and nursing care. *Nursing Clinics of North America*, 52(1), 83–113. doi: 10.1016/j.cnur.2016.11.005.

Bauer, C. Gerlach, M. A., & Doughty, D. (2000). Care of metastatic skin lesions. *Journal of Wound, Ostomy, and Continence Nursing*, 27(4), 247–251.

Beamer, L. C., & Grant, M. (2018). Longitudinal trends in skin-related and global quality of life among women with breast radiodermatitis: A pilot study. *European Journal of Oncology Nursing*, 33, 22–27.

Boulanger, J., Ducharme, A., Dufour, A., et al. (2015). Management of the extravasation of anti-neoplastic agents. *Supportive Care in Cancer*, 23, 1459–1471 doi: 10.1007/s00520-015-2635-7.

Bower, M., Stein, R., Evans, T. R. J., et al. (1992). A double-blind study of the efficacy of metronidazole gel in the treatment of malodorous fungating tumours. *European Journal of Cancer*, 28A(4/5), 888–889.

Carpenter, P. A., Kitko, C. L., Elad, S., et al. (2015). National Institutes of Health consensus development project on criteria for clinical trials in chronic graft-versus-host disease: V. The 2014 ancillary therapy and supportive care working group report. *Biology of Blood and Marrow Transplantation*, 21, 1167–1187. doi: 10.1016/j.bbmt.2015-03-024.

Chen, A. P., Setser, A., Anadkat, M. J., et al. (2012). Grading dermatologic adverse events of cancer treatments: The common terminology criteria for adverse events Version 4.0. *Journal of the American Academy of Dermatology*, 67(5), 1025–1039.

Clabbers, J. M. K., Boers-Doets, C. B., Gelderblom, H., et al. (2016). Xerosis and pruritus as major EGFRI-associated adverse events. *Supportive Care in Cancer*, 24, 513–521. doi: 10.1007/s00520-015-2781-y.

Cochran, S., & Jakubek, P. R. (2010). Malignant cutaneous disease. In M. L. Haas & G. J. Moore-Higgs (Eds.), *Principles of skin care and the oncology patient* (pp. 77–100). Pittsburgh, PA: Oncology Nursing Society.

Costa Santos, C. M., de Mattos Pimenta, C. A., & Nobre, M. R. C. (2010). A systematic review of topical treatments to control the odor of malignant fungating wounds. *Journal of Pain and Symptom Management*, 39(6), 1065–1076.

Coyle, C. E., Griffie, J., & Czaplewski, L. M. (2014). Eliminating extravasation events: A multidisciplinary approach. *Journal of Infusion Nursing*, 37(3), 157–164. doi: 10.1097/NAN.0000000000000034.

Feight, D., Baney, T., Bruce, S., et al. (2011). Putting evidence into practice: Evidence-based interventions for radiation dermatitis. *Clinical Journal of Oncology Nursing*, 15(5), 481–492.

Ferreira, E. B., Vasques, C. I., Gadia, R., et al. (2017). Topical interventions to prevent acute radiation dermatitis in head and neck cancer patients: A systematic review. *Supportive Care in Cancer*, 25, 1001–1011. doi: 10.1007/s00520-016-3521-7.

Foss, F. M., & Girardi, M. (2016). Mycosis fungoides and sezary syndrome. *Hematology/Oncology Clinics of North America*, 31, 297–315. doi: 10.1016/j.hoc.2016.11.008.

George, R., Prasoona, T. S., Kandasamy, R., et al. (2017). Improving malodour management in advanced cancer: A 10-year retrospective study of topical, oral and maintenance metronidazole. *BMJ Supportive & Palliative Care*, 7, 286–291. doi: 10.1136/bmjspcare-2016-001166.

Guggina, L. M., Choi, A. W., & Choi, J. N. (2017). EGFR inhibitors and cutaneous complications: A practical approach to management. *Oncology and Therapy, 5*(2), 135–148. doi: 10.1007/s40487-017-0050-6.

Hack, E., Thachil, T., & Karanth, N. (2018). Pectoralis major radiation recall. *Journal of Medical Radiation Sciences, 66*, 62–65. doi: 10.1002/jmrs.303.

Hegedus, F., Mathew, L. M., & Schwartz, R. A. (2017). Radiation dermatitis: An overview. *International Journal of Dermatology, 56*, 909–914. doi: 10.1111/ijd.13371.

Helm, T. N., & Elston, D. M. (2019). Dermatologic manifestations of metastatic carcinomas. *Medscape*. Retrieved from https://emedicine.medscape.com/article/1101058-overview

Hofheinz, R., Deplanque, G., Komatsu, Y., et al. (2016). Recommendations for the prophylactic management of skin reactions by epidermal growth factor receptor inhibitors inpatients with solid tumors. *The Oncologist, 21*, 1483–1491. doi: 10.1634/theoncologist.2016-0051.

Hofheinz, R., Segaert, S., Safont, M. J., et al. (2017). Management of adverse events during treatment of gastrointestinal cancers with epidermal growth factor inhibitors. *Critical Reviews in Oncology/Hematology, 114*, 102–113. doi: 10.1016/j.critrevonc.2017.03.032.

Hopewell, J. W. (1990). The skin: Its structure and response to ionizing radiation. *International Journal of Radiation Biology, 57*(4), 751–773.

Huang, Z., Chen, Y., Chen, W., et al. (2018). Clinical evidence of prevention strategies for capecitabine-induced hand-foot syndrome. *International Journal of Cancer, 142*, 2567–2577. doi: 10.1002/ijc.31269.

Hymes, S. R., Strom, E. A., & Fife, C. (2006). Radiation dermatitis: Clinical presentation, pathophysiology, and treatment 2006. *Journal of the American Academy of Dermatology, 54*(1), 28–46.

Jackson-Rose, J., Groman, A., Dial, L. S., et al. (2017). Chemotherapy extravasations: Establishing a national benchmark for incidence among cancer centers. *Clinical Journal of Oncology Nursing, 21*(4), 438–445. doi: 10.1188/17CJON.438-445.

Jawed, S. I., Myskowski, P. L., Horwitz, S., et al. (2014). Primary cutaneous T-cell lymphoma (mycosis fungoides and Sézary syndrome) Part II. Prognosis, management, and future directions. *Journal of the American Academy of Dermatology, 70*(2), 223.e1–223.e17.

Kalemikerakis, J., Vardaki, Z., Fouka, G., et al. (2012). Comparison of foam dressings with silver versus foam dressings without silver in the care of malodorous malignant fungating wounds. *Journal of B.U.ON.: official journal of the Balkan Union of Oncology, 17*(3), 560–564.

Kang, Y., Lee, S. S., Yoon, D. H., et al. (2010). Pyridoxine is not effective to prevent hand-foot syndrome associated with capecitabine therapy: Results of a randomized, double-blind, placebo-controlled study. *Journal of Clinical Oncology, 28*(24), 3824–3829.

Kavand, S., Lehman, J. S., Hashmi, S., et al. (2017). Cutaneous manifestations of graft-versus-host disease: Role of the dermatologist. *International Journal of Dermatology, 56*(2), 131–140. doi: 10.1111/ijd.13381.

Kimmel, J., Fleming, P., Cuellar, S., et al. (2018). Pharmacological management of anticancer agent extravasation: A single institutional guideline. *Journal of Oncology Pharmacy Practice, 24*(4), 129–138.

Kubo, A., Hashimoto, H., Takahaski, N., et al. (2016). Biomarkers of skin toxicity inducted by anti-epidermal growth factor receptor antibody treatment in colorectal cancer. *World Journal of Gastroenterology, 22*(2), 887–894. doi: 10.3748/wjg.v22.i2.887.

Lacouture, M., & Sibaud, V. (2018). Toxic side effects of targeted therapies and immunotherapies affecting the skin, oral mucosa, hair and nails. *American Journal of Clinical Dermatology, 19*(Suppl 1), S31–S39. doi: 10.1007/s40257-018-0384-3.

Lacouture, M. E., Anadkat, M. J., Bensadoun, R. J., et al.; MASCC Skin Toxicity Study Group. (2011). Clinical practice guidelines for the prevention and treatment of EGFR inhibitor-associated dermatologic toxicities. *Supportive Care in Cancer, 19*(8), 1079–1095.

Lacouture, M. E., Anadkat, M., Jatoi, A., et al. (2018). Dermatologic toxicity occurring during anti-EGFR monoclonal inhibitor therapy in patients with metastatic colorectal cancer: A systematic review. *Clinical Colorectal Cancer, 17*(2), 85–96. doi: 10.1016/j.dcc.2107.12.004.

Lewis, L., Carson, S., Bydder, S., et al. (2014). Evaluating the effects of aluminum-containing and non-aluminum containing deodorants on axillary skin toxicity during radiation therapy for breast cancer: A 3-armed randomized controlled trial. *International Journal of Radiation Oncology Biology Physics, 90*(4), 765–771.

Lucas, A. S., Lacouture, M., Thompson, J., et al. (2018). Radiation dermatitis: A prevention protocol for patients with breast cancer. *Clinical Journal of Oncology Nursing, 22*(4), 429–437. doi: 10.1188/18.CJON.429-437.

Lucey, P., Zouzias, C., Franco, L., et al. (2017). Practice patterns for prophylaxis and treatment of acute radiation dermatitis in the United States. *Supportive Care in Cancer, 25*, 2857–2862. doi: 10.1007/s00520-017-3701-0.

Lund-Nielsen, B., Adamsen, L., Kolmos, H. J., et al. (2011). The effect of honey-coated bandages compared with silver-coated bandages on treatment of malignant wounds—A randomized study. *Wound Repair and Regeneration, 19*, 664–670.

Macdonald, J. B., Macdonald, B., Golitz, L. E., et al. (2015). Cutaneous adverse effects of targeted therapies: Part I: Inhibitors of the cellular membrane. *Journal of the American Academy of Dermatology, 72*(2), 203–218. doi: 10.1016/j.jaad.2014.07.032.

Mahalingam, M., & Reddy, V. B. (2015). Mycosis fungoides, then and now...have we travelled? *Advances in Anatomic Pathology, 22*(6), 376–383. doi: 10.1097/PAP.0000000000000092.

McLellan, B., Ciardiello, F., Lacouture, M. E., et al. (2015). Regorafenib-associated hand-foot skin reaction: Practical advice on diagnosis, prevention and management. *Annals of Oncology, 26*, 2017–2026. doi: 10.1093/annonc/mdv244.

McQuestion, M. (2011). Evidence-based skin care management in radiation therapy: Clinical update. *Seminars in Oncology Nursing, 27*(2), e1–e17.

Meghrajani, C. G., Co, H. C., Ang-Tiu, C. M., et al. (2013). Topical corticosteroid therapy for the prevention of acute radiation dermatitis: A systematic review of randomized controlled trials. *Expert Review of Clinical Pharmacology, 6*(6), 641–649. doi: 10.1586/17512433.2013.841079.

National Cancer Institute. (2019a). Radiation therapy to treat cancer. Retrieved September 24, 2019, from https://www.cancer.gov/about-cancer/treatment/types/radiation-therapy#HRTWAC

National Cancer Institute. (September 23, 2019b). Targeted cancer therapies. Retrieved October 13, 2019, from https://www.cancer.gov/about-cancer/treatment/types/targeted-therapies/targeted-therapies-fact-sheet#what-are-targeted-cancer-therapies

National Cancer Institute. (n.d.). NCI dictionary of cancer terms: Fungating lesion. Retrieved November 11, 2019, from http://www.cancer.gov/dictionary?CdrID=367427

National Comprehensive Cancer Network (NCCN). (2018). NCCN clinical practice guidelines in oncology: Primary cutaneous lymphomas. Retrieved November 11, 2019, from https://www.nccn.org/professionals/physician_gls/default_nojava.aspx#site

Neumann, J. (2017). Nursing challenges caring for bone marrow transplantation patients with graft versus host disease. *Hematology/Oncology and Stem Cell Therapy, 10*, 192–194. doi: 10.1016/j.hemonc.2017.06.001.

Nikolaou, V., Syrigos, K., & Saif, M. W. (2016). Incidence and implication of chemotherapy related hand-foot syndrome. *Expert Opinion on Drug Safety, 15*(12), 1625–1633. doi: 10.1080/14740338.2016.1238067.

Onesti, M. G., Carella, S., Fioramonti, P., et al. (2017). Chemotherapy extravasation management. *Annals of Plastic Surgery, 79*(5), 450–456. doi: 10.1097/SAP.0000000000001248.

Parker, J. J., Rademaker, A., Donnelly, E. D., et al. (2017). Risk factors for the development of acute radiation dermatitis in breast cancer patients. *International Journal of Radiation Oncology Biology Physics, 99*(2), E40–E41. doi: 10.1016/j.ijrobp.2017.06.688.

PDQ® Adult Treatment Editorial Board. *PDQ Mycosis Fungoides (including Sézary syndrome) treatment*. Bethesda, MD: National Cancer Institute. Updated 9/20/2019. Retrieved December 6, 2020, from https://www.cancer.gov/types/lymphoma/hp/mycosis-fungoides-treatment-pdq

Pérez Fidalgo, J. A., García Fabregat, L., Cerbantes, A., et al. (2012). Management of chemotherapy extravasation: ESMO-EOPNS clinical practice guidelines. *Annals of Oncology, 23*(Suppl 7), vii167–vii173.

Peterson, E., Weed, J., Lo Sicco, K., et al. (2019). Cutaneous T cell lymphoma: A difficult diagnosis demystified. *Dermatologic Clinics, 37*(4), 455–469. doi: 10.1016/j.det.2019.05.007.

Ramasubbu, D. A., Smith, V., Hayden, F., et al. (2017). Systemic antibiotics for treating malignant wounds. *Cochrane Database of Systematic Reviews, 8,* CDO011609. doi: 10.1002/14651858.CD011609.pub2.

Reguiai, Z., Bachet, J. B., Bachmeyer, C., et al. (2012). Management of cutaneous adverse events induced by anti-EGFR (epidermal growth factor receptor): A French interdisciplinary therapeutic algorithm. *Supportive Care in Cancer, 20*(7), 1395–1404.

Rodrigues, K. S., Oliveira-Ribeiro, C., de Abreu Fiuza Gomes, S., et al. (2018). Cutaneous graft-versus-host disease: Diagnosis and treatment. *American Journal of Clinical Dermatology, 19,* 33–50. doi: 10.1007/s40257-017-0306-9.

Rolz-Cruz, G., & Kim, C. C. (2008). Tumor invasion of the skin. *Dermatologic Clinics, 26,* 89–102.

Russi, E. G., Moretto, F., Rampino, M., et al. (2015). Acute skin toxicity management in head and neck cancer patients treated with radiotherapy and chemotherapy or EGFR inhibitors: Literature review and consensus. *Critical Reviews in Oncology/Hematology, 96,* 167–182. doi: 10.1016/j.critrevonc.2015.06.001.

Sibaud, V. (2018). Dermatologic reactions to immune checkpoint inhibitors: Skin toxicities and immunotherapy. *American Journal of Clinical Dermatology, 19,* 345–361. doi: 10.1007/s40257-017-0336-3.

Singh, M., Alavi, A., Wong, R., et al. (2016). Radiodermatitis: A review of our current understanding. *American Journal of Clinical Dermatology, 17,* 277–292. doi: 10.1007/s40257-016-0186-4.

Spalek, M. (2016). Chronic radiation-induced dermatitis: Challenges and solutions. *Clinical, Cosmetic and Investigational Dermatology, 9,* 473–482. doi: 10.2147/CCID.S94320.

Tandler, S., & Stephen-Haynes, J. (2017). Fungating wounds: Management and treatment options. *British Journal of Nursing, 26*(12), S6–S14. doi: 10.12968/bjon.2017.26.12.S6.

Tilley, C., Lipson, J., & Ramos, M. (2016). Palliative wound care for malignant fungating wound: Holistic considerations at end-of-life. *Nursing Clinics of North America, 51*(3), 513–531. doi: 10.1016/j.cnur.2016.05.006.

Tsichlakidou, A., Govina, O., Vasilopoulos, G., et al. (2019). Intervention for symptom management in patients with malignant fungating wounds—A systematic review. *Journal of B.U.ON.: Official journal of the Balkan Union of Oncology, 24*(3), 1301–1308.

Turajlic, S., & Swanton, C. (2016). Metastasis as an evolutionary process. *Science, 352*(6282), 169–175. doi: 10.1126/science.aaf2784.

Valentine, J., Belum, V. R., Duran, J., et al. (2015). Incidence and risk of xerosis with targeted anticancer therapies. *Journal of the American Academy of Dermatology, 72*(4), 656–666. doi: 10.1016/j.jaad.2014.12.010.

Villarreal, C. D., Alanis, J. C., Pérez, J. C., et al. (2016). Cutaneous graft-versus-host disease after hematopoietic stem cell transplant—A review. *Anais Brasileiros de Dermatologia, 91*(3), 336–343. doi: 10.1590/abd1806-4841.20164180.

Villela-Castro, D. L., Santos, V. L., & Woo, K. (2018). Polyhexanide versus metronidazole for odor management in malignant (fungating) wounds. *Journal of Wound, Ostomy, and Continence Nursing, 45*(5), 413–418. doi: 10.1097/WON.0000000000000460.

Wang, C. X., Anadkat, M. J., & Musiek, A. C. (2019). Dermatologic conditions of the early post-transplant period in hematopoietic stem cell transplant recipients. *American Journal of Clinical Dermatology, 20,* 55–73. doi: 10.1007/s40257-018-0391-4.

Watanabe, K., Shimo, A., Tsugawa, K., et al. (2016). Safe and effective deodorization of malodorous fungating tumors using topical metronidazole 0.75% gel (GK567): A multicenter open-label, phase III study (RDT.07.SRE.27013). *Supportive Care in Cancer, 24,* 2583–2590. doi: 10.1007/200520-015-3067-0.

Wei, F., Shin, D., & Cai, X. (2018). Incidence, risk and prognostic role of anti-epidermal growth factor receptor-induced skin rash in biliary cancer: A meta-analysis. *International Journal of Clinical Oncology, 23,* 443–451. doi: 10.1007/s10147-017-1231-x.

Wilcox, R. A. (2017). Cutaneous T-cell lymphoma: 2017 update on diagnosis, risk-stratification, and management. *American Journal of Hematology, 92,* 1085–1102. doi: 10.1002/ajh.24876.

Wolf, J. R. (2019). UpToDate: Radiation dermatitis. Retrieved November 9, 2019, from https://www.uptodate.com/contents/radiation-dermatitis?search=radiation%20dermatitis&source=search_result&selectedTitle=1~33&usage_type=default&display_rank=1

Wong, R. K. S., Bensadoun, R. J., Boers-Doets, C. B., et al. (2013). Clinical practice guidelines for the prevention and treatment of acute and late radiation reactions for the MASCC Skin Toxicity Study Group. *Supportive Care in Cancer, 21,* 2933–2948.

CASE STUDY

Mrs. R is a 76-year-old female with a diagnosis of Stage IV breast cancer, with a fungating tumor wound, who has been admitted to the hospital inpatient unit with neutropenic fever. The patient has never been seen by a wound care nurse in the past. She is newly diagnosed with her breast cancer and has not undergone a mastectomy or radiation due to her advanced disease. She received her first course of chemotherapy (paclitaxel, pertuzumab, and trastuzumab) 12 days ago.

The wound care nurse is consulted by the oncology team for wound care recommendations. The patient reports her usual care of her wound involves dabbing it with hydrogen peroxide once per day and then covering the area with paper towels. She states she has had the wound on her breast for about 6 months. She states she was afraid to go to the doctor, so she did not tell anyone about her wound. She states that since her chemotherapy, she has had an increase in odor from the wound.

On exam, the patient presents with a large fungating tumor on her left breast. The wound is 6 cm (l) × 5 cm (w) and located in the lateral aspect of the breast. The wound bed is 50% dry yellow slough tissue that is firmly adherent. The remainder of the wound is 50% pink tissue. The periwound skin is firm but not erythematous. There is foul odor noted from the wound bed.

The patient's social history includes a history of smoking 1 ppd × 50 years. She also reports recent weight loss of 20 lb over the past 6 months.

Pertinent lab values include HBG of 6.8, WBC of 2.1, and PLT of 38. No nutritional lab values have been drawn. Cefepime 1 g q8h IV has been ordered to address her neutropenic fever.

WOUND CARE NURSE INTERVENTIONS

The goal of care for this patient is control of symptoms including wound odor:

- Wound care order: Irrigate wound with 250 mL of normal saline under pressure. Apply metronidazole crushed tablets 250 mg, and cover with petrolatum gauze dressing. Top with bulky dressing and secure in nonadherent fashion twice daily.

OUTCOME

On reevaluation 2 days later, no odor is noted in the patient's room. The patient reports she feels more comfortable. She states she thinks she can do the procedure at home independently. On hospital discharge, the patient was instructed to decrease wound care to daily and clean the wound in the shower if able rather than doing irrigations to the wound bed.

QUESTIONS

1. Which prevention strategy for radiation dermatitis is recommended based on the available evidence?
   A. Apply ice packs daily after the treatment for 20 minutes.
   B. Shave daily in the treatment field using a straight razor.
   C. Apply moisturizers to the treatment field that contain lanolin.
   D. Clean the skin twice daily with a pH-balanced cleanser.

2. A wound care nurse is caring for cancer patients receiving radiation treatment. Which patient factor does NOT place the patient at greater risk for radiation dermatitis?
   A. Diabetes mellitus as a comorbid condition
   B. Age <50 years
   C. Diagnosis of renal failure
   D. History of smoking

3. A wound care nurse is describing the clinical presentation of radiation dermatitis to a patient receiving radiation for breast cancer. Which statement accurately describes the development of this condition?
   A. "There is frequently erythema developing following the first treatment that disappears within a few hours but returns with subsequent treatments."

   B. "Persistent erythema typically becomes manifest at about treatment day 4 to 5, assuming 1.8 to 2 Gy per treatment (single-dose fraction)."
   C. "Hyperpigmentation may develop at weeks 1 to 2 due to overactivity of the melanocytes."
   D. "Moist desquamation may develop once the total dose reaches 30 to 40 Gy, resulting in partial-thickness skin loss with exposure of the dermis."

4. Your patient is receiving an EGFR inhibitor. The bedside nurse asks you to explain why the patient's leg ulcer is not improving despite optimum therapy. What is your best response?
   A. The patient has impaired nutrition, which is preventing the wound from healing.
   B. The patient has a biofilm that is preventing wound healing.
   C. EGFR inhibitors block cellular pathways and processes essential to cell growth and survival.
   D. EGFR inhibitors prevent the patient from mounting an inflammatory response.

5. What is the role of the wound care nurse in the management of extravasation injuries related to chemotherapy?
   A. Stop the infusion immediately and notify the prescribing health professional.
   B. Aspirate any residual vesicant from the IV device using a 1- to 3-mL syringe.
   C. Assist with surgical debridement.
   D. Recommend topical therapy once initial rescue treatment has been provided.

6. A patient receiving targeted chemotherapy with an EGRF inhibitor presents with scaly, pruritic skin. She reports that she initially had a rash but that has now resolved. The patient's current skin condition should be documented as which of the following?
A. Xerosis
B. Hand–foot skin reaction
C. Paronychia
D. Papulopustular rash

7. A wound care nurse is caring for a patient diagnosed with grade 1 hand–foot skin reaction. What is a recommended treatment for this condition?
A. Chemotherapy treatment interruption until severity is Grade 0
B. Pain management with systemic medications
C. Clobetasol 0.05% daily
D. Antiseptic baths with povidone–iodine

8. A patient is diagnosed with Stage III cutaneous T-cell lymphoma (mycosis fungoides and Sézary syndrome). What finding is characteristic of this stage of the syndrome?
A. Skin patches and plaques that cover <10% body surface area
B. Lymphadenopathy without nodal infiltration
C. Pathologically positive lymph nodes
D. The presence of generalized erythroderma

9. What treatment is a recommended intervention used to manage a patient with malignant skin lesions?
A. Providing vigorous wound cleansing
B. Irrigating the wound with normal saline or warm tap water
C. Managing bleeding with warm compresses to the wound
D. Increasing the frequency of dressing changes

10. Which of the following is true regarding GVHD?
A. Graft versus host disease is usually associated with allogeneic transplants, may be either acute or chronic, and frequently results in skin pathology.
B. Classic acute GVHD is defined as reactions occurring after day 100.
C. Skin manifestations of GVHD typically present in the first 2 to 5 days posttransplant with a rash that begins acrally but becomes generalized in distribution.
D. Acute GVHD usually affects the endovascular system.

ANSWERS AND RATIONALES

1. D. Rationale: Instruct patients undergoing radiation therapy to clean the skin twice daily with pH-balanced cleansers paying particular attention to areas with skin-to-skin contact. Pat the skin dry; do not rub.

2. B. Rationale: These factors are similar to those known to result in impaired wound healing and include smoking, poor nutritional status, older age, obesity, race, comorbid conditions (e.g., diabetes, renal failure), and problems with skin integrity prior to initiation of radiation therapy. Previous sun exposure and normal skin care routines (e.g., use of harsh soaps, perfumed soap, or lotions or scrubbing the skin) can also affect the risk for radiation dermatitis.

3. A. Rationale: Common early skin changes include a transient erythema, seen within a few hours of irradiation, which subsides after 24 to 48 hours but recurs with subsequent treatments.

4. C. Rationale: Since EGFR is essential to normal keratinocyte function, including the vital functions of the skin cell, such as the ability to proliferate, differentiate, and migrate; wound healing; and carcinogenesis, inhibition of this pathway causes the characteristic skin changes associated with this drug class.

5. D. Rationale: The wound care nurse's role in management of extravasation injuries is to recommend topical therapy once initial treatment has been provided. Principles of moist wound healing should be followed, with recommendations based on the characteristics of the wound.

6. A. Rationale: In the 2nd month, the papulopustular rash resolves, but there is persistent erythema, xerosis, and formation of telangiectasias in the areas previously affected by the rash.

7. C. Rationale: For grade 1 reactions, current recommendations include keratolytics including urea cream 1% to 40% or salicylic acid 5% to 10% on hyperkeratotic areas only. Lidocaine gel or other topical analgesics can help to relieve pain. Topical corticosteroids such as clobetasol 0.05% applied twice daily are recommended with use of thick socks at night. If oozing lesions are present, these may be treated with antiseptic baths. Agents recommended include potassium permanganate, chlorhexidine gluconate, or diluted bleach.

8. D. Rationale: SS is characterized by the combination of circulating neoplastic T cells and erythroderma, with or without lymphadenopathy. In MF, the presence of generalized erythroderma is characteristic of Stage III disease.

9. B. Rationale: Wound cleansing should be gentle to avoid causing increased pain or bleeding. Showering is a common and simple approach to cleansing these wounds. If the patient is unable to shower, irrigation with normal saline or warm tap water is also an acceptable method of cleansing.

10. A. Rationale: Graft versus host disease is usually associated with allogeneic transplants, may be either acute or chronic, and frequently results in skin pathology.

CHAPTER 32

THERMAL WOUNDS: BURN AND FROSTBITE INJURIES

Yvette Mier

OBJECTIVES

1. Describe the pathology of burn injuries.
2. Define the following terms and discuss implications for management: zone of coagulation, zone of stasis, and zone of hyperemia.
3. Identify the criteria for referral to a burn center.
4. Describe the principles of topical therapy for thermal injuries.
5. Explain the pathology of frostbite injury and recommended management.

TOPIC OUTLINE

● INTRODUCTION

Thermal wounds are unique in terms of pathophysiology and overall wound management. Wound care nurses must possess a basic knowledge of thermal wound assessment and management, which is based on the location and mechanism of injury and the percentage of total body surface area (TBSA) involved. The wound care nurse should be familiar with the indications for referring injured patients to a regional burn center to avoid a potentially devastating delay in appropriate care.

● BURN WOUNDS

Major burn injuries are one of the most complex injuries the body can sustain. They create intense emotional responses in most people including health care professionals. Associations with severe pain, sepsis, and death versus survival accompanied by gross disfigurement have been the images presented by the media for many years. Due to advances in burn care, this perception is now inaccurate. Survival as the primary goal in burn care has essentially been achieved. The major goal of burn care is to address and maximize quality of life (Herndon, 2012). This goal is best achieved with specialized care provided by a multidisciplinary team that includes burn surgeons, nurses (including the wound care nurse), physical, occupational and respiratory therapists, dieticians, social workers, case managers, pharmacists, and psychologists. Effective teams assure an equal voice for each team member, and all members understand each other's overlapping role in treating the patient as they move from acute injury through recovery into long-term rehabilitation. This type of specialized, cohesive team is typically found in regional burn centers (Connor-Ballard, 2009; Simko & Culleton, 2013).

KEY POINT

Survival as a goal of burn care has essentially been achieved. The major goals relate to maximizing quality of life.

EPIDEMIOLOGY

The most current burn data from the American Burn Association Burn Incidence Fact Sheet indicates that in 2016, 486,000 people sustained a burn injury significant enough to seek treatment in a hospital emergency department in the United States. Forty thousand of those individuals required hospital admission, and 30,000 required treatment at specialized burn centers. Prevalence of burn injuries differentiates by age, gender, and ethnicity. Twenty-four percent of all burn injuries occur in children under age 15. Children under the age of 5 are 2.5 times more likely to be burned than the general population. Fifty-five percent of burned patients are between the ages of 20 and 59. Seniors account for the remaining 21%. Males are more likely to be burned than females (68% male, 32% female). Ethnic disparities are as follows: Caucasian 59%, African American 20%, Hispanic 14%, and Other 7%. Most burn injuries occur in the home (75%) with flames being the most common cause unless the patient is under age 5, where scald injury is the most common type of burn. Work-related burn injuries account for 13% of all burn trauma patients. Almost all burn injuries are preventable (American Burn Society, 2016; Greenhalgh, 2019).

KEY POINT

Seventy-five percent of burn injuries occur in the home. Flame and scald injuries are the most common types of burns.

The annual health care cost associated with burn injuries is $1.5 billion; adding indirect costs raises that sum to over $5 billion (McDermott & Weiss, 2016). Current survival rate is 96.8% for adults and 99% for children. Death is more likely when the burn is associated with anoxic brain injury from a concurrent inhalation injury (Antoon, 2020; American Burn Association, 2016; Fire Deaths, n.d.; McDermott &Weiss, 2016).

RISK FACTORS

Groups at increased risk of burn injury include children <4 years of age, adults older than 65 years of age, individuals living in poverty, and individuals living in rural areas. Smoking is the leading causative agent in residential fires, and 37% of fire-related deaths occur in homes without working smoke detectors. Alcohol consumption is associated with 40% of all residential fire deaths (Fire Deaths, n.d.).

MECHANISMS OF BURN INJURY

Sources of burn injury include thermal burns, chemical burns, electrical burns, and radiation burns. The pathophysiology involved in each of these injuries is similar. Each also has important considerations that guide treatment and recovery.

Thermal Burns

Thermal burns occur as the result of heat transfer, specifically through conduction, radiation, or convection. Conduction injuries occur when an object has direct contact with a heat source, such as touching a hot stove or being submerged in boiling water. Radiation involves the conversion of kinetic energy to electromagnetic energy, which then travels in space until it reaches an object and is converted back to kinetic energy. Examples of radiation-induced burn injuries would include those from a tanning bed or a heat lamp. Convection injuries involve heat carried by air currents. A burn caused by a flash explosion would be an example of this type of thermal burn (Carrougher, 1998).

Two factors determine the severity of a thermal burn injury: the temperature to which the tissue is heated and length of exposure to the elevated temperature (Carrougher, 1998). For example, water heated to 140°F will produce a full-thickness burn in 3 seconds. Water heated to 156°F will produce the same full-thickness burn in 1 second. In contrast to water, substances of a thicker consistency, such as grease or hot oil, will naturally have a longer contact time with the skin and will produce a deeper injury. Moving further along the same progressive viscosity spectrum, substances such as tar or candle wax would have the longest contact time with the skin and would produce the deepest burn. Of interest in this example, tar itself is not harmful and poses no health risks after it has cooled. Often by the time the burn-injured patient reaches a medical facility for treatment, the tar has cooled and is no longer contributing to the severity of the burn. Tar is very difficult to remove, and its painful debridement is not immediately necessary. It can be left in place and removed over several days. The best approach to tar removal is with the use of petrolatum jelly dressings changed every few hours. Of course, if the tar burn covers a large surface area, the burn surgeon may elect to surgically remove the tar and associated devitalized tissue more quickly. While the depth of the burn cannot be ascertained until all of the tar is removed, these burns are almost always full thickness (American Burn Association, 2018; Herndon, 2012).

> **KEY POINT**
>
> The severity of a thermal burn is determined by the temperature to which the tissue is heated and the length of exposure. Burns caused by viscous liquids are typically worse than those caused by water due to the greater time of exposure.

Chemical Burns

Chemical burns are caused by tissue exposure to noxious substances. The severity of the burn is directly proportional to the concentration and quantity of the agent, the length of time exposed, and the cutaneous toxicity of the agent. Chemical burns tend to progress until the agent is inactivated, either through tissue dissipation or dilution with sufficient amounts of water (Carrougher, 1998). Health care workers treating chemical burns should wear full personal protective equipment to prevent accidental self-exposure. Substances that cause chemical burns are classified based on pH, as either alkalis or acids.

> **KEY POINT**
>
> Chemical burns tend to progress until the agent is inactivated (e.g., via copious irrigation with water). Health care workers should wear full personal protective equipment when treating patients with chemical burns.

Alkali Burns

Alkalis are commonly found in industrial cleaning agents, oven cleaners, fertilizers, and cement. They generally produce more severe burns because they bind with cutaneous lipids to cause a reaction characterized by destruction of proteins and progressive necrosis and liquefaction of tissues, which permits the chemical to penetrate more deeply into the tissue (Evans, 2016). Copious irrigation with water is the initial treatment for this type of burn injury. Within this category of burn injury, wet cement burns can be particularly challenging. Spills into a worker's boots or gloves do not become symptomatic for several hours; by that time, the injury is extensive and treatment often requires surgical debridement and grafting (Herndon, 2012).

Acid Burns

Acids are commonly found in household bathroom cleansers, swimming pool chemicals, and industrial drain cleaners. These burn injuries are characterized by coagulation necrosis and protein precipitation. These tissue reactions create a barrier within the exposed tissue that self-limits further penetration of the acid. Hydrofluoric acid (HF) burns constitute a major exception to this rule of thumb in management of acid burns. HF is the strongest known inorganic acid. It rapidly penetrates deeply into the tissue and acts as a metabolic poison that binds calcium and magnesium, which can produce cardiac dysrhythmias. As is true of cement burns, there is frequently a delay between exposure to HF and the onset of symptoms. When the patient does present for treatment, it is imperative to identify the concentration of the acid. The concentration can usually be found on the label of the container or on a Material Safety Data

Sheet (MSDS). Treatment of low-concentration HF burns involves copious irrigation with water and topical application of calcium gluconate gel. In burns involving higher concentrations, treatment can be as extreme as amputation or urgent surgical excision of the burned site (Evans, 2016; Herndon, 2012). Burns as small as 2% TBSA, with an HF concentration of 10%, can be potentially life threatening due to systemic hypocalcemia.

Vesicant Burns

Vesicant burns are typically associated with military injuries or terrorist attacks and are considered a possible threat in the United States following the attacks on the World Trade Center on September 11, 2001. Vesicant agents include sulfur mustard, nerve gas, lewisite, and phosgene oxime. The exact mechanism of action for these agents is not completely understood. It is believed that they damage cellular DNA, causing progressive cellular necrosis. Clinical presentation usually involves pain, severe pruritus, and blister formation. When the blisters rupture, amber fluid is released and shallow ulcerations remain. Treatment is lavage with copious amounts of water. Injuries associated with vesicant-induced burns would be triaged in community hospitals prior to transfer to burn units (Atiyeh & Hayek, 2010; Carrougher, 1998; Herndon, 2012).

Electrical Burns

Electrical burn injuries are divided into four separate groups: high voltage (more than 1,000 V), low voltage (<1,000 V), lightning strikes, and electric arc injuries. The severity of an electrical burn is dependent on the type of current, the pathway of the flow, the resistance of the tissue involved, and the duration of contact. If the current flows through the heart, brain, or visceral organs, the damage can be devastating. It is important to note that complications associated with electrical burns can be immediate or delayed (Carrougher, 1998; Evans, 2016).

Voltage Injuries

Voltage injuries are the most common type of electrical burn and are usually associated with alternating current (AC). With AC, the electricity flows back and forth between the power source and the entry point on the patient's body. This can cause cardiac dysrhythmias and skeletal muscle and diaphragmatic tetany. Direct current (DC) injuries are most commonly associated with lightning strikes. The use of DC can also be found in industrial settings. DC injuries flow in one direction (Carrougher, 1998; Evans, 2016).

Electrical current always follows the path of least resistance through the body. It flows from the point of contact (entry wound) to the ground (exit wound). Tissue resistance is the most important factor in determining direction of flow and amount of heat generated. Different tissues offer different levels of resistance; the greater the resistance, the greater the amount of heat generated. Skin resistance varies based on the condition of the skin; thicker, callused, and even dirty skin has higher resistance than clean, wet skin. The path followed by the electrical current is usually along the nerves and blood vessels. The path can also be along the bones. As the electricity travels under the intact skin, heat is dissipated, which causes necrosis of the underlying tissue. If the heat is dissipated along the very dense bone, it causes necrosis of the adjacent muscle (Carrougher, 1998; Evans, 2016; Herndon, 2012).

Arc Burns

Arc burns occur when electricity flows alongside but external to the body; as the electricity jumps from the point of contact to the ground, it causes the air between the two points to become superheated. Arc burns are most commonly associated with high-tension wires. Since the body is never in contact with the actual current, there are no systemic electrical consequences (heart dysrhythmia). The joints in close proximity to the superheated air are at highest risk for injury. Arc burns most frequently occur when the elbow is in a flexed position and present as visible burn wounds on the volar aspect of the wrist and the antecubital fossa (Carrougher, 1998; Evans, 2016; Herndon, 2012).

Compartment Syndrome

Electrical burns frequently require early surgical intervention due to the development of compartment syndrome secondary to edema in the fascial compartments. Peripheral pulses must frequently be assessed. The patient must also be monitored for symptomatic progressive neuropathy and pain, which typically precedes pulse loss. Deep tissue necrosis following electrical injury must quickly be identified and treated to avoid life-threatening metabolic acidosis and myoglobinuria resulting in acute renal failure. Wide tissue debridement, fasciotomies, and even limb amputation may be necessary for survival (Carrougher, 1998; Evans, 2016; Herndon, 2012).

KEY POINT

The severity of an electrical burn is determined by the type of current, direction of flow, tissue resistance, and duration of contact. If the current flows through the heart, brain, or visceral organs, the damage can be devastating.

KEY POINT

When treating a burned extremity, vascular assessment is imperative. The wound care nurse needs to be creative in the application of a dressing to this area so that the bedside nurse can check pulses and sensory function regularly without doing a complete dressing change.

Neurologic Symptoms

Neurologic symptoms occur in more than 50% of all cases involving electrical burns. Immediate symptoms can include paraplegia or quadriplegia and an altered level of consciousness. These symptoms usually resolve within a few days. Delayed symptoms can begin a few days after injury or several years later. Delayed symptoms include seizures, headaches, and memory loss. If the electrical burn involves the head, there is a high risk of ocular disorders, most commonly cataracts (Evans, 2016).

KEY POINT

Electrical burns are commonly associated with compartment syndrome, neurologic symptoms, and delayed complications.

Radiation Burns

Radiation burns are the rarest kind of burn. They occur with exposure to ionizing radiation. Tissue damage occurs when radiant energy is transferred to the body, stimulating the formation of highly reactive chemicals. When these chemicals interact with normal body chemicals, they form cellular toxins that target rapidly growing cells. The areas of the body with the most rapidly growing cells involve the skin, GI tract, and bone marrow. The severity of radiation damage is commensurate to the amount of exposed body surface and length of time exposed. Treatment involves decontamination and wound care (Carrougher, 1998; Herndon, 2012).

INHALATION INJURY

Inhalation injury is the most common and lethal concomitant injury associated with burn injuries. The three types of inhalation injuries include carbon monoxide poisoning, upper airway inhalation injury, and lower airway inhalation injury. Carbon monoxide poisoning causes asphyxiation and is responsible for the majority of deaths associated with fires. Asphyxiation occurs prior to the burn injury, if a burn injury occurs at all (Evans, 2016).

Inhalation injuries involving the upper airway are heat related. Edema above the glottis develops rapidly and causes airway obstruction. Patients admitted with facial burns, singed nasal hairs, dyspnea, carbonaceous sputum, disorientation, anxiety, and hoarseness should be monitored closely for airway edema. Intubation with mechanical ventilation is required until the edema is resolved (Carrougher, 1998; Evans, 2016).

KEY POINT

Inhalation injury is the most common and lethal concomitant injury associated with burn injury. The wound care nurse should closely monitor any patient with facial burns, singed nasal hairs, dyspnea, disorientation, anxiety, or hoarseness for airway edema.

Inhalation injuries involving the lower airway are usually the result of noxious chemicals produced from combustion reactions that occur during the normal course of a fire. This commonly occurs when the fire is located in a small, enclosed space. The noxious chemicals cause damage to the mucosa in the distal airways, which results in sloughing of the damaged mucosa 1 to 3 days post injury. Clinically, the patient presents with distal airway obstruction, atelectasis, pneumonia and respiratory failure requiring mechanical ventilation with aggressive pulmonary toileting (Evans, 2016).

PATHOPHYSIOLOGY AND MANAGEMENT OF BURN INJURY

There are numerous medical conditions that, as a result of their pathophysiology, result in significant tissue loss. These include necrotizing fasciitis, Stevens-Johnson syndrome, epidermolysis bullosa, toxic epidermal necrolysis, and staphylococcal scalded skin syndrome. In all these conditions, there is a period of acute physiologic stress, inflammation, edema, hypermetabolism, hemodynamic instability, core body temperature variations, glycolysis, proteolysis, and lipolysis. It can also be correctly argued that these responses are present in all critically ill trauma and surgical patients. Burn injuries differentiate themselves from these cases based on the severity, length, and overall amplitude of the physiologic response (Jeschke & Herndon, 2017).

The pathophysiology and management of a thermal injury can be conceptualized as an ongoing process involving three stages: emergent, acute wound management and rehabilitative. The first 72 hours is considered the emergent phase. The focus of this phase is hemodynamic stabilization through fluid resuscitation and early wound management. This is followed by the acute wound management phase. As the name implies, the focus of this phase is wound management, which includes debridement and skin grafting along with general support for wound healing. When the wounds are healed, the final phase begins. The rehabilitative phase can last for months or years depending on the severity of the burn. The focus in this phase is on maximizing functional capacity and psychosocial adaptation and returning the patient to the highest quality of life possible (Evans, 2016).

KEY POINT

The major phases of burn injury and care are the emergent phase (fluid resuscitation and initial wound care), acute wound management (debridement and skin grafting along with nutritional support and glycemic control), and rehabilitation (physical and psychosocial support for resumption of lifestyle to greatest extent possible).

Generally, burns smaller than 30% TBSA produce a local response only. However, burns larger than 30% TBSA produce both a local and systemic pathologic response.

Local Response

The local response to injury is unique to burns and includes three zones of injury: zone of coagulation, zone of stasis, and zone of hyperemia (**Fig. 32-1**). The zone of coagulation is the point of the most severe damage. Tissue destruction in this area is irreversible due to the coagulation of cells and the denaturing of proteins. If damage extends through the dermis, it is a full-thickness burn injury. If the damage is confined to the tissue above the dermal appendages, the burn is a partial-thickness injury (Evans, 2016; Hettiaratchy & Dziewulski, 2004).

> ### KEY POINT
>
> Small burns (<30% TBSA) usually trigger only a local response. Larger burns trigger both local and systemic responses.

Surrounding the zone of coagulation is the zone of stasis. This area is characterized by decreased tissue perfusion due to vessel constriction and thrombus formation producing transient ischemia. Tissue damage in this area is potentially reversible with appropriate fluid resuscitation, which promotes tissue perfusion. It is for this reason that the initial management of a burn injury focuses on this zone to preserve as much tissue as possible. Preexisting medical conditions can have a significant impact on the clinical course of the burn injury. Comorbidities such as diabetes mellitus, COPD, CHF, morbid obesity, and hypertension, as well as potential burn complications, such as infection, prolonged hypotension, and edema, can all further compromise tissue perfusion and lead to irreversible tissue necrosis (Evans, 2016; Herndon, 2012; Hettiaratchy & Dziewulski, 2004; Ogawa & Orgill, 2013).

> ### KEY POINT
>
> There are three zones of burn injury: the central zone of coagulation (irreversible damage); a surrounding zone of stasis, which may progress to tissue loss or may recover, depending on management; and an outer zone of hyperemia, which heals in <21 days if managed appropriately.

The zone of hyperemia is the outermost area of burn injury. This area is characterized by vasodilation and inflammation, which manifests clinically as an outer zone of erythema. This zone is usually a partial-thickness injury and will heal in <21 days unless complicated by infection or prolonged hypoperfusion (**Fig. 32-2**) (American Burn Association, 2018; Evans, 2016; Hettiaratchy & Dziewulski, 2004).

Systemic Response

Systemic responses to burns >30% TBSA occur in both the emergent and acute phases of burn management. In the emergent phase, there is a release of cytokines and other inflammatory mediators by the damaged tissues. These mediators cause initial vasoconstriction followed by vasodilation and increased capillary permeability. The increased permeability permits plasma proteins to leak into the surrounding tissue, leading to changes in

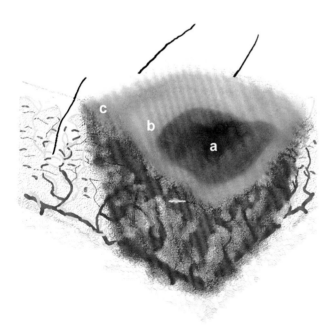

FIGURE 32-1. Zones of Injury Correlate to the Depth of Injury. "*a*" is the zone of necrosis. "*b*" is the zone of stasis. "*c*" is the zone of hyperemia. (Reprinted with permission from Mulholland, M. W., Maier, R. V., et al. (2006). *Greenfield's surgery scientific principles and practice* (4th ed.). Philadelphia, PA: Lippincott Williams & Wilkins.)

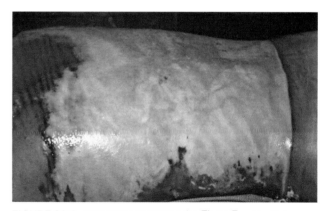

FIGURE 32-2. This Photo Illustrates the Three Zones of Injury. The center of the burn, which appears tan and leathery, is the zone of necrosis. Surrounding that zone, notice the moist, pale, *pink* tissue. This is the zone of stasis. The outermost rim, which appears bright *red*, is the zone of hyperemia. (Reprinted with permission from Mulholland, M. W., Maier, R. V., et al. (2006). *Greenfield's surgery scientific principles and practice* (4th ed.). Philadelphia, PA: Lippincott Williams & Wilkins.)

osmotic pressure that cause a significant loss of plasma into the tissues. The result is third spacing and the anasarca associated with burn injury, as well as the potential for severe hypovolemia and multisystem organ failure. Edema not only occurs at the site of injury but is generalized throughout the body (anasarca). Pulmonary edema can be a serious complication. Even in the absence of an inhalation injury, the lungs are susceptible to edema following a major burn (American Burn Association, 2018; Antoon, 2020; Evans, 2016; Herndon, 2012).

Fluid Resuscitation

Adequate fluid resuscitation during the emergent phase of burn management is imperative to prevent multisystem organ failure. Loss of plasma volume (hypovolemia) translates into generalized hypoperfusion of all tissues including the heart, which results in decreased cardiac output. Decreased cardiac output in turn causes decreased blood flow to the kidneys and GI tract. Decreased blood flow to the kidney reduces glomerular filtration and, if left untreated, leads to tubular necrosis and acute renal failure. Decreased blood flow to the GI system causes mucosal atrophy, which limits the ability to absorb nutrients, and reduces peristalsis. Decreased peristalsis predisposes the patient to ileus and a type of stress ulcer known as a Cushing's ulcer. Diminished blood flow to the bowel mucosa also causes increased intestinal permeability, which adversely affects the function of the immune system. A healthy immune system is vital to surviving a major burn injury (Evans, 2016; Herndon, 2012). Fluid resuscitation is calculated based on the TBSA involved, age of the patient, presence or absence of inhalation injury, and preburn comorbidities.

KEY POINT

Prompt and adequate fluid resuscitation is essential to prevention of multisystem failure; aggressive nutritional support and glycemic control are also important elements of systemic support because burn injuries result in a hypermetabolic state and impaired glucose metabolism.

Nutritional Support

As hemodynamic stability returns, and the patient moves from the emergent phase to the acute phase of burn management, there is a consistent release of catecholamines, glucocorticoids, glucagon, and dopamine. This slowly propels the patient into a hypermetabolic state, which ultimately leads to a catabolic state. It is for this reason that aggressive nutrition protocols are paramount to survival (Herndon, 2012).

Burn-injured patients sustain extreme metabolic stress, which persists for up to 3 years post-injury. This means that nutritional needs must be continually monitored and met to avoid malnutrition. Patients who are unable to consume enough protein, fat, carbohydrate,

vitamins (vitamin C and zinc), trace minerals, and amino acids (glutamine and arginine) will require supplemental nutrition. This is important because nutritional deficiencies impede fibroblast proliferation, collagen synthesis, and ultimately epithelial migration. When supplemental nutrition is required, as is the case in most large burns, enteral nutrition is preferred to parenteral nutrition. Enteral nutrition helps maintain the structural and functional integrity of the gastrointestinal tract and is started early to prevent atrophy of the villi within the GI tract. If enteral nutrition is delayed, the intervening atrophy of the villi results in reduced absorption and poor tolerance, which is manifested by diarrhea. There are many formulas that exist to calculate the specific needs of each patient which take into account age, preburn or dry weight, depth of the burn, and percentage of the TBSA affected (Carrougher, 1998; Evans, 2016; Kavalukas & Barbul, 2011).

KEY POINT

The wound care nurse managing a patient with a burn wound in an outpatient setting needs to monitor the patient for weight loss and to intervene as needed to manage the hypermetabolic state and to assure sufficient support for healing.

Management Hyperglycemia

Other postburn metabolic phenomena include impaired glucose metabolism and insulin sensitivity which can last up to 12 months post injury. This is a difficult problem to manage in any patient but an even bigger problem in patients with a comorbid diagnosis of diabetes or prediabetes. There is a 10- to 50-fold elevation in corticosteroid levels that persist up to 3 years after burn injury. This increases the risk of hyperglycemia which also contributes to the patient being more susceptible to disease (Somerset et al., 2014; Jeschke & Herndon, 2017).

Persistent hypermetabolism and associated hyperglycemia are areas of ongoing research in burn management. The beta-adrenergic blocker, propranolol, is currently providing the most effective management of burn-induced catabolism. The optimal target for glucose control in burn-injured patients is elusive and a source of controversy. Maintaining blood glucose levels below 110 mg/dL through the administration of insulin reduces mortality, infection, and sepsis. It has also been proven to assist in the resolution of acute kidney injuries and in the weaning of patients from mechanical ventilation. Research suggests that tight glucose control results into better outcomes in long-term rehabilitation. Attempts to maintain glucose levels below 110 mg/dL are associated with four times the number of serious hypoglycemic episodes and associated adverse events. Maintaining blood glucose levels below 150 mg/dL is the more accepted target at present (Jeschke & Herndon, 2017).

BURN WOUND EVALUATION

The classification of burn injury severity is largely based on the size and depth of the injury. The location is also an important factor to consider when determining severity.

Size

The size or extent of a burn injury is expressed in terms of the percentage of TBSA affected. Accurate assessment is essential as it guides initial management. TBSA is used both to calculate adequate fluid resuscitation and to predict the physiologic response. There are several methods of calculating TBSA. The most common method is known as the rule of nines (**Fig. 32-3**). The rule of nines divides the body into sections, with each section corresponding to a percentage of TBSA for an average adult. Because a child's body sections are proportioned differently than an adult's, a modified TBSA chart must be used. There is a child-specific chart based on the rule of nines. The pediatric Lund-Browder chart is more accurate and is more commonly used in assessing TBSA for a child (**Fig. 32-4**). If the burn pattern involves scattered, small areas, calculating TBSA can be more challenging. As a general rule, the area from the crease of the wrist to the crease of the base of the fingers (palm) on the patient's hand is considered 1% and total TBSA

can be crudely calculated with this method. Accuracy of TBSA assessment varies, depending on the method chosen and the experience of the clinician (American Burn Association, 2018; Antoon, 2020; Connor-Ballard, 2009; Evans, 2016; Herndon, 2012; Kliegman et al., 2011).

> **KEY POINT**
>
> Burn wounds are classified based on size (percent of TBSA) and depth (epidermal, partial thickness, or full thickness). In classifying a wound based on thickness, the wound care nurse must remember that burn wounds continue to evolve over the first 72 hours. Follow-up assessment is critical.

Burns involving <15% TBSA in adults and burns involving <10% TBSA in children are classified as minor burns. In adults, burns involving 15% to 25% TBSA (where <10% TBSA is full thickness) are classified as moderate burns. In children under 10 years of age, partial-thickness burns affecting 10% to 20% TBSA are considered moderate burns. Major burns include all burns >25% TBSA in adults and 20% TBSA in children (Herndon, 2012).

> **KEY POINT**
>
> Burns involving <15% TBSA in adults and <10% TBSA in children are classified as minor burns. Burns involving >25% TBSA in adults or >20% TBSA in children are considered major burns.

Depth

Burn depth is based on clinical examination. It may involve the epidermis only, part or all of the dermis, or may extend through the subcutaneous tissue into the muscle and bone. Nomenclature remains a source of confusion in the medical literature when describing burn injuries. This is important to rectify so that a common vocabulary can be applied to all burn injuries. This would not only facilitate accurate communication among providers but also be important in training and education programs (Kearns et al., 2013).

Historically, the description of a burn was based on degree of injury (first, second, third, or fourth). This is no longer the standard of care. Burns are now classified based on the level of tissue involvement: epidermal, partial thickness, or full thickness (Herndon, 2012).

Burns involving the epidermis only are not counted when calculating TBSA. They are red, hot, and painful, but do not blister and do not involve skin loss. They typically heal in 3 to 4 days. Sunburn is an example that falls into this category. Treatment is focused primarily on comfort measures: gentle cleansing, mild analgesics for pain management, loose clothing, and use of moisturizers (Evans, 2016; Helvig, 2002; Herndon, 2012).

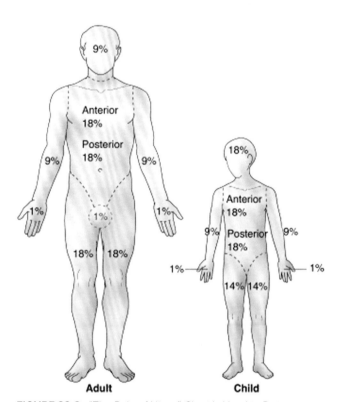

FIGURE 32-3. "The Rule of Nines" Chart Is Used to Determine Percentage of TBSA Affected in Adults. The modified pediatric chart can be used to assess children; however, the pediatric Lund-Browder chart is preferred. (Reprinted with permission from Mulholland, M. W., Lillemoe, K. D., Doherty, G. M., et al. (Eds.) (2011). *Greenfield's surgery: Scientific principles & practice* (5th ed.). Philadelphia, PA: Lippincott Williams & Wilkins.)

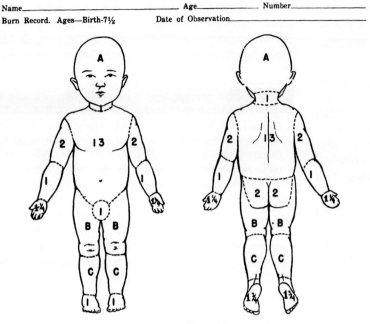

BURN SHEET

Name_____ Age_____ Number_____
Burn Record. Ages—Birth-7½   Date of Observation_____

RELATIVE PERCENTAGES OF AREAS AFFECTED BY GROWTH

Area	Age 0	1	5
A = ½ of Head	9½	8½	6½
B = ½ of One Thigh	2¾	3¼	4
C = ½ of One Leg	2½	2½	2¾

% BURN BY AREAS

Probable 3rd° Burn { Head_____ Neck_____ Body_____ Up. Arm_____ Forearm_____ Hands_____
{ Genitals_____ Buttocks_____ Thighs_____ Legs_____ Feet_____

Total Burn { Head_____ Neck_____ Body_____ Up. Arm_____ Forearm_____ Hands_____
{ Genitals_____ Buttocks_____ Thighs_____ Legs_____ Feet_____

Sum of All Areas_____ Probably 3rd°_____ Total Burn_____

FIGURE 32-4. The Pediatric Lund-Browder Chart Is Used to Determine Percentage of TBSA Affected in Infants and Small Children. (Reprinted with permission from Harwood-Nuss, A., Wolfson, A., & Linden, C. (1996). *The clinical practice of emergency medicine* (p. 1207). Philadelphia, PA: Lippincott-Raven.)

KEY POINT

Burns involving only the epidermis (e.g., a nonblistering sunburn) are not counted when calculating TBSA.

Partial-Thickness Burns

Partial-thickness burns extend into but not through the dermis. They are divided into two categories: superficial and deep partial-thickness burns. In the first 72 hours post burn, it can be difficult to distinguish between superficial and deep injuries due to the dynamic evolution of the burn injury. Ongoing assessment is important (American Burn Association, 2018; Herndon, 2012).

Superficial partial-thickness burns are erythematous, very painful, and blanchable to touch. They are characterized by edema, blister formation, and weeping. Superficial partial-thickness burns heal spontaneously with moist wound care within 2 weeks. A scald or flash burn would be likely examples of this type of injury. Blisters < 2 cm should be left intact. Large blisters should be unroofed. It is only when a large blister is unroofed that depth can be determined as

larger blisters are often deep partial-thickness injuries (**Fig. 32-5**) (Evans, 2016; Helvig, 2002; Herndon, 2012; Jeschke & Herndon, 2017).

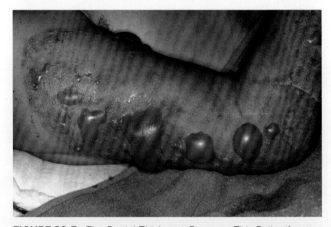

FIGURE 32-5. The Partial-Thickness Burns on This Patient's Upper Arm Display the Characteristic Blisters Common in This Injury. In the area just below the elbow, loss of the epidermis is evident revealing a *pink*, moist wound bed. This is also consistent with a superficial partial-thickness burn. (Reprinted with permission from Britt, L. D., Peitzman, A., Barie, P., et al. (2012). *Acute care surgery*. Philadelphia, PA: Wolters Kluwer Health.)

Deep partial-thickness burns appear paler and drier and do not blanch to the touch. Some blistering may or may not be present as these wounds are frequently inter-mixed with superficial partial-thickness burns (**Fig. 32-6**). These injuries are treated with moist wound care and typi-cally heal in <21 days. Burns that heal within 14 to 21 days exhibit reduced cohesion between the epidermis and dermis for up to 3 months. Intermittent formation of blis-ters in response to shearing from minor trauma is com-mon during this time. If the injury takes longer than 21 days to heal, excision and grafting should be considered to prevent issues with hypertrophic scarring. This is partic-ularly true if the injury is in proximity to a joint (Evans, 2016; Helvig, 2002; Herndon, 2012; Jeschke & Herndon, 2017).

Full-Thickness Burns

Full-thickness burns involve necrosis of the entire dermis and extend, at a minimum, into the subcuta-neous tissue. The associated devitalized tissue is called eschar. Eschar can have different appearances depending on the depth and mechanism of the injury. Eschar appears dry, waxy, and white in thermal injuries producing coagulation of vessels in the subcutaneous tissue. If the burn extends into the deeper tissues (e.g., muscle), the appearance of the eschar may be brown, dry, leathery, and charred. The presentation is often associated with prolonged flame contact. Noncharred full-thickness burn eschar can have a mottled appear-ance (chemical burns) or a dry, cherry-red appear-ance (severe scald injuries). As burn-induced edema worsens, the eschar typically becomes very firm. If the eschar involves an extremity and is circumferential or close to circumferential, an emergent escharotomy is required to prevent acute arterial occlusion (**Fig. 32-7**). Full-thickness burns involve complete destruction of the nerves. This fact has led to the commonly held belief that full-thickness burns are not painful. Burns are rarely of uniform depth so what appears to be a full-thickness injury may include areas of painful, par-tial-thickness injury. The wound care nurse must always assess the patient for pain as opposed to assuming that the wound is not painful. Full-thickness burns are treated with early excision and skin grafting to avoid secondary complications, such as infection and hyper-trophic scarring (American Burn Association, 2018; Evans, 2016; Helvig, 2002; Herndon, 2012; Jeschke & Herndon, 2017).

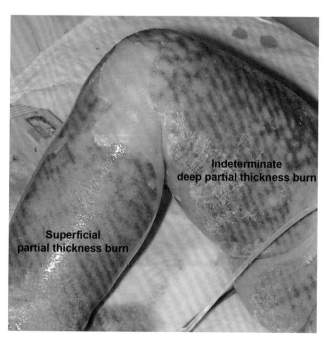

FIGURE 32-6. This Photo Illustrates Both Superficial and Deep Partial-Thickness Burns. Note the white, dry, patchy appearance on the deep partial-thickness burn compared to the consistent, moist pink appearance on the superficial partial-thickness burn. (Reprinted with permission from Mulholland, M. W., Maier, R. V., et al. (2006). *Greenfield's surgery scientific principles and practice* (4th ed.). Philadelphia, PA: Lippincott Williams & Wilkins.)

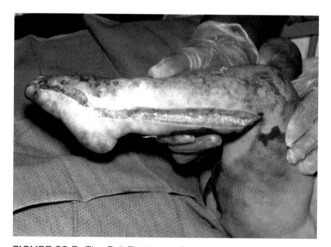

FIGURE 32-7. The Full-Thickness Burns on the Left Leg and Foot of This Child Display the Leathery, Dry Eschar Characteristic of Full-Thickness Burns. Edema beneath the circumferential eschar necessitated the escharotomy incision evident in the midlateral line of the burned leg and the lateral aspect of the foot. (Reprinted with permission from Britt, L. D., Peitzman, A., Barie, P., et al. (2012). *Acute care surgery*. Philadelphia, PA: Wolters Kluwer Health.)

Location

The location of a burn injury is also of critical importance. Burns involving the face require special care to prevent scarring and loss of function (**Fig. 32-8**). If the hands or feet are involved in the burn, care must be taken to preserve function and blood supply. Perineal burns require fastidious care. They are at high risk for infection due to the presence of GI flora, which could cause the burn to evolve in depth. Grafting is extremely difficult in this area, and graft failure rates are high. Burn injuries involving any joint require complex management. Grafting is almost always the best treatment because any scarring across the joint could lead to contractures. These patients need appropriate splinting, positioning, and range of motion exercises to ensure that function of the joint is preserved (Helvig, 2002).

Nonaccidental Injury

The abuse of children, the elderly, and dependent adults is a universal problem. It is not limited to any socioeconomic class, race, or religion. Abusers can include caregivers, family members, or institutional staff. It is estimated that up to 10% of all pediatric burns are the result of abuse (Hettiaratchy & Dziewulski, 2004). When evaluating a burn injury, the health care provider must consider whether the story told about how the injury occurred and the actual pattern of the burn correlate with one another.

Nonaccidental burn injuries can be the result of neglect or violent assault. Scald, flame, and thermal contact burns are the types of burns most commonly associated with abuse. Scald burns that appear symmetrical, lack splash marks, and are on the buttocks and perineum should be concerning for abuse (**Fig. 32-9**). When an individual is intentionally submerged into hot liquid, there is a clear line of demarcation between the injured and healthy skin. Thermal burns caused as a result of

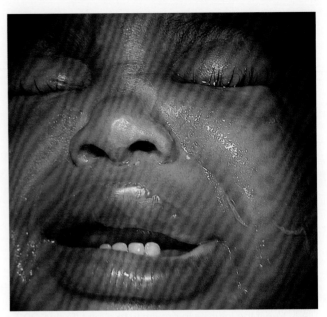

FIGURE 32-8. This Facial Burn Is Superficial Partial Thickness as Evidenced by Weeping, Blistering, and Edema. This child would need close monitoring of the airway; progressive edema could cause obstruction requiring mechanical ventilation. (Reprinted with permission from Fleisher, G. R., Ludwig, S., & Baskin, M. N. (2004). *Atlas of pediatric emergency medicine*. Philadelphia, PA: Lippincott Williams & Wilkins.)

intentional contact with a hot object, such as an iron, will match the exact shape of the object. An intentional burn from a cigarette appears deep and round. An accidental cigarette burn does not appear round because the natural reflex is to pull away. Any suspicion of nonaccidental injury should immediately trigger hospital admission and notification of social services (Hettiaratchy & Dziewulski, 2004; Mok, 2008).

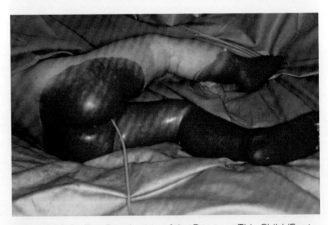

FIGURE 32-9. The Distribution of the Burns on This Child (Feet, Legs, Posterior Thighs, Buttocks, and Perineum) Is Characteristic of Abuse Caused by Intentional Immersion Scalding. Note the absence of splash burns. (Reprinted with permission from Britt, L. D., Peitzman, A., Barie, P., et al. (2012). *Acute care surgery*. Philadelphia, PA: Wolters Kluwer Health.)

When evaluating a burn injury, the wound care nurse must remember that abuse of children, elders, and dependent individuals is common, and must determine whether the clinical presentation of the burn injury matches the story being told.

REFERRAL CRITERIA

The American Burn Association (ABA) has established and maintained criteria to guide providers in making appropriate decisions regarding referral of a patient to a specialized burn center. Criteria for referral to a burn center are listed in **Box 32-1**. Despite these guidelines, retrospective studies continue to suggest that nearly 50% of all burn patients who meet the established criteria are never transferred to a burn center (Fish & Bezuhly, 2012). Another retrospective study looking at accuracy of TBSA percentage measurements between referring hospitals and burn centers showed the ratio of overestimation to underestimation exceeded 19:1 (Bettencourt et al., 2019). These studies point out that first responders and ED physicians need more education and support when making decisions regarding burn management (Stiles, 2018). Utilizing telehealth could bridge this problem so that patients with burn injuries are assessed and transferred to a regional burn center to assure optimal outcomes. The financial, physical, emotional, and spiritual costs associated to patients and facilities when over or under estimation of TBSA occurs and patients are transferred or not transferred appropriately could be improved (Bettencourt et al., 2019). Wound care nurses can safely treat burn injuries that fall outside the ABA referral guidelines in local hospitals, and partial-thickness burns <10% TBSA can be treated in an outpatient setting (Jeschke & Herndon, 2017).

BOX 32-1   CRITERIA FOR REFERRAL TO BURN CENTER

1. Partial-thickness burns >10% TBSA
2. Burns that involve the face, hands, feet, genitalia, perineum, or major joints
3. Full-thickness burns in any age group
4. Electrical burns, including lightning injury
5. Chemical burns
6. Inhalation injury
7. Burn injury in patients with preexisting medical disorders that could complicate management, prolong recovery, or affect mortality
8. Any patient with burns and concomitant trauma (such as fractures) in which the burn injury poses the greatest risk of morbidity or mortality
9. Burn-injured children in hospital without qualified personnel or equipment for the care of the children
10. Burn injury in patients who will require special social, emotional, or rehabilitative intervention

American Burn Association (ABA). (2018). *Advanced Burn Life Support Course Provider Manual.* Chicago, IL: ABA. Retrieved from http://ameriburn.org/wp-content/uploads/2019/08/2018-abls-providermanual.pdf

KEY POINT

The wound care nurse must be knowledgeable about the criteria for referral to a burn center to assure that all patients who meet the criteria are appropriately referred and transferred. Wound care nurses can safely treat burns that do not meet the criteria for referral.

BURN WOUND CARE

The key elements of local burn wound care include pain management, wound cleansing, and dressing selection.

Pain Management

Before the start of any wound care procedure, premedication with pain management is important. Pain associated with wound care is the shared experience of all burn-injured patients. In addition to the effect on the patient's quality of life, the physiologic stress response to pain can compromise wound healing and prolong the recovery process. Because pain is a subjective sensation that is experienced differently by each patient, and because response to pain relief measures and medications is also variable, it is not possible to establish a universal protocol for managing pain in all burn patients. This has led to inconsistency in the treatment of pain and to the potential for under treatment in the burn patient. The wound care nurse needs to make pain assessment and management a top priority when caring for burn patients.

KEY POINT

Preemptive pain management is a top priority in burn care. Pain management specialists should be consulted when needed for complex patients, such as those with a history of drug abuse.

Opioids are the drug of choice in treating pain during the acute phase, specifically intravenous (IV) morphine. Supplemental benzodiazepines given prior to dressing change procedures can promote relaxation and potentiate the effects of the morphine. Aspirin and nonsteroidal anti-inflammatory agents are avoided due to potential adverse effects on coagulation and the high risk of gastric ulcers (Connor-Ballard, 2009; Evans, 2016; Helvig, 2002).

As the wound heals, IV narcotics are slowly replaced with oral pain medications. Adequate pain management with oral medications alone must be achieved prior to discharge from the acute care setting. Once in the outpatient setting, hydromorphone and hydrocodone are commonly prescribed medications. Patients are given instructions to take the medication 30 minutes to 1 hour prior to the dressing change procedure to reduce pain. Short acting oral benzodiazepines are prescribed to be taken prior to dressing change as necessary (Connor-Ballard, 2009; Evans, 2016; Helvig, 2002). New research in pain management using distraction through virtual reality simulations is promising and may be helpful in titrating down doses of opioids (Furness et al., 2019).

Physicians and nurses who are inexperienced in treating burn wounds may confuse opioid tolerance with addiction and may be reluctant to prescribe or administer higher doses of narcotics. The reluctance is often more often when the patient has a history of drug or alcohol abuse. Many clinicians fail to realize that these patients have accelerated systemic clearance of narcotics and require significantly higher doses of medications to achieve pain control; not a recreational high. The burn care team must recognize that ineffective pain management leads to increased anxiety surrounding the dressing change procedure leading to a negative spiral in which anxiety further limits the effectiveness of any prescribed medication. Uncontrolled pain can also have long-term psychological consequences (Connor-Ballard, 2009; Helvig, 2002). Pain management specialists should be consulted as they can be very helpful in assuring appropriate pain management for these complex patients.

Cleansing

The goal of wound care is to maintain a clean, moist environment and prevent infection. Wound cleansing should be kept as simple as possible. Burn wounds are not sterile. Meticulous attention to maintaining a clean environment while doing dressing changes is important to prevent infection. Therapy rooms where dressing changes are done should be kept warm as the burn-injured patient has difficulty regulating core body temperature secondary to skin loss. Burn wounds may be cleaned with saline or a commercial wound cleanser. Larger burns can be gently washed in a clean shower with running water and mild soap. In the hospital setting, immersion hydrotherapy has largely been eliminated due to the risk of cross contamination and infection. Nonimmersion hydrotherapy using a table and shower head remains in use in many facilities. This technique is also associated with risks related to infection control, and protocols to minimize risk must be instituted. Loose, necrotic tissue can be trimmed away during the cleansing procedure (Helvig, 2002; Langschmidt et al., 2014; Slaviero et al., 2018).

Silver Dressings

Silver-based dressings have a long history in topical burn treatment. Silver is a broad-spectrum bactericidal agent that works by disrupting DNA replication. It is effective against both aerobic and anaerobic organisms, gram-positive and gram-negative bacteria, fungi, and some viruses. Older formulations include silver nitrate and silver sulfadiazine (SSD). These dressings were considered the gold standard for decades and were effective in preventing infection. The major drawback in use of these agents is that they are rapidly inactivated by substances in the wound environment. Frequent dressing changes are necessary to maintain therapeutic levels of bactericidal activity. SSD remains the most widely recognized and commonly used topical burn-specific antimicrobial agent (Cambiaso-Daniel et al., 2018; Fish & Bezuhly, 2012; Gravante et al., 2009).

KEY POINT

Silver sulfadiazine is the most commonly used topical burn-specific antimicrobial agent. Frequent dressing changes are needed to maintain therapeutic levels of bactericidal activity. Nanocrystalline silver dressings can maintain therapeutic antimicrobial levels for 3 to 7 days.

Nanocrystalline silver is the gold standard in topical burn treatment with the level of evidence supporting its use is robust. Silver in this form is more effective than SSD as it allows for the rapid yet sustained release of the silver ions into the wound bed. Dressings can provide therapeutic antimicrobial levels for 3 to 7 days, depending on the specific formulation and the amount of exudate. These dressings have been associated with reduced numbers of infections, reduced levels of pain related to dressing changes, and reduced length of hospital stay, all of which translate into improved clinical outcomes. Studies comparing SSD and nanocrystalline silver reveal a cost savings when costs are calculated based on overall wound care (including the cost of primary and secondary dressings, labor, and medications involved in the dressing change procedure) (Caruso et al., 2006). Nanocrystalline silver dressings are manufactured in a variety of forms such as high-density polyurethane mesh, hydrofiber, high performance fabric, or soft silicone foam. The effectiveness of one form versus another may depend on the property of the dressing in relation to the characteristics of the wound. For example, some research studies suggest that hydrofiber nanocrystalline dressings are more effective in highly exudative burn wounds as compared to high-density polyurethane mesh nanocrystalline dressings. Other studies comparing various forms of silver dressings report no difference in days to healing, or infection. They do report differences in cost, ease of use, and patient comfort related to specific dressings. A current study on animal models demonstrates that silver ions can be absorbed into the blood stream potentially causing liver toxicity, especially with 7-day silver dressings. The benefit of silver dressings outweighs the risk of liver damage in patients. The risk can be mitigated with blood work to monitor liver function (Abboud et al., 2014; Besner et al., 2007; Caruso et al., 2006; Gravante et al., 2009; Karimi et al., 2020; Kee et al., 2017; Rick et al., 2004; Sheckter et al., 2020; Verbelen et al., 2014).

Medical Grade Honey Dressings

Honey is one of the oldest documented wound care dressings. Its beneficial effects appear to be due in part to its high osmolality, which inhibits bacterial growth. It is supported in the literature as effective against a broad spectrum of bacterial species, including *Pseudomonas aeruginosa*. This virulent and opportunistic species is often a problem in burn wounds. There is a high correlation between *Pseudomonas* burn colonization and skin graft failure. Evidence suggests that honey may be a useful agent in the treatment of burn wounds infected with or at risk of infection with *Pseudomonas* (Aziz & Hassan, 2017; Fish & Bezuhly, 2012; Molan et al., 2002; Norman et al., 2017).

Sulfamylon Dressings

Mafenide acetate (Sulfamylon) cream or solution has limited use on burn wounds. Sulfamylon use is based on the fact that it is a broad-spectrum antimicrobial agent, which has the ability to penetrate eschar. Application to any area of a burn wound with intact nerve endings may cause the patient additional pain. It cannot be used on large wounds because systemic absorption can lead to metabolic acidosis. It is most commonly used to treat deep partial or full-thickness burns to the ears or nose. These cartilaginous areas, which are not very vascular, may benefit from the penetrating antimicrobial effects this agent provides (Jeschke & Herndon, 2017).

Bromelain-Based Enzymatic Dressing

Bromelain-based enzymatic dressing (trade name Nexo-Brid®) has been used in the European Union and other international markets since the 1980s. This product is currently under FDA review for safety and efficacy for possible use in the U.S. market in the near future. Nexo-Brid is clinically indicated for use as a debriding agent in deep partial and full-thickness burns. Randomized control trials describe benefits as decreased time to complete debridement with or without surgery, decreased time to wound closure, and improved scar appearance (Loo et al., 2018). One published case study expressed concern about possible coagulation abnormalities following the use of NexoBrid but could not make a definitive claim (Martín et al., 2017).

Biologic and Biosynthetic Dressings

Biologic and biosynthetic dressings are used to provide temporary coverage for wounds in which autografting is planned for definitive closure. They decrease the risk of infection, assist in regulation of core body temperature, decrease loss of fluid and proteins, and decrease overall metabolic stress. Commonly used biologic burn dressings include xenografts (pig skin) and allografts (fresh or cryopreserved cadaver skin). Xenografts are more readily available. Allografts are considered superior since they more closely reproduce normal human skin function. Xenografts must be removed or allowed to slough prior to grafting. Allografts can act as a dermal substrate if the epithelium is removed or allowed to slough prior to grafting. Wound care involving these dressings includes daily gentle cleansing, coverage with a nonadherent gauze, and monitoring for rejection and signs of infection (Evans, 2016; Fish & Bezuhly, 2012; Jeschke & Herndon, 2017).

> **KEY POINT**
>
> Biologic and biosynthetic dressings are used to provide temporary coverage for burns in which grafting is planned for definitive closure.

Biosynthetic dressings are part biologic (usually animal) and part synthetic. The biosynthetic dressing most commonly used in burn management is Biobrane®. It is composed of porcine dermal collagen chemically bound to a nylon and silicone membrane. It is a flexible, temporary dressing used to treat partial-thickness burns and donor sites or excised full-thickness burns. It mimics the function of the skin with good fluid exchange and barrier protection. It is very flexible, which means it can be used in joint areas to allow for range of motion and normal function. Wound care is minimal. Following placement of the Biobrane®, a fluffed dressing and gauze wraps are applied and secured with elastic bandages to provide a moderate-level compression. The dressing should be left in place and undisturbed for 48 hours. At that point, the Biobrane® is adherent to the wound bed and dressings are no longer needed. The area is monitored for infection until the Biobrane® is removed approximately 14 days later when the autograft is applied (Evans, 2016; Falanga and Lazic, 2011; Feng et al., 2018; Fish and Bezuhly, 2012).

BURN WOUND CLOSURE

Early excision and closure of burn wounds leads to improved outcomes including reduced length of hospital stay, reduced infections, reduced incidence of hypertrophic scars (HTSs), and reduced time for rehabilitation.

Autografts

The optimal closure of a burn wound is achieved with the patient's own skin (autologous grafting), which ideally occurs 3 to 4 days after injury. Split-thickness skin grafts (STSGs) are harvested from healthy skin, with an average thickness of 0.008 to 0.0012 inches. STSG include the epidermis and a thin layer of the dermis. They can be applied as intact sheets or can be meshed to cover larger areas. Sheet grafts are used in locations that require better functional and cosmetic outcomes, such as the hands, feet, joints, face, and neck. Sheet grafts are frequently managed without a dressing in the initial postoperative period, since it is important to closely monitor the newly placed graft for fluid collection between the graft and the underlying wound bed. If fluid collects, it causes separation of the graft and the wound bed with failure of the graft. Any fluid accumulation must be removed to promote graft adherence. This can be done through aspiration or by carefully rolling a cotton-tipped applicator over the top of the graft to express the fluid (Antoon, 2020; Evans, 2016; Jeschke & Herndon, 2017).

KEY POINT

The optimal closure of a burn wound is achieved with the patient's own skin (autologous grafting), which ideally occurs 3 to 4 days after injury. The graft must be carefully monitored for any fluid accumulation between the graft and wound bed, which must be removed.

Meshed autologous skin grafts are used on larger burns; meshing facilitates coverage of a greater surface area. If the grafted area is an extremity or a joint, splints are applied to maintain a functional position. Postoperatively the meshed graft is dressed with a nonadherent layer to prevent shearing and a bolster dressing composed of fluffed gauze soaked in 5% Sulfamylon solution; the solution is reapplied every 2 to 3 hours to maintain efficacy. The bolster component of the dressing is designed to maintain approximation of the wound bed with the graft and is important for normal healing and take of the graft. The graft will survive only if it gets adequate blood supply from the wound bed through the ingress of capillary loops, which requires close adherence of the graft to the wound bed. The initial dressing is typically left undisturbed for 5 to 7 days, at which time the dressings are removed to allow examination of the graft. Dressing changes at this time usually involve nonadherent products that support moist wound healing. Graft donor sites are treated as superficial partial-thickness burns. Dressing choice for donor sites varies greatly and ranges from petrolatum gauze to alginates to biosynthetic dressings (Evans, 2016; Ogawa & Orgill, 2013).

Full-thickness skin grafts (FTSG) are used only on small full-thickness burns, usually for reconstructive purposes. They are obtained from a full-thickness donor site where the donor skin is excised down to the subcutaneous tissue layer. Because they are thicker grafts, they are less prone to contractures and hypertrophic scarring. Donor sites are sutured closed and allowed to heal through primary intention or with placement of an STSG (Evans, 2016).

Negative pressure wound therapy (NPWT) has become a widely used treatment for acute and chronic wounds. Some studies validate its use for certain aspects of burn care. NPWT has proven beneficial in its use as a dressing that bolsters skin grafts, promotes integration of bilaminate dermal substitutes, promotes

reepithelialization of skin graft donor sites, and potentially reduces the zone of stasis (Kantak et al., 2017).

Cultured Epithelial Autografts

Cultured epithelial autografts (CEAs) have been used for many years in burns with >50% TBSA due to the limited availability of healthy donor sites. In this procedure, autologous keratinocytes are harvested and sent to a tissue lab to replicate over 3 to 4 weeks before transplantation. The epithelial cells are placed on a petrolatum-based dressing and applied to a wound bed. Reported success rates with CEAs alone are variable. Recent literature reports high success rates when CEAs are used in conjunction with acellular dermal matrices. Wound care for CEAs is easy. The surgeon secures the CEA-impregnated dressing with staples and covers it with gauze. The dressing is left undisturbed for 7 to 10 days. Care must be taken to avoid friction and mechanical stress at the fragile graft site. Afterward, wound care is the same as previously described for STSG (Evans, 2016; Fang et al., 2014; Fish & Bezuhly, 2012).

Staged Closure

In burns involving more than 30% TBSA, autologous skin grafting is not always an immediate option due to limited availability of uninjured skin. In these cases, wound closure is completed in staged procedures. The full-thickness burns are excised and, if autologous skin is not available for grafting, the open wound is covered with an acellular matrix dressing that replaces the lost dermis. This acellular dressing supports ingrowth of new blood vessels and formation of healthy granulation tissue. When autologous skin becomes available, the skin grafting procedure is completed. There are several products that are used in this capacity. The two most commonly used are Integra® and AlloDerm® (Evans, 2016; Fish & Bezuhly, 2012; Paul et al., 2001; Jeschke & Herndon, 2017).

Integra is a meshed bilayer matrix dressing that promotes neogenesis and collagen synthesis. The inner layer is composed of bovine collagen and chondroitin-6-sulfate. The outer layer is silicone sheeting, which is removed approximately 2 weeks following initial application. If there is skin appropriate for an autograft or a CEA is available at the time of removal of the Integra, then grafting is done which is usually successful. Integra is advantageous because it can replace the entire dermis and can be applied directly over muscle or bone. Integra is particularly effective when used in combination with NPWT. If the peri-wound skin integrity is insufficient to maintain NPWT, the Integra dressing is managed in the same manner as a fresh STSG (Evans, 2016; Fang et al., 2014; Fish & Bezuhly, 2012).

AlloDerm is an acellular matrix dressing derived from cryopreserved cadaver allograft. Because all of the epidermal and dermal cells are removed during processing, the final product is acellular and nonimmunogenic. Like Integra, it works as a scaffold to promote neoangiogenesis and collagen synthesis. It does have one major limitation, the STSG must be placed immediately following AlloDerm placement. Wound care associated with AlloDerm is the same as wound care associated with a newly placed STSG. If a patient has limited donor skin availability and CEA is not available, this product may not be appropriate (Evans, 2016; Fish & Bezuhly, 2012).

PRESSURE INJURIES AND BURN PATIENTS

All patients with limited mobility are at risk for pressure injury. While no burn-specific literature exists, it is suspected that pressure injuries are more problematic in the burn population due to initial hypovolemic shock followed by edema, hypermetabolism, nutritional deficits, wet dressings, and splinting with immobilization post-grafting procedures. An aggressive pressure injury prevention program must be implemented. Education and involvement of the entire multidisciplinary team is important. When the patient is too hemodynamically unstable to tolerate turning, it should be documented, and repositioning should be resumed as soon as tolerated. Precautions to avoid friction and shearing should be implemented, including low shear surfaces and use of appropriate lifting and repositioning devices. Physical and occupational therapists must be cognizant of pressure injury risk when constructing splints. Low or high air loss surfaces can be used to reduce pressure and promote evaporation of excessive moisture. When the patient is able to get out of bed, pressure redistribution chair cushions should be used (EPUAP/NPIAP/PPPIA, 2019; Richard et al., 2004).

KEY POINT

Burn patients are thought to be at high risk for pressure injuries. A comprehensive program of risk assessment and preventive interventions should be implemented.

SCAR FORMATION

Full-thickness burn injuries heal through scar formation. Immediately after reepithelialization, healed skin appears pink, soft, and flat. With normal remodeling, the scar tissue remains flat. Burn wounds are high risk for excessive scarring, either HTS or keloid. The likelihood of this increases as the depth of the burn increases. Hypertrophic or keloid scars become visible after a period of time that ranges from weeks to months (Bloemen et al., 2009; Carrougher, 1998).

KEY POINT

Burn wounds are high risk for excessive scarring, either hypertrophic scar (HTS) or keloid. The likelihood of this increases as the depth of the burn increases.

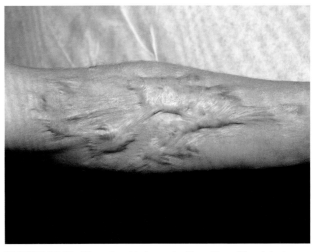

FIGURE 32-10. Hypertrophic Irregular Burn Scar. (Reprinted with permission from Lugo-Somolinos, A., et al. (2011). *VisualDx: Essential dermatology in pigmented skin*. Philadelphia, PA: Wolters Kluwer Health.)

Hypertrophic Scar Formation

HTS formation is more common postburn injury as compared to other types of wounds. Risk factors that predict the formations of HTSs include age, with children being at greater risk than adults. Individuals with darker skin tones and lighter skin tones are at greater risk. Additional risk factors include increased depth of burn injury, increased incidence of infection, and a prolonged number of days to healing. Vitamin D deficiency is a contributing factor for HTS formation. HTSs present as raised, thickened, firm scars that are reddish in color and that do not extend beyond the borders of the original injury (**Fig. 32-10**). Related complaints of pain and excessive pruritus are common (Cho et al., 2019; Herndon, 2012; Holland et al., 2012).

Treatment of HTS is most effective if initiated early. The use of custom pressure garments has been the standard of care for many years (**Fig. 32-11**). Although

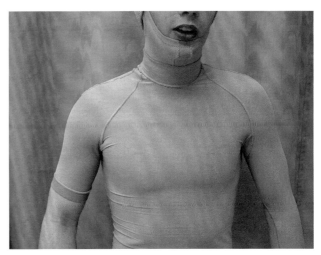

FIGURE 32-11. Custom, Elastic Pressure Garments. Application of pressure garments helps prevent hypertrophic burn scarring. (Used with permission of Jobst Institute, Inc., Toledo, OH.)

there is little published evidence as to the exact mechanism of action for pressure garments, they have been shown to reduce scar thickness and redness as well as pruritus. Pressure garment therapy is associated with reduced time to scar maturation. Garments should be worn 23 hours/day, which makes compliance with therapy sometimes challenging, especially with children. Patients and parents of children with burns should be educated and encouraged to be compliant with therapy and should understand the potential long-term ramifications of noncompliance (Antoon, 2020; Evans, 2016; Herndon, 2012; Jones et al., 2008). Additional options for management of HTS include topical silicone gel and silicone gel sheets, and intralesional injections of corticosteroid, all of which have been shown to be of benefit. In extreme cases, surgical excision may be necessary for either cosmetic or functional improvement (Bloemen et al., 2009; Jones et al., 2008).

Keloid Formation

Keloid formation can occur spontaneously or in response to trauma. It is more common in individuals with darker skin tones compared to lighter skin tones. Keloid scars appear as raised, firm, hyperpigmented nodules. They extend, sometimes dramatically, beyond the borders of the original injury. Treatment of keloids is difficult at best. There are reports of limited success with corticosteroid injection, chemotherapy agents, radiation, lasers, and surgical removal where a rim of keloid scar is left in place. Surgical removal is usually not done unless the keloid becomes pendulous (Bloemen et al., 2009; Jones et al., 2008).

PRURITUS

Itching is an irritating and often persistent occurrence associated with healing and healed burn wounds. The exact etiology of the pruritus is not known though there are several theories as to the cause. Increased histamine production is believed to be the primary source of itching and is thought to be related to inflammatory mediators produced during healing. Itching sensations are most intense immediately after the burn wound has healed and peak 2 to 6 months later. Complaints of pruritus can last up to 18 months. Itching that persists beyond that point is thought to have a psychogenic component. Treatment includes oral antihistamines, use of moisturizers to minimize dry skin, a cool air-conditioned environment, application of cool cloths, massage, and compression garments (which are thought to decrease inflammation). Another less common measure is the administration of penicillin. This is based on evidence that most HTS are colonized with *Staphylococcus aureus* and beta-hemolytic streptococcus when compared to non-HTS (Herndon, 2012).

KEY POINT

Itching is an often persistent occurrence associated with burn wounds. Management includes moisturizers, antihistamines, pressure garments, cool cloths, massage, and sometimes penicillin.

TRAUMATIC BLISTERS IN REEPITHELIALIZED BURN WOUNDS

Newly healed epithelium is thin and very fragile with reduced cohesion between the epidermal and dermal layers. Minor trauma can cause small blisters to form. This can be very stressful to the patient as they are often emotionally vulnerable and fear setbacks. Patients need to be educated about blisters and reassured that the tensile strength of the epithelium will increase over time. Ruptured blisters should be treated with moist wound care (Herndon, 2012).

PSYCHOSOCIAL ADAPTATION FOLLOWING BURN INJURY

The traumatic nature of burn injuries has lasting physical and psychological consequences. The burn patient's emotional and mental health needs are often obscured by the physical needs associated with survival. Long term, most of these patients need help in coming to terms with their changed body and psychological distress is common. Acute stress disorder, post-traumatic stress disorder (PTSD) and depression are observed in 45% of adult survivors. Risk factors for psychological disorders include the percentage of TBSA affected, length of hospital stay, preburn anxiety or depression disorders, and being female. There does not seem to be a correlation between the visibility of burn scars and psychological distress, but the literature suggests that the degree of distress is related to the individual's subjective perception of how others see them. Those with a higher self-esteem, preburn injury are much more likely to do well emotionally in the rehabilitative phase (Fish & Bezuhly, 2012; Logsetty et al., 2013).

KEY POINT

Acute stress disorder, post-traumatic stress disorder, and depression are observed in 45% of adult survivors.

Psychosocial adaptation in the rehabilitation phase must be multifaceted and must address patient concerns. These concerns usually center on the ability to return to work, issues related to sexual function and sexual relationships, and the ability to return to preburn roles within the family. Adaptation is best supported through formal counseling, burn-specific support groups, and vocational retraining. In pediatric populations, a school reentry program is necessary. These programs should be specific to the child's developmental level and educational needs. School staff and children should have the opportunity, before the patient returns to school, to obtain accurate information and to ask questions to reduce anxiety (Antoon, 2020; Fish & Bezuhly, 2012).

> ### KEY POINT
>
> The Phoenix Society for Burn Survivors and the World Burn Congress can offer invaluable support and resources for burn survivors. The wound care nurse should encourage the individual to utilize available resources to optimize their mental health and adaptation.

MARJOLIN'S ULCERS

The incidence of Marjolin's malignant ulcers ranges from 1% to 2% of all burn scars, with squamous cell cancers as the most common histology type. Pathogenesis is not well understood, and it is possible that multiple mechanisms play a role. The biologic behavior of these malignancies is frequently more virulent than other types of skin cancers. Malignant transformation is most frequently associated with burn scars but can also occur in scars associated with other chronic wounds. There is always a dormant period between the offending injury and the development of the ulcer. The average time to malignant transformation is 35 years post injury. Although rare, acute onset can occur in weeks post injury. Treatment must be aggressive and usually includes radical excision in conjunction with radiation therapy (Copcu, 2009; Kawilarang, 2020).

> ### KEY POINT
>
> Healed burns and donor sites are more susceptible to melanoma, and burn scars can also undergo malignant transformation (Marjolin's ulcer). Instruction in sun protection should be a standard component of discharge teaching, and any nonhealing or deteriorating wound should be biopsied, as should recurrent wounds in previously healed burn sites.

RESEARCH AND NEW DIRECTIONS IN BURN CARE

The Multicenter Trial Group is a group established by the ABA, with the objective of providing best practice data to guide burn management. Most of the studies published involve retrospective reviews of burn care in North America (Fish & Bezuhly, 2012). The ABA participates in federally funded studies to improve burn care and collaborates with burn centers across the country.

The ability to accurately and expeditiously diagnose burn depth has a significant impact on clinical management and resultant outcomes. Literature suggests that assessment based on clinical observation is only 70% accurate even among experienced burn surgeons. Noncontact laser Doppler imaging has been shown to augment clinical assessment. This technology provides a color perfusion map of the burn wound, which, in conjunction with physical examination, can improve accuracy in depth assessment. The imaging can be done daily during the emergent phase of burn management to evaluate dynamic changes in wound bed perfusion. The major barrier to implementing this technology is the associated high cost (Fish & Bezuhly, 2012; Herndon, 2012; Shin & Yi, 2016).

Expeditious closure of burn wounds is a major contributor to burn survival. Not only is closure vital, but the speed at which closure occurs affects the risk for life-threatening complications during the acute phase. Speed of closure also has long-term effects, specifically on the degree of scarring and on psychosocial adaptation in the rehabilitative phase. An ongoing area of research is identification of best and earliest approaches to burn closure. There are reports of success with cultured skin substitutes, platelet-rich plasma, and amniotic membranes (Boyce et al., 2006; Mohammadi et al., 2013; Schlanser et al., 2017).

Giving the patient the best cosmetic and functional outcome is a major focus when treating burn injuries. In reconstructive surgery, fat has been used as filler for many years. Research suggests that fat grafting could have additional benefits. Stem cells derived from fat cells are regenerative, and in vitro studies reveal a significant improvement in the texture, thickness, and contours of the skin when treated with fat grafts (Ranganathan et al., 2013).

> ### KEY POINT
>
> Patients see themselves in the eyes of their caregivers and family members before they ever see a mirror. The wound care nurse must monitor their facial expressions and counsel the family regarding burn wound appearance when they begin to assist with dressing changes.

LONG-TERM SEQUELAE OF BURNS

A burn injury that occurred in the 1950s was associated with a high mortality rate despite medical treatment. The current burn injury survival rate is 96.8% for adults and 99% for children. Using the largest, long-term data collected in the Burn Model System National Database, there is a movement to reclassify a burn injury as an acute condition that becomes a chronic condition. The physical sequelae of medical problems post burn injury include paresthesia, pruritis, ongoing musculoskeletal problems (contractures, heterotopic ossification, joint pain), memory recall impairment, hot and cold intolerance, chronic fatigue, hypertrophic scarring, depression, anxiety, insomnia, palpitations, chest pain, weight loss and gain, dysphagia, pulmonary embolus, and PTSD. While some of these are commonly known post-burn phenomenon, others are not readily recognized as a complication of a burn injury. It is important to acknowledge the burn injury as a chronic disease to provide a framework for treatment with the development of long-term practice guidelines to enable primary care providers to better assist in meeting the long-term needs of burn survivors (Kelter et al., 2020).

FROSTBITE

Frostbite is a traumatic injury that occurs when tissue temperature falls below freezing. It is a relatively common injury in the United States in the homeless population and among individuals living in lower socioeconomic urban areas. Frostbite is on the rise in association with increasing popularity of outdoor winter recreational activities. It is a local injury that usually is seen on the extremities or the face. Predisposing factors include alcohol and drug use, mental illness, and motor vehicle accident or failure of a motor vehicle (Carceller et al., 2019; Herndon, 2012; Koljonen et al., 2004; Vuola, 2004; Woo et al., 2013).

KEY POINT

Frostbite is a relatively common injury in the homeless population and those living in lower socioeconomic urban areas. It is most likely to involve the face or extremities.

PATHOPHYSIOLOGY

The pathophysiology of frostbite has 4 overlapping pathologic phases. The first stage is the pre-freeze stage. It is the cooling of tissue causing vasoconstriction and ischemia but no ice crystals form. The second stage is the freeze-thaw stage. At this stage of exposure, cellular damage and death occur to the formation of ice crystals both intra- and extracellularly. The third stage is known as the vascular stasis stage. In this stage, vessels alternate between constriction and dilation. This can result in thrombus formation. The fourth and final stage is the late ischemic stage. This is a progressive stage that results in destruction of the microcirculation and leads to total cellular death (McIntosh et al., 2019).

CLASSIFICATION OF INJURY

Frostbite classification is based on depth and resembles burn classifications. It is classified as frostnip, superficial frostbite, and deep frostbite.

Frostnip

When a frostnip injury occurs, the skin becomes very pale and sensation is slowly lost. When rewarming occurs, the skin becomes hyperemic. Paresthesia can persist for several weeks, but there is no significant tissue damage with frostnip (Herndon, 2012; Koljonen et al., 2004).

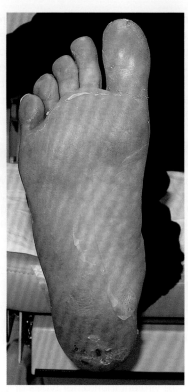

FIGURE 32-12. Superficial Frostbite Injury. (Reprinted with permission from The Podiatry Institute. (2012). *McGlamry's comprehensive textbook of foot and ankle surgery, 2-Volume Set* (4th ed.). Philadelphia, PA: Wolters Kluwer.)

Superficial Frostbite

Superficial frostbite is subdivided into first- and second-degree frostbite. With first-degree frostbite, there is partial freezing limited to the superficial layers of the epidermis; initial characteristics of first-degree frostbite include erythema, edema, and hyperemia. Superficial skin desquamation may occur 5 to 10 days post injury (**Fig. 32-12**), but there is no long-term tissue damage. With second-degree frostbite, there is freezing of the entire epidermis. These wounds are characterized by significant edema, erythema, and the formation of vesicles filled with clear fluid (**Fig. 32-13**). As these wounds evolve, there is skin loss (desquamation) and eschar formation.

KEY POINT

First-degree frostbite is manifested by erythema, edema, and superficial skin desquamation 5 to 10 days post injury, but no long-term damage. Second-degree frost bite is manifested by edema, erythema, and blister formation. These wounds evolve to skin loss and possible eschar formation.

Deep Frostbite

Deep frostbite is subdivided into third- and fourth-degree classifications. Third-degree frostbite involves freezing

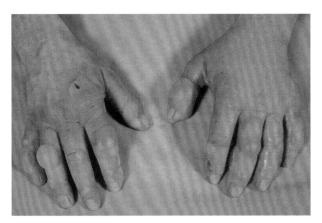

FIGURE 32-13. Frostbite with Bullae Formation. (Reproduced with permission from Berg, D., & Worzala, K. (2006). *Atlas of adult physical diagnosis*. Philadelphia, PA: Lippincott Williams & Wilkins.)

injury of the entire skin, with extension into the subcutaneous tissue. It is manifested initially by the presence of violet-hued, hemorrhagic blisters. Skin necrosis ensues and appears blue-gray. Fourth-degree frostbite involves freezing of the skin, subcutaneous tissue, muscle, tendon, and bone. There is rarely any edema. It initially appears mottled, cyanotic, or deep red. As the injury progresses, the involved area appears dry, black, and mummified (**Fig. 32-14**) (Koljonen et al., 2004).

TREATMENT

Initial treatment of a frostbite injury is to prevent further injury. For many years, field first aid recommended rubbing the injured area with snow. This is now known to cause further damage.

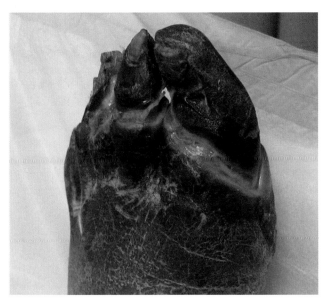

FIGURE 32-14. Demarcated Fourth-Degree Frostbite with Necrosis of the Toes. (Photo courtesy of Scott Sherman, MD.)

On-Site Interventions

Current recommendations for on-site interventions include removal of any jewelry (which conducts cold), placing involved extremity in the axilla of a first responder for 10 minutes and covering the patient in blankets until transport to a medical facility can be accomplished (Carceller et al., 2019; Herndon, 2012; Koljonen et al., 2004).

Rewarming

The next phase of treatment involves rewarming. This is a painful procedure, and the patient should be medicated accordingly. Rewarming should be carried out in a circulating water bath at a recommended temperature of 37°C to 39°C. The patient is kept in the bath for approximately 30 minutes or until sensation returns and flushing is seen on the most distal aspect of the involved tissue. Prevention of intravascular thrombosis should be attempted with the use of antithromboxane agents, ibuprofen being the most common, and topical aloe vera gel (Herndon, 2012; Koljonen et al., 2004).

Post-Thaw Management

Post-thaw management involves standard wound care for the injured tissue. There is evidence in the literature that hyperbaric oxygen therapy may be useful, even if there is a significant time lapse between the injury and initiation of hyperbaric oxygen therapy (HBOT). Surgery may be required but is delayed until there is a clear line of demarcation between the viable and devitalized tissue. This may take 1 to 3 months (Herndon, 2012; Kemper et al., 2014; Koljonen et al., 2004).

KEY POINT

Post-thaw management of third- and fourth-degree frostbite involves standard wound care. HBOT may also be helpful. Debridement is delayed until there is a clear line of demarcation between viable and devitalized tissue, which may take 1 to 3 months.

 CONCLUSION

Many wound care nurses will be asked to consult on a burn wound or frostbite injury. Regardless of the severity of the injury, the wound care nurse will be expected to write wound care protocols and direct basic wound management. It is essential for the wound care nurse to be knowledgeable regarding the referral criteria to a burn center. Wound care recommendations should be made on an understanding of the underlying pathophysiology of the wound, accurate assessment of the tissue layers involved, and an understanding of the three phases of burn management. Effective management of thermal injuries requires a multidisciplinary and holistic approach if optimal long-term outcomes are to be achieved.

CASE STUDIES

CASE STUDY #1

A 24-year-old male presents 72 hours post flash explosion involving gasoline. He was treated immediately after the incident in an urgent care center. He was instructed to change the dressing daily with silver sulfadiazine (SSD) and told to follow up in the wound center.

Wound Assessment: The patient is out of the emergent phase and is in the acute wound care phase of management. His only comorbidity is tobacco abuse. Arm burns are not circumferential. Chest burn is epidermal only and not counted in TBSA assessment. TBSA is estimated at 9% with depth assessment categorized as superficial partial thickness. Patient has palpable radial pulses. He is afebrile with stable vital signs. PO intake is reported as fair. It is safe to treat this patient on an outpatient basis. He will follow up in 3 days.

Wound Care Recommendations: Shower with mild soap and water. The possibility of any gasoline on the skin must be addressed. SSD is not the best choice, but it is not a wrong choice. The patient who has no insurance has already purchased several jars. Continue daily SSD dressing changes. Education regarding nutrition and smoking cessation provided. Patient is given instructions to start high-protein diet and add a multivitamin and vitamin C 1,000 mg daily.

Day 6 (see figure):

Wound Assessment: Burn is not larger but more visible. Note intact hair follicles apparent in the arms. Patient is doing well. Oral intake improved.

Wound Care Recommendations: Continue with current plan of care.

Day 9 (see figure):

Wound Assessment: Burns are largely healed.

Wound Care Recommendations: Moist wound care and protection from trauma. Patient will change dressing daily with wound gel and nonstick gauze.

Day 14 (see figure):

Wound Assessment: Burn is healed. Skin needs continued protection from trauma and routine application of moisturizing agents. No long-term compression therapy needed.

Wound Care Recommendations: Patient discharged with instructions: gentle skin care with moisturizer applied at least twice daily and protection from sun with use of protective clothes. Daily use of sunscreen starting in 2 weeks (skin too sensitive at present) for a minimum of 3 months.

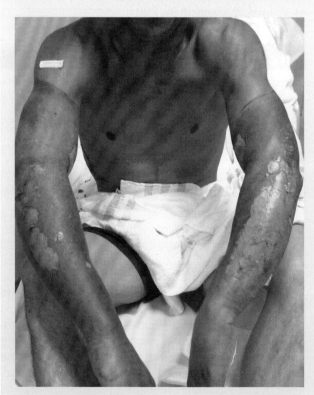

Day 6 Post Injury.

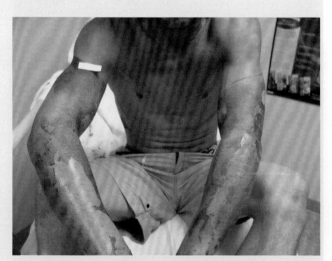

Day 9 Post Injury.

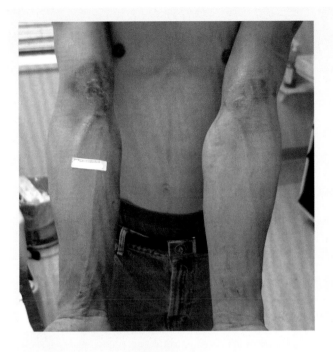

Day 14 Post Injury.

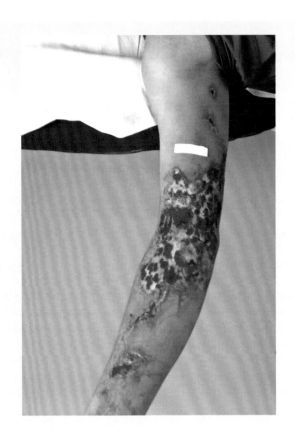

CASE STUDY #2

A 17-year-old male involved in motor vehicle accident. Left arm with thermal burn. Patient was admitted to a local hospital and stabilized. Wound care nurse consulted 3 days after injury.

Wound Assessment: Patient is out of the emergent phase and is in the acute wound care phase. He has no comorbidities. The wound appears dry with white, leathery patches surrounded by red tissue indicating full thickness intermixed with deep partial thickness. TBSA is approximately 4%. The injury occurs over a major joint in an extremity. Patient has a palpable radial pulse. Patient meets criteria for transfer to a burn center.

Wound Care Recommendations: Wound cleansed with normal saline (NS) and a nanocrystalline silver dressing applied. Formal recommendation to transfer patient to a burn center was made to attending physician who agreed and patient was transferred within 24 hours. Follow-up report provided by the burn unit indicated that the patient was treated with surgical excision of the burn-injured tissue and placement of STSG.

CASE STUDY #3

A 47-year-old female is referred from her primary care provider to an outpatient wound center for evaluation of burns to her feet. The burns occurred 5 days prior when she fell asleep in front of a space heater. Medical history includes non–insulin-dependent diabetes (A1c 6.2) and hypertension. She denies any history of tobacco use or alcohol use.

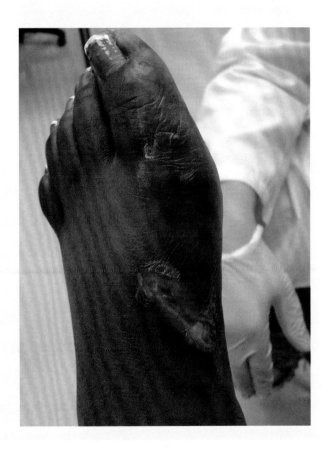

Wound Assessment: This patient is out of the emergent phase and in the acute wound care phase. TBSA is 1% per foot. Burns in individuals with darker skin tones are more difficult to evaluate than burns in individuals with lighter skin tones. Note the discoloration of the great toe—appears blistered—unable to determine accurate depth at this time. There is a similar burn to the right foot (not pictured). The burn to the left dorsal midfoot is characterized by eschar surrounded by pink tissue. This burn is full thickness. Bilateral lower extremities are noted to have 1+ edema. Bilateral dorsalis pedal and posterior tibial pulses are identified with Doppler only. Weinstein monofilament test reveals loss of protective sensation (LOPS).

Wound Care Recommendations: Vascular status is unclear, and immediate referral to a vascular surgeon for ABI/PVR of the lower extremities was made. In the interim, toe blisters were painted with povidone–iodine. Midfoot burn wounds were treated with nanocrystalline silver dressing. Patient is placed in offloading shoe. Education is provided regarding the role of nutrition and glucose control in wound healing.

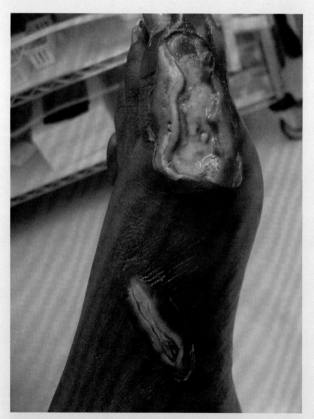

Postburn Injury Day 12. Arterial study revealed bilateral lower extremities with an ABI of 0.6. Vascular surgeon believes healing potential is marginal and would like to be reconsulted if wound does not progress within the next week.

Day 12 (see figure):

Wound Assessment: Right foot burns appear unchanged (not pictured). Left great toe foot blister now appears as dry pink tissue surrounding adherent slough. Depth of this burn is deep partial thickness.

Wound Care Recommendations: Wounds cleansed with NS and treated with nanocrystalline silver dressings. Due to ABI, recommended evaluation for adjunctive HBOT. Continue to educate patient regarding the role of nutrition and glucose control in wound healing.

Postburn day 14:

Patient went for HBOT evaluation and $TCPO_2$ testing, which indicated patient was a good candidate for HBOT. The facility recommended 5 treatments per week for the next 6 to 7 weeks. Patient reported that she could not afford her per dive copay and declined therapy. No change in appearance of wounds.

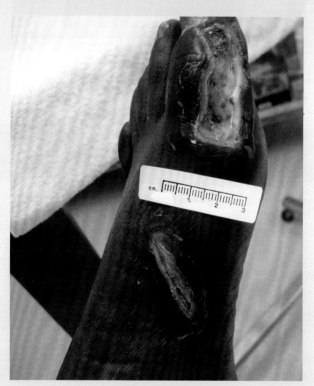

Postburn Day 19.

Day 19 (see figure):

Wound Evaluation: Deterioration of left great toe burn wound. Appearance is dry and leathery. No change in right foot burn wounds (not pictured).

Wound Care Recommendations: Reconsult vascular surgery. Wounds cleansed with NS and treated with nanocrystalline silver dressings.

Ultimate Outcome: Patient was admitted into the hospital for an arteriogram, and a stent was placed to left leg to improve blood flow. Unfortunately, the small vessels feeding the left great toe were calcified secondary to pathology associated with diabetes.

Two days after discharge from the hospital, the patient's blood sugar spiked to 350. She was again admitted into the hospital for treatment. While there, the left foot became gangrenous and a life-saving below-the-knee amputation was done. The patient has since adapted well and has returned to her normal life with the aid of a prosthetic limb. The right foot healed completely.

REFERENCES

Abboud, E. C., Legare, T. B., Settle, J. C., et al. (2014). Do silver-based wound dressings reduce pain? A prospective study and review of the literature. *Burns, 40*(Suppl 1), S40–S47. doi: 10.1016/j.burns.2014.09.012.

American Burn Association. (2016). *Burn incidence fact sheet.* Chicago, IL: ABA. Retrieved from http://ameriburn. org/who-we-are/media/burn-incidence-fact-sheet

American Burn Association (ABA). (2018). *Advanced Burn Life Support Course Provider Manual.* Chicago, IL: ABA. Retrieved from http://ameriburn.org/wp-content/uploads/2019/08/2018-abls-provider-manual.pdf

Antoon, A. Y. (2020). Burn injuries. In R. M. Kliegman & J. W. St. Geme. *Nelson Textbook of Pediatrics* (21st ed.). Philadelphia, PA: Elsevier Inc.

Atiyeh, B. S., & Hayek, S. N. (2010). Management of war-related burn injuries: Lessons learned from recent ongoing conflicts providing exceptional care in unusual places. *Journal of Craniofacial Surgery, 21*, 1529–1537.

Aziz, Z., & Hassan, B. A. R. (2017). The effects of honey compared to silver sulfadiazine for the treatment of burns: A systematic review of randomized controlled trials. *Burns, 43*(1), 50–57.

Besner, G. E., Paddock, H., Fabia, R., et al. (2007). Silver impregnated antimicrobial dressing reduces hospital length of stay for pediatric patients with burns. *Journal of Burn Care & Research, 28*, 409–411.

Bettencourt, A. P., Carter, J., Cartotto, R., et al. (2019). Bringing burn referral criteria into the 21st century: A structured expert consensus project to update and refine recommendations for transfer and consultation. *Journal of Burn Care & Research, 40*(Suppl 1). doi: 10.1093/jbcr/irz013.024.

Bloemen, M. C., van der Veer, W. M., Ulrich, M. M., et al. (2009). Prevention and curative management of hypertrophic scar formation. *Burns, 35*(4), 463–475.

Boyce, S. T., Kagan, R. J., Greenhalgh, D. G., et al. (2006). Cultured skin substitutes reduce requirements for harvesting of skin autograft for closure of excised, full-thickness burns. *Journal of Trauma and Acute Care Surgery, 60*, 821–824.

Cambiaso-Daniel, J., Boukovalas, S., Bitz, G. H., et al. (2018). Topical antimicrobials in burn care: Part I–topical antiseptics. *Annals of Plastic Surgery.* doi: 10.1097/SAP.0000000000001297. Accessed on April 16, 2020.

Carceller, A., Javierre, C., Ríos, M., et al. (2019). Amputation risk factors in severely frostbitten patients. *International Journal of Environmental Research and Public Health, 16*(8), 1351. doi: 10.3390/ijerph16081351.

Carrougher, G. J. (1998). *Burn care and therapy.* St. Louis, MO: Mosby.

Caruso, D. M., Foster, K. N., Blome-Eberwein, S. A., et al. (2006). Randomized clinical study of hydrofiber dressing with silver or silver sulfadiazine in the management of partial-thickness burns. *Journal of Burn Care & Research, 27*, 298–309.

Cho, Y. S., Seo, C. H., Joo, S. Y., et al. (2019). The association between postburn vitamin D deficiency and the biomechanical properties of hypertrophic scars. *Journal of Burn Care & Research, 40*(3), 274–280. doi: 10.1093/jbcr/irz028.

Connor-Ballard, P. (2009). Understanding and managing burn pain: Part 1. *American Journal of Nursing, 109*, 48–56.

Copcu, E. (2009). Marjolin's ulcer: A preventable complication of burns? *Plastic and Reconstructive Surgery, 124*, 156e–161e.

European Pressure Ulcer Advisory Panel, National Pressure Injury Advisory Panel, and Pan Pacific Pressure Injury Alliance [EPUAP/NPIAP/PPPIA]. (2019). In E. Haesler (Ed.), *Prevention and treatment of pressure ulcers/injuries: Clinical Practice Guideline. The International Guideline..*

Evans, J. (2016). Burns. In R. Bryant & D. Nix (Eds.), *Acute and chronic wounds: Current management concepts* (5th ed.). St. Louis, MO: Elsevier Inc.

Falanga, V., & Lazic, T. (2011). Bioengineered skin constructs and their use in wound healing. *Plastic and Reconstructive Surgery, 127*, 75S–90S.

Fang, T., Lineaweaver, W., Sailes, F., et al. (2014). Clinical application of cultured epithelial autografts on acellular dermal matrices in the treatment of extended burn injuries. *Annals of Plastic Surgery, 73*(5), 509–515.

Feng, J. J., See, J. L., Choke, A., et al. (2018). Biobrane™ for burns of the pubic region: Minimizing dressing changes. *Military Medical Research, 5*(1), 29. doi: 10.1186/s40779-018-0177-2.

Fire Deaths and Injuries. (n.d.). Fact sheet. Retrieved April 21, 2014, from https://www.cdc.gov/HomeandRecreationsSafety/Fire-Prevention/fires-factsheet.html

Fish, J. S., & Bezuhly, M. (2012). Acute burn care. *Plastic and Reconstructive Surgery, 130*, 349e–358e.

Furness, P. J., Phelan, I., Babiker, N. T., et al. (2019). Reducing pain during wound dressings in burn care using virtual reality: A study of perceived impact and usability with patients and nurses. *Journal of Burn Care & Research, 40*(6), 878–885. doi: 10.1093/jbcr/irz106.

Gravante, G., Caruso, R., Sorge, R., et al. (2009). Nanocrystalline silver: A systematic review of randomized trials conducted on burned patients and an evidenced-based assessment of potential advantages over older silver formulations. *Annals of Plastic Surgery, 63*, 201–205.

Greenhalgh, D. G. (2019). Management of burns. *New England Journal of Medicine, 380*(24), 2349–2359.

Helvig, E. I. (2002). Managing thermal injuries within WOCN practice. *Journal of Wound, Ostomy, and Continence Nursing, 29*, 76–82.

Herndon, D. N. (2012). *Total burn care* (4th ed., p. 2,6,10,17,40,42,46). Retrieved from https:www.clinicalkey.com/

Hettiaratchy, S., & Dziewulski, P. (2004). Pathophysiology and types of burns. *British Medical Journal, 328*, 1427–1429.

Holland, A. J., Chan, Q. E., Harvey, J. G., et al. (2012). The correlation between time to skin grafting and hypertrophic scarring following an acute contact burn in a porcine model. *Journal of Burn Care & Research, 33*, e43–e48.

Jeschke, M. G. & Herndon, D. N. (2017). Burns. In C. M. Townsend, R. D. Beauchamp, B. M. Evers, et al. (Eds.), *Sabiston Textbook of Surgery* (20th ed.). Philadelphia, PA: Elsevier.

Jones, I. S., Berman, B., Viera, M. H., et al. (2008). Prevention and management of hypertrophic scars and keloids after burns in children. *Journal of Craniofacial Surgery, 19*, 989–1006.

Kantak, N. A., Mistry, R., Varon, D. E., et al. (2017). Negative pressure wound therapy for burns. *Clinics in Plastic Surgery, 44*(3), 671–677.

Karimi, H., Latifi, N. A., Mehrjerdi, A. Z., et al. (2020). Histopathological changes of organs (lungs, liver, kidney, and brain) after using two types of AgiCoat and Acticoat nanosilver dressings on deep second-degree burn in rat. *Journal of Burn Care & Research, 41*(1), 141–150.

Kavalukas, S., & Barbul, A. (2011). Nutrition and wound healing: An update. *Plastic and Reconstructive Surgery, 127*, 38S–43S.

Kawilarang, B. (2020). Marjolin's ulcer: A malignant complication of burn wound. *Recent Advances in Biology and Medicine, 6*(2020), 12034.

Kearns, R., Holmes, J., & Cairns, B. (2013). Burn injury: What's in a name? Labels used for burn injury classification: A review of the data from 200-2012. *Annals of Burns and Fire Disasters, 26*, 115–120.

Kee, E. G., Stockton, K., Kimble, R. M., et al. (2017). Cost-effectiveness of silver dressings for paediatric partial thickness burns: An economic evaluation from a randomized controlled trial. *Burns, 43*(4), 724–732.

Kemper, T. C., de Jong, V. M., Anema, H. A., et al. (2014). Frostbite of both first digits of the foot treated with delayed hyperbaric oxygen: A case report and review of literature. *Undersea & Hyperbaric Medicine, 41*(1), 65–70.

Kelter, B. M., Holavanahalli, R., Suman, O. E., et al. (2020). Recognizing the long-term sequelae of burns as a chronic medical condition. *Burns, 46*(2), 493–496. https://doi: 10.1016/j.burns.2019.10.017

Koljonen, V., Andersson, K., Mikkonen, K., et al. (2004). Frostbite injuries treated in the Helsinki area from 1995 to 2002. *Journal of Trauma and Acute Care Surgery, 57*(6), 1315–1320.

Langschmidt, J., Caine, P. L., Wearn, C. M., et al. (2014). Hydrotherapy in burn care: A survey of hydrotherapy practices in the UK and Ireland and literature review. *Burns, 40*(5), 860–864.

Logsetty, S., Hunter, T. A., Medved, M. I., et al. (2013). "Put on your face to face the world": Women's narratives of burn injury. *Burns, 39*, 1588–1598.

Loo, Y. L., Goh, B. K. L., & Jeffery, S. (2018). An overview of the use of bromelain-based enzymatic debridement (Nexobrid®) in deep partial and full thickness burns: Appraising the evidence. *Journal of Burn Care & Research, 39*(6), 932–938. doi: 10.1093/jbcr/iry009.

Martín, N., Guilabert, P., Abarca, L., et al. (2017). Coagulation abnormalities following NexoBrid® use: A Case Report. *Journal of Burn Care & Research, 39*(6), 1067–1070. doi: 10.1093/jbcr/irx044.

McDermott, K. W., Weiss, A. J., & Elixhauser, A. (2016). *Burn-Related Hospital Inpatient Stays and Emergency Department Visits, 2013.* Rockville, MD: Agency for Healthcare Research and Quality AHRQ.

Mcintosh, S. E., Freer, L., Grissom, C. K., et al. (2019). Wilderness medical society practice guidelines for the prevention and treatment of frostbite: 2019 update. *Wilderness & Environmental Medicine, 30*(4S), S19–S32. doi: 10.1016/j.wem.2019.05.002.

Mohammadi, A., Johari, H., & Eskandari, S. (2013). Effects of amniotic membrane on graft take in extremity burns. *Burns, 39*, 1137–1141.

Mok, J. Y. (2008). Non-accidental injury in children—An update. *Injury, 39*, 978–985.

Molan, P. C., Cooper, R., & Halas, E. (2002). The efficacy of honey in inhibiting strains of *Pseudomonas aeruginosa* from infected burns. *The Journal of Burn Care & Rehabilitation, 23*, 366–370.

Norman, G., Christie, J., Liu, Z., et al. (2017). Antiseptics for burns. *The Cochrane Database of Systematic Reviews, 7*(7), CD011821. doi: 10.1002/14651858.CD011821.pub2.

Ogawa, R., & Orgill, D. (2013). Current methods of burn reconstruction. *Plastic and Reconstructive Surgery, 131*, 827e–836e.

Paul, C. N., Hansen, S. L., Voight, D. W., et al. (2001). Using skin replacement products to treat burns and wounds. *Advances in Skin & Wound Care, 14*, 37–46.

Ranganathan, K., Wong, V. C., Krebsbach, P. H., et al. (2013). Fat grafting for thermal injury: Current state and future directions. *Journal of Burn Care & Research, 34*, 219–226.

Richard, R. L., Gordon, M. D., Gottschlich, M. M., et al. (2004). Review of evidenced-based practice for the prevention of pressure sores in burn patients. *The Journal of Burn Care & Rehabilitation, 25*, 388–410.

Rick, C., Caruso, D. M., Foster, K. N., et al. (2004). Aquacel Ag in the management of partial-thickness burns: Results of a clinical trial. *The Journal of Burn Care & Rehabilitation, 25*, 89–97.

Schlanser, V., Dennis, A., Ivkovic, K., et al. (2017). Placenta to the rescue: Limb salvage using dehydrated human amnion/chorion membrane. *Journal of Burn Care & Research, 39*(6), 1048–1052. doi: 10.1093/jbcr/irx031.

Sheckter, C. C., Meyerkord, N. L., Sinskey, Y. L., et al. (2020). The optimal treatment for partial thickness burns—A cost utility analysis of skin allograft vs. topical silver dressings. *Journal of Burn Care & Research, 41*(3), 450–456. doi: 10.1093/jbcr/iraa003.

Shin, J. Y., & Yi, H. S. (2016). Diagnostic accuracy of laser Doppler imaging in burn depth assessment: Systematic review and meta-analysis. *Burns, 42*(7), 1369–1376.

Simko, L. M., & Culleton, A. (2013). Caring for patients with burn injuries. *Nursing, 43*, 26–34.

Slaviero, L., Avruscio, G., Vindigni, V., et al. (2018). Antiseptics for burns: A review of the evidence. *Annals of Burns and Fire Disasters, 31*(3), 198.

Somerset, A., Coffey, R., Jones, L., et al. (2014). The impact of prediabetes on glycemic control and clinical outcomes postburn injury. *Journal of Burn Care & Research, 35*, 5–10.

Stiles, K. (2018). Emergency management of burns: Part 1. *Emergency Nurse, 26*(1), 37–42. doi: 10.7748/en.2018.e1623.

Verbelen, J., Hoeksema, H., Heyneman, A., et al. (2014). Aquacel® Ag dressing versus Acticoat™ dressing in partial thickness burns: A prospective, randomized, controlled study in 100 patients. Part 1: burn wound healing. *Burns, 40*(3), 416–427.

Vuola, J. (2004). Frostbite injuries treated in the Helsinki area from 1995 to 2002. *Journal of Trauma and Acute Care Surgery, 57*, 1315–1320.

Woo, E., Lee, J., Hur, G., et al. (2013). Proposed treatment protocol for frostbite: A retrospective analysis of 17 cases based on a 3-year single institution experience. *Archives of Plastic Surgery, 40*, 510–516.

QUESTIONS

1. The wound care nurse is caring for a patient who was exposed to a product containing 10% hydrofluoric acid and has burns on 3% of his body. For what life-threatening condition would the wound care nurse monitor this patient?

A. Hypocalcemia
B. Hyperkalemia
C. Hypophosphatemia
D. Hyponatremia

2. A patient is admitted to an acute care facility with electrical burns on 40% of his body caused by alternating current. This patient would be at risk for which of the following serious complications?

A. Cellular necrosis
B. Atelectasis
C. Compartment syndrome
D. Hypometabolism

3. A patient admitted to a burn unit with thermal injuries is in the emergent phase of the injury. What would be the primary focus of care during this phase of recovery?

A. Debridement
B. Hemodynamic stabilization
C. Skin grafting
D. Maximizing functional capacity

4. The burn team initially focuses on the zone of stasis when planning wound care. What is the rationale for this strategy?
   A. Tissue damage in this area is potentially reversible.
   B. Prevention of denaturing of proteins may prevent tissue damage.
   C. Full-thickness burns in this area must be treated first.
   D. The outermost area of burn injury requires the most aggressive therapy.

5. An adult sustained major burns in a home fire. What are the criteria for this classification of burns?
   A. Burns involve <10% TBSA.
   B. Burns involve <15% TBSA.
   C. Burns involve <15% to 25% TBSA with <10% full-thickness burns.
   D. Burns involve >25% TBSA.

6. A wound care nurse caring for a patient with burns documents the following: Burns are erythematous, painful, and blanchable to touch, with edema, blister formation, and weeping present. What stage of burns is the wound care nurse describing?
   A. Superficial burns
   B. Superficial partial-thickness burns
   C. Deep partial-thickness burns
   D. Full-thickness burns

7. Which burn injury can safely be treated in an outpatient setting based on the ABA referral guidelines?

   A. Burns that involve the hands
   B. Full-thickness burns
   C. Partial-thickness burns <10%
   D. Patients with partial-thickness burns and concomitant trauma

8. What drug of choice would the wound care nurse recommend to treat pain during the acute phase of burn treatment?
   A. Intravenous morphine
   B. Aspirin
   C. Nonsteroidal anti-inflammatory agents
   D. Oral pain medications

9. Which type of graft, used for reconstructive purposes, would the wound care nurse recommend for a small, full-thickness burn?
   A. Meshed autologous skin graft
   B. Full-thickness skin graft
   C. Cultured epithelial autograft
   D. Split-thickness skin graft

10. The wound care nurse suggests a meshed autologous skin graft for a large burn on a patient's knee area. Which action is performed correctly in this procedure?
   A. Preoperatively, the wound is dressed with a nonadherent layer to prevent shearing.
   B. Postoperatively, a bolster dressing is applied to the meshed graft composed of gauze soaked in 10% saline solution.
   C. Since the grafted area is a joint, a splint is applied to maintain a functional position.
   D. The initial dressing is usually left undisturbed for 10 to 14 days, at which time dressings are removed to examine the graft.

ANSWERS AND RATIONALES

1. A. Rationale: HF is the strongest known inorganic acid. It rapidly penetrates deeply into the tissue and acts as a metabolic poison that binds calcium and magnesium, which can produce cardiac dysrhythmias.

2. C. Rationale: Edema occurs at the fascial level causing compartment syndrome.

3. B. Rationale: Without hemodynamic stability, achieved through appropriate fluid resuscitation, the patient develops multisystem organ failure and dies.

4. A. Rationale: Tissue in the zone of stasis can be salvaged with appropriate management. Goal is to save as much tissue as possible.

5. D. Rationale: The ABA defines major burns as burns >25% TBSA.

6. B. Rationale: ABA definition of superficial partial-thickness burn injury.

7. C. Rationale: Partial-thickness burns less measuring <10% TBSA can be treated in an outpatient wound center safely.

8. A. Rationale: IV morphine is the optimal pain medication in the acute phase. Aspirin and nonsteroidal anti-inflammatory agents are known to produce stomach ulcers in burn patients.

9. B. Rationale: Full-thickness skin grafts have more flexibility and provide better functional reconstruction.

10. C. Rationale: Failure to splint would result in contracture and loss of function. The current goal of burn management is to maximize quality of life, which in this case would be to maintain function of the knee joint for ambulation.

CHAPTER 33

TRAUMATIC WOUNDS: ASSESSMENT AND MANAGEMENT

David R. Crumbley and Lizabeth E. Andrew

OBJECTIVES

1. Describe the mechanisms of injury associated with common traumatic injuries.

2. Outline key considerations in management of traumatic wounds.

3. Describe the role of NPWT in management of traumatic wounds.

4. Explain the significance of compartment syndrome and management options.

TOPIC OUTLINE

● INTRODUCTION

Traumatic injuries occur when an external or foreign object strikes the body. These injuries are commonly caused by motor vehicle accidents (MVAs), gunshots, natural disasters, explosive blasts, falls, and industrial accidents (Nelson et al., 2016). Traumatic wounds may involve damage to bone and internal organs, are not created surgically, and always are viewed as contaminated and at risk for infection. This chapter presents an overview of the major causes of traumatic wounds, the

management of these wounds, and complications that may arise.

● CAUSES OF TRAUMATIC WOUNDS

MOTOR VEHICLE ACCIDENTS

Crashes and pedestrian accidents involving automobiles, trucks, and motorcycles cause multiple blunt force and deceleration injuries that may result in open and closed fractures, and injuries to the head, internal organs and blood vessels, spinal cord, and soft tissues. Blunt force trauma occurs when the body is propelled against objects within or outside the vehicle. Penetrating injuries cause skin or muscle damage and may involve bones, vessels, and internal organs.

Those who suffer blunt force injuries from an MVA may also have open wounds related to surgical intervention. In the event of a crush injury or fracture, the patient may undergo a fasciotomy to prevent or mitigate compartment syndrome of an extremity. Abdominal surgery may be required to control hemorrhage, repair damaged organs, prevent or treat abdominal compartment syndrome, and allow tissue swelling to resolve. Compartment syndrome and fasciotomy management are discussed later in this chapter.

BULLET/GUNSHOT WOUNDS

When a bullet (also known as a missile or projectile) strikes tissue, the tissue is lacerated and crushed along the trajectory of the projectile (Cubano et al., 2018). As the projectile interacts with the tissue, it produces both a smaller permanent cavity and a larger temporary cavity. The permanent cavity involves an area of tissue necrosis proportionate to the size of the projectile. It can extend the length of the projectile's travel through the tissue. The temporary cavity is created by the lateral transfer of tissue as the projectile passes through it (Cubano et al., 2018) (**Fig. 33-1**). Elastic tissue such as muscle, blood vessels, skin, and fat are pushed aside but usually rebound after the passage of the projectile. Contusions and hemorrhaging of the muscle tissue may occur. In contrast, nonelastic tissues like bone and liver may fracture (Cubano et al., 2018; Lichte et al., 2010). Bone involvement can result in severe injury as the pieces of fractured bone create secondary missiles that cause additional trauma to surrounding tissues.

KEY POINT

Bullets and similar projectiles create both a smaller permanent cavity and a larger temporary cavity; the tissues involved in the temporary cavity may rebound and recover (soft tissue) or may fracture (bone and liver).

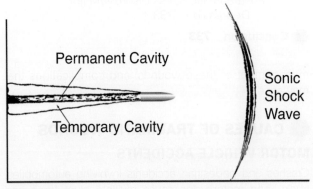

FIGURE 33-1. Projectile–Tissue Interaction, Showing Components of Tissue Injury. (Courtesy of Borden Institute Fort Sam Houston, TX.)

Injuries caused by firearms are often classified by the velocity of the projectile. The rule of thumb for care providers is to treat the wound, not the weapon (Cubano et al., 2018). Handguns cause low-velocity wounds; hunting rifles or military weapons cause high-velocity wounds (Lichte et al., 2010). Velocity alone cannot predict tissue trauma. The potential for tissue trauma depends on the tissue involved, low-energy transfer versus high-energy transfer, and the nature of the projectile. In gunshot wounds, especially high-energy transfer wounds, tissue damage can be extensive, and the extent of damage may not be fully determined until 4 days after the initial injury (Edlich et al., 2010). The difficulty in determining the full extent of tissue damage is due to the fact that energy is transferred from the high-energy projectile to tissue adjacent to the area of initial impact. This tissue may appear to be healthy on initial examination but may become necrotic over subsequent hours and days. This delayed necrosis can be caused by vascular damage or by massive edema that compromises blood flow and tissue oxygenation. It can also be a result of bacterial contamination. This phenomenon is often termed wound evolution by military physicians. The wound evolves over the first few days following injury.

Conversely, tissue that initially appears ischemic may improve over the first few days following injury, a phenomenon known in trauma and burn care as tissue resuscitation. Tissue resuscitation involves recovery of tissue adjacent to the primary site. This tissue sustains trauma but may recover without progression to necrosis, depending on the care provided following the injury. Prompt and effective management of soft tissue edema can prevent the vascular compression that would cause tissue necrosis.

In summary, there is both direct injury that is irreversible, and indirect injury of the adjacent tissue and vasculature related to tissue transfer and to soft tissue swelling. This indirect injury may cause progressive tissue necrosis or may be reversed by prompt management of edema.

KEY POINT

In high-energy gunshot wounds, tissue damage can be extensive, and the extent of the damage may not be evident for several days postinjury.

BLAST INJURIES

Blast injuries can be caused by military explosive munitions, improvised explosive devices (IEDs), or industrial accidents. Blast injuries can be categorized into four types: (1) primary, (2) secondary, (3) tertiary, and (4) quaternary injuries (Cubano et al., 2018). Proximity to the blast epicenter is a major determinant of the type of injury and the severity of injury (**Fig. 33-2**). Victims may experience

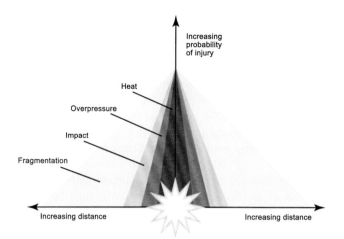

FIGURE 33-2. The Probability of Sustaining a Given Trauma is Related to the Distance from the Epicenter of the Detonation. (Courtesy of Borden Institute Fort Sam Houston, TX.)

all four types of injury depending upon the device and the proximity of the victim to the explosion. Musculoskeletal extremity injuries are the most frequently occurring blast injuries (Cubano et al., 2018; Hayda et al., 2004).

Primary blast injuries are caused by the sonic shockwave of the blast striking the body. These injuries take place relatively close to the source of explosion. This shockwave or overpressure force causes damage to hollow organs such as the lung, the gastrointestinal tract, and the ear. Secondary blast injuries occur when device fragments or debris are propelled through the air by the blast causing penetrating trauma, fragmentation injuries, and blunt trauma. Fragments from a terrorist's IED may contain objects such as marbles, nails, and glass. **Figure 33-3** shows the mechanism of injury from a landmine and the propulsion of debris into the deep tissue. In blasts that occur in or near a building, penetrating wounds may be caused by fragments from the glass blown out of windows, or other debris from the building structure (Hayda et al., 2004). Tertiary blast injuries occur when the victim is thrown by the blast and strikes surrounding objects. Victims may suffer blunt and penetrating injuries, fractures, and traumatic amputations. Quaternary blast injuries are all other injuries including thermal injuries, injuries from toxic exposure, and any postincident events or exacerbations of chronic conditions (Centers for Disease Control and Prevention, 2012; Cubano et al., 2018; Ramasamy et al., 2009).

WOUNDS CAUSED BY NATURAL DISASTERS

Earthquakes, tornadoes, and hurricanes are natural disasters that collapse buildings and create falling debris. The debris and falling structures can cause serious injuries with extensive orthopedic trauma (fractured extremities) as well as internal damage. The most common injuries associated with earthquakes include open and closed fractures, crush injuries, and wound infections (Hotz et al., 2011; Sonshine et al., 2012). Tornadoes and hurricanes can generate flying debris that causes penetrating wounds, especially near the storms' strong epicenters. Wounds caused by natural disasters may be contaminated with debris, soil, or contaminated water, and crush injuries and fractures may result in compartment syndrome. When large-scale natural disasters occur, especially in underdeveloped nations, the potential for wound complications is even greater, because the time from injury to treatment may extend from hours to days.

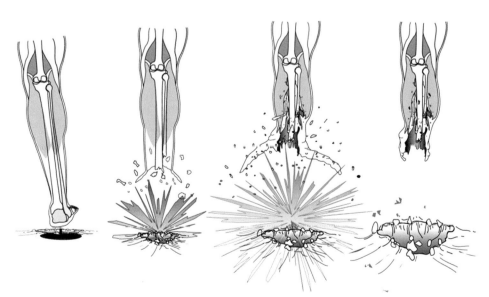

FIGURE 33-3. Mechanisms of Injuries Caused by Antipersonnel Landmines. (Courtesy of Borden Institute Fort Sam Houston, TX.)

MANAGEMENT OF TRAUMATIC WOUNDS

MANAGEMENT OF BACTERIAL CONTAMINATION

Bacterial contamination is a serious concern in the management of traumatic wounds. All traumatic wounds, regardless of mechanism of injury, should be considered contaminated due to the nonsterile nature of their occurrence and the environment where the injury occurs.

Bacterial contamination can occur in any environment where damaged soft tissue comes in contact with soil or debris. Wounds may be contaminated by bacteria from soil, especially when a blast projects soil deeply into soft tissue. Gunshot wounds and blast wounds may be contaminated with clothing, fragments from projectiles, or soil, and fecal contamination can occur when the bowel is perforated.

A number of U.S. Service Members in Afghanistan who sustained significant blast injuries caused by IEDs were subsequently diagnosed with cutaneous mucormycosis, an aggressive fungal infection caused by soil contaminants projected deeply into the soft tissue by IEDs buried in the soil (Lewandowski et al., 2013). Mucormycosis is a serious but rare fungal infection caused by a group of molds called mucormycetes. It may cause a life-threatening angioinvasive fungal infection that is difficult to eradicate. Following the Joplin, Missouri tornado in 2011, 13 victims developed mucormycosis; 5 of the 13 died. Since all victims were located in the area that sustained storm damage, their infections were associated with penetrating soft tissue trauma and multiple wounds caused by deadly tornadic winds (Fanfair et al., 2012).

A wound caused by glass or sharp metal exhibits less tissue damage and is more resistant to infection than a wound caused by blunt trauma (Edlich et al., 2010; Thacker et al., 1977). Sharp objects create less tissue damage, and less energy is necessary to create the wound. In contrast, blunt trauma wounds exhibit more damage to the wound edges because more force is needed to cause the tissue failure. The blunt trauma wound is created through compression and tension of the tissue rather than through shearing, which is the mechanism of injury with a sharp object. Because the object is blunt and not sharp, more tissue comes in contact with the wounding object and more damage is caused to the surrounding tissue (Edlich et al., 2010).

INITIAL ACUTE MANAGEMENT AND HEMORRHAGE CONTROL

The initial acute management of traumatic injuries focuses on life-threatening conditions that involve the patient's airway, breathing, and circulation; care is dictated by advanced trauma life support (ATLS) guidelines, with the goals of ensuring correct management and preventing complications (Committee on Trauma, 2018). Controlling hemorrhage is critical because it is a leading cause of death from trauma, second only to central nervous system injury (Oyeniyi et al., 2017). Hemorrhage from extremities is the leading preventable cause of mortality in combat casualties (Beekley et al., 2008; Bellamy et al., 1986; Day, 2016), and internal bleeding caused by blunt and penetrating injury is a life-threatening complication for any trauma patient. Surgical intervention is necessary if the patient with active internal bleeding is hemodynamically unstable. Since surgery can increase the risk of mortality, surgical intervention may be postponed if the patient with internal bleeding is hemodynamically stable (Lichte et al., 2010).

Direct pressure is the best initial intervention if the source of bleeding is external. A hemostatic dressing may be used with direct pressure to provide additional hemostasis. For severe extremity wounds where direct pressure is not effective and bleeding cannot be controlled, a tourniquet should be applied to prevent possible death from exsanguination. Attention must be paid to the placement and timing of the tourniquet because applying a tourniquet puts the patient at risk for hypoperfusion, ischemia, and necrosis of the tissue underneath and distal to the tourniquet placement. The patient will be at risk for compartment syndrome if the tourniquet is in place for more than 90 minutes (Beekley et al., 2008; Kam et al., 2001).

Tourniquet use has historically been controversial due to the potential for complications such as those listed above. Findings related to prehospital tourniquet use by military health care providers in recent conflicts indicate that the appropriate use of tourniquets in patients with severe extremity injury and hemorrhage is a potentially lifesaving intervention with limited adverse outcomes (Beekley et al., 2008). Safe and effective prehospital tourniquet protocols include the following: (1) use only a commercial tourniquet with a wide band that is specifically designed to function as a tourniquet, (2) gradually tighten the tourniquet just to the point of hemorrhage control, (3) limit application to extremity injuries with severe bleeding and apply the tourniquet proximal to the site of injury, (4) leave the tourniquet in place if transport time to a higher level of care is <30 minutes, (5) reassess tourniquet use after 30 minutes for possible removal and placement of a pressure dressing to prevent pain and tissue ischemia (when transport time >30 minutes), (6) leave the tourniquet in place if the patient is unstable and in circulatory shock, (7) if tourniquet removal is advised, loosen carefully, apply pressure dressing, and leave the tourniquet in place in case of recurrent hemorrhage, (8) do not remove the tourniquet from an amputated or near amputated extremity, and (9) in mass casualty settings when tourniquet use is required, mark "TK" and application time clearly on patient's forehead or other prominent location (Doyle & Taillac, 2008).

OBTAINING WOUND HISTORY

Recording a thorough wound history is essential once life-threatening conditions have been mitigated and the patient is stable. A wound history should include the mechanism of injury as well as the time of injury. This information provides insight into the extent of injury and the potential for infection. The time from injury to initial treatment can impact the susceptibility of the wound to infection. Even a 3-hour delay initiating antibiotics can have a negative impact on the effectiveness of both topical and systemic antibiotics (Edlich et al., 1971). This is partly because the vascular permeability and inflammatory changes that occur in response to injury can reduce the effectiveness of either systemic or topical antibiotic therapy by creating a coagulum that surrounds the bacteria and prevents penetration by the antibiotic (Edlich et al., 1971).

> ### KEY POINT
>
> The time from initial injury to initiation of antibiotic therapy has a major impact on outcomes; a delay of 3 hours can significantly reduce the effectiveness of topical and systemic antibiotics.

A review of the patient's wound history and their immunization status informs the need for tetanus prophylaxis. In traumatic wounds, the anaerobic bacterium *Clostridium tetani* (*C. tetani*) enters the body through the broken skin. *C. tetani* infection can occur through puncture wounds or penetrating injuries, bites, burns, frostbite, or crush injuries or through necrotic tissue contaminated with soil, feces, or saliva (Afshar et al., 2011; Finkelstein et al., 2017; Wood, 2004). Tetanus is a rare disease in the United States and Western Europe because of rigorous immunization programs. Individuals who have had a tetanus booster within the 5 years preceding injury may not require prophylaxis. Tetanus immunization is recommended if immunization status cannot be determined or if the wound is heavily contaminated. Tetanus prophylaxis is recommended for (1) wound management if the patient's most recent tetanus vaccination is >5 years or if the patient's immunization status cannot be determined; (2) wounds contaminated with soil, feces, or saliva; (3) puncture wounds or avulsions; and (4) wounds caused by missiles, crush injuries, burns, and frostbite (Havers et al., 2020; Kretsinger et al., 2006). When working with populations outside the United States or Western Europe, tetanus prophylaxis is extremely important. Limited active immunization programs in underdeveloped countries are one cause for the high incidence of tetanus worldwide (Finkelstein et al., 2017).

WOUND DEBRIDEMENT AND IRRIGATION

After initial trauma management and mitigation of life-threatening injuries and the completion of a thorough wound history, the wound should be debrided and irrigated. Debridement is paramount in establishing a healthy wound healing environment (Haury et al., 1978). Surgical debridement is necessary to remove nonviable tissue (skin, fat, fascia, bone, muscle, or tendon), which can harbor bacteria or may be heavily contaminated with soil or foreign bodies (**Fig. 33-4**). This nonviable tissue serves as a medium for anaerobic organisms, compromising the body's ability to fight infection, and potentially contaminating healthy tissue (Joint Theatre Trauma System Clinical Practice Guideline, 2012).

For larger and/or heavily contaminated wounds, debridement and irrigation are performed in the operating room under anesthesia to prevent additional pain for the patient and to permit wound exploration. Understanding the mechanism of injury and environment of the injury will help the surgeon to determine the degree of debridement and irrigation necessary. The extent of debridement required is determined by the surgeon's assessment of the wound and surrounding tissue. Copious irrigation of the wound removes the foreign material and increases the accuracy of the assessment.

There are a variety of acceptable approaches to irrigation, including bulb irrigation, pulsatile lavage, gravity irrigation, and high-pressure syringe irrigation using a 35-mL syringe and 19-gauge catheter (Gross et al., 1972; Joint Theatre Trauma System Clinical Practice Guideline, 2012; Nelson et al., 2016; Stevenson et al., 1976). Sterile normal saline, sterile water, sterile antibiotic solution, or potable water may be used for wound irrigation (Fernandez et al., 2004; Hall, 2007; Storer et al., 2012). Potable water may be used for irrigation outside of the operating room but would never be used within the operating room. A sterile isotonic solution is the preferred solution for irrigating large traumatic wounds (Joint Theatre Trauma System Clinical Practice Guideline, 2012).

Military medicine uses the term wound evolution to describe the changes in tissue viability that occur in traumatic large soft tissue injuries over the first 4 to 7 days following injury (Edlich et al., 2010; Joint Theatre Trauma System Clinical Practice Guideline, 2012). This change in tissue viability calls for a more frequent schedule of debridement and irrigation in the acute phase (<72 hours) and a less frequent debridement and irrigation schedule during the subacute phase (3 to 7 days) (Joint Theatre Trauma System Clinical Practice Guideline, 2012). This frequent debridement and irrigation schedule of every 24 to 48 hours allows for a more accurate assessment of tissue evolution. High-energy traumatic wounds have a greater amount of soft tissue damage and require more extensive debridement (Lichte et al., 2010).

COMPARTMENT SYNDROME

Compartment syndrome can occur in patients who have suffered extremity fractures, crush injuries, contusions from blunt trauma, arterial or venous injuries, or burns, and in patients whose wounds were acutely managed with

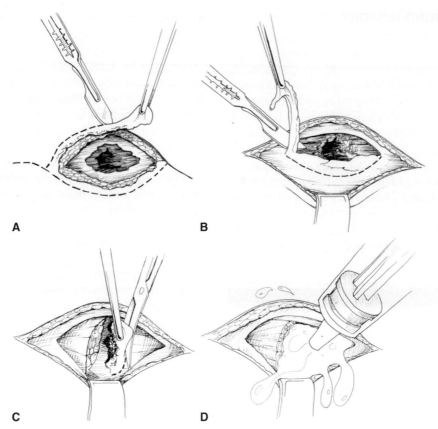

A   **B**

C   **D**

FIGURE 33-4. (A) Skin excision, **(B)** removal of fascia, **(C)** removal of avascular tissue, and **(D)** irrigation. (Courtesy of Borden Institute Fort Sam Houston, TX.)

tourniquets or pneumatic antishock garments. Acute limb compartment syndrome is an emergent limb-threatening syndrome caused by increased pressure in a closed fascial space that results in high intracompartmental pressures that reduce capillary perfusion and compromise tissue viability (Gourgiotis et al., 2007). In the conscious and unsedated patient, the hallmark sign of compartment syndrome is pain disproportionate to injury. Other clinical signs include paresthesia, pallor, and pulselessness. Early detection and treatment are critical to prevent muscle necrosis, amputation, or death. The patient may require a fasciotomy, which is a surgical incision into the affected muscular fascia. The incision opens the fascial compartment, which reduces intracompartmental pressures and restores perfusion to the muscle tissue (Gourgiotis et al., 2007; Joint Trauma System Clinical Practice Guideline, 2016a, 2016b). Fasciotomy incisions are not closed primarily. They are usually closed 3 to 7 days later, once the swelling has resolved (Gourgiotis et al., 2007; Pollak, 2008).

KEY POINT

Compartment syndrome is a common complication of traumatic injury and requires emergent intervention (such as fasciotomy) to prevent tissue necrosis caused by severe edema and vessel compression.

The critically injured trauma patient who suffers blunt or penetrating intra-abdominal injuries and requires massive resuscitation efforts is at risk for developing abdominal compartment syndrome, a life-threatening condition with a high mortality rate (Harrell & Melander, 2012). Treatment involves surgical decompressive laparotomy, which is the abdominal equivalent of fasciotomy (Anand & Ivatury, 2011). The fascia of the abdomen is not reapproximated immediately; a temporary abdominal closure (TAC) is performed instead. This TAC may consist of (1) a skin-only closure (fascia is not closed), (2) use of a commercially available abdominal closure system, or (3) a system fashioned from sterile irrigation bags placed over the bowel with the use of negative pressure. Military medicine uses the term temporizing to describe this process of temporarily closing the abdominal compartment until bowel edema resolves and the fascia can be reapproximated (Anand & Ivatury, 2011; De Laet et al., 2020; Navsaria et al., 2013; Vertrees et al., 2017).

THE OPEN TRAUMATIC WOUND

A myriad of topical therapies are available for the management of traumatic wounds, and the selection of specific therapies and dressings should be grounded in wound healing principles (Pollak, 2008). This chapter focuses on the therapies used most frequently to manage the complex traumatic wound. Please refer to Chapters 8 and 9 for more in-depth discussions of the principles for topical therapy and dressing selection.

Primary closure of traumatic soft tissue injuries is not recommended due to contamination, risk of infection, and concern regarding tissue viability. Traumatic soft tissue injuries are typically left open to heal by delayed primary closure or secondary intention (Edlich et al., 2010; Joint Theatre Trauma System Clinical Practice Guideline, 2012; Lichte et al., 2010; Nelson et al., 2016). Wounds complicated by compartment syndrome are also left open to allow edema to resolve following fasciotomy or decompressive laparotomy (Cubano, et al., 2018).

KEY POINT

Wounds complicated by infection or compartment syndrome should be left open until infection and edema are controlled.

Primary closure is reserved for wounds without contamination, wounds with limited tissue loss, and wounds to the face. Complex traumatic wounds with extensive tissue loss are frequently managed with delayed primary closure, a skin graft, or tissue flap (Edlich et al., 2010; Joint Theatre Trauma System Clinical Practice Guideline, 2012; Lichte et al., 2010; Nelson et al., 2016). Wounds left to heal by secondary intention are generally smaller, well approximated, and located in an area where cosmesis is less important (e.g., the trunk). Wounds healing by secondary intention take longer to heal as they must first fill with granulation tissue and then must undergo epithelial migration from the wound edges. Secondary intention wound healing also produces more scar tissue than does primary closure.

In delayed primary closure, wound closure is delayed allowing time for elimination of infection and management of edema (Edlich et al., 2010). The exact time for closure varies but may be as soon as 3 to 5 days after initial surgery (Edlich et al., 2010; Joint Theatre Trauma System Clinical Practice Guideline, 2012). Wounds with extensive soft tissue loss will require a skin graft or tissue flap to cover the defect (Nelson et al., 2016). If open traumatic wounds are complicated by concomitant fractures, the fractures must be stabilized with either internal or external fixation prior to or at the time of wound closure (**Fig. 33-5**).

To ensure the wound bed is free of contaminants and nonviable tissue, serial debridements and wound irrigations are continued until the wound bed is clean and the wound can be closed surgically. If the wound cannot be closed primarily, temporary coverage must be implemented to (1) protect and prepare the wound bed, (2) prevent contamination and desiccation of the wound, and (3) manage exudate. The technique of temporarily covering the wound awaiting delayed primary closure,

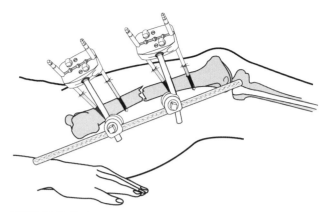

FIGURE 33-5. Frame Applied and Fracture Grossly Reduced. Lateral placement of stabilizing rod is preferred. (Courtesy of Borden Institute, Fort Sam Houston, TX.)

skin graft, or tissue flap is often referred to as temporizing the wound.

TEMPORIZATION OF THE OPEN SOFT TISSUE INJURY/NEGATIVE PRESSURE WOUND THERAPY

Following thorough debridement of the traumatic wound, the surgeon may choose to cover the wound with fluffed moistened sterile gauze (antimicrobial or plain gauze) or may use a negative pressure wound therapy (NPWT) system with reticulated open cell foam dressings (NPWT/ROCF). A moistened sterile gauze dressing may be used in wounds where there is questionable tissue viability or extreme contamination necessitating frequent returns to the operating room every 24 hours for debridement and irrigation. Cavitary wounds should never be packed in a manner that would obstruct fluid egress from the wound. Rather, they should be lightly filled, so that the gauze serves to wick the fluid out of the wound (Cubano et al., 2018). This approach is especially important when managing traumatic wounds with small openings.

NPWT/ROCF is the preferred coverage for the patient who will undergo less frequent debridement and irrigation, for example, every 48 to 72 hours (Cubano et al., 2018; Joint Theatre Trauma System Clinical Practice Guideline, 2012). Over the past 20 years, NPWT/ROCF has become the treatment of choice for military surgeons and trauma surgeons managing complex soft tissue wounds, penetrating trauma, open fractures, and fasciotomy incisions (Blum et al., 2012; Jeffery 2016; Krug et al., 2011; Pollak, 2008). This approach is based on case studies, anecdotal evidence, and the demonstrated mechanisms of action and clinical benefits of NPWT: (1) reduction of wound fluid and edema, which enhances blood flow to the wound, (2) promotion of granulation tissue formation, (3) removal of inflammatory cytokines, (4) reduction of cross-contamination in the hospital, (5) reduction in time to definitive closure, and (6) reduction in frequency of painful dressing changes (Crumbley & Perciballi, 2007; Ma et al., 2016; Morykwas et al., 1997; Pollak, 2008; Venturi et al., 2005). These qualities make NPWT an important adjunct in the management of complex soft tissue injuries with significant tissue loss resulting in wounds that are contaminated, edematous, painful, and heavily exudative, and that often have irregularly shaped edges. NPWT bridges the wound until definitive closure is performed, simplifies the process of soft tissue coverage, and may reduce the need for major soft tissue reconstructive procedures (Bernabe et al., 2014; Dedmond et al., 2007; Stannard et al., 2010). Chapters 12 and 34 provide additional details regarding indications, contraindications, and guidelines for use of NPWT.

KEY POINT

NPWT has become the treatment of choice for military surgeons and trauma surgeons managing complex soft tissue wounds, penetrating trauma, open fractures, and fasciotomy incisions.

NPWT dressings are changed every 48 to 72 hours in the complex soft tissue wound until the wound is clean and stable and ready for closure. Dressing changes usually are scheduled to coincide with routine debridements and irrigations in the operating room. This approach provides for effective pain control during dressing changes (Tarkin, 2008). Settings for NPWT range from 75 to 125 mm Hg of negative pressure. Continuous suction may be better tolerated than intermittent in the complex open wound as the switching off and on of negative pressure may be painful and may cause loss of an effective seal in wounds with a large surface area or high-volume exudate. In complex traumatic wounds with exposed bone, tendons, nerves, or vessels, it is important to prevent injury and desiccation of these structures. This can be done by applying a nonadherent layer over the structure that provides protection from the ROCF dressing (Baharestani et al., 2009; Nelson et al., 2016). A nonadherent layer should be used whenever there is concern for tissue adherence to the ROCF dressing during removal.

When using NPWT in wounds with high bacterial loads, consideration should be given to the use of a silver-impregnated ROCF dressing or a silver wound contact layer to assist in reducing bacterial burden (Nelson et al., 2016; Stinner, et al., 2011; Tarkin, 2008). Some silver dressings may cause staining of the wound producing a dark appearance similar to that of necrotic tissue (Schlatterer, & Hirshorn, 2008). This discoloration due to silver is known as argyria (Trop et al., 2006). It is important to communicate the use of silver dressings to the surgical team to prevent misidentification of healthy tissue as necrotic tissue.

An alternative method for reducing bioburden in the heavily contaminated wound is the application of NPWT with instillation and dwell time (NPWTi-d) (Anghel et al., 2016; Giovinco et al., 2010; Lewandowski et al., 2013). NPWTi-d is NPWT with the periodic instillation and dwelling of a topical solution onto the wound bed with postulated benefits being cleansing the wound of bioburden and facilitating removal of devitalized tissue (Gupta et al., 2016; Kim et al., 2018). Instillation solutions used with NPWTi-d include wound cleansers, antiseptics, and normal saline. There is no consensus on the antimicrobial benefit of one NPWTi-d solution over another. A recent study indicates that normal saline may be as effective as an antiseptic solution (Kim et al., 2015). U.S. military surgeons use dilute Dakin® solution (0.025% sodium hypochlorite) with NPWTi-d successfully in the management of an invasive fungal infections in the combat wounded (Joint Trauma System Clinical Practice Guideline, 2016a, 2016b; Lewandowski et al., 2013; Lewandowski et al., 2016). The use of wound instillation is not advised until staff has been trained and policies are in place to prevent the inadvertent delivery of wound solutions via alternative routes (IV, IM, or PO).

ANTIBIOTIC BEADS

Antibiotic-impregnated polymethyl methacrylate (PMMA) beads are commonly placed in high-risk traumatic wounds with concomitant orthopedic injury. The beads are placed into the wound bed near the site of the orthopedic injury to prevent or mitigate osteomyelitis or other infectious processes (Large et al., 2012). NPWT with ROCF is also frequently used in these wounds, and there have been concerns that the concomitant use of NPWT might reduce the effectiveness of the beads. Large and colleagues (2012) conducted a study and found that antibiotic concentration in the wound was reduced by NPWT if there was no fascia or tissue between the NPWT dressing and the antibiotic beads. It is recommended that a nonadherent dressing or tissue coverage be placed between the beads and the NPWT foam to prevent a reduction in antibiotic concentration (Joint Theatre Trauma System Clinical Practice Guideline, 2012).

SPLIT-THICKNESS SKIN GRAFTS

Large soft tissue wounds healing by second intention may require a split-thickness skin graft for final closure of the wound. Skin grafting is delayed until the wound bed is healthy and free of nonviable tissue and infection and has granulated to near skin level. NPWT has replaced traditional bolster dressings as the preferred method for maintaining close adherence between the split-thickness graft and the underlying wound bed for complex wounds (Baharestani et al., 2009; Moisidis et al., 2004; Scherer et al., 2002; Yin et al., 2018). NPWT/ROCF is beneficial because it (1) provides downward pressure

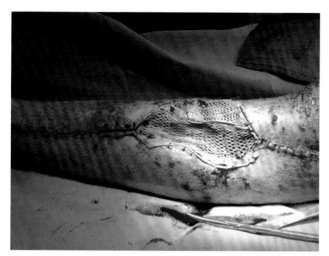

FIGURE 33-6. Split-Thickness Skin Graft Placed on Open Wound and Secured with Staples.

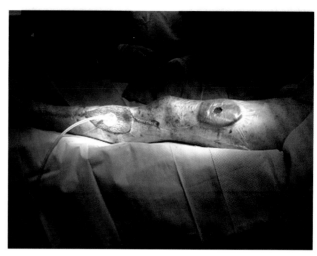

FIGURE 33-8. NPWT/ROCF Dressing Applied over Skin Graft.

onto the graft promoting apposition to the wound bed, (2) prevents wound fluid from accumulating under the graft, (3) promotes a moist environment, and (4) seals the wound from outside contamination (Tarkin, 2008). Use of NPWT also protects the graft from shearing forces and works well in irregular areas. Once the skin graft has been harvested, it is passed through a meshing device. The graft is then placed onto the wound bed and secured in place, typically with circumferential staples (**Fig. 33-6**). A nonadherent dressing is placed over the split-thickness skin graft as an interface between the NPWT/ROCF dressing and the skin graft (**Fig. 33-7**). This is done to prevent adherence of the foam to the graft and subsequent lifting of the graft during dressing removal (**Fig. 33-8**). Removal of the dressing most frequently occurs about 3 to 5 days postoperatively or when there is adequate graft take (Baharestani et al., 2009; Tarkin, 2008). Leaving the NPWT/ROCF dressing in place longer

than 5 days is not recommended, since this may result in formation of hypergranulation tissue between the interstices of the meshed graft.

KEY POINT

Split-thickness skin grafts may be needed for coverage of large soft tissue defects, and NPWT is commonly used to maintain close adherence between the graft and the wound bed. A contact layer should be placed between the graft and the foam to prevent adherence of the graft to the foam.

FASCIOTOMY WOUNDS

Following a fasciotomy to an extremity, the incision or wound is left open to allow for the muscle edema to resolve (**Fig. 33-9**). If the wound edges are well approximated, the fasciotomy wound can be closed through delayed primary closure within 3 to 7 days postoperatively (Gourgiotis et al., 2007; Pollak, 2008). If the wound edges are not well approximated and delayed primary closure is not possible, the wound is closed by placing a skin graft over the defect. In all circumstances, the fasciotomy wound is initially left open and requires temporary

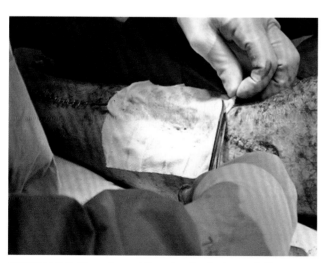

FIGURE 33-7. Nonadherent Dressing Applied over Split-Thickness Skin Graft.

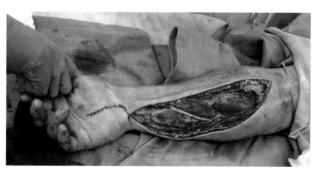

FIGURE 33-9. Fasciotomy Performed Due to Compartment Syndrome of Forearm.

coverage or bridging until the wound can be closed, through either delayed primary closure or a split-thickness skin graft. Temporary management of the open fasciotomy wound is frequently provided by NPWT/ROCF. NPWT/ROCF provides temporary coverage, a moist healing environment, less frequent dressing changes, and removal of excess fluid while the edema resolves (Blonska-Staniec et al., 2016; Morykwas et al., 2002; Tarkin, 2008; Yang et al., 2006). The surgeon may use a crossed rubber band technique with the NPWT system to keep the wound edges more closely approximated (**Fig. 33-10**). This process may improve the potential for delayed primary closure and reduce the need for skin grafting (Tarkin, 2008). This technique involves use of crossed rubber bands stapled to the wound edges to hold the wound edges in closer approximation. In this case, a nonadherent NPWT foam dressing is placed over the fasciotomy wound prior to application of the crossed rubber bands. If the nonadherent type NPWT foam dressing is not available, a nonadherent contact layer may be used as an interface between the fascia and the standard NPWT foam dressing. When the wound is ready for closure, the rubber bands and the NPWT nonadherent foam dressing are removed and the wound is closed primarily (Baharestani et al., 2009; Tarkin, 2008). If the fasciotomy wound is to be closed using a skin graft, then the NPWT/ROCF dressing may be used without a contact layer or nonadherent NPWT dressing. This approach may enhance granulation tissue formation over the muscle, which facilitates skin graft take (Stone et al., 2004).

Fasciotomy wounds of the abdomen, like fasciotomy wounds of the extremity, are left open to allow intrafascial edema to resolve. Management of the open abdominal fasciotomy wound commonly involves TAC by use of an NPWT system (Navsaria et al., 2013). NPWT systems allow for TAC by (1) providing a closed environment that prevents desiccation of the abdominal contents, (2) removing excess wound fluid, and (3) reducing the amount of fascial retraction (Navsaria et al., 2013; Nelson et al., 2016; Vertrees et al., 2017). NPWT systems designed specifically for management of the complex open abdomen are commercially available. These commercially available systems consist of a fenestrated nonadherent film that is placed directly over the abdominal viscera, a foam layer

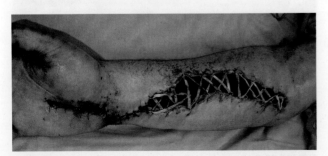

FIGURE 33-10. Vessel Loop and Staples Used to Approximate the Tissues and Minimize the Area Requiring A Skin Graft.

that is placed on top of the nonadherent film, an occlusive dressing covering the wound, and a negative pressure pump. The purpose of the fenestrated nonadherent film is to serve as a base layer that prevents adherence of the abdominal organ tissue to the ROCF dressing. This reduces the risk of fistula development. The fenestrations permit free egress of excess fluid out of the abdomen (Wang et al., 2019). When a commercial system is not available, fenestrated IV bags can be used as the nonadherent base layer. A layer of moistened gauze or sterile surgical towels are placed on the nonadherent base to fill the wound space. Drainage tubes are placed on top of the moistened gauze/sterile towels and an occlusive cover dressing is used to create a seal. Negative pressure is then delivered by attaching low wall suction to the drainage tubes that originate from underneath the edges of the occlusive dressing (Barker et al., 2007; Cubano et al., 2018; Vertrees et al., 2017). These dressings will be used until abdominal edema resolves and delayed primary closure can be performed.

● COMPLICATIONS OF TRAUMATIC WOUNDS

INFECTION

Due to the nature of the high-risk traumatic wound, wound infection and osteomyelitis are always potential complications. High-risk wounds include grossly contaminated wounds; wounds with retained foreign material; wounds contaminated with organic material; wounds with devitalized tissue; wounds with delayed presentation; wounds to the foot or mouth; wounds with open fractures; wounds involving joint, tendon, or cartilage; and wounds involving an immunocompromised host (Moran et al., 2008). The concept of wound bed preparation is important in these cases. Comprehensive care that prepares a wound to heal and involves the foundational elements of wound care should be carried out at every wound encounter as follows: cleansing, debridement of necrotic or nonviable tissue with attention to wound edges, and management and prevention of infection (Moore et al., 2019).

Adequate cleansing and meticulous debridement technique are the most beneficial interventions to prevent wound infections (Haury et al., 1978; Moran et al., 2008). It is important to assess for signs and symptoms that could indicate infection in these high-risk wounds. Purulent drainage, fever, erythema, edema, pain, nonhealing wounds or fractures, and unexplained elevated blood glucose levels in the patient with diabetes are all indicators of infection and warrant further assessment. Treatment requires PO or IV antibiotics that are guided by wound or tissue culture findings. The adjunctive use of antimicrobial dressings or antiseptic wound irrigation solutions may also be necessary. Early administration of antibiotics is important as a delay in treatment lasting longer than 6 hours may allow bacteria to proliferate to levels sufficient to cause infection, and even a 3-hour delay may inhibit the effectiveness of systemic or topical antibiotics (Edlich, 1989; Edlich et al., 1971). Antibiotics administered via the IV route are preferred for contaminated wounds (Edlich et al., 2010).

HETEROTOPIC OSSIFICATION

Heterotopic ossification (HO) is the formation of mature bone in nonosseous tissue or deposition of bone in soft tissues (Melcer et al., 2011; Potter et al., 2006). Signs and symptoms of HO may include fever, chills, inflammation, impaired joint mobility, a palpable mass or bony spurs in soft tissue, and pain along pressure-sensitive areas of the injured or residual limb (Adams, 2014). HO is readily visible on radiograph and is most commonly found in the extremities of patients who have suffered traumatic injuries including blunt trauma, fractures, burns, traumatic brain injury, and spinal cord injury (Barfield et al., 2017; Kaplan et al., 2004; Polfer et al., 2013). The exact etiopathogenesis of HO is unclear. HO has become more common with the increase in combat-related blast injuries and amputations occurring from recent conflicts. A few explanations for this recent increase in HO include (1) the intensification of primary and secondary blast forces related to advancements in weaponry and explosives, (2) medical advances allowing patients to survive injuries that have previously been fatal, and (3) amputation close to or within the zone of injury, with the goal of preserving as much of the injured extremity as possible (Potter et al., 2006). Complications of HO formation include pain at the injury or amputation site, neurovascular entrapment, and skin breakdown caused by the use of prosthetics (Melcer et al., 2011; Polfer et al., 2013). HO can be limiting to the amputee by preventing prosthesis wear due to pain and skin breakdown. Resolution of symptoms may be managed conservatively through prosthetic adjustments, or in severe cases may require surgical excision of the offending bony formation (Melcer et al., 2011). Prophylactic nonsteroidal anti-inflammatory drug therapy and low-dose local radiation therapy may be beneficial in preventing HO formation ((Barfield et al., 2017; Potter et al., 2006).

KEY POINT

Complications of traumatic wounds include infection, heterotopic ossification (HO), posttraumatic stress disorder (PTSD), and major depression.

POSTTRAUMATIC STRESS DISORDER/MAJOR DEPRESSION

Posttraumatic stress disorder (PTSD) and major depression are prevalent among individuals suffering from major traumatic injury. In a large trauma center study, more than 40% of patients hospitalized following a traumatic injury suffered from PTSD or major depression, or both (Shih et al., 2010; Warren et al., 2014). PTSD and major depression place the trauma patient at risk for poor long-term outcomes that include physical disability, an increased risk for alcohol misuse, and a lower perceived quality of life (Heltemes et al., 2014; Shih et al., 2010). Early intervention is imperative to prevent and mitigate the effects of PTSD and depression in the trauma patient and provide the opportunity for a full recovery. Patients suffering from significant trauma and their family members should be screened for PTSD and depression and referred to the appropriate provider. The Primary Care PTSD screening tool (PC-PTSD) is an easy-to-use screening device for PTSD that has been used effectively in both military and civilian trauma patients (Reese et al., 2012). The most recent version of the PC-PTSD tool, the PC-PTSD-5 tool, has shown significant diagnostic accuracy with veterans in the primary care setting (Prins et al., 2016). The PC-PTSD-5 consists of five questions concerning recent nightmares, avoidance of situations, watchfulness or hypervigilance, feelings of numbness or detachment from others or activities, and feelings of guilt related to the event (Prins et al., 2016).

CONCLUSION

The major mechanisms for traumatic injury include MVAs, gunshots, blasts, and natural disasters. Initial management of traumatic injury must focus on stabilizing the patient using measures dictated by ATLS guidelines. After the trauma patient is stabilized, it is important to obtain a through history regarding the nature of the wounding: time of injury, environment in which the injury occurred, and tetanus immunization status. The wound history will guide the treatment team in developing their initial management of the wound. In the acute traumatic wound, debridement of all nonviable tissue and thorough irrigation are critically important interventions for prevention of wound infection. Multiple debridements may be necessary in the first 4 to 7 days following a traumatic wound to ensure that all nonviable tissue is removed from the wound. These multiple debridements are necessary because the wound evolves over time and nonviable tissue will continue to declare itself during this time period. Patients who suffer crush injuries, fractures, arterial injuries, or burns and require application of tourniquets to control bleeding may also require fasciotomies to prevent compartment syndrome. Initially, most traumatic wounds must be left open because of the contaminated nature of these wounds. A temporary coverage for open traumatic wounds may be provided via NPWT/ROCF. NPWT/ROCF has become the standard for the management of open wounds until these wounds can safely be closed by delayed primary closure, skin graft, or tissue flap.

REFERENCES

Adams, L. (2014). Heterotopic ossification. *Radiation Therapist, 23*(1), 27–48.

Afshar, M., Raju, M., Ansell, D., et al. (2011). Narrative review: Tetanus—a health threat after natural disasters in developing countries. *Annals of Internal Medicine, 154*(5), 329–335.

Anand, R., & Ivatury, R. (2011). Surgical management of intra-abdominal hypertension and abdominal compartment syndrome. *The American Surgeon, 77*(Suppl 1), S42–S45.

Anghel, E., Kim, P., & Attinger, C. (2016). A solution for complex wounds: the evidence for negative pressure wound therapy with instillation. *International Wound Journal, 13*(Suppl 3), 19–24.

Baharestani, M., Amjad, I., Bookout, K., et al. (2009). V.A.C. Therapy in the management of paediatric wounds: Clinical review and experience. *International Wound Journal, 6*(Suppl 1), 1–26.

Barfield, W. R., Holmes, R. E., & Hartsock, L. A. (2017). Heterotopic ossification in trauma. *Orthopedic Clinics of North America, 48*(1), 35–46. doi: 10.1016/j.ocl.2016.08.009.

Barker, D, Green, J., Maxwell, R., et al. (2007). Experience with vacuum-pack temporary abdominal wound closure in 258 trauma and general and vascular surgical patients. *Journal of the American College of Surgeons, 204*(5), 784–792.

Beekley, A., Sebesta, J., Blackbourne, L., et al.; 31st Combat Support Hospital Research Group. (2008). Prehospital tourniquet use in Operation Iraqi Freedom: Effect on hemorrhage control and outcomes. *Journal of Trauma, 64*(2), S28–S37.

Bellamy, R., Maningas, P., & Vayer, J. (1986). Epidemiology of trauma: Military experience. *Annals of Emergency Medicine, 15*(12), 1384–1388.

Bernabe, K., Desmarais, T., & Keller, M. (2014). Management of traumatic wounds and a novel approach to delivering wound care in children. *Advances in Wound Care, 3*(4), 335–343.

Blonska-Staniec, M. K., Barczak, A. E., Garus, A., et al. (2016). The use vacuum therapy in wound healing after fasciotomy in compartment syndrome—Case report and literature review. *Acta Angiologica, 22*(4), 158–163.

Blum, M., Esser, M., & Richardson, M. (2012). Negative pressure wound therapy reduces deep infection rate in open tibial fractures. *Journal of Orthopaedic Trauma, 26*(9), 499–505.

Centers for Disease Control and Prevention (CDC). (2012). *Blast injuries: Fact sheets for professionals*. National Center for Injury Prevention and Control Division of Injury Response. Retrieved from https://stacks.cdc.gov/view/cdc/21571

Committee on Trauma. (2018). *Advanced trauma life support® (ATLS®) student course manual*. Chicago, IL: American College of Surgeons.

Crumbley, D., & Perciballi, J. (2007). Negative pressure wound therapy in a contaminated soft tissue wound. *Journal of Wound, Ostomy, and Continence Nursing, 34*(5), 507–512.

Cubano, M., et al. (2018). *Emergency war surgery* (5th ed.). Fort Sam Houston, TX: Borden Institute. Retrieved from https://www.cs.amedd.army.mil/borden/bookDetail.aspx?ID=cb88853d-5b33-4b3f-968c-2cd95f7b7809

Day, M. (2016). Control of traumatic extremity hemorrhage. *Critical Care Nurse, 36*(1), 40–51. doi: 10.4037/ccn2016871.

De Laet, I. E., Malbrain, M. L., & De Waele, J. J. (2020). A clinician's guide to management of intra-abdominal hypertension and abdominal compartment syndrome in critically ill patients. *Critical Care, 24*(1), 1–9.

Dedmond, B., Kortesis, B., Punger, K., et al. (2007). The use of negative-pressure wound therapy (NPWT) in the temporary treatment of soft-tissue injuries associated with high-energy open tibial shaft fractures. *Journal of Orthopaedic Trauma, 21*(1), 11–17.

Doyle, G., & Taillac, P. (2008). Tourniquets: A review of current use with proposals for expanded prehospital use. *Prehospital Emergency Care, 12*(2), 241–256.

Edlich, R. (1989). General requirements for controlled clinical trials of antibiotic treatment of soft tissue lacerations. *Annals of Emergency Medicine, 18*(8), 900.

Edlich, R., Madden, J., Prusak, M., et al. (1971). Studies in the management of the contaminated wound: VI. The therapeutic value of gentle scrubbing in prolonging the limited period of effectiveness of antibiotics in contaminated wounds. *The American Journal of Surgery, 121*(6), 668–672.

Edlich, R. F., Rodeheaver, G. T., Thacker, J. G., et al. (2010). Revolutionary advances in the management of traumatic wounds in the emergency department during the last 40 years: Part I. *Journal of Emergency Medicine, 38*(1), 40–50.

Fanfair, R., Benedict, K., Bos, J., et al. (2012). Necrotizing cutaneous mucormycosis after a tornado in Joplin, Missouri, in 2011. *New England Journal of Medicine, 367*(23), 2214–2225.

Fernandez, R., Griffiths, R., & Ussia, C. (2004). Effectiveness of solutions, techniques and pressure in wound cleansing. *JBI Reports, 2*(7), 231–270.

Finkelstein, P., Teisch, L., Allen, C. J., et al. (2017). Tetanus: A potential public health threat in times of disaster. *Prehospital and Disaster Medicine, 32*(3), 339–342.

Giovinco, N., Bui, T., Fisher, T., et al. (2010). Wound chemotherapy by the use of negative pressure wound therapy and infusion. *Eplasty, 10*, e9.

Gourgiotis, S., Villias, C., Germanos, S., et al. (2007). Acute limb compartment syndrome: A review. *Journal of Surgical Education, 64*(3), 178–186.

Gross, A., Cutright, D., & Bhaskar, S. (1972). Effectiveness of pulsating water jet lavage in treatment of contaminated crushed wounds. *American Journal of Surgery, 124*(3), 373–377.

Gupta, S., Gabriel, A., Lantis, J., et al. (2016). Clinical recommendations and practical guide for negative pressure wound therapy with instillation. *International Wound Journal, 13*(2), 159–174.

Hall, S. (2007). A review of the effect of tap water versus normal saline on infection rates in acute traumatic wounds. *Journal of Wound Care, 16*(1), 38–41.

Harrell, B. R., & Melander, S. (2012). Identifying the association among risk factors and mortality in trauma patients with intra-abdominal hypertension and abdominal compartment syndrome. *Journal of Trauma Nursing, 19*(3), 182–189.

Haury, B., Rodeheaver, G., Vensko, J., et al. (1978). Debridement: An essential component of traumatic wound care. *American Journal of Surgery, 135*(2), 238–242.

Havers, F. P., Moro, P. L., Hunter, P., et al. (2020). Use of tetanus toxoid, reduced diphtheria toxoid, and acellular pertussis vaccines: Updated recommendations of the advisory committee on immunization practices—United States, 2019. *MMWR. Morbidity and Mortality Weekly Report, 69*(3), 77. doi: 10.15585/mmwr.mm6903a5external icon.

Hayda, R., Harris, R., & Bass, C. (2004). Blast injury research: Modeling injury effects of landmines, bullets, and bombs. *Clinical Orthopaedics and Related Research*, (422), 97–108.

Heltemes, K., Clouser, M., MacGregor, A., et al. (2014). Co-occurring mental health and alcohol misuse: Dual disorder symptoms in combat injured veterans. *Addictive Behaviors, 39*(2), 392–398.

Hotz, G., Ginzburg, E., Wurm, G, et al. (2011). Post-earthquake injuries treated at a field hospital—Haiti, 2010. *Morbidity and Mortality Weekly Report, 59*(51/52), 1673–1677.

Jeffery S. L. (2016). The management of combat wounds: The British Military Experience. *Advances in Wound Care, 5*(10), 464–473. doi: 10.1089/wound.2015.0653.

Joint Theatre Trauma System Clinical Practice Guideline. (2012). Initial management of war wounds: Wound debridement and irrigation. Retrieved from https://jts.amedd.army.mil/assets/docs/cpgs/JTS_Clinical_Practice_Guidelines_(CPGs)/Wounds_Debridement_Irrigation_25_Apr_12_ID31.pdf

Joint Trauma System Clinical Practice Guideline. (2016a). Acute extremity compartment syndrome and the role of fasciotomy in extremity war wounds. Retrieved from https://jts.amedd.army.mil/assets/docs/cpgs/JTS_Clinical_Practice_Guidelines_(CPGs)/Extremity_Compartment_Syndrome-Fasciotomy_Extremity_War_Wounds_25_Jul_2016_ID17.pdf

Joint Trauma System Clinical Practice Guideline. (2016b). Invasive fungal infection in war wounds. Retrieved from https://jts.amedd.army.mil/assets/docs/cpgs/JTS_Clinical_Practice_Guidelines_(CPGs)/Invasive_Fungal_Infection_04_Aug_2016_ID28.pdf

Kam, P. C. A., Kavanaugh, R., & Yoong, F. F. Y. (2001). The arterial tourniquet: Pathophysiological consequences and anaesthetic implications. *Anaesthesia, 56*(6), 534–545.

Kaplan, F., Glaser, D., Hebela, N., et al. (2004). Heterotopic ossification. *Journal of the American Academy of Orthopaedic Surgeons, 12*(2), 116–125.

Kim, P., Applewhite, A., Dardano, A., et al. (2018). Use of a novel foam dressing with negative pressure wound therapy and instillation: recommendations and clinical experience. *Wounds, 30*(3 Suppl), S1–S17.

Kim, P., Attinger, C., Oliver, N., et al. (2015). Comparison of outcomes for normal saline and an antiseptic solution for negative pressure wound therapy with instillation. *Plastic and Reconstructive Surgery, 136*(5), 657e–664e.

Kretsinger, K., Broder, K. R., Cortese, M. M., et al. (2006). Infection Control Practices Advisory Committee (HICPAC) for use of Tdap among health-care personnel. *MMWR. Morbidity and Mortality Weekly Report, 55*(RR-17), 1–36.

Krug, E., Berg, L., Lee, C., et al. (2011). Evidence-based recommendations for the use of negative pressure wound therapy in traumatic wounds and reconstructive surgery: Steps towards an international consensus. *Injury, 42*(Suppl 1), S1–S12.

Large, T., Douglas, G., Erickson, G., et al. (2012). Effect of negative pressure wound therapy on the elution of antibiotics from polymethylmethacrylate beads in a porcine simulated open femur fracture model. *Journal of Orthopaedic Trauma, 26*(9), 506–511.

Lewandowski, L., Purcell, R., Fleming, M., et al. (2013). The use of dilute Dakin's solution for the treatment of angioinvasive fungal infection in the combat wounded: A case series. *Military Medicine, 178*(4), e503–e507.

Lewandowski, L., Weintrob, A., Tribble, D., et al. (2016). Early complications and outcomes in combat injury–related invasive fungal wound infections: a case-control analysis. *Journal of Orthopaedic Trauma, 30*(3), e93–e99.

Lichte, P., Oberbeck, R., Binnebösel, M., et al. (2010). A civilian perspective on ballistic trauma and gunshot injuries. *Scandinavian Journal of Trauma, Resuscitation and Emergency Medicine, 18*, 35. doi: 10.1186/1757-7241-18-35.

Ma, Z., Shou, K., Li, Z., et al. (2016). Negative pressure wound therapy promotes vessel destabilization and maturation at various stages of wound healing and thus influences wound prognosis. *Experimental and Therapeutic Medicine, 11*(4), 1307–1317. doi: 10.3892/etm.2016.3083.

Melcer, T., Belnap, B., Walker, G., et al. (2011). Heterotopic ossification in combat amputees from Afghanistan and Iraq wars: Five case histories and results from a small series of patients. *Journal of Rehabilitation Research and Development, 48*(1), 1–12.

Moisidis, E., Heath, T., Boorer, C., et al. (2004). A prospective, blinded, randomized, controlled clinical trial of topical negative pressure use in skin grafting. *Plastic and Reconstructive Surgery, 114*(4), 917–922.

Moore, Z., Dowsett, C., Smith, G., et al. (2019). TIME CDST: an updated tool to address the current challenges in wound care. *Journal of Wound Care, 28*(3), 154–161.

Moran, G., Talan, D., & Abrahamian, F. (2008). Antimicrobial prophylaxis for wounds and procedures in the emergency department. *Infectious Disease Clinics, 22*(1), 117.

Morykwas, M., Argenta, L., Shelton-Brown, E., et al. (1997). Vacuum-assisted closure: A new method for wound control and treatment: Animal studies and basic foundation. *Annals of Plastic Surgery, 38*(6), 553–562.

Morykwas, M., Howell, H., Bleyer, A., et al. (2002). The effect of externally applied subatmospheric pressure on serum myoglobin levels after a prolonged crush/ischemia injury. *Journal of Trauma, 53*(3), 537–540.

Navsaria, P., Nicol, A., Hudson, D., et al. (2013). Negative pressure wound therapy management of the "open abdomen" following trauma: A prospective study and systematic review. *World Journal of Emergency Surgery, 8*(1), 4.

Nelson, V., Crumbley, D., & Elster, E. (2016). Traumatic wounds: Bullets, blasts, and vehicle crashes. In R. Bryant & D. Nix (Eds.), *Acute and chronic wounds: current management concepts* (5th ed.). St Louis, MO: Elsevier Mosby.

Oyeniyi, B., Fox, E. E., Scerbo, M., et al. (2017). Trends in 1029 trauma deaths at a level 1 trauma center: Impact of a bleeding control bundle of care. *Injury, 48*(3), 5–12.

Polfer, E., Forsberg, J., Fleming, M., et al. (2013). Neurovascular entrapment due to combat-related heterotopic ossification in the lower extremity. *Journal of Bone and Joint Surgery, 95*(24), e195.

Pollak, A. (2008). Use of negative pressure wound therapy with reticulated open cell foam for lower extremity trauma. *Journal of Orthopaedic Trauma, 22*(10), S142–S145.

Potter, B., Burns, T., Lacap, A., et al. (2006). Heterotopic ossification in the residual limbs of traumatic and combat-related amputees. *Journal of the American Academy of Orthopaedic Surgeons, 14*(10), S191–S197.

Prins, A., Bovin, M., Smolenski, D., et al. (2016). The primary care PTSD screen for DSM-5 (PC-PTSD-5): development and evaluation within a veteran primary care sample. *Journal of General Internal Medicine, 31*(10), 1206–1211.

Ramasamy, A., Hill, A., Hepper, A., et al. (2009). Blast mines: Physics, injury mechanisms and vehicle protection. *Journal of the Royal Army Medical Corps, 155*(4), 258–264.

Reese, C., Pederson, T., Avila, S., et al. (2012). Screening for traumatic stress among survivors of urban trauma. *Journal of Trauma and Acute Care Surgery, 73*(2), 462–468.

Scherer, L., Shiver, S., Chang, M., et al. (2002). The vacuum assisted closure device: A method of securing skin grafts and improving graft survival. *Archives of Surgery, 137*(8), 930–934.

Schlatterer, D., & Hirshorn, K. (2008). Negative pressure wound therapy with reticulated open cell foam-adjunctive treatment in the management of traumatic wounds of the leg: a review of the literature. *Journal of Orthopaedic Trauma, 22*(10), S152–S160.

Shih, R., Schell, T., Hambarsoomian, K., et al. (2010). Prevalence of posttraumatic stress disorder and major depression after trauma center hospitalization. *Journal of Trauma, 69*(6), 1560–1566.

Sonshine, D., Caldwell, A., Gosselin, R., et al. (2012). Critically assessing the Haiti earthquake response and the barriers to quality orthopaedic care. *Clinical Orthopaedics and Related Research, 470*(10), 2895–2904.

Stannard, J., Singanamala, N., & Volgas, D. (2010). Fix and flap in the era of vacuum suction devices: What do we know in terms of evidence-based medicine? *Injury, 41*(8), 780–786.

Stevenson, T., Thacker, J., Rodeheaver, G., et al. (1976). Cleansing the traumatic wound by high pressure syringe irrigation. *Journal of the American College of Emergency Physicians, 5*(1), 17–21.

Stinner, D., Waterman, S. M., Masini, B. D., et al. (2011). Silver dressings augment the ability of negative pressure wound therapy to reduce bacteria in a contaminated open fracture model. *Journal of Trauma and Acute Care Surgery, 71*(1), S147–S150.

Stone, P., Prigozen, J., Hofeldt, M., et al. (2004). Bolster versus negative pressure wound therapy for securing split-thickness skin grafts in trauma patients. *Wounds, 16*(7), 219–223.

Storer, A., Lindauer, C., Proehl, J., et al. (2012). Emergency nursing resource: Wound preparation. *Journal of Emergency Nursing, 38*(5), 443–446.

Tarkin, I. (2008). The versatility of negative pressure wound therapy with reticulated open cell foam for soft tissue management after severe musculoskeletal trauma. *Journal of Orthopaedic Trauma,* *22*(10), S146–S151.

Thacker, J., Stalnecker, M., Allaire, P., et al. (1977). Practical applications of skin biomechanics. *Clinics in Plastic Surgery, 4*(2), 167–171.

Trop, M., Novak, M., Rodl, S., et al. (2006). Silver-coated dressing Acticoat® caused raised liver enzymes and argyria-like symptoms in burn patient. *Journal of Trauma and Acute Care Surgery, 60*(3), 648–652.

Venturi, M., Attinger, C., Mesbahi, A., et al. (2005). Mechanisms and clinical applications of the vacuum-assisted closure (VAC) device: A review. *American Journal of Clinical Dermatology, 6*(3), 185–194.

Vertrees, A., Shriver, C. D., & Salim, A. (2017). To close or not to close: Managing the open abdomen. In M. J. Martin, A. C. Beekley & M. J. Eckert, (Eds.), *Front line surgery: A practical approach* (2nd ed.). Cham, Switzerland: Springer International.

Wang, Y., Alnumay, A., Paradis, T., et al. (2019). Management of open abdomen after trauma laparotomy: A comparative analysis of

dynamic fascial traction and negative pressure wound therapy systems. *World Journal of Surgery, 43*(12), 3044–3050.

Warren, A., Foreman, M., Bennett, M., et al. (2014). Posttraumatic stress disorder following traumatic injury at 6 months: Associations with alcohol use and depression. *Journal of Trauma and Acute Care Surgery, 76*(2), 517–522.

Wood, M. J. (2004). Toxin-mediated disorders: Tetanus, botulism, and diphtheria. In J. Cohen, et al. (Eds.), *Infectious diseases.* Philadelphia, PA: Mosby.

Yang, C., Chang, D., & Webb, L. (2006). Vacuum-assisted closure for fasciotomy wounds following compartment syndrome of the leg. *Journal of Surgical Orthopaedic Advances, 15*(1), 19–23.

Yin, Y., Zhang, R., Li, S., et al. (2018). Negative-pressure therapy versus conventional therapy on split-thickness skin graft: a systematic review and meta-analysis. *International Journal of Surgery, 50,* 43–48.

QUESTIONS

1. Wound care nurses implement care for patients with various types of traumatic wounds. Which statement accurately describes the effect of these wounds on the human body?
   A. Blunt trauma injuries cause skin or muscle damage but do not usually affect bones, vessels, and internal organs.
   B. As a bullet interacts with the tissue, it produces both a smaller permanent cavity and a larger temporary cavity.
   C. Elastic tissue, such as muscle, blood vessels, skin, and fat may fracture and result in secondary injury.
   D. Handguns cause high-velocity wounds; hunting rifles or military weapons cause low-velocity wounds.

2. The wound care nurse documents that tissue adjacent to a gunshot wound that appeared healthy on examination has become necrotic 8 hours later. What is the term for this phenomenon?
   A. Tissue resuscitation
   B. Hidden necrosis
   C. Wound evolution
   D. Boomerang effect

3. A wound care nurse working in a VA hospital cares for patients with various types of blast injuries. Which statement accurately describes the effect of a tertiary blast injury?
   A. The victim is thrown by the blast and strikes surrounding objects.
   B. The sonic shockwave of the blast strikes the body.
   C. Device fragments are propelled through the air and cause trauma.
   D. Thermal injuries and injuries from toxic exposure occur.

4. The wound care nurse is caring for patients who sustained significant blast injuries caused by a tornado. For what life-threatening secondary condition would the nurse monitor these patients?
   A. Delayed wound healing
   B. Viral infections
   C. Fungal infections
   D. Dehydration

5. A patient presents with hemorrhaging from a wound located on a lower extremity. What is the best initial intervention for this type of external bleeding?
   A. Tourniquet
   B. Bandages
   C. Surgical closure of the wound
   D. Direct pressure

6. In which case would wound management with tetanus prophylaxis be recommended?
   A. The patient's most recent tetanus vaccination is >2 years.
   B. The wound is contaminated with soil, feces, or saliva.
   C. The wound is a closed wound caused by blunt trauma.
   D. The wound is a pressure ulcer that becomes infected.

7. The wound care nurse monitors patients with traumatic wounds for signs of compartment syndrome. Which of the following is a sign of this condition?

A. Rapid pulse
B. Cyanosis
C. Pain that is disproportionate to injury
D. Neurological changes

8. For which type of wounds is primary closure the treatment of choice?

A. Wounds to the face
B. Soft tissue injuries
C. Infected wounds
D. Wounds complicated by compartment syndrome

9. What is one benefit of negative pressure wound therapy (NPWT)?

A. Reduction of granulation tissue formation
B. Increase in inflammatory cytokines
C. Prevention of infection
D. Reduction in time to definitive closure

10. The wound care nurse assesses a patient with a large soft tissue wound that is healing by secondary intention. Final closure of this wound is generally accomplished by:

A. Antibiotic beads
B. Split-thickness skin grafts
C. NPWT with ROCF
D. Fasciotomy

ANSWERS AND RATIONALES

1. B. Rationale: Bullets and similar projectiles create both a smaller permanent cavity and a larger temporary cavity; the tissues involved in the temporary cavity may rebound and recover (soft tissue) or may fracture (bone and liver).

2. C. Rationale: Military medicine uses the term wound evolution to describe the changes in tissue viability that occur in traumatic large soft tissue injuries over the first 4 to 7 days following injury.

3. A. Rationale: Tertiary blast injuries occur when the victim is thrown by the blast and strikes surrounding objects. Victims may suffer blunt and penetrating injuries, fractures, and traumatic amputations.

4. C. Rationale: Blast injuries may be complicated by cutaneous mucormycosis, an aggressive fungal infection caused by soil contaminants projected deeply into the soft tissue. It may cause a life-threatening angioinvasive fungal infection that is difficult to eradicate.

5. D. Rationale: Direct pressure is the best initial intervention for hemorrhage if the source of bleeding is external.

6. B. Rationale: *Clostridium tetani* infection (tetanus) can occur through puncture wounds or penetrating injuries, bites, burns, frostbite, or crush injuries or through necrotic tissue contaminated with soil, feces, or saliva.

7. C. Rationale: In the conscious and unsedated patient, the hallmark sign of compartment syndrome is pain disproportionate to injury.

8. A. Rationale: Primary closure is reserved for wounds without contamination, wounds with limited tissue loss, and wounds to the face.

9. D. Rationale: One of the demonstrated mechanisms of action and clinical benefits of NPWT is reduction in time to definitive closure.

10. B. Rationale: Large soft tissue wounds healing by second intention require a split-thickness skin graft for final closure of the wound.

CHAPTER 34

MANAGEMENT OF SURGICAL WOUNDS

Tod Brindle and Sue Creehan

OBJECTIVES

1. Describe the phases of healing for a closed surgical wound and implications for assessment of these wounds.

2. Discuss guidelines for prevention, prompt detection, and management of surgical wound complications, to include infection, dehiscence, and compartment syndrome.

3. Explain situations in which a surgical wound cannot be closed primarily and options for the management of these open surgical wounds.

4. Explain indications for use of mesh in closure of abdominal wounds, the differences in unmodified and modified mesh, and implications for assessment and management of wounds with exposed mesh.

5. Describe assessment and management of open abdominal or chest wounds, to include modifications in standard wound care and in use of NPWT.

TOPIC OUTLINE

● INTRODUCTION

According to the Centers for Disease Control and Prevention (CDC), approximately 51.4 million inpatient surgical procedures are performed annually in the United States (CDC, 2009). The most recent outpatient statistics indicate that an additional 25.7 million procedures are performed in hospital-based ambulatory surgical clinics and 22.5 million procedures are performed in free standing ambulatory surgery centers (Hall et al., 2017). The number of acute surgical wounds far exceeds that of chronic wounds, yet chronic wound healing carries the burden of higher cost and greater impact on quality of life. Acute surgical wounds typically proceed normally through the phases of healing. Surgical wounds are sometimes complicated by impaired healing and dehiscence due to intrinsic and extrinsic risk factors. The major goal in the management of surgical wounds is to prevent complications and eliminate deterrents to healing (Franz et al., 2008).

Individuals undergo surgical procedures for a variety of reasons such as for the management of complications related to acute disease and for repair of an injury. The reason for and timing of surgery can impact the outcome in terms of wound healing. With elective surgeries, the date of surgery can be selected when the patient's health is in optimal condition. The patient who undergoes emergent surgery related to acute illness or injuries is at risk for impaired healing from physiologic stressors affecting the body. Tissue that is already diseased, inflamed, or traumatized does not heal as well as healthy tissue.

● HEALING PROCESS FOR SURGICAL WOUNDS

Acute full-thickness injuries heal in a predictable manner through the overlapping stages of hemostasis, inflammation, proliferation, and remodeling. This also is the classic pathway for surgical wound healing. In humans, the repair of tissue and organs after surgery occurs almost entirely by replacement with scar tissue and regeneration (Phillips, 2000). Surgical wounds proceed through the phases of repair in an orderly and timely manner when obstacles to healing are minimized and the host response is maximized. Healed surgical wounds are characterized by restoration of skin integrity through re-epithelialization of the incision and full-thickness restoration (not maturation) in the tissue layers beneath. If an acute surgical wound has not adhered to normal healing sequence within a 4- to 6-week time frame, most authors agree that it is then labeled chronic (Lee & Hansen, 2009; Widgerow, 2013). The time point at which a surgical wound becomes chronic has been a long-standing topic of discussion. According to Widgerow (2013), although many attempts have been made to define the chronic wound concept, it is perhaps most logical to label a wound as chronic when it does not adhere to normal sequence in terms of symptoms, signs, or time to heal.

Acute surgical wounds undergo uncomplicated healing and rapid closure. The trajectory toward healing is affected by intrinsic and extrinsic host factors as well as surgical skill and technique. Not all surgical wounds are located in healthy tissue, and the poor integrity of the tissue can cause delays in healing to occur. Surgical wounds located in areas of significant trauma, such as crush injuries, or grossly contaminated wounds may require a longer than anticipated time to heal (Widgerow, 2013). A surgical wound that has not matured to its anticipated healing end point of closure and displays characteristics such as bleeding, exudate, and pain after a 4-week time period may be considered to be a chronic surgical wound (Widgerow, 2013).

A brief overview of the normal healing sequence for a surgical wound follows.

HEMOSTASIS AND INFLAMMATION

Acute wound healing begins with establishment of hemostasis and initiation of inflammation. Skin cell toll-like receptors respond to both damage-associated molecular patterns and pathogen-specific molecular patterns activating leukocyte-mediated chemokine signaling (Sorg et al., 2017). The coagulation cascade is activated by vessel disruption and involves platelet aggregation to form a clot and vasoconstriction to control hemorrhaging and reduce blood loss. Surgeons augment these physiologic reflexes through use of the Bovie® and other electrocauterization tools beginning with skin incision. Vasoconstriction of the vessels in the surgical field is the immediate response to a surgical injury. Platelet activation produces two key results that are critical to both hemostasis and the inflammatory phase of repair: (1) fibrin clot formation, which seals the vessels to prevent bacterial invasion and serves as a temporary scaffolding for cell migration, and (2) the release of growth factors and cytokines that recruit the leukocytes needed for bacterial control and elimination of any damaged tissue. Once hemostasis is accomplished, the wound moves into the inflammatory phase of repair. This phase is supported by vasodilatation, which occurs within minutes following the initial vasoconstrictive response. The increased blood flow that accompanies the inflammatory phase is the basis for the edema, erythema, warmth, and pain that is characteristic of this phase of healing (Doughty & Sparks, 2016). The key cells during the initial phase of repair (hemostasis and inflammation) include platelets, neutrophils, and macrophages.

KEY POINT

The repair process for a surgical wound begins with platelet activation and clot formation, which seals the vessels to prevent bacterial invasion, provides a temporary scaffolding for cell migration, and releases the growth factors and cytokines that recruit the cells needed for repair.

Neutrophils are phagocytic leukocytes that migrate by an increasing cytokine and chemokine gradient to the area of injured tissue. These cells both secrete additional proinflammatory cytokines and reactive oxygen species in response to tissue injury to enhance microorganism

removal and simultaneously facilitate proliferative cell activation. Macrophages arrive in the wound 2 to 3 days postinjury and are another key cell in the inflammatory phase as well as a transitional cell to the proliferative phase. Pathogen-specific molecular patterns result in macrophage phenotypic differentiation into M1 or M2 subsets, which have phagocytic and proliferative roles. Macrophages carry out a number of key functions: they secrete elastase and collagenase to break down damaged tissue, they destroy microorganisms through phagocytosis and release of nitric oxide, and they attract fibroblasts to the wound bed by chemotactic signaling. For example, M2 macrophages are associated with extracellular matrix (ECM) production, down-regulate the inflammatory response, and signal fibroblast proliferation (Sorg et al., 2017).

PROLIFERATIVE PHASE

In a surgical wound in which the wound edges are approximated with staples, sutures, or fibrin glue, the proliferative phase begins within 24 hours of injury and overlaps the inflammatory phase. The first component of the proliferative phase is epithelial resurfacing. Keratinocytes respond to cytokines released from neutrophils and advance from the wound edges to resurface the minor disruption in skin integrity (Chin et al., 2007). Because the epithelial defect is very small in an approximated wound, initial epithelialization is complete within 2 days. Once epithelial resurfacing is complete, the bacterial barrier has been restored and wound dressings become optional. The presence of a closed skin incision after epithelialization does not guarantee underlying healing of the subcutaneous tissues. Proliferation is a complex process involving the coordination of endothelial cells, fibroblasts, and keratinocytes resulting in scar formation, angiogenesis, peripheral nerve, and vessel repair.

KEY POINT

In a surgical wound closed primarily, the proliferative phase of repair begins within 24 hours and overlaps the inflammatory phase. The first component of the proliferative phase is epithelial resurfacing, followed by formation of sufficient granulation tissue to knit the underlying tissue layers together.

The second component of the proliferative phase is granulation tissue formation, which begins on days 3 to 5 postinjury, following and overlapping the inflammatory phase. The goal of the proliferative phase is to synthesize new tissue to fill the defect in the soft tissues (suture line). Granulation tissue formation involves the simultaneous production of new blood vessels and the synthesis of new connective tissue proteins (creation of an ECM). Angiogenesis is dominated by the regulation of cell interaction with the M2 macrophage. Due to local tissue hypoxia during the wounding process and secondary to increased metabolic demand for oxygen, major proangiogenic mediators including VEGF, VEGFA, FGF2, PDGF, TGF-β1 are released resulting in neovascularization. This neovascular network is responsible for delivery of oxygen rich blood and nutrients to the wound. Simultaneously, a collagen matrix is being formed that provides the supportive architecture for the new vessels (Cañedo-Dorantes & Cañedo-Ayala, 2019). The fibroblasts are responsible for synthesis of collagen and other connective tissue proteins that form the ECM (Chin et al., 2007). Deposition of collagen early in the healing process is important for successful wound closure as wound dehiscence is most likely to occur by post-op days 5 to 8 (Whitney, 2016). The newly formed collagen is type III, which lacks tensile strength. During the remodeling phase, the type III collagen is converted to type I collagen, which provides tensile strength.

In open wounds, contraction of the wound occurs at the same time that granulation tissue is being formed. Deposition of ECM components leads to increased mechanical wound stress, which stimulates activation of fibroblasts, pericytes, adipocytes, resident mesenchymal progenitor cells, and bone marrow–derived mesenchymal stem cells leading to contraction of the wound edges (Karppinen et al., 2019). Contraction is beneficial in open wounds. If the open wound is located over a joint, contraction could result in limitation of mobility and function and scar deposition (Greer et al., 2007). Contraction does not occur in surgical wounds where the edges are approximated.

REMODELING PHASE

Each phase of wound healing overlaps and happens simultaneously. The remodeling phase begins during the final days of the proliferative phase and involves breakdown of the type III collagen and replacement with organized parallel patterns of type I collagen (Chin et al., 2007). The remodeling phase lasts from 3 weeks to 2 years postinjury.

KEY POINT

The maturation phase lasts from 3 weeks to 2 years post-surgery and involves breakdown of the type III collagen with replacement with type I collagen, which provides tensile strength.

SURGICAL WOUND CLASSIFICATIONS

Surgical wounds are classified as class I to IV based on the degree of sterility or contamination (Chupp & Edhayan, 2018). The classification may guide the surgeon's decision for primary, delayed primary, or secondary intention closure. Appropriate classification impacts interhospital ratings, reimbursement, and perspectives

of quality of care, requiring accuracy in diagnosis and documentation (Chupp & Edhayan, 2018). The definitions are as follows:

Class I/clean: An uninfected operative wound with no inflammation observed and no entry into respiratory, alimentary, genital, or uninfected urinary tract. Incision is closed primarily and if necessary drained with a closed drainage apparatus.

Class II/clean-contaminated: An operative wound in which the respiratory, alimentary, genital, or urinary tract were entered under controlled conditions and without unusual contamination. No evidence of infection or major break in technique was encountered. The incision is closed primarily and if necessary drained with a closed drainage apparatus.

Class III/contaminated: An open, fresh, accidental wound. Includes surgeries with major breaks in techniques or gross spillage from the GI tract <4 hours old, and incisions in which acute, nonpurulent inflammation occurs. These wounds are left open initially and later closed through delayed primary closure or left open to heal by secondary intention.

Class IV/dirty-infected: Old traumatic wounds with retained devitalized tissue and those that involve existing clinical infection or perforated viscera >4 hours old. Microorganism(s) causing the infection were present in operative field before surgery. These wounds are left open to heal by secondary intention.

KEY POINT

Surgical wounds are classified based on the degree of contamination (from class I to class IV). Clean wounds can usually be closed primarily, while dirty wounds and those with heavy bacterial loads are usually managed with delayed closure or left open to heal by secondary intention.

⬤ METHODS OF CLOSURE

PRIMARY CLOSURE

Primary closure of a wound occurs when the edges of the wound are approximated by a surgeon and held in place by staples, sutures, or skin adhesives (**Fig. 34-1**). Primary closure implies each tissue layer is approximated and closed, including the dermis, subcutaneous layer, fascia, and muscle. Primary closure typically occurs at the conclusion of a surgical procedure, although it is a wound closure technique used for clean traumatic injuries as well. Placement of sutures or staples for tissue approximation is an additional form of injury. Sutures and staples are an intentionally placed foreign body. If the foreign body becomes infected or causes irritation, the wound rarely heals until the material is extruded or removed.

Primary repair should approximate the wound edges without causing strangulation of vessels within the wound

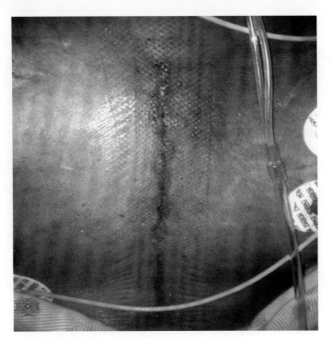

FIGURE 34-1. Wound Closed by Primary Intention.

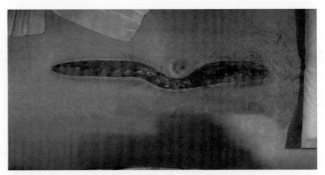

FIGURE 34-2. Wound Ready for Delayed Primary Closure.

adhesive or suture secured anchoring devices with approximating plastic strips or elastic strips, which provide mechanical creep or the elongation of skin, and skin relaxation principles. Evidence is insufficient to suggest which technique for primary closure is most advantageous. Delayed closure may also be used prior to graft application. The delay is used to create a healthy bed of granulation tissue that will support the graft (**Fig. 34-2**).

> **KEY POINT**
>
> Delayed primary closure is used for heavily contaminated wounds. The wound is left open until bacterial loads have been controlled, at which point the wound edges are approximated and closed with sutures, staples, or skin adhesives.

(Franz et al., 2008). Lee and Hansen (2009) stress the importance of atraumatic tissue handling, selective cauterization of blood vessels, and avoidance of excessive tension at the suture/staple line in the prevention of skin and soft tissue necrosis. Skin necrosis from vascular disruption or excessive closure tension leads to impaired healing and eventually a chronic open wound (Lee & Hansen, 2009).

Primary closure is the preferred method of closure for clean wounds and wounds involving repair of injured structures such as nerves, tendons, and blood vessels when the zone of injury is small and the wound is clean. Primary closure is contraindicated in the presence of tension, potential infection, and when the extent of injury is unclear (Lee & Hansen, 2009). Contaminated or infected wounds should not be primarily closed (Franz et al., 2008).

DELAYED PRIMARY CLOSURE (TERTIARY INTENTION WOUND MANAGEMENT)

Delayed primary closure was developed during World War II in an effort to reduce infection rates in traumatic war injuries (Wechter et al., 2005). Wounds were debrided and left open with packing for several days, then sutured closed. This practice change reduced the incidence of wound infections from 23% to 2% (Wechter et al., 2005). Currently, delayed primary closure is used when there is a high level of contamination. The wound is left open until topical therapy has reduced the bacterial load and the likelihood of soft tissue infection (typically 2 to 5 days). At that point, the wound edges are approximated and closed with sutures, staples, or skin adhesives. For large defects, or for progressive closure during the reduction of tissue edema and tension, topical tension relief systems are available. Many of these systems involve

SECONDARY INTENTION

Surgical wounds not closed primarily or with delayed primary closure are left open to heal by secondary intention (**Fig. 34-3**). These wounds are treated with topical wound care to optimize the body's ability to fill the cavity or deficit with scar. This approach is indicated for heavily contaminated wounds, poorly perfused wounds, malignant wounds, wounds with necrosis or known infection, and wounds with extensive tissue loss in which attempted approximation would create excessive tension and increased risk for dehiscence (Greer et al., 2007). Surgical wounds most commonly left open to heal by secondary intention involve GI perforations, penetrating trauma wounds, perforated appendix, and compartment syndrome. Aggressive or serial debridement of necrotic tissue, elimination of malignant tissue, and eradication of infection may permit eventual surgical closure of wounds initially left open.

> **KEY POINT**
>
> Wounds left open to heal by secondary intention include those involving bowel perforation, penetrating trauma, and compartment syndrome. The focus in management of these wounds is on wound care to promote granulation tissue formation and epithelial resurfacing.

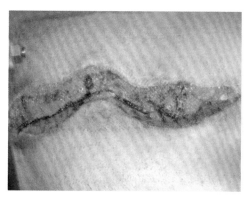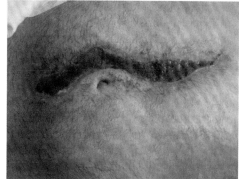

FIGURE 34-3. Wounds Healing by Secondary Intention.

FLAP OR GRAFT

Another method of surgical closure involves placement of a graft or flap. Grafting can involve donor tissue from another species (biologics, heterograft, or xenograft), from another human being (allograft), or from the patient (autograft). Autografts can be split thickness (epidermis and part of the dermis), full thickness (epidermis and dermis), or composite (skin and underlying tissue). Flaps involve closure of the defect with skin and soft tissue from another area of the body and include random flaps, axial/arterial flaps, musculocutaneous flaps, fasciocutaneous flaps, and free flaps. Grafts and flaps are reserved for large tissue defects and a functional inability to close the tissue primarily. The flap or graft serves to provide immediate coverage of the wound base, which may provide protection and coverage for exposed muscles, tendons, and bones or organs. Even though the decision to apply a graft or flap resides with the provider, the wound care nurse may be consulted to assist in developing the plan of care for a grafted patient. It is important to assure stabilization of the graft, use of atraumatic dressings, exudate management, and to monitor for graft adherence and flap viability.

SURGICAL CLOSURE COMPLICATIONS

Common complications involving surgically closed wounds include hematomas and seromas, incisional separation, and dehiscence. Evisceration is a less common event.

Hematomas or seromas involve collections of clotted blood or serum between the tissue layers of the surgical wound and can exert pressure to interfere with perfusion of the adjacent tissue. Hematomas are of concern because blood is an excellent medium for bacterial growth. Hematomas that are not reabsorbed should be evacuated to avoid a fluid collection of microorganisms (Franz et al., 2008). The evacuation of the hematoma can be accomplished by needle aspiration or placement of a drain. Franz and colleagues (2008) noted that wound hematomas are increasing due to the increased use of prophylactic and therapeutic anticoagulation and antiplatelet therapy in surgical patients (Nutescu et al., 2011).

> **KEY POINT**
>
> Hematomas provide an excellent medium for bacterial growth. Hematomas that are not quickly reabsorbed should be evacuated by aspiration or placement of a drain.

Incisional separation is superficial. The skin edges are separated, but the deeper tissues remain approximated. The term dehiscence refers to separation of the skin and soft tissue layers and can be further classified as complete or incomplete. Complete dehiscence involves disruption of the fascia and often the peritoneum, whereas incomplete dehiscence is a separation of the epidermis, dermis, and subcutaneous tissue but not the fascia. Evisceration is protrusion of the intestine into the wound and requires an emergent response to maintain bowel viability (Whitney, 2016).

> **KEY POINT**
>
> Dehiscence refers to separation of the skin and soft tissue layers and can be further classified as complete or incomplete. Evisceration is protrusion of the intestine into the wound and requires an emergent response to maintain bowel viability.

SURGICAL WOUND ASSESSMENT

Ongoing assessment of the surgical wound is an important element of postoperative nursing management. Visual assessment of the incision and surrounding tissue and gentle palpation are key to determining progress in healing. Acute surgical wounds should proceed in an orderly and timely fashion though the phases of healing. Aligning surgical site assessment with the physical manifestations of the wound healing phases of inflammation, proliferation, and remodeling will help determine if the wound is healing.

DAY 1 TO DAY 4: INFLAMMATION AND EPITHELIAL RESURFACING OF CLOSED WOUND

The incision should be well approximated, skin edges touching, red in color. Periwound skin may appear inflamed, may feel warm to the touch, and may be tender on palpation. Edema and erythema in the surrounding soft tissue is normal. If staples or sutures are present, mild inflammation of the staple and/or suture insertion sites is normal since they are intentionally placed foreign bodies (Bates-Jensen & Williams, 2012). Often, a continuous halo of erythema may be seen around the wound margins. The erythema should not extend >2 cm from the wound edges and should steadily decrease in intensity.

A close look at the incision will reveal a new epithelial layer covering the incision at 48 to 72 hours postoperatively. This is referred to as epithelial resurfacing and indicates that the wound is closed, and the protective skin barrier function has been restored (Bates-Jensen & Williams, 2012).

> **KEY POINT**
>
> In assessing a closed surgical wound, the wound care nurse should correlate clinical findings with physiologic events. At 48 to 72 hours postoperatively, the incision is normally closed at the surface, and by 5 to 8 days postoperatively, a healing ridge should be palpable.

Any exudate will be sanguineous, progressing to serosanguinous as vessel leakage subsides, and extracellular serous fluid mixes with residual bloody serum. The amount of exudate should be minimal.

DAY 5 TO DAY 9: PROLIFERATIVE PROCESS

The redness of the incision fades to pink as capillary beds regress beneath the newly epithelialized surface, which is thickening to become the five keratinocyte cell layers normally found in the skin. In normal healing, the epithelium is intact with no breaks in its integrity. Any pre-existing inflammation, edema, or erythema in the periwound skin area should have dissipated. Exudate should not be present (Bates-Jensen & Williams, 2012).

Beneath the surface, a collagen matrix is being established. Palpation along the entire length of the incision should reveal a stiffness or firmness to the tissue up to 1 cm on either side of the incision (Phillips, 2000). This is known as a healing ridge and is a normal expected outcome. Lack of a healing ridge is an indicator of high risk for dehiscence or infection (Lee & Hansen, 2009). Wound dehiscence most often occurs by post-op days 5 to 8 and is linked to delayed or inadequate collagen deposition (Whitney, 2016).

DAYS 10 TO 14: CONTINUED PROLIFERATION AND EARLY REMODELING

As the proliferative phase continues, the sutures and staples can safely be removed and wound closure strips may or may not be applied. The epithelial resurfacing is visible, the healing ridge is palpable, and surrounding tissue remains normal. There is no exudate at this point of surgical wound healing (Bates-Jensen & Williams, 2012).

BEYOND DAY 15

As capillary regression continues, the color of the incision continues to pale and the incision takes on a pearly gray appearance. As the collagen converts to type I and reorganizes in a patterned fashion, the healing ridge softens (Bates-Jensen & Williams, 2012). The final tensile strength of the healed incision is approximately 80% compared to its preinjured state.

GUIDELINES FOR INCISIONAL CARE

The primary purpose of a postoperative incisional dressing is to act as a barrier to external contamination, absorb, exudate, and keep it away from the skin and provide a moist environment to promote epithelization. These principles may be reflected in a variety of advanced wound dressings, antimicrobial wound dressings, skin sealants such as cyanoacrylate monomers, and incisional negative pressure wound therapy. There are more than 35 variables that influence the risk of surgical site infection (SSI), and a dressing is not capable of mitigating all of these risk factors. A dressing is likely to aid in the prevention or management of an SSI versus an organ space or deep SSI. A 2016 Cochrane systematic review indicated that overall there were low-quality studies to suggest a specific dressing (transparent film, hydrocolloid, silver dressings, contact dressings, etc.) to prevent SSI following clean or contaminated cases (Dumville et al., 2016). Several randomized controlled trials (RCTs) have been published demonstrating the benefit of postoperative antimicrobial dressings compared to nonantimicrobial standard dressings for the prevention of superficial SSI (Kuo et al., 2017; Stanirowski et al., 2016). In surgical procedures such as caesarean section and orthopedic procedures, the use of postoperative antimicrobial dressings has become standard of care. The effectiveness of these dressings has not been demonstrated as significant in all surgical procedures (Biffi et al., 2012; Struik et al., 2018). For the prevention of superficial SSI, patients at high risk of dehiscence; those with prolonged drainage from the incision; and those with comorbidities such as advanced age, smoking, diabetes, obesity and immune suppression, which increase overall risk of infection, the use of antimicrobial dressings should be considered. Most authors and clinical experts agree that primary incisional wounds should be protected by a sterile occlusive dressing that provides protection against bacterial invasion. There remains insufficient evidence to determine the appropriate time a dressing should be removed postoperatively (Toon et al., 2015). Often the dressing applied in the OR is left in place for the first 48 hours. If there is a need to change this dressing due to soiling, dislodgement, or drainage, sterile supplies and technique are recommended. This first postoperative sterile dressing change should be performed by the health care provider that hospital policy or physician's order dictates. After 48 to 72 hours, the patient may have the dressing removed and may be allowed to shower so long as epithelial resurfacing is complete. If epithelial resurfacing has not occurred, reapplication of a sterile dressing with characteristics to promote re-epithelialization is appropriate and may aid in reducing the risk of SSI.

KEY POINT

Clinical experts agree that primary incisional wounds should be protected by a sterile occlusive dressing that provides protection against bacterial invasion for the first 48 hours and until re-epithelialization has occurred.

There is general agreement that a postoperative incision should be covered by a sterile dressing and cared for using sterile technique for the first 48 hours postoperatively, but there is a lack of evidence supporting the use of one dressing over another. When choosing a postoperative dressing, the wound care nurse should also consider the potential for medical adhesive–related skin injury (MARSI), blister formation secondary to epidermal stabilization with dermal shift related to postoperative edema, pain on dressing removal, and any history of allergies to the dressing ingredients.

Sterile technique and dressings should be used when caring for fresh post-op wounds healing by delayed primary closure. The principles of moist wound healing covered in Chapter 3 should be followed. Since the goal of delayed primary closure is to reduce the bioburden of the wound, thorough irrigation with normal saline or a noncytotoxic wound cleanser should occur with each dressing change. Dressings should be selected that will provide an optimum environment for granulation tissue formation. Once the surgeon primarily closes the wound, the procedure for primary closure wounds should be followed.

Class III and IV surgical wounds are typically left open to heal by secondary intention. Wounds left open heal by formation of granulation tissue, wound contraction, and epithelial resurfacing. Topical therapy for these wounds is based on the principles of wound bed preparation with the optimal dressing determined by the wound's characteristics, wound bed tissue type, absence or presence of undermining or tunneling, and the type and amount of exudate.

INDICATIONS AND GUIDELINES FOR THE MANAGEMENT OF COMPLEX WOUNDS

Wound care nurses are frequently asked to recommend management for acute surgical wounds and are expected to provide the evidence to support the use of advanced therapies.

NEGATIVE PRESSURE WOUND THERAPY

First described by Kostiuchenok et al. (1986) and later popularized for clinical practice in 1997, negative pressure wound therapy (NPWT) has proven to be a major tool in the management of complex wounds (Argenta & Morykwas, 1997; Morykwas et al., 1997). The application of controlled subatmospheric (negative) pressure to open wounds has been shown to promote healing through its effects on the microcirculation, endothelial cell activation (Borgquist et al., 2011; Chen et al., 2005; Wackenfors et al., 2004), removal of wound exudate and debris, stimulation of angiogenesis and collagen synthesis, and reduction in levels of proinflammatory cytokines and bacterial colony counts (Anesäter et al., 2011; Weigand & White, 2013). The beneficial effects are the basis for use of NPWT in wounds healing by delayed primary closure or secondary intention and for wounds involving grafts and flaps.

CLOSED INCISION NPWT
Benefits of Closed Incision NPWT

There has been an increase in the use of NPWT on closed incisions following surgery for the prevention of infection and associated complications. Closed incision negative pressure wound therapy (ciNPWT) is becoming common practice in many facilities due to the effectiveness of the therapy and the availability of disposable ciNPWT devices. Compared to traditional NPWT systems, these devices are unable to manage large surface area wounds and copious exudate but provide benefit to patients and providers through increased mobility, concealment, decreased noise, ease of use, and cost reduction compared to traditional NPWT systems by avoiding insurance coverage issues and allowing for decreased length of stay (LOS) (Wells et al., 2019). There are a variety of devices available including electric powered, mechanically powered, all-in-one-dressing apparatuses, and foam- and gauze-based kits. Each system has its own differentiating factors that may persuade a provider to select a particular device due to practical considerations such as ease of use and exudate management capabilities. In most cases, product decisions will be based on contractual arrangements through procurement.

Following surgery, patients are at risk for surgical complications such as dehiscence, infection, seroma, or hematoma. Risk factors that are direct correlates to these complications may include edema, prolonged incisional drainage, and underlying comorbid conditions, for example diabetes, immunosuppression, obesity, which compromise wound healing and the development of tensile strength (Karlakki et al., 2013). The use of ciNPWT is suggested to directly address these concerns. The application of subatmospheric pressure on intact tissue surrounding the closed incision has been demonstrated to result in a significant increase in vascular endothelial growth factor (VEGF) expression after 8 days of therapy in preclinical in vivo porcine studies (Shah et al., 2019). Human cohort studies in bariatric patients have demonstrated improved oxygen saturation and tissue perfusion surrounding the wound closure when ciNPWT is utilized. It is suspected that ciNPWT prevents bacterial inoculation before closure and improves lymphatic clearance and perfusion of the tissues, while limiting edema, hematoma, and seroma formation.

Factors affecting the risk for dehiscence include the host's ability to synthesize collagen, the strength of the suture material, the closure technique, and factors that increase stress on the incision such as obesity, coughing. One benefit of ciNPWT is a reduction in lateral tension. An in vitro study by Wilkes and colleagues (2012) demonstrated a 50% reduction in lateral stress and 50% improvement in the tensile strength of the incision. This translates into reduced risk of dehiscence. They found that ciNPWT altered the distribution of forces to the tissue in a way consistent with normal intact skin. Without the ciNPWT, there was a tendency for the lines of stress to be directed toward the sutures, resulting in a bowing effect, increased stress on the incision, and a possible increase in risk of hematoma as well as dehiscence (Wilkes et al., 2012).

Strugala and Martin (2017) conducted the first systematic review and meta-analysis of all known studies on the impact of prophylactic use of a specific design of NPWT device on surgical site complications. They found a significant reduction in SSI, wound dehiscence, and length of stay (LOS) on the basis of pooled data from 16 studies showing a benefit of a single-use NPWT system compared with standard care in closed surgical incisions.

Colorectal surgeries have been studied for the potential benefit of ciNPWT on SSI and secondary wound complications. A systematic review and meta-analysis of ciNPWT on closed laparotomy incisions following general and colorectal surgery was performed by Sahebally and colleagues (2018). Nine studies including 1,266 patients demonstrated significantly lower rate of SSI compared with standard dressings but no difference in rates of complications including seroma or wound dehiscence.

Zwanenburg and colleagues (2020) performed a meta-analysis of randomized and nonrandomized studies that compared ciNPWT with control dressings to evaluate the efficacy of ciNPWT for the prevention of postoperative wound complications such as SSI. There is strong evidence that ciNPWT reduced SSI. There is less evidence that ciNPWT reduces the risk of wound dehiscence, skin necrosis, and seroma.

NPWT may prevent subcutaneous fluid accumulation in a closed wound and subsequently reduce SSI. In a meta-analysis of ciNPWT on closed abdominal incisions, Wells and associates (2019) found that use of ciNPWT may reduce the incidence of superficial SSI but has no effect on deep or organ space SSI, wound dehiscence, or hospital LOS.

A meta-analysis conducted by Svensson-Björk et al. (2019) assessed the effects of incisional NPWT on the incidence of SSI in closed groin incisions after arterial surgery. They found that ciNPWT after groin incisions for arterial surgery reduced the incidence of SSI compared with standard wound dressings. The risk of bias highlighted the need for a high-quality RCT with cost-effectiveness analysis.

An RCT of ciNPWT for the reduction of SSI in primarily closed incisions after open and laparoscopic-converted colorectal surgery was conducted. Murphy et al. (2019) included patients undergoing segmental subtotal and total colectomies as well as low or ultra-low anterior resections. They found that the 30-day incidence of SSI was not different between gauze dressing and ciNPWT. There was no difference in SSI in a subgroup analysis of those patients who did and did not receive ostomies.

Grauhan and colleagues (2013) conducted a prospective RCT involving obese cardiac surgery patients. The authors found that ciNPWT used over clean, closed incisions for the first 6 to 7 postoperative days significantly reduces the incidence of SSI after median sternotomy in a high-risk group of obese patients.

Selection of ciNPWT

Many of the early studies utilizing NPWT on closed incisions utilized traditional NPWT foam- or gauze-based systems with a contact layer to protect the skin. New developments in ciNPWT technology give the clinician more options. Single-use (disposable) negative pressure therapy units are available from multiple manufacturers in both powered and nonpowered versions. In the above study by Grauhan and colleagues (2013) as well as a previous study by Colli (2011), a significant benefit of disposable ciNPWT systems in the prevention of postoperative infection was reported, as well as a reduction in wound seroma (Pachowsky et al., 2011). An in vitro comparative analysis was performed by Malmsjö and colleagues (2014) in which a disposable, battery-operated ciNPWT device was compared to a traditional NPWT system utilizing a variety of foam and gauze combinations. The authors reported no significant differences in wound contraction, wound microvascular blood flow, or the delivery of the measured levels of pressure to the tissues. The selection of a specific NPWT system should be based on clinical practice considerations.

Indications

Indications for ciNPWT should be based on the available evidence as well as assessment of individual patient comorbidities and risk for wound complications. Surgical patients undergoing vascular, cardiac surgery, obstetrics, and closed laparotomy incisions have shown the greatest reduction in infection, seroma, and dehiscence rates. Considerations may be made for patients at risk for delayed healing such as obese patients or patients at risk for prolonged incisional drainage. They should be considered for ciNPWT. Wound care nurses should utilize their clinical judgment as to whether routine use of ciNPWT is beneficial following contaminated procedures and colorectal surgeries. Many of the studies compared ciNPWT to standard gauze or nonantimicrobial dressings. Wound care nurses should consider a method for differentiating the use of standard closure, advanced incisional dressings, and surgical procedures with evidence for ciNPWT utilization to trend SSI incidence and cost. The use of ciNPWT on all incisions may not be financially feasible. Regardless of surgical procedure, secondary considerations for ciNPWT include exudate levels, cost, mobility, and discretion.

KEY POINT

In selecting a specific system for ciNPWT, the wound care nurse must consider amount of exudate, cost, and the patient's need for mobility and discretion.

Exudate

Exudate levels are a key consideration in selection of traditional versus disposable systems. Disposable ciNPWT systems manage exudate through evaporative loss, an absorptive dressing, or a small external canister. They are intended for the management of wounds with minimal to moderate exudate. Large or copiously draining wounds would overwhelm the capacity of these dressings and their associated canisters. The wound care nurse should consider the anticipated volume of drainage and the probable duration of drainage when determining the best system to use. The wound care nurse should consider that large amounts of continued drainage may be indicative of developing complications. The wound care nurse should review manufacturers' guidelines for each system used in the facility to include the volume of drainage accommodated by the dressing or canister and whether the canister can be changed independent of the dressing.

Cost

Cost is another consideration and is significantly decreased with the use of disposable systems. In a wound with minimal exudate, the one-time fee and up to 7-day wear time is of major benefit, especially in the ambulatory surgery setting and the outpatient setting. The ability to discharge a patient following ambulatory surgery and to schedule the first postoperative dressing change for the outpatient setting eliminates the need for home health and frequent dressing changes. Cost is also a key consideration in selection of ciNPWT for an indigent patient who requires, but does not qualify for, traditional NPWT at home.

Mobility and Discretion

Mobility and discretion of the disposable systems are popular features and another reason for selection when there is limited exudate. The disposable systems are considerably smaller and may either fit into a pocket or be secured to the body by an arm or leg strap. These systems have shorter drainage tubing lengths and can often be applied in a manner that minimizes or eliminates visibility to others. Traditional NPWT systems are bulky and require a shoulder or cross body sling. Better mobility and discretion may facilitate compliance, especially among teens and young adults, who may be sensitive to therapy that is visible in social situations.

Selection between a powered versus nonpowered ciNPWT systems is a matter of personal choice, as there is no evidence to suggest any difference in clinical performance between the two systems. Ease of use or comfort level may be the deciding factor. Some nonpowered versions offer a variety of suction settings to allow for customization of the NPWT setting, where powered disposables often have only one default pressure setting. Since these systems vary in their design, wound care nurses should determine and consider the expected battery life versus the projected length of pressure delivery in spring-loaded nonpowered versions.

Complications and Contraindications for ciNPWT

Traditional NPWT had complications reported primarily related to bleeding, infection, and retained dressing material. Although there are different levels of risk related to use of NPWT for closed incisions, the wound care use should be aware of potential risk factors and contraindications for ciNPWT (Netsch et al., 2016).

Relative contraindications to the use of ciNPWT include signs and symptoms of active infection or hematoma. Wound care nurses must always carefully assess the wound and patient to determine appropriateness of ciNPWT.

MANAGEMENT OF COMPLEX SURGICAL WOUNDS: ABDOMINAL WOUNDS

Understanding the Abdominal Wall, Loss of Domain, and Muscle Disruption

The abdominal wall is a dynamic and intricate system of muscle and connective tissue. Any alteration in the physical structure of the abdominal wall will result in a change in muscle physiology and function. The centrally located rectus abdominis muscle is divided vertically by a thick band of connective tissue known as the linea alba, which serves as the primary insertion site for the muscles of the abdominal wall; the external oblique, internal oblique, and transversus abdominis muscles. Multiple layers of fascia encase the abdominal wall, primarily the anterior and posterior rectus fascia (**Fig. 34-4**).

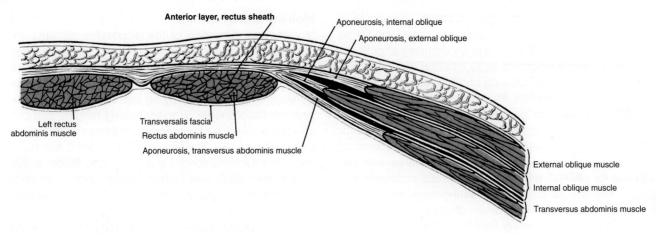

Anterior layer, rectus sheath

Aponeurosis, internal oblique

Aponeurosis, external oblique

Left rectus abdominis muscle

Transversalis fascia

Rectus abdominis muscle

Aponeurosis, transversus abdominis muscle

External oblique muscle

Internal oblique muscle

Transversus abdominis muscle

FIGURE 34-4. Cross Section of the Abdominal Wall.

KEY POINT

The abdominal wall is a dynamic and intricate system of muscle and connective tissue. Any alteration (such as occurs with laparotomy) results in altered muscle physiology and function. For example, primary closure delayed more than 7 to 10 days may result in lateralization requiring abdominal wall reconstruction (AWR).

Impact of Muscle Disruption

The abdominal wall has multiple functions: maintenance of upright posture, spine stabilization, complex movements, protection of the abdominal viscera, respiration, and Valsalva maneuver (Brown et al., 2011). The function of the abdominal muscles is greatly affected by entry into the abdominal cavity during laparotomy. When an incision is made through the linea alba, the release of the weight causes lateralization of the rectus muscle and corresponding fascia. Lateralization of the abdominal wall is defined as movement of the rectus muscle and its associated fascia away from the midline over time. Lateralization causes a marked reduction in load applied to the oblique muscles, which eventually results in atrophy (Criss et al., 2014). The main goal following open abdominal procedures is to approximate the rectus and fascia in order to reestablish abdominal wall structure and function. In patients with abdominal wall defects (congenital, traumatic, or postoperative), simple approximation is not possible and it is necessary to reconstruct the abdominal wall. This requires use of structures capable of replicating the function of skin, fascia, and muscle whenever possible. Criss and colleagues (2014) used dynamometry to demonstrate a physiologic return of abdominal wall function 6 months following abdominal wall reconstruction (AWR) with a corresponding statistically significant increase in patient quality of life. Positive outcomes of AWR are largely dependent upon surgeon technique, proper selection of reinforcing mesh, and the patient's comorbidities and inherent ability to heal.

Management of the Open Abdomen

In situations in which approximation of the abdominal wall is not possible at the time of surgery, effective management of the open abdomen is important. Situations in which the abdomen must be left open include prevention or treatment of abdominal compartment syndrome (ACS), control of life-threatening intra-abdominal bleeding, and management of severe intra-abdominal sepsis (Atema et al., 2015). Specific approaches to management of the open abdomen are driven by the surgeon and are beyond the scope of this chapter. It should be noted that the longer the abdomen remains open, the greater the risk of complications. Kaplan and colleagues (2005) found that leaving the abdomen open for 7 to 10 days usually resulted in sufficient lateralization and adhesion formation to prevent primary closure. This is consistent with the findings of Rausei and colleagues (2014) who reported that reducing the time that the abdomen remained open was associated with a greater likelihood of closure and a decrease in complications. Conditions resulting in prolonged bowel edema, such as peritonitis and sepsis, are associated with increased risk of ACS if the rectus is closed prematurely. These patients may require a significant delay in wound closure, which results in a chronic open abdomen. NPWT has been used effectively to reduce edema and inflammation, permitting primary closure at a much earlier point (Plaudis et al., 2012). In some cases, the rectus cannot be approximated, and the resulting muscle atrophy will necessitate future AWR to reestablish normal function. Many techniques are used to reconstruct the abdominal wall, including advanced techniques such as separation of components, use of biologic materials, mesh traction, zipper closures, and dynamic sutures (Burlew et al., 2012).

KEY POINT

NPWT has been used effectively to reduce edema and inflammation associated with open abdominal wounds, permitting primary closure at a much earlier point.

INCISIONAL FAILURE FOLLOWING PRIMARY CLOSURE

Incisional failure is a common and significant postoperative complication, and risk of incisional failure is influenced by surgical technique, for example, material used to approximate the tissues and by the patient's comorbidities and ability to heal normally. In a wound left open to the fascia, incisional failure may result in evisceration. In an abdominal wound that is closed to the skin level, failure ranges from superficial skin dehiscence (partial dehiscence), to dehiscence down to the fascia (full dehiscence), to dehiscence of the fascia, to obvious evisceration. Failure may also be manifest as postoperative hernia formation. The linea alba is the most common site for hernia formation in the laparotomy patient. Incisional failure is related to either mechanical or biological risk factors.

Mechanical Risk Factors

Mechanical risk factors for incisional failure include conditions that result in application of excessive force to the newly approximated rectus and fascia. These forces include the weight of the abdominal pannus in a morbidly obese individual, intra-abdominal hypertension, sudden increases in intra-abdominal pressure, or ineffective suture technique. Sources of excessive abdominal pressures include benign activities, such as endotracheal suctioning, coughing, and deep breathing, or changes in position from lying to sitting. Excessive pressures may also result from abnormal bowel wall edema, intra-abdominal hypertension, and ACS. To manage these risks, surgeons may elect to use either synthetic or biologic mesh to support and reinforce the abdominal wall, with the goal of preventing incisional failure and hernia formation or recurrence. Evidence is inconclusive as to whether primary suture closure may be inferior to mesh repair in prevention of incisional failure. Hernia recurrence is higher when mesh is not utilized (Burns et al., 2020). The creation of an ostomy has been shown to create a midline shift toward the contralateral side, which alters rectus muscle thickness and innervation and increases mechanical stress on the suture line. Ostomy creation is also thought to increase the risk of incisional hernia.

Biologic Risk Factors

Biologic risk factors for incisional failure include comorbidities that alter fibroblast function and collagen synthesis, for example, ischemia, smoking, corticosteroid use, chronic obstructive pulmonary disease, morbid obesity, and infection. Obesity can be viewed as both a mechanical and biologic risk factors for incisional failure. This is concerning given the increase in the percentage of children and adults who are obese or morbidly obese. According to the Centers for Disease Control and Prevention (CDC), from 2015 to 2017, 8.1% of infants and toddlers, 18.5% of 2- to 19-year-olds, and 35.7% of adults 20 to 39 years of age and 42.8% of adults 40 to 59 were reported to be obese (Hales et al., 2017). Obesity is found to be highest in Hispanics (28.0%), non-Hispanic Blacks (19%), followed by non-Hispanic Whites (14.6%) and may vary according to socioeconomic status (Hales et al., 2020). Obesity increases the mechanical stress on the incision. Many obese individuals are found to have protein malnutrition, which compromises their ability to synthesize new connective tissue proteins. Malnutrition not only impedes wound healing and increases the risk of wound infection but has also been shown to increase the risk of pulmonary complications in abdominal surgery patients secondary to expiratory muscle weakness (Lunardi et al., 2012). Nutritional assessment and the involvement of a registered dietitian nutritionist (RDN) in the care of any patient at risk for nutritional compromise are important. Less common risk factors include congenital collagen disorders leading to reduced ability to produce collagen of normal tensile strength. This leads to a postoperative scenario where dehiscence may occur despite the best surgical technique. Another risk factor is severe abdominal trauma causing ischemic injury to the abdominal wall musculature, which requires excision and creates a permanent defect.

KEY POINT

Risk factors for incisional failure include mechanical factors that increase stress on the suture line such as morbid obesity, coughing, suctioning, or position changes and biologic risk factors that impair healing such as smoking, malnutrition, and steroid use.

MANAGING THE CHRONIC OPEN ABDOMEN AND FROZEN ABDOMEN

When consulted regarding the management of an open abdominal wound, the wound care nurse must conduct a focused history and physical, with specific attention paid to the operative note. In reviewing the operative note, the wound care nurse should note the type of surgery performed, any impact to the abdominal organs, reports of any complications, and the type of closure (closure to fascia level, approximation of all tissue and skin layers, or skin-only closure). It is important to correlate the structures visualized in the wound base with an understanding of the type of closure. In abdominal wounds that have been closed to the fascia, the wound care nurse should see intact, well-approximated fascial sutures in the wound base, as well as healthy subcutaneous tissue and dermis along the sidewalls of the wound (**Fig. 34-5**). In the presence of an intact fascial closure with no evidence of dehiscence or suture line tension, the underly-

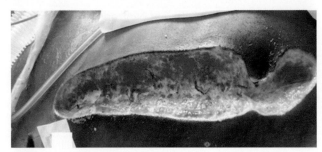

FIGURE 34-5. Wound Closed to Fascia Level.

ing abdominal organs are effectively protected. A fascial closure that is only partially intact due to areas of dehiscence can result in exposure of the bowel (**Fig. 34-6**). In progressive incisional failure and dehiscence, obvious evisceration may occur (**Fig. 34-7**) or there may be abdominal wall dehiscence with exposure of underlying abdominal organs (**Fig. 34-8**).

Each situation requires a different approach to wound management. Skin-only closure can look identical to primary closure, but they are very different and require different management (**Fig. 34-9**). A skin-only closure is used when primary fascial closure is not possible. Skin flaps are raised to provide superficial coverage of the large wound defect to decrease the risk of postoperative complications such as enteroatmospheric fistula formation. In these two examples, therapy options and expectations are inherently different based upon the anatomy underlying the skin incision. A request to manage an at-risk incision with ciNPWT would require appropriate assessment of the incision in a skin-only closure for any signs of bowel exposure (**Fig. 34-10**) to determine the safety of such therapy and to provide protection of any sensitive structures during wound care.

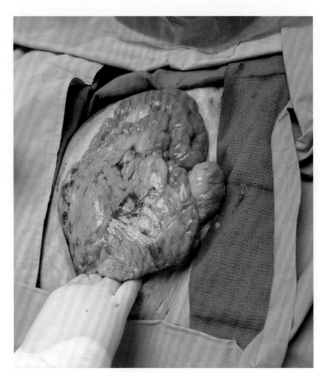

FIGURE 34-7. Evisceration.

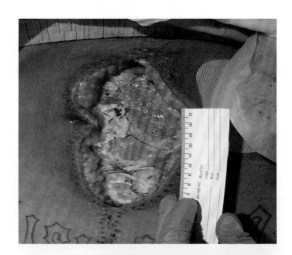

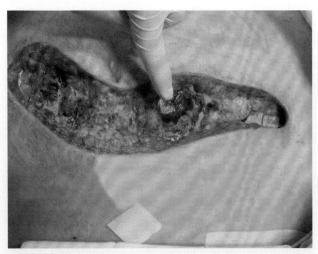

FIGURE 34-6. Wound Closed to Fascia Level with Partial Dehiscence.

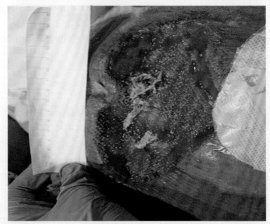

FIGURE 34-8. Abdominal Wound Dehiscence with Partial Organ Exposure.

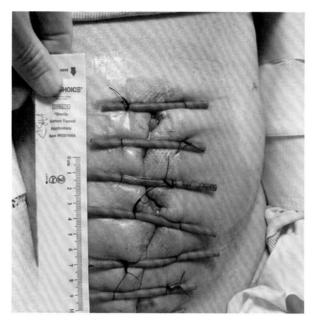

FIGURE 34-9. Skin-Only Closure.

KEY POINT

In assessing an open abdominal wound and making recommendations for care, it is important to correlate the structures visualized in the wound base with the type of closure.

Plan of Care

Before providing wound care recommendations on the postoperative abdominal wound, the wound care nurse should ensure that there is communication with the surgeon regarding any structures exposed in the wound

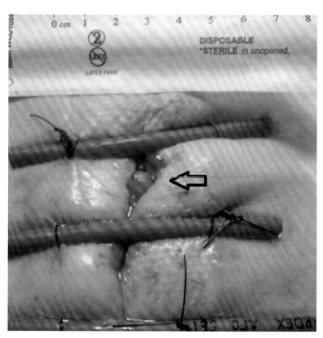

FIGURE 34-10. Skin-Only Closure with Bowel Exposure.

bed and the plan of care for the patient. When complex wounds are presented, a bedside meeting for discussion and visualization of the structures is recommended.

Depending on the specific wound and type of abdominal wall closure (AWC), the plan of care may include one or more of the following:

1. Primary closure of all tissue/skin layers: Support for healing and prevention of complications, either via advanced incisional dressings or ciNPWT.

2. Primary fascial and skin closure with the use of synthetic or biologic mesh: The wound care nurse should be aware of common complications with both synthetic and biologic mesh to enhance assessment of the closed incision. The location of placement of the mesh should be known so that in the case of incisional failure and mesh exposure, the anatomy can be more readily identified. Supportive wound care may involve either ciNPWT or advanced incisional dressings.

3. Delayed primary fascial closure: Use of a temporary open abdomen technique such as intra-abdominal NPWT (e.g., ABTHERA®) may be utilized to achieve a rapid reduction in edema and enhanced neoangiogenesis in preparation for delayed primary closure (**Fig. 34-11**).

4. Closure of the abdominal wall to fascia level using reinforced biologic mesh or bridged biologic mesh: the patient returns from surgery with an open abdominal wound to the layer of the reinforced mesh closure. The goal is to promote ingrowth of granulation tissue and incorporation of the mesh into the granulation tissue, which will allow for secondary or delayed primary closure of the skin and subcutaneous tissues. The mesh placement location should be known so that the wound care nurse can accurately identify any separation or disintegration of the mesh and can distinguish the mesh from other underlying structures. Management frequently involves traditional NPWT with careful attention to protection of any exposed mesh.

5. Open abdominal wound with exposed abdominal organs (viscera) and omentum, due to inability to close the abdominal wall: Inflammatory adhesions and granulation may result in the exposed organs (small and large intestine, liver) becoming one large visceral mass without distinguishable anatomy (known as a frozen abdomen). Goal is either a skin-only closure or granulation over the exposed structures with or without absorbable mesh in preparation for eventual skin graft closure. Direct topical therapy over exposed organs requires coordination with surgical team with focus on patient safety, maintenance of acceptable levels of moisture and core body temperature, and complication prevention.

6. NOTE: In the case of no. 4 or 5 above, the wound care nurse and the patient should be aware that

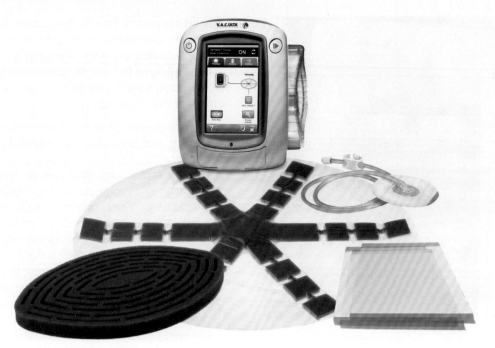

FIGURE 34-11. Intra-abdominal NPWT. (ABTHERA® open abdomen dressing. Used with Permission. Courtesy of 3M.)

without correction of the abdominal wall defect and achievement of a complete fascial closure, the patient will likely need a subsequent surgery 3 to 6 months in the future for definitive AWR.

Specific considerations for the provision of topical therapy for open abdominal wounds include the anatomical structures involved and the presence of exposed mesh. There is a correlation between the load strain achieved by the closure of the abdominal wall and reestablishment of normal anatomical alignment and wound healing outcomes. Mechanotransduction is the process that allows living organisms to respond to their mechanical environment. The principles of mechanotransduction are where normal mechanical forces impact cellular signaling and the proliferative response of fibroblasts. In the case of incisional failure and hernia development, this alteration in normal mechanical load may interfere with normal cell signaling and may impair normal wound healing.

KEY POINT

Specific considerations in providing care for open abdominal wounds include identification and protection of the anatomical structures involved and of exposed mesh.

For abdominal wounds that are open to the fascial sutures, assessment is focused on the continued approximation of the fascial closure, the viability of the tissue, any signs of abdominal distention, and the presence of developing necrosis or signs and symptoms of infection. Patients with intact fascial closures may be managed

with the principles of wound bed preparation and attention to systemic factors affecting healing (**Fig. 34-12**). Certain principles of wound bed preparation should be modified dependent upon wound presentation. Instrumental debridement should never be performed when it involves the fascial suture line as this may cause dehiscence or evisceration. Unless warranted by the surgeon's evaluation, noninstrumental approaches to debridement, such as autolysis, and dressings to reduce bacterial loads are usually more appropriate. Signs of dehiscence should be reported to the surgeon immediately to determine the plan of care. The wound care nurse should reassess the appropriateness of current topical therapy recommendations based upon the possible exposure of underlying structures such as bowel (**Fig. 34-13**).

KEY POINT

Patients with intact fascial structures can be managed with principles of wound bed preparation. Instrumental debridement of the fascial suture line should never be performed due to the risk for dehiscence or evisceration.

Since the underlying viscera is protected in these wounds, wound care follows the principles of wound bed preparation and support of granulation tissue. While there is limited evidence to support its use in all cases, an abdominal binder is often recommended following primary closure in at-risk patients to provide support to the patient especially during activities associated with increased intra-abdominal pressure.

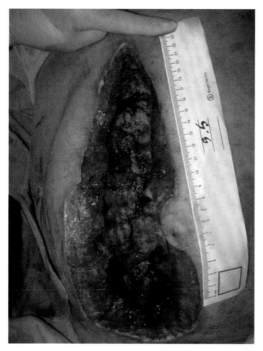
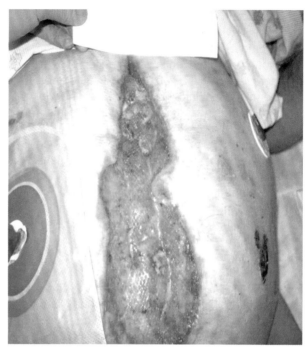

FIGURE 34-12. Tension-Free Fascial Closure with Granulation.

The wound care nurse should assess tension exerted on the wound edges as well as viability of the tissue present in the wound and the quantity of granulation tissue.

Following contaminated surgeries, such as colorectal surgery or laparotomy following a perforation, ostomy creation, or bowel resection, the wound is often left open to heal by secondary intention to monitor for signs and

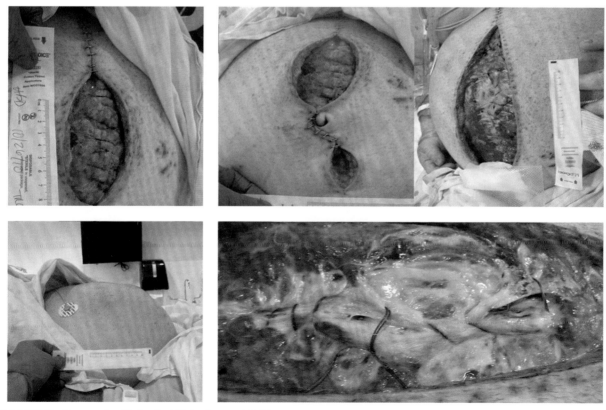

FIGURE 34-13. Progressive Abdominal Distention and Dehiscence.

symptoms of infection and viability of the subcutaneous tissues. As opposed to healing with granulation, techniques that promote approximation of the edges of the granulating wound while preventing the creation of dead space can improve both clinical and aesthetic outcomes. Once it is determined that the wound is proliferating well with granulation tissue and there is no evidence of infection, either delayed primary closure or a variety of surgical wick techniques should be considered. **Figure 34-14** shows an example of interrupted incisional closure in the OR combined with use of NPWT sponges as wicks. The sponges were dipped into antimicrobial solutions and packed into the full-thickness openings down to the fascial closure, to minimize wound size while allowing for continued wound monitoring. **Figure 34-15** shows a wick technique used for a morbidly obese patient following heart transplantation. This patient underwent 1 week of standard NPWT to produce adequate granulation tissue followed by interrupted incisional closure and use of NPWT sponges as wicks. The wicks were changed routinely with reduction in depth as the wound filled with granulation tissue. While this was not an abdominal wound, the management technique was the same. This

technique promotes granulation as well as closure of the wound edges, while managing exudate and providing ongoing monitoring for infection. A multitude of options for wound bed management are available that are based on the principles of moist wound healing. The specific option should be selected based on wound characteristics and individualized patient assessment.

KEY POINT

In managing large open wounds, techniques that promote wound edge approximation while preventing the creation of dead space can improve both clinical and aesthetic outcomes.

Critical Assessment Factors

Before assessing and making recommendations for chronic open abdominal wound management, one of the most important questions to ascertain is if there were any new anastomoses or enterotomies created during the surgery. The question is important in the prevention of the enteroatmospheric and enterocutaneous

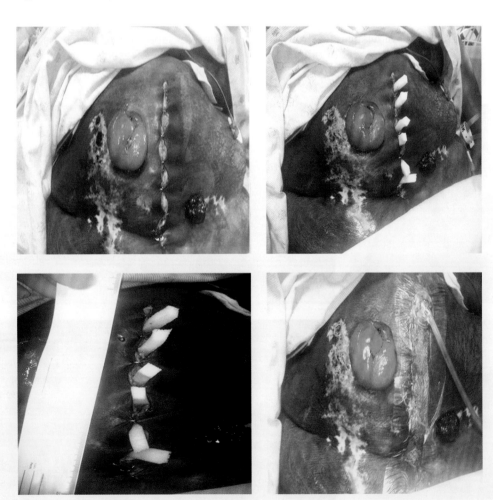

FIGURE 34-14. Interrupted Surgical Technique with "Wicks."

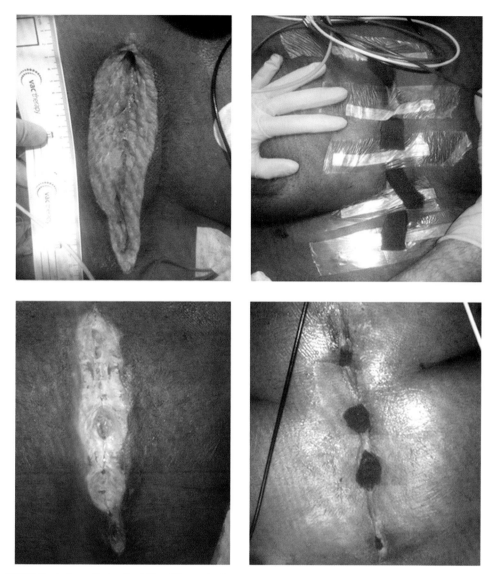

FIGURE 34-15. "Wick" Technique Status Post Heart Transplant.

fistula (ECF). Despite the many causes of fistula known in the literature, 85% of fistulas occur as the result of an anastomotic leak. The wound care nurse should discuss the location of any new anastomosis or the existence of any incidental enterotomies created and closed during surgery. The goal is to determine if they are buried or superficial. The surgeon will attempt to protect these sites by placing them deep in the abdominal cavity if the bowel is sufficiently mobile. In situations where there is omental covering for protection of the new anastomosis or closed enterotomy or where the involved area of bowel has been placed in the depth of the cavity away from the wound surface, more advanced therapies such as NPWT may be utilized (**Fig. 34-16**). Multiple studies show that with proper understanding and application of NPWT, there is relatively low risk for a NPWT-induced ECF. When there is a superficial anastomosis or enterotomy, NPWT is usually considered contraindicated due

to risk of fistula formation. If NPWT is used in this type of situation, it is important to use low-pressure settings and to protect the wound surface with a contact layer (or several nonadherent contact layers) or a nonadherent layer of foam.

KEY POINT

When managing an open abdominal wound, the wound care nurse must determine whether there are any new anastomoses or repaired enterotomies that lie close to the wound surface. If so, NPWT should be avoided or used with contact layers and low pressure settings.

When working with exposed bowel or organ structures, there is no evidence-based, dressing-specific topical therapy recommendations. The wound care nurse should keep the following principles in mind: atraumatic, autolytic,

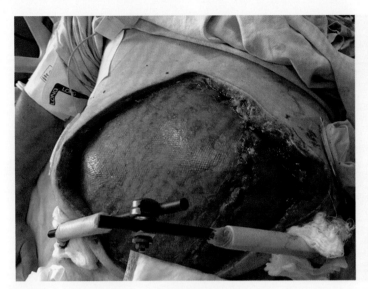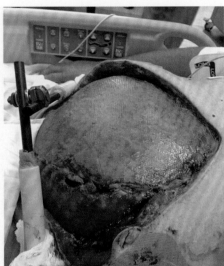

FIGURE 34-16. Open Abdomen with Residual Omentum under Vicryl Mesh.

normothermic wound care or atraumatic, autolytic, antimicrobial, normothermic wound care, with attention to minimizing the frequency of dressing changes. The wound care nurse should never perform sharp debridement over organ structures secondary to the risk of inadvertent trauma, enterotomy, or bleeding. Due to the excellent perfusion of the abdominal viscera, autolysis usually provides sufficient debridement of any necrotic tissue. In cases of the chronic open abdomen, multiple strategies exist: advanced wound dressings, NPWT with atraumatic application technique and nonadherent contact layer, and wound pouching. Due to the high moisture vapor transmission rate and poor insulation and barrier function of gauze-based products, advanced dressings are often preferred. Specific therapy decisions must be based on thorough patient and wound assessment. A moist warm wound environment is important if organs are exposed, to prevent serosal inflammation and wound bed desiccation. This can be accomplished with many products. Volume of exudate and exposed structures are the key factors to be considered in product selection. Transparent film dressings are selected as the cover dressing due to their ability to trap ambient moisture and maintain wound bed temperature. Contact layers must be used in the wound base to prevent trauma to exposed organs. Silicone contact layers are preferred as they will not change their structure or function over time. Some petrolatum-based products may actually adhere to the wound bed over time, with dehydration or dilution of the petrolatum. Between the contact layer and the secondary dressing, appropriate packing materials include roll gauze or large sheets of alginate or hydrofiber. In wounds with very little exudate, hydrogels may be the most appropriate option. The wound care nurse must consider safety issues when selecting products for wound care. When selecting filler and wicking agents for wounds with extensive undermining, the goal is to reduce the number of dressing pieces used and to clearly communicate

with care providers how many dressing pieces have been placed into the wound.

The chronic open or frozen abdomen is often managed with NPWT due to the ability to create granulation tissue in a relative short amount of time. This therapy should only be chosen if there are no known superficial anastomoses or enterotomy closure sites present and following discussion with the surgeon. If NPWT is used in this situation, it is important to use nonadherent dressings in the wound bed and to assure atraumatic dressing or sponge removal. In determining the level of protection needed, the wound care nurse must consider the presence of omental coverage and the amount of granulation tissue covering the wound bed and the underlying organs. In addition to assuring appropriate use of nonadherent contact layers or foam, whenever there are exposed organs or anastomoses close to the surface of the wound, the wound care nurse should initiate negative suction at settings much lower than the standard settings recommended by the manufacturer. Initial settings of −25 to −50 mm Hg should be utilized, with slow titration to higher levels based upon wound presentation and amount of granulation.

In the event that NPWT is not recommended due to the presence of anastomoses or enterotomies, and advanced topical dressings are complicated by a large wound surface area, the use of wound pouches or fistula pouches should be considered. Benefits include the moist environment created by the pouch, along with the ability to manage high levels of exudate and to access the wound frequently for assessment if necessary. Some of these pouches have multiple port sites that can be placed to bedside drainage systems to manage large volumes of exudate. Another option is to connect the pouching system to wall suction on a low setting. If this is contraindicated for any reason, it must be clearly communicated to the staff. An additional advantage provided by pouching systems is protection of the periwound skin and prevention of periwound moisture–associated skin damage (PMASD) and the associated increase in risk of infection (Colwell et al., 2011). One negative consideration in use of pouching systems for chronic open abdomen management is that sterile packaging may or may not be available. The use of a clean pouch should be discussed with the surgeon to determine appropriateness of use. In most cases, this is not a problem since an open abdomen is already colonized with bacteria. In extreme cases involving massive bowel wall edema secondary to peritonitis and ACS, a large pouching system may be used to accommodate the eviscerated organs (**Fig. 34-17**). Complex patients requires definitive collaboration between the wound care nurse and the surgical team.

THE ENTEROATMOSPHERIC FISTULA

ECFs are characterized by the connection of an internal organ to the skin, whereas enteroenteric fistulas involve two or more organs such as an ileocolonic fistula, and enteroatmospheric fistulas (EAF) are a connection between an organ system and the air, such as with a complex open abdomen (Brindle, 2012). Fistula management is discussed in detail in Chapter 36. The discussion in this chapter will be limited to description of a technique for isolating the fistula and the enteric output from the wound bed, permitting use of NPWT to the wound if indicated.

KEY POINT

Enterocutaneous fistulas (ECF) are characterized by connection of the bowel to the skin, while enteroatmospheric fistulas (EAF) involve connection of the bowel to an open wound.

Multiple techniques for EAF isolation have been described in the literature (Brindle, 2012; Brindle & Blankenship, 2009; Heineman et al., 2015; Reider, 2017). An early technique based on the ability to provide complete fecal stream diversion allows for skin grafting in the presence of a high-output small bowel EAF. It is referred to as the Brindle and Whelan glove isolation technique. Brindle and Whelan technique has been shown to provide up to 1 week of fecal diversion at a time, while allowing for repetitive dressing changes of the surrounding wound. The technique is best created in the operating room using a latex orthopedic glove to create a platform for pouching (**Fig. 34-18**).

Commercially available fistula isolation devices include Wound Crown®, Fistula Funnel®, and Isolator Strips®. These devices are used in conjunction with NPWT and ostomy pouches to contain effluent, promote wound closure, and reduce frequency of dressing changes (NSWOCC, 2018) (**Fig. 34-19**). For detailed step-by-step instructions, see Nurses Specializing in Wound Ostomy Continence Canada (NSWOCC) best practice recommendations at http://www.flipbookserver.com/?PID=1000959.

KEY POINT

Effective management of an enteric fistula emptying into an open wound bed frequently requires isolation of the fistula. This allows for the containment and quantification of effluent and promotes wound closure with reduced frequency of dressing changes.

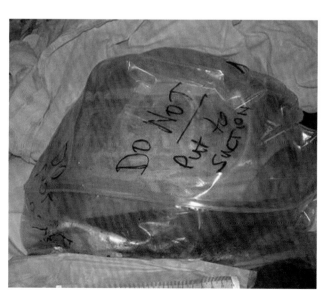

FIGURE 34-17. Open Abdominal Wound Managed with Large Wound Pouch.

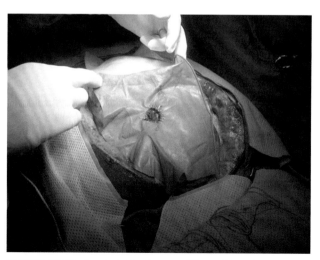

FIGURE 34-18. Surgical Attachment of Open Glove Square to Os of Fistula.

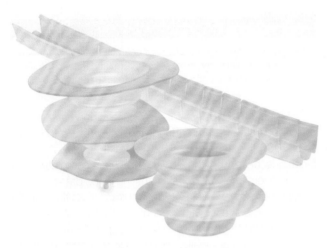

FIGURE 34-19. Commercial Fistula Isolation Devices.

⬤ MANAGEMENT OF WOUNDS CLOSED WITH MESH

Synthetic and biologic mesh products are occasionally used to provide abdominal closure intending to prevent hernia formation. There is no evidence to support the use of biologic or biosynthetic meshes in the prevention of incisional and parastomal hernias. In complex abdominal wall hernia repairs (incarcerated hernia, parastomal hernia, infected mesh, open abdomen, ECF, and component separation technique), biologic and biosynthetic meshes do not provide a superior alternative to synthetic meshes (Köckerling et al., 2018). International guidelines do not recommend routine use of biologic or biosynthetic meshes in early closure of the open abdomen in favor of alternate techniques, for example, NPWT, mechanical closure devices, or primary closure.

Factors influencing hernia recurrence were reported by Satterwhite et al. (2012) and include the following: history of more than two prior hernia repairs, postoperative complications such as infection, over-lay mesh placement, use of human-derived allograft, and surgeon technique. While potentially reducing the risk of incisional failure and hernia recurrence, mesh is not without its own inherent risks. Wound infections were found to be more frequent in patients undergoing mesh repair than in patients closed with primary suture repair (Köckerling et al., 2018).

Both synthetic and biologic mesh products are utilized to strengthen/support the abdominal wall, to close a defect in the rectus abdominis that cannot be primarily approximated, or to serve as a bridge between large rectus defects in order to protect the underlying viscera. Selection of the specific mesh to be used is largely surgeon specific. The evidence supporting mesh selection is variable with some of the data available are limited to animal studies. Evidence-based guidance is conflicting. Biologics are frequently selected rather than synthetics in the following situations: when there is contamination, when there are concerns regarding injury to the bowel,

when the patient has comorbidities that increase the risk of infection or impaired healing, or when large surface areas are involved (Köckerling et al., 2018).

There are no data regarding the best options for topical therapy in wounds with mesh products. Exposure of synthetic mesh is usually indicative of impaired healing and infection, and surgical excision may be warranted. The surgeon should be notified if there is suspected mesh exposure within a dehisced abdominal wound.

TYPES OF MESH

In order to discuss wound assessment, topical therapy selection, and management of abdominal wounds with exposed biologics, the wound care nurse must first understand what a biologic mesh is and the expected response of the host to an implanted biologic.

Biologic meshes are acellular ECM products. The matrix is composed of collagen, elastin, glycoproteins, and retained vascular channels from either cadaveric, bovine, or porcine sources. The source of the ECM, the method in which the tissue was harvested, and any chemical modifications made by the manufacturer all impact the response of the host. An implanted biologic is compatible with the host tissue and provides support for regeneration and remodeling of the host tissue. The product should not cause a significant inflammatory response, resulting in resorption of the biologic secondary to protease degradation. A determinant of how the body will respond to these products is the level of antigenicity that remains following product preparation and preservation.

There are two important assessment factors: surgical location of the mesh and the name brand of mesh used. The wound care nurse may find the brand name of mesh used in the operative note. Knowing this information will provide guidance in terms of anticipated time until granulation and what to expect from both a visual and olfactory presentation of the mesh. There are no studies to determine which product is better suited for AWR, and in most institutions, surgeons have a variety of options and select these products based on the needs of the individual patient.

ASSESSMENT GUIDELINES

When a mesh is exposed in the wound bed, the wound care nurse should contact the surgeon to determine the type of mesh implanted. This information will provide guidance in terms of expectations and assessment parameters. Some types of mesh will typically show evidence of granulation within 7 to 14 days, while others may take >4 weeks to show signs of granulation. As a mesh begins to granulate, it often appears to be disintegrating or breaking down within the wound bed. If the mesh has small areas of granulation and areas of apparent disintegration (resembling slough), this would be indicative of normal progression (**Fig. 34-20**). All biologic meshes

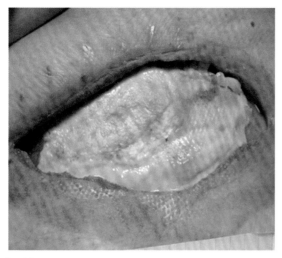
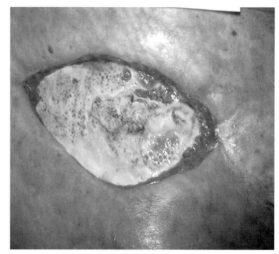

FIGURE 34-20. Progressive Vascularization of Mesh.

produce an odor, which is sometimes strong and often mistaken for fistula formation. Thorough assessment is necessary to determine if there are any other signs or symptoms of infection associated with the wound and whether antimicrobial therapy is required. The mesh should appear flat and taut in the wound bed, with no evidence of buckling. When the mesh buckles or folds, it is no longer adherent to the underlying wound bed and cannot be appropriately vascularized. This separation of the mesh from the wound bed can lead to seroma or

abscess formation under the mesh, which may result in mesh destruction and removal (**Fig. 34-21**). If buckling is seen, this should be reported to the surgeon.

TOPICAL THERAPY FOR EXPOSED BIOLOGIC MESH

Biologic mesh was designed to either provide secondary structural support to a wound managed with primary closure or to provide primary coverage of an abdominal wall defect. The intent is to cover the mesh with granu-

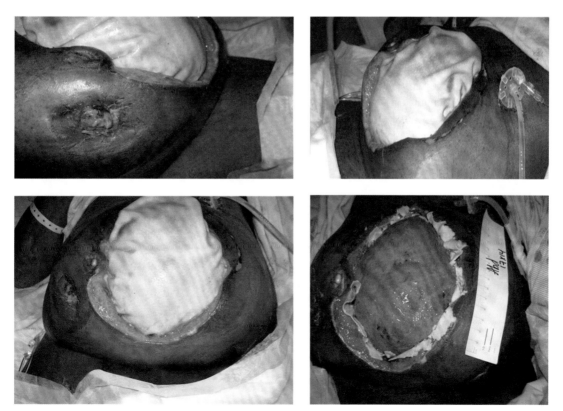

FIGURE 34-21. Mesh that is Buckling and has to be Removed.

lation, while managing moisture and protecting against infection. Management of exposed mesh requires creation of an environment that prevents mesh desiccation, controls bioburden, and protects against trauma. The wound care nurse needs to assess the mesh for the amount of surface area exposed and drainage present, as larger areas of exposure will require attention to maintaining adequate levels of moisture.

Biologic mesh may be considered preferable to synthetic mesh in contaminated wounds because of its greater resistance to infection. Biologic mesh may still get infected. As the biologic mesh begins to granulate, there may be residual areas that never become viable, and these areas will ultimately slough out of the wound. During this process, the nonviable mesh looks very similar to necrotic slough. In the postoperative period, the wound care nurse should never use conservative sharp debridement since the underlying mesh may be adherent to bowel, and debridement may result in accidental enterotomy. Debridement of any nonviable or nongranulating mesh should be accomplished conservatively by autolytic techniques (**Fig. 34-22**).

There are no evidence-based recommendations for appropriate topical therapy to be utilized with biologic mesh. The following recommendations are based upon principles of wound care and biology of the mesh.

Biologic mesh is composed of connective tissue proteins, and since ingrowth of granulation tissue is dependent on fibroblast activity, cytotoxic and debriding products should be avoided. Examples of products to avoid would be the application of topical endogenous collagenases, cytotoxic concentrations of antimicrobials such as ¼, ½, or full-strength Dakin solution, hydrogen peroxide, acetic acid, etc. The focus of wound bed preparation with exposed mesh is on irrigation, maintenance of a moist wound surface, minimizing the frequency of dressing changes, reducing the risk of trauma, and

reducing bioburden. NPWT continues to be used in the management of open wounds with biologic mesh. The wound care nurse may modify standard procedures to assure maintenance of sufficient moisture at the wound surface and to prevent trauma with dressing removal. For example, large areas of exposed biologic mesh may either require hydrophilic foam or moisture retentive contact layers utilizing petrolatum. Wounds with large volumes of exudate or wounds involving small areas of exposed mesh may benefit from NPWT using hydrophobic foam or gauze. Suction settings are typically set between –75 and –125 mm Hg to manage exudate.

> ### KEY POINT
>
> When managing a wound with exposed mesh, the wound care nurse should avoid use of any products that could cause breakdown of connective tissue proteins. This includes enzymes (collagenase) and antiseptics (e.g., Dakin solution or acetic acid).

Irrigation with 500 to 1,000 cc of normal saline should be used to decrease bioburden and removed using suction. If high levels of bioburden are suspected, irrigation should continue, either with saline or a noncytotoxic solution such as hypochlorous acid (HOCl) or polyhexamethylene biguanide. The use of these products should be short term as their use with biologic mesh has not been studied. Dry wounds with mesh exposure and possible infection may benefit from use of a wound pouching system to maintain moisture or use of hydrogel applied daily with a moisture retentive dressing. For wounds with moderate to high volumes of exudate, either alginates or hydrofibers may be selected. High release silver dressings have the potential of staining the mesh, which may interfere with assessment. Alternatives to silver

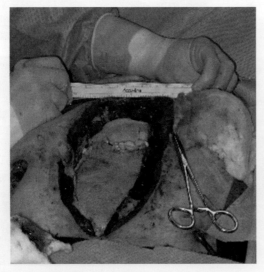
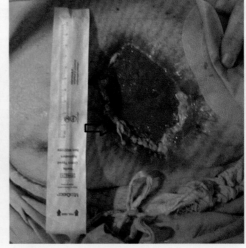

FIGURE 34-22. Nonviable Residual Mesh.

could be any noncytotoxic broad-spectrum topical such as cadexomer iodine, dialkylcarbomoyl chloride (DACC)-coated dressings, Manuka honey, or products known to be bacteriostatic such as hydroconductive nonadherent dressing with LevaFiber technology or methylene blue–gentian violet foams. There are no evidence-based guidelines to determine the most appropriate product. Additional options include NPWT with instillation. Benefits of instillation include reports of antibiofilm activity and enhanced promotion of granulation tissue as compared to NPWT (Gupta et al., 2016). Its use with exposed biologic mesh has not been sufficiently studied. Standard moist wound healing provides adequate support for both autolysis and granulation tissue formation. Management of all biologic meshes involves the avoidance of wet-to-dry dressings due to the risk of desiccation.

KEY POINT

In management of any open abdominal wound with exposed mesh, topical therapy should include 500 to 1,000 mL irrigation with saline to reduce bacterial loads.

 ## MANAGEMENT OF THE POSTSTERNOTOMY WOUND AND OPEN CHEST

Care of the patient poststernotomy from cardiothoracic surgery involves similar considerations as described above in the management of the open abdomen. In the case of the poststernotomy wound, the surgeon must close and stabilize the sternum, followed by either a primary closure of the muscle, soft tissues, and skin or by closure to fascia level followed by delayed secondary closure of the full-thickness wound. In selected cases involving surgical complications, the surgeon may opt to leave the chest open and provide delayed sternal closure following stabilization of the patient. Each clinical situation will be addressed from the standpoint of important assessment and management principles.

PRIMARY CLOSURE

Primary closure is achieved by the closure of the sternum, fascia, muscle, subcutaneous tissue, and skin. Protocols for incisional management include sterile dressing application in the operating room with removal after 48 to 72 hours of the operative procedure. Daily cleansing either with tap water, saline or with antimicrobials such as chlorhexidine gluconate (CHG). Patients at risk for wound dehiscence may benefit from the application of ciNPWT after surgery. Assessment criteria for the closed sternal incision involves evaluation of epithelialization, signs of underlying complications such as seroma or hematoma, or signs of infection. Examples of infection may include increasing erythema, induration, warmth, pain, and drainage; elevated white blood cell count; and elevated protein C. Devascularized tissues, such as adipose tissue in obese populations or to the sternum itself after left internal mammary artery harvesting, may be present. Following complete epithelialization of the incision, a natural biologic barrier to bacterial invasion is reestablished. Epithelialization does not signify complete healing, as there may be failure to form sufficient granulation tissue for healing of the underlying soft tissues and/or failure of bony union of the sternum.

Sternal Healing

The sternum itself may take upward of 3 to 6 months to heal despite adequate soft tissue closure (Cohen & Griffin, 2002), making sternal approximation and reinforcement the most important aspect of wound management long term; if the sternum does not heal appropriately, the patient experiences long-term instability of the chest wall. Sternal dehiscence is most often due to infectious complications but can also be caused by noninfectious impediments to wound healing. A factor leading to noninfectious dehiscence is sternal motion and instability occurring following surgery. Sternal closure technique has also been identified as a contributing factor, though controversy exists as to the best technique for ensuring stability of the sternum and preventing late nonunion, reoperation, or mediastinitis.

KEY POINT

Assessment of a closed sternal wound must include inspection and palpation to detect indicators of sternal closure breakdown. For example, sternal movement during respiration and coughing, sternal click, sudden onset of increasing pain, bubbling along the closure line, and exudate indicate wound healing problems. The wound care nurse should avoid any aggressive probing of undermined or tunneled areas.

Assessment of Sternal Healing

Due to the significance of sternal separation and failure to heal, manual palpation of the sternum is recommended in addition to the standard assessment for evidence of skin or soft tissue infection. The wound care nurse should place one finger on each side of the sternal incision and should feel for sternal movement during inspiration/expiration and coughing. The wound care nurse should also listen and feel for an audible sternal click, which indicates that the sternal edges are moving against each other. Sudden onset of increasing pain is another potential indicator of sternal separation. Any indicators of sternal movement should be reported to the surgeon. The ability to express seropurulent exudate, clear amber exudate, or old bloody drainage should be reported to the surgeon since these findings are indicators of infection, seroma, or necrotic fat. If there is partial skin dehiscence, the wound care nurse should assess for signs of underlying air movement, bubbling, or disappearance of any irrigated saline. The wound care nurse should strictly avoid aggressive probing of any undermined or tunneled areas, as forceful exploration could result in subsequent dehiscence or entrance into a deeper cavity. The wound care nurse should use caution in placing wicking material into blind tunnels, as the difference between barometric pressure and intrathoracic pressure in wounds with sternal separation may result in a sucking chest wound, which could cause the packing strip to be sucked into the deep recesses of the wound or chest cavity and out of the visual field of the wound care nurse.

Sternal dehiscence may heal on its own or may require surgical intervention. In a retrospective study by Nazerali and colleagues (2014), investigators found complete sternal healing with no evidence of mediastinitis in 57 high-risk patients who underwent rigid sternal fixation using a variety of sternal fixation-plate devices. The results suggest that prophylactic use of rigid fixation may safely be considered in high-risk cases, especially those prone to mediastinitis. In the case of chronic dehiscence and nonunion, debridement with rewiring or debridement with muscle flaps is often required (Olbrecht et al., 2006).

STERNAL CLOSURE WITH OPEN CHEST WOUND

Sternal closure to the fascia leaving an open full-thickness wound may be the best surgical approach for patients at high risk for impaired healing or infection or the patient who has undergone multiple sternotomies (**Figs. 34-23 and 34-24**). The approach allows the surgical team to monitor the patient for any signs or symptoms of infection, necrosis, or wound deterioration and provides for immediate intervention. The goal in the management of the wound is establishment of sufficient granulation tissue to allow for secondary closure or delayed primary

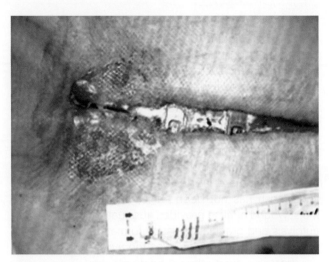

FIGURE 34-24. Chest Wound Open to the Sternum with Talon Exposure.

closure. When managing the wounds, the wound care nurse must provide appropriate wound bed preparation and moist wound healing and must also monitor for sternum closure. In many cases, the sternum and sternal wires are exposed, necessitating sterile technique for dressing changes in addition to assessment for proper sternal approximation and any signs of sternal nonunion or dehiscence. The wound care nurse should provide several minutes of direct visualization of the sternum during normal breathing or any episodes of coughing and should be alert to any signs of fluctuation. If any evidence of sternal fluctuation is found, the surgeon should be notified so that the plan of care can be reviewed.

NPWT is selected in these situations to provide sternal stability, prevent frequent changes in intrathoracic pressure changes, and decrease the risk of retained wound exudate in the thoracic cavity. Some modifications in standard wound care that should be incorporated when there is sternal separation: gentle cleansing with normal saline and avoidance of high-volume irrigations, to prevent retention of fluid in the chest cavity. As with all filler dressings, documentation of the number, type, and location of packing materials to prevent retention of dressings is needed. When NPWT is not recommended (e.g., in wounds complicated by infection or necrosis), the wound care nurse should recommend a filler dressing that provides sufficient absorptive capacity to meet the wound's needs, while allowing for ease of removal and prevention of retained dressings.

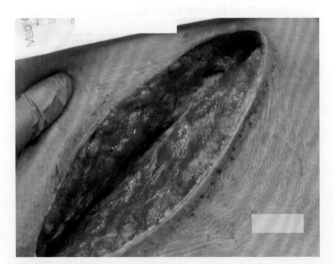

FIGURE 34-23. Chest Wound Closed to Fascia Level.

KEY POINT

NPWT may be indicated for wounds with sternal separation, to provide increased stability, and to reduce the risk of retained exudate in the thoracic cavity.

When no sternal fluctuation is seen, and the primary sternal closure is stable, the wound care nurse can implement wound healing principles. One exception to recommendations for wound bed preparation would be to avoid sharp debridement along the sternal closure. There is often a layer of fascia over the wires that may be mistaken for necrosis. Inappropriate debridement of the sternal closure may result in sternal wire rupture, debridement of the fascia, and increased risk of sternal dehiscence.

Patients with full-thickness wounds after hardware insertion experience pain. Patients undergoing implantation of a ventricular access device (VAD, LVAD, RVAD, BiVAD) or total artificial heart (TAH) report little to no pain with sternal wound dressing changes but exhibit hypersensitivity of the periwound skin, especially in response to adhesive removal. Measures should be implemented to reduce the risk of pain and MARSI (McNichol et al., 2013) such as the use of contact layers, liquid skin protectants to the periwound skin, use of silicone-based or gel-based adhesive removers, and limiting the skin surface covered by adhesive products.

Cardiac surgery patients are also at higher risk for bleeding because they are typically anticoagulated. Their coagulation levels can change suddenly, and they may require repeated laboratory studies prior to wound care. The wound care nurse may need to consult with the surgeon about delaying or postponing NPWT dressing change due to concerns over bleeding. The wound care nurse should always have a plan for establishing hemostasis in the event of acute bleeding, such as the use of kaolin impregnated gauze agents (Quick Clot®), cellulose-based products (Surgicel®/Surgifoam®), or cautery agents such as silver nitrate. Primary dressings should be selected based on their nonadherent quality. Options include nonadherent contact layers with and without NPWT, alginates, hydrofibers, hydrogels, and avoidance of wet-to-dry dressings. Patients who are status post heart transplantation require systemic immunosuppressive agents and are at greater risk for infection. Malnutrition delays wound healing and increases the risk of infection. For these patients, advanced dressings may be indicated earlier in the management process to minimize the effects of the proinflammatory and antiangiogenic wound environment. Complex therapies such as noncontact low-frequency ultrasound have also been shown to be beneficial by reducing inflammation and promoting angiogenesis.

OPEN CHEST WITH DELAYED STERNAL CLOSURE

While the closed, superficial, and deep open wound care are within the scope of practice for the wound care nurse, but open chest management (OCM) is the surgeon's domain. Wound care nurses are often asked for recommendations regarding management of these complex wounds and must be knowledgeable regarding the principles underlying appropriate management. In cases where the sternum cannot be closed with usual surgical techniques, plastic surgery will be consulted. Bota et al. (2019) in a retrospective cohort study including 58 patients who received standardized latissimus dorsi flap coverage of a sternum defect wound after post-sternotomy mediastinitis found that all patients showed complete wound healing on follow-up. They found that the latissimus dorsi pedicled flap is a safe, reproducible technique for coverage of deep sternal wounds, with few relevant perioperative complications (Bota et al., 2019). Sears et al. (2017) found that a delay in flap closure was associated with greater mortality and resource use. The wound care nurse should be knowledgeable regarding the following: reasons for delayed sternal closure; principles of sternal stabilization, sternal padding, and ventricular protection; and the principles underlying successful use of NPWT for OCM.

The incidence of OCM has been reported between 1% and 4% in adult cardiac surgery and as high as 50% following ventricular assist device surgeries (Wong et al., 2017). Medium duration of OCM was 3 days, with the following comorbid conditions including male gender, diabetes mellitus, cardiac dysfunction, and postoperative complications.

A retrospective study found no difference in infectious complications between a primary sternal closure control and an OCM group, despite the fact that the OCM group were higher acuity and required frequent reentries for bleeding. Additional studies should be conducted given the projected increased use of ventricular assist devices (VAD). The number of patients with heart failure in the United States is expected to exceed 8 million people by 2030 and be the leading cause of disability in the country. It is estimated that <10% of patients will qualify for heart transplant given the current shortages in donor organs (Colvin et al., 2016). With VAD and TAH procedures becoming the standard of care for advanced heart failure (44.9% of all patients in 2014), providers will need to manage OCM especially with the high reported rates of postoperative bleeding in these patients (Aissaoui et al., 2018; Allen et al., 2013; Silva Enciso, 2016). A study of trauma patients undergoing emergent thoracotomy found no difference in the rate of infections or survival between temporary OCM versus definitive closure. However, the open chest patients had significantly lower peak inspiratory pressures compared to their closed counterparts (Lang et al., 2011).

Neonatal and pediatric studies support similar indications for the use of an open chest technique following cardiac surgery. Because of the small size of their chests, newborns are at risk for decompensation related to tamponade-like effects. Vojtovič and colleagues (2009) evaluated 23 neonates following biventricular correction surgery and found that chest closure decreased stroke volume, arterial blood pressure, cardiac output, and oxygenation secondary to decreased lung compliance. These risks are compounded by the relative difficulty of assessing for subtle changes that may develop days after closure. Delayed sternal closure is not without its risks in this population. In an 8-year retrospective study of neonates undergoing primary sternal closure versus delayed closure using either skin-only or membrane-assisted closure, mortality was higher in the delayed sternal closure groups than the primary skin closure. While there were no reported differences in sternal wound complications among the three groups, the overall postoperative course was found to be far more complex in the delayed sternal closure group. The results may be more indicative of the critical patient condition that necessitated delayed sternal closure than the technique itself.

In all cases of delayed sternal closure, the surgical team must monitor the patient daily for indications that the patient is ready for closure. Most often, the patient is assessed for hemodynamic stability, blood gas studies reflecting appropriate oxygenation without the need for aggressive respiratory support, decreasing lactate levels, no evidence of bleeding or sepsis, sufficient mean arterial pressure and systolic arterial pressures, and a total negative fluid balance. If the patient does not meet these indicators, or if sudden decompensation occurs following attempted closure, the sternum may be again left open. Safely temporizing this wound becomes a priority.

Management Guidelines

Principles for safe management of the open chest involve stabilization of the open sternal edges, sternal padding, and myocardial protection. Specific recommendations for management have not been established, and surgeon preference often guides the plan of care. A mesh membrane is frequently placed temporarily to provide myocardial protection and to reduce the development of adhesions to the pericardium. It is important to keep the often jagged edges of the cut sternum stabilized and separated. Inadvertent downward movement or contact with the myocardium may result in ventricular laceration. If ventricular laceration is not treated immediately, death may result secondary to profuse bleeding or massive air embolism (Spain, 2004). Methods for stabilizing the sternum vary, but include rigid plastic stents, sometimes created from large-gauge syringes (Hashemzadeh & Hashemzadeh, 2009; Ozker et al., 2012). In pediatric patients, multiple techniques have been described including the use of rib spreaders, stents, or struts (Pye & McDonnell, 2010). When sternal supports are chosen, the pericardial cavity is typically not packed with other materials; this permits ongoing visualization during any emergent events.

KEY POINT

Principles for safe management of the open chest involve stabilization of the open sternal edges, sternal padding, and myocardial protection.

If the sternal bone is too poor quality to accommodate a rigid support, or the surgeon believes temporary skin-only closure is not feasible, chest packing may be utilized. Multiple contact layers are utilized with or without an underlying membrane to provide protection of the myocardium, and the chest is then packed with sterile gauze. This provides multiple layers of protection between the sternal edges and the underlying organs to prevent trauma. The patient does need to be monitored for signs of tamponade, which can occur should the pericardial space be packed too tightly or when packing is required because of active bleeding. In the event of bleeding, radiopaque hemostatic gauze rolls are typically utilized (Combat Gauze®). Newer devices have been developed to provide progressive approximation of the sternum. They capitalize on the ability to stabilize the sternum. Santini et al. (2012) described their experience with an implantable, temporary sternal spreader, which allowed for progressive closure using a rotating wire mechanism outside of the chest. They reported safe and effective closure in all patients, although the small sample size limits the impact of these findings.

NPWT has been utilized in the management of the open chest, and the wound care nurse may be asked to provide advice regarding safe application and suction settings for adult and pediatric patients. It is important to ascertain the safety of NPWT use when there is exposed myocardium and to provide protection against ventricular laceration or heart rupture.

Multiple porcine studies have been conducted to test the impact of NPWT on open chest wounds. In a study evaluating the effects of NPWT on normal, reperfused, and ischemic myocardium following lower anterior descending (LAD) coronary artery occlusion, NPWT was found to significantly increase microvascular blood flow (Lindstedt et al., 2007). In this porcine model, a sternal spreader was used to maintain open chest status while NPWT foam was directly applied to the myocardium at a setting of −50 mm Hg. Investigators found a statistically significant increase in myocardial blood flow following NPWT in all situations, including the ischemic myocardium. When applying NPWT to an open chest, the wound care nurse should be cognizant of findings regarding the impact of NPWT on the thoracic cavity and the heart. Torbrand and colleagues (2008) described two major findings: (1) only the anterior aspect of the myocardium in direct contact with the NPWT system is impacted and pressure readings on the posterior aspect of the heart and the pleura space are unaffected and (2) this difference in anterior and posterior pressure causes the right ventricle to be pulled upward toward the sternum where it might be exposed to the sharp sternal edges and at risk for potential rupture (Torbrand et al., 2008). The researchers state that this does not preclude NPWT use but does indicate a need for cautious application of this therapy to the open chest. Multiple contact layers are suggested to separate the sternal edges from any underlying structures. In clinical studies in humans, NPWT has demonstrated benefit in the management of the open chest associated with delayed sternal closure and in clearance of mediastinitis.

Bleeding is a potential complication of NPWT in patients with open chest wounds since most of these patients are anticoagulated with elevated international normalized ratio (INR) levels. Clinical staff caring for the patient with NPWT need to be educated on the signs and symptoms of active bleeding and appropriate response such as immediate cessation of therapy along with measures to accomplish hemostasis. Bleeding in the open chest wound may be due to venous bleeding from the wound margins, periosteal bleeding from the sternum, or arterial bleeding from graft failure or ventricular injury. Additionally, hidden bleeding is a concern. In a case series comparing the effectiveness of gauze-based versus foam-based NPWT fillers, a blood clot that developed between the contact layers and the gauze resulted in cardiac tamponade necessitating emergent dressing change. The authors concluded that gauze-based NPWT seemed to be as clinically effective as foam-based NPWT but noted a greater risk for over packing the chest cavity with gauze as compared to foam (Rajakaruna & Marchbank, 2011).

The safety and effectiveness of NPWT was reported in a 15-year study of 47,325 sternotomy patients, which were managed with noninfected OCM using 218 cases of NPWT compared to 238 traditional wound packing cases. Reoperations for bleeding were found to be less common in NPWT compared to packing. None of the patients in the study experienced NPWT-related cardiovascular injuries, and among matched patients, the NPWT was associated with better early survival at 6 months. The authors report use of sternal stabilizing bar, silicone contact layer, and reticulated foam NPWT packing material to fill the open chest (Bakaeen et al., 2019).

KEY POINT

There are multiple case series that demonstrate the benefit and safety of NPWT for adults or neonates undergoing delayed primary closure of chest wounds due to congenital anomalies or mediastinitis. Modifications in standard techniques may be required to prevent complications such as bleeding.

There are multiple case series that demonstrate the benefit and safety of NPWT for neonates undergoing delayed primary closure due to congenital anomalies or mediastinitis. Lower suction settings are usually recommended for these patients. One case report describes deterioration of cardiac parameters when pressure was increased to −75 mm Hg, which was alleviated when the pressure was reduced to −25 mm Hg (Oeltjen et al., 2009). This underscores the importance of individualizing suction settings for both adults and children based on the patient's hemodynamic response. With children and adults, complete protection of the myocardium with multiple contact layers is important. The periwound skin must be thoroughly protected since recommendations include sizing the foam larger than the wound so that it overlaps onto the skin to provide greater stability for the wound. The NPWT suction setting may need to be titrated to avoid interference with the function of percutaneous chest tubes. In cardiac surgery, there are often at least three chest tubes inserted: mediastinal, pleural, and myocardial. Chest tubes are placed to low wall suction (typically −20 mm Hg) via the use of Pleur-evac® to evacuate blood and serous fluid from the chest cavity. In the presence of an open chest wound or open communication in a primarily closed sternal wound, NPWT may interfere with delivery of suction to the chest tubes. The NPWT suction setting should be reduced until acceptable chest tube function is achieved in coordination with the cardiothoracic surgeon or intensivist. When the connection between the wound and the thoracic space has closed, or when the chest tubes are no longer necessary, the NPWT suction may be increased to appropriate levels.

SURGICAL WOUND COMPLICATIONS

SURGICAL SITE INFECTION AS A QUALITY OF CARE INDICATOR

SSIs are the most common hospital-acquired infection (HAI) in the United States, impacting 160,000 to 300,000 patients annually, costing the U.S. health care system between $3.5 and $10 billion dollars. The incidence of SSI is between 2% and 5% of all inpatient surgeries with an associated 3% mortality and 2 to 11 times higher risk of death and long-term disability. SSI increases the LOS in an additional 7 to 10 days and increases readmission rates (Berríos-Torres et al., 2017). Of importance to the wound care nurse, 60% of SSI are estimated to be preventable with the use of evidence-based measures (Anderson et al., 2014; Ban et al., 2017). Given SSI is a pay-for-performance effort, the wound care nurse should be a part of an organization's quality improvement team to help drive SSI efforts. Without focused prevention, a 2% value-based purchasing (VBP) and 1% hospital-acquired condition penalty can be leveed on the hospital (Centers for Medicare & Medicaid Services, 2017).

KEY POINT

SSIs are the most commonly reported hospital-acquired infection in the United States and are associated with increase in risk of death or long-term disability.

SSI has become a national quality indicator due to the costs, morbidity, and mortality associated with an infection. SSI surveillance and prevention initiatives have evolved since the 1980s with a focus worldwide on decreasing the rates of SSI via adherence to best practices for prevention. One issue related to use of SSI as a quality indicator is the complexity surrounding risk for and development of infection and the difficulty in accurately measuring adherence to prevention guidelines. Biscione (2009) stated that for SSI rates to accurately reflect the quality of care provided by different facilities and surgeons, reporting measures must be able to adjust for risk based on case mix and acuity of patient populations. There is disagreement as to the percentage of HAIs that could be achieved with the implementation of all available prevention initiatives. Despite these issues, the responsibility of the wound care nurse is to implement best practices to achieve the lowest SSI rate.

Guidelines for SSI Prevention

There are many resources available to aid facilities and wound care nurses to decrease SSIs. Professional societies such as the Society for Healthcare Epidemiology of America (SHEA), the Infectious Diseases Society of America (IDSA), the Association for Professionals in Infection Control and Epidemiology (APIC), The Joint Commission (TJC), and the Institute of Healthcare Improvement (IHI) provide excellent resources and guidelines for decreasing HAIs (Bates et al., 2014; Yokoe et al., 2014). One of the most widely utilized tools is the Surgical Care Improvement Project (SCIP) guidelines. In 2006, the Centers for Medicare & Medicaid Services and Centers for Disease Control and Prevention collaborated to develop the SCIP (Bratzler & Hunt, 2006). SCIP guidelines focus on the prevention of four major surgical complications: SSI, venous thromboembolism, cardiac events, and respiratory complications (Rosenberger et al., 2011). For SSI, SCIP recommendations included the following:

- Prophylactic antibiotic administration within 1 hour of surgical procedure or, for vancomycin, within 2 hours of procedure.
- Proper antibiotic is selected.
- Discontinuation of antibiotics within 24 hours after surgery (48 hours in the case of cardiac surgery).
- Controlling postoperative 6 AM glucose levels in cardiac surgery patients.
- No hair removal or hair removal at the site of surgery with clippers or depilatory (no razors).
- Urinary catheter removal 1 to 2 days after surgery.
- Appropriate perioperative temperature management.

These measures focus on process measures for the prevention of SSI and on preoperative, intraoperative, and postoperative interventions. Studies fail to show a consistent relationship between adherence to SCIP measures and SSI rates, which is troublesome as SCIP measure compliance is publicly reported and tied to hospital reimbursement (Cataife et al., 2014; Haynes et al., 2009; Tillman et al., 2013). Awad (2012) concluded that the SCIP guidelines are not all-inclusive, may produce invalid rates or comparisons, and subsequently do not accurately guide the public in choosing where to receive their care. Despite the debate on these measures, there is continued focus on pay-for-performance and pay-for-value initiatives including SCIP. A program that has been validated and shown to improve care delivery through outcomes assessment and clinician feedback is the National Surgical Quality Improvement Program (NSQIP). NSQIP offers program support including data collection and analysis for all facility types. The data are risk and case adjusted, based on direct medical chart information, and include 30-day outcomes (http://site.acsnsqip.org). Multiple studies have shown that adherence to the NSQIP program resulted in improved outcomes, decreased lengths of stay, reduced mortality by 27%, decreased complications by 45%, and provided a financial cost savings (Guillamondegui et al., 2012; Hall et al., 2009; Ingraham et al., 2010; McNelis & Castaldi, 2014).

Additional guidelines and recommendations for the prevention of SSI can be found on the CDC Web site (http://www.cdc.gov/HAI/ssi/ssi.html), which includes resources such as the National Healthcare Safety Network (www.cdc.gov/nhsn/), the nation's widely used health care–associated infection tracking system. SSI prevention is as important in ambulatory surgery as in acute care settings. Owens and colleagues (2014) provided a retrospective analysis of outpatient surgical procedures complicated by SSI that required a postsurgical acute care visit within 14- and 30-day follow-up periods. The researchers found that the overall rate of significant infections were low in the databases queried. Considering the number of outpatient surgeries performed each year, the numbers of SSIs may be significantly higher than initially appreciated (Owens et al., 2014).

Infection Classification and Risk

Prevention and identification of SSIs is predicated on understanding that infections occur in three distinct areas: organ space, deep tissue, and superficial tissues, and that the causative factors, preventive measures, clinical presentation, and treatment vary based on location. The criteria for specific classification of each infection as determined by the CDC may be found at http://www.cdc.gov/nhsn/pdfs/pscmanual/9pscssicurrent.pdf.

The pathogens responsible for infection arise from one of two sources, endogenous or exogenous. Endogenous organisms are the patient's own flora and originate from the skin, mucous membranes, or gastrointestinal system; they usually cause infection in the areas where they normally reside. Infection from a distant source can result in a secondary infection at the surgical site. When the source of the infection is not from the host itself, the source is considered exogenous. Exogenous sources include medical personnel, breaks in surgical technique, the physical environment (including ventilation), and the equipment utilized during the surgical procedure (CDC, 2020).

Patient risk factors are another important consideration in the prevention and management of SSIs. Patient factors that increase the risk for infection include increased age, obesity, poor nutrition, diabetes mellitus, previous surgical infection, duration of surgery, excessive blood loss, chronic obstructive pulmonary disease, connective tissue disease, steroid use, smoking, peripheral vascular disease, renal insufficiency, and noncompliance with appropriate antibiotic prophylaxis. Risk factors have been found to differ considerably based on the type of operative procedure, age, and procedure duration. A list of these risk factors published by the National Healthcare Safety Network by standardized infection ration (SIR) is available at https://www.cdc.gov/nhsn/pdfs/ps-analysis-resources/nhsn-sir-guide.pdf.

Smokers are reported to have a higher incidence of both infectious and noninfectious wound healing complications across all surgical specialties when compared to nonsmokers. In a study involving orthopedic patients, Jain and colleagues (2015) found diabetes and smoking to be most predictive of SSIs. Laparoscopic procedures are associated with a decreased SSI rate when compared with open procedures in colon and gastric surgery (Imai et al., 2008) and in gynecological surgeries for cancer. Using the NSQIP database, 6,854 laparoscopic patients were studied with 5.4% incidence of SSI; open laparotomy presented a 3.5 times higher risk of infection, and the major risk factors were identified as obesity, ascites, preoperative anemia, American Society of Anesthesiologists score of Class of 3 or greater, hypoalbuminemia, preoperative weight loss, and respiratory comorbidities (Mahdi et al., 2014). Even the technique for wound closure and the materials used to approximate the tissues have been identified as having a significant impact on infection development.

Preoperative Skin Preparation and Daily Bathing

An important strategy for infection prevention is consistent and appropriate hand hygiene on the part of all health team members. Despite advancing technology, no single intervention has more impact than routine hand hygiene both before and after any patient encounter.

Appropriate use of topical antimicrobial agents for presurgical bathing, site preparation, and postoperative site care are also important in reducing SSI rates. CHG is widely used due to its documented ability to reduce the levels of pathogens on the skin surface. CHG's molecular design allows this cationic molecule to readily bind

to organic structures, providing a prolonged antimicrobial benefit (Wilson et al., 2004). CHG has replaced traditional antiseptics such as povidone–iodine (PVI) and alcohol with studies showing benefit across a variety of surgical procedures. In a systematic review by Lee and colleagues (2010), CHG outperformed PVI in prevention of SSIs in over nine RCTs and was also more cost-effective. Darouiche et al. (2010) found SSI rates in PVI cases to be consistently higher than their CHG comparator. Borer and colleagues (2007) found that a body wash with 4% CHG could effectively reduce the levels of the most virulent organisms such as *Acinetobacter baumannii*. The reduction in HAI associated with use of CHG was not limited to SSI but included a reduction in central line–associated blood stream infections (CLABSI), catheter-associated urinary tract infections (CAUTI), and multidrug-resistant organism (MDRO) ventilator-associated pneumonia (VAP) (Evans et al., 2010; Montecalvo et al., 2012; Timsit et al., 2009). Climo and colleagues (2013) conducted a large multicenter, cluster-randomized trial comparing bathing with a 2% no-rinse CHG daily bathing cloth to bathing with the same manufacturer's non-CHG bathing cloth. They found a 23% lower rate of MDRO acquisition, 28% reduction in CLABSI, and a 53% reduction in central catheter–associated bloodstream infections.

Because of the evidence supporting use of CHG in adults and in children over the age of 2 months, CHG has become the product of choice for preoperative bathing and decolonization, surgical site preparation, and daily skin cleansing in ICU settings. While the majority of studies show minimal adverse events associated with daily use of an antiseptic such as CHG, the long-term effects of daily bathing with CHG are unknown. This is typically not a problem for the short stay acute care patient; long-term care and long-term acute care patients could have longer exposure times. It should be noted that while CHG is universally recommended for the reduction of SSI, it should not be used on the face or in areas where contact with mucous membranes could occur. It is not recommended for use in the perineal area and is not indicated for CAUTI prevention. Both the APIC and CDC guidelines recommend early catheter removal, gentle meatal cleansing, stabilization of the catheter, meticulous management of the drainage system and spout, and maintenance of a closed system as elements in a CAUTI prevention program.

KEY POINT

CHG has become the product of choice for preoperative bathing and decolonization and surgical site preparation for adults and children over the age of 2 months.

Patients and clinicians frequently ask about the time frame for safely showering or bathing after surgery related to postoperative showering and subsequent SSI development. In a Cochrane review, Toon et al. (2015) examined the impact of early postoperative bathing within the first 48 hours and delayed bathing or showering after 48 hours; studies involving dirty, contaminated, or open wounds were excluded. They found only 1 RTC involving patients who had undergone minor skin excision procedures. There was no statistically significant difference in infection rates between those patients who showered or bathed in the initial 48 hours and those who delayed showering or bathing until >48 hours postop. Copeland-Halperin et al. (2020) found similar results. Published literature demonstrated no increase in the overall rate of wound infections or complications when patients showered within 48 hours versus on post-op day 3 or later. Surgical patients are commonly instructed to avoid submerging their wounds in any body of water until closure is complete. Many surgeons prefer the use of occlusive surgical dressings until epithelialization is complete around 48 hours postoperatively. These preferences and recommendations have not been fully validated by research.

Dressings

The recommended guidelines for SSI prevention include the application of a sterile dressing over the closed incision in the operating room and maintaining this dressing until 48 hours postoperatively at which time it can be discontinued. The specific postoperative dressing is not specified, and there is no evidence to support use of dressings beyond 48 hours. As patients become increasingly vulnerable, the focus on SSI prevention becomes more intense. The number and features of antimicrobial dressings continue to increase. The effectiveness of a topically applied dressing to prevent SSI has not been determined.

The National Institute of Health and Clinical Excellence (NICE, 2019) released guidelines that addressed the use of dressings for SSI prevention. Over eight RTCs were presented, representing a variety of topical dressings, and none of them were found to have any significant difference in the incidence of SSI related to specific dressings. None of the RCTs evaluated antimicrobial dressings. They compared moist wound healing products such as alginates, petrolatum gauze, and transparent films to either sterile gauze dressings or leaving the wound open to air. Use of an antimicrobial barrier dressing to prevent postoperative bacterial penetration may be helpful. Similar strategies have been found to be successful in the prevention of other HAIs. CLABSI rates have been reduced by the use of CHG-impregnated topical dressings (Timsit et al., 2009). As organ space and deep SSIs are typically related to factors such as skin preparation or intraoperative technique, dressings may be most beneficial in supporting epithelial resurfacing and preventing postoperative contamination.

Epithelialization is complete within 48 to 72 hours, which reduces the risk of bacterial invasion. Dressings are typically discontinued at the second to third postoperative day. Multiple comorbid conditions affect healing. Incomplete epithelialization and persistent drainage are indicators of increased risk for infection. Antimicrobial dressings may be warranted in these patients. Incisions located within a skin fold, such as the abdomen or groin, may also present increased risk for infection and incisional breakdown and may also benefit from use of an antimicrobial dressing. A systematic review of the addition of cyanoacrylate glue in addition to standard closure to prevent SSI was performed in accordance to PRISMA guidelines and GRADE assessment. Three articles were identified with low study quality overall. No difference between cyanoacrylate glue and control was reported in a single RCT, while a nonrandomized trial demonstrated statistically significant reduction. There was not sufficient evidence overall to suggest cyanoacrylate specifically for SSI reduction (Machin et al., 2019). Siah and Yatim (2011) evaluated 166 patients managed either with an occlusive antimicrobial dressing or with their incisions left open to air. There were significant differences found between the two groups in bacterial colonization at days 5 to 7 postoperatively. The control group was 4.1 times more likely to be contaminated with bacteria than patients managed with antimicrobial incision dressings. In a study by Kuo and colleagues (2017), a silver-impregnated postoperative dressing was an independent risk factor for the reduction of SSI compared to standard dressing. With normal healing, the benefits of antimicrobial dressings may be negligible. In at-risk patients and those with persistent drainage or delayed epithelialization, antimicrobial dressings may reduce the bioburden at the incision and may help to reduce superficial SSIs. Patients who will experience delayed wound healing and may benefit from an antimicrobial dressing cannot be predicted at the time of surgery. Routine use of these dressings is associated with increases in the cost of care. Given the lack of evidence, antimicrobial dressing use is likely best reserved for high-risk patients and those with evidence of delayed healing. The use of prophylactic antimicrobial dressings may be beneficial with severely immunocompromised patients, genital wounds, poorly perfused wounds, or patients with an MDRO. International consensus recommendations support the use of antimicrobials on wounds up to 2 weeks even in the absence of any signs of infection (Cutting et al., 2009; Dumville et al., 2016; International Consensus, 2012). Options for antimicrobial dressings and the advantages and disadvantages of each are discussed in detail in Chapter 11. Reduction in wound healing complications including infection has been associated with use of ciNPWT (Adogwa et al., 2014; Grauhan et al., 2014).

COMPARTMENT SYNDROME

The bilateral upper extremities, shoulders, and bilateral lower extremities have multiple compartments of connective tissue and muscle that encase neurovascular structure. The fascial sheaths of the upper and lower extremity compartments are tightly wrapped around these muscle systems, creating individual tissue compartments surrounded by inelastic covers. These compartments are very susceptible to changes in pressure, due either to exterior forces such as overly tight circumferential dressings or interior forces such as bleeding or edema. When pressure within the compartment rises, the vessels are compressed. The end result is ischemia leading to tissue necrosis, neurologic deficits, muscle necrosis, ischemic contractures, infection, delayed healing, and possibly amputation (Egro et al., 2014). Risk factors for compartment syndrome include fracture, vascular lesions, crush injuries, blunt trauma causing contusions, peritonitis, burns, and prolonged muscular effort. Compartment syndrome of the gluteus muscles due to pressure injury has also been reported, typically following long surgical procedures (Osteen & Haque, 2012). While the development of compartment syndrome generally involves the lower extremities and the forearms, compartment syndrome may occasionally develop in the hands following intravenous medication administration.

KEY POINT

While compartment syndrome usually involves the lower extremities and forearms, this complication occasionally develops in the abdomen.

Presentation and Diagnosis

Symptoms of compartment syndrome include disproportionate pain in relation to the trauma, pain that increases and is not relieved by the administration of pain medication, tight, painful presentation of the muscle compartment, and the development of sensory deficits distal to the site of injury (Uzel et al., 2013). Compartment syndrome has been reported to be atraumatic. The wound care nurse should be alert to the development of new-onset, localized, and severe edema coupled with any other indicators for compartment syndrome. In the presence of third-degree burns or intra-abdominal hypertension, the presentation may also involve profound hemodynamic instability. In addi-

tion to physical assessment, direct measurement of compartment pressures and serologic laboratory evaluations may be indicated. Compartment pressures are frequently used in diagnosis, especially when the clinical picture is unclear. Studies have shown that one-time compartment pressure recordings have a high false-positive rate and cannot be used as the sole diagnostic criterion (Whitney et al., 2014). In the case of ACS, continuous pressure measurements may be utilized in the intensive care unit and can provide trending data that help determine the need for surgical intervention. Specifically, an increase in intra-abdominal pressures (IAP) >20 mm Hg is associated with the development of organ failure, and readings >30 mm Hg are associated with a fourfold increase in the risk of sepsis and death in burn patients (Strang et al., 2014). Laboratory analysis includes measurement of lactate, myoglobin, and uric acid levels since these correlate to the metabolically induced changes associated with increasing compartment pressures (Mitas et al., 2014). Lactate levels >3.0 mm/L are indicative of increasing tissue hypoxia and may indicate the need for fasciotomy, and elevated uric acid levels are associated with advanced ischemic damage. Myoglobin and bilirubin levels may also be elevated, but these levels are dependent upon the scope of the injury and therefore do not function as independent variables. Evaluation of blood chemistries reflecting end-organ dysfunction, such as renal failure, is used to guide management (Long et al., 2019).

KEY POINT

Patients experiencing compartment syndrome often require fasciotomy, which results in large, copiously draining wounds with exposed musculature.

Treatment

Treatment for compartment syndrome varies depending on severity and may involve conservative monitoring or noninvasive testing, intravenous hypertonic mannitol, or surgical intervention. In severe cases, immediate intervention is required to reduce pressures in the affected compartment (Ross, 2001). A fasciotomy is a surgical incision to divide the fascia encasing the muscle compartment. It is typically performed to accommodate distention of the edematous musculature and for removal of blood or accumulating fluids. The surgery typically results in a large open wound, with copious drainage. Depending on location, there may also be muscle and organ exposure. Initial management typically involves the use of highly absorptive dressings and frequent assessment of the musculature. The muscle should be beefy red and should contract if tapped or flicked. If there is minimal muscular contraction, or a dusky, blue or gray appearance, the surgeon should be notified immediately. Vascular evaluation is required, and an extension of the fasciotomy may be needed. Once muscle viability has been established, dressing selection should be based on the need for edema reduction and exudate control. NPWT is commonly used for the management of compartment syndrome (Rimawi & Gonzalez, 2019). Following reduction of tissue edema and resolution of the acute event, the wounds may either be primarily closed or allowed to granulate with subsequent application of a skin graft.

 CONCLUSION

The management of surgical wounds requires collaboration and coordination between all members of the health care team to improve patient outcomes. Care recommended or provided by the wound care nurse ranges from simple to complex but always includes systemic measures for support of wound healing and topical therapy based on the principles of moist wound healing. Common complications of surgical wounds include infection and incisional breakdown. Some complicated surgical procedures result in open abdominal or open chest wounds that present multiple challenges in management. Management of these wounds requires an interdisciplinary team and understanding of the surgical procedure and the structures exposed in the wound bed. Advanced therapies such as NPWT and biologic dressings may be indicated to protect exposed structures and minimize the risk of fistula formation while promoting wound healing.

REFERENCES

Adogwa, O., Fatemi, P., Perez, E., et al. (2014). Negative pressure wound therapy reduces incidence of post-operative wound infection and dehiscence after long-segment thoracolumbar spinal fusion: A single institutional experience. *The Spine Journal, 14*, 2911–2917. doi: 10.1016/j.spinee.2014.04.011.

Aissaoui, N., Jouan, J., Gourjault, M., et al. (2018). Understanding left ventricular assist devices. *Blood Purification, 46*(4), 292–300. doi: 10.1159/000491872.

Allen, L. A., Smoyer Tomic, K. E., Wilson, K. L., et al. (2013). The inpatient experience and predictors of length of stay for patients hospitalized with systolic heart failure: Comparison by commercial, Medicaid, and Medicare payer type. *Journal of Medical Economics, 16*(1), 43–54. doi: 10.3111/13696998.2012.726932.

Anderson, D. J., Podgorny, K., Berrios-Torres, S. I., et al. (2014). Strategies to prevent surgical site infections in acute care hospitals: 2014 update. *Infection Control & Hospital Epidemiology, 35*(S2), S66–S88.

Anesäter, E., Borgquist, O., Hedstrom, E., et al. (2011). The influence of different sizes and types of wound fillers on wound contraction and tissue pressure during negative pressure wound therapy. *International Wound Journal, 8*(4), 336–342.

Argenta, L. C., & Morykwas, M. J. (1997). Vacuum-assisted closure: A new method for wound control and treatment: Clinical experiences. *Annals of Plastic Surgery, 38*, 563–577.

Atema, J. J., Gans, S. L., & Boermeester, M. A. (2015). Systematic review and meta-analysis of the open abdomen and temporary abdominal closure techniques in non-trauma patients. *World Journal of Surgery, 39*(4), 912–925. doi: 10.1007/s00268-014-2883-6.

Awad, S. S. (2012). Adherence to surgical care improvement project measures and post-operative surgical site infections. *Surgical Infections, 13*(4), 234–237.

Bakaeen, F. G., Haddad, O., Ibrahim, M., et al. (2019). Advances in managing the noninfected open chest after cardiac surgery: Negative-pressure wound therapy. *The Journal of Thoracic and Cardiovascular Surgery, 157*(5), 1891–1903.

Ban, K. A., Minei, J. P., Laronga, C., et al. (2017). American College of Surgeons and Surgical Infection Society: Surgical site infection guidelines, 2016 update. *Journal of the American College of Surgeons, 224*(1), 59–74. doi: 10.1016/j.jamcollsurg.2016.10.029.

Bates-Jensen, B., & Williams, J. (2012). Management of acute surgical wounds. In C. Sussman & B. Bates-Jensen (Eds.), *Wound care: A collaborative practice manual for health professionals* (4th ed., pp. 215–229). Baltimore, MD: Lippincott Williams & Wilkins.

Bates, O. L., O'Connor, N., Dunn, D., et al. (2014). Applying STAAR interventions in incremental bundles: Improving post-CABG surgical patient care. *Worldviews on Evidence-Based Nursing, 11*(2), 89–97.

Berríos-Torres, S. I., Umscheid, C. A., Bratzler, D. W., et al. (2017). Centers for disease control and prevention guideline for the prevention of surgical site infection, 2017. *JAMA Surgery, 152*(8), 784–791.

Biffi, R., Fattori, L., Bertani, E., et al. (2012). Surgical site infections following colorectal cancer surgery: A randomized prospective trial comparing common and advanced antimicrobial dressing containing ionic silver. *World Journal of Surgical Oncology, 10*, 94.

Biscione, F. M. (2009). Rates of surgical site infection as a performance measure: Are we ready? *World Journal of Gastrointestinal Surgery, 1*(1), 11–15.

Borer, A., Gilad, J., Porat, N., et al. (2007). Impact of 4% chlorhexidine whole-body washing on multidrug-resistant *Acinetobacter baumannii* skin colonisation among patients in a medical intensive care unit. *Journal of Hospital Infection, 67*(2), 149–155.

Borgquist, O., Anesäter, E., Hedström, E., et al. (2011). Measurements of wound edge microvascular blood flow during negative pressure wound therapy using thermodiffusion and transcutaneous and invasive laser Doppler velocimetry. *Wound Repair and Regeneration, 19*(6), 727–733.

Bota, O., Josten, C., Borger, M. A., et al. (2019). Standardized musculocutaneous flap for the coverage of deep sternal wounds after cardiac surgery. *Annals of Thoracic Surgery, 107*(3), 802–808.

Bratzler, D. W., & Hunt, D. R. (2006). The surgical infection prevention and surgical care improvement projects: National initiatives to improve outcomes for patients having surgery. *Clinical Infectious Diseases, 43*(3), 322.

Brown, S. H., Ward, S. R., Cook, M. S., et al. (2011). Architectural analysis of human abdominal wall muscles: Implications for mechanical function. *Spine, 36*(5), 355.

Brindle, C. T. (2012). Enterocutaneous fistulas. Current concepts in management. In A. Losen & J. E. Janis (Eds.), *Advances in abdominal wall reconstruction.* St Louis, MO: Quality Medical Publishing.

Brindle, C. T., & Blankenship, J. (2009). Management of complex abdominal wounds with small bowel fistulae: Isolation techniques and exudate control to improve outcomes. *Journal of Wound Ostomy & Continence Nursing, 36*(4), 396–403.

Burlew, C. C., Moore, E. E., Biffl, W. L., et al. (2012). One hundred percent fascial approximation can be achieved in the postinjury open abdomen with a sequential closure protocol. *The Journal of Trauma and Acute Care Surgery, 72*(1), 235–241. doi: 10.1097/TA.0b013e318236b319.

Burns, F. A., Heywood, E. G., Challand, C. P., et al. (2020). Is there a role for prophylactic mesh in abdominal wall closure after emergency laparotomy? A systematic review and meta-analysis. *Hernia, 24*, 441–447. doi: 10.1007/s10029-019-02060-1.

Cañedo-Dorantes, L., & Cañedo-Ayala, M. (2019). Skin acute wound healing: A comprehensive review. *International Journal of Inflammation, 2019*, 3706315. doi: 10.1155/2019/3706315.

Cataife, G., Weinberg, D. A., Wong, H. H., et al. (2014). The effect of Surgical Care Improvement Project (SCIP) compliance on surgical site infections (SSI). *Medical Care, 52*(2 Suppl), 266–273.

Centers for Disease Control and Prevention. (2009). U.S. outpatient surgeries on the rise. Retrieved from http://www.cdc.gov/nchs/pressroom/09newsreleases/outpatientsurgeries.htm

Centers for Disease Control and Prevention (CDC). (2020). Surgical site infection (SSI) event. Retrieved from https://www.cdc.gov/nhsn/pdfs/pscmanual/9pscssicurrent.pdf

Centers for Medicare and Medicaid Services. (2017). Hospital value-based purchasing, In Medicare Learning Network, ICN 907664. Retrieved April 5, 2020, from https://www.cms.gov/Outreach-and-Education/Medicare-Learning-Network-MLN/MLNProducts/downloads/Hospital_VBPurchasing_Fact_Sheet_ICN907664.pdf

Chen, S. Z., Li, J., Li, X. Y., et al. (2005). Effects of vacuum assisted closure on wound microcirculation: An experimental study. *Asian Journal of Surgery, 28*(3), 211–217.

Chin, G., Schultz, G., Diegelmann, R., et al. (2007). Biochemistry of wound healing in wound care practice. In P. Sheffield & C. Fife (Eds.), *Wound care practice* (2nd ed., pp. 53–78). Flagstaff, AZ: Best Publishing Company.

Chupp, R. E., & Edhayan, E. (2018). An effort to improve the accuracy of documented surgical wound classifications. *The American Journal of Surgery, 215*(3), 515–517.

Climo, M. W., Yokoe, D. S., Warren, D. K., et al. (2013). Effect of daily chlorhexidine bathing on hospital-acquired infection. *New England Journal of Medicine, 368*(6), 533–542.

Cohen, D. J., & Griffin, L. V. (2002). A biomechanical comparison of three sternotomy closure techniques. *Annals of Thoracic Surgery, 73*, 563–568.

Colli, A. (2011). First experience with a new negative pressure incision management system on surgical incisions after cardiac surgery in high risk patients. *Journal of Cardiothoracic Surgery, 6*, 160. Retrieved from http://www.cardiothroacicsurgery.org/content/6/1/160

Colvin, M., Smith, J. M., Skeans, M. A., et al. (2016). Heart. *American Journal of Transplantation, 16*(Suppl 2), 115–140. doi: 10.1111/ajt.13670.

Colwell, J. C., Ratliff, C. R., Goldberg, M., et al. (2011). MASD Part 3: Peristomal moisture–associated dermatitis and periwound moisture–associated dermatitis: A consensus. *Journal of Wound Ostomy & Continence Nursing, 38*(5), 541–553.

Copeland-Halperin, L. R., Rada, M. L. R. V., Levy, J., et al. (2020). Does the timing of postoperative showering impact infection rates? A systematic review and meta-analysis. *Journal of Plastic, Reconstructive & Aesthetic Surgery, 73*, 1306–1311. doi: 10.1016/j.bjps.2020.02.007.

Criss, C. N., Petro, C. C., Krpata, D. M., et al. (2014). Functional abdominal wall reconstruction improves core physiology and quality-of-life. *Surgery, 156*(1), 176–182.

Cutting, K., White, R., & Hoekstra, H. (2009). Topical silver-impregnated dressings and the importance of the dressing technology. *International Wound Journal, 6*, 396–402.

Darouiche, R. O., Wall, M. J., Itani, K. M. F., et al. (2010). Chlorhexidine-alcohol versus povidone-iodine for surgical-site antisepsis. *New England Journal of Medicine, 362*, 18–26.

Doughty, D., & Sparks, B. (2016). Wound healing physiology and factors that affect the repair process. In R. Bryant & D. Nix (Eds.), *Acute & chronic wounds: Current management concepts* (5th ed.). St. Louis, MI: Elsevier Inc.

Dumville, J. C., Gray, T. A., Walter, C. J., et al. (2016). Dressings for the prevention of surgical site infection. *Cochrane Database of Systematic Reviews*, (12), CD003091. doi: 10.1002/14651858.CD003091.pub4.

Egro, F. M., Jaring, M. R., & Khan, A. F. (2014). Compartment syndrome of the hand: Beware of innocuous radius fractures. *Eplasty, 14*, 46–51.

Evans, H. L., Dellit, T. H., Chan, J., et al. (2010). Effect of chlorhexidine whole-body bathing on hospital-acquired infections among trauma patients. *Archives in Surgery, 145*(3), 240–246.

Franz, M., Robson, M., Steed, D., et al. (2008). Guidelines to aid healing of acute wounds by decreasing impediments of healing. *Wound Repair and Regeneration, 16*, 723–748.

Grauhan, O., Arashes, N., Tutku, B., et al. (2014). Effect of surgical incision management on wound infection in a post sternotomy patient population. *International Wound Journal*, (Suppl 1), 6–9.

Grauhan, O., Navasardyan, A., Hofmann, M., et al. (2013). Prevention of poststernotomy wound infections in obese patients by negative pressure wound therapy. *The Journal of Thoracic and Cardiovascular Surgery, 145*(5), 1387–1392.

Greer, D., Smith, J., & McCorvey, D. (2007). Principles of surgical wound management. In P. Sheffield & C. Fife (Eds.), *Wound care practice* (2nd ed., pp. 251–275). Flagstaff, AZ: Best Publishing Company.

Guillamondegui, O. D., Gunter, O. L., Hines, L., et al. (2012). Using the national surgical quality improvement program and the Tennessee surgical quality collaborative to improve surgical outcomes. *Journal of American College of Surgery, 214*(4), 709–714.

Gupta, S., Gabriel, A., Lantis, J., et al. (2016). Clinical recommendations and practical guide for negative pressure wound therapy with instillation. *International Wound Journal, 13*(2), 159–174.

Hales, C. M., Carroll, M. D., Fryar, C. D., et al. (2017). Prevalence of obesity among adults and youth: United States, 2015–2016. *NCHS Data Brief*, (288), 1–8. Retrieved April 14, 2020, from http://www.cdc.gov/nchs/data/databriefs/db288.pdf

Hales, C. M., Carroll, M. D., Fryar, C. D., et al. (2020). Prevalence of obesity and severe obesity among adults: United States, 2017–2018. *NCHS Data Brief*, (360), 1–8. Retrieved April 14, 2020, from http://www.cdc.gov/obesity/data/adult.html

Hall, B. L., Hamilton, B. H., Richards, K., et al. (2009). Does surgical quality improve in the American College of Surgeons National Surgical Quality Improvement Program: An evaluation of all participating hospitals. *Annals of Surgery, 250*(3), 363–376.

Hall, M. J., Schwartzman, A., Zhang, J., et al. (2017). Ambulatory surgery data from hospitals and ambulatory surgery centers: United States, 2010. *National Health Statistics Reports*, (102), 1–15.

Hashemzadeh, K., & Hashemzadeh, S. (2009). In hospital outcomes of delayed sternal closure after open cardiac surgery. *Journal of Cardiac Surgery, 24*, 30–33.

Haynes, A. B., Weiser, T. G., Berry, W. R., et al. (2009). A surgical safety checklist to reduce morbidity and mortality in a global population. *New England Journal of Medicine, 360*(5), 491–499.

Heineman, J. T., Garcia, L. J., Obst, M. A., et al. (2015). Collapsible enteroatmospheric fistula isolation device: A novel, simple solution to a complex problem. *Journal of the American College of Surgeons, 221*(2), e7–e14.

Imai, E., Ueda, M., Kanao, K., et al. (2008). Surgical site infection risk factors identified by multivariate analysis for patient undergoing laparoscopic, open colon, and gastric surgery. *American Journal of Infection Control, 36*, 727–731.

Ingraham, A. M., Richards, K. E., Hall, B. L., et al. (2010). Quality improvement in surgery: The American College of Surgeons national Surgical Quality Improvement Program approach. *Advances in Surgery, 44*(1), 251–267.

International Consensus. (2012). *Appropriate use of silver dressings in wounds. An expert working group consensus*. London: Wounds International. Retrieved from www.woundsinternational.com

Jain, R. K., Shukla, R., Singh, P., et al. (2015). Epidemiology and risk factors for surgical site infections in patients requiring orthopedic surgery. *European Journal of Orthopaedic Surgery & Traumatology, 25*(2), 251–254. doi: 10.1007/s00590-014-1475-3

Kaplan, M., Banwell, P., Orgill, D. P., et al. (2005). Guidelines for the management of the open abdomen: Recommendations from a multidisciplinary expert advisory panel. *Wounds, 17*(Suppl), S1–S24.

Karlakki, S., Brem, M., Giannini, S., et al. (2013). Negative pressure wound therapy for management of the surgical incision in orthopaedic surgery: A review of evidence and mechanisms for an emerging indication. *Bone & Joint Research, 2*(12), 276–284.

Karppinen, S. M., Heljasvaara, R., Gullerg, D., et al. (2019). Toward understanding scarless skin wound healing and pathological scaring. *F1000 Research, 8*, F1000. doi: 10.12688/f1000research.18293.1.

Köckerling, F., Alam, N. N., Antoniou, S. A., et al. (2018). What is the evidence for the use of biologic or biosynthetic meshes in abdominal wall reconstruction? *Hernia, 22*(2), 249–269.

Kostiuchenok, I. I., Kolker, V. A., & Karlov, V. A. (1986). The vacuum effect in the surgical treatment of purulent wounds. *Vestnik Khirurgii, 9*, 18–21.

Kuo, F. C., Chen, B., Lee, M. S., et al. (2017). AQUACEL® Ag surgical dressing reduces surgical site infection and improves patient satisfaction in minimally invasive total knee arthroplasty: A prospective, randomized, controlled study. *BioMedical Research International, 2017*, 1262108. doi: 10.1155/2017/1262108.

Lang, J. L., Gonzalez, R. P., Aldy, K. N., et al. (2011). Does temporary chest wall closure with or without chest packing improve survival for trauma patients in shock after emergent thoracotomy? *Journal of Trauma and Acute Care Surgery, 70*(3), 705–709.

Lee, C., & Hansen, S. (2009). Management of acute wounds. *Surgical Clinics of North America, 89*, 659–676. doi: 10.1016/j.suc.2009.03.005.

Lee, I., Agarwal, R. K., Lee, B. Y., et al. (2010). Systemic review and cost analysis comparing use of chlorhexidine with use of iodine for preoperative skin antisepsis to prevent surgical site infection. *Infection Control and Hospital Epidemiology, 31*(12), 1219–1229.

Lindstedt, S., Malmsjo, M., & Ingemansson, R. (2007). No hypoperfusion is produced in the epicardium during application of myocardial topical negative pressure in a porcine model. *Journal of Cardiothroacic Surgery, 2*, 53. Retrieved from http://www.cardiothoracic-surgery.org/content/2/1/53

Long, B., Koyfman, A., & Gottlieb, M. (2019). Evaluation and management of acute compartment syndrome in the emergency department. *The Journal of Emergency Medicine, 56*(4), 386–397.

Lunardi, A. C., Miranda, C. S., Silva, K. M., et al. (2012). Weakness of expiratory muscles and pulmonary complications in malnourished patients undergoing upper abdominal surgery. *Respirology, 17*(1), 108–113.

Machin, M., Liu, C., Coupland, A., et al. (2019). Systematic review of the use of cyanoacrylate glue in addition to standard wound closure in the prevention of surgical site infection. *International Wound Journal, 16*(2), 387–393.

Mahdi, H., Gojayev, A., Buechel, M., et al. (2014). Surgical site infection in women undergoing surgery for gynecologic cancer. *International Journal of Gynecologic Cancer, 24*(4), 779–786.

Malmsjö, M., Huddleston, E., & Martin, R. (2014). Biological effects of a disposable, canisterless negative pressure wound therapy system. *Eplasty, 2*(14), e15.

McNelis, J., & Castaldi, M. (2014). The National Surgery Quality Improvement Project (NSQIP): A new tool to increase patient safety and cost efficiency in a surgical intensive care unit. *Patient Safety in Surgery, 8*, 19. doi: 10.1186/1754-9493-8-19.

McNichol, L., Lund, C., Rosen, T., et al. (2013). Medical adhesives and patient safety: State of the science consensus statements for the assessment, prevention, and treatment of adhesive-related skin injuries. *Journal of Wound Ostomy & Continence Nursing, 40*(4), 365–380.

Mitas, P., Vejrazka, M., Hruby, J., et al. (2014). Prediction of compartment syndrome based on analysis of biochemical parameters. *Annals of Vascular Surgery, 28*(1), 170–177.

Montecalvo, M. A., McKenna, D., Yarrish, R., et al. (2012). Chlorhexidine bathing to reduce central venous catheter-associated bloodstream infection: Impact and sustainability. *The American Journal of Medicine, 125*(5), 505–511.

Morykwas, M. J., Argenta, L. C., Shelton-Brown, E. I., et al. (1997). Vacuum-assisted closure: A new method for wound control and treatment: Animal studies and basic foundation. *Annals of Plastic Surgery, 38*(6), 553–562.

Murphy, P. B., Knowles, S., Chadi, S. A., et al. (2019). Negative pressure wound therapy use to decrease surgical nosocomial events in colorectal resections (NEPTUNE): A randomized controlled trial. *Annals of Surgery, 270*(1), 38–42. doi: 10.1097/SLA.0000000000003111.

National Institute for Health and Care Excellence (NICE). (2019). *Surgical site infection: prevention and treatment.* Retrieved December 15, 2019, from https://www.nice.org.uk/guidance/ng125

Nazerali, R. S., Hinchcliff, K., & Wong, M. S. (2014). Rigid fixation for the prevention and treatment of sternal complications: A review of our experience. *Annals of Plastic Surgery, 72*, S27–S30.

Netsch, D. S., Nix, D. P., & Haugen, V. (2016). Negative pressure wound therapy. In R. A. Bryant & D. P. Nix (Eds.), *Acute & chronic wounds: Current management concepts* (5th ed.). St. Louis, MI: Elsevier Inc.

Nurses Specialized in Wound, Ostomy and Continence Canada (NSWOCC). (2018). *Nursing best practice recommendations: Enterocutaneous fistulas (ECF) and enteroatmospheric fistulas (EAF)* (2nd ed.). Ottawa, ON: Nurses Specialized in Wound, Ostomy and Continence Canada.

Nutescu, E. A., Bathija, S., Sharp, L. K., et al. (2011). Anticoagulation patient self-monitoring in the United States. *Pharmacotherapy, 31*(12), 1161–1174.

Oeltjen, J. C., Panos, A. L., Salerno, T. A., et al. (2009). Complete vacuum-assisted sternal closure following neonatal cardiac surgery. *Journal of Cardiac Surgery, 24*, 748–750.

Olbrecht, V. A., Barreiro, C. J., Bonde, P. N., et al. (2006). Clinical outcomes of noninfectious sternal dehiscence after median sternotomy. *The Annals of Thoracic Surgery, 82*(3), 902–907.

Osteen, K. D., & Haque, S. H. (2012). Bilateral gluteal compartment syndrome following right total knee revision: A case report. *The Ocshner Journal, 12*, 141–144.

Owens, P. L., Barrett, M. L., Raetzman, S., et al. (2014). Surgical site infections following ambulatory surgery procedures. *JAMA, 311*(7), 709–716.

Ozker, E., Saritas, B., Vuran, C., et al. (2012). Delayed sternal closure after pediatric cardiac operations: Single center experience: A retrospective study. *Journal of Cardiothoracic Surgery, 7*, 102.

Pachowsky, M., Gusinde, J., Klein, A., et al. (2011). Negative pressure wound therapy to prevent and treat surgical incisions after total hip arthroplasty. *International Orthopaedics, 36*, 719–722.

Phillips, S. (2000). Physiology of wound healing and surgical wound care. *ASAIO Journal, 46*, S2–S5.

Plaudis, H., Rudzats, A., Melberga, L., et al. (2012). Abdominal negative-pressure therapy: A new method in countering abdominal compartment and peritonitis-prospective study and critical review of literature. *Annals of Intensive Care, 2*(1), S23.

Pye, S., & McDonnell, M. (2010). Nursing considerations for children undergoing delayed sternal closure after surgery for congenital heart disease. *Critical Care Nurse, 30*(3), 50–61.

Rajakaruna, C., & Marchbank, A. (2011). Gauze-based negative pressure wound therapy to infected deep sternotomy wound complicated by cardiac tamponade: A case report. *International Wound Journal, 8*(1), 96–98.

Rausei, S., Dionigi, G., Boni, L., et al. (2014). Open abdomen management of intra-abdominal infections: Analysis of a twenty-year experience. *Surgical infections, 15*(3), 200–206.

Reider, K. E. (2017). Fistula isolation and the use of negative pressure to promote wound healing. *Journal of Wound, Ostomy and Continence Nursing, 44*(3), 293–298.

Rimawi, M., & Gonzalez, J. M. (2019). *Bedside or surgical fasciotomy: Which would you choose for treatment of compartment syndrome?*

Retrieved December 15, 2019, from https://pdfs.semanticscholar.org/dde7/0502b94e9fa667b8a075ccccb3691a52624f.pdf

Rosenberger, L. H., Politano, A. D., & Sawyer, R. G. (2011). The surgical care improvement project and prevention of post-operative infection, including surgical site infection. *Surgical Infections, 12*(3), 163–168.

Ross, D. (2001). Compartment syndrome. In P. L. Swearingen & J. H. Keen (Eds.), *Manual of critical care nursing* (4th ed.). St. Louis, MO: Mosby.

Sahebally, S. M., McKevitt, K., Stephens, I., et al. (2018). Negative pressure wound therapy for closed laparotomy incisions in general and colorectal surgery: A systematic review and meta-analysis. *JAMA Surgery, 153*(11), e183467.

Santini, F., Onorati, F., Telesca, M., et al. (2012). Preliminary experience with a new device for delayed sternal closure strategy in cardiac surgery. *International Journal of Artificial Organs, 35*(6), 471–476.

Satterwhite, T. S., Miri, S., Chung, C., et al. (2012). Outcomes of complex abdominal herniorrhaphy: Experience with 106 cases. *Annals of Plastic Surgery, 68*(4), 382–388.

Sears, E. D., Momoh, A. O., Chung, K. C., et al. (2017). A national study of the impact of delayed flap timing for treatment of patients with deep sternal wound infection. *Plastic and Reconstructive Surgery, 140*(2), 390–400. doi: 10.1097/PRS.0000000000003514.

Shah, A., Sumpio, B. J., Tsay, C., et al. (2019). Incisional negative pressure wound therapy augments perfusion and improves wound healing in a swine model pilot study. *Annals of Plastic Surgery, 82*(4S), S222–S227.

Siah, C. J., & Yatim, J. (2011). Efficacy of total occlusive ionic silver-containing dressing combination in decreasing risk of surgical site infections: An RCT. *Journal of Wound Care, 20*(12), 561–568.

Silva Enciso, J. (2016). Mechanical circulatory support: current status and future directions. *Progress in Cardiovascular Diseases, 58*(4), 444–454. doi: 10.1016/j.pcad.2016.01.006.

Sorg, H., Tilkorn, D. J., Hager, S., et al. (2017). Skin wound healing: An update on the current knowledge and concepts. *European Surgical Research, 58*(1–2), 81–94.

Spain, K. (2004). Use of deep hypothermic circulatory arrest following ventricular laceration: A case report. *AANA Journal, 72*(3), 193–195.

Stanirowski, P. J., Bizoń, M., Cendrowski, K., et al. (2016). Randomized controlled trial evaluating dialkylcarbamoyl chloride impregnated dressings for the prevention of surgical site infections in adult women undergoing cesarean section. *Surgical Infections, 17*(4), 427–435.

Strang, S. G., Van Lieshout, E. M., Breederveld, R. S., et al. (2014). A systematic review on intra-abdominal pressure in severely burned patients. *Burns, 40*, 9–16.

Strugala, V., & Martin, R. (2017). Meta-analysis of comparative trials evaluating a prophylactic single-use negative pressure wound therapy system for the prevention of surgical site complications. *Surgical Infections, 18*(7), 810–819. doi: 10.1089/sur.2017.156.

Struik, G. M., Vrijland, W. W., Birnie, E., et al. (2018). A randomized controlled trial on the effect of a silver carboxymethylcellulose dressing on surgical site infections after breast cancer surgery. *PLoS One, 13*(5), e0195715.

Svensson-Björk, R., Zarrouk, M., Asciutto, G., et al. (2019). Meta-analysis of negative pressure wound therapy of closed groin incisions in arterial surgery. *British Journal of Surgery, 106*(4), 310–318.

Tillman, M., Wehbe-Janek, H., Hodges, B., et al. (2013). Surgical care improvement project and surgical site infections: Can integration in the surgical safety checklist improve quality performance and clinical outcomes? *Journal of Surgical Research, 184*(1), 150–156.

Timsit, J. F., Schwebel, C., Bouadma, L., et al. (2009). Chlorhexidine-impregnated sponges and less frequent dressing changes for prevention of catheter-related infections in critically ill adults: a randomized controlled trial. *JAMA, 301*(12), 1231–1241.

Toon, C. D., Sinha, S., Davidson, B. R., et al. (2015). Early versus delayed post-operative bathing or showering to prevent wound complications. *Cochrane Database of Systematic Reviews*, (7), CD010258. doi: 10.1002/14651858.CD010258.pub3.

Torbrand, C., Ingemansson, R., Gustafsson, L., et al. (2008). Pressure transduction to the thoracic cavity during topical negative pressure therapy of a sternotomy wound. *International Wound Journal, 5*, 579–584.

Uzel, A. P., Bulla, A., & Henri, S. (2013). Compartment syndrome of the thigh after blunt trauma: A complication not to be ignored. *Musculoskeletal Surgery, 97*(1), 81–83.

Vojtovič, P., Reich, O., Selko, M., et al. (2009). Haemodynamic changes due to delayed sternal closure in newborns after surgery for congenital cardiac malformations. *Cardiology in the Young, 19*(6), 573–579.

Wackenfors, A., Sjögren, J., Gustafsson, R., et al. (2004). Effects of vacuum-assisted closure therapy on inguinal wound edge microvascular blood flow. *Wound Repair and Regeneration, 12*(6), 600–606.

Wechter, M., Pearlman, M., & Hartmann, K. (2005). Reclosure of the disrupted laparotomy wound: A systematic review. *Obstetrics & Gynecology, 106*(2), 376–383. doi: 10.1097/01.AOG.000017114.75338.06.

Weigand, C., & White, R. (2013). Microdeformation in wound healing. *Wound Repair and Regeneration, 21*, 793–799.

Wells, C. I., Ratnayake, C. B., Perrin, J., et al. (2019). Prophylactic negative pressure wound therapy in closed abdominal incisions: A meta-analysis of randomised controlled trials. *World Journal of Surgery, 43*(11), 2779–2788. doi: 10.1007/s00268-019-05116-6.

Whitney, J. (2016). Surgical wounds and incision care. In R. Bryant & D. Nix (Eds.), *Acute & chronic wounds current management concepts* (5th ed.). St. Louis, MI: Elsevier Mosby.

Whitney, A., O'Toole, R. V., Hui, E., et al. (2014). Do one-time intracompartmental pressure measurements have a high false-positive rate in diagnosing compartment syndrome? *Journal of Trauma and Acute Care Surgery, 76*(2), 479–483.

Widgerow, A. (2013). Surgical wounds. In M. Flanagan, (Ed.), *Wound healing and skin integrity: Principles and practice* (pp. 224–241). West Sussex, UK: Wiley-Blackwell.

Wilkes, R. P., Kilpad, D. V., Zhao, Y., et al. (2012). Closed incision management with negative pressure wound therapy (CIM) biomechanics. *Surgical Innovation, 19*(1), 67–75.

Wilson, C. M., Gray, G., Read, J. S., et al. (2004). Tolerance and safety of different concentrations of chlorhexidine for peripartum vaginal and infant washes: HIVNET025. *Journal of Acquired Immune Deficiency Syndromes, 35*(2), 138.

Wong, J. K., Joshi, D. J., Melvin, A. L., et al. (2017). Early and late outcomes with prolonged open chest management after cardiac surgery. *The Journal of Thoracic and Cardiovascular Surgery, 154*(3), 915–924.

Yokoe, D. S., Anderson, D. J., Berenholtz, S. M., et al. (2014). A compendium of strategies to prevent healthcare-associated infections in acute care hospitals: 2014 updates. *Infection Control & Hospital Epidemiology, 35*(S2), S21–S31.

Zwanenburg, P. R., Tol, B. T., Obdeijn, M. C., et al. (2020). Meta-analysis, meta-regression, and GRADE assessment of randomized and non-randomized studies of incisional negative pressure wound therapy versus control dressings for the prevention of postoperative wound complications. *Annals of Surgery, 272*, 81–91. doi: 10.1097/SLA.0000000000003644. Retrieved December 15, 2019, from https://europepmc.org/article/med/31592899

QUESTIONS

1. A surgical wound that is beginning to develop granulation is in what phase of wound healing?
A. Hemostasis
B. Inflammatory
C. Proliferative
D. Remodeling

2. The wound care nurse is assessing an open surgical abdominal wound. The surgical record indicates that there was nonpurulent inflammation related to gross spillage from the colon. This wound would fall into which of the following classifications?
A. Class I
B. Class II
C. Class III
D. Class IV

3. Which type of wound would be most likely to heal by primary intention?
A. Appendectomy for perforated appendix
B. Total knee replacement
C. Repair of gunshot wound
D. Fasciotomy for compartment syndrome

4. Which of the following is a known benefit of closed incision negative pressure wound therapy (ciNPWT)?
A. Endothelial cell deactivation
B. Increase in levels of proinflammatory cytokines
C. Increase in lateral tension
D. Increased tissue perfusion in the periwound tissues

5. Which factor is a key consideration in the selection of traditional versus disposable ciNPWT system?
A. Cost
B. Exudate
C. Patient preference
D. Wound appearance

6. What is the most common cause of fistula formation in wounds?
A. Anastomotic leak
B. Debridement of the wound
C. Infection
D. Trauma

7. Which management strategy would the wound care nurse recommend for a patient with a chronic open abdominal wound where underlying structures are unknown?
A. NPWT used on a high-pressure setting
B. Autolytic atraumatic wound care methods
C. Sharp debridement of necrotic tissue
D. Strict avoidance of wound or fistula pouches

8. The wound care nurse is caring for a patient whose surgeon used a biologic mesh when closing the surgical incision. Mesh lowers the risk of
A. Infection
B. Granulation tissue growth
C. Hernia development
D. Incisional pain

9. Which topical therapy would the wound care nurse recommend when biologic mesh is used in a wound bed?
A. Use of debriding agents
B. Application of topical endogenous collagenases
C. Use of hydrogen peroxide or acetic acid
D. Thorough irrigation with saline

10. Which of the following is a Surgical Care Improvement Project (SCIP) recommendation for the prevention of surgical site infection (SSI)?
A. Prophylactic antibiotic administration within 1 hour of surgical procedure
B. Continuation of antibiotics for 5 days postoperatively
C. Hair removal at the surgical site using a razor
D. Urinary catheter placement for at least 1 week postoperatively

ANSWERS AND RATIONALES

1. C. Rationale: The second component of the proliferative phase is granulation tissue formation, which begins on days 3 to 5 postinjury, following and overlapping the inflammatory phase.

2. C. Rationale: Class III/contaminated: Open, fresh, accidental wounds. Includes surgeries with major breaks in techniques or gross spillage from the GI tract <4 hours old, and incisions in which acute, nonpurulent inflammation occurs.

3. B. Rationale: Primary closure is the preferred method of closure for clean wounds and wounds involving repair of injured structures such as nerves, tendons, and blood vessels when the zone of injury is small and the wound is clean. Primary closure is contraindicated in the presence of tension, potential infection, and when the extent of injury is unclear.

4. D. Rationale: Human studies in bariatric patients have demonstrated improved oxygen saturation and tissue perfusion surrounding the wound closure when ciNPWT is utilized.

5. B. Rationale: Exudate levels are a key consideration in selection of traditional versus disposable systems.

6. A. Rationale: Despite the many causes of fistula known in the literature, 85% of fistulas occur as the result of an anastomotic leak.

7. B. Rationale: When caring for a patient with an chronic open abdominal wound where underlying structures are unknown, the wound care nurse should keep the following principles in mind: atraumatic, autolytic, normothermic wound care with or without antimicrobial, with attention to minimizing the frequency of dressing changes.

8. C. Rationale: Synthetic and biologic mesh products are frequently used to reduce the risk of incisional failure and hernia development or recurrence.

9. D. Rationale: The focus of wound bed preparation with the presence of biologic mesh exposure is on thorough irrigation with saline or other noncytotoxic wound cleanser.

10. A. Rationale: For SSI, SCIP recommendations included the following:

- Prophylactic antibiotic administration within 1 hour of surgical procedure, or, for vancomycin, within 2 hours of procedure.
- Proper antibiotic is selected.
- Discontinuation of antibiotics within 24 hours after surgery (48 hours in the case of cardiac surgery).
- Controlling postoperative 6 AM glucose levels in cardiac surgery patients.
- No hair removal or hair removal at the site of surgery with clippers or depilatory (no razors).
- Urinary catheter removal 1 to 2 days after surgery.
- Appropriate perioperative temperature management.

CHAPTER 35

PALLIATIVE WOUND CARE

Kevin R. Emmons and Barbara A. Dale

OBJECTIVES

1. Explain the similarities and differences in hospice care and palliative care.

2. Describe the philosophy of palliative care and the implications for care.

3. Discuss modifications in standard pressure injury prevention protocols that may be indicated for the palliative care patient.

4. Explain skin changes that are common at end of life and that increase the risk for skin breakdown.

5. Describe principles of management for wounds commonly found in the palliative care population, to include pressure injuries, malignant wounds, skin tears, and leg ulcers.

TOPIC OUTLINE

● INTRODUCTION

In most situations, the goal of wound management is wound healing, and each aspect of assessment and treatment is geared toward that outcome. This healing goal and expectation is reflected in the common caveat that a wound that fails to show measurable improvement in the first 2 to 4 weeks of therapy must be reevaluated and management must be changed. From this perspective, a nonhealing wound represents a failure of wound management. This focus on healing is appropriate in most cases. For some patients and situations, it is inappropriate and can compromise appropriate care. There are many patients whose wound care is better approached from a palliative care perspective. This requires the wound care nurse to shift their approach from a singular goal of wound healing to a comprehensive focus on patient-centered goals such as improved quality of life, stabilization of the wound, or a decrease in odor, pain, and exudate. It is important to clarify that palliative wound care is not a singular protocol or care pathway devoid of wound healing outcomes. Rather palliative wound care is a concept and approach that can be integrated and applied across the care continuum.

> **KEY POINT**
>
> Palliative care requires the wound nurse to shift their approach from a singular goal of wound healing to a more comprehensive focus on patient-centered goals such as improved quality of life.

 PALLIATIVE CARE OVERVIEW

In an updated fact sheet, the World Health Organization (2018) describes palliative care as "an approach that improves the quality of life of patients (adults and children) and their families who are facing problems associated with life-threatening illness. It prevents and relieves suffering through the early identification, correct assessment and treatment of pain and other problems, whether physical, psychosocial or spiritual." The Worldwide Hospice and Palliative Care Alliance (WHPCA) adds further clarification, stating that (1) palliative care is needed for long-term as well as life-threatening or life-limiting conditions, (2) there is no time or prognostic limit on the delivery of palliative care, (3) palliative care is needed at all levels and settings of care, and (4) palliative care should be integrated alongside curative care (Connor & Gwyther, 2018).

In a comprehensive analysis on palliative care, it was concluded that palliative care should be thought of early within a chronic disease trajectory (Hui et al., 2013).

Nurses play an integral role in providing palliative care. Palliative care competencies that all nurses should possess include symptom management, communication, and advocacy (Hagan et al., 2018). Sekse et al. (2017) identified the following themes that encompass a nurse's role in providing palliative care: being available, coordinating care, anticipating needs, being dedicated, and being supportive in demanding situations. All nurses should have knowledge of palliative care principles to empower them to provide comprehensive patient-centered care.

PALLIATIVE VERSUS HOSPICE CARE

Palliative care is often confused with hospice care. Hospice care is limited to patients at the end of life, while palliative care has a broader application (Meghani, 2004). The confusion between palliative care and hospice care has resulted in negative perceptions and stigma. Many people interpret palliative care as meaning loss of hope or withdrawal of active treatment. These inaccurate and negative perceptions have limited the acceptance and implementation of the palliative care framework and philosophy. Hui and colleagues (2012) recommended use of the alternative term, supportive care, for palliative care provided during early stages of chronic diseases. It has been proposed that supportive care precedes both early palliative care and end-of-life care, addressing potential lifelong complications in patients cured of the underlying disease (Klastersky et al., 2015). The authors also suggest that supportive care does not cease at death but continues into the bereavement phase providing care for loved ones. This change in nomenclature may be an important nuance that promotes patient, family, and provider acceptance over an entire course of illness and continues after death. At this time, the accepted term is palliative care, and this chapter addresses concepts and strategies for palliative wound care.

> **KEY POINT**
>
> Hospice care is limited to end-of-life care, while palliative care has much broader application and is not limited to end of life.

PRINCIPLES OF PALLIATIVE CARE

The concept of palliative care is dynamic and will continue to evolve over time (Meghani, 2004). The concept of palliative wound care will also evolve as science progresses. Several articles describing palliative wound care emphasize the importance of symptom management, wound stabilization, measures to reduce suffering, and strategies to improve quality of life as important aspects of palliative wound care (Ennis & Meneses, 2005; Hughes et al., 2005; Langemo et al., 2007). Ferris et al. (2007) concluded that palliative wound care includes therapies aimed at (1) effective communication, decision making, and care delivery; (2) stabilization of the wound; (3) minimizing risk of infection and wound progression; (4) managing issues that cause patient and family suffering; and (5) optimizing function and quality of life as long as possible. A comprehensive concept analysis on the evolution of palliative wound care defined it as a holistic and integrated approach to care that provides symptom management, improves psychosocial well-being, is multidisciplinary, is driven by patient/family goals, and is integrated into everyday care practice (Emmons & Lachman, 2010).

INDICATIONS FOR PALLIATIVE CARE

A common challenge is determining when to implement a palliative wound care approach in the non–terminally ill patient. Emmons and Lachman (2010) suggest that a palliative approach is appropriate whenever outcomes shift from a primary focus on wound healing to a focus on symptom control and relief of suffering, with the goal of improving quality of life and psychosocial well-being. They note that it is not necessary to abandon the goal of healing (Emmons & Lachman, 2010). Excellence in palliative wound care promotes healing to the extent that repair is possible (Ching et al., 2019; Maida et al., 2012). Scenarios in which palliative wound care may be beneficial include challenging symptom management, chronic debilitating disease or advanced illness, severe malnutrition and dehydration, unknown etiology when the diagnostic workup is inconsistent with goals of care, chronic long-standing or large wounds for which healing is unlikely, and when surgery or other treatments are not an option or are against patient and family wishes (Ching et al., 2019; Emmons & Lachman, 2010; Letizia et al., 2010; Maida, 2013).

Palliative Wound Care

Palliative care is the best approach for wounds with limited potential for healing. Wound care nurses have no objective measures for identifying these wounds. A Wound Healing Probability Tool was developed to aid wound care nurses to determine the likelihood of wound healing (**Table 35-1**) (Letizia et al., 2010). The greater the number of items selected on the 20 item Wound Healing Probability Tool, the less likely the wound is to heal. While the tool has not been validated, wound care nurses may use it to guide decision making. With many impediments, palliation might be a better focus than an emphasis on wound healing. The tool also aids in providing the wound care nurse with standard language to communicate with other health care providers, patients, and family members on factors impeding wound healing. It also provides specifics for documenting the rationale for a plan of care.

TABLE 35-1 FRAIL HEALING PROBABILITY ASSESSMENT TOOL

- Wound(s) is over 3 months old or is a reoccurrence of a preexisting breakdown
- The patient spends 20 or more hours of a day in a dependent position (chair or bed)
- The patient is incontinent of urine
- The patient is incontinent of feces
- The patient has lost >5% of baseline weight, or 10 pounds, in the past 90 days
- The patient does not eat independently
- The patient does not walk independently
- The patient has a history of falls within last 90 days
- The patient is unable/unwilling to avoid placing weight over wound(s) site(s)
- Wound is associated with complications of diabetes mellitus
- Wound is associated with peripheral vascular disease (PVD)
- Severe chronic obstructive pulmonary disease (COPD)
- End-stage renal, liver, or heart disease
- Wound is associated with arterial disease
- The patient has diminished range of motion (ROM) status nonresponsive to rehabilitative services
- The patient has diminished level of mental alertness demonstrated by muted communication skills and inability to perform activities of daily living (ADLs) independently
- Wound is full thickness with presence of tunneling
- Blood values indicate a low oxygen-carrying capacity
- Blood values indicate an exhausted or decreasing immune capacity (i.e., low lymphocyte count)
- Blood values indicate below normal visceral protein levels that have not responded to nutritional support efforts (i.e., low prealbumin, transferrin, retinol-binding protein, and albumin)

From Letizia, M., Uebelhor, J., & Paddack, E. (2010). Providing palliative care to seriously ill patients with nonhealing wounds. *Journal of Wound, Ostomy, and Continence Nursing, 37*(3), 277–282.

Wounds have been shown to negatively impact the individual's quality of life, with degree of impact determined by symptom presence and severity as well as psychosocial responses (Emmons, 2012). Common wound-related symptoms that impact quality of life include chronic or episodic wound pain, odor, drainage, itching, and bleeding (Alvarez et al., 2007; Emmons, 2012; Langemo et al., 2007; Woo et al., 2018). Poorly controlled wound-related symptoms may result in psychosocial responses that further impair quality of life, such as fear, anxiety, depression, anger, and concerns regarding burden on others (Alvarez et al., 2007; Eisenberger & Zeleznik, 2003; Woo et al., 2018). The HOPPES acronym has been developed as a simple aid to remembering symptom assessment. The letters represent **h**emorrhage, **o**dor control, **p**ain, **p**ruritus, **e**xudate management, and **s**uperficial infection (Woo et al., 2018). The presence of a superficial infection can increase both physical and psychosocial symptoms. One aspect of palliative wound care is effective symptom control, which improves quality of life and psychosocial well-being (Graves & Sun, 2013).

Palliative Wound Care Patient Exemplar

An example of a non–terminally ill patient who is considered for palliative wound care is a patient on a ventilator with a nonhealing wound who is not a surgical candidate, has severe malnutrition, and has a highly exudative wound. In this case, the wound care nurse should document that wound healing is unlikely at the present time, due to the presence of multiple concomitant factors that impair wound healing. The wound care plan should focus on stabilizing the wound, preventing infection, controlling symptoms (exudate), and optimizing the patient physiologically. When and if the patient improves, wound improvement is likely to be seen, and goals may be modified to include a focus on healing. This scenario highlights the need for realistic and clearly articulated care goals and a plan of care that emphasizes symptom management but does not abandon the goal of healing.

● DEVELOPING A PALLIATIVE PLAN OF CARE

An essential aspect of palliative wound care is the focus on the whole patient rather than a focus solely on the wound. When developing a plan of care, the wound care nurse must collect all pertinent information to create a comprehensive clinical picture. This provides the foundation for discussions that involve the patient, family, and other members of the health care team and that result in informed rational decisions regarding the plan of care. In addition to the current and past medical history, laboratory data, physical exam, and wound assessment, the wound care nurse must collect scenario-specific information that addresses the patient's quality of life, wound-related symptomatology and concerns, and patient and family preferences, goals, and values.

The process of developing a palliative plan of care is designed to be patient centered.

Patients are experts in their care and should be empowered to participate in treatment decision making, monitor treatment responses, and actively communicate with the health care team (Woo et al., 2015). An open conversation exploring the impact of the illness and the wound and the patient's and family's perceptions and concerns helps to elicit important information for goal setting and care planning. Specific questions should be asked regarding wound-related symptoms, such as "What is bothering you the most (pain, odor, drainage, bleeding, frequent dressings, etc.)?" The family should be queried as well, since their concerns may be somewhat different; for example, the patient may be most concerned about pain, while the family may be very distressed by odor

and drainage. In addition to physical symptomatology, the wound care nurse should ask about factors such as cosmesis, social isolation, functional impairment or limitations related to the wound, and burden of care. Once the wound care nurse has developed an understanding of the issues and concerns of most importance to the patient and family, those concerns can be prioritized in order of importance to the patient and family and probable responsiveness to interventions. It is important to help the patient and family establish realistic goals with achievable outcomes. For example, if the patient and family identify wound healing as a high-priority goal but the wound care nurse knows that healing is not likely at the present time due to ongoing chemotherapy and nutritional compromise, the wound care nurse should explain the conditions required for healing. They should redirect the goals to wound stabilization and symptom management until blood counts and nutritional status return to normal, when the care focus can be shifted to wound healing. Goals and interventions will change in response to the disease trajectory and patient response to medical and surgical management. It is important for the wound care nurse to explain that the wound care provided will be evidence based and will support healing but will be modified based on the patient's condition and the patient's and family's priorities at any given point in time. Wound healing may be one of the goals, but it is not the primary goal of palliative wound care.

● SKIN CHANGES AT END OF LIFE

Palliative wound care is associated with end-of-life care. With advanced illness and at end of life, significant changes in bodily systems occur, each of which has an impact on skin integrity. Although skin changes at the end of life were documented over 100 years ago (Charcot, 1877), it was not until recently that this issue received more focus among clinicians and in the literature. The Kennedy terminal ulcer (KTU), Trombley-Brennan terminal tissue injury (TB-TTI), and Skin Changes At Life's End (SCALE) have become common concepts used to describe skin changes at end of life (Ayello, et al., 2019). For example, the KTU was first described in 1989 as unavoidable skin breakdown that occurs at end of life. The characteristics of KTU include (1) location on the sacrococcygeal area, (2) sudden onset of deeply discolored skin in the shape of a butterfly or pear, (3) rapid progression despite appropriate management (from deep purple, red, black, or blue area to clearly necrotic

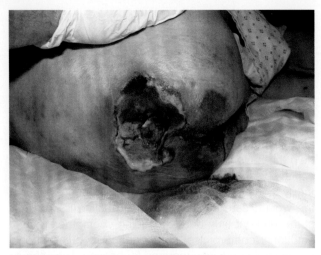

FIGURE 35-1. A Rapidly Evolving Unstageable Pressure Injury with Deep Tissue Pressure Injury (DTPI) on Sacrum.

wound), and (4) irregular borders (Kennedy, 1989). The KTU was the first wound hypothesized to be the result of hypoperfusion associated with multiorgan failure such as occurs during the dying process. Once these ulcers develop, there is rapid enlargement within a short window of time; a moist necrotic area forms over the center of the well-demarcated area, regardless of pressure-redistributing interventions (Langemo & Black, 2010; Yastrub, 2010) (**Fig. 35-1**). In contrast to the KTU, the TB-TTI has been described as spontaneous bruise-like lesions, is located over bony prominences and in areas not exposed to pressure, and typically presents within 72 hours of death (Ayello, et al., 2019; Trombley, et al., 2012). TB-TTIs should not be confused with deep tissue pressure injuries (Ayello, et al., 2019).

KEY POINT

Kennedy Terminal Ulcer was first described in 1989 as unavoidable skin breakdown that occurs at end of life and is characterized by rapid onset and progression despite appropriate preventive care.

In 2008, an interdisciplinary panel of 18 wound experts convened to develop a consensus statement on the changes that occur at the end of life (Skin Changes at Life's End [SCALE]) (Sibbald et al., 2010). SCALE can be attributed to reduced soft tissue perfusion, decreased tolerance to external insults, and impaired removal of metabolic wastes. Risk factors and signs and symptoms associated with SCALE include suboptimal nutrition, loss of appetite, weight loss, cachexia and wasting, low serum albumin and prealbumin, low hemoglobin, and dehydration. At end of life, the dying process may compromise the homeostatic mechanisms of the body, including perfusion. When cardiac output is reduced, the body attempts to protect vital organs by shunting blood away

from the skin resulting in peripheral tissue hypoperfusion (White-Chu & Langemo, 2012). Diminished tissue perfusion is the most significant risk factor for SCALE. Most of the skin has collateral vascular supply, but the most distal locations (fingers, toes, ears, and nose) lack collaterals. These areas are more susceptible to hypoperfusion and to pressure damage, even if the pressure is of minimal intensity and limited duration. Mechanical insults that would normally be well tolerated (limited pressure, shear, and friction) can lead to skin hemorrhage, gangrene, infection, skin tears, and pressure injuries (Sibbald et al., 2010). An important aspect of SCALE is the inclusion of factors, in addition to pressure, such as equipment or devices, incontinence, chemical irritants, chronic exposure to body fluids, skin tears, shear, friction, or infections that contribute to loss of skin integrity (Ayello, et al., 2019). A major conclusion from the SCALE consensus panel was that not all pressure injuries are avoidable (Sibbald et al., 2010, 2011).

Skin changes at end of life are now being described as skin failure for consistency with terminology related to other end-of-life changes such as cardiac and renal failure. Organ failure of other systems is well accepted, and as the largest organ system in the body, it is reasonable that the skin can fail too. Skin failure as a concept is developing as more literature examines the phenomena. Skin failure has been defined as an event in which the skin and underlying tissue die due to hypoperfusion that occurs concurrent with severe dysfunction or failure of other organ systems (Langemo & Brown, 2006). Levine (2017) has expanded this definition as the state in which tissue tolerance is so compromised that cells can no longer survive in zones of physiologic impairment such as hypoxia, local mechanical stresses, impaired delivery of nutrients, and buildup of toxic metabolic by-products. The severity and impact of skin failure can manifest according to the trajectory of illness such as acute onset or a more insidious chronic development, as for other organ systems. Acute skin failure has been defined as tissue death because of hypoperfusion concurrent with a critical illness (Cohen et al., 2017), as a pressure-related injury concurrent with critical illness that manifests as a result of hemodynamic instability and major organ system compromise (Delmore et al., 2015). In the dermatology literature, skin failure is described as a cutaneous state characterized by erythema and scaling of >90% of the body's surface (Guerry & Lemyze, 2012).

There is no widely accepted standard definition of skin failure, and the onset can be acute or chronic. The precise mechanisms of skin failure are unknown, and there are no standard tests to determine when skin failure occurs. This ambiguity often presents the wound care nurse with difficulties in determining how to document wound etiology, such as in the case of a pressure injury in a severely compromised patient or in someone who is actively dying. At the current time it would not be appropriate to document the primary wound etiology as skin failure. With the limited scientific knowledge on skin failure, the development of a wound in the presence of pressure is presumed to be a pressure injury and pressure injury staging should be documented. This does not preclude the wound care nurse from documenting all of the factors that may have contributed to wound development in the likely setting of skin failure. This is similar to the long-term care setting model of documenting avoidable versus unavoidable pressure injuries or KTUs in Long-Term Acute Care (LTAC). Both of these must be accompanied by thorough documentation. In the setting of suspected skin failure, documentation of the trajectory of illness, factors that significantly impact other organ systems, and factors that may contribute to the skin failing can create a clinical picture of why a person was at greater risk for developing a wound. This is in addition to documenting all of the preventative measures that may have been implemented to mitigate wounds that could have been reasonably prevented (Black et al., 2011; Edsberg et al., 2014; WOCN, 2016).

> ### KEY POINT
>
> Skin changes at end of life are also sometimes classified as skin failure, for consistency with terminology relating to other organ systems at end of life (e.g., cardiac failure or renal failure).

● COMMON WOUNDS IN THE PALLIATIVE CARE POPULATION

PRESSURE INJURIES

Pressure injuries are the most commonly reported wound in hospice and palliative care (Maida et al., 2012). The prevalence and incidence of pressure injuries varies depending on the setting. A recent systematic review of pressure injuries in patients receiving palliative care, Ferris and colleagues (2019) reported that home palliative care had the lowest prevalence of pressure injuries of 12.4% with an incidence rate between 10.2% and 11%, the inpatient setting had prevalence of 27% with an incidence rate between 13.8% and 19%, and nursing home—managed palliative care patients had the highest prevalence rate of 54.7%, while the incidence rates ranged from 6.9% to 16.2% depending on length of nursing home stay. These numbers are not surprising, given the fact that hospice and palliative care patients are high risk due to the disease trajectory and, for hospice patients, the impact of terminal illness on perfusion status. Factors contributing to pressure injury risk among all palliative care patients include deteriorating physical condition, increasing frailty, immobility, decreased nutritional and fluid intake, fecal and urinary incontinence, changes in sensory perception and levels of conscious-

ness, and alterations in hemodynamic status (Ayello et al., 2015; Coleman et al., 2013). Neurological or non-cancer diagnosis, previous pressure injuries, older age, and caregiver frailty have also been shown to increase risk for the development of new pressure injuries in home health and hospice palliative care patients (Burt, 2013; Reifsnyder & Magee, 2005). In addition to being higher risk for pressure injury development, palliative care and hospice care patients are at risk for impaired healing, due to the same factors that contribute to injury development.

> ### KEY POINT
>
> Pressure injuries are the most commonly reported wound among palliative care and hospice patients. In addition to being high risk for pressure injury development, these patients are high risk for impaired healing.

Risk Assessment

The Braden Scale for Predicting Pressure Sore Risk is a reliable validated tool and has been shown to positively reflect risk in the palliative care patient (Bolton, 2007). The Braden scale does not consider other physiologic conditions that may increase risk in palliative care or in patients with severe organ failure. Additional risk factors for pressure injury development in addition to those included in the Braden scale have been identified in the critical care population. These include factors that may not be easily mitigated due to the severity of illness: presence of septic shock, use of vasopressor agents, sedation, and prolonged mechanical ventilation (Cox et al., 2018). In contrast to the Braden scale, the Hunters Hill Marie Curie Center pressure sore risk assessment tool (Hunters Hill Tool) was designed specifically for use in the palliative care setting (Chrisman, 2010). The Hunters Hill Tool includes the primary risk factors addressed by the Braden and Norton Scales but also considers existing skin condition. This tool has not been tested for interrater reliability, and there is limited research regarding its validity. Further research is needed in regard to the impact of reduced tissue perfusion on pressure injury development in this population, and the implications for risk assessment and prevention.

Prevention

Pressure injury prevention is important in palliative care. The specific components of the program must be modified to meet the needs of the individual patient. Information gained from the overall patient assessment, the total risk assessment score, and the risk assessment subscale scores should be used to formulate a specific prevention program that addresses the individual's needs and priorities (Bolton, 2007). For example, a typical prevention program for the patient with a low mobility subscale score would include a pressure redistribution support surface and routine turning and repositioning (EPUAP/NPIAP/PPPIA, 2019; VandenBosch et al., 1996).

In the general patient population, these measures are usually sufficient to protect the tissues against ischemic damage. However, in palliative care patients who have compromised tissue perfusion, pressure injuries may develop despite these interventions, because lower levels of applied pressure may be sufficient to induce ulceration (Lyder & Ayello, 2008).

Palliative care and hospice care patients must be recognized as a high-risk group for whom accepted preventive measures may be insufficient. In addition, specific aspects of preventive care may be inconsistent with the patient's care goals and priorities. These will be discussed individually.

Turning and Positioning

It is widely accepted that keeping the head of the bed at or lower than 30 degrees reduces pressure in the sacrococcygeal area and helps to protect the vulnerable tissues in this anatomic region and that regular turning and repositioning are key pressure injury prevention measures (WOCN, 2016). Patients may require higher degrees of head of bed elevation due to pain or compromised pulmonary or cardiovascular status and may refuse turning due to pain and the desire to be left undisturbed once they get comfortable. Turning and repositioning recommendations have changed in recent literature to reflect a schedule that is patient centered and reflects a person's individual status and risk factors (EPUAP/NPIAP/PPPIA, 2019; WOCN, 2016). Appropriate interventions might include obtaining a higher-level pressure redistribution support surface, reducing turning frequency, and augmenting the turning program with small weight shifts or use of pillows to reduce pressure over vulnerable areas (Krapfl & Gray, 2008). Pharmacologic and nonpharmacologic modalities prior to scheduled position changes may be helpful in meeting the dual goals of pressure injury prevention and maintenance of patient comfort (Langemo et al., 2015). When pain precludes routine turning and repositioning, nursing documentation should include a notation regarding reasons for not turning the patient and compensatory interventions, for example, "Patient refused turning 10 PM till 6 AM due to pain and unwillingness to be disturbed—verbalizes awareness that failure to turn increases risk of skin breakdown. Will contact MD regarding adjustments in pain medication; minor weight shifts provided every 2 hours in attempt to minimize ischemic damage. The patient remains on high-level air support surface."

KEY POINT

Measures to prevent pressure injury development are important for the palliative care or hospice patient. Specific interventions (such as turning frequency and nutritional management) may require modification if comfort goals have been determined higher priority than skin care goals.

Support Surfaces

Support surfaces should be selected based on the patient's mobility in bed and willingness to be turned, comfort factors, need for microclimate control, and environmental factors. All patients found to be at risk for developing pressure injuries should be placed on a pressure redistribution support surface. Those who cannot be turned and repositioned frequently should be placed on an alternating pressure overlay or mattress if tolerated. Some patients find the shifts in position produced by alternating pressure surfaces to be uncomfortable and may prefer a nonpowered surface. Repositioning should occur at least every 4 hours if on a pressure redistribution support surface or viscoelastic foam and every 2 hours on a regular mattress (Langemo et al., 2015). Regardless of the type of support surface being used, heels should be suspended using heel protectors or pillows under the calves (WOCN, 2016).

Nutrition

In general, a low nutrition subscale score on the pressure injury risk assessment tool prompts the wound care nurse to implement supportive interventions that will increase intake of the fluids, calories, protein, and vitamins necessary for wound healing and pressure injury prevention. In the palliative care setting, aggressive nutritional interventions may not be appropriate. Nausea, anorexia, and weight loss are common manifestations in palliative care individuals and at end of life. Families and caregivers may see their family member deteriorating and not understand that loss of appetite and reduced food and fluid intake is common with chronic illness and at end of life. They may request or demand supplemental nutrition such as tube feedings. Open communication with caregivers should include information about the use of alternatives such as hand feeding and oral supplements as preferable to enteral feedings, even if the overall intake is poor. Enteral nutrition can provide for basic nutritional needs and would seem to be the ideal solution to situations in which oral intake is inadequate; however, there are a number of complications associated with enteral feedings. Studies on patients with advanced dementia have shown little to no benefit in reducing risk or promoting healing of pressure injuries (Hanson, 2013; Teno et al., 2012). Hand feeding or comfort feeding can help reduce symptoms such as dry mouth, hunger, and thirst as well as providing an opportunity for patient caregiver interaction. Oral care aids in reducing mouth pain and improving taste (Langemo & Black, 2010). Small frequent meals and lifting of any dietary restrictions (such as glucose or salt restriction) has been shown to be beneficial in improving nutritional intake. It may not always be possible to assure adequate intake of fluids and nutrients, and the patient's goals must determine the priorities in care, including nutritional management (EPUAP/NPIAP/PPPIA, 2019; Posthauser, 2007).

In summary, pressure injury prevention is important in the palliative care setting for a number of reasons. Skin breakdown can add to the patient's discomfort, level of morbidity, and risk of mortality. Pressure injury development increases the level of skilled and formal care required, which can adversely affect the patient's quality of life (Brink et al., 2006). Caregivers often see the development of a pressure injury as an indicator of poor care by themselves or staff. In most cases, use of appropriate support surfaces, routine use of heel elevation devices, and attention to modified repositioning programs is effective in maintaining skin integrity. The basic concept of palliative care is holistic care directed by patient and caregiver goals. In some situations, pressure injuries may be unavoidable (e.g., situations in which the patient is cachectic, the tissues are poorly perfused, and the patient and family elect comfort as a higher priority than maintenance of skin integrity). It is important to document decisions regarding care priorities and reasons for modified positioning. There should be ongoing documentation of skin status; staff and caregivers should be taught to incorporate skin inspection into routine care and activities of daily living. Any observation of impending or actual breakdown should be reported to the patient and family, with further discussion as to care priorities (aggressive skin care vs. comfort care). Consistent priorities in care are to (1) comply with patient wishes and overall goals, (2) help to maintain or improve quality of life, and (3) facilitate reduction of burdensome symptoms.

MALIGNANT WOUNDS

In some patients with advanced cancer, the tumor extends to and invades the skin (**Figs. 35-2 to 35-4**). In 2017, about 30% of hospice patients had a primary diagnosis of cancer (National Hospice and Palliative Care Organization, 2019), and it is estimated that 5% to 19% of all patients with a malignant neoplasm diagnosis will develop a skin lesion (Sibbald et al., 2011). Thirty percent of patients with metastatic breast cancer develop cutaneous lesions (Ladizinski et al., 2014), with 62% of fungating wounds found on the breast. Head and neck cancers account for another 24% (Bergstrom, 2011).

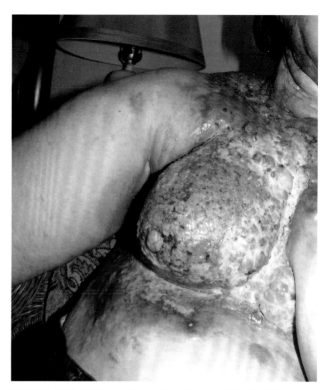

FIGURE 35-2. Malignant Fungating Wound of the Right Breast with Associated Lymphedema.

A fungating wound is defined as the infiltration and proliferation of malignant cells into the skin and its supporting blood and lymph vessels (Bergstrom, 2011). These cutaneous malignant wounds can be further classified as either ulcerative or fungating depending on the growth pattern. Ulcerative tumors form craters while proliferative tumors form a nodular fungus or cauliflower-type lesion referred to as fungating (Langemo, 2012). All malignant wounds produce both physical and emotional stress for patients and caregivers due to the symptoms and the appearance of the wound. The most reported symp-

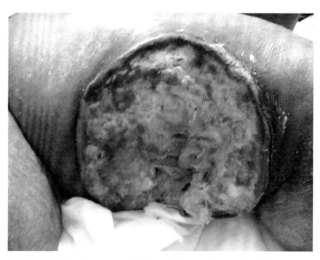

FIGURE 35-3. Ulcerative Malignant Wound on the Left Inner Thigh.

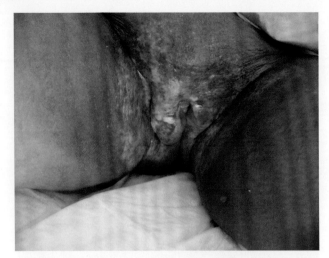

FIGURE 35-4. Malignant Fungating Wound of the Vulva.

toms associated with malignant wounds are malodor and infection, drainage, bleeding, and pain (Tsichlakidou et al., 2019). Managing symptoms is essential to improving quality of life. Management of these symptoms can be easily adapted and applied in the care of other wound etiologies such as pressure injuries and leg ulcers.

Odor

A common and very distressing symptom reported by patients and caregivers is wound odor. Patients typically report feeling embarrassed and stigmatized because of wound odor, which leads to social isolation increasing feelings of hopelessness and depression (Lo et al., 2012). Both indirect and direct methods can be used for odor control. Indirect odor control can be attained by reducing the necrotic tissue and bacterial loads within the wound (Akhmetova et al., 2016). Reducing the overall bacterial load is particularly helpful in reducing wound odor by addressing the cause. Thorough irrigation of the wound with copious amounts of potable (drinkable) water can help reduce bacterial counts in the wound. If the patient is able to shower, allowing free indirect flow of water across the wound bed is another effective approach to reduction of bacterial loads (Bergstrom, 2011). Dressings such as cadexomer iodine, gentian violet, honey, and silver products can help reduce odor by providing an antimicrobial effect (Akhmetova et al., 2016). These dressings may be cost-effective since most can stay in place for a longer period of time. Antiseptic solutions are highly effective at reducing odor-causing bacteria. Sodium hypochlorite and acetic acid are inexpensive and effective, but they can cause burning or tingling at the site and periwound irritation and discomfort (due to pH levels). In addition, they add to caregiver burden because they must be changed daily (Merz et al., 2011). To reduce the risk of periwound irritation and pain at the site, a contact layer or base layer of moist saline gauze can be used with the sodium hypochlorite or acetic acid–moistened

gauze as a secondary layer. Sodium hypochlorite is thrombolytic and may increase topical bleeding and should be used cautiously with friable wounds (Ayello et al., 2015). Polyhexamethylene biguanide (PHMB) (0.2%) and superoxide water with hypochlorous acid solutions are less caustic antiseptic choices and are effective at reducing bacteria and odor (Akhmetova et al., 2016; Beers, 2019). Antiseptic solutions should be used for a short period of time to quickly reduce bacterial loads, reducing symptom burden. The use of advanced antimicrobial dressings with longer wear time can be implemented for sustained bacterial suppression. Advanced antimicrobial and moisture-retentive dressings may also contribute to reduced bacterial loads and reduced odor, by supporting autolytic debridement and through direct antimicrobial action unless there is significant immune dysfunction.

Topical metronidazole and antimicrobial dressings are first-line approaches to management of odor with fungating malignant wounds; antiseptics such as dilute Dakin solution may also be used on a short-term basis.

Metronidazole is the most commonly studied intervention for the management of wound odor. Topical metronidazole has shown to reduce and control wound odor within 4 to 14 days and is comparable to some antiseptics (Alexander, 2009; Finlayson et al., 2017; Villela-Castro et al., 2018). Metronidazole is commercially available with a prescription as a gel, powder, paste, cream, or tablet. The gel, paste, or creams can be applied directly to the malignant wound in a thick layer, which promotes a moist wound healing environment, decreases dry cracking lesions, reduces trauma with removal of the dressing, and promotes autolytic debridement of nonviable tissue. Tablets can be dissolved in potable water and used to irrigate the wound, or the solution can be used to soak gauze used to pack or cover the wound. Tablets can also be crushed and sprinkled on the wound surface and then covered with petrolatum gauze and a dry bulky dressing. If the wound care nurse crushes a tablet, he or she should wear a mask or crush the tablets in a bag, as metronidazole particles are harmful to pleural tissue. There is insufficient evidence to determine the efficacy of oral metronidazole on controlling wound odor (Ramasubbu et al., 2017).

Direct methods of odor control are aimed at trapping unpleasant volatile organic compounds or gasses before they are inhaled (Akhmetova et al., 2016). Charcoal dressings are available but are infrequently used due to cost and the need to secure the dressing circumferentially with tape so that the odor molecules are forced through the charcoal as opposed to being allowed to escape from the sides of the dressing. Room deodorizers and other types of aromatherapy can also be used to mask any odors, such as essential oils (peppermint, lavender, lemon, etc.), scented candles, or charcoal. Kitty litter or coffee grounds placed in containers around the home or under the patient's bed have also been cited as a useful adjunct for odor control (Merz et al., 2011).

Drainage

Drainage from malignant wounds is frequently copious, and with odor, is frequently embarrassing for the patient. Copious amounts of drainage may cause periwound moisture-associated skin damage (PWMASD). The periwound skin should be routinely protected with moisture barrier creams or ointments or with liquid barrier films. Measures to reduce bacterial bioburden and to eliminate necrotic tissue help to reduce drainage. Once bioburden is reduced and odor is controlled, exudate can be managed with a variety of dressings that are nonadherent, conformable, and absorptive. Unfortunately, malignant wounds are frequently located in difficult to dress areas such as the chest wall, axilla, or head and neck region. Silicone adhesive foam dressings are a good choice for smaller wounds with low-to-moderate volumes of exudate. Larger wounds with higher-volume drainage may require alginate or Hydrofiber dressings as the primary dressing with secondary gauze dressings for additional absorption. Stockinette-like tube bandages or binders can be useful for securing dressings when tape is not appropriate. Wounds with especially high output may benefit from the use of an ostomy or wound pouching system.

Bleeding

The fear of bleeding and/or hemorrhage can be worrisome to the palliative care patient, their caregivers, and health care providers as bleeding is often difficult to manage. Bleeding occurs frequently in malignant wounds because cancer cells stimulate angiogenesis, thus increasing vascularity. In addition, associated pathologies (e.g., thrombocytopenia, disseminated intravascular coagulopathy [DIC], and malnutrition) are common and can also increase the risk of bleeding. These wounds are friable because the quality of the new vasculature is poor (Recka et al., 2012). Slight trauma to the wound bed caused by dressing changes, cleansing, stretching or cracking of the skin and wound, and frequent movement can all contribute to bleeding. Major bleeding episodes are usually due to the wound's proximity to large vessels, such as in head and neck wounds. Tumor growth can cause pressure on vessels, leading to erosion and leaks or to major bleeding episodes.

KEY POINT

Bleeding is a common and frightening complication associated with fungating malignant wounds. Calcium alginate dressings can be used to control minor oozing, but major bleeding usually requires hemostatic foams or gauze.

Prevention of bleeding should be a priority in management of malignant wounds. Maintaining a moist wound surface using nonadherent topical products reduces the risk of trauma and reduces the incidence of episodic bleeding. Selection of methods to control bleeding is dependent on access to specific products and medications. Common topical agents to treat bleeding include natural hemostatic agents, coagulants, sclerosing agents, vasoconstrictors, fibrinolytic inhibitors, and astringents (Woo & Sibbald, 2010). Control of minor generalized oozing can be achieved with calcium alginate dressings. The calcium found within these dressings helps promote the clotting cascade and thereby eliminates bleeding. Most brands of calcium alginate can also be found in a rope structure that easily accommodates the often irregular contours of malignant and fungating wounds. Considerations when using alginates for hemostasis is that the coagulation of blood may cause the dressing to stick to the wound bed, which can lead to recurrent bleeding upon alginate removal. It is best to leave the base layer of alginate in the wound during subsequent dressing changes and to allow the alginate to gradually separate from the wound and to be removed with gentle wound irrigations. For large areas of active bleeding, gelling hemostatic foams and hemostatic surgical gauze are better options, though more expensive and not as readily available. These hemostatic dressings can be applied in layers and left in place. Epinephrine-soaked gauze can also be applied topically; it causes vasoconstriction of vessels, helping to control bleeding. The topical application of zinc chloride paste (Mohs paste) as a chemical hemostatic agent has been documented in several wound etiologies. In a small study, bleeding was controlled in malignant wounds; however pain associated with the initial application was noted (Kakimoto et al., 2010). Antifibrinolytic medication (e.g., tranexamic acid and aminocaproic acid) can be taken orally or in some cases applied topically (Recka et al., 2012) for management of low-pressure bleeding. These medications are more costly and require a prescription. For minor bleeding, silver nitrate is a quick and easy intervention that cauterizes exposed vessels. In severe cases that may cause significant distress, surgical and radiologic procedures can be performed. In some scenarios when bleeding cannot be stopped, the implementation of nonpharmacologic and comfort measures to reduce distress are imperative. Collection devices such as wound or ostomy pouching systems can contain large amounts of blood and can be easily emptied. Finally, patients and their caregivers can be instructed to keep dark towels and dark sheets on hand to mask the color and to reduce anxiety associated with bleeding or hemorrhage.

Pain

Pain can be difficult to manage, and wound-related pain is no exception. The principles of wound-related pain management have been discussed in Chapter 8, and these principles and strategies are equally effective for management of pain in palliative care patients. Use of the World Health Organization (WHO) pain control ladder may be beneficial in management of any patient with chronic pain. Persons who would benefit from palliative care often have concurrent conditions requiring effective pain management with long-acting and breakthrough pain medications. Uncontrolled general chronic pain can exacerbate and potentiate other pain such as wound-related pain. A thorough pain assessment to determine triggering and relieving factors is the first step in determining whether the pain is persistent or associated primarily with procedures or dressing changes. Persistent pain is managed with around-the-clock analgesics. Procedure-related pain can be reduced with premedication, use of nonadherent dressings, gentle technique, less frequent dressing changes, and allowing the patient to call time-outs during dressing changes if needed. Patients and providers alike often look for topical solutions to reduce wound-related pain. Morphine in hydrogel can be an effective pain reliever, and it has little to no systemic absorption (Emmons et al., 2014). Other topical anesthetics (lidocaine and EMLA cream) may provide intermittent pain relief but can be accompanied by transient burning and systemic absorption with chronic use.

> **KEY POINT**
>
> A thorough pain assessment and aggressive pain management are critical components of care for the palliative care patient.

SKIN TEARS

Prevention of skin tears in palliative care involves the same principles and strategies as skin tear prevention for the general population. Most skin tears occur as a result of falls, adhesive removal, assistance with activities of daily living (bathing, dressing, turning, and repositioning), and trauma incurred during transfers (e.g., bumping the extremities against side rails or wheelchair parts). Interventions to prevent skin tears are the same for palliative care and usual care patients. Palliative care patients are usually higher risk and require greater awareness and more attentive preventive care. Meticulous skin care with pH-balanced cleansers, routine use of emollients and lotions, gentle handling techniques to reduce friction and shear, and proper transfer and reposition techniques are some of the interventions that can be implemented. Instructing caregivers to keep the patient's and their own nails trimmed is an often overlooked measure. Protective sleeves and leggings are commercially available and very beneficial. Simple alternatives include stockinette, and athletic socks with the toes cut out can be used. Tape should be avoided whenever possible. Devices and dressings should be secured with wrap gauze, binders, stretch net, stockinette, mastectomy

bras, or nonadhesive self-adherent wrap. In providing topical care, the wound care nurse should avoid dressings with aggressive adhesives. Good options for management include use of contact layer dressings covered by dry gauze and secured with roll gauze (extremity wounds), or silicone adhesive foam dressings (trunk wounds) (LeBlanc & Baranoski, 2011).

> **KEY POINT**
>
> In providing topical care, the wound care nurse should avoid use of aggressive adhesives and should use wrap gauze to secure dressings on extremity wounds.

LOWER LEG ULCERATIONS

A history of leg ulcers or active lower limb ulcers is not uncommon in the palliative care population. Simple preventive measures should be continued for those with a history of lower-extremity ulcers and those known to be at risk. Active wounds should be managed based on symptomatology. Differential assessment is important in the management of any lower leg ulcers to confirm etiology because management of these wounds differs based on the causative factors. For example, venous ulcers are typically best managed by elevation and compression, whereas arterial ulcers are best managed with activity and positioning as tolerated. Neuropathic ulcers are most often seen on the plantar surface of the foot in an individual with diabetes. Elements of management when the goal is healing include consistent off-loading along with tight glucose control. For the palliative care patient, the primary goals in the management of a foot or leg ulcer are pain control and prevention of infection. Pain is the most often reported symptom with venous and arterial ulcers (Pieper et al., 2009). Measures to relieve the pain differ based on etiology. For example, arterial ulcer pain is relieved in part by dependency, while patients with venous ulcers find relief with elevation. Patients with neuropathic ulcers may have nighttime or rest pain (paresthesias) that may require pharmacologic management. Interventions to address pain in each of these individuals would vary greatly. Differential assessment is important.

Venous Leg Ulcers

Patients with venous leg ulcers can experience pain related to the underlying venous insufficiency, pain caused by the ulcer itself, or skin irritation and discomfort caused by the high-volume exudate associated with a venous leg ulcer. Standard pain management therapies for venous leg ulcers can be utilized in the palliative care patient unless contraindicated (compression, leg elevation, and oral analgesics if needed). The large amount of drainage can be managed with highly absorptive dressings and use of moisture barrier ointments or liquid barrier films for periwound skin protection. Patients with respiratory diagnoses and patients with heart failure often cannot tolerate compression therapy due to the risk of increased pulmonary distress caused by increased venous return. To control drainage and edema, a trial of modified low-level compression bandaging may be implemented (WOCN, 2019). Short-stretch bandages may be a good alternative to multilayer compression if the patient is unable to tolerate normal compression levels; however, short-stretch bandages are only effective in the ambulatory patient (WOCN, 2019). It should be noted that long-stretch bandages, such as ACE-type bandages, do not require the patient to be ambulatory but do not provide consistent effective compression. Tubular elasticated dressings provide 10 mm Hg compression with each layer and are generally more effective than Ace bandages and easier for the home caregiver to apply. If the patient's status improves over time to the point where he or she can tolerate higher compression, then more traditional methods and levels of compression therapy can be provided.

Arterial and Gangrenous Wounds

Pain associated with arterial or developing gangrenous leg ulcers is typically treated systemically. As ischemia progresses, the pain can become intense. Topical care is based on the status of the wound. If the wound is open and most of the wound bed is viable, principles of moist wound healing should be utilized. Maintenance of a moist wound bed prevents tissue desiccation, which causes increased pain. In contrast, the wound that is primarily covered with dry stable eschar or dry gangrene should be dressed with dry dressings or kept open to air to keep the area dry (WOCN, 2014) to prevent infection or progression from dry gangrene to wet gangrene. When managing dry eschar or dry gangrene, some wound care nurses advocate daily application of povidone–iodine solution or a liquid film barrier and allowing it to dry, with the goal of reducing topical bacteria while maintaining dry stable eschar (WOCN, 2016). The wound care nurse

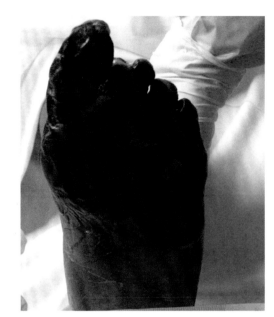

FIGURE 35-5. Dry Gangrene of the Left Foot.

should be aware that the appearance of dry eschar or gangrene is often overwhelming to the patient or caregiver. Simply covering the area with loose dry dressings is appropriate and can reduce the emotional pain associated with visualizing a necrotic area (**Fig. 35-5**).

● CONCLUSION

The emergence of palliative wound care is due in part to the fact that people are living longer with more severe and chronic diseases. The plan of care frequently needs to shift to palliative goals rather than healing. Healing goals are not abandoned; they are reprioritized within the context of palliation first and healing second. Wound care nurses must have the knowledge to develop a plan of care that is appropriate within the context of the person's health status.

CASE STUDIES

PALLIATIVE WOUND CARE CASE

A 43-year-old female with a primary diagnosis of HIV/AIDS was admitted to home health hospice. A wound care consult was requested for assessment and management of wound odor related to a neck wound. Upon physical examination, a large fungating wound was noted on the left side of the neck. Significant odor was noted upon exam. The malignant wound deeply invaded into the neck cavity and had significant white, yellow, and black necrosis. There was a 3-cm tunnel

noted at about 7 o'clock. Exudate was minimal and able to be contained with daily gauze dressings prior to assessment. The periwound assessment revealed previous radiation burns and dry desquamation.

Wound odor was the primary reason for this consult. After speaking with patient and family, it became clear that the problems were more extensive. Our conversation started with questions asking about how this wound had affected the patient and her family. This revealed that the patient was embarrassed to be seen

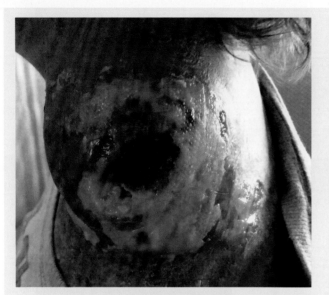

Malignant Fungating Wound on the Neck.

outside with gauze wrapped around her neck and with a terrible strong odor. As a result, this patient became socially isolated in her house. We then explored other things that bothered her such as the drainage and the burden of dressing changes and trying to keep them in place. The discussion then transitioned into the patient's and family's goals. We listed and prioritized them as follows: (1) control odor, (2) have cosmetically appealing dressing, (3) find dressings that are easy to apply and painless upon removal, and (4) regain ability to go to a restaurant and movie without feeling embarrassed about the wound. During this time, we discussed the fact that tumor wounds would not shrink without treatment (which had been stopped). We explored the possibility of the wound continuing to grow and the potential for other issues such as itching and the possibility of bleeding.

A plan was developed for each of the goals. Cleansing lightly in the shower was recommended. A topical metronidazole cream was chosen as the antimicrobial and deodorizing agent. This was chosen because the wound did not have significant drainage, and this product was available through the providing pharmacy. The metronidazole cream would provide a cooling sensation, a moist environment that would support autolytic debridement (to the extent physiologically possible), and atraumatic removal of the cover dressing. The cover dressing selected was a thin foam dressing with a silicone adhesive. This dressing reduced the topical layer to a single thin layer as opposed to a bulky gauze wrap; the silicone adhesive foam dressing also reduced the flaky irritated skin that had developed following radiation. An elastic loose-fitting head band was used to keep the dressing in place during frequent movement and to provide a final appealing look for the patient. She could choose any color to match her outfit. Options were also discussed for the management of bleeding (both oozing and major bleeding) and for management of increasing odor and drainage (should this become a problem).

FOLLOW-UP

Within 4 days, the odor had almost completely subsided. The patient reported that she frequently left the house with family, and she no longer had fears related to uncontrolled wound symptoms.

As the patient's disease process progressed and she became homebound, the plan of care changed until her death. Drainage had increased, and a silver alginate was chosen as the topical dressing with silicone adhesive foam cover dressings, which contained both odor and drainage.

This case exemplifies the need to explore what is important to the patient and family. Here, social isolation was the main issue and was caused by wound odor and the need for bulky conspicuous dressings. The plan of care was driven by the patient and family with the collaboration of the wound care nurse. Fears regarding healing and wound progress were discussed, and options were developed to alleviate concerns. This plan of care focused on improving quality of life by giving the patient back the freedom to leave the house without the burden of uncontrolled symptoms.

REFERENCES

Akhmetova, A., Saliev, T., Allan, I. U., et al. (2016). A comprehensive review of topical odor-controlling treatment options for chronic wounds. *Journal of Wound, Ostomy, and Continence Nursing, 43*(6), 598–609.

Alexander, S. (2009). Malignant fungating wounds: managing pain, bleeding and psychosocial issues. *Journal of Wound Care, 18*(10), 418–425.

Alvarez, O. M., Kalinski, C., Nusbaum, J., et al. (2007). Incorporating wound healing strategies to improve palliation (symptom management) in patients with chronic wounds. *Journal of Palliative Medicine, 10*(5), 1161–1189.

Ayello, E. A., Levine, J. M., Langemo, D., et al. (2019). Reexamining the literature on terminal ulcers, SCALE, skin failure, and unavoidable pressure injuries. *Advances in Skin & Wound Care, 32*(3), 109–121.

Ayello, E. A., Sibbald, R. G., Woo, K. Y., et al. (2015). Skin alterations. In M. Matzo, & D. W. Sherman (Eds.), Palliative care nursing: quality care to the end of life (4th ed., pp. 627–647). New York, NY: Springer.

Beers, E. H. (2019). Palliative wound care: Less is more. *The Surgical Clinics of North America, 99*(5), 899–919.

Bergstrom, K. (2011). Assessment and management of fungating wounds. *Journal of Wound, Ostomy, and Continence Nursing, 38*(1), 31–37.

Black, J. M., Edsberg, L. E., Baharestani, M. M., et al. (2011). Pressure ulcers: Avoidable or unavoidable? Results of the national pressure ulcer advisory panel consensus conference. *Ostomy/Wound Management, 57*(2), 24–37.

Bolton, L. (2007). Which pressure ulcer risk assessment scales are valid for use in the clinical setting? *Journal of Wound, Ostomy, and Continence Nursing, 34*(4), 368–381.

Brink, P., Smith, T. F., & Linkewich, B. (2006). Factors associated with pressure ulcers in palliative home care. *Journal of Palliative Medicine, 9,* 1369–1375.

Burt, T. (2013). Palliative care of pressure ulcers in long-term care. *Annals of Long-Term Care, 21*(3), 20–28.

Charcot, J. M. (1877). *Lectures on the diseases of the nervous system* (Vol. 1). London, UK: New Sydenham Society.

Ching, A. H., Le, N., Norwich-Cavanaugh, A., et al. (2019). Evidence-based gardening: using palliative approaches to cure complex wounds. *Annals of Plastic Surgery, 83*(4S), S45–S49.

Chrisman, C. A. (2010). Care of chronic wounds in palliative care and end-of-life patients. *International Wound Journal, 7*(4), 214–235.

Cohen, K. E., Scanlon, M. C., Bemanian, A., et al. (2017). Pediatric skin failure. *American Journal of Critical Care, 26*(4), 320–328.

Coleman, S., Gorecki, C., Nelson, E. A., et al. (2013). Patient risk factors for pressure ulcer development: Systematic review. *International Journal of Nursing Studies, 50*(7), 974–1003.

Connor, S. R., & Gwyther, E. (2018). The worldwide hospice palliative care alliance. *Journal of Pain and Symptom Management, 55*(2S), S112–S116. https://doi.org/10.1016/j.jpainsymman.2017.03.020

Cox, J., Roche, S., & Murphy, V. (2018). Pressure injury risk factors in critical care patients. *Advances in Skin & Wound Care, 31*(7), 328–334.

Delmore, B., Cox, J., Rolnitzky, L., et al. (2015). Differentiating a pressure ulcer from acute skin failure in the adult critical care patient. *Advances in Skin & Wound Care, 28*(11), 514–524.

Edsberg, L. E., Langemo, D., Baharestani, M. M., et al. (2014). Unavoidable pressure injury: State of the science and consensus outcomes. *Journal of Wound, Ostomy, and Continence Nursing, 41*(4), 313–334. doi: 10.1097/WON.0000000000000050.

Eisenberger, A., & Zeleznik, J. (2003). Pressure ulcer prevention and treatment in hospices: A qualitative analysis. *Journal of Palliative Care, 19*(1), 9–14.

Emmons, K. R. (2012). Wounds at the end of life: Wound symptoms and severity, quality of life, and patient-reported symptoms and preferences for care (Doctoral Dissertation). Drexel libraries e-repository and archives. Retrieved from http://hdl.handle.net/1860/3757

Emmons, K. R., Dale, B., & Crouch, C. (2014). Palliative wound care part 2: Application of principles. *Home Healthcare Nurse, 32*(4), 201–222.

Emmons, K. R., & Lachman, V. L. (2010). Palliative wound care: A concept analysis. *Journal of Wound, Ostomy, and Continence Nursing, 37*(6), 639–644.

Ennis, W. J., & Meneses, P. (2005). Palliative care and wound care: 2 emerging fields with similar needs for outcomes data. *Wounds, 17*(4), 99–104.

European Pressure Ulcer Advisory Panel, National Pressure Injury Advisory Panel, and Pan Pacific Pressure Injury Alliance [EPUAP/NPIAP/PPPIA]. (2010). In E. Haesler (Ed.), *Prevention and treatment of pressure ulcers/injuries: Clinical Practice Guideline.* The International Guideline.

Ferris, F. D., Al Khateib, A. A., Fromantin, I., et al. (2007). Palliative wound care: Managing chronic wounds across life's continuum: A consensus statement from the International Palliative Wound Care Initiative. *Journal of Palliative Medicine, 10*(1), 37–39.

Ferris, A., Price, A., & Harding, K. (2019). Pressure ulcers in patients receiving palliative care: A systematic review. *Palliative Medicine, 33*(7), 770–782.

Finlayson, K., Teleni, L., & McCarthy, A. L. (2017). Topical opioids and antimicrobials for the management of pain, infection, and infection-related odors in malignant wounds: A systematic review. *Oncology Nursing Forum, 44*(5), 626–632.

Graves, M. L., & Sun, V. (2013). Providing quality wound care at the end of life. *Journal of Hospice & Palliative Nursing, 15*(2), 66–74.

Guerry, M. M. J., & Lemyze, M. (2012). Acute skin failure. *The British Medical Journal, 345,* e5028.

Hagan, T. L., Xu, J., Lopez, R. P., et al. (2018). Nursing's role in leading palliative care: A call to action. *Nurse Education Today, 61,* 216–219.

Hanson, L. C. (2013). Tube feeding versus assisted oral feeding for persons with dementia: Using evidence to support decision-making. *Annals of Long-Term Care, 21*(1), 16–28.

Hughes, R. G., Bakos, A. D., O'Mara, A., et al. (2005). Palliative wound care at the end of life. *Home Health Care Management & Practice, 17*(3), 196–202.

Hui, D., De La Cruz, M., Mori, M., et al. (2013). Concepts and definitions for "supportive care," "best supportive care," "palliative care," and "hospice care" in the published literature, dictionaries, and textbooks. *Supportive Care in Cancer, 21*(3), 659–689.

Hui, D., Mori, M., Parsons, H. A., et al. (2012). The lack of standardized definitions in the supportive and palliative oncology literature. *Journal of Pain and Symptom Management, 43*(3), 582–592.

Kakimoto, M., Tokita, H., Okamura, T., et al. (2010). A chemical hemostatic technique for bleeding from malignant wounds. *Journal of Palliative Medicine, 13*(1), 11–13.

Kennedy, K. L. (1989). The prevalence of pressure ulcers in an intermediate care facility. *Decubitus, 2*(2), 44–45.

Klastersky, J., Libert, I., Michel, B., et al. (2015). Supportive/palliative care in cancer patients: quo vadis? *Supportive Care in Cancer, 24*(4), 1883–1888.

Krapfl, L. A., & Gray, M. (2008). Does regular repositioning prevent pressure ulcers? *Journal of Wound, Ostomy, and Continence Nursing, 36*(6), 571–577.

Ladizinski, B., Alavi, A., Jambrosic, J., et al. (2014, July). Cancers mimicking fungal infections. *Advances in Skin & Wound Care, 27*(7), 301–309.

Langemo, D. K. (2012). General principles and approaches to wound prevention and care at end of life: An overview. *Ostomy/Wound Management, 58*(5), 24–34.

Langemo, D. K., Anderson, J., Hanson, D., et al. (2007). Understanding palliative wound care. *Nursing, 37*(1), 65–66.

Langemo, D. K., & Black, J. (2010). Pressure ulcers in individuals receiving palliative care: A National Pressure Ulcer Advisory Panel White Paper. *Advances in Skin & Wound Care, 23*(2), 59–72.

Langemo, D. K., & Brown, G. (2006). Skin fails too: Acute, chronic, and end-stage skin failure. *Advances in Skin & Wound Care, 19*(4), 206–211.

Langemo, D., Haesler, E., Naylor, W., et al. (2015). Evidence-based guidelines for pressure ulcer management at the end of life. *International Journal of Palliative Nursing, 21*(5), 225–232.

LeBlanc, K., & Baranoski, S. (2011). Skin tears: State of the science: Consensus statements for the prevention, prediction, assessment, and treatment of skin tears. *Advances in Skin & Wound Care, 24*(S9), 2–15.

Letizia, M., Uebelhor, J., & Paddack, E. (2010). Providing palliative care to seriously ill patients with nonhealing wounds. *Journal of Wound, Ostomy, and Continence Nursing, 37*(3), 277–282.

Levine, J. M. (2017). Unavoidable pressure injuries, terminal ulceration, and skin failure. *Advances in Skin & Wound Care, 30*(5), 200–202.

Lo, S. F., Hayter, M., Hu, W. Y., et al. (2012). Symptom burden and quality of life in patients with malignant fungating wounds. *Journal of Advanced Nursing, 68*(6), 1312–1321.

Lyder, C. H., & Ayello, E. A. (2008). Pressure ulcers: A patient safety issue. In R. G. Hughes (Ed.), *Patient safety and quality: An evidence-based handbook for nurses* (pp. 1–33). Rockville, MD: Agency for Healthcare Research and Quality. Retrieved from http://www.ncbi.nlm.nih.gov/books/NBK2650/

Maida, V. (2013). Wound management in patients with advanced illness. *Current Opinion in Supportive and Palliative Care, 7*(1), 73–79.

Maida, V., Ennis, M., & Corban, J. (2012). Wound outcomes in patients with advanced illness. *International Wound Journal, 9*(6), 683–692.

Meghani, S. H. (2004). A concept analysis of palliative care in the United States. *Journal of Advanced Nursing, 46*(2), 152–161.

Merz, T., Klein, C., Uebach, B., et al. (2011). Fungating wounds-multidimensional challenge in palliative care. *Breast Care (Basel), 6,* 21–24.

National Hospice and Palliative Care Organization. (2019). *NHPCO's facts and figures. Hospice Care in America* (2019 ed.). Alexandria, VA: National Hospice and Palliative Care Organization.

Pieper, B., Vallerand, A. H., Nordstrom, C. K., et al. (2009). Comparison of bodily pain. Persons with and without venous ulcers in an indigent care clinic. *Journal of Wound, Ostomy, and Continence Nursing, 36*(5), 493–502.

Posthauser, M. E. (2007). The role of nutritional therapy in palliative care. *Advances in Skin & Wound Care, 20*(1), 32–33.

Ramasubbu, D., Smith, V., Hayden, F., et al. (2017). Systemic antibiotics for treating malignant wounds. *The Cochrane Database of Systematic Reviews, 8*(8), CD011609.

Recka, K., Montagnini, M., & Vitale, C. A. (2012). Management of bleeding associated with malignant wounds. *Journal of Palliative Medicine, 15*(8), 952–954.

Reifsnyder, J., & Magee, H. (2005). Development of pressure ulcers in patients receiving home hospice care. *Wounds, 17*(4), 74–79.

Sekse, R. J. T., Hunskår, I., & Ellingsen, S. (2017). The nurses' role in palliative care: A qualitative meta-synthesis. *Journal of Clinical Nursing, 27*(1–2), e21–e38.

Sibbald, R. G., Goodman, L., Woo, K. Y., et al. (2011). Special considerations in wound bed preparation 2011: An update. *Advances in Skin & Wound Care, 24*(9), 415–438.

Sibbald, R. G., Krasner, D. L., & Lutz, J. (2010). SCALE: Skin Changes at Life's End Final Consensus Statement: October 1, 2009©. *Advances in Skin & Wound Care, 23*(5), 225-236.

Teno, J. M., Gozalo, P., Mitchell, S. L., et al. (2012). Feeding tubes and the prevention or healing of pressure ulcers. *Archives of Internal Medicine, 172*(9), 697–701.

Trombley, K., Brennan, M. R., Thomas, L., et al. (2012). Prelude to death or practice failure? Trombley-Brennan Terminal Tissue Injuries. *Journal of Hospice & Palliative Medicine, 29*(7), 541–545.

Tsichlakidou, A., Govina, O., Vasilopoulos, G., et al. (2019). Intervention for symptoms management in patients with malignant fungating wounds—a systematic review. *Journal of the Balkan Union of Oncology, 24*(3). 1301–1308.

VandenBosch, T., Montoye, C., Satwicz, M., et al. (1996). Predictive validity of the Braden Scale and nurse perception in identifying pressure ulcer risk. *Applied Nursing Research, 9*(2), 80–86.

Villela-Castro, D. L., de Gouveia Santos, V. L. C., & Woo, K. (2018). Polyhexanide versus metronidazole for odor management in malignant (fungating) wounds. *Journal of Wound, Ostomy, and Continence Nursing, 45*(5), 413–418.

White-Chu, E. F., & Langemo, D. (2012). Skin failure: Identifying and managing an underrecognized condition. *Annals of Long-Term Care, 20*(7), 28–32.

Woo, K., Conceição, V. L., & Alam, T. (2018). Optimizing quality of life for people with non-healing wounds. *Wounds International, 9*(3), 6–14.

Woo, K. Y., Krasner, D. L., Kennedy, B., et al. (2015). Palliative wound care management strategies for palliative patients and their circles of care. *Advances in Skin & Wound Care, 28*(3), 130–140.

Woo, K. Y., & Sibbald, R. G. (2010). Local wound care for malignant palliative wounds. *Advances in Skin & Wound Care, 23*(9), 417–428.

World Health Organization. (2018). *Fact Sheets: Palliative Care.* Geneva, Switzerland: World Health Organization.

Wound Ostomy Continence Nurses Society. (2014). *Guideline for management of wound in patients with lower-extremity arterial disease.* Mount Laurel, NJ: WOCN.

Wound, Ostomy, Continence Nurses Society. (2016). *Guideline for prevention and management of pressure ulcers (injuries).* Mt Laurel, NJ: WOCN.

Wound Ostomy Continence Nurses Society. (2019). *Guideline for management of wounds in patients with lower-extremity venous disease. WOCN Clinical Practice Guideline Series No. 4.* Mount Laurel, NJ: WOCN.

Yastrub, D. J. (2010). Pressure or pathology: Distinguishing pressure ulcers from the Kennedy Terminal Ulcer. *Journal of Wound, Ostomy, and Continence Nursing, 37*(3), 249–250.

QUESTIONS

1. A wound care nurse recommends palliative care for a patient with terminal cancer who has a nonhealing pressure injury. Which statement accurately describes a principle of palliative wound care?

A. Palliative care is applicable only to life-threatening conditions.

B. Palliative care is limited to the long-term care setting.

C. Palliative care is applicable early within a course of chronic illness.

D. The focus of palliative care is wound healing.

2. What is the biggest difference between palliative care and hospice care?

A. Hospice care is limited to end-of-life care.

B. Palliative care focuses on wound healing.

C. Hospice care is more appropriate for patients with chronic conditions.

D. Palliative care denotes the withdrawal of active treatment.

3. Which of the following meets the Kennedy Terminal Ulcer criteria for unavoidable skin breakdown occurring at the end of life?
   A. Location on the extremities
   B. Slow progression from pink color to clearly necrotic tissue
   C. Circular shape
   D. Rapid progression despite appropriate care

4. Which end-of-life condition is the most significant risk factor for SCALE (Skin Changes at Life's End)?
   A. Undernutrition
   B. Hypoperfusion
   C. Impaired removal of metabolic wastes
   D. Cachexia

5. Which type of wound occurs most frequently in hospice and palliative care?
   A. Pressure injuries
   B. Malignant wounds
   C. Skin tears
   D. Lower leg ulcerations

6. Which of the following measures to prevent pressure injury development is appropriate for the palliative or hospice patient?
   A. Keeping the head of the bed higher than 30 degrees
   B. Avoiding the use of pillows or folded towels to reduce pressure
   C. Using higher-level pressure redistribution support systems
   D. Increasing turning frequency

7. Pressure injury prevention is of great importance in the palliative care setting. Which measure helps to accomplish this goal?
   A. Use enteral feedings instead of hand feeding to improve healing ability.
   B. Reposition patients on pressure redistributing support surfaces every 4 hours.
   C. Reposition patients on regular mattresses every hour.
   D. Avoid floating heels with heel protectors or pillows.

8. Which of the following is a first-line approach to the management of odor with fungating wounds?
   A. Charcoal dressings
   B. Topical metronidazole and antimicrobial dressings
   C. Long-term irrigation with antiseptic solutions
   D. Soaking the wound in a basin of potable water

9. The wound care nurse is providing palliative care to a patient with a small very shallow pressure injury that has a low volume of exudate. What dressing would be the best choice?
   A. Alginate or Hydrofiber dressing + gauze and tape
   B. Dry gauze dressings
   C. Silicone adhesive foam dressing
   D. Wet-to-dry gauze dressings

10. The wound care nurse is choosing a dressing for a leg ulcer with a large area of active bleeding. What would be the best choice?
   A. Silver nitrate followed by wet-to-dry gauze
   B. Hydrofiber dressing + wrap gauze
   C. Adhesive foam dressing
   D. Gelling hemostatic foam

ANSWERS AND RATIONALES

1. C. Rationale: In a comprehensive analysis on palliative care, it was concluded that palliative care should be thought of early within a chronic disease trajectory

2. A. Rationale: Hospice care is limited to patients at the end of life, while palliative care has a broader application.

3. D. Rationale: The characteristics of KTU include (1) location on the sacrococcygeal area, (2) sudden onset of deeply discolored skin in the shape of a butterfly or pear, (3) rapid progression despite appropriate management (from deep purple, red, black, or blue area to clearly necrotic wound), and (4) irregular borders.

4. B. Rationale: Diminished tissue perfusion is the most significant risk factor for SCALE.

5. A. Rationale: Pressure injuries are the most commonly reported wound in hospice and palliative care.

6. C. Rationale: Appropriate interventions might include obtaining a higher-level pressure redistribution support surface, reducing turning frequency, and augmenting the turning program with small weight shifts or use of pillows to reduce pressure over vulnerable areas.

7. B. Rationale: Repositioning should occur at least every 4 hours if on a pressure redistribution support surface or viscoelastic foam and every 2 hours on a regular mattress.

8. B. Rationale: Topical metronidazole and antimicrobial dressings are first-line approaches to management of odor with fungating malignant wounds. Metronidazole is the most commonly studied intervention for the management of wound odor.

9. C. Rationale: Silicone adhesive foam dressings are a good choice for smaller wounds with low-to-moderate volumes of exudate.

10. D. Rationale: For large areas of active bleeding, gelling hemostatic foams and hemostatic surgical gauze are appropriate options, though more expensive and not as readily available.

CHAPTER 36

FISTULA MANAGEMENT

Denise Nix and Ruth A. Bryant

OBJECTIVES

1. Describe causative and contributing factors to fistula development.
2. Describe management of the patient with an enterocutaneous fistula.
3. Describe management of the patient with an enteroatmospheric fistula.
4. Outline criteria and guidelines for promotion of spontaneous fistula closure.
5. Explain the significance of pseudostoma formation in the patient with a fistula.
6. Discuss indications for surgical closure of a fistula.
7. Develop and implement individualized management plan for the fistula patient that provides for containment of drainage and odor while protecting perifistular skin.

TOPIC OUTLINE

INTRODUCTION

A *fistula* (*plural fistulas or fistulae*) is an abnormal passage between two or more epithelialized surfaces that results in communication between one body cavity or hollow organ and another hollow organ or the skin (Bryant & Best, 2015). An *enterocutaneous fistula* (*ECF*) is an abnormal connection between the gastrointestinal tract and the skin. An *enteroatmospheric fistula* (*EAF*) is an abnormal connection between the gastrointestinal tract and the atmosphere (e.g., a fistula that develops in an open surgical wound (Nurses Specialized in Wound, Ostomy and Continence Canada [NSWOCC] [formerly CAET], 2018). ECF and EAF are difficult complications that most often arise after abdominal surgical procedures. Although fistulas *can* be located *within* a wound, they should not be confused with a draining wound, surgically placed drain site, or wound dehiscence.

The mortality rates for patients with a fistula range from 5.5% to 30% (Parli et al., 2018; Quinn et al., 2017; Willcutts et al., 2015). Death is most often due to sepsis but also malnutrition, fluid and electrolyte imbalance, and multiorgan failure (Juárez-Oropeza & Román-Ramos, 2012; Wercka et al., 2016). Cost impact is significant. Teixeira and colleagues (2019), compared outcome data of patients with and without an ECF among level 1 trauma center patients who required acute trauma laparotomies. During the 9-year period, 36 of 2,373 (1.5%) patients undergoing a laparotomy developed an ECF. After matching age, gender, and severity scores of patients with ECF to patients without ECF, results showed a statistically significant increase in ICU length of stay and hospital length of stay in patients with ECFs ($p < 0.001$). Hospital charges for patients with an ECF averaged $539,309 as compared to $126,996 in similar patients without an ECF.

An interprofessional approach is needed to meet the needs of the patient with a fistula. Essential team members often include the WOC nurse, dietitian, pharmacist, clinical nurse, social worker, surgeon, provider, radiologist, physiotherapist, occupational therapist, spiritual advisor, radiation therapist, and interventional radiologist (Heimroth et al., 2018; NSWOCC, 2018; Rahman & Stavas, 2015). Management for this patient population requires a clear understanding of the underlying pathophysiology, astute assessment skills, knowledge about management alternatives and options, competent technical skills, diligent follow-up, and persistence (Bryant & Best, 2015).

CLINICAL PRESENTATION AND CLASSIFICATION

Clinical indications for potential ECF or EAF formation include postoperative abdominal pain, tenderness, distention, prolonged ileus, disruption in intestinal peristalsis, and wound infection. The definitive indicator of an ECF or EAF is the passage of gastrointestinal (GI) secretions into an open wound bed or through an unintentional opening onto the skin. Associated complications in patients with a fistula include fever, tachycardia, increased respiratory rate, fluid and electrolyte imbalance, perifistular skin breakdown, malnutrition, and sepsis (NSWOCC, 2018; Whelan & Ivatury, 2011).

Manifestations of a fistula tract terminating in the vagina include passage of urine (vesicovaginal fistula) or passage of gas, feces, and/or purulent and extremely malodorous drainage (rectovaginal or enterovaginal fistula). Irradiation-induced rectovaginal fistulas often are preceded by diarrhea, passage of mucus and blood rectally, a sensation of rectal pressure, and a constant urge to defecate (Zelga et al., 2017). Fistulas between the intestinal tract and the urinary bladder (e.g., colovesical fistula) present with passage of gas or stool-stained urine through the urethra. Diagnostic tests to confirm presence of a fistula include computed tomography (CT) scan, contrast radiography of the GI Tract, fistulogram, ultrasonography, and plain radiography (NSWOCC, 2018; Whelan & Ivatury, 2011).

KEY POINT

The definitive indicator of an ECF or EAF is the passage of GI secretions into an open wound bed or through an unintentional opening onto the skin.

Most clinicians describe and classify fistulas according to location, involved structures, and volume of effluent. Although less frequently used, fistulas may also be classified by complexity (see **Table 36-1**). Mucous fistulas

TABLE 36-1 FISTULA CLASSIFICATION

	DESIGNATION	CHARACTERISTICS
Location	Internal	Tract contained within body
	External	Tract exits through skin
Involved structures (not inclusive)	Colon to vagina	Colovaginal
	Intestine to skin	Enterocutaneous
	Bladder to vagina	Vesicovaginal
	Colon to skin	Colocutaneous
	Rectum to vagina	Rectovaginal
Volume	High output	>500 mL/24 h
	Moderate output	200–500 mL/24 h
	Low output	<200 mL/24 h
Complexity	Simple	Short direct tract, no abscess, no other organ involvement
	Complex	Type 1—abscess, multiple organ involvement
		Type 2—opens into the base of a wound

Modified from Bryant, R., & Best, M. (2015). Management of draining wounds and fistulas. In R. Bryant & D. Nix (Eds.), *Acute and chronic wounds: Current management concepts* (5th ed.). St. Louis, MO: Mosby.

are intentionally created surgical openings in which a defunctionalized section of bowel is secured to the abdomen. These produce mucus only and are managed with dressings or pouches; the mucous fistula does not increase morbidity or mortality (Bryant & Best, 2015). The mucous fistula is not further discussed in this chapter (see Chapter 9).

> **KEY POINT**
>
> Fistulas are typically "named" for the organ of origin and the organ of termination; for example, an ECF is one from the bowel to the skin, and a colovesical fistula is one from the colon to the bladder.

ETIOLOGIC FACTORS

Approximately 25% of fistulas develop spontaneously and are associated with an intrinsic intestinal disease such as inflammatory bowel disease (most common), cancer, radiation enteritis, ischemic bowel, diverticulitis, appendicitis, perforated duodenal ulcers, or external trauma (Haack et al., 2014). Spontaneous fistulas are generally resistant to spontaneous closure. Patients treated for a pelvic cancer are particularly vulnerable to ECFs due to radiation damage; the fistula may develop immediately following radiation or years later (Heimroth et al., 2018; Tran & Thorson, 2008). Irradiation-induced ECFs are more likely to occur in patients who receive higher radiation doses (>5,000 cGy), smoke cigarettes, or have atherosclerosis, hypertension, diabetes mellitus, advanced age, pelvic inflammatory disease, or previous pelvic surgery (Hollington et al., 2004; Tran & Thorson, 2008).

> **KEY POINT**
>
> Most ECF and EAFs occur postoperatively as a result of anastomotic breakdown; however, fistulas may also develop spontaneously as a result of inflammatory bowel disease (e.g., diverticulitis, Crohn's disease, radiation enteritis) or trauma.

The majority of ECF and EAFs (75% to 85%) are iatrogenic (inadvertently induced from a medical procedure); these fistulas develop postoperatively due to anastomotic breakdown (Gribovskaja-Rupp & Melton, 2016; Heimroth et al., 2018; Nussbaum & Fischer, 2006). With respect to postoperative small bowel fistulae, about half are from an anastomotic leak, with the other half occurring from inadvertent injury to the small bowel during dissection (Gribovskaja-Rupp & Melton, 2016). Surgery-related risk factors include poor nutrition, inadequate blood supply, poor suture technique, inadequate bowel prep (e.g., emergency surgery), extensive lysis of adhesions, and trauma surgery (Kassis & Makary, 2008; Nussbaum & Fischer, 2006; Telem et al., 2010; Wong et al., 2004).

Systemic reviews continue to indicate that the method of anastomosis (stapled or hand-sewn) is not a predictor of ECF following surgery for trauma (Neutzling et al., 2017).

Patients scheduled for elective surgical procedures should have risk factors addressed to minimize the risk of anastomotic breakdown. When emergency surgery is necessary, prevention strategies include adequate intravenous (IV) fluids, circulatory support, keeping the patient warm, and broad-spectrum antibiotics (Causey et al., 2012; Kassis & Makary, 2008). Historically, a diverting temporary stoma was commonly performed following bowel resection and anastomosis in trauma patients. However, studies indicate that diversion following colonic anastomosis for penetrating colonic injury did not reduce the incidence of septic complications, including abscess and fistula and thus practice is no longer standard of care (Causey et al., 2012; Chamieh et al., 2018).

MEDICAL MANAGEMENT

Spontaneous closure of a fistula is defined as closing with medical management within 6 to 8 weeks (Teixeira et al., 2009). Spontaneous closure rates in the era of advanced wound care and parenteral nutrition vary considerably with most studies demonstrating closure rates in the 20% to 40% range when sepsis is controlled and appropriate nutritional support is provided (Gribovskaja-Rupp & Melton, 2016; Kassis & Makary, 2008; Nussbaum & Fischer, 2006). According to Wong et al. (2004), 90% of simple fistulas close spontaneously, whereas <10% of complex fistulas close spontaneously.

Historically, 90% of spontaneous closure has been reported to occur in the 1st month after sepsis resolution, with an additional 10% closing in the 2nd month. More recently, case studies report fistulae closure in the second and third month with use of negative pressure wound therapy (NPWT) to promote wound healing (Gribovskaja-Rupp & Melton, 2016). The use of NPWT in fistula management will be discussed later in this chapter.

Favorable conditions for spontaneous closure (Gribovskaja-Rupp & Melton, 2016) include

- Transferrin >200 mg/dL
- No obstruction, bowel in continuity
- No inflamed intestine, infection, or sepsis
- Balanced electrolytes
- Timely referral to tertiary care center and subspecialty care
- Output <200 mL/24 h

Reducing fistula output has been shown to positively impact fluid and electrolyte balance; similarly, nutritional needs are more easily met as fistula output decreases (Polk & Schwab, 2012). However, there is no statistical evidence to support the concept of an inverse relationship between spontaneous closure and fistula output (Davis & Johnson, 2013; NSWOCC, 2018).

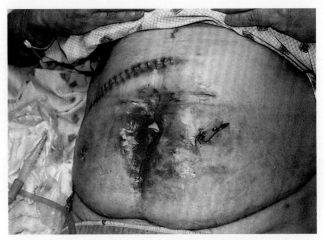

FIGURE 36-1. ECF (Small Bowel to Skin); Extensive Skin Damage Due to Enzymatic Drainage; Drain in Place for Abscess Management. (Reproduced with permission from Davis, M., Dere, K., & Hadley, G. (2000). Options for managing an open wound with draining enterocutaneous fistula. *Journal of Wound, Ostomy & Continence Nursing, 27*(2), 118–123.)

> **KEY POINT**
>
> Reducing fistula output has been shown to positively impact fluid and electrolyte balance and allow for nutrition needs to be more easily met. However, an association between increased rate of spontaneous fistula closure and decreased fistula output has not been proven.

Objectives of fistula management are described below and include (1) definition of the fistula tract; (2) maintenance of fluid and electrolyte balance; (3) nutritional support; (4) measures to minimize fistula output; (5) control of infection; and (6) skin protection and containment of effluent (Bryant & Best, 2015). The literature sometimes refers to a protocol called "SNAP," which stands for management of *s*kin and sepsis, *n*utrition, definition of fistula *a*natomy, and proposing a *p*rocedure to address the fistula (Kaushal & Carlson, 2004; Samad et al., 2015). An interdisciplinary team implements the SNAP protocol by early identification and treatment of the sepsis, oral and parenteral nutrition, identifying the type of fistula and optimal management.

DEFINITION OF THE FISTULA TRACT

Once the patient is stabilized, definition of the fistula tract should be undertaken. The fistula should be assessed for point of origin, condition of adjacent bowel, presence of abscess, and any distal obstruction or bowel discontinuity. This can be accomplished with a range of radiological examinations: fistulagram, ultrasonography, and plain radiography, magnetic resonance imaging (MRI), positive emission tomography (PET) scan, or computerized tomography (Arebi & Forbes, 2004; NSWOCC, 2018; Schecter et al., 2009; Whelan & Ivatury, 2011). During diagnostic workup, it is important that the patient receive nothing by mouth for the first couple days in order to accurately quantify the fistula output and complete diagnostic testing to determine the origin of the fistula (Kumpf et al., 2017; Willcutts, 2015).

CONTROL OF INFECTION

Uncontrolled sepsis and sepsis-associated malnutrition have been shown to be important determinants of mortality in the patient with a fistula (Dubose & Lundy, 2010; Lynch et al., 2004; NSWOCC, 2018). Patients with an intra-abdominal abscess may present with abdominal pain, fever, anorexia, tachycardia, or prolonged ileus. The presence of a palpable mass may or may not be present. Abdominal abscess may be difficult to detect in postoperative patients as analgesia and antibiotics may mask signs of infection (Mehta & Copelin, 2019).

Blood work is not specific for an intra-abdominal abscess but may reveal signs of infection such as leukocytosis, abnormal liver function, anemia, or thrombocytopenia. CT scan remains the most definitive test to rule out an intra-abdominal abscess. A CT scan can reveal the location, size, and presence of bowel thickening, thumb printing, and ileus. Intra-abdominal abscess almost always requires IV antibiotics. If the abscess is localized, CT-guided aspiration can be performed to drain the abscess (Li et al., 2018). This can obviate the need for early operative intervention. As seen in **Figure 36-1**, if a fistula develops, a definitive procedure can be deferred with the drain left in place to control further abscess formation (Davis et al., 2000; Lynch et al., 2004). Abscess contents should be cultured following percutaneous or surgical drainage, to assure appropriate antibiotic therapy (Wong et al., 2004).

MAINTENANCE OF FLUID AND ELECTROLYTE BALANCE

Fluid and electrolyte imbalance increases mortality and morbidity in patients with ECF/EAF (NSWOCC, 2018). Each day 8 to 10 L of fluid flows through the jejunum, depending on oral intake. In the intact functioning intestine, 98% of this fluid is (re) absorbed, leaving only 100 to 200 mL of fluid to be excreted in the stool. Development of a fistula permits abnormal fluid losses, with volume of loss determined in part by size of the fistulous opening and in part by anatomic location within the bowel. For example, fistulas located in the proximal small bowel are generally high output, while fistulas occurring in the colon are typically low output.

When providing fluid replacement, the provider must consider both the volume and the composition of the fistulous drainage, both of which are impacted by fistula location within the GI tract. Severe metabolic disturbances have been noted with fistula output >200 mL/day due to loss of hydrogen, chloride, sodium, and potassium ions (Arebi & Forbes, 2004; Makhdoom et al., 2000). Careful monitoring of tissue perfusion, weight, urine, and fistula output is necessary to evaluate fluid balance. Adequate fluid and electrolyte replacement is critical to prevent hypovolemia and circulatory failure in the patient with a high-output fistula (Makhdoom et al., 2000). As previously mentioned, while fluids need to be replaced during diagnostic workup, oral ingestion should be curtailed until tests are completed so that quantification of fistula output is as accurate as possible (Kumpf et al., 2017; Willcutts, 2015).

NUTRITIONAL SUPPORT

Once fluid levels and electrolyte balance have been stabilized and sepsis is managed, nutritional support is required. The goals of nutrition management are to provide adequate nutrition, maintain fluid levels and electrolyte balance, and support spontaneous closure of the ECF whenever possible (Kumpf et al., 2017). The route of nutritional support depends on the patient's ability to ingest sufficient quantities, the location of the fistula tract, the absorptive capacity of the bowel mucosa, and the patient's tolerance.

In the past, the use of total parenteral nutrition (TPN), accompanied by simultaneous "bowel rest," revolutionized the care of the patient with a fistula (Dubose & Lundy, 2010). However, TPN is associated with an appreciable rate of bacteremia and line sepsis. In one study conducted by Wong and colleagues (2004), positive blood cultures were obtained from 24.6% of 88 catheters utilized to deliver TPN to patients undergoing nonoperative management of enteric fistulas. Additionally, there is insufficient evidence to demonstrate that parenteral nutrition is associated with improved spontaneous closure rates (David & Johnson, 2013; NSWOCC, 2018).

Today, there has been a return to enteral nutrition (utilizing the GI tract for direct nutritional support) for prevention and management of fistulas. Enteral intake maintains the health and integrity of the intestinal mucosa, prevents translocation of bacteria, and maintains the normal structural, immunologic, and hormonal integrity of the GI tract. In addition, enteral nutrition can be provided at a lower cost as compared to TPN (Dubose & Lundy, 2010). During a small retrospective study, Collier and colleagues (2007) noted that early postoperative initiation of enteral nutrition (≤4 days) resulted in a lower fistula formation rate than did nutritional approaches involving later initiation of enteral feedings (9% vs. 26%, respectively). Researchers also noted that the use of early enteral nutrition resulted in earlier primary abdominal closure and lower hospital charges (Collier et al., 2007; Dubose & Lundy, 2010).

Four feet of healthy small intestine (in the adult) are needed to meet nutritional needs via the enteral route (Knechtges & Zimmermann, 2009). Therefore, enteral nutrition may be feasible for the patient whose fistula is located in the most proximal or distal portion of a functional GI tract. When the fistula is located in the most proximal segment of the bowel, the enteral feeding must be administered distal to the fistula. Many types of enteral solutions are available, and a dietician should be consulted to recommend the most appropriate solution and administration procedure so that GI intolerance (e.g., diarrhea, abdominal distention) can be avoided.

Fistuloclysis refers to the infusion of enteral nutrition via the distal stoma of an ECF or EAF with or without reinfusion of the output. The distal opening of the fistula is used for access for a catheter or tube, and enteral nutrition or fistula output is infused (Kumpf et al., 2017). Effective fistuloclysis requires effective pouching and catheter stabilization (Polk & Schwab, 2012). Refeeding enteroclysis is the reinfusion of fistula output (also known as chyme). Refeeding enteroclysis is usually performed in conjunction with enteral nutrition. In select patients with a proximal enteric fistula, however, water, electrolyte, and nutritional requirements can be met by simple refeeding without supplementary enteral nutrition. This technique has not gained widespread popularity (Coetzee et al., 2014).

Depending on the location of the fistula tract, the absorptive capacity of the bowel mucosa, and the patient's tolerance, parenteral nutrition remains an important option for prevention and management of fistulas. Many patients continue to be successfully treated exclusively through bowel rest and parenteral nutrition. In most cases, however, it is an important bridge to, or supplement for, enteral feeds (Polk & Schwab, 2012). A dietician is vital to the prevention and treatment of fistulas and may also recommend vitamins and trace minerals often deficient in malnourished patients with ECF/EAF (NSWOCC, 2018).

MEASURES TO MINIMIZE FISTULA OUTPUT

Reducing fistula output has been shown to reduce the loss of fluids, electrolytes, and nutrients and protect the perifistula skin (NSWOCC, 2018). This may be done with medications or by limiting oral and/or enteral intake to the amount needed to keep the intestinal mucosa healthy. Significantly reduced oral/enteral intake minimizes fistula output by decreasing luminal contents, GI stimulation, and pancreaticobiliary secretion. Medications used to decrease fistula output include antidiarrheals, antimotility agents, and proton pump inhibitors (Bailey & Glasgow, 2016; de Vries et al., 2017; Haack et al., 2014; Polk & Schwab, 2012; Williams et al., 2010). Consultation with a pharmacist is beneficial to understand their risk and benefits of these medications.

The relationship between medications closure of non-matured fistulas is not known. However, three separate meta-analyses reported the effectiveness of somatostatin and its analog, octreotide, in reducing closing time and increasing the number of fistulas closed without surgery (Coughlin et al., 2012; Rahbour et al., 2012; Stevens et al., 2011). Mortality, however, was not reduced. Finally, the odds of spontaneous closure and time till closure were improved in patients who received continuous infusion of somatostatin. Somatostatin is administered through continuous IV infusion due to its short half-life of 1 to 2 minutes. Octreotide's half-life is almost 2 hours, and it is administered three times daily subcutaneously (Makhdoom et al., 2000). Octreotide is not recommended for routine use due to reports of precipitated villous atrophy, interruption of intestinal adaptation, and acute cholecystitis. Some authors recommend a 5- to 8-day trial, with discontinuation of the octreotide if there is no significant reduction in fistula output within that time frame (Draus et al., 2006).

SKIN PROTECTION AND CONTAINMENT

Establishing and maintaining skin protection and containment of the fistula effluent can be a challenging and yet rewarding experience. When managing a patient with a fistula, it is beneficial to be guided by four general principles presented by Rolstad and Wong (2004).

1. Assess the pouching system and seal frequently; expect to make changes in the management system.
2. Build flexibility into the care plan.
3. Innovate, using the easiest, most practical approach first.
4. Recognize that inexperienced caregivers frequently provide care of the patient.

Skin protection and effluent containment should be initiated as soon as the fistula develops and is not contingent upon medical diagnosis. Goals for topical management of a fistula are listed in **Box 36-1** (Bryant & Best, 2015). Methods and techniques for skin protection and containment will be described in the intervention section of the chapter.

KEY POINT

Skin protection and effluent containment should be initiated as soon as the fistula develops and is not contingent upon medical diagnosis nor the medical plan of care.

 ## FISTULA MANAGEMENT FOR THE WOC NURSE

Methods and strategies for fistula management are guided by a thorough assessment; the parameters first described by Irrgang and Bryant (1984) remain the standard for fistula assessment today (Bryant & Best, 2015).

ASSESSMENT

In addition to determining the type of fistula, assessment must include abdominal contours, fistula opening,

---

BOX 36-1   GOALS FOR TOPICAL MANAGEMENT OF THE ECF

- Perifistular skin protection
- Containment of effluent
- Odor control
- Patient comfort
- Accurate measurement of effluent
- Patient mobility
- Ease of care
- Cost containment

---

effluent characteristics, and the condition of the perifistular skin. Each dressing or pouch change represents an opportunity to reevaluate the fistula and to modify the care plan accordingly. All assessments, reassessments, interventions, responses to interventions, and management and follow-up plans should be documented (see **Box 36-2**).

BOX 36-2   DOCUMENTATION FOR THE WOC NURSE

Focused Assessment
- Fistula source (see **Table 36-1**)
- Pain
- Fistula opening
  - Location
  - Length and width
  - Height (retracted, skin level, protruding)
- Perifistular skin integrity
  - Intact
  - Impaired (erythema, maceration, candidiasis, denudement)
- Abdominal contours and proximity of fistula to scars, skin folds, bony prominences, drains, or ostomies
- Output/effluent
  - Volume
  - Consistency
  - Color
  - Odor
- Containment system and frequency of changes

Interventions
- Emotional support
- Changes in containment method/procedure with rationale (if any change required)
- Education of patient/family
  - Normal versus impaired skin
  - Signs of infection
  - Containment procedure

Evaluation
- Indicators of progress in closure (or impediments, such as pseudostoma formation)
- Effectiveness of containment system
  - Wear time without leakage
  - Perifistular skin intact or improved
  - Odor control
  - Effects on patient mobility
  - Ease of care
- Patient/family response to interventions
  - Patient satisfaction
  - Comfort
  - Level of activity
  - Learning

Follow-up Plan
- Approximate day of next visit
- Instruction for staff between visits (including what to do if questions/concerns arise)

Progress toward/Impediments to Spontaneous Closure

A critical aspect of assessment is evaluation of progress toward and impediments to spontaneous closure (see **Box 36-3**). Progress in closure is evidenced by reduced output through the fistula tract along with increased fecal output through the distal bowel (rectum or stoma); thus, fistula output should be monitored, as should the output from any stoma, and the patient with an intact distal bowel should be routinely queried regarding bowel movements. Any indicators of abscess formation (e.g., increasing abdominal tenderness, fever, or purulent drainage mixed with the fecal output) must be promptly reported so that intervention can be initiated. The nurse must also be alert to development of a stomatized fistula, also known as a pseudostoma or an epithelialized stoma; this occurs when the anterior wall of the bowel becomes adherent to the abdominal wall and the fistula tract undergoes mucosal eversion. The end result is a permanent opening into the bowel that must be closed surgically; thus, the surgeon or provider should be made aware when a "stoma" is observed in the wound bed (see **Fig. 36-2**).

KEY POINT

Assessment of the individual with a fistula must include the volume and characteristics of the output, the contours of the abdominal wall and fistula opening, and indicators of progress toward or impediments to spontaneous closure.

Abdominal Contours and Fistula Opening

The fistula opening and abdominal contours should be assessed while the patient is standing, sitting, and lying down if possible. If the pannus is large, more positions may be necessary to observe the changes in perifistular contours that occur with shifts in position of the pannus. Skin

---

BOX 36-3   FACTORS THAT PREVENT SPONTANEOUS CLOSURE

- Compromised distal suture line/anastomosis (i.e., tension on suture line, improper suturing technique, inadequate blood supply to anastomosis)
- Distal obstruction
- Foreign body in fistula tract or suture line
- Epithelium-lined tract contiguous with skin (pseudostoma)
- Presence of tumor or disease in site
- Previous irradiation to site
- Crohn's disease
- Abscess
- Hematoma

Adapted from Bryant, R., & Best, M. (2015). Management of draining wounds and fistulas. In R. Bryant & D. Nix (Eds.), *Acute and chronic wounds: Current management concepts* (5th ed.). St. Louis, MO: Mosby. (In Print.)

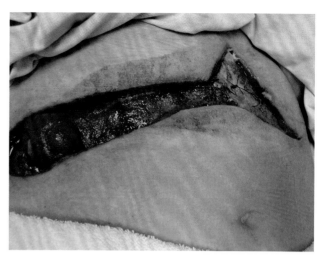

FIGURE 36-2. Pseudostoma in Deep Wound.

contours should be noted, and the abdomen should be inspected for irregular skin surfaces that are created by scars, creases, bony prominences, or other obstacles such as sutures/staples, incisions (dehisced or intact), or stomas. The location of the fistula should be identified, and visible openings should be measured (length and width in cm) and documented. The level at which the fistula empties in relation to the skin (or wound) surface is of critical importance. The fistula opening may be retracted (lower than skin level), level with the skin, above the level of the skin, or in a deep wound (see **Fig. 36-2**). If the fistula empties directly onto the skin and is level with the skin, a convex pouching system is usually required; in contrast, a fistula that has undergone mucosal maturation (pseudostoma formation) and that protrudes above the level of the skin may enable a better pouch seal. The opening might also contain a drain, as seen in **Figure 36-1**, for drainage of an abscess.

KEY POINT

A "pseudostoma" occurs when the anterior wall of the bowel becomes adherent to the abdominal wall, and the fistula tract undergoes mucosal eversion to create an epithelium-lined tract. Pseudostoma development requires physician notification because it means the fistula will have to be closed surgically.

Assessment of all these parameters will help determine the level of skin protection required, as well as the flexibility, size, and shape of adhesive barrier needed for effective protection of the perifistular skin and avoidance of any areas that could compromise the adhesion of the pouching system or cause discomfort to the patient.

Effluent Characteristics

Assessment of fistula effluent (source, volume, odor, consistency, composition) influences topical management selection by providing insight into the degree of risk for perifistular skin breakdown and odor as well as the type of pouch closure needed. For example, an odorous fistula producing effluent with semi-formed consistency is most likely originating from the left transverse or descending colon. Effluent from the transverse or descending colon will be less damaging to the skin than is output from the small intestine or stomach. (See **Fig. 36-1** for illustration of skin damage related to small bowel drainage.) Thus, the primary goals of topical management for that patient would be containment of effluent and odor control.

Fistula output volumes >100 mL over 24 hours usually require a pouch or suction or both. In contrast, the fistula with minimal output can often be managed with the application of a perifistular moisture barrier and an absorptive dressing. However, in the presence of odor, even the patient with a low-output fistula may prefer a containment pouch for odor control. It should be noted that odor may originate from numerous sources, including fecal drainage, exudate, necrotic or infected tissue, soiled dressings, and/or chemicals used during treatment.

KEY POINT

There are multiple options for containment of fistula effluent and perifistular skin protection; the best option for an individual patient is determined by the volume and characteristics of the output and the abdominal contours.

Consistency of effluent is particularly important to selection of a pouching system because it influences the type of skin barriers needed as well as the type of drainage outlet required to efficiently empty the pouch. For example, liquid effluent is much more corrosive than is thick effluent and is much more likely to result in premature erosion of the skin barrier; thus, liquid effluent requires the most durable skin barrier/protectant. Liquid effluent is easier to empty from a spout rather than clamp type closure.

Constant exposure of the epidermis to moisture, enzymes, extremes in pH, and mechanical trauma frequently leads to perifistular skin damage. Denudation of perifistular skin is a common complication in fistula patients and often is present when the patient is first seen with the fistula. Perifistular skin is also at risk for fungal infection as a consequence of moisture entrapment against the skin and antibiotic precipitated changes in the normal skin flora. Candidiasis is a common secondary perifistular skin complication and requires treatment with a topical antifungal agent. See Chapter 16 to learn more about moisture-associated skin damage (MASD).

In addition to visual inspection, valuable information can be obtained from the patient and nursing staff. For example, patient reports of burning or stinging sensations around the fistula commonly indicate denudation or erosion of the epidermis, and the patient who requires frequent dressing or pouch changes is at risk for skin damage from mechanical injury in addition to damage from exposure to the effluent.

INTERVENTIONS AND CONTAINMENT STRATEGIES

Fistulas can be managed with skin protection and either dressings or containment devices (pouches, suction, negative pressure). There are a wide number of products available, and the appropriate selection is based on patient assessment. Principles of management warrant repetition: begin with the easiest approach based on assessment and sound rationale, reassess frequently and be flexible, and expect that needs will change. Interventions should be based on established principles and rationale, should include measures for skin protection and containment as well as patient and family support and education, and should be thoroughly documented (see **Box 36-2**). **Tables 36-2 and 36-3** present factors to consider when selecting containment methods.

KEY POINT

The recommended approach to determining the best system for effluent containment and skin protection is to begin with the simplest approach and modify as needed.

Skin Protectants and Barriers

Skin protectant products are available in many types and forms (**Table 36-2**). Major types include moisture barrier skin protectant creams, ointments, or pastes; solid pectin-based adhesive wafers, rings, or strips; hydrocolloid or karaya-formulated rings; barrier (ostomy) paste formulated with or without alcohol; barrier powder; and liquid barrier film products (previously known as skin sealant), which are available as wipes, wands, and sprays with or without alcohol. As previously stated, product selection must always be based on assessment and a clear understanding of the patient's needs and the properties and indications for use of the various products. For example, moisture barrier products are appropriate only for low-output fistulas managed with dressings. Pectin-based barrier wafers, rings, strips, and paste are widely used to protect the skin and improve adhesion of pouching systems and NPWT systems. Barrier powder is used to treat denuded skin. Liquid barrier film products are primarily used to protect the skin against adhesive trauma. **Table 36-2** provides indications and contraindications for use of each type of barrier product.

KEY POINT

Moisture barrier products are used to protect the skin against moisture and drainage but are appropriate only for low-output fistulas managed with absorptive products; barrier films are used primarily to protect against adhesive trauma; and pectin-based pouches, rings, and pastes are used to promote an effective pouching system and to protect the skin against enzymatic drainage.

TABLE 36-2 FISTULA PRODUCTS AND THEIR INDICATIONS

PRODUCT/ACCESSORY	ACTION	INDICATIONS
Liquid skin barrier wipes, wands, or sprays	Provides a protective film to skin	**Low-output fistulae**—provides protective layer to skin. Used in combination with dressings **High-output fistulae**—used in combination with pouches, suction systems, and NPWT to protect against adhesive trauma
Moisture barrier creams, ointments, or pastes	Repels moisture and protects skin	**Low-output fistulae**—provides protection to skin around fistula. May be used in combination with dressings **High-output fistulae**—not indicated. Does not provide enough protection with high-output effluent. Contraindicated with the use of any adhesive products (i.e., pouches), as creams will not allow products to adhere to skin
Skin barrier rings, strips, and pastes	Provides physical barrier to effluent/stool	**Low-output fistulae**—provides skin protection against effluent **High-output fistulae**—used to fill in uneven surfaces for pouching or as a part of the pouching system
Pouches	Contain effluent/stool and odor from fistula	**Low-output fistulae**—where odor is a problem or the patient prefers to change pouch as opposed to dressings **High-output fistulae**—used to contain stool and odor
Suction systems	Contain effluent in combination with low intermittent suction and dressings or pouches	**Low-output fistulae**—not indicated **High-output fistulae**—where pouching systems to gravity drainage are not effective due to large amounts of liquid effluent. Not a long-term solution
NPWT	Direct pressure closure	**Low-output fistulae**—not indicated **High-output fistulae**—where closure is a possibility. No abscess can be present. The patient must receive bowel rest and nutritional support, e.g., TPN. There should be no evidence of epithelial cells on opening of fistula (no evidence of pseudostoma formation).
Dressings	Absorb drainage	**Low-output fistulae**—used in combination with other skin protectants such as liquid skin barrier wipes, barrier creams and pastes, and skin barrier wafers **High-output fistulae**—not indicated

NPO, nothing by mouth; NPWT, negative pressure wound therapy; TPN, total parenteral nutrition.

TABLE 36-3 FISTULA CONTAINMENT OPTIONS BASED ON OUTPUT AND NEED FOR ACCESS

OUTPUT VOLUME	<100 mL	<100 mL	>100 mL OR DRESSING CHANGE > EVERY 4 h	>100 mL OR DRESSING CHANGE > EVERY 4 h
Need for odor control	No	Yes	Yes or no	Yes or no
Need for frequent access	Yes/no	Yes/no	Yes	No
Containment options	Absorptive dressings and perifistular skin protectant (e.g., ointment, paste barrier)	Charcoal cover dressing (placed over absorptive dressings) with environmental deodorants and frequent dressing changes OR Ostomy pouch	Wound management system with window, emptied frequently or attached to a dependent bedside drainage collector OR Two-piece ostomy pouch emptied frequently Two piece urostomy pouch urostomy emptied frequently or attached to a dependent bedside drainage collector (urinary or fecal spout)	Pouching systems OR Closed systems with suction or attached to straight drainage NPWT

Pectin-Based Barrier Products

Most containment pouches have an integrated solid skin barrier attached to the pouch by the manufacturer. Barrier pastes, strips, or rings are frequently needed accessory products that are used to fill skin defects and create a flat pouching surface, add convexity, or provide caulking to ensure an effective pouch seal. If the skin is denuded and moist, a barrier powder may be lightly applied (sprinkled on the skin, gently rubbed in, and the excess brushed off) (as shown in **Fig. 36-3**) to absorb moisture and improve adhesion of the barrier and pouch to the damaged skin. It is important to realize that application of excessive amounts of powder will impair adhesion. When the skin is extremely denuded, application of the powder can be followed by application of an alcohol-free liquid barrier film; these steps can be repeated up to three times to create a dry surface or crust. This technique is known as "crusting." When applied and removed appropriately, most of these pectin barrier products are safe to use on damaged skin. It should be noted that liquid barrier films must be allowed to dry so solvents can escape before other products are applied. Some barrier films and barrier pastes contain alcohol and can cause great discomfort when used on damaged skin. Clear protocols and ongoing staff education are essential to assure that alcohol-free products are the "standard of care" for damaged skin. Great care must be taken to prevent medical adhesive–related skin damage (MARSI) as described in Chapter 16.

> **KEY POINT**
>
> Skin barrier powder can be dusted onto areas of denuded skin to create a gummy protective layer, to avoid excessive powder application, and to prevent interference with pouch adhesion.

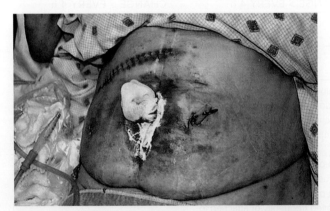

FIGURE 36-3. Pectin Powder Dusted onto Weeping Damaged Skin; Excess Powder Removed to Avoid Compromised Adhesion of Pouch. (Reproduced with permission from Davis, M., Dere, K., & Hadley, G. (2000). Options for managing an open wound with draining enterocutaneous fistula. *Journal of Wound, Ostomy & Continence Nursing, 27*(2), 118–123.)

Absorptive Dressings and Moisture Barriers

Fistulas that are nonodorous with low-volume output (<100 mL/day) or located in deep creases or anatomical locations that make pouching impossible may require management with dressings and moisture barriers. In these situations, the perifistular skin may be protected with a liquid barrier film or a moisture barrier ointment (petrolatum, dimethicone, or zinc oxide–based ointment or paste) or solid skin barrier, over which absorptive dressings are applied. The frequency of changes and reapplication of dressings and barriers is determined by the volume of drainage and the specific products being used. Absorptive dressings include gauze (sponges or strip packing), alginates, hydrofibers, foams, and combinations. When packing is required (e.g., wounds with depth, tunnels, or undermined areas), a dressing must be selected that can be completely retrieved from the wound. If the volume of drainage is such that the dressing must be changed more frequently than every 4 to 8 hours, pouching or closed suction should be considered.

Closed Suction

Closed suction systems can provide skin protection, drainage containment, and odor control and have been used for years as a reliable and cost-effective method for managing high-output fistulas or fistulas that are too difficult to pouch (Jeter et al., 1990; Jones & Harbit, 2003; Kordasiewicz, 2004). The wound and surrounding skin are gently cleansed; the periwound skin is then protected with a liquid barrier film and/or hydrocolloid barrier strips. Any major skin defects adjacent to the wound can be filled with barrier strips or paste to improve adhesion of the dressing. The wound base is covered by several layers of moistened gauze to prevent damage to the wound surface by the suction catheter; the suction catheter is then placed near the fistula orifice and stabilized with additional layers of moistened gauze. The entire wound is then covered with a transparent adhesive dressing, and paste is applied around the suction catheter where it exits the wound, if needed to obtain a secure seal. The suction catheter is connected to wall suction at a low level of continuous suction (see **Fig. 36-4A–C**). A Hemovac can provide the suction for short periods to increase the patient's mobility. Effluent must be liquid if suction is to be effective; thick or particulate effluent will occlude the catheter. Typically, these systems are changed every 2 to 3 days to prevent leakage and to permit wound assessment.

> **KEY POINT**
>
> Closed suction may be a good option for the patient who is not a candidate for pouching; it provides effective drainage containment and skin protection but is used only short term because it severely limits patient mobility.

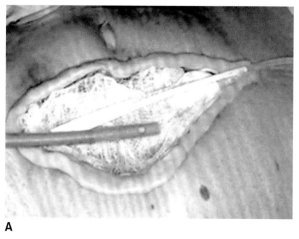

A

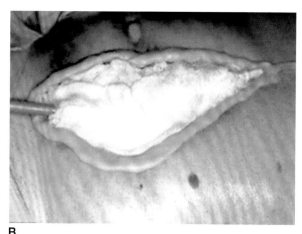

B

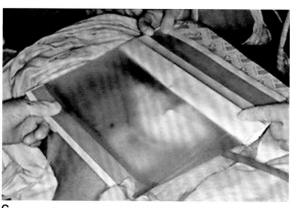

C

FIGURE 36-4. A–C. Closed Suction Procedure.

It must be emphasized that a catheter that is inserted into the fistula tract will act as a foreign body and may interfere with healing and even increase fistula output. On the other hand, a catheter coiled in a defect above the orifice or in the open wound surrounding the fistula opening will not inhibit closure. Because firm tubes can injure fragile tissue, only soft, flexible suction catheters should be used with fistulas. Suction systems should be considered a short-term intervention because of the limitations placed on patient mobility and the time-intensive nature of the care (Dearlove, 1996; Nishide, 1997; Pontieri-Lewis, 2005).

KEY POINT

A catheter inserted into the fistula tract acts as a foreign body and prevents wound closure.

Negative Pressure Wound Therapy

NPWT incorporates foam or gauze and subatmospheric pressure (suction) to promote closure of fistula tracts, the removal and containment of effluent, and/or wound healing. The mechanisms involved in promotion of wound healing include reduction in edema (with associated improvement in perfusion), and mechanical deformation of cells, which has been shown to stimulate the wound repair process. NPWT systems have built-in sensors to alert caregivers to potential and actual breaches in the integrity of the system.

Although there are no large studies comparing NPWT fistula management with traditional pouching techniques, its use with fistula management is widespread because surgeons are familiar with the technology from the use with problematic wounds. Wainstein and colleagues (2008) reported their 10-year experience with a vacuum-assisted device in management of 179 fistulas in 91 patients. Forty-two patients (46%) achieved spontaneous closure within 90 days of initiating vacuum-assisted therapy. Among the others, the closure rate after operation was 84%. Overall mortality rate was 16%.

NPWT can be used with fistulas located in open wounds so long as the following conditions are met: the fistula exhibits the potential for spontaneous closure (i.e., no evidence of pseudostoma formation); there is no evidence of exposed bowel in the wound base; and there is no evidence of abscess or distal obstruction. Caution should be used to prevent any additional fistula formation, that is, a contact layer or the nonporous "white" foam should be used in contact with the wound bed. If the effluent is too thick for suction, or if the fistula has "stomatized" but the wound still needs NPWT for promotion of granulation tissue formation, there are techniques and devices that segregate the fistula for management with pouching while permitting continued use of NPWT for promotion of wound healing (Bruhin et al., 2014; Heineman et al., 2015; Reed et al., 2006; Reider, 2017) (see **Box 36-4 and Fig. 36-5**). The NSWOCC (2018) Nursing Best Practice Recommendations for ECF and EOF presents pictorial step-by-step procedures for isolating fistulas with and without the use of commercially available devices and can be accessed at http://nswoc.ca/ecf-best-practices/. Further information about the application and use of NPWT is presented in Chapter 12 of the wound core curriculum.

KEY POINT

NPWT can be used to promote wound healing and fistula closure so long as there are no impediments to spontaneous closure; a contact layer or nonporous foam should be used in contact with the wound bed to prevent any additional trauma.

Pouching Systems

Fistula pouches, ostomy pouches (pediatric or adult), retracted penis pouches, and fecal incontinence collectors have all been used for fistula management. Most are attached to a skin barrier. Additional skin barrier products may be required to caulk edges, fill creases, and/or add convexity (see **Table 36-2**).

When the fistula is located adjacent to an incision, the skin barrier of the pouch sometimes needs to be placed over the incision to prevent leakage onto the incision. When applied and removed appropriately, these products will protect rather than harm an incision. A simple strategy for protection of the incision is to place steri-strips or tape strips over the suture line or staple line prior to application of the pouching system.

Strategies to promote adhesion of the pouch to the perifistular skin include assurance of a dry surface; a moist surface will impair pouch adhesion. Skin barrier powders (NOT talc or corn starch) may be used to absorb moisture from denuded skin and to create a dry surface that supports pouch adherence. The amount of skin barrier powder used should be just enough to absorb the moisture and create a gummy or dry surface; too much powder will impair the adhesion of the pouch. Severely denuded skin may benefit from the "crusting" procedure, as described previously.

KEY POINT

If a pouching system or NPWT dressing extends over the suture or staple line, steri-strips or tape strips may be placed over the incision for protection prior to application of the dressing or pouching system.

BOX 36-4   PROCEDURE FOR ISOLATING A FISTULA FOR NPWT

1. Assemble equipment: Ostomy pouch and supplies, NPWT supplies, skin barrier ring, skin barrier paste, transparent dressing.
2. Prepare ostomy/fistula pouch as described in **Box 36-5**. Apply bead of paste to back of pouch around opening.

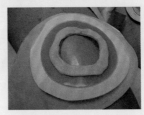

3. Cut a ring out of NPWT sponge dressing material slightly larger than the stomatized fistula; place into wound bed around fistula opening.

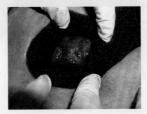

4. Optional: Place skin barrier ring right around fistula and over the NPWT sponge ring; apply bead of paste directly around fistula to caulk area between fistula and barrier ring.
5. Proceed to dress the wound utilizing NPWT procedure/protocol. Initiate suction and assure secure seal.

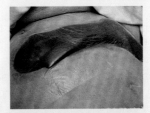

6. Cut an opening in the transparent dressing over fistula.

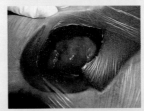

7. Apply the pouch over the fistula on top of the NPWT dressing; close the end of the pouch.

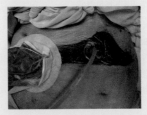

Photos courtesy of Terri Reed and Diana Economon.

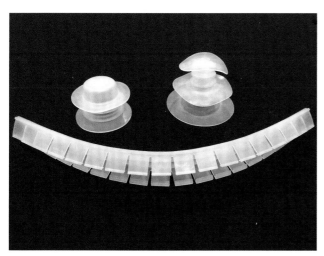

FIGURE 36-5. Example of a Commercially Available Device for Isolating a Fistula, Stoma, or Drain to Diverting Effluent Away from Wounds. One piece devices are compressible and customizable for different sizes and number of fistulas. (Photo courtesy of Mary Anne Obst.)

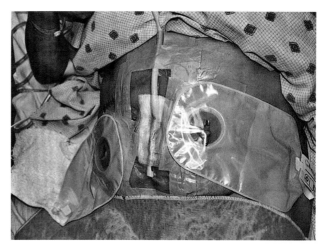

FIGURE 36-6. Two Pouches Used for Separate Fistulas. (Reproduced with permission from Davis, M., Dere, K., & Hadley, G. (2000). Options for managing an open wound with draining enterocutaneous fistula. *Journal of Wound, Ostomy & Continence Nursing, 27*(2), 118–123.)

Medical adhesive products approved for the skin should be used according to manufacturers' instructions and only when needed. Medical adhesives can be used to enhance the tack of an existing adhesive, to extend the adhesive surface on a pouch, or to compensate for the reduced adhesion caused by the application of skin barrier powder onto denuded perifistular skin. Medical adhesives are formulated as liquids/cements, medical adhesive sprays, and adhesive strips, rings, and sheets. Some adhesive products contain potential irritants or allergens, such as latex and/or alcohol; therefore, it is critical for the WOC nurse to carefully evaluate any adhesive product being considered for use in terms of indications, contraindications, and guidelines for use. Adhesive liquids and sprays must be allowed to dry completely in order for solvents to evaporate and the adhesive product to become tacky (Bryant, 1992; Bryant & Best, 2015).

If two drainage/fistula sites are too far apart to be included in one pouching system, two pouches may be necessary (see **Fig. 36-6**) (Davis et al., 2000). When the fistula is located in a deep wound (see **Fig. 36-2**), it may be helpful to select a pouching system with an integrated window/access cap that facilitates adjunct use of wound filler dressing such as an alginate or antimicrobial or saline-moistened gauze. A pattern and procedure for preparation, removal, and application of the pouching system should be created, dated, and kept in the patient's room with instructions and supplies. **Figure 36-7** and **Box 36-5** present examples of a pattern and pouch change procedure.

Pouching System Adaptations

There are situations in which adaptations of standard pouching techniques are required. Pouching system adaptations (e.g., bridging, saddle bagging, and troughing) have been previously described and illustrated by Bryant (1992) and are recognized internationally over two decades later (NSWOCC, 2018). These techniques will be briefly described and illustrated (**Figs. 36-8 to 36-10**).

Troughing (**Fig. 36-8**) is a very effective management technique when the fistula is located within an open wound and routine pouching procedures are ineffective. The periwound skin is first protected with overlapping strips of skin barrier or hydrocolloid sheets and/or barrier paste. The wound is then covered with a transparent adhesive dressing; prior to application of the transparent dressing, an opening is cut into the most dependent portion of the dressing and a pouch is applied over the opening. The opening in the pouch/transparent dressing

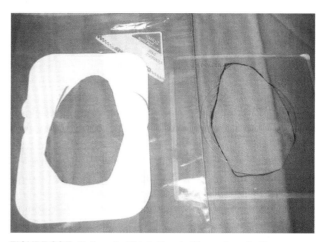

FIGURE 36-7. Pattern for Fistula Pouch. (Reproduced with permission from Davis, M., Dere, K., & Hadley, G. (2000). Options for managing an open wound with draining enterocutaneous fistula. *Journal of Wound, Ostomy & Continence Nursing, 27*(2), 118–123.)

BOX 36-5 FISTULA POUCH CHANGE PROCEDURE

1. Assemble equipment: Pouch with integrated skin barrier, pattern, skin barrier paste, scissors, closure device, or attachment for bedside bag, water, and soft gauze.
2. Prepare pouch.
   a. Trace pattern onto skin barrier surface of pouch. Note: the pattern should provide at least ¼ inch "clearance" of the wound edges (to prevent undermining of drainage under edge of pouch).
   b. Pull the anterior pouch surface away from posterior surface to avoid accidentally cutting hole in pouch surface.
   c. Cut out skin barrier surface according to tracing.
   d. Remove protective backing(s) from the pouch.
5. Remove and apply the pouch.
   a. Remove the pouch, using "push–pull" technique; gently press down on skin with one hand while pulling up on the pouch with the other.
   b. Discard the pouch and save closure clip or attachment device for bedside bag.
   c. Control any discharge with soft gauze.
   d. Clean the skin with water or gentle skin cleanser (without emollients that may impair adhesion of the pouch).
   e. Dry gently and thoroughly.
   f. Position the patient so abdomen has minimal wrinkles and folds (usually supine).
   g. Apply paste around the fistula. Fill in any uneven skin surfaces with paste, barrier rings, or skin barrier strips as needed.
   h. Apply a new pouch, centering fistula/wound site in opening.
   i. Close the bottom of the pouch with clip or attach to bedside bag.

unit must be placed at the junction between the skin and the inferior aspect of the wound and must be wider than the diameter of the wound at that point. Since most wounds for which the trough procedure is required are very large, it is helpful to apply the transparent adhesive dressing in overlapping strips. (Typically the strips are applied from "bottom" to "top"; the bottom strip is the one with the opening and the pouch.) Since most of these fistulas are high output, it is helpful to select a pouch with a spout that can be connected to gravity drainage (or to wall suction if needed) (Bryant, 1992; Hoedema & Suryadevara, 2010).

Troughing can frequently be used to provide effective skin protection and containment of effluent for patients in whom a secure pouch seal cannot be maintained. A common concern in management of fistulas located within open wounds and managed either by pouching or troughing is the impact of small bowel drainage on the healing process. Fortunately, the enzymes in small bowel fluid do not attack the newly formed collagen and blood vessels that comprise granulation tissue, and the very low bacterial counts in small bowel fluid minimize the risk of infection. Clinicians observe that wounds with fistulas continue to heal at the expected rate despite exposure to small bowel effluent.

Bridging (**Fig. 36-9**) may be used when the fistula is located at the inferior aspect of a long vertically oriented wound or at the most lateral aspect of an extensive horizontally oriented wound. The goal is to isolate the fistula from the remainder of the wound so that the fistula can be managed with pouching or troughing and the wound can be managed with moist wound healing or packing. Steps in the bridging procedure are as follows: (1) Identify a point slightly above (or medial to) the fistula at which the bridge will be "built." (2) Apply 1-inch strips of skin barrier or hydrocolloid wafer in layers to create a structure that fills the wound at that point and extends slightly above skin level. (The white foam used for NPWT therapy can also be used to create a bridge that fills the wound and extends slightly above the skin surface.) (3) Cut a strip of skin barrier or hydrocolloid wafer that is 1-inch wide (to match the width of the bridge) and long enough to cover the diameter of the wound and 2 inches of skin on either side of the wound. Place the covering strip over the bridge and onto the surrounding skin. (4) Proceed with pouching or troughing of the fistula and management of the remaining wound according to moist wound healing principles (Bryant, 1992; Hoedema & Suryadevara, 2010).

KEY POINT

Wounds continue to heal at the expected rate despite exposure to small bowel effluent.

Saddlebagging (**Fig. 36-10**) is a technique in which two pouches are attached at the skin barrier adhesive edges of each pouch to create one pouch with a larger adhesive surface than standard pouches (Bryant, 1992; Bryant & Best, 2015). This technique may be necessary for larger fistulas or fistulas within a large wound that need to be pouched.

EDUCATION AND EMOTIONAL SUPPORT

The development of a fistula is associated with a significant reduction in the health-related quality of life for the patient and their family (Hoeflok et al., 2015). Education and emotional support are critical aspects of the plan of care and its effectiveness. Patients report feelings of loss of control, frustration, embarrassment, hopelessness, isolation, and demoralization due to prolonged hospitalization, financial concerns, alterations in body image, and uncertain outcomes (Kaushal & Carlson, 2004; Kozell & Martins, 2003; Lloyd et al., 2006; Renton et al., 2006). Feelings may be exacerbated by the inability to eat

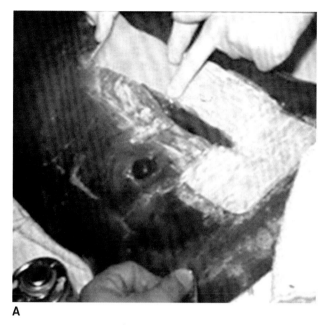

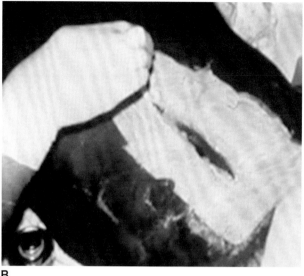

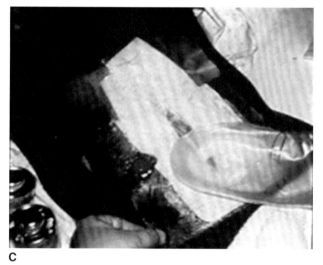

FIGURE 36-8. A–C. Troughing Procedure.

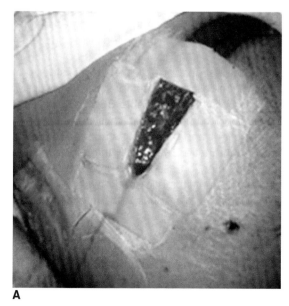

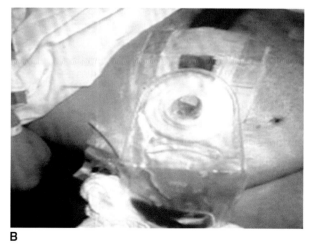

FIGURE 36-9. A, B. Bridging.

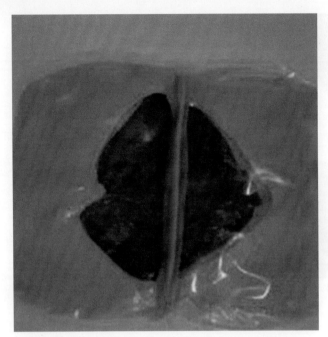

FIGURE 36-10. Saddlebagging: Example of Two Fistula Pouches Connected Together along the Adhesive Surface to Make One Larger Adhesive Surface.

normally, the possibility of additional procedures, the trial and error process so often required to achieve adequate skin protection and containment of effluent, and the prolonged care trajectory (Kozell & Martins, 2003).

KEY POINT

Education and emotional support are critical aspects of care for the patient with a fistula and his/her family.

Open communication with the patient and family will decrease anxiety, increase trust, and facilitate independence (Cobb & Knaggs, 2003; Kaushal & Carlson, 2004; Kozell & Martins, 2003). Education should be individualized based on goals of care, specific management approaches, and the patient's needs and learning style. Whenever possible, the patient should learn by participating in his/her care to gain back his/her independence and sense of control. It is important for the WOC nurse to help the patient and family to establish realistic goals and expectations and to understand that fistula management and educational needs change over time (Burch & Buchan, 2004; Kozell & Martins, 2003).

SURGICAL CLOSURE

Given few fistulas close spontaneously, surgical intervention is required for closure of most fistulas. Surgical procedures may also be indicated for palliation (Nussbaum & Fischer, 2006). Factors known to prevent spontaneous closure are listed in **Box 36-3** (Bryant & Best, 2015).

Systemic review and meta-analysis conducted by de Vries and colleagues (2017) found that postponing surgery for enteric fistula closure is associated with lower recurrence. Because of the wide range of time to definitive surgery within each study, optimal timing of surgery could not be defined. Researchers estimate between 6 and 12 months after the last laparotomy may be needed to resolve abdominal infection, restore nutritional state and homeostasis, softening of adhesions, and provide adequate wound care and muscle strength. This bridging-to-surgery approach has become standard practice in Intestinal Failure (IF) centers (de Vries et al., 2017; ESCP, 2016).

Surgical interventions for ECF and EAFs either divert the fecal stream (without resection of the fistula) or provide definitive resection of the fistula tract. Diversion techniques divert the stool away from the fistula site without removal of the fistula by creating a stoma proximal to the fistula or by anastomosing (end-to-end or side-to-side) the two segments of bowel on each side of the fistula. This approach is required when resection of the fistula is not possible or appropriate, such as in the presence of extensive or recurrent malignancy or inadequate perfusion in the vicinity of the fistula due to previous surgery, scar formation, or prior irradiation. The process of resection involves removal of the diseased tissue and fistula tract followed by end-to-end anastomosis of the intestine. To protect the anastomosis, diversion of the fecal stream through a temporary stoma may be indicated. If the fistula involves the colon and the distal colon and rectum are not suitable for anastomosis or the anal sphincters are not competent, a permanent stoma with a Hartmann's pouch may be the safest procedure. Enteric fistulas communicating with the urinary tract will always require diversion of the fecal stream proximal to the fistula site to prevent urinary tract infections and pyelonephritis. Timing of surgery depends on the patient's status. Surgery for a type 1 fistula (see **Table 36-1**) is appropriate when the patient is nutritionally and metabolically stable, the fistula tract has been free of infection for 6 to 8 weeks, and the abdominal wall and peritoneal cavity have returned to a relatively soft, supple, pliable state; the goal is to maximize the potential for successful closure of the fistula and to minimize the potential for additional complications, including recurrent fistula formation. Judicious timing is warranted for surgical closure of complex type 2 fistulas (see **Table 36-1**); surgery is usually delayed for 3 to 6 months, which is extremely frustrating for the patient and family. It is important to be able to explain to the patient and family that the extensive intra-abdominal infection associated with the original bowel perforation or anastomotic breakdown resulted in formation of extensive scar tissue within the abdominal cavity (obliterative peritonitis) and that it takes a number of months for the scar tissue to soften enough for the surgeon to separate the loops of bowel and remove the fistula tract without risking additional injury to the bowel and additional fistula formation. Nutritional, metabolic, and immunologic status should be restored prior to surgery (Wong et al., 2004); for the patient with an ECF or EAF, this usually means that TPN will be required until the fistula is closed. However, the restrictions on oral intake are usually liberalized once it is clear that the fistula will not close spontaneously and that surgical intervention will be required; typically patients are allowed to eat and drink small amounts for pleasure and to keep the bowel mucosa healthy, as discussed earlier.

> **KEY POINT**
>
> Surgical closure is required for fistulas with known impediments to healing and for those that "fail" medical management (i.e., fail to close within 5 to 6 weeks of comprehensive management); surgical intervention is usually delayed for several months to permit softening of intra-abdominal adhesions.

VESICOVAGINAL, RECTOVAGINAL, OR ENTEROVAGINAL FISTULAS

While the vast majority of fistulas involve openings between two loops of bowel or between the bowel and the skin, fistulous openings can also develop between the bladder, rectum, or small bowel and the vagina. Vesicovaginal fistulas (between the bladder and vagina) are typically managed initially by urinary diversion with indwelling urethral or suprapubic catheter or nephrostomy tubes, followed by surgery to close the fistula tract. The urine draining continually from the vagina is usually managed with absorptive pads; alternatively, a balloon-tipped catheter can be placed in the vagina and connected to a leg bag. (If the diameter of the vaginal vault exceeds the diameter of the inflated balloon, causing the catheter to constantly slip out of place, the catheter can be threaded through a baby nipple so that the tip of the catheter rests just above the base of the nipple; the baby nipple/catheter unit is then folded and gently inserted into the vagina so that the base of the nipple rests within the introitus to minimize leakage.) This technique can also be used for management of enterovaginal fistulas; because the drainage is thicker, it is necessary to use a large diameter catheter. Rectovaginal fistulas are typically managed by fecal diversion to permit healing of the fistula tract. For the patient who is not a candidate for surgical intervention, the focus of management should be measures to minimize vaginal contamination, specifically, titration of fiber and fluid intake to maintain soft formed stool that will not pass through the narrow fistulous tract. The patient can also be counseled to use mild antiseptics approved for intravaginal use to reduce or eliminate odor (e.g., TrimoSan)

CONCLUSIONS

Caring for a patient with a fistula is one of the most challenging, and rewarding, situations the WOC nurse will encounter. Effective management requires a clear understanding of the anatomy of the fistula tract and

plan of care, ongoing assessment regarding progress in closure or evidence of failure to close, creativity in developing an effective strategy for containment of effluent and odor, and consistent support and education for the patient and family. The key ingredients to positive outcomes when managing a patient with a fistula are patience; persistence; interdisciplinary collaboration; close surveillance; excellent communication with the patient, family, and colleagues; and a little ingenuity.

REFERENCES

Arebi, N. & Forbes, A. (2004). High output fistula. *Clinics in Colon and Rectal Surgery, 7*(2), 89–98.

Bailey, E. H., & Glasgow, S. C. (2016). Challenges in the medical and surgical management of chronic inflammatory bowel disease. *Surgical Clinics of North America, 95,* 1233–1244.

Bryant, R. (1992). Management of drain sites and fistulas. In R. Bryant (Ed.), *Acute and chronic wounds: Nursing management.* St. Louis, MO: Mosby.

Bryant, R., & Best, M. (2015). Management of draining wounds and fistulas. In R. Bryant, & D. Nix (Eds.), *Acute and chronic wounds: Current management concepts* (5th ed.). St. Louis, MO: Mosby.

Bruhin, A., Ferreira, F., Chariker, M., et al. (2014). Systematic review and evidence based recommendations for the use of negative pressure wound therapy in the open abdomen. *International Journal of Surgery, 12*(10), 1105–1114.

Burch, J., & Buchan, D. (2004). Support and guidance for failure and enterocutaneous fistula care. *Gastrointestinal Nursing, 2*(7), 25–32.

Causey, M. W., Rivadeneira, D. E., & Steele, S. R. (2012). Historical and current trends in colon trauma. *Clinics in Colon and Rectal Surgery, 25*(4), 189–199.

Chamieh, J., Prakash, P., & Symons, W. J. (2018). Management of destructive colon injuries after damage control surgery. *Clinics in Colon and Rectal Surgery, 31*(1), 36–40. doi: 10.1055/s-0037-1602178.

Cobb, A., & Knaggs, E. (2003). The nursing management of enterocutaneous fistulae: A challenge for all. *British Journal of Community Nursing, 8*(9), S32–S38.

Coetzee, E., Rahim, Z. et al. (2014). Refedding enteroclysis as an alternative to parenteral nutrition for enteric fistula. *Colorectal Disease, 16*(10), 823–830.

Collier, B., Guillamondegui, O., Cotton, B., et al. (2007). Feeding the open abdomen. *Journal of Parenteral and Enteral Nutrition, 31*(5), 410–415.

Coughlin, S., Roth, L., Lurati, G., et al. (2012). Somatostatin analogues for the treatment of enterocutaneous fistulas: A systematic review and meta-analysis. *World Journal of Surgery, 36*(5), 1016–1029.

Davis, M., Dere, K., Hadley, G., et al. (2000). Options for managing an open wound with draining enterocutaneous fistula. *Journal of Wound, Ostomy, and Continence Nursing, 27*(2), 118–123.

Davis, K. G., & Johnson, E. K. (2013). Controversies in the care of the Enterocutaneous fistula. *Surgical Clinics of North America, 93,* 231–250.

Dearlove, J. L. (1996). Skin care management of gastrointestinal fistulas. *Surgical Clinics of North America, 76*(5), 1095–1109.

de Vries, F. E. E., Reeskamp, L. F., van Ruler, O., et al. (2017). Systematic review: Pharmacotherapy for high output enterostomies or enteral fistulas. *Alimentary Pharmacology & Therapeutics, 46*(3), 266–273.

Draus, J. M. Jr., Huss, S. A., Harty, N. J., et al. (2006). Enterocutaneous fistula: Are treatments improving? *Surgery, 140*(4), 570–576; discussion 576–578.

Dubose, J., & Lundy, J. (2010). Enterocutaneous fistulas in the setting of trauma and critical illness. *Clinics in Colon and Rectal Surgery, 23*(3), 182–189.

ESCP Intestinal Failure Group; Vaizey, C. J., Maeda, Y., Barbosa, E., et al. (2016). ESCP consensus on the surgical management of intestinal failure in adults. *Colorectal Disease, 18,* 535–548.

Gribovskaja-Rupp, I., & Melton, G. (2016). Enterocutaneous fistula: Proven strategies and updates. *Clinics in Colon and Rectal Surgery, 29*(2), 130–137.

Haack, C. I., Galloway, J. R., & Srinivasan, J. (2014). Enterocutaneous fistulas: A look at causes and management. *Current Surgery Reports, 2*, 71.

Heimroth, J., Chen, E., & Sutton, E. (2018). Management approaches for enterocutaneous fistulas. [Review] *The American Surgeon, 84*(3), 326–333.

Heineman, J. T., Garcia, L. J., Obst, M. A., et al. (2015). Collapsible enteroatmospheric fistula isolation device: A novel, simple solution to a complex problem. *Journal of the American College of Surgeons, 221*, e7–e14.

Hoedema, R. & Suryadevara, S. (2010). Entrostomal therapy and wound care of the fistula patient. *Clinic Colon Rectal Surgery, 23*(3), 161–168.

Hoeflok J, Jaramillo M, Li T, et al. (2015). Health-related quality of life in community-dwelling persons living with enterocutaneous fistulas. *Journal of Wound, Ostomy, and Continence Nursing, 42*(6), 607–613.

Hollington, P., Maurdsley, J., Lim, W., et al. (2004). An 11 year experience of enterocutaneous fistulae. *British Journal of Surgery, 91*, 1046–1051.

Irrgang, S., & Bryant, R. (1984). Management of the enterocutaneous fistula (continuous education credit). *Journal of Enterostomal Therapy, 11*(6), 211–228.

Jeter, K. F., Tintle, T. E., & Chariker M. (1990). Managing draining wounds and fistulae: New and established methods. In D. Krasner (Ed.), *Chronic wound care: A clinical source book for healthcare professionals* (pp. 240–246). King of Prussia, PA: Health Management.

Jones, E. G., & Harbit, M. (2003). Management of an ileostomy and mucous fistula located in a dehisced wound in a patient with morbid obesity. *Journal of Wound, Ostomy, and Continence Nursing, 30*(6), 351.

Juárez-Oropeza, M. A., & Román-Ramos, R. (2012). Factors predictive of recurrence and mortality after surgical repair of enterocutaneous fistula. *Journal of Gastrointestinal Surgery, 16*(1), 156–163, discussion 163–164.

Kassis, E. S., & Makary, M. A. (2008). Enterocutaneous fistula. In J. S. Cameron (Ed.), *Current surgical therapy* (9th ed.). St. Louis, MO: Mosby.

Kaushal, M., & Carlson, G. L. (2004). Management of enterocutaneous fistulae. *Clinics in Colon and Rectal Surgery, 17*(2), 79–87.

Knechtges, P., & Zimmermann, E. M. (2009). Intra-abdominal abscesses and fistulae. In T. Yamada, et al. (Eds.), *Textbook of gastroenterology* (Vol II, 6th ed.). Philadelphia, PA: Lippincott Williams & Wilkins.

Kordasiewicz, L. M. (2004). Abdominal wound with fistula and large amount of drainage status after incarcerated hernia repair. *Journal of Wound, Ostomy, and Continence Nursing, 31*(3), 150.

Kozell, K., & Martins, L. (2003). Managing the challenges of enterocutaneous fistulae. *Wound Care Canada, 1*(1), 10–14.

Kumpf, V. J., de Aguilar-Nascimento, J. E., Diaz-Pizarro Graf, J. I., et al. (2017). ASPEN-FELANPE clinical guidelines. *JPEN Journal of Parenteral and Enteral Nutrition, 41*(1), 104–112.

Li, P. H., Tee, Y. S., Fu, C. Y., et al. (2018). The role of noncontrast CT in the evaluation of surgical abdomen patients. *The American Surgeon, 84*(6), 1015–1102.

Lloyd, D. A. J., Gabe, S. M., & Windsor, A. C. J. (2006). Nutrition and management of enterocutaneous fistula. *British Journal of Surgery, 93*, 1045–1055.

Lynch, A. C., Delaney, C. P., Senagore, A. J., et al. (2004). Clinical outcome and factors predictive of recurrence after enterocutaneous fistula surgery. *Annals of Surgery, 240*(5), 825–831.

Makhdoom, Z. A., Komar, M. J., & Still, C. D. (2000). Nutrition and enterocutaneous fistulas. *Journal of Clinical Gastroenterology, 31*(3), 195.

Mehta, N. Y., Copelin, E. L. II. (Updated 31 July 2019). Abdominal abscess. In *Stat Pearls [Internet]*. Treasure Island, FL: Stat Pearls Publishing. Retrieved from https://www.ncbi.nlm.nih.gov/books/NBK519573

Neutzling, C. B., Lustosa, S. A. S., Proenca, I. M., et al. (2017). Stapled versus handsewn methods for colorectal anastomosis surgery. *Cochrane Database of Systematic Reviews*, (2), CD003144. doi: 10.1002/14651858.CD003144.pub2.

Nishide, K. (1997). Development of closed-suction pouch drainage for giant fistulae: A report on two cases. *WCET Journal, 17*(1), 16–19.

Nurses Specialized in Wound, Ostomy and Continence Canada (NSWOCC) (formally CAET). (2018). *Nursing best practice recommendations: Enterocutaneous fistulas (ECF) and enteroatmospheric fistulas (EAF)* (2nd ed.) Retrieved December 15, 2019, from Ottawa Web site at http://nswoc.ca/ecf-best-practices.

Nussbaum, M. S., & Fischer, D. R. (2006). Gastric, duodenal and small intestinal fistulas. In C. J. Yeo, et al. (Eds.), *Shackelford's surgery of the alimentary tract* (6th ed.). St. Louis, MO: Saunders.

Parli, S. E., Pfeifer, C. Oyler, D. R., et al (2018). Redefining "bowel regimen": Pharmacologic strategies and nutritional considerations in the management of small bowel fistulas [Review]. *American Journal of Surgery, 216*(2), 351–358.

Polk, T. M., & Schwab, C. W. (2012). Metabolic and nutritional support of the enterocutaneous fistula patient: A three-phase approach. *World Journal of Surgery, 36*(3), 524–533.

Pontieri-Lewis, V. (2005). Management of gastrointestinal fistulae: A case study. *Medical-Surgical Nursing, 14*(1), 68–72.

Quinn, M., Falconer, S., & McKee, R. F. (2017). Management of enterocutaneous fistula: Outcomes in 276 patients. *World Journal of Surgery, 41*(10), 2502–2511.

Rahman, F. N., & Stavas, J. M. (2015). Interventional radiologic management and treatment of enterocutaneous fistulae [Review]. *Journal of Vascular & Interventional Radiology: JVIR, 26*(1), 7–19.

Rahbour, G., Sci, B. M., & Siddiqui, M. R. (2012). Systematic review and meta analysis a meta-analysis of outcomes following use of somatostatin and its analogues for the management of enterocutaneous fistulas. *Annals of Surgery, 256*(6), 946–954.

Reed, T., Economon, D., & Wiersema-Bryant, L. (2006). Colocutaneous fistula management in a dehisced wound: A case study. *Ostomy/Wound Management, 52*(4), 60–64, 66.

Reider, K. (2017). Fistula isolation and the use of negative pressure to promote wound healing. A case study. *Journal of Wound, Ostomy, and Continence Nursing, 44*(3), 293–298.

Renton, S., Robertson, I., & Speirs, M. (2006). Alternative management of complex wounds and fistulae. *British Journal of Nursing, 15*(16), 851–853.

Rolstad, B., & Wong, W. D. (2004). Nursing considerations in intestinal fistulas. In P. A. Cataldo & J. M. MacKeigan (Eds.), *Intestinal stomas: Principles, techniques, and management* (2nd ed.). New York, NY: Marcel Dekker.

Samad, S., Anele, C., Akhtar, M., et al (2015). Implementing a pro-forma for multidisciplinary management of an enterocutaneous fistula: A case study. *Ostomy/Wound Management, 61*(6), 46–52.

Schecter, W. P., Hirshberg, A., Chang, D. S., et al. (2009). "Enteric fistula" principles of management. *Journal of the American College of Surgeons, 209*(4), 484–491.

Stevens, P., Foulkes, R. E., Hartford-Beynon, J. S., et al. (2011). Systematic review and meta-analysis of the role of somatostatin and its analogues in the treatment of enterocutaneous fistula. *European Journal of Gastroenterology & Hepatology, 23*(10), 912–922.

Teixeira, P. G., Inaba, K., Dubose, J., et al. (2009). Enterocutaneous fistula complicating trauma laparotomy: A major resource burden. *The American Surgeon, 75*(1), 30–32.

Telem, D. A., Chin, E. H., Nguyen, S. Q., et al. (2010). Risk factors for anastomotic leak following colorectal surgery: A case–control study. *Archives of Surgery, 145*(4), 371–376.

Tran, N. A., & Thorson, A. G. (2008). Rectovaginal fistula. In J. L. Cameron (Ed.), *Current surgical therapy* (9th ed.). St. Louis, MO: Mosby.

Wainstein, D. E., Fernandez, E., Gonzalez, D., et al. (2008). Treatment of high output enterocutaneous fistulas with a vacuum-compaction device. A ten-year experience. *World Journal of Surgery, 32*, 430–435.

Wercka, J., Cagol, P. P., Melo, A. L., et al. (2016). Epidemiology and outcome of patients with postoperative abdominal fistula. *Revista do Colégio Brasileiro de Cirurgiões, 43*(2), 117–123.

Whelan, J. F. Jr., & Ivatury, R. R. (2011). Enterocutaneous fistulas: An overview. *European Journal of Trauma and Emergency Surgery, 37*(3), 251–258.

Willcutts, K., Mercer, D., & Ziegler, J. (2015). Fistuloclysis: An interprofessional approach to nourishing the fistula patient. *Journal of Wound, Ostomy, and Continence Nursing, 42*(5), 549–553.

Williams, L. J., Zolfaghari, S., & Boushey, R. P. (2010). Complications of enterocutaneous fistulas and their management. *Clinics in Colon and Rectal Surgery, 23*(3), 209–220.

Wong, W. D., et al. (2004). Management of intestinal fistulas. In P. A. Cataldo & J. M. MacKeigan (Eds.), *Intestinal stomas: Principles, techniques, and management* (2nd ed.). New York, NY: Marcel Dekker.

Zelga, P., Tchórzewski, M., Zelga, M., et al. (2017). Radiation-induced rectovaginal fistulas in locally advanced gynecological malignancies-new patients, old problem? *Langenbeck's Archives of Surgery, 402*(7), 1079–1088.

QUESTIONS

1. The WOC nurse suspects that a patient's surgical wound is developing a fistula. Which of the following is the definitive indicator of an enterocutaneous fistula?
   A. Fever and infection in the wound bed
   B. Abdominal pain and wound dehiscence
   C. Blood migrating from a wound bed to the gastrointestinal tract
   D. Passage of gastrointestinal secretions or urine into an open wound bed

2. A patient is diagnosed with an enterocutaneous fistula with a high-output volume. Which statement correctly defines this diagnosis?
   A. A passage is created from the intestine to the skin, and the volume is >500 mL/24 h.
   B. A passage is created from the colon to the vagina, and the volume output is >500 mL/24 h.
   C. A passage is created from the bladder to the vagina, and the volume output is 200 to 500 mL/24 h.
   D. A passage is created from the colon to the skin, and the volume output is <200 mL/24 h.

3. The WOC nurse is assessing the wound of a patient diagnosed with a type 1 complex fistula. What data regarding the fistula would the nurse document in the patient record?
   A. Fistula with a short direct tract, no abscess, no other organ involvement
   B. Fistula with an abscess, with multiple organ involvement
   C. Fistula that opens into the base of the wound
   D. Fistula with a tract that is contained within the body

4. What is the etiology of the majority of enterocutaneous fistulas (ECFs)?
   A. Bowel disease
   B. Diverticulitis
   C. Surgical procedures
   D. External trauma

5. The WOC nurse is planning care for a patient with an enterocutaneous fistula (ECF). What is a key initial step in managing a patient with ECF?
   A. Administer H_2 antagonists to decrease ECF closure time.
   B. Use a 2-week trial of octreotide to reduce fistula output.
   C. Limit oral or enteral intake to amount keeping intestinal mucosa healthy.
   D. Force fluids to decrease gastric, biliary, and pancreatic secretions.

6. A patient is diagnosed with an intra-abdominal abscess following a CT scan. What is the initial management of choice for this patient?
   A. CT-guided drainage
   B. Surgical intervention
   C. Pharmacological management
   D. Keeping the patient NPO for 3 days

7. Which of the following assessment findings indicates that the patient will require surgical closure?
   A. Output exceeding 750 mL/24 h.
   B. Evidence of mucosal eversion/pseudostoma formation.
   C. History indicates fistula has been present >14 days.
   D. Hypertrophic granulation tissue in wound bed.

8. The WOC nurse is recommending products for patients with fistulas. Which product is used correctly?
   A. Moisture barrier cream for a high-output fistula
   B. Negative pressure wound therapy (NPWT) for a low-output fistula
   C. Suction system for a low-output fistula
   D. Pouch for a high- or low-output fistula

9. A patient presents with a fistula that has an output volume <50 mL with a need for odor control. What would be a good containment option for this patient?
   A. Wound management system with window emptied frequently
   B. Closed system with suction
   C. Charcoal dressings over dressings with environmental deodorants

   D. Absorptive dressings (e.g., calcium alginate dressings)

10. The WOC nurse is teaching a patient how to change a fistula pouch. Which of the following is a recommended step in this procedure?
   A. Trace the pattern onto the skin barrier surface of the pouch providing at least ¼ inch clearance of wound edges.
   B. Trace the pattern onto the skin barrier of the pouch being careful to size the opening to match the contours of the wound exactly.
   C. Remove the pouch by pulling off the skin quickly while applying gentle pressure on skin with one hand.
   D. Clean the skin with an alcohol wipe or skin cleanser with an emollient and dry gently and thoroughly.

ANSWERS AND RATIONALES

1. D. Rationale: Fever, infection, abdominal pain, wound dehiscence, and blood migrating from a wound bed to the gastrointestinal tract may occur with a fistula. However, passage of gastrointestinal secretions or urine into an open wound bed is a definitive indicator.

2. A. Rationale: An enterocutaneous fistula is a passage from the GI or GU tract to this skin, a passage from the GI or GU tract to the vagina is called a colo or vestico vaginal fistula. High-output volume is defined as >500 mL/24 h.

3. B. Rationale: A simple fistula does not involve abscess or organ while a complex fistula type 1 involves abscess and multiple organs or opens to the wound base.

4. C. Rationale: ECFs can occur spontaneously, as a result of inflammatory bowel disease, cancer, or diverticulitis. However, they most commonly develop postoperatively, due to anastomotic breakdown.

5. C. Rationale: Reduced oral/enteral intake minimizes fistula output by decreasing luminal

contents, GI stimulation, and pancreaticobiliary secretions. H_2 receptors have not been shown to affect either the number of ECFs that close spontaneously or the time to ECF closure. Octreotides decrease intestinal output in some situations and may be appropriate as a short-term adjunctive therapy.

6. A. Rationale: CT-guided drainage is the initial management of choice in patients presenting with spontaneous or postoperative intra-abdominal abscess. This can obviate the need for early operative intervention.

7. B. Rationale: A fistula with high output or duration >14 days can spontaneously close under the right conditions. Evidence of mucosal eversion/pseudostoma formation, however, will not close spontaneously and will require surgical closure. Hypertrophic granulation tissue in wound bed does not impact fistula closure.

8. D. Rationale: The high-output fistula is best managed with pouches, suction systems, or NPWT. Moisture barrier creams provide skin protection for the low-output fistula.

9. C. Rationale: Charcoal dressings are better designed for odor control than other absorbent dressings and can manage the low-output fistula with the proper skin protection and change frequency. A wound management system with a window emptied frequently or a closed system with suction may control odor but are indicated for the high-output fistula.

10. A. Rationale: Prepare a fistula pouch by tracing the pattern onto the skin barrier surface of the pouch providing at least ¼ inch clearance of wound edges, matching contours of the wound exactly does not allow enough adhesive surface. Pulling adhesive off the skin quickly can cause skin injury. Alcohol can be caustic to perifistula skin. Skin cleanser with emollient can impair adhesion of the pouch.

CHAPTER 37

NURSING MANAGEMENT OF THE PATIENT WITH PERCUTANEOUS TUBES

Jane Fellows and Michelle Rice

OBJECTIVE

Apply assessment and nursing management techniques to address the complex care needs of a patient with percutaneous tubes.

TOPIC OUTLINE

INTRODUCTION

Percutaneous tube placement into body organs or spaces is a means for drainage of fluids, maintaining an opening into an organ where obstruction exists, or providing for instillation of fluids, medication, or feeding through the tube. The tubes are usually placed by a health care provider in surgery, via endoscopy or interventional radiology. The WOC nurse is often consulted for management of these tubes and the complications that may occur with them. Knowledge of the location, purpose, and desired outcome of the tube placement is essential to effectively manage the care of patients with these tubes. The use of percutaneous tubes is common in the adult and pediatric patient populations across acute care, long-term care, and home care settings. Increasingly they are being used for pain relief and symptom management in palliative care (Requarth, 2011).

Common types of these tubes are gastrostomy, jejunostomy, biliary, and nephrostomy.

GASTROSTOMY AND JEJUNOSTOMY TUBES

Nasogastric tubes (NGTs) are the simplest to insert in the gastrointestinal (GI) tract and the least invasive, but they carry a higher risk for dislodgment and aspiration leading to pneumonia (Boullata et al., 2017). When feeding through the tube or decompression of the GI tract is needed for more than a few weeks, a percutaneous tube is inserted. NGT are indicated for short-term use. Common indications for gastrostomy tube (GT) insertion are obstructing head and neck cancer, benign and malignant esophageal disease, neurologic dysfunction, trauma, and respiratory failure.

GTs have been reported in the literature since the 1800s. Dr. Martin Stamm developed a surgical procedure for placement of a tube directly into the stomach, which is still used today. The standard Stamm gastrostomy involves circumferential purse-string sutures to stabilize the tube within the lumen of the stomach and affix the stomach to the anterior abdominal wall. A later technique developed by Witzel involves creating a serosal tunnel as well as an abdominal wall tunnel through which the tube passes. This is useful when the stomach has been altered so that it cannot be secured to the abdominal wall such as after a gastric bypass surgery or resection of esophageal cancer. Variations on these open surgical procedures remained the standard of care for feeding or gastric decompression until the 1980s when a procedure for percutaneous endoscopic gastrostomy (PEG) was developed. PEG is a method of placing a tube into the stomach through the skin, aided by endoscopy (**Fig. 37-1**). A PEG with a jejunal extension tube can be placed through a preexisting PEG to facilitate more distal feeding while also providing an avenue for gastric decompression when necessary.

PEG is often considered the method of choice for enteral access due to the simplicity, effectiveness, and lower cost of the procedure, but it is important to do a complete assessment of the patient's GI anatomy and comorbid conditions before deciding which type of enteral access will be best for the patient (Boullata et al., 2017). PEG is not always clinically appropriate, and some of the possible contraindications include the following:

- Uncorrected coagulopathy or thrombocytopenia
- Upper tract obstruction or malformation
- Severe ascites
- Hemodynamic instability
- Sepsis
- Intra-abdominal perforation
- Active peritonitis
- Abdominal wall infection at the selected site of placement
- Gastric outlet obstruction (if PEG tube is being placed for feeding)
- Severe gastroparesis (if PEG tube is being placed for feeding)
- History of total gastrectomy

When a PEG is not feasible for the patient, radiologic placement is a possible alternative. This was first described in the literature in the mid-1980s (Kim et al., 2010) and avoids the use of an endoscope and is not contraindicated in the presence of upper tract obstruction. It uses fluoroscopy and ultrasound to identify the stomach, and a GT with a balloon is secured against the gastric mucosa with an external bumper on the skin (**Fig. 37-2**). If gastroesophageal reflux or delaying gastric emptying is a problem, another feeding tube option is a percutaneous gastrojejunal tube (**Fig. 37-3**). This tube has a balloon and an external skin bumper. There is an extension that is guided through the duodenum and into the jejunum for feeding. These tubes will have a gastric port that can be used for medication or fluid administration or decompression of the stomach and one port for the jejunal feeding. A study of 124 patients requiring conversion

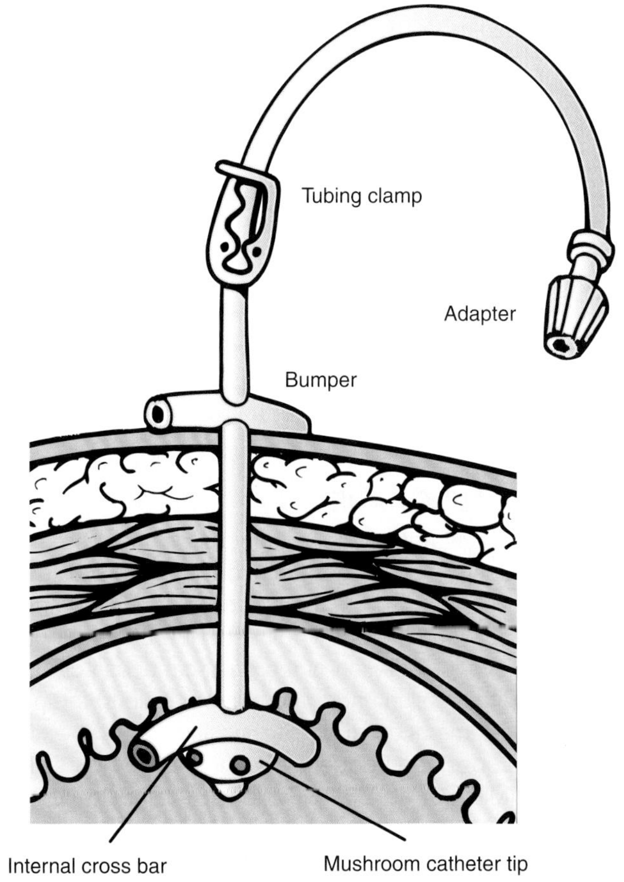

Tubing clamp

Adapter

Bumper

Internal cross bar   Mushroom catheter tip

FIGURE 37-1. PEG Tube with Internal and External Bumper. (Published in (2015). *Essentials for nursing practice* (8th ed., pp. 926–926), copyright Elsevier.)

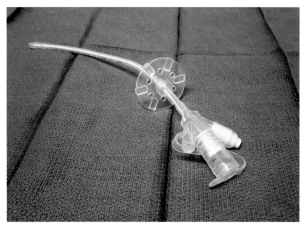

FIGURE 37-2. Balloon-Tipped Gastrostomy Tube. (Courtesy of Jane Fellows, MSN, RN, CWOCN.)

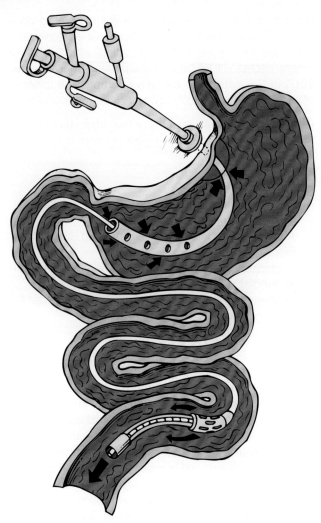

FIGURE 37-3. PEG with Jejunal Extension. (Published in (2015). *Essentials for nursing practice* (8th ed., pp. 926–926), copyright Elsevier.)

from a GT to gastrojejunal tube showed a significantly higher success rate using the radiologic placement procedure rather than nonradiologic procedures (Kim et al., 2010). These radiologic procedures require providers with training in interventional radiology, which is not always an option in all facilities.

Both the PEG and radiologic procedures can be done with sedation rather than anesthesia making the procedure safer for the patient, and the time for initial feedings is not delayed. If feeding in the stomach is not possible due to surgical absence of the organ, severe gastroparesis, or gastric outlet obstruction, radiologic intervention is used to place a feeding tube directly into the jejunum. This tube is initially secured with a stabilizer sutured to the skin.

For those patients who are not candidates for PEG or radiologic procedures, surgical approaches offer the advantage of direct visualization of tube placement into the intended organ (stomach or jejunum). An open laparotomy or laparoscopy is done by a surgeon in the operating room, and the patient receives general anesthesia. During the surgical approach, the stomach or jejunum is identified following a laparotomy incision or insertion of the laparoscope. The laparoscopic approach offers smaller incision size, less pain, and decreased risk of incisional hernia (Mizrahi et al., 2014). The appropriate feeding tube is secured within the lumen of the targeted organ and brought out through a separate stab incision. If a patient is scheduled for an open or laparoscopic abdominal surgery and it is expected that a feeding tube may be needed, it should be placed at the time of the surgery.

COMPARATIVE COMPLICATION RATES

There are many potential complications with these procedures, and most of the patients are malnourished and have significant comorbidities. However, the complication rates are relatively low. The complication rates reported in the literature vary, but it seems generally accepted to be 1% to 3% for PEG placement, 8% to 10% with radiologic procedures, and 7% to 15% with surgical procedures (Miller et al., 2014). Complications associated with percutaneous endoscopic approaches include endoscopic trauma and perforation of the GI tract, bleeding, skin and soft tissue infection, injury to intra-abdominal viscera such as the liver or colon, tube dislodgment, and fistula creation. Radiologic placement has many of the same risks as do endoscopically placed tubes, but there is no risk of upper tract trauma from the endoscope. Surgically placed tubes are associated most commonly with skin and soft tissue infection, incisional hernia, bleeding, inadvertent removal of the tube, and complications associated with general anesthesia. Issues with inadvertent injury to surrounding intra-abdominal viscera are very rare due to the better visibility during the procedure. In a study comparing laparoscopic versus open laparotomy, the laparoscopic surgery took longer to perform, but the complication rate was higher in the open surgery group (Mizrahi et al., 2014).

ROUTINE TUBE CARE

Following placement of percutaneous gastric tubes, the external bolster should generally be left in place for at least 4 days. After 4 days, there should be 1/2 to 1 cm of laxity left between the entry point and the bumper of the tube to prevent ulceration of the gastric mucosa or pressure injury to the skin under the bumper. Due to the possibility of edema at the tube site, positioning of the tube should be observed frequently for the first 48 hours after insertion (Miller et al., 2014). Evidence for most effective site care is lacking, but patient education materials recommend that the site be washed with mild soap and water, rinsed well with water, and dried daily. One gauze drain sponge may be placed under the bumper unless it sutured in place to absorb any drainage from the site. The use

BOX 37-1 PROCEDURE FOR POUCH APPLICATION AROUND THE GASTROSTOMY TUBE

Equipment:
Ostomy pouch: One piece
Scissors
Skin barrier powder
Wet and dry cloths
No sting skin prep
Cotton-tipped applicators
Gloves
Catheter holder device
Water-resistant tape

Directions:
1. Clamp tube and turn off feeding.
2. Remove the pink tape from around the tube where it exits the pouching system and gently remove the pouch using adhesive remover or warm water. Be careful not to pull or dislodge the tube.
3. Clean the skin with water and pat dry. Cleanse the area under the tube bumper by inserting a cotton-tipped applicator between sutures. Sprinkle skin barrier powder under the bumper to protect the skin.

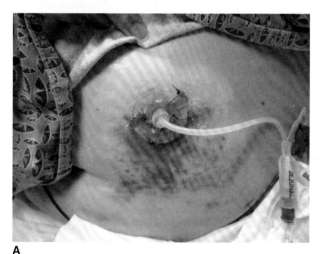

A

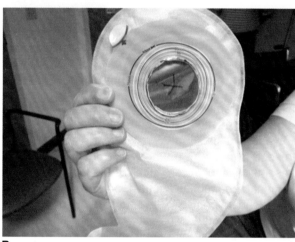

B

4. If there is any skin breakdown (**A**), sprinkle skin barrier powder on the skin, rub in, and seal with alcohol-free liquid skin barrier.
5. Cut an opening in the skin barrier of the one-piece pouching system to fit around the bumper. Cut an X-shaped opening on the front of the pouch so the gastrostomy tube can be pulled through (**B**).
6. Place catheter holder device over X cut in front of the pouch to secure the tube and avoid leakage (**C**). Instructions come with each device. Cut a hole in the nipple large enough to pull the tube through (**D**).

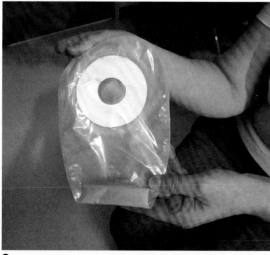

C

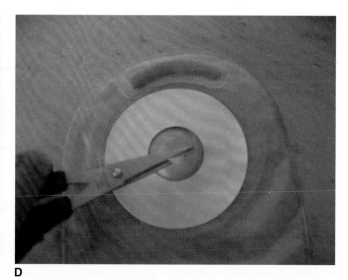

D

BOX 37-1   PROCEDURE FOR POUCH APPLICATION AROUND THE GASTROSTOMY TUBE *(Continued)*

7. Pull tube through the opening and place the pouch on the skin. Make sure the skin is dry before placing the pouch (**E**). Use water resistant tape around the tube where it exits the pouch to seal the opening in the nipple (**F**).

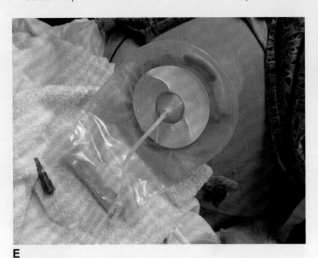

E

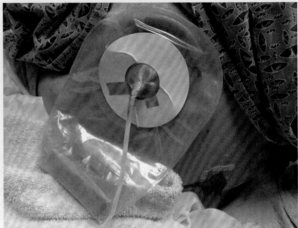

F

patients. The remaining patients received a silver alginate under a foam dressing, and if that did not resolve the hypergranulation, a steroid cream was applied (Warriner & Spruce, 2014). When hypergranulation tissue is present, it is important to stabilize the tube to reduce movement of the tube in the tract. Silver nitrate applicator sticks should be used with care to avoid getting the silver nitrate on intact skin as this may cause a burning sensation. More than one application may be needed. In extreme cases, surgical excision of the tissue may be required (Roveron & Antonini, 2018).

TUBE REPLACEMENT

GTs may become accidentally dislodged for a variety of reasons. The stabilizer may have loosened, water may have leaked from the balloon, inadvertent traction is placed on the tube, or the patient may have pulled it out. The latter cause is usually secondary to an altered mental state. In these patients, a low-profile tube may be appropriate (**Fig. 37-5**). The low-profile tube may also be used as a replacement tube when the patient wishes to have one for convenience and ease of concealing the tube under clothing. It is required to measure the stoma tract; there are measuring devices that determine the size tract for low-profile tube needed. This is especially important in pediatric patients as a child is growing and may need to have another size tube. GT replacement may be done by a nurse, but verification of workplace policies and regulations of the state board of nursing should guide the decision to do this. In a healthy person, the tract in which the GT is placed would be healed

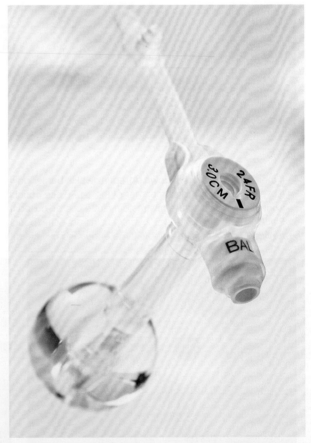

FIGURE 37-5. Low-Profile Gastrostomy Tube. MIC-KEY™ G Feeding Tube is a Registered Trademark or Trademark of Halyard Health, Inc. or its affiliates. (Image copyright © 2014 HYH. All rights reserved.)

in 2 to 3 weeks. The patients requiring enteral access for feeding are usually malnourished and have chronic conditions that may interfere with healing, so it is advisable to wait 4 to 6 weeks before a nurse should attempt tube replacement (Boullata et al., 2017). There is a risk of inserting the tube in the peritoneum if the tract is not healed. When a tube is dislodged unexpectedly after 6 weeks from original placement, it must be replaced as soon as possible before the tract and the opening in the skin begins to close (**Box 37-2**). For patients at home, a family member may be taught to do this to avoid loss of access. Placing a tube into the opening will solve the immediate problem of maintaining the tract, but the tube should not be used until proper placement has been ascertained by radiographic study or return of gastric fluid through the tube (Boullata et al., 2017). Replacement GTs are preferred, but a Foley catheter may be used temporarily if a GT is not available. The only reason for using a tube not designed for the GI tract is to keep the tract open until a GT can be obtained and inserted (Boullata et al., 2017).

KEY POINT

The patient should understand that when the tube falls out, they should replace the tube immediately or seek medical attention for replacement.

PEDIATRIC CONSIDERATIONS

The use of enteral feeding tube is a widely used, effective, and standard means of meeting the nutritional needs of child with a dysfunctional GI tract or who is unable to take oral nutrition. Enteral tubes are common in pediatric patients with neurological disorders as well as diseases resulting in malnutrition including cancer, short gut syndrome, cystic fibrosis, cardiac illness, and metabolic illness (Pars & Cavusoglu, 2019). The procedure is considered minimally invasive, and patients are discharged a short time after the procedure (Rollins et al., 2013). However, the procedure is not without risks and complications. A review of the literature demonstrates that patients with GTs have significant number of complications and emergency department (ED) visits for nonurgent tube issues. According to Pars and Cavusoglu (2019), the frequency of common minor complications ranges from 2% to 55% and includes tube blockage, dislocation, and peristomal skin infections. Major complications including aspiration, bleeding, pneumoperitoneum, and peritonitis range in frequency from 5% to 25%. Other common complications include leakage, peristomal skin breakdown, enlarged tracts, medical device–related pressure injuries, and hypergranulation tissue.

The management of these complications is the same as for adult patients with a feeding tube. Tube

---

BOX 37-2 PROCEDURE FOR CHANGING A GASTROSTOMY TUBE

Equipment:
Gastrostomy tube of the same size as the one being removed
Water-based lubricant
Empty 10-mL syringe
10-mL syringe filled with water
60-mL catheter-tipped syringe
Gauze pads
Gloves

Directions:
1. Inform the patient of the purpose of the procedure.
2. Place the patient in supine position or elevate the head 30 degrees, as the patient prefers.
3. Test the balloon on the new tube by filling it with water and ascertain that there is no leak. Remove the water from the balloon.
4. Slide the bumper up the tube to make sure it moves easily.
5. If the old tube is in place (i.e., it has not been inadvertently removed), use an empty syringe to remove the water from the balloon through the aspiration port. Reaspirate to be sure the balloon is empty.
6. Pull the tube gently out. Note the length of the tube from skin level to the tip.
7. Use gauze to wipe away any gastric contents that come out with the tube. The insertion site and 5 cm beyond the site should be cleansed with normal saline and dried well.
8. Lubricate the replacement tube. Do not use a petroleum-based lubricant.
9. Insert the lubricated tube into the stoma opening a couple of centimeters past the length of the tube that was removed.
10. Fill the balloon with the required amount of water.
11. Pull the tube up until you feel resistance against the stomach wall.
12. Slide the bumper down the tube so that there is only 2 to 3 mm of space between the bumper and the skin. No dressing is required. The tube should be able to be turned around freely in the opening. Rotate the tube 360 degrees to confirm the tube has free rotation.
13. Use the 60-mL syringe to aspirate gastric contents to affirm correct placement.
14. If no gastric contents can be aspirated, connect the tube to a bedside drainage bag and wait 20 minutes to see if the contents drain.
15. If there is no drainage in 20 minutes, tube placement should be confirmed with an abdominal radiograph in the oblique position using contrast.
16. Do not start feeding or flush the tube until there is confirmation of intragastric placement.
17. Document the size of tube and the amount of water that was used to inflate the balloon.

---

dislodgment may be decreased with a low-profile tube, and these are used frequently in pediatric patients. A retrospective study by Novotny et al. (2009) of 223 young children who received a standard PEG (*n* = 110) versus a low-profile PEG (*n* = 113) showed a significant decrease in tube dislodgment with the low-profile tube and no difference in infection rate. There was also a significantly decreased length of hospital stay in the low-profile tube group. There was not a difference in ED visits for minor complications with the tubes. Use of a silicone foam dressing can be used as a pressure injury prevention strategy for patients at risk. Silver impregnated moisture wicking fabric can also be used for moisture management and treatment of hypergranulation tissue. It is important to wrap the fabric upward around the tube if the goal is moisture management. This will allow the moisture to be wicked away from the skin (Singh, 2016). According to a 4-year prospective study by Goldberg et al. (2010), infection developed in 37% of patients with the majority of infections occurring during the first 15 days after placement. Hypergranulation tissue was noted in 68% of children with a recurrence in 17% of patients after receiving treatment. A 2009 retrospective cross-sectional descriptive study by Saavedra et al. (2009) showed that over a 23-month period, 77 patients had 181 ED visits for complaints related to the GT. Dislodgment of the GT occurred in 62% of the patients, and 75% of the visits were for GT replacement. In a study of 247 patients treated at a tertiary children's hospital, Correa et al. (2014) found that 20% of patients accounted for 44 ED visits within the first 30 days of discharge for complaints of leaking, mild clogs, and hypergranulation (hyperplasia) tissue. During the time period of 31 to 365 days post discharge, 40 additional patients returned to the ED a total of 71 times for potentially avoidable visits.

It is clear that care of these children creates substantial stress for family caregivers specific education on recognizing potential complications and how to manage them must be provided to the patients and their families in order to decrease the number of avoidable visits to the clinic, ED or rehospitalizations. It is important to assess the learning style of the family, engage an interdisciplinary approach, and incorporate multimedia into family education. Families that are confident in their knowledge and ability to provide needed care may have a decrease in anxiety and increase in satisfaction (Schweitzer et al., 2014). In addition, the use of patient messaging and uploading of patient's photos via the electronic health record (HER) is a secure way for families to obtain answers and a plan of care for minor issues. This is an area in which a WOC nurse can have tremendous impact on patient and caregiver quality of life.

NEPHROSTOMY TUBES

Percutaneous nephrostomy tubes are inserted through the skin and into the renal pelvis of the kidney. The purpose of percutaneous nephrostomy tubes is to facilitate drainage of urine after a partial or complete obstruction has occurred or if a urine leak is present (diverting the urine away from the leak to allow healing). Indications for use include tumors, strictures, dilations, and kidney stone removal. The tube exits through the flank and is connected to extension tubing and drains into a leg or bedside drainage bag. Important factors in the management of this tube include tube stabilization to prevent pulling, kinking, or dislodgment; possible tube flushing with MD order; prevention of skin irritation; and signs of infection (Martin & Baker, 2019).

Tube stabilization can be accomplished with the use of a commercial catheter holder. Tape may also be used if commercial devices are not available. When securing the tube, consider the tube angle to prevent kinking.

In some instances, flushing of the tube may be needed if there is an absence of urine; persistent flank pain; or presence of clots, debris, or sediment (Seladi-Shulman, 2018). Consult facility protocols and/or health care provider guidelines for this practice. Generally, 5 to 10 mL of sterile, normal saline is flushed into the tube. Do not force the saline into the tube. After saline is instilled, reconnect to straight drainage. If unable to instill saline, the health care provider must be notified.

During the first 2 weeks post procedure, sterile gauze nephrostomy dressings should be kept dry and be changed daily and as needed for drainage. For sensitive skin, consider the use of adhesive remover or releaser to loosen the dressing. If a sterile transparent dressing is in use, it must be changed every 3 days. After the initial 2-week period, the dressing should be changed twice per week and if wet or lifting off (Martin & Baker, 2019). If skin irritation occurs, consider the use of an alcohol-free liquid skin barrier to protect the area. If a fungal rash appears to be present, use an antifungal powder rather than an ointment or cream. If there appears to be sensitivity to the adhesive, consider a dressing with a silicone backing.

Patient and family education includes how to flush the tube if ordered by health care provider, signs of infection, skin care, how to use and care for a leg or bedside drainage bag, and how often the nephrostomy tube will be changed (usually every 2 to 3 months).

⬤ BILIARY TUBES

Biliary tubes are necessary when an alternate method of draining bile from the hepatobiliary system is needed. Often, the bile ducts are blocked, resulting in a buildup of bile in the liver that can lead to jaundice, nausea, vomiting, itching, fever, dark urine, and infection; see **Box 37-3**. Blockages are caused by tumors, strictures, and gallstones. The thin tube is inserted through the skin into the bile ducts by an interventional radiologist and is connected to a small drainage bag.

Management of the biliary tube includes adequate securement of the tube to prevent kinking or dislodgment, flushing of the tube with MD order, dressing changes, and keeping the drain bag below the waist to facilitate proper drainage (MSKCC, 2017).

REFERENCES

Boullata, J, Correra, A., Harvey, L., et al. (2017). ASPEN safe practices for enteral nutrition therapy. *Journal of Parenteral and Enteral Nutrition, 41*(1), 15–103.

Correa, J. A., Fallon, S. C., Murphy, K. M., et al. (2014). Resource utilization after gastrostomy tube placement: Defining areas of improvement for future quality improvement projects. *Journal of Pediatric Surgery, 49*(11), 1598–1601. doi: 10.1016/j.jpedsurg.2014.06.015.

Goldberg, E., Barton, S., Xanthopoulos, M. S., et al. (2010). A descriptive study of complications of gastrostomy tubes in children. *Journal of Pediatric Nursing, 25*(2), 72–80. doi: 10.1016/j.pedn.2008.07.008.

Kim, C. Y., Patel, M. B., Miller, M. J., et al. (2010). Gastrostomy-to-gastrojejunostomy tube conversion: Impact of the method of original gastrostomy tube placement. *Journal of Vascular and Interventional Radiology, 21*(7), 1031–1037.

Martin, R., & Baker, H. (2019). Nursing care and management of patients with a nephrostomy. *Nursing Times, 115*(11), 40–43.

Memorial Sloan Kettering Cancer Center (MSKCC). (2017). About your biliary drainage catheter. https://www.mskcc.org/cancer-care/patient-education/about-your-biliary-drainage-catheter

Miller, K. R., McClave, S. A., Kiraly, L. N., et al. (2014). A tutorial on enteral access in adult patients in the hospitalized setting. *Journal of Parenteral and Enteral Nutrition, 38*(3), 282–294.

Mizrahi, I., Garg, M., Divino, C. M., et al. (2014). Comparison of laparoscopic vs open approach to gastrostomy tubes. *JSLS: Journal of the Society of Laparoendoscopic Surgeons, 18*(1), 28–33.

Novotny, N. M., Vegeler, R. C., Breckler, F. D., et al. (2009). Percutaneous endoscopic gastrostomy buttons in children: Superior to tubes. *Journal of Pediatric Surgery, 44*(6), 1193–1196.

Pars, H., & Cavusoglu, H. (2019). A literature review of percutaneous endoscopic gastrostomy. *Gastroenterology Nursing, 42*(4), 351–359.

Requarth, J. (2011). Image-guided palliative care procedures. *Surgical Clinics of North America, 91*(2), 367–402.

Rollins, H., Nathwani, N., & Morridson, D. (2013). Optimizing wound care in a child with an infected gastrostomy exit site. *British Journal of Nursing, 22*, 1275–1279.

Roveron, G., & Antonini, M. (2018). Clinical practice guidelines for nursing management of percutaneous endoscopic gastrostomy and jejunostomy (PEG/PEJ) in adult patients. *Journal of Wound, Ostomy, and Continence Nursing, 45*(4), 326–334.

Saavedra, H., Loske, J. D., Shanley, L., et al. (2009). Gastrostomy tube related complaints in the pediatric emergency department identifying opportunities for improvement. *Pediatric Emergency Care, 25*(11), 728–732.

Schweitzer, et al., 2014. Evaluation of a discharge education protocol for pediatric patients with gastrostomy tubes. *Journal of Pediatric Health Care, 28*(5), 420–428.

Seladi-Shulman, J. (2018). Caring for your nephrostomy tube. https://www.healthline.com/health/nephrostomy-tube-care

Singh, C.D. (2016). Use of a moisture wicking fabric for prevention of skin damage around drains and parenteral access lines. *Journal of Wound, Ostomy and Continence Nursing, 43*(5), 551–553.

Warriner, L., & Spruce, P. (2014). Managing over granulation tissue around gastrostomy sites. *British Journal of Nursing, 21*(5), S20–S25.

BOX 37-3 SIGNS AND SYMPTOMS OF BILIARY TUBE BLOCKAGE

Leakage at exit site
Decrease in bile drainage output
Inability to flush the tube
Fever, chills, nausea, and increased jaundice

(Source: Memorial Sloan Kettering Cancer Center [MSKCC]. (2017). About your biliary drainage catheter. Retrieved from https://www.mskcc.org/cancer-care/patient-education/about-your-biliary-drainage-catheter)

Dressing changes should be done weekly and whenever wet or soiled. For sensitive skin, consider the use of adhesive remover or releaser to loosen the dressing. If skin irritation develops, an alcohol-free liquid skin barrier may be used to protect the area. Flushing the tube is done twice daily with 10 mL or other prescribed amount of sterile saline. Never force the saline into the tube. If there is inability to instill, pain occurs, or leakage at the exit site occurs, the health care provider must be notified (MSKCC, 2017).

KEY POINT

Patient and caregiver education must include routine care of the catheter, assessment of catheter integrity, signs of infection, and signs and symptoms of a blockage.

 ## CONCLUSIONS

The provision of adequate nutrition support in the hospital setting is the standard of care. The use of the gastrointestinal tract for feeding that is provided through enteral access is preferred to the use of parenteral nutrition whenever possible (Boullata et al., 2017). It carries benefits physiologically for the patient as well as decreases the significant risks associated with parenteral nutrition. Patients with higher acuity are candidates for enteral access through endoscopic, radiologic, and surgical techniques available in various care settings. The WOC nurse must know what procedures may be done in his or her practice setting to be prepared for managing the care of these patients and those with other types of percutaneous tubes. Caregiver support and patient education are essential for those patients leaving the hospital with percutaneous tubes, and the WOC nurse can play an important role in preparing both patients and caregivers for discharge (see Care of Feeding Tubes, Appendix I).

1. The nurse is assessing a patient who has a nasogastric tube (NGT) in place following gastric surgery. What complication should the patient be monitored for?
   A. Fluid and electrolyte imbalance
   B. Aspiration pneumonia
   C. Constipation
   D. Gastroesophageal reflux

2. A patient is scheduled for placement of a feeding tube in interventional radiology. What potential complication is avoided by using this method instead of the endoscopic method?
   A. Bleeding
   B. Soft tissue infection
   C. Upper tract trauma
   D. Liver trauma

3. What intervention is most likely to prevent hypergranulation tissue from forming around a gastrostomy tube?
   A. Cleaning the area around the tube with hydrogen peroxide
   B. Stabilizing the tube to reduce movement of the tube in the tract
   C. The use of several gauze pads to absorb drainage
   D. Maintenance of the external bumper at least one inch above the skin

4. The nurse is teaching a patient routine tube care for a newly placed percutaneous endoscopic gastrostomy (PEG) tube. What statement follows recommended guidelines for this care?
   A. Following placement of the tube, the external bolster will be left in place for 1 week.
   B. A water-resistant dressing should be placed over the tube and insertion site and left in place for 48 hours.
   C. The site of the tube should be washed with mild soap and water, rinsed well with water, and dried daily.
   D. One gauze drain sponge may be placed under the bumper of a tube that is sutured in place to absorb any drainage from the site.

5. The nurse is providing care for a patient with a gastrostomy tube. What is a recommended intervention when using the tube to administer medication?
   A. Flush the tube with 15 mL water before and after each medication.
   B. Flush the tube with 60 mL water before giving medication.
   C. Cut tablets in half before administering through the tube.
   D. Do not give any medications that do not come in liquid form.

6. What would be the first intervention when a feeding tube becomes clogged?
   A. Insert a brush into the tube to remove any mechanical obstruction.
   B. Aspirate fluid from the tube and instill 20 mL of cranberry juice into the tube.
   C. Use pancreatic enzymes and sodium bicarbonate tablets crushed and mixed in water.
   D. Use a 60-mL catheter-tipped syringe filled with lukewarm water and pull back and forth on the plunger to dislodge the obstruction.

7. If a G tube leaks with feedings, what is the most common skin complication that is likely to occur?
   A. Irritant dermatitis
   B. Candidiasis
   C. Cellulitis
   D. Allergic reactions

8. When using a low profile G tube, it is important to measure the tract to select the correct g tube length. Ongoing monitoring of the size is especially important in which population of patients?
   A. Geriatric
   B. Terminally ill
   C. Pediatric
   D. Young adults

9. A patient has a percutaneous nephrostomy tube. Which condition describes the most likely reason it was placed?
   A. It is an alternative to dialysis for urinary drainage.
   B. The patient has experienced frequent urinary tract infections.
   C. The patient has urinary incontinence.
   D. Urine cannot pass into the bladder because of an ureteral obstruction.

10. A patient has a percutaneous biliary tube for malignant obstruction of the bile duct. The caregiver reports a 24-hour history of leakage of bile fluid around the tube that has saturated several 4 × 4 gauze pads. There is very little fluid in the drainage bag. What is the first action the nurse should take to resolve this problem?
    A. Protect the skin from the bile drainage with a skin barrier cream.
    B. Flush the tube to see if there is blockage causing the fluid to leak around the tube.
    C. Call the health care provider to arrange for removal of the tube.
    D. Instruct the caregiver to change the dressings more frequently to avoid contact of the fluid with the skin.

ANSWERS AND RATIONALES

1. B. Rationale: Dislodgement of the tube could result in fluid going into the lungs causing aspiration pneumonia.

2. C. Rationale: There is no need for the use of an endoscope to ascertain placement with the radiologic procedure, so the upper GI tract is not at risk for trauma.

3. B. Rationale: A tube that is not stabilized can move in the tract and can damage the tissue around the tube; thus, stabilizing the tube may prevent hypertrophic granulation tissue formation.

4. C. Rationale: While evidence for care is lacking, the generally accepted standard for tube site care is daily cleansing with mild soap and water.

5. A. Rationale: 15 mL of water is adequate to ensure patency of the tube and clear the tube of residual medication after completing administration.

6. D. Rationale: Using a push-pull technique with warm water in a catheter tip syringe is the first method used to dislodge a tube blockage.

7. A. Rationale: If leakage occurs around the tube, the fluid may contain both the formula mixed with the gastric fluid. Gastric fluid and formula will cause skin breakdown, irritant dermatitis.

8. C. Rationale: The tube length is critical for a good fit of the low profile tube and because pediatric patients frequently have low profile tubes, and as they grow, the length between the skin and the stomach will change necessitating a new tube length.

9. D. Rationale: Nephrostomy tubes are used to prevent hydronephrosis resulting from the inability of the kidney to drain into the bladder due to ureteral obstruction.

10. B. Rationale: Obstruction of the tube is the most likely cause of this problem. Skin protection is very important but, first, the tube function needs to be assessed. The health care provider will need to be notified if the tube is unable to be flushed, but exchange, not removal of the tube, would be the likely result.

Venous, Arterial, and Neuropathic Lower-Extremity Wounds: Clinical Resource Guide

The Wound, Ostomy and Continence Nurses Society™ suggests the following format for bibliographic citations:

Wound, Ostomy and Continence Nurses Society. (2019). *Venous, arterial, and neuropathic lower-extremity wounds: Clinical resource guide.* Mt. Laurel, NJ: Author.

CONTRIBUTORS

Originated By:

Wound Committee, WOCN Society

Original Publication Date: November 2009

Updated/Revised:

April 2013: Wound Committee, WOCN Society

September 2017: Phyllis A. Bonham, PhD, MSN, RN, CWOCN, DPNAP, FAAN Clinical Editor, WOCN Society

Chair, Wound Guidelines Task Force, WOCN Society

November 2019: Phyllis A. Bonham, PhD, MSN, RN, CWOCN, DPNAP, FAAN Chair, Wound Guidelines Task Force, WOCN Society

INTRODUCTION

This Clinical Resource Guide (CRG) updates the previous document, *Venous, Arterial, and Neuropathic Lower-Extremity Wounds: Clinical Resource Guide* (WOCN®, 2017). The guide is a synopsis of content derived from the WOCN Society's Clinical Practice Guideline Series for managing lower-extremity wounds due to venous, arterial, or neuropathic disease. The relevant section of the CRG is updated along with each publication of a new/updated Clinical Practice Guideline.

Refer to the complete version of each of the WOCN Society's Clinical Practice Guidelines for more detailed, evidence-based information about the management of wounds in patients with lower-extremity venous, arterial, or neuropathic disease (WOCN, 2012, 2014, 2019): The guidelines are available in print or as an electronic mobile app from the WOCN Society's Bookstore (www.wocn.org/bookstore):

- *Guideline for Management of Wounds in Patients with Lower-Extremity Neuropathic Disease* (2012).
- *Guideline for Management of Wounds in Patients with Lower-Extremity Arterial Disease* (2014).
- *Guideline for Management of Wounds in Patients with Lower-Extremity Venous Disease* (2019).

PURPOSE

This guide provides an overview of common assessment findings and key characteristics of the three most common types of lower-extremity wounds (i.e., venous, arterial, neuropathic). In addition, it includes a summary of the following information: measures to improve venous return and tissue perfusion; measures to prevent trauma; goals, considerations, and options for topical therapy; adjunctive therapies; and indications for referral to other health care providers for additional evaluation and treatment.

LOWER-EXTREMITY VENOUS DISEASE (LEVD) WOUNDS (WOCN, 2019)	LOWER-EXTREMITY ARTERIAL DISEASE (LEAD) WOUNDS (WOCN, 2014)	LOWER-EXTREMITY NEUROPATHIC DISEASE (LEND) WOUNDS (WOCN, 2012)
Assessment: History/Risk Factors		
• Older age (>50 years of age). • High BMI; obesity. • Female sex; pregnancies (multiple or close together). • Simultaneous insufficiency of two out of three venous systems; venous reflux/obstruction. • Previous leg surgery; leg fractures. • Impaired calf muscle pump. • Restricted range of motion of the ankle; greater dorsiflexion of the ankle. • Varicose veins. • Family history of venous disease. • Previous venous leg ulcer (VLU). • Systemic inflammation. • Venous thromboembolism (VTE): pulmonary embolus (PE), deep vein thrombosis (DVT), thrombophlebitis, postthrombotic syndrome. • Injection drug use. • Sedentary lifestyle or occupation; reduced mobility; prolonged sitting or standing. • Triggers for VLUs: Cellulitis; trauma (penetrating injury, burns); contact allergic dermatitis; rapid onset of leg edema; dry skin/itching; insect bites.	• Advanced age. • Tobacco use. • Diabetes. • Hyperlipidemia. • Hypertension. • Elevated homocysteine. • Chronic renal insufficiency. • Family history of cardiovascular disease. • Ethnicity. • Persistent *Chlamydia pneumoniae* infection. • Periodontal disease.	• Advanced age; heredity. • Alcoholism. • Diabetes mellitus (diabetes) longer than 10 years; poor diabetes control; impaired glucose tolerance. • Hansen disease (leprosy); Charcot-Marie-Tooth (Charcot) disease. • Tobacco use. • Human immunodeficiency virus/acquired immunodeficiency syndrome and related drug therapies. • Hypertension. • Obesity. • Raynaud disease; scleroderma. • Hyperthyroidism; hypothyroidism. • Chronic obstructive pulmonary disease. • Spinal cord injury; neuromuscular diseases. • Abdominal, pelvic, and orthopedic procedures. • Paraneoplastic disorders. • Acromegaly/height. • Exposure to heavy metals (e.g., lead, mercury, arsenic). • Malabsorption syndrome due to bariatric surgery; celiac disease; vitamin deficiency (B_{12}, folate, niacin, thiamine); pernicious anemia. • Loss of protective sensation; rigid foot deformities; gait abnormalities; history of previous ulcer/amputation.
Assessment: Comorbid Conditions		
• Cardiovascular disease. • Hypertension. • Lymphedema. • Rheumatoid arthritis. • Lower-extremity arterial disease (LEAD). • Diabetes.	• Cardiovascular disease; cerebrovascular disease; vascular procedures or surgeries. • Sickle cell anemia. • Obesity; metabolic syndrome. • Arthritis. • Spinal cord injury. • Migraine. • Atrial fibrillation. • Human immunodeficiency virus. • Low testosterone.	• Lower-extremity arterial disease (LEAD). • Kidney disease.
Assessment: Wound Location		

The most typical location is superior to the medial malleolus, but wounds can be anywhere on the lower leg including back of the leg/posterior calf.	Areas exposed to pressure, repetitive trauma, or rubbing from footwear are the most common locations:
	• Lateral malleolus.
	• Mid-tibial area (shin).
	• Phalangeal heads, toe tips, or web spaces.
	• Heels.
		• Plantar foot surface is the most typical location.
		• Other common locations include
		  o Pressure points/sites of painless trauma/repetitive stress, over bony prominences (e.g., heels).
		  o Metatarsal head (e.g., first metatarsal head and interphalangeal joint of great toe).
		  o Dorsal and distal aspects of toes, interdigital areas, interphalangeal joints.
		  o Midfoot or forefoot: Collapse of midfoot structures with "rocker-bottom foot" suggests Charcot fracture.

LOWER-EXTREMITY VENOUS DISEASE (LEVD) WOUNDS (WOCN, 2019)	LOWER-EXTREMITY ARTERIAL DISEASE (LEAD) WOUNDS (WOCN, 2014)	LOWER-EXTREMITY NEUROPATHIC DISEASE (LEND) WOUNDS (WOCN, 2012)
Assessment: Wound Characteristics		
• Base: Ruddy red; granulation tissue and/or yellow adherent fibrin or loose slough may be present. • Size: Variable; can be large. • Depth: Usually shallow. • Edges: Irregular; epibole (rolled edges) may be present; undermining or tunneling are uncommon. • Exudate: Moderate to heavy; character of exudate varies. • Infection: Not common.	• Base: Pale; granulation rarely present; necrosis common; eschar may be present. • Size: Variable; often small. • Depth: May be deep. • Edges: Rolled; smooth; punched-out appearance; undermining may be present. • Exudate: Minimal. • Infection: Frequent (signs may be subtle). • Pain: Common. • Nonhealing; wound often precipitated by minor trauma.	• Base: Pale or pink; necrosis/eschar may be present. • Size: Variable. • Depth: Varies from shallow to exposed bone/tendon. • Edges: Well defined; smooth; undermining may be present. • Shape: Usually round or oblong. • Exudate: Usually small to moderate; foul odor and purulence indicate infection.
Assessment: Surrounding Skin		
• Edema: Pitting or nonpitting; worsens with prolonged standing or sitting with legs dependent. • Scarring from previous wounds. • Ankle flare; varicose veins. • Hemosiderosis (i.e., brown staining); hyperpigmentation • Lipodermatosclerosis. • Atrophie blanche (smooth white plaques). • Maceration; crusting; scaling; itching. • Temperature: Normally warm to touch. • Localized elevation of skin temperature (1.2°C higher), measured with a noncontact infrared thermometer, may indicate inflammation.	• Pallor on elevation. • Dependent rubor. • Shiny, taut, thin, dry, and fragile. • Hair loss over lower extremity. • Atrophy of skin, subcutaneous tissue, and muscle. • Edema: Atypical of arterial disease; localized edema may indicate infection. • Temperature: Skin feels cool to touch.	• Normal skin color. • Anhidrosis; xerosis; fissures; maceration; tinea pedis. • Callus over bony prominences (might cover a wound) and periwound; hemorrhage into a callus indicates ulceration underneath. • Musculoskeletal/structural foot deformities. • Erythema and induration may indicate infection/cellulitis. • Edema: Unilateral edema with increased erythema, warmth, and a bounding pulse may indicate Charcot fracture. • Temperature: Skin warm to touch; localized elevation of skin temperature >2°C indicates inflammation. • Diabetic skin markers: Dermopathy, necrobiosis lipoidica, acanthosis nigricans, bullosis diabeticorum.
Assessment: Nails		
N/A	• Dystrophic.	• Dystrophic; hypertrophy. • Onychomycosis; paronychia.
Assessment: Complications		
• Venous eczema/dermatitis (e.g., erythema, itching, vesicles, weeping, scaling, crusting, afebrile). • Infection/Cellulitis (e.g., pain, erythema, swelling, induration, bullae, desquamation, fever, leukocytosis); tinea pedis. • Variceal bleeding. • VTE, DVT. • Mixed venous and arterial disease.	• Infection/Cellulitis (e.g., pain, edema, periwound fluctuance; or only a faint halo of erythema around the wound). • Osteomyelitis (e.g., probe to bone). • Gangrene (wet or dry).	• Infection/Cellulitis. • Arterial ischemia. • Osteomyelitis. • Charcot fracture (e.g., swelling, pain, erythema, localized temperature elevation of 3°C–7°C compared to an unaffected area). • Gangrene.

(Continued)

LOWER-EXTREMITY VENOUS DISEASE (LEVD) WOUNDS (WOCN, 2019)	LOWER-EXTREMITY ARTERIAL DISEASE (LEAD) WOUNDS (WOCN, 2014)	LOWER-EXTREMITY NEUROPATHIC DISEASE (LEND) WOUNDS (WOCN, 2012)

Assessment Perfusion/Sensation of the Lower Extremity: Pain

• Leg pain may be variable (e.g., severe, throbbing).
  o Pain may be accompanied by complaints of leg heaviness, tightening, or aching.
  o Leg pain worsens with dependency.
  o Elevation relieves pain.
• Differentiate venous claudication from arterial, ischemic claudication:
  o Venous claudication: Exercise-related leg pain due to venous outflow obstruction; occurs in the absence of arterial disease; is relieved by leg elevation.
  o Arterial, ischemic claudication/pain: Reproducible cramping, aching, fatigue, weakness, and/or frank pain in the calf, thigh, or buttock that occurs after walking/exercise, and is typically relieved with 10 minutes' rest; pain is increased by leg elevation and alleviated by dependency of the limb.
	• Intermittent claudication is a classical sign and indicates that 50% of the vessel is occluded (i.e., cramping, aching, fatigue, weakness, and/or pain in the calf, thigh, or buttock that occurs after walking/exercise and typically is relieved with 10 minutes' rest).
	• Resting, positional, or nocturnal pain may be present; resting pain indicates that 90% of the vessel is occluded.
	• Elevation exacerbates pain.
	• Dependency relieves pain.
	• Neuropathy and paresthesia may occur from ischemic nerve dysfunction.
	• Acute limb ischemia: A sudden onset of the 6 Ps (i.e., pain, pulselessness, pallor, paresthesia, paralysis, and polar [coldness]) indicates an acute embolism; warrants an immediate referral to a vascular surgeon.
	• Critical limb ischemia (CLI): Chronic rest pain; rest pain of the forefoot/toes. Ischemic nonhealing wounds or gangrene are limb threatening with a high mortality rate and warrant referral to a vascular surgeon.
		• Pain may be superficial, deep, aching, stabbing, dull, sharp, burning, or cool.
		• Decreased or altered sensitivity to touch occurs.
		• Altered sensation not described as pain (e.g., numbness, warmth, prickling, tingling, shooting, pins and needles; "stocking-glove pattern") may be present.
		• Pain may be worse at night.
		• Allodynia (i.e., intolerance to normally painless stimuli such as bedsheets touching feet/legs) may occur.

Assessment Perfusion/Sensation of the Lower Extremity: Peripheral Pulses

• Pulses are present and palpable.	• Pulses are absent or diminished (i.e., dorsalis pedis, posterior tibial). • Femoral or popliteal bruits may be heard.	• Pulses are present and palpable. • If coexisting LEAD is present: Pulses are absent or diminished (i.e., dorsalis pedis, posterior tibial); and femoral or popliteal bruits may be heard.

Assessment Perfusion/Sensation of the Lower Extremity: Common Noninvasive Vascular Tests

• Capillary refill: Delayed capillary refill may be present (>3 seconds).
• Venous refill time may be prolonged (>20 seconds).
• Ankle–brachial index (ABI): Commonly within normal limits (1.0–1.3).
• Duplex scanning with ultrasound: Most reliable noninvasive test to diagnose anatomical and hemodynamic abnormalities and detect venous reflux.
	• Capillary refill: Abnormal (>3 seconds).
	• Venous refill time: Prolonged (>20 seconds).
	• ABI values/interpretation:
	  o Noncompressible arteries: Unable to obliterate the pulse signal at cuff pressure >250 mm Hg.
	  o Elevated: >1.30.
	  o Normal: ≥1.00.
	  o LEAD: ≤0.90.
	  o Borderline perfusion: ≤ 0.60–0.80.
	  o Severe ischemia: ≤ 0.50.
	  o Critical ischemia: ≤ 0.40.
	• Transcutaneous oxygen ($TcPO_2$): <40 mm Hg is hypoxic; <30 mm Hg is CLI.
	• Toe–brachial index (TBI): <0.64 indicates LEAD.
	• Toe pressure (TP): <30 mm Hg (<50 mm Hg if diabetes present) indicates CLI.
	• Assess light pressure sensation using a 5.07/10 g Semmes-Weinstein monofilament.
		• Capillary and venous refill times: Normal.
		• ABI: LEAD, which often coexists with neuropathic disease and diabetes, should be ruled out.
		• The ABI can be elevated >1.30 or arteries can be noncompressible (i.e., unable to obliterate the pulse signal at cuff pressure >250 mm Hg), which indicates calcified ankle arteries. In such cases, a TP or TBI is indicated.
		  o TBI: <0.64 indicates LEAD.
		  o TP: <50 mm Hg (if diabetes is present) indicates CLI and failure to heal.
		• $TcPO_2$: <40 mm Hg is hypoxic; <30 mm Hg is CLI.

LOWER-EXTREMITY VENOUS DISEASE (LEVD) WOUNDS (WOCN, 2019)	LOWER-EXTREMITY ARTERIAL DISEASE (LEAD) WOUNDS (WOCN, 2014)	LOWER-EXTREMITY NEUROPATHIC DISEASE (LEND) WOUNDS (WOCN, 2012)

Assessment Perfusion/Sensation of the Lower Extremity: Screen for Loss of Protective Sensation

• Assess light pressure sensation using a 5.07/10 g Semmes-Weinstein monofilament. • Assess vibratory sensation using a 128-Hz tuning fork. • Check deep tendon reflexes at the ankle and knee with a reflex/percussion hammer. • Inability to feel the monofilament, diminished vibratory perception, and diminished reflexes indicate a loss of protective sensation and an increased risk of wounds.	• Assess vibratory sensation using a 128-Hz tuning fork. • Check deep tendon reflexes at the ankle and knee with a reflex/percussion hammer. • Inability to feel the monofilament, diminished vibratory perception, and diminished reflexes indicate a loss of protective sensation and an increased risk of wounds.	• Assess light pressure sensation using a 5.07/10 g Semmes-Weinstein monofilament. • Assess vibratory sensation using a 128-Hz tuning fork. • Check deep tendon reflexes at the ankle and knee with a reflex/percussion hammer. • Inability to feel the monofilament, diminished vibratory perception, and diminished reflexes indicate a loss of protective sensation and an increased risk of wounds.

Measures to Improve Venous Return	**Measures to Improve Tissue Perfusion**	

• Use compression therapy: 30–40 mm Hg compression at the ankle if ABI is equal to/ or >0.80:
  o Multicomponent compression systems are more effective than single-component systems.
  o Multicomponent systems with an elastic bandage are more effective than those with only inelastic components.
  o Use highest level of compression that patients can tolerate and with which they can comply.
  o Use lifelong compression to reduce/ prevent VLUs and VLU recurrence.
  o Consider intermittent pneumatic compression for patients who are immobile, need higher levels of compression than can be provided by wraps or stockings, or are intolerant of stockings or bandaging systems.
  o Do not rely on antiembolism stockings or hose that provide low pressure (≤20 mm Hg) and are not designed for therapeutic compression to prevent or treat LEVD or VLUs.
• Elevate legs above heart level: 30 minutes, 4 times per day; increase exercise (e.g., walking, calf muscle exercise, toe lifts, ankle flexion).
• Avoid constricting garments, crossing legs, prolonged standing, and high-heeled shoes.
• Stop tobacco use.
• Manage weight; healthy nutrition.
• Consider medications to promote VLU healing: pentoxifylline, simvastatin, sulodexide, or doxycycline.
• Consider invasive and noninvasive surgical procedures to improve VLU healing and reduce VLU recurrence (i.e., surgery; subendoscopic perforator surgery; skin grafts; biological dressings; human skin equivalents; hair follicle grafts; thermal or nonthermal ablation of varicose veins).
	• Revascularize if possible.
	• Change lifestyle: Stop tobacco use; avoid secondhand smoke, restrictive garments, and cold temperatures.
	• Maintain proper hydration/nutrition.
	• Maintain legs in a neutral or dependent position.
	• Increase physical activity: Walking; supervised exercise 30–45 minutes, 3 times per week.
	• Use medications to control hypertension, hyperlipidemia, homocysteine levels, and diabetes; antiplatelets to improve blood cell movement through narrowed vessels.
	• Control or reduce weight if obese.
		• Revascularize if ischemic.
		• Stop tobacco use.
		• Maintain tight glucose/glycemic control; control hypertension.
		• Engage in exercise that is adapted to prevent injury.
		• Consider medications, as indicated.

(Continued)

LOWER-EXTREMITY VENOUS DISEASE (LEVD) WOUNDS (WOCN, 2019)	LOWER-EXTREMITY ARTERIAL DISEASE (LEAD) WOUNDS (WOCN, 2014)	LOWER-EXTREMITY NEUROPATHIC DISEASE (LEND) WOUNDS (WOCN, 2012)
Measures to Prevent Trauma		

• Screen patients for LEAD by Doppler-derived ABI prior to application of compression stockings/bandages/wraps.
• Mixed venous/arterial disease:
  o Use reduced compression (23–30 mm Hg) for patients with LEVD, wounds, and edema if ABI is <0.80 and equal to/or >0.50.
  o Do not apply compression if ABI is <0.50, ankle pressure is <70 mm Hg, or TP is <50 mm Hg.
	• Use proper footwear; wear socks/stockings with shoes; obtain professional nail/callus care.
	• Use pressure redistribution/off-loading products/devices for heels, toes, and bony prominences, especially if bedbound or chairbound.
	• Avoid chemical, thermal, and mechanical injury (e.g., no bare feet even in the house; no hot soaks or heating pads; no medicated corn pads).
	• Self-inspect the lower extremities daily; promptly report injuries to the health care provider.
	• Use reduced compression (23–30 mm Hg) for mixed venous/arterial disease if the ABI is <0.80.
	• Do not apply compression if ABI is <0.50, ankle pressure is <70 mm Hg, or TP is <50 mm Hg.
		• Reduce shear stress and offload the at-risk neuropathic foot, and/or foot with wounds (e.g., bed rest, total contact casts, walking splints, orthopedic shoes); use assistive devices for support, balance, and additional offloading.
		• Use proper footwear; obtain routine professional nail/callus care.
		• Use pressure redistribution/offloading products/devices for heels, toes, and bony prominences, especially if in bed or chairbound.
		• Avoid chemical, thermal, and mechanical injury (e.g., no bare feet even in the house; no hot soaks or heating pads; no medicated corn pads; wear socks/stockings with shoes).
		• Self-inspect the lower extremities on a daily basis.

Topical Therapy: Goals		
• Reduce and control edema. • Promote wound healing. • Maintain moist wound surface. • Attain/maintain intact skin: Protect the periwound skin from drainage; absorb/manage exudate. • Prevent trauma/injury. • Prevent, promptly identify, and manage complications (e.g., venous eczema/dermatitis, infection/cellulitis, variceal bleeding, etc.). • Reduce pain. • Improve functional status and quality of life. • Prevent VLU recurrence.	• Prevent trauma/injury. • Prevent, promptly identify, and manage complications (e.g., infection/cellulitis, etc.). • Promote wound healing. • Minimize pain. • Preserve limb.	• Prevent trauma/injury. • Prevent, promptly identify, and manage complications (e.g., infection/cellulitis, osteomyelitis, etc.). • Promote wound healing. • Keep the periwound dry while maintaining a moist wound bed. • Minimize pain. • Preserve limb.
Topical Therapy: Considerations/Options		

• Treat infection: Use culture-guided antibiotic/antimicrobial therapy.
  o Consider topical antimicrobial/antiseptics for localized, superficial infection (i.e., silver-based dressings; cadexomer iodine).
  o Deep tissue infection/cellulitis warrants culture-guided systemic treatment.
• Remove devitalized tissue with an appropriate method of debridement.
• Consider debridement if biofilm is suspected.
• Cleanse wound and skin with noncytotoxic cleansers.
• Use absorptive dressings to control exudate.
• Avoid known skin irritants and allergens, tapes, and adhesives in patients with venous eczema/dermatitis.
	• Avoid occlusive dressings: Use dressings that permit easy, frequent visualization of the wound.
	• Aggressively treat infection.
	• Dry, noninfected wounds with stable, fixed eschar, necrosis; or a stable blister:
	  o Maintain, keep dry, protect, no debridement.
	  o Assess perfusion status and signs of infection.
	• Infected, necrotic wounds:
	  o Refer for revascularization/surgical removal of necrotic tissue and antibiotic therapy.
	  o Do not rely on topical antibiotics as the sole therapy to treat infected, ischemic wounds.
		• Use dressings that maintain a moist surface, absorb exudate, and allow easy visualization.
		• Use occlusive dressings cautiously.
		• Aggressively treat infection/cellulitis, including fungal infection.
		• Do not rely on topical antimicrobials alone to treat cellulitis, but they could be used in conjunction with systemic antimicrobials; use of antimicrobials should be culture guided.
		• Debride focal callus to reduce pressure.
		• Debride avascular/necrotic tissue in nonischemic wounds.

LOWER-EXTREMITY VENOUS DISEASE (LEVD) WOUNDS (WOCN, 2019)	LOWER-EXTREMITY ARTERIAL DISEASE (LEAD) WOUNDS (WOCN, 2014)	LOWER-EXTREMITY NEUROPATHIC DISEASE (LEND) WOUNDS (WOCN, 2012)

• Patch test individuals with known sensitivities and delayed healing prior to use of new products.
• Consider use of barrier products to protect the periwound skin from excessive drainage and maceration.
• Identify and treat venous eczema/dermatitis (i.e., topical steroid 1–2 weeks).
• Use emollients to manage dry, scaly skin.
• Consider topical anesthetics for painful wound care/debridement (i.e., lidocaine; lidocaine and prilocaine mixture).
• Consider use of analgesic-containing dressings to reduce wound pain such as ibuprofen-releasing dressings.
	• Promptly institute culture-guided systemic antibiotics for patients with CLI and evidence of limb infection or cellulitis, and/or infected wounds.
	• Open/draining wounds with necrotic tissue:
	  o Consider a closely monitored trial of autolytic or enzymatic debridement.
	• Open/draining wounds with exposed bones or tendons:
	  o Consider a carefully monitored trial of moist, nonocclusive, absorbent, dressings.
	• Open/draining, nonnecrotic wounds:
	  o Consider moist wound healing with nonocclusive, absorbent dressings.	

Adjunctive Therapy

• Electrical therapy. • Negative pressure wound therapy. • Ultrasound (high-frequency ultrasound; noncontact low-frequency ultrasound).	• Arterial flow augmentation (i.e., intermittent pneumatic compression). • Electrotherapy. • Low-frequency ultrasound. • Hyperbaric oxygen therapy. • Spinal cord stimulation, lumbar sympathectomy, or peridural anesthesia for intractable pain in patients not suitable for surgery. • Bone marrow–derived, mononuclear cell therapy for pain relief/limb salvage in patients not suitable for surgery. • Immune modulation therapy for patients with claudication or CLI.	• Hyperbaric oxygen therapy. • Skin substitutes. • Negative pressure wound therapy. • Growth factor therapy. • Surgery to correct structural deformities. • Surgical debridement/implantation of antibiotic beads, spacers, or gels. • Pain management specialists.

Indications for Referral to Other Health Care Providers for Additional Evaluation and Treatment

• Dermatology referral for unresponsive eczema/dermatitis after 1–2 weeks of treatment with a topical steroid.
• Vascular/surgical referral for:
  o Infection/Cellulitis.
  o Nonhealing wound after 4 weeks of appropriate therapy.
  o VTE, DVT.
  o Variceal bleeding.
  o Intractable pain.
  o Atypical appearance or location of wound.
	• Vascular/surgical referral:
	  o Infected, ischemic wounds: Clinical signs of infection/cellulitis or suspected osteomyelitis.
	  o Atypical appearance or location of wound.
	  o Intractable pain.
	  o Wounds and/or edema in mixed venous/arterial disease that fail to respond to compression therapy or worsens.
	  o Absence of both dorsalis pedis and posterior tibial pulses.
	  o ABI <0.90 plus one or more of the following: Wound fails to improve with 2–4 weeks of appropriate therapy; severe ischemic pain; and/or intermittent claudication.
	  o ABI <0.50.
	  o ABI >1.30 or noncompressible arteries.
	• Urgent vascular/surgical referral for symptoms of acute limb ischemia; CLI (ABI <0.40; ankle pressure <50 mm Hg; TP <30 mm Hg or <50 mm Hg if diabetes present; $TcPO_2$ <30 mm Hg); and/or gangrene.
		• Refer patients who use tobacco and have a loss of protective sensation to foot care specialists and for tobacco cessation education/counseling.
		• Refer patients with gait abnormalities to a qualified pedorthic professional for shoe or device customization.
		• Vascular/surgical referral:
		  o Infection/Cellulitis or suspected osteomyelitis (i.e., probe to the bone).
		  o Atypical appearance or location of wound.
		  o Symptoms/new onset of Charcot fracture.
		  o Musculoskeletal/structural foot deformities.
		  o ABI <0.90 and no response to 2–4 weeks of conservative wound care.
		  o ABI <0.50.
		  o ABI >1.30 or noncompressible arteries.
		• Urgent vascular/surgical referral for symptoms of acute limb ischemia, CLI, and/or gangrene.

REFERENCES

Wound, Ostomy and Continence Nurses Society. (2012). *Guideline for management of wounds in patients with lower-extremity neuropathic disease*. WOCN Clinical Practice Guideline Series 3. Mt. Laurel, NJ: Author.

Wound, Ostomy and Continence Nurses Society. (2014). *Guideline for management of wounds in patients with lower-extremity arterial disease*. WOCN Clinical Practice Guideline Series 1. Mt. Laurel, NJ: Author.

Wound, Ostomy and Continence Nurses Society. (2017). *Venous, arterial, and neuropathic lower-extremity wounds: Clinical resource guide*. Mt. Laurel, NJ: Author.

Wound, Ostomy and Continence Nurses Society. (2019). *Guideline for management of wounds in patients with lower-extremity venous disease*. WOCN Clinical Practice Guideline Series 4. Mt. Laurel, NJ: Author.

Procedure for Measuring and Calculating the ABI

ACTION	PROCEDURE
Prepare equipment and supplies	1. Gather equipment and supplies for the ABI. • Portable continuous wave Doppler with 8–10 MHz probe (5 MHz if a large amount of edema is present at the ankle). • Aneroid sphygmomanometer and pressure cuff. • Ultrasound transmission gel. • Alcohol pads to clean the Doppler and gauze, tissue, or pads to remove the transmission gel from the patient's skin. • Towels, sheets, or blankets to cover the trunk and extremities. • Paper and pen for recording test results; calculator. • Inspect the equipment and check the batteries if a battery-operated Doppler is used, and replace equipment that is damaged or not calibrated. 2. Pressure cuffs for arms and ankles should be long enough to fully encircle the limb. The width of the cuff's bladder should be 40% of the limb's circumference and the length sufficient to cover 80% of the limb's circumference. • Typically, 12-cm-wide cuffs are used for arms and 10-cm-wide cuffs at the ankles. • Extra-large adult cuffs might be needed (14 cm).
Prepare patient and environment	1. Inquire about recent use of tobacco, caffeine, or alcohol; recent heavy activity, and presence of pain. Note: When possible, advise the patient to avoid stimulants or heavy exercise for an hour prior to the test. 2. Perform the ABI in a quiet, warm environment to prevent vasoconstriction of the arteries (21–23 ± 1°C). 3. The best ABI results are obtained when the patient is relaxed, is comfortable, and has an empty bladder. 4. Explain the procedure to the patient. 5. Remove shoes, socks, and tight clothing to permit placement of the pressure cuff and access to the pulse sites by the Doppler probe. 6. Place the patient in a flat, supine position. Place one small pillow behind the patient's head for comfort. 7. Cover the trunk and extremities to prevent cooling. 8. Ensure the patient is comfortable and have the patient rest for a minimum of 10 minutes prior to the test to allow pressures to normalize. 9. After the rest period, measure the arm and ankle pressures.
Measure brachial pressures with Doppler	1. The arm should be relaxed, supported, and at heart level. 2. Prior to placement of the cuff, apply a protective barrier (e.g., plastic wrap) on the extremity if any wounds or alterations in skin integrity are present. 3. Place the pressure cuff with the bottom of the cuff ~2–3 cm above the cubital fossa on the arm. 4. The cuff should be wrapped without wrinkles and placed securely to prevent slipping and movement during the test. 5. Palpate the brachial pulse to determine the location to obtain an audible pulse. 6. Apply transmission gel over the pulse site. 7. Place the tip of the Doppler probe at a 45-degree angle pointed towards the patient's head until an audible pulse signal is obtained. 8. Inflate the pressure cuff 20–30 mm Hg above the point where the pulse is no longer audible. 9. Deflate the pressure cuff at a rate of 2 3 mm Hg per second, noting the manometer reading at which the first pulse signal is heard and record that systolic value. 10. Cleanse/remove gel from the pulse site. 11. Repeat the procedure to measure the pressure on the other arm. 12. If a pressure needs to be repeated, wait 1 minute before reinflating the cuff. 13. Use the higher of the brachial pressures from the right or left arm to calculate the ABI for both legs.

(Continued)

ACTION	PROCEDURE
Measure ankle pressures with Doppler	1. Prior to placing the cuff, apply a protective barrier (e.g., plastic wrap) on the extremity if there are any wounds or alterations in skin integrity.
	2. Place the cuff on the patient's lower leg with the bottom of the cuff ~2–3 cm above the malleolus.
	3. The cuff should be wrapped without wrinkles and placed securely to prevent slipping and movement during the test.
	4. Measure both dorsalis pedis and posterior tibial pulses on each leg.
	5. Locate the pulses by palpation or with the Doppler probe.
	6. Apply transmission gel to the pulse site.
	7. Place the tip of the Doppler probe at a 45-degree angle pointed towards the patient's knee until an audible pulse signal is obtained.
	8. Inflate the pressure cuff 20–30 mm Hg above the point where the pulse is no longer audible.
	9. Deflate the cuff slowly at a rate of 2–3 mm Hg per second noting the manometer reading at which the first pulse signal is heard and record that systolic value.
	10. Cleanse/remove gel from the pulse site.
	11. Repeat the procedure to measure pressures on the other ankle.
	12. If a pressure needs to be repeated, wait 1 minute before reinflating the cuff.
	13. Use the higher of the ankle pressures of each leg to calculate the ABI for each leg.
Calculate the ABI	1. Divide the higher of the dorsalis pedis or posterior tibial systolic pressure for each ankle by the higher of the right or left brachial pressures to obtain the ABI for each leg.

$$ABI = \frac{\text{Higher of either the dorsalis pedis or posterior tibial pressures}}{\text{Higher of the brachial pressures}}$$

	2. Interpret and compare the ABI values from each leg.
	3. Refer the patient for further testing and evaluation if the ABI is <0.90, >1.30, or unmeasurable due to noncompressible vessels; and/or if the patient's clinical symptoms and ABI are inconsistent.
	4. Document findings, follow-up plans, and referrals.

Note. Table adapted with permission from: Wound, Ostomy and Continence Nurses Society. (2011). *Ankle brachial index: Quick reference guide for clinicians*. Mt. Laurel, NJ: Author.

INTERPRETATION OF ANKLE–BRACHIAL INDEX (ABI)

ABI	INTERPRETATION
Unable to obliterate the pulse signal at cuff pressure >250 mm Hg	Noncompressible arteries
>1.30	Elevated
≥1.00	Normal
≤0.90	LEAD
≤0.60–0.80	Borderline perfusion
≤0.50	Severe ischemia
≤0.40	Critical limb ischemia (limb threatened)

Note. Table reprinted with permission from: Wound, Ostomy and Continence Nurses Society. (2014). *Guideline for management of wounds in patients with lower-extremity arterial disease. WOCN clinical practice guideline series1* (p. 60). Mt. Laurel, NJ: Author.

Demonstration of Ankle-Brachial Index (ABI) Procedure. (Source: WOCN Society's Wound Treatment Associate (WTA) Program.): https://youtu.be/CPfVMa9s9c0

WOCN Society Position Statement: Role and Scope of Practice for Wound Care Providers

Originated By: Wound Treatment Associate Task Force
Date Completed: June 1, 2011
Revised: March–April, 2017
Date Approved by the WOCN Board of Directors: April 18, 2017

STATEMENT OF POSITION

The Wound, Ostomy, and Continence Nurses Society (WOCN) is a clinician-based, professional organization whose members treat individuals with wounds, ostomies, and incontinence and are committed to cost-effective, outcome-based health care (WOCN & Wound, Ostomy Continence Nursing Certification Board [WOCNCB], 2008). The WOCN Society is dedicated to assuring that appropriate care is available for individuals with wounds, ostomies, and incontinence, because patients deserve health care that assists them in maximizing their functional status (WOCN & WOCNCB, 2008).

The WOCN Society recognizes that to fulfill its mission of ensuring access to quality care to patients with acute and chronic wounds, there is a need to extend education to other providers.

The WOCN Society recognizes the following levels of wound care providers: wound, ostomy, and continence (WOC) specialty nurses (i.e., WOC registered nurses [baccalaureate prepared]; WOC graduate-level prepared registered nurses; WOC advanced practice registered nurses [WOCN, 2017]); and wound treatment associates. The WOCN Society endorses the appropriate utilization of each level of wound care provider.

PURPOSE (RATIONALE FOR POSITION)

The primary purpose of this position statement is to clarify the roles of the different levels of wound care providers: WOC registered nurses, WOC graduate-level prepared registered nurses, WOC advanced practice registered nurses, and wound treatment associates. Brief descriptions of the role and scope of practice for each level of provider are included in this document.

HISTORY/BACKGROUND

WOCN Society Mission, Philosophy, Goals, and Strategic Plans

Mission. "The WOCN Society is a professional nursing society, which supports its members by promoting educational, clinical, and research opportunities to advance the practice and guide the delivery of expert health care to individuals with wounds, ostomies, and incontinence" (WOCN, 2016, p. 6).

Philosophy. The philosophy of the WOCN Society includes the following beliefs:

The WOCN Society believes that nursing as a profession enhances health care services to a multifaceted society and includes prevention, health maintenance, therapeutic intervention, and rehabilitation. Wound, ostomy and continence (WOC) nursing is an area of specialty practice within the framework of nursing that strives to advance the health care and quality of life of all affected individuals.

The WOCN Society believes that continuing education and research provide the basis for current, comprehensive nursing practice for patients with wounds, ostomies, and incontinence. Learning may occur on a basic, advanced, or continuing educational level and combines the acquisition of theoretical knowledge and clinical expertise. The WOCN Society provides quality continuing education for its members and for other health care professionals to enhance and improve WOC nursing practice.

By a process of accreditation, the WOCN Society promotes high standards of education and requires a minimum baccalaureate degree as the entry level for Wound, Ostomy, and Continence Nursing Education Programs (WOCNEPs).

WOCNEPs may provide a trispecialty education program for wound, ostomy, and continence care and/or any of the specialty practice areas individually (WOCN, 2016, p. 2).

Goals. The WOCN Society has established the following goals:

1. Provide standards of practice for the WOC nurse to ensure quality patient care services.
2. Provide continuing nursing education for the professional development of the WOC specialty nurse.
3. Represent and promote WOC specialty nursing practice to the public, to allied health care professionals, the community, and governmental groups.
4. Accredit Wound, Ostomy, and Continence Nursing Education Programs (WOCNEPs).
5. Provide quality continuing education in the field of WOC specialty nursing to other health care providers.
6. Promote ongoing development of the profession and the Society through research and long-range planning activities (WOCN, 2016, p. 8).

Strategic plans. The WOCN Society's 2009 strategic plan included the following vision, goal, and objective for education (WOCN, 2009, 2011):

- **Vision.** The WOCN Society will be the premier provider of WOC nursing education.
- **Goal.** The WOCN Society will be the premier provider of education for all levels of nurses providing WOC services.
- **Objective.** Increase educational outreach/offerings for nurses providing wound, ostomy, and/or continence care who do not have baccalaureate degrees, such as nurses with an associate degree or diploma and licensed practical/vocational nurses.

The strategy to meet the objective was to develop a WOCN Society–endorsed educational program for nurses who were providing wound and ostomy care and did not have a baccalaureate degree. Pursuant to the 2009 strategic plan, the WOCN Society developed a position paper to clarify the role and scope of practice for each level of wound care provider (WOCN, 2011), and a continuing education program was developed and implemented for the education of wound treatment associates.

WOC Nursing Specialty Scope of Practice

WOC nursing was recognized as a specialty nursing practice in 2010 by the American Nurses Association (ANA), and the scope and standards of practice for WOC nursing were published (WOCN, 2010). The Society is currently preparing an update to the 2010 WOC nursing scope and standards of practice to maintain recognition by the ANA (WOCN, 2017). WOC specialty nurses can specialize in all three areas of WOC nursing or focus on one or more areas of specialization.

WOC nursing is a multifaceted, evidence-based practice that incorporates a unique body of knowledge to enable nurses to provide excellence in prevention, health maintenance, therapeutic intervention, and rehabilitative and palliative nursing care to persons with select disorders of the gastrointestinal, genitourinary, and integumentary systems. WOC nursing directs

its efforts at improving the quality of care, life, and health of health care consumers with wound, ostomy, and/or continence care needs (hereafter, referred to as health care consumers). This complex nursing specialty encompasses the care of individuals of all ages, in all health care settings, and across the continuum of care.

WOC nurses influence and guide the delivery of optimal care for health care consumers directly through the provision of hands-on care and indirectly through their roles as educators, consultants, researchers, or administrators throughout the health care community (WOCN, 2017, p. 6).

Current Issues and Trends

"Major trends in the American healthcare system present endless opportunities and challenges for WOC nursing. WOC specialty practice is influenced by shifts in population demographics, legislative initiatives, and rising health care costs as well as patient safety and quality concerns" (WOCN, 2010, p. 20). WOC nurses provide care to individuals with multiple types of wounds due to pressure, venous, arterial, or neuropathic disease; trauma; surgery; and/or other disease processes such as cancer and infection (WOCN, 2017). Wounds are costly and are a large burden for society and the health care community. On an annual basis, wounds due to pressure affect more than 2.5 million people in the United States at a cost of $9.1 to $11.6 billion, and 60,000 of those individuals die (Berlowitz et al., n.d.). "Key factors that influence the outcomes for patients with acute or chronic wounds are the availability and accessibility of evidence-based, specialized care to meet the growing need for prevention and treatment of complex wounds" (WOCN, 2017, p. 7).

As the population ages, it is expected that increasing numbers of individuals will suffer from acute and chronic wounds, which will require more health care providers with specialized skills to manage the wounds. In addition, there are increasing numbers of military service personnel requiring expert wound care, and there are few high-level educational programs available to the Armed Services.

Therefore, there is a need to extend education to non-specialty nursing providers who can collaborate with WOC nurses and other health care providers to meet the needs of individuals with acute and chronic wounds. The following recommendation provides a description of the role and scope of practice for each level of wound care provider, which includes a brief overview of the criteria and competencies for each level of provider.

RECOMMENDATION

Role and Scope of Practice for Wound Care Providers: WOC Registered Nurse, WOC Graduate-Level Prepared Registered Nurse, WOC Advanced Practice Registered Nurse, and Wound Treatment Associate

Note: Practice limits are defined by each state. Each nurse is accountable to practice in accordance with the specific requirements of the licensing board in the state(s) in which the nurse practices.

1. **Criteria and competencies for the WOC registered nurse.**
   a. *Education.* Minimum baccalaureate degree.
   b. *Licensure.* Licensed as a registered nurse by the State Board of Nursing (SBON) in the state(s) where the nurse practices.
   c. *Specialty Education/Certification.* Completion of a WOCN Society–accredited educational program in wound management and/or certification by the WOCNCB in wound care (i.e., certified wound, ostomy, and continence nurse [CWOCN]; certified wound care nurse [CWCN]; certified wound and ostomy nurse [CWON]).
   d. *Level of autonomy.* Functions under the guidance of a physician or advanced practice registered nurse.
   e. *Selected competencies for wound care and management* (WOCN, 2017). The WOC registered nurse:
      • Provides expert hands-on care for individual patients with acute or chronic wounds (e.g., advanced treatment modalities; conservative sharp instrumental wound debridement of devitalized tissue or chemical cauterization per physician order, etc.).
      • Serves as a consultant to provide insight and potential solutions for complex clinical cases to improve patient care and outcomes.
      • Uses judgment and critical thinking skills to assess, diagnose, and identify outcomes; develop and implement an individualized care plan; and evaluate care of the patient with an acute or chronic wound.
      • Uses evidence-based assessment techniques, instruments, tools, and available data and information to identify problems and needs of the patient with an acute or chronic wound.
      • Collects pertinent data (e.g., biological, physical, functional, psychosocial, etc.) using a systemic process to identify the patient's needs.
      • Synthesizes and prioritizes assessment data to provide focused care for the patient with an acute or chronic wound.
      • Assesses the impact of family dynamics and cultural and religious beliefs on the patient's care needs.
      • Formulates culturally sensitive, expected outcomes based on the assessment and diagnosis.
      • Uses evidence-based knowledge and research findings to guide practice and develop strategies/interventions to manage care to achieve appropriate goals and outcomes for patients with acute or chronic wounds.
      • Assists the patient with an acute or chronic wound to identify options for care.
      • Conducts an ongoing evaluation of the goals and outcomes for management of the patient with an acute or chronic wound, and uses assessment data to revise/modify the diagnosis, outcomes, plans, and strategies as warranted.
      • Engages the patient with an acute or chronic wound in self-care to maximize independence and achieve goals for quality of life.
      • Articulates the role and responsibilities of the WOC nurse to team members.
      • Leads interprofessional teams to communicate, collaborate, and consult effectively; and ensure that safe, effective, efficient, timely, patient-centered, and equitable care is provided for the patient with an acute or chronic wound.
      • Coordinates care for the prevention and management of complications.
      • Develops and implements evidence-based educational programs for patients, staff, and other health care providers.
      • Evaluates processes, policies, procedures, and protocols/guidelines for care of patients with acute or chronic wounds; and recommends revisions when warranted.
      • Provides leadership in the design of quality improvement initiatives to optimize outcomes of care for patients with acute or chronic wounds.
      • Advocates for the patient with an acute or chronic wound (and for the specialty and professional practice) to ensure the availability and access for the patient to specialty care services, resources, and supplies including insurance coverage.
      • Facilitates/coordinates use of systems and community resources to implement and enhance care of patients with acute or chronic wounds across the continuum of care.
      • Engages consumer alliance and advocacy groups in health teaching and health promotion activities for patients.

2. **Criteria and competencies for the WOC graduate-level prepared registered nurse.**
   a. *Education.* Master's degree or higher.
   b. *Licensure.* Licensed as a registered nurse by the State Board of Nursing (SBON) in the state(s) where the nurse practices.
   c. *Specialty Education/Certification.* Completion of a WOCN Society accredited educational program in wound management and/or certification by the WOCNCB in wound care (i.e., CWOCN, CWCN, CWON).

d. ***Level of autonomy.*** Has advanced knowledge, skills, abilities, and judgment; functions in an advanced level as determined by the nurse's position; and is not required to have additional regulatory oversight (ANA, 2015).

e. ***Selected competencies for wound care and management*** (WOCN, 2017). In addition to competencies of the WOC registered nurse, the WOC graduate-level prepared registered nurse:

- Applies knowledge from advanced preparation, current research, and evidence when making clinical decisions to achieve optimal outcomes for the patient with an acute or chronic wound.
- Uses available benchmarks to evaluate practice at the individual, departmental, or organizational level.
- Uses data and theory-driven approaches to effect organizational or system changes to improve practice and outcomes for patients with acute or chronic wounds, and determine if plans are effective or need revision.
- Critically critiques evidence from databases for applicability to practice.
- Evaluates tools, instruments, and services for diverse populations who need care for acute or chronic wounds.
- Designs quality improvement studies, research initiatives, and other programs to improve health care and outcomes for patients with acute or chronic wounds in diverse settings.
- Contributes to WOC nursing knowledge and other evidence by conducting, critically appraising, or synthesizing research and other evidence to improve health care practices.
- Synthesizes relevant research, empirical evidence, and frameworks when designing and implementing educational programs for patients, staff, and other health care providers.
- Incorporates theories and research in generating strategies to promote health and healthy lifestyles of populations who need care for acute or chronic wounds.
- Mentors colleagues for the acquisition of advanced clinical knowledge, skills, abilities, and judgment.
- Creates evaluation strategies to address cost effectiveness, cost benefits, clinical effectiveness, and efficiency of WOC nursing practice.
- Analyzes outcomes, related to organizational care delivery and populations served, to make recommendations for improvements in the delivery systems for care of patients with acute or chronic wounds across care settings.

3. **Criteria and competencies for the WOC advanced practice registered nurse (APRN).**

   a. ***Education.***
      - Master's degree or higher.
      - Completion of a graduate-level educational program that is accredited by a national nursing or nursing-related accrediting body that is recognized by the Department of Education or the Council for Higher Education Accreditation, and prepares the APRN in a specific role (i.e., clinical nurse specialist, certified nurse practitioner, certified registered nurse anesthetist, certified nurse–midwife) with population-focused competencies (ANA, 2015; APRN Consensus Work Group & National Council of State Boards of Nursing [NCSBN] APRN Advisory Committee, 2008; Stanley, 2012).

   b. ***Licensure.*** Licensed to practice as an APRN in a specific role by the State Board of Nursing (SBON) in the state(s) where the nurse practices (ANA, 2015; APRN Consensus Work Group & the NCSBN-APRN Advisory Committee, 2008; Stanley, 2012).

   c. ***Specialty Education/Certification.***
      - Completion of a WOCN Society accredited educational program in wound management and/or specialty certification or advanced practice (AP) certification by the WOCNCB in wound care (i.e., CWOCN, CWCN, CWON, CWOCN-AP, CWCN-AP, CWON-AP; WOCN, 2017).
      - Certification as an APRN by a nationally recognized certification board such as the American Nurses Credentialing Center or the American Academy of Nurse Practitioners (ANA, 2015; APRN Consensus Work Group & the NCSBN-APRN Advisory Committee 2008; Stanley, 2012).

   d. ***Level of autonomy.*** Functions independently or in collaboration with a physician, which is dependent on the SBON where the APRN practices.

   e. ***Selected competencies for wound care and management*** (WOCN, 2017). In addition to competencies of the WOC registered nurse and WOC graduate-level prepared registered nurse, the WOC advanced practice registered nurse:
      - Serves as a provider of WOC nursing services in accordance with state and federal laws and regulations.
      - Provides consultation to patients and professionals to improve care and outcomes for patients with complex clinical cases due to acute or chronic wounds.
      - Initiates diagnostic tests and procedures relevant to the current status of the patient.

- Formulates a differential diagnosis based on the history, physical examination, and diagnostic test results.
- Uses advanced assessment, knowledge, and skills to make clinical decisions for care of the patient with an acute or chronic wound.
- Develops plans of care that integrate assessment, diagnostic strategies, and therapeutic interventions; and reflect current, evidence-based knowledge, and best practice for care of patients with acute or chronic wounds.
- Uses prescriptive authority, procedures, referrals, treatments, and therapies in accordance with state and federal laws and regulations.
- Prescribes evidence-based pharmacological agents, treatments, supplies (e.g., topical therapies, dressings), and durable medical equipment according to clinical indicators and results of diagnostic and laboratory tests; and in accordance with state and federal laws and regulations.
- Synthesizes evaluation data from the patient, community, population, and/or institution to determine the effectiveness of plans for attainment of goals and outcomes for the patient with an acute or chronic wound.
- Uses evaluation data to make or recommend changes in process, policy, procedures, or protocols for care when warranted.
- Defines expected outcomes that integrate evidence, best practice, and input from inter-professional team members to address cost and clinical effectiveness of care for patients with acute or chronic wounds.
- Provides leadership to promote communication and collaboration to assure safe and quality patient care.
- Engages in comparison evaluations and in partnerships with patients to determine the effectiveness of diagnostic tests, clinical procedures, therapies, and treatment plans; and optimize the health and quality of care for patients with acute or chronic wounds.

4. **Criteria and competencies for the wound treatment associate.**
   a. ***Education.*** Minimum of a nursing diploma, associate degree, practical/vocational nurse education; or successful completion of military medic training.
   b. ***Licensure.*** Licensed as a registered nurse or practical nurse/vocational nurse by the SBON in the state(s) where the nurse practices. (Licensure is not required for military medics.)
   c. ***Continuing Education.*** Certificate of completion from a WOCN Society–endorsed Wound Treatment Associate Program.

d. ***Certification.*** Certification as a wound treatment associate (WTA-C) is available for nurses from the WOCNCB. Certification may be preferred or required by some employers.
e. ***Level of autonomy.*** Functions under the direction of the supervising WOC specialty nurse (i.e., WOC registered nurse, WOC graduate-level prepared registered nurse, WOC advanced practice registered nurse); a physician, physician's assistant, or nurse practitioner; or other qualified health care providers, experienced in wound care, such as a clinical nurse specialist or a certified wound specialist (CWS).
f. ***Selected competencies for wound care and management.*** The wound treatment associate:
   - Collaborates with the supervising WOC specialty nurse or other health care provider and team members, and in accordance with established protocols:
     o Identifies patients at risk for developing pressure injury and/or wound complications.
     o Implements preventive care per established protocols and monitors skin status.
     o Implements treatment plans established by the supervising WOC specialty nurse or physician, and uses topical therapies and products as outlined in the plan.
     o Provides routine care that promotes optimal outcomes for the patient with an acute or chronic wound.
     o Provides ongoing monitoring of the wound and the patient's response to the established plan to include observation and measurement of the wound.
   - Notifies the supervising WOC specialty nurse or other health care provider when the wound deteriorates or fails to make progress.
   - Identifies patients who require referral to a WOC specialty nurse and/or other health care provider.
   - Assists with providing individualized education to patients, caregivers, and team members regarding prevention of pressure injuries and management of wounds.
   - Participates in quality improvement programs.

CONCLUSION

To meet the needs of individuals with acute or chronic wounds, the WOCN Society has recognized there is a need to extend education to nonspecialty nursing providers who can collaborate with WOC specialty nurses and other health care providers. The WOCN Society recognizes four levels of wound care providers and endorses the appropriate utilization of each level of provider (i.e., WOC registered nurse, WOC graduate-level prepared registered nurse, WOC advanced practice registered nurse, and wound treatment associate). A description of the role and scope of practice for each level of wound care provider has been developed. The description includes a brief overview of the criteria and competencies for each provider as a basis for developing and providing educational programs and clarifying the differences in the preparation, role functions, and duties of the different providers.

REFERENCES

American Nurses Association. (2015). *Nursing: Scope and standards of practice* (3rd ed.). Silver Spring, MD: Author.

APRN Consensus Work Group & National Council of State Boards of Nursing APRN Advisory Committee. (2008). *Consensus model for APRN regulation: Licensure, accreditation, certification, & education.* Retrieved February 16, 2017, from www.aprnlace.org

Berlowitz, D., Vandeusen Lukas, C., Parker, V., et al. (n.d.). *Preventing pressure ulcers in hospitals: A toolkit for improving quality care.* Retrieved February 16, 2017, from http://www.ahrq.gov/sites/default/files/publications/files/putoolkit.pdf

Stanley, J. M. (2012). Impact of new regulatory standards on advanced practice registered nursing: The APRN consensus model and LACE.

Nursing Clinics of North America, 47(2), 241–250. doi: 10.1016/j.cnur.2012.02.001.

Wound, Ostomy and Continence Nurses Society. (2009). *The Wound, Ostomy and Continence Nurses Society strategic plan 2009–2011.* Mt. Laurel, NJ: Author. Retrieved April 24, 2011, from http://www.wocn.org/pdfs/About_Us/2010_Strategic_Plan.pdf

Wound, Ostomy and Continence Nurses Society. (2010). *Wound, ostomy and continence nursing: Scope & standards of practice.* Mt. Laurel, NJ: Author.

Wound, Ostomy and Continence Nurses Society. (2011). *Position statement about the role and scope of practice for wound care providers.* Mt. Laurel, NJ: Author. Retrieved February 16, 2017, from http://www.wocn.org/?page=RoleScopeWTA

Wound, Ostomy and Continence Nurses Society. (2016). *WOCN policy & procedure manual.* Mt. Laurel, NJ: Author. Retrieved February 16, 2017, from http://www.wocn.org/?page=WOCNPPManual

Wound, Ostomy and Continence Nurses Society. (2017). *Wound, ostomy and continence nursing: Scope & standards of practice* (2nd ed.). Mt. Laurel, NJ: Author. Manuscript in preparation.

Wound, Ostomy and Continence Nurses Society & Wound, Ostomy and Continence Nursing Certification Board. (2008). *Position statement: Entry level wound, ostomy and continence nurse education and certification.* Mt. Laurel, NJ: Wound, Ostomy and Continence Nurses Society. Retrieved February 16, 2017, from http://www.wocn.org/?page=EntryWOCNurse

Abscess: a localized collection of pus surrounded by inflamed tissue, usually due to an infectious process.

Acral skin: nonhairy skin located primarily on the hands, feet, and parts of the face.

AFO: an ankle–foot orthosis. A splint used to control the position of the foot relative to the tibia.

Air plethysmography (APG): measures venous reflux, obstruction, and poor calf muscle pump function, which are associated with poor venous return. Air plethysmograph consists of a 35-cm-long polyurethane tubular air chamber that surrounds the entire leg. The air chamber is inflated with air at 6 mm Hg and connected to a pressure transducer/amplifier and a recorder or computer. Changes in volume of the leg as a result of filling or emptying of veins produce corresponding changes in the pressure of the air chamber.

Allodynia: a painful response to a normally innocuous stimulus (as in an intolerance to bedsheets touching legs).

Ambulatory venous hypertension: develops when abnormalities occur in any part of the system (i.e., calf muscle pump dysfunction and/or incompetent valves and perforating veins in the superficial, perforator, or deep vein systems). This leads to reflux of blood through this incompetent system.

Angiography: diagnostic or therapeutic radiography of the heart and blood vessels using a radiopaque contrast medium.

Angioplasty: use of a balloon to open or enlarge the lumen in a blood vessel. It is commonly done to treat stenosis of arteries due to atherosclerosis. Often, during the procedure, atherectomy and/or insertion of a stent may be performed.

Ankle–brachial index (ABI): a noninvasive vascular assessment technique providing an objective indicator of arterial perfusion to a lower extremity. The ABI is a ratio obtained by dividing the higher of each ankle's systolic pressure by the higher of the brachial systolic pressures. If blood flow is normal, the pressure in the ankle should equal or be slightly higher than that in the arm.

Ankle flare: see malleolar flare.

Antibacterial: an agent that inhibits the growth of bacteria.

Antibiotic: a natural or synthetic agent with the capacity to destroy or inhibit bacterial growth.

Antimicrobial: an agent that acts directly on a microbe to either kill the organism or hinder the development of new colonies.

Antiseptic: a nonselective, topical agent that inhibits multiplication of microorganism, or it may kill microorganisms.

Arterial insufficiency: lack of sufficient blood flow via the arteries to the extremities, which can be caused by cholesterol deposits (atherosclerosis), clots (emboli), or damaged, diseased, or weak vessels.

Arteriogram or angiogram: a diagnostic or therapeutic radiographic test of using radiopaque contrast medium.

Arteriosclerosis: a common disorder of the arteries marked by thickening, hardening, and loss of elasticity of the walls of blood vessels.

Atherosclerosis: plaques of cholesterol, fats, and other elements that are deposited in the walls of large- and medium-sized arteries. The walls of the vessels become thick and hardened, leading to narrowing, which reduces circulation to organs and other areas normally supplied by the artery.

Athlete's foot (*tinea pedis*): dermatophyte infection of feet characterized by erythema, chronic peeling of skin, fissuring of web spaces between toes, maceration, and blistering.

Atrophie blanche: smooth, plaques that resemble scar tissue and are often surrounded by regions of skin hyperpigmentation.

Autonomic dysreflexia: a syndrome in which there is a sudden onset of excessively high blood pressure. It is more common in people with spinal cord injuries.

Autonomic neuropathy: causes changes in digestion, bowel and bladder function, sexual response, and perspiration. It can also affect nerves that serve the heart and control blood pressure. It can cause hypoglycemia unawareness, a condition in which people no longer experience warning signs of hypoglycemia.

Avascular: lacking in blood supply; synonyms are dead, devitalized, necrotic, and nonviable. Specific types include slough and eschar.

Bacteremia: presence of bacteria in the blood.

Bioburden: degree or load of microorganisms (i.e., bacteria, virus, fungi) that contaminate a wound, which is influenced by the quantity and virulence of microbes.

Biofilm: a structured community of microorganisms embedded in a protective matrix that is adherent to the surface of the wound and is resistant to antimicrobials.

Biological wound coverings: human or animal tissue used as temporary wound coverings.

Biological dressings include:

> **Allograft:** Skin from another individual.
>
> **Autograft:** Skin from the patient.
>
> **Cadaver skin:** Skin from a cadaver.
>
> **Xenograft:** Skin from another species (e.g., pig skin).
>
> **Amniotic membrane:** From the amniotic tissue of a fetus.
>
> **Artificial skin:** Tissue engineered skin, bioengineered skin, skin substitutes, human skin equivalents [single epidermal layer or epidermal and dermal layer].

Body mass index (BMI): a mathematical formula to assess relative body weight. BMI is calculated as weight in kilograms divided by the square of the height in meters (kg/m^2).

Bony prominences: a bony elevation or projection on an anatomical structure.

Bottoming out: the state of support surface deformation beyond critical immersion whereby effective pressure redistribution is lost.

Bowel management system: a pouch or indwelling system designed to collect fecal effluent.

Bunion/bunionette: a localized swelling at either the medial or dorsal aspect of the first joint of the big toe, caused by an inflamed bursa due to pressure, shear, and friction. (Bunionette involves localized swelling at the lateral aspect of the 5th toe.)

C-reactive protein (CRP): CRP is a protein found in the blood. It is a marker for inflammation.

Calf muscle pump dysfunction: varying degrees of dysfunction of the calf muscle pump as it sends venous blood back to the heart.

Cellulitis: a diffuse, acute inflammation and infection of the skin and subcutaneous tissue that signifies a spreading infectious process.

Charcot deformity, neuropathic fracture, neuropathic osteoarthropathy: a Charcot joint is a progressive condition of the musculoskeletal system characterized by joint dislocations, pathologic fractures, and debilitating deformities. This disorder results in progressive destruction of bone and soft tissues at weight-bearing joints and may cause significant disruption of the bony architecture in its most severe form. Charcot arthropathy can occur at any joint; however, it occurs most commonly in the lower extremity at the foot and ankle.

Charcot-Marie-Tooth disease: usually characterized by weakness of the peroneal leg muscles and commonly resulting in a high-arched foot with marked claw toes.

Chronic venous insufficiency: characterized by symptoms or signs produced by venous hypertension as a result of structural or functional abnormalities of veins.

Claudication: consistent and reproducible, lower-extremity symptoms that are usually confined to the calf muscles (can affect the thigh or buttocks) and are brought on by exercise and only relieved by rest.

Claw toes: deformity caused by flexion contractures involving both proximal and distal interphalangeal joints.

Colonization: presence and limited proliferation of microorganisms on/or within a wound that does not provoke a host response or impair wound healing.

Complete decongestive therapy (CDT): also known as comprehensive decongestive therapy, complex physiotherapy, and complex decongestive physiotherapy, is the gold standard for treatment for lymphedema that includes manual lymph drainage (MLD), compression bandaging, compression garments, therapeutic exercises, meticulous skin care, and patient education.

Compression therapy: application of sustained, external pressure to the affected lower extremity to control edema and aid the return of venous blood to the heart. Compression therapy is achieved by stockings, wraps or bandages (e.g., multilayer single component, multilayer multicomponent, elastic and/or inelastic, products or systems), or other devices such as pneumatic compression pumps. Some wraps are reusable. Multilayer systems combine elastic and inelastic layers. Compression may be classified as inelastic/short stretch or elastic.

Contamination: presence of nonproliferating microorganisms on/or within a wound at a level that does not provoke a host reaction.

Corns: (clavus) a small conical callosity caused by pressure over a bony prominence, usually on a toe. A hyperkeratosis, that is, a thickening of normal keratin of the skin.

Critical limb ischemia (CLI): CLI is defined as limb pain occurring at rest or impending limb loss due to severely compromised blood flow in the affected limb. The term should be used for all patients with chronic ischemic rest pain (inadequate resting perfusion), ulcers, or gangrene attributable to objectively proven arterial occlusive disease. Term CLI implies chronicity and is to be distinguished from acute limb ischemia, which is commonly due to an embolism.

Dermatitis: inflammation of the epidermis and dermis.

Dressing Techniques:

Continuously moist saline gauze: A technique whereby gauze is moistened with normal saline to maintain a moist environment.

Wet-to-dry saline gauze: A technique whereby gauze is moistened with normal saline, applied wet to the wound and allowed to dry, and then removed when adhered to the wound bed. As the dressing is removed, the wound is nonselectively debrided.

Edema: a local or generalized condition that involves the abnormal pooling of fluid in body tissues.

Electrical stimulation: the use of an electrical current to transfer energy to a wound. The type of electricity that is transferred is controlled by the electrical source.

Electromagnetic therapy: application of electromagnetic radiation or pulsed electromagnetic fields (PEMF) to the body.

Epibole: also clinically referred to as rolled-over edges, is often seen in chronic wounds with poor healing dynamics.

Epithelialization: the process of becoming covered with or converted to epithelium.

Erysipelas: type of skin infection (cellulitis).

Erythema: a redness of the skin due to dilation of the superficial capillaries. Types of erythema are as follows:

Blanchable erythema: Reddened area that temporarily turns white or pale when pressure is applied with a fingertip. Blanchable erythema over a pressure site is usually due to a normal reactive hyperemic response.

Nonblanchable erythema: Redness that persists when fingertip pressure is applied. Nonblanchable erythema over a pressure site is a symptom of a stage 1 pressure injury.

Eschar: black or brown necrotic devitalized tissue; tissue can be loose or firmly adherent, hard, or soft.

Extrinsic factor: a factor outside body that contributes to the development of a pressure injury.

Exudate: any fluid that has been extruded from a tissue or its capillaries, such as fluid, cells, or cellular debris, which has escaped from blood vessels and has been deposited in tissue surfaces. It is characteristically high in protein and white blood cells.

Fibrinogen: a protein involved in coagulation. Fibrinogen reacts with other molecules to produce blood clots.

Fissure: any cleft or groove, normal or otherwise, especially a crack-like break in the skin.

Fistula: an abnormal passage from an internal organ to the body surface or between two internal organs.

Friction: the force of two surfaces moving across one another, such as the mechanical force exerted when skin is dragged across a coarse surface such as traditional bed linens.

Full-thickness tissue loss: ulceration extending through dermis to involve subcutaneous tissue and possibly muscle/bone.

Hallux: the big toe, or great toe.

Hammer toe: a toe that is permanently flexed downward, due to a flexion contracture involving the proximal interphalangeal joint.

Hemosiderin staining: reddish/brown/black discoloration of the lower legs and ankles in patients with LEVD, which develops from extravasation of red blood cells (RBCs) into the subcutaneous tissue; as the RBCs break down the pigment is released and causes discoloration of the skin.

Heterotopic bone formation: heterotopic ossification (HO) is the formation of lamellar bone where bone does not usually form, such as in soft tissues. May mature with time. May be a complication of pressure injuries or traumatic injury.

Irrigation: mechanical removal of wound debris by irrigation with fluid at 8 to 15 pounds per square inch (psi).

Hyperalgesia: an increased response to a painful stimulus.

Hyperbaric oxygenation: the administration of oxygen under greater than normal atmospheric pressure (usually two to three times absolute atmospheric pressure).

Hypergranulation hyperplasia: of granulation tissue is believed to occur as a result of an extended inflammatory response, recognized by its friable red appearance.

Hyperkeratosis: thickening of the horny layer of the epidermis or mucous membrane.

Incidence: the proportion of at-risk persons who develop a pressure injury over a specific period.

Induration: abnormal hardening of tissues.

Infection: microorganisms invade deep into wound tissue, proliferate, and provoke a host response including delayed healing and/or tissue damage. Quantitative measures of wound infection have been defined as >105 CFU/g of biopsied tissue. Localized infection is contained in one location, system, or structure; spreading infection occurs when the infecting organisms invade the tissue surrounding the wound, which can include the muscle, fascia, organs, or body cavities. Typical overt signs and symptoms of infection in an acute wound include purulent exudate, increasing odor, erythema, warmth, tenderness, edema/swelling, new or increasing pain, and delayed healing. In chronic wounds or in individuals who are immunocompromised or have poor arterial perfusion, the classical signs of infection may be absent. Chronic wounds often display subtle signs and symptoms, such as friable/bleeding granulation tissue, hypergranulation tissue, epithelial bridging, pocketing in granulation tissue, increased odor, delayed wound healing, wound breakdown and enlargement, and new ulcerations of the periwound tissue.

Insensate foot: loss of protective sensation due to peripheral neuropathy.

Intertriginous: an area where opposing skin surfaces touch and may rub, such as skin folds of the groin, axilla, and inframammary area.

Intertrigo: an inflammation of the top layers of skin caused by moisture, bacteria, or fungi in the folds of the skin.

Ischemia: poor blood supply to an organ or part, often marked by pain and organ dysfunction.

Ischemic rest pain: ischemic pain is often described as a throbbing pain, dull ache, or numbness that typically worsens when the patient elevates the leg and in the evenings or nights while lying supine. The pain is relieved by lowering the leg to a dependent position due to mild improvement in the arteriolar blood flow caused by the effects of gravity. Ischemic rest pain might also be described as a burning pain in the arch or distal foot that occurs while the patient is recumbent and is relieved when the feet/legs are returned to a dependent position.

Keratolytic agents: soften, separate, and cause desquamation of the cornified epithelium or horny layer of skin.

Lipodermatosclerosis: induration and hyperpigmentation of the lower third of the leg that is related to chronic inflammation in LEVD; may present clinically with an "apple-core" or "inverted champagne bottle" appearance to the lower leg. Acute lipodermatosclerosis may occur, which is characterized by pain, tenderness, and hardening of the skin in the lower legs; and is thought to be the acute counterpart of chronic lipodermatosclerosis.

Loss of protective sensation (LOPS): degree of neuropathy beyond which the patient has a measurably increased risk for diabetic foot ulceration.

Lymphangitis: inflammation of the lymphatic vessels, commonly seen as red streaks on skin near a focus of infection.

Lymphedema: swelling of the subcutaneous tissues caused by obstruction of the lymphatic system. Is a result of fluid accumulation and may arise from surgery, radiation, or the presence of a tumor in the area of the lymph nodes. Over time, this results in firming or hardness of the tissue that is characterized by fibrosis and scarring.

Malleolar flare (ankle flare): visible capillaries from distension of small veins around the malleolar area.

Manual lymphatic drainage (MLD): a component of CDT for treatment of lymphedema; involves gentle, manual movement of the skin with light hand and finger movements to direct lymph flow out of compromised areas to healthy functioning areas of the lymphatic system.

Marjolin ulcer: cutaneous malignancy arises in the setting of previously injured skin, long-standing scars, and chronic wounds. Most common type is squamous cell carcinoma.

Medical adhesive–related skin damage (MARSI): damage to the skin resulting from the use of medical adhesives. Includes contact dermatitis, allergic dermatitis, maceration, folliculitis, and mechanical damage such as skin tears, friction blisters, and epidermal stripping.

Metabolic syndrome: a cluster of conditions that increase the risk of heart disease, stroke, and diabetes including high blood pressure, high blood sugar, abnormal cholesterol levels, and excess body fat around the waist.

Metatarsalgia: a cramp-like burning pain that focuses in the region of the metatarsal bones of the foot.

Metatarsals: long bones of the midfoot proximal to the toes (phalanges). They are numbered from one to five, five being behind the little toe.

Moisture-associated skin damage (MASD): injury to the skin caused by repeated or sustained exposure to moisture in the form of water, urine or stool, perspiration, mucus, or saliva.

Moisture-retentive dressings: dressings that allow wounds to remain moist.

Moisture vapor transmission rate (MVTR): a measure of the passage of water vapor through a substance.

Monofilament: Semmes-Weinstein monofilaments are calibrated nylon monofilaments. These monofilaments produce a characteristic force perpendicular to the contacting surface and are identified by manufacturer-assigned numbers.

Motor neuropathy: biomechanical and muscle alteration leading to anatomic deformity.

Negative pressure wound therapy (NPWT): assists in wound closure by applying localized negative pressure to the surface and margins of the wound. This negative pressure therapy is applied to a special dressing positioned in the wound cavity or over a flap or graft. The negative pressure helps in removing fluids from the wound.

Neuroma: a benign growth of nerve tissue; can cause nerve compression and significant pain.

Neuropathy: see peripheral neuropathy.

Nongranulating: absence of granulation tissue; wound surface appears smooth as opposed to granular. For example, in a wound that is clean but nongranulating, the wound surface appears smooth and red as opposed to cobblestone.

Off-loading: the effective reduction of pressure and stress from repetitive walking at areas of highest foot pressure such as over the plantar surfaces and the bony areas of the forefoot.

Onychomycosis: fungal infection of the fingernails or toenails that results in thickening, roughness, and splitting of the nails, usually due to *Trichophyton rubrum*.

Orthotic: an externally applied device (e.g., splint or insole) used to control the position and/or function of a body part.

Osteomyelitis: inflammation of bone and marrow, usually caused by pathogens entering the bone during an injury or surgery.

Panniculitis: acute inflammation of the subcutaneous layer of fat.

Paresthesia: abnormal neurological sensations described as pins and needles, electric-like, numb aching feet, knife-like, or shooting pains.

Partial-thickness wound: confined to the superficial skin layers; damage does not penetrate below the dermis and may be limited to the epidermal layers only.

Paronychia: infection at the edge of the nail, usually the result of an ingrown toenail.

Pedorthist: specialist in prescription footwear.

Peripheral neuropathy: a syndrome where muscle weakness, paresthesias, impaired reflexes and autonomic symptoms of the hands and feet are common. Pain, numbness, or tingling in the extremities may progress to an inability to feel heat, cold, pain or any sensation in the affected areas.

> *Sensory neuropathy:* A common disorder characterized by tingling, aching, burning, and searing discomfort beginning in the toes and spreading to the soles of the feet and then to the tops of the feet, the ankles, and, on occasion, the knees. Numbness of the feet, which is usually also painful, frequently occurs. There may be loss of protective sensation and impaired temperature perception.

> *Motor neuropathy:* Biomechanical and muscle alteration results in weakened intrinsic foot muscles leading to anatomic deformity.

Plantar fasciitis: inflammation involving the fascia of the sole of the foot.

Plantar ulcer: a full-thickness breakdown on the plantar surface of the foot.

Point prevalence: the method used most commonly to measure prevalence. It measures the proportion of people who have a pressure ulcer at a specific point in time.

Pressure redistribution: ability of a support surface to distribute load over the contact areas of the human body to reduce the overall pressure and avoid areas of focal pressure.

Proprioceptive sense: the biofeedback from the extremities, which tells the brain where and in what position the body is. Proprioception is critical in balance.

Pulsatile lavage: a delivery of irrigation fluid in rapid, discrete pulses. Disposable, battery-powered units deliver variable irrigation pressures and concurrent suction. The pulsing of the irrigation fluid may increase the amount of debris removed. Concurrent suction immediately removes irrigation fluid, which has been contaminated by contact with the wound.

Purpura: a disorder with bleeding beneath the skin or mucous membranes that causes black and blue spots (ecchymosis) or pinpoint bleeding.

Reliability: the consistency of a set of measurements or measuring instrument.

Reticular veins: reticular veins are slightly bulging veins (1 to 3 mm), darker in color, that form bluish networks that crisscross over the thighs and lower legs.

Ringworm: any of a number of contagious fungal skin diseases characterized by ring-shaped scaly itching patches on the skin.

Risk assessment: assessment to determine which, if any, risk factors are present that might contribute to the development of skin ulceration.

Sclerotherapy: a strong solution (the sclerosant) is injected directly into the venules, causing inflammation of the walls of the vessel to make them disappear over a few weeks to months.

Segmental pressure measurements: similar to the ABI test, with the addition of two or three additional blood pressure cuffs. A Doppler measures the blood pressure at each cuff location on the leg. A significant drop in pressure between two adjacent cuffs indicates a narrowing of the artery or blockage along the arteries in this portion of the leg.

Sepsis: a condition in which the body is fighting a severe infection that has spread via the bloodstream.

Shear: the mechanical force that is parallel rather than perpendicular to an area. Shear may play a role in triangularly shaped or tunneled sacral pressure ulcers. Force per unit magnitude of the area acting parallel to the surface of the body. This parameter is affected by pressure, the coefficient of friction between the materials contacting each other, and how much the body interlocks with the support surface.

Sinus tract: course or path of tissue destruction occurring in any direction from the surface or edge of the wound; results in dead space with potential for abscess formation. Also sometimes called tunneling.

Slough: soft moist avascular (devitalized) tissue; may be white, yellow, tan, or green; may be loose or firmly adherent.

Subfascial endoscopic perforator surgery (SEPS): a minimally invasive surgical technique for the ablation of incompetent perforator veins in the lower leg.

Support surfaces: surfaces that are used to widely distribute body weight pressure over the dependent surface.

Surfactants: a surface-active agent that reduces the surface tension of fluids to allow greater penetration.

Telangiectasia (telangiectases): tortuous, spidery distended, blue to red capillary veins visible under skin.

Transepidermal water loss (TEWL): the amount of water that passes through the skin to the external environment. The average TEWL is approximately 300 to 400 mL/day.

Thrombus: blood that has clotted in the heart or a blood vessel.

Tinea pedis (athlete's foot): dermatophytic infection of the feet with erythema, chronic peeling of skin, fissuring of web spaces between toes, maceration, and possibly blistering.

Toe–brachial index (TBI): TBI is an index calculated by dividing the systolic blood pressure in the great toe by the higher of the brachial systolic blood pressures from the right or left arms.

Toe pressure: a toe pressure is a systolic pressure that is measured on the great toe (or second toe if the great toe is absent or cannot be used due to pain or wounds). The toe pressure is typically measured by PPG using a small digital cuff. Toe pressures may be more accurate in patients with calcified ankle arteries.

Total contact cast (TCC): a casting technique that is used to heal diabetic foot ulcers and to protect the foot during the early phases of Charcot fracture dislocations. The cast is used to heal diabetic foot ulcers by distributing weight along the entire plantar aspect of the foot.

Transcutaneous oxygen pressure (TcPO$_2$): this pressure reflects the amount of oxygen coming out through the skin, which, in turn, reflects the amount of oxygen delivered to the skin by the blood.

Transcutaneous oxygen measurement/transcutaneous oximetry (TCOM): transcutaneous oximetry evaluates the delivery of oxygen to tissue by measuring oxygen pressure at the skin surface over a localized area of heat-induced hyperemia and provides a functional assessment of ischemia.

Tunneling: see sinus tract.

Undermining: area of tissue destruction extending under intact skin along the periphery of a wound; commonly seen in shear injuries. Can be distinguished from sinus tract by the fact that undermining involves a significant portion of wound edge.

Unna's boot: static inelastic zinc-impregnated bandage with or without calamine.

Validity: concerned with the study's success at measuring what the researchers set out to measure.

Varicose veins: swollen and twisted veins that appear blue and appear close to the surface of the skin. They may bulge, throb, and cause the legs to feel heavy and to swell. Varicose veins may occur in almost any part of the body but are most often seen in the back of the calf or the inside of the leg between the groin and the ankle.

Vascularization: the process where body tissues develop small blood vessels (capillaries). It can be a natural occurrence or the result of surgical intervention.

Vein ablation: radiofrequency ablation and endovenous laser ablation. Laser ablation is performed by making a tiny puncture (percutaneous) through the skin through which a laser is passed into the saphenous vein. The laser is activated and applies very localized heat to the inner vein wall inducing thermal damage that permanently blocks the vein and it becomes closed. Saphenous reflux is eliminated.

Vein stripping: a surgical procedure done under general or local anesthetic to remove varicose veins. The surgery involves making one or more incisions upon the desired area, usually the groin and ankle, followed by insertion of a thin wire-like instrument at the incision into the vein. The instrument then removes or "strips" the vein by pulling it out through the incision.

Venous dermatitis: a red itchy rash on the lower legs of patients with LEVD due to increased permeability of capillary walls, which allows proteins to infiltrate the interstitial spaces causing irritation and inflammation.

Venous eczema: the resulting increased permeability of capillary walls with LEVD allows proteins to infiltrate the interstitial spaces, which is irritating. This irritant reaction causes eczema, with or without the presence of an ulcer. Erythema is often a feature of venous eczema due to the dilation of capillaries in response to the irritant effect.

Venous insufficiency: a condition in which the veins do not efficiently return blood from the lower limbs back to the heart. It usually involves one or more veins. The valves in the veins usually channel the flow of blood towards the heart. When these valves are damaged, the blood leaks and pools in the legs and feet. Symptoms include swelling of the legs and pain in the extremities (i.e., dull aching, heaviness, or cramping).

Venous leg ulcer (VLU): also known as varicose or stasis ulcer; may be full or partial-thickness skin loss caused by varicose veins, CVI and inflammation due to damaged valves and veins of the legs with subsequent leakage of fluid into the interstitial space.

INDEX

Note: Page numbers followed by "*f*" refer to figures; page numbers followed by "*t*" refer to tables.